Instructional
Course Lectures

Volume 47 1998

American Academy
of Orthopaedic Surgeons

Instructional Course Lectures

Volume 47 1998
including index for 1997 and 1998

Edited by
W. Dilworth Cannon, Jr, MD
Professor of Clinical Orthopaedic Surgery and
Director of Sports Medicine
University of California, San Francisco
San Francisco, California

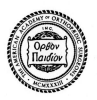

American Academy
of Orthopaedic Surgeons
6300 North River Road
Rosemont, IL 60018

American Academy of Orthopaedic Surgeons
Instructional Course Lectures
Volume 47

Vice President, Educational Programs: Mark W. Wieting
Director, Department of Publications: Marilyn L. Fox, PhD
Senior Editor: Bruce A. Davis
Associate Senior Editors: Joan Abern, Lisa Moore
Production Manager: Loraine Edwalds
Production Coordinators: David Stanley, Sophie Tosta
Production Assistants: Geraldine Dubberke, Jana Ronayne

Contributors

Brian D. Adams, MD, Professor, Department of Orthopedic Surgery, University of Iowa, Iowa City, Iowa

John P. Albright, MD, Professor, Director, Sports Medicine Service, Department of Orthopaedic Surgery, University of Iowa College of Medicine, Iowa City, Iowa

David W. Altchek, MD, Assistant Attending Orthopaedic Surgeon, Sports Medicine and Shoulder Service, The Hospital for Special Surgery, New York, New York

Deborah J. Ammeen, BS, Research Associate, Anderson Orthopaedic Research Institute, Arlington, Virginia

Richard D. Angliss, MB, BS, FRACS, Department of Orthopaedic Surgery, London Health Science Center, London, Ontario, Canada

Sue D. Barber-Westin, BS, Director of Clinical Studies, Cincinnati Sportsmedicine Research and Education Foundation, Cincinnati, Ohio

David M. Bell, MD, Fremont Orthopaedic Medical Group, Fremont, California

Robert H. Bell, MD, Assistant Professor of Orthopaedic Surgery, Northeastern Ohio Universities College of Medicine, Crystal Clinic, Akron, Ohio

Pedro K. Beredjiklian, MD, Resident, Department of Orthopaedic Surgery, Hospital of the University of Pennsylvania, Philadelphia, Pennsylvania

Richard A. Berger, MD, PhD, Associate Professor of Orthopedic Surgery and Anatomy, Mayo Foundation, Rochester, Minnesota

Daniel J. Berry, MD, Assistant Professor of Orthopedics, Mayo Medical School, Consultant in Orthopedic Surgery, Mayo Clinic, Rochester, Minnesota

Louis U. Bigliani, MD, Professor, Department of Orthopaedic Surgery, Columbia University, College of Physicians and Surgeons, Chief of the Shoulder Service, Columbia-Presbyterian Medical Center, New York, New York

J. Mark Blue, MD, Department of Orthopaedic Surgery, Union Memorial Hospital, Baltimore, Maryland

Mathias P.G. Bostrom, MD, Assistant Attending Orthopaedic Surgeon, Hospital for Special Surgery, New York, New York

Andrew W. Brown, MD, Sports Medicine Fellow, Orthopaedic Surgery, University of Iowa College of Medicine, Iowa City, Iowa

Joseph A. Buckwalter, MD, Professor, Department of Orthopaedics, University of Iowa, Iowa City, Iowa

Pieter Buma, PhD, Department of Orthopaedics, Orthopaedic Research Laboratory, Academic Hospital Nijmegen, Nijmegen, The Netherlands

Stephen S. Burkhart, MD, Clinical Associate Professor, University of Texas Health Science Center at San Antonio, San Antonio Orthopaedic Group, San Antonio, Texas

David L. Butler, PhD, Professor, Department of Aerospace Engineering and Engineering Mechanics, University of Cincinnati, Cincinnati, Ohio

Miguel E. Cabanela, MD, MS, Professor of Orthopedic Surgery, Mayo Medical School, Rochester, Minnesota

John J. Callaghan, MD, Professor, Department of Orthopaedics, University of Iowa College of Medicine, Iowa City, Iowa

Eric W. Carson, MD, The Emory Clinic/Emory University School of Medicine, Assistant Professor, Department of Orthopedics, Section of Sports Medicine, Decatur, Georgia

Hugh P. Chandler, MD, Assistant Clinical Professor, Harvard Medical School, Boston, Massachusetts

Frank A. Cordasco, MD, Assistant Clinical Professor, Department of Orthopaedic Surgery, Columbia University, College of Physicians and Surgeons, New York, New York

Clive P. Duncan, MD, MSc, FRCSC, Professor and Chairman, Department of Orthopaedics, Faculty of Medicine, University of British Columbia, Vancouver, British Columbia, Canada

James Dunwoody, MD, Chief Resident, Department of Orthopaedics, Faculty of Medicine, University of British Columbia, Vancouver, British Columbia, Canada

Gerard A. Engh, MD, President, Anderson Orthopaedic Research Institute, Arlington, Virginia

Peter J. Evans, MD, PhD, FRCSC, Sports Medicine Program, Division of Orthopaedic Surgery, University of Toronto, Toronto, Ontario, Canada

Diego L. Fernandez, MD, Associate Professor of Orthopaedic Surgery, University of Berne, Berne, Switzerland

Donald C. Fithian, MD, Assistant Clinical Professor, Department of Orthopedic Surgery, University of California, San Diego, San Diego, California

Evan L. Flatow, MD, Professor of Orthopaedic Surgery, Associate Chief, The Shoulder Service, New York Orthopaedic Hospital, Columbia-Presbyterian Medical Center, New York, New York

Peter J. Fowler, MD, FRCSC, Medical Director, Fowler Kennedy Sport Medicine Clinic, University of Western Ontario, London, Ontario, Canada

Gerard T. Gabel, MD, Assistant Professor, Department of Orthopedic Surgery, Baylor College of Medicine, Houston, Texas

Donald S. Garbuz, MD, FRCSC, Clinical Instructor, Division of Reconstructive Surgery, Department of Orthopaedics, University of British Columbia, Vancouver Hospital and Health Sciences Centre, Vancouver, British, Columbia, Canada

Jean W.M. Gardeniers, MD, PhD, Department of Orthopaedics, Academic Hospital Nijmegen, Nijmegen, The Netherlands

John C. Garrett, MD, Resurgens, PC, Atlanta, Georgia

Gary M. Gartsman, MD, Texas Orthopedic Hospital, Houston, Texas

Andrew Green, MD, Assistant Professor of Orthopaedic Surgery, Brown University School of Medicine, Providence, Rhode Island

Patrick E. Greis, MD, Shoulder Service, Assistant Professor of Orthopaedic Surgery, University of Pittsburgh, Pittsburgh, Pennsylvania

Allan E. Gross, MD, FRCSC, Head, Division of Orthopaedic Surgery, Mount Sinai Hospital, University of Toronto, Toronto, Ontario, Canada

Carl T. Hasselman, MD, Resident, Department of Orthopedic Surgery, University of Pittsburgh, Pittsburgh, Pennsylvania

Richard J. Herzog, MD, Associate Professor of Radiology, University of Pennsylvania Medical Center, Philadelphia, Pennsylvania

Robert N. Hotchkiss, MD, Hospital for Special Surgery, New York, New York

Joseph P. Iannotti, MD, PhD, Associate Professor, Department of Orthopaedic Surgery, Chief of Shoulder and Elbow Service, University of Pennsylvania Medical Center, Philadelphia, Pennsylvania

Stan L. James, MD, Orthopaedic Healthcare Northwest, Eugene, Oregon

Donald C. Jones, MD, Orthopedic Healthcare Northwest, Orthopedic Consultant, University of Oregon Athletic Department, Clinical Instructor, OHSU, Eugene, Oregon

Jesse B. Jupiter, MD, Director, Orthopaedic Hand Service, Massachusetts General Hospital, Boston, Massachusetts

Evan H. Karas, MD, Fellow, Shoulder Surgery and Sports Medicine, University of Pennsylvania Medical Center, Philadelphia, Pennsylvania

Michael A. Kelly, MD, Insall-Scott-Kelly Institute for Orthopaedics and Sports, New York, New York

Kenneth A. Krackow, MD, Professor of Orthopaedic Surgery, State University of New York at Buffalo, The Buffalo General Hospital, Buffalo, New York

Joseph M. Lane, MD, Professor Orthopaedic Surgery, Director, Division Metabolic Bone Disease, Hospital for Special Surgery, Cornell University Medical College, New York, New York

Joseph P. Leddy, MD, Clinical Professor, Department of Surgery, Orthopaedics, Chief, Hand Surgery Service, Robert Wood Johnson University Medical School, New Brunswick, New Jersey

David G. Lewallen, MD, Associate Professor, Mayo Graduate School of Medicine, Consultant, Department of Orthopedic Surgery, Mayo Clinic/Mayo Foundation, Rochester, Minnesota

Peter L. Lewis, FRACS, Department of Orthopaedic Surgery, London Health Sciences Center, London, Ontario, Canada

Scott R. Lipson, MD, West Penn Orthopaedics, Clarion, Pennsylvania

Ian K.Y. Lo, MD, University of Western Ontario, London, Ontario, Canada

William J. Maloney, MD, Associate Professor, Washington University School of Medicine, Chief, Orthopaedic Surgery, Barnes Jewish Hospital, St. Louis, Missouri

Henry J. Mankin, MD, Professor of Orthopaedics, Harvard Medical School, Chief, Orthopaedic Oncology, Massachusetts General Hospital, Boston, Massachusetts

Bassam A. Masri, MD, FRCSC, Clinical Assistant Professor, Vancouver General Hospital and Health Sciences Centre, Department of Orthopaedics, Vancouver, British Columbia, Canada

Eric L. Masterson, BSc, MCh, FRCS (Orth), Fellow in Adult Reconstruction, Vancouver General Hospital and Health Sciences Centre, Department of Orthopaedics, Vancouver, British Columbia, Columbia

Leslie S. Matthews, MD, Chief, Department of Orthopaedic Surgery, Union Memorial Hospital, Baltimore, Maryland

David S. Menche, MD, Associate Director of Sports Medicine, Medical Director of Physical Therapy and Occupational Therapy, The Hospital for Joint Diseases Orthopaedic Institute, New York, New York

Anthony Miniaci, MD, FRCSC, Director, Sports Medicine, The Toronto Hospital, University of Toronto, Toronto, Ontario, Canada

Bernard F. Morrey, MD, Professor, Department of Orthopedic Surgery, Mayo Medical School, Rochester, Minnesota

Tom R. Norris, MD, Department of Orthopaedics, California-Pacific Medical Center, San Francisco, California

Tom F. Novacheck, MD, Director, Motion Analysis Laboratory, Assistant Professor of Orthopaedics, University of Minnesota, Gillette Children's Specialty Healthcare, St. Paul, Minnesota

Frank R. Noyes, MD, Adjunct Professor, Department of Aerospace Engineering, and Engineering Mechanics, University of Cincinnati, Cincinnati, Ohio

Regis J. O'Keefe, MD, Associate Professor, University of Rochester Medical Center, Rochester, New York

Guy D. Paiement, MD, Associate Professor of Clinical Orthopedics, University of California at San Francisco, San Francisco, California

Wayne G. Paprosky, MD, FACS, Associate Professor, Department of Orthopaedic Surgery, Rush Medical College, Chicago, Illinois

Lars Peterson, MD, PhD, Associate Professor, Department of Orthopaedics, University of Göteborg, Gothenburg, Sweden

Matthew J. Phillips, MD, Assistant Clinical Professor of Orthopaedic Surgery, State University of New York at Buffalo, The Buffalo General Hospital, Buffalo, New York

Mark I. Pitman, MD, Chief of Sports Medicine, Hospital for Joint Diseases, New York, New York

Arthur C. Rettig, MD, Orthopaedic Surgeon, Methodist Sports Medicine Center, Indianapolis, Indiana

Robin R. Richards, MD, FRCSC, Head, Division of Orthopaedic Surgery, St. Michael's Hospital, Associate Professor, Division of Orthopaedic Surgery, University of Toronto, Toronto, Ontario, Canada

Cecil H. Rorabeck, MD, FRCSC, Professor and Chair, University of Western Ontario, University Hospital, London, Ontario, Canada

Randy N. Rosier, MD, PhD, Professor of Orthopaedics, Oncology, and Biophysics, University of Rochester Medical Center, Rochester, New York

Harry E. Rubash, MD, Associate Professor and Clinical Vice Chairman, Chief, Division of Adult Reconstructive Surgery, Department of Orthopaedic Surgery, University of Pittsburgh Medical Center, Pittsburgh, Pennsylvania

Felix H. Savoie III, MD, Director, Upper Extremity Service, Mississippi Sports Medicine and Orthopaedic Center, Jackson, Mississippi

B. Willem Schreurs, MD, PhD, Department of Orthopaedics, Academic Hospital Nijmegen, Nijmegen, The Netherlands

Arun S. Shanbhag, PhD, Associate Professor, Department of Orthopaedic Surgery, University of Pittsburgh, Pittsburgh, Pennsylvania

Walter H. Short, MD, Associate Professor, Department of Orthopedic Surgery, State University of New York, Health Science Center, Syracuse, New York

Peter T. Simonian, MD, Hospital for Special Surgery, Sports Medicine and Shoulder Service, New York, New York

Raj K. Sinha, MD, PhD, Joint Reconstruction Fellow, Department of Orthopaedic Surgery, University of Pittsburgh Medical Center, Pittsburgh, Pennsylvania

viii

Tom J.J.H. Slooff, MD, PhD, Professor of Orthopaedics, University Hospital St. Badboud, Nijmegen, The Netherlands

Mark J. Spangehl, MD, FRCSC, Clinical Fellow in Adult Reconstruction, Department of Orthopaedics, Mayo Clinic, Rochester, Minnesota

Carl L. Stanitski, MD, Chief, Department of Orthopaedic Surgery, Childrens Hospital of Michigan, Professor, Wayne State University, Detroit, Michigan

George T. Stollsteimer, MD, Fellow, Mississippi Sports Medicine and Orthopaedic Center, Jackson, Mississippi

Russell G. Tigges, MD, Orthopedic Associates, Poughkeepsie, New York,

C. Thomas Vangsness, Jr, MD, Associate Professor, Department of Orthopaedic Surgery, USC School of Medicine, Los Angeles, California

Steven F. Viegas, MD, Professor and Chief, Division of Hand Surgery, Department of Orthopaedics and Rehabilitation, Professor, Department of Anatomy and Neurosciences, University of Texas Medical Branch, Galveston, Texas

Jon J.P. Warner, MD, Director, Shoulder Service, Associate Professor of Orthopaedic Surgery, University of Pittsburgh, Pittsburgh, Pennsylvania

Russell F. Warren, MD, Surgeon-in-Chief, Hospital for Special Surgery, Professor of Orthopaedic Surgery, Cornell Medical College, New York, New York

Terry L. Whipple, MD, Clinical Associate Professor of Orthopaedic Surgery, University of Virginia, Charlottesville, Virginia

Thomas L. Wickiewicz, MD, Chief, Sports Medicine and Shoulder Service, Hospital for Special Surgery, Associate Professor, Cornell Medical College, New York, New York

Ross M. Wilkins, MD, MS, Institute for Limb Preservation, Denver, Colorado

Alastair S.E. Younger, MB, MSc, FRCSC, Clinical and Research Fellow, Department of Orthopaedics, Faculty of Medicine, University of British Columbia, Vancouver, British Columbia, Canada

David J. Zaleske, MD, Chief, Pediatric Orthopaedics, Massachusetts General Hospital, Boston, Massachusetts

Brad Zwahlen, MS, Mayo Clinic, Rochester, Minnesota

Preface

This 47th volume of the Instructional Course Lectures is composed of articles from a group of outstanding Instructional Course lecturers, drawing predominantly from the 165 courses presented in San Francisco at the American Academy of Orthopaedic Surgeons Annual Meeting in 1997. Articles were also solicited from a select group of symposia presenters from the Annual Meeting program. The editor has the flexibility to emphasize specific areas of orthopaedic surgery. We try not to repeat articles that have been published in ICL volumes over the past 5 years. Because of the current strong interest in the following subjects, I have chosen to emphasize the shoulder, and articular cartilage injury and repair in this volume. Many other high-quality, pertinent articles from other areas of orthopaedics balance out the volume. Orthopaedic surgeons who missed specific Instructional Courses now have the opportunity to find and review subjects of interest, covered in more depth in this volume than when originally presented at the Annual Meeting.

I would like to thank the other members of the Instructional Course Committee for assembling an outstanding group of courses of general interest to the majority of the fellowship, including an increasing number of international registrants. I also appreciate the help provided me by Clive P. Duncan, MD, in soliciting an interesting group of articles on hip surgery, and by Louis U. Bigliani, MD, in obtaining the articles on shoulder surgery. I would also like to thank Bruce Davis for his advice and help in soliciting and editing of this volume, along with other members of the publications staff: Sophie Tosta, Joan Abern, Lisa Moore, and David Stanley. I also want to extend my gratitude to Edmond Young, MD, who helped me edit several manuscripts.

W. Dilworth Cannon, Jr, MD
San Francisco, California

Contents

Section 5 Knee, Ankle, and Foot

Shoulder

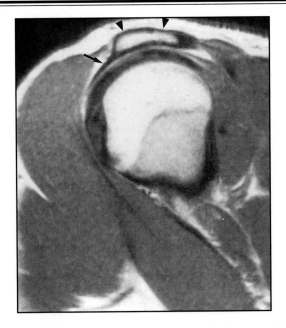

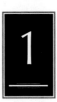

Magnetic Resonance Imaging of the Shoulder

Richard J. Herzog, MD

The foundation of successful patient care is an accurate clinical diagnosis. The accomplishment of this goal begins with a complete history and physical examination. If the initial evaluation does not provide the information needed to explain the symptoms, additional diagnostic testing is usually needed. The additional data provided by these tests become useful clinical information only when they are integrated with the patient's history and the results of the physical examination and other ancillary tests. Imaging studies may also be part of the preoperative workup in order to confirm the presence of a pathologic condition and to determine its extent. In the past, radiographic imaging studies, such as plain radiography and computed tomography, and radionuclide studies have played a major role in the diagnostic evaluation of patients who have a musculoskeletal disorder. These studies focused mainly on the detection of osseous abnormalities. With the recent development and implementation of magnetic resonance imaging (MRI), it is now possible to evaluate noninvasively the soft-tissue structures of the body, such as muscles, tendons, and ligaments, which are the structures frequently responsible for most of the symptoms in patients who have musculoskeletal dysfunction.

The goal of any imaging study is to define accurately the pathomorphologic changes in a specific tissue, organ, or part of the body. Whenever possible, objective diagnostic criteria should be employed when the findings of an imaging study are reported. Objective categorization of pathologic changes facilitates the interpretation and communication of abnormalities detected on a test, and these same criteria can then be used when follow-up tests are performed to assess the effects of different forms of therapy, such as surgical intervention or nonsurgical rehabilitation. The reproducibility and reliability of all objective diagnostic criteria must be evaluated rigorously in prospective, blinded studies before they are implemented.[1]

Magnetic Resonance Imaging

Complete assessment of all of the soft tissues and osseous structures of the shoulder girdle is mandatory to achieve a comprehensive evaluation of dysfunction of the shoulder. MRI studies should be performed in three orthogonal planes for all patients. The images are made with the arm comfortably positioned at the side in slight abduction and neutral or slight external rotation.[2] The axis of the different scan planes is determined by the orientation of the scapulohumeral axis, which is defined by an initial axial localizing sequence. The coronal sequence is oriented parallel to the long axis of the body of the scapula and the supraspinatus tendon and perpendicular to the glenoid fossa. The coronal sequence extends from the coracoid process through the entire rotator cuff mechanism—that is, the tendinous cuff and the muscles. The sagittal sequence is oriented perpendicular to the coronal sequence and extends from the suprascapular notch through the rotator cuff and into the adjacent deltoid muscle. Both the coronal and the sagittal sequences are oriented obliquely to the true coronal and sagittal planes of the body because of the normal rotation of the scapula on the chest wall. Therefore, these sequences are correctly designated oblique coronal and oblique sagittal. The axial sequence is oriented perpendicular to the glenoid fossa and extends from the superior margin of the acromioclavicular joint through the quadrilateral space.

The MRI sequences typically used to evaluate the musculoskeletal system are the spin-echo, gradient-echo, and short tau inversion recovery (STIR) sequences. They provide excellent contrast and spatial resolution for the evaluation of normal anatomic structures and pathologic changes within the body. Spin-echo T1-weighted sequences (a short relaxation time and a short echo time) are optimum to display tissues containing fat or blood and provide excellent anatomic detail. Spin-echo proton-density-weighted sequences (a long relaxation time and a short echo time) are also used to assess soft-tissue and osseous anatomy. Spin-echo T2-weighted sequences (a long relaxation time and a long echo time) are used to delineate tissue containing fluid or edema. STIR and spin-echo fat-saturated T2-weighted sequences are particularly sensitive to fluid or edema in soft tissues and osseous structures.

The high signal intensity in cancellous bone on T1-weighted sequences is due to the large amount of fat within the cancellous bone. Any process that replaces this fat results in decreased signal intensity on the spin-echo T1-weighted sequence. If

Table 1
Routine protocol for magnetic resonance imaging of the shoulder

Plane*	Relaxation Time(msec)	Echo Time (msec)	No. of Excitations	Image Matrix	Thickness (mm)	Skip (mm)	Comments
Oblique coronal							Parallel to long axis of body of scapula, including soft tissues anterior and posterior to humeral head
1	2,500	Dual-echo minimum/70	1	256 by 192	4	0.5	Classic multi-echo
Oblique sagittal							Perpendicular to long axis of scapula from base of coracoid through humeral head
1	1,500	Minimum	1	256 by 192	4	0.5	
2	4,000	Approximately 90	2	256 by 192	4, same location as 1	0.5	Fast spin echo-echo train length-8; fat-saturated band width, 32 kHz
Axial							From superior to acromioclavicular joint through glenoid and humeral neck
1	1,500	Minimum	1	256 by 192	3	0.5	
2	4,000	Approximately 90	2	256 by 192	3, same location as 1	0.5	Fast spin echo-echo train length-8; fat-saturated band width, 32 kHz

* 1 = made with the upper extremity in neutral or slight external rotation, and 2 = a field of view of 16 cm for all sequences

the abnormal process contains increased free water (as with an inflammatory focus or malignant cells), there is increased signal intensity in the cancellous bone on spin-echo T2-weighted and STIR sequences. If the process replacing the marrow fat contains fibrous tissue or additional mineralization, there is low signal intensity on all of the MRI sequences.

With MRI, it is now possible to follow noninvasively the evolution of injury, repair, and remodeling of tissue as well as the changes of tissue aging. Acute injury to vascularized tissue incites an inflammatory response, with an increase in tissue hydration that is detected on spin-echo T2-weighted and STIR sequences as a focus of high signal intensity. With tissue-healing, remodeling, and fibrosis, the signal intensity on the T2-weighted and STIR sequences decreases because of the increased amount of collagen and the decreased amount of fluid in the tissue. Aging involves changes in both the cellular and the extracellular components of tissue.[3] Tissue-aging that is accompanied by desiccation of the tissue demonstrates decreased signal intensity on spin-echo T2-weighted sequences. Tissue-aging that is accompanied by fatty infiltration

demonstrates increased signal intensity on spin-echo T1-weighted sequences, and that accompanied by myxoid degeneration of collagen demonstrates increased signal intensity on spin-echo T2-weighted or STIR sequences because of the increased hydration of the degenerated tissue.

Recent advances in MRI, including faster imaging sequences and improved surface coil design, have markedly increased the amount of information provided by these images. Our routine imaging examination of the shoulder, performed with a 1.5-tesla MRI system, is different for each plane (Table 1). The type of equipment employed markedly affects the quality of the images and their potential usefulness. While patients tolerate some low-field-strength open MRI systems better than they do high-field-strength systems because they are not enclosed closely by the low-field-strength unit, the quality of the images generated by these open systems is typically poorer than that achieved with high-field-strength systems.

The MRI sequences used for most musculoskeletal evaluation, including that of the shoulder, are similar. A com-

plete discussion of the physics of MRI and the different sequences that are currently used are outside the scope of this paper.[4-6] Absolute contraindications to MRI include the presence of a cardiac pacemaker, a metallic foreign body in the eye or spine, a cerebral aneurysm clip, some types of infusion pumps, bone or nerve stimulators, and an ocular or cochlear implant.[7] It is the responsibility of both the clinician who orders the MRI study and the facility that performs it to screen patients adequately before the examination.

Rotator Cuff and Impingement

The rotator cuff is one of the largest tendinous structures in the body and, because of the functional demands placed on it, it is prone to overload and failure. Rotator cuff disease represents a spectrum of pathologic changes within the cuff, including microscopic or macroscopic failure of fibers associated with tissue edema, hemorrhage, and fibrosis. These conditions are superimposed on the normal changes in the cuff due to aging. The primary mechanisms of injury to the cuff appear to be extrinsic impingement and intrinsic overload. A patient who has impingement syndrome has pain on attempted use of the shoulder, particularly with overhead activities. The pain is precipitated by entrapment or abrasion of the rotator cuff and the peritendinous bursa and soft tissue. This may occur under a degenerated acromioclavicular joint or subjacent to the coracoacromial arch (the arch formed by the coracoid process, the coracoacromial ligament, and the acromion). In the supraspinatus outlet (the space between the humeral head and the coracoacromial arch), the rotator cuff mechanism may impinge against a thickened coracoacromial ligament; an osseous ridge projecting off the anteroinferior margin of the acromion at the insertion of the coracoacromial ligament; or a curved, tilted, or hooked acromion. With the arm abducted and externally rotated, the undersurface of the cuff may also impinge against the posterosuperior margin of the glenoid labrum and the rim of the glenoid. Repetitive abrasion of the rotator cuff mechanism may precipitate bursal or peritendinous inflammation or failure of the cuff. Such failure represents a continuum of pathologic changes within the cuff, beginning with hemorrhage and edema, followed by inflammation and fibrosis, and possibly ending with a partial or full-thickness tear.[8]

Disruption of the fibers secondary to abrasion is associated with edema or hemorrhage, or both, in the cuff and in the peritendinous tissues. If an inflammatory reaction is incited within the cuff by failure of the collagen fibers, then the term tendinitis is appropriate to describe the pathologic condition. The response of the cuff to the initial injury depends on the functional demands placed on the shoulder as well as on the reparative capacity of the cuff. There is still controversy concerning the ability of a cuff to heal and how the aging process affects this ability. Recent investigation suggests that the vascularity of a cuff may be maintained with aging[9] but the altered struc-

ture of the collagen and proteoglycans in the aging cuff may affect its response to chronic microtrauma or acute macrotrauma.

As failure of the cuff evolves from acute or subacute tendinitis into a more chronic condition, possibly associated with a partial or full-thickness tear, biopsy of the cuff may demonstrate hyaline or myxoid degeneration of the collagen fibers, fibrovascular proliferation, and few or no inflammatory cells. The term tendinosis and not tendinitis is probably appropriate to describe such a cuff.[10] Tendinosis may represent an abortive healing response of a tendon from chronic extrinsic impingement or intrinsic overload. Tendinitis may be superimposed on tendinosis if there is new failure of the fibers in a weakened, degenerated cuff.

While this spectrum of abnormalities may cause similar problems about the shoulder, including pain, decreased strength, and a limited range of motion, the prognoses and therapeutic options vary widely depending on the degree of the pathologic changes within the cuff. The optimum role of an imaging study is to define the nature and extent of these pathologic changes and to provide a comprehensive assessment of all of the structures of a shoulder that may precipitate or perpetuate failure of the cuff.

With MRI, it is possible to define precisely the morphology of the acromioclavicular joint, the coracoacromial arch, and the rotator cuff. MRI demonstrates the location at which a cuff may be impinging on an area of osseous proliferation (Fig. 1).[11] It is also possible to detect bursal inflammation, which is typically associated with tears of the rotator cuff, including partial-thickness tears of the articular surface and intratendinous tears.[12] Impingement—that is, pushing against—is a physical phenomenon and can be detected on MRI. However, the diagnosis of impingement syndrome, which is a painful symptom complex sec-

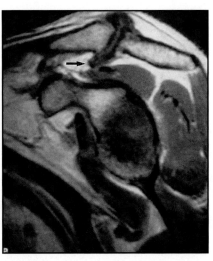

Fig. 1 Proton-density-weighted oblique sagittal image showing an osseous proliferation projecting off the inferior margin of the acromioclavicular joint (arrow) and impinging on the anterosuperior margin of the supraspinatus myotendinous junction.

ondary to the repetitive abrasion and inflammation of the rotator cuff or the peritendinous tissue, or both, as a result of impingement, can only be made clinically. MRIs are typically made with the patient's arm slightly abducted and in neutral or slight external rotation. This position does not precipitate symptoms of impingement in most patients; therefore, until dynamic MRI studies can be performed with the arm abducted or in forward elevation and internal rotation it is not possible to assess completely the dynamic relationships of the cuff to the acromioclavicular joint and the coracoacromial arch.

Changes in the width and configuration of the subacromial space with scapular protraction and retraction were studied with MRI by Solem-Bertoft and associates.[13] In a limited number of normal subjects, the anterior opening of the subacromial space became smaller with scapular protraction. In young patients, degenerative changes of the acromioclavicular joint or the acromion are rare. A torn cuff is more likely to be due to

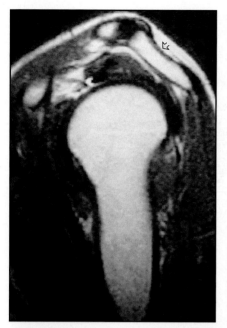
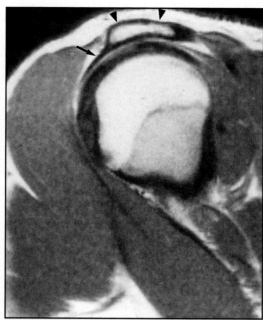
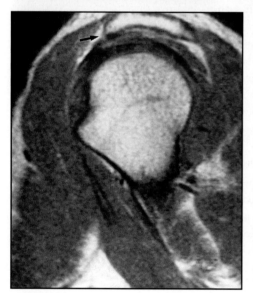
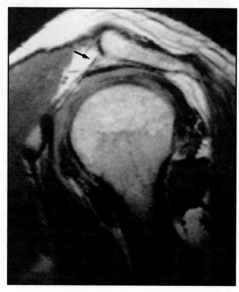

Fig. 2 Proton density-weighted oblique sagittal images. **Top left,** A type-I acromion (arrow) and no impingement on the cuff. **Top right,** A type-II acromion (arrowheads) and a mildly thickened coracoacromial ligament (arrow) associated with moderate narrowing of the supraspinatus outlet. **Bottom left,** A type-III acromion with a hook of the anteroinferior margin (arrow). **Bottom right,** A large osseous ridge (arrow) projecting off the anteroinferior margin of a type-I acromion. This represents an acquired deformity of the acromion that results in narrowing of the supraspinatus outlet similar to that seen with a type-III acromion.

impingement of the cuff against the glenoid labrum or rim or to be related to chronic tensile overload and secondary fatigue failure of the cuff fibers. With decreased tensile strength of the cuff, additional stress may precipitate a partial or full-thickness tear. Direct-impaction injuries of the rotator cuff may also occur in athletes who engage in contact sports.[14] If biomechanical imbalance results from a torn rotator cuff or is secondary to primary instability of the shoulder, sec-

ondary impingement on the cuff may occur and elicit symptoms. Impingement may also result from a decrease in the functional area of the supraspinatus outlet due to post-traumatic changes of the humeral head or the acromion or to hypertrophy of the myotendinous unit of the rotator cuff secondary to physical conditioning.

Before ultrasound and MRI were developed, plain radiography was the primary diagnostic imaging study used to

evaluate pain in the shoulder. While plain radiographs are helpful in the evaluation of osseous anatomy and abnormalities, they provide only indirect evidence of pathologic changes of the rotator cuff. The best indicator of a torn rotator cuff on an anteroposterior radiograph of the shoulder made with the upper extremity in neutral rotation is a distance of less than 6 mm between the humeral head and the acromion.[15] Unfortunately, this is a very late finding in the natural history of degeneration of the cuff and, when present, usually indicates a very large or massive tear. The supraspinatus outlet radiograph has recently been used to assess the shape of the acromion, but because a plain radiograph represents a two-dimensional projection image of a three-dimensional structure it is frequently difficult to determine the true shape of the acromion. Interobserver variability in the assessment of the shape also makes it difficult to interpret this radiograph.[16]

With the direct multiplanar capabilities of MRI, it is possible to depict all of the osseous and soft-tissue structures that make up the coracoacromial arch and that may encroach on the supraspinatus outlet. It is important to assess the morphology of the acromial process. The precise shape of the acromion can be determined on the oblique sagittal image immediately lateral to the acromioclavicular joint and is defined as straight (type I), curved (type II), or hooked (type III). In addition to assessing the shape of the acromion (Fig. 2), it is important to determine whether there is an abnormal tilt of the acromion inferolaterally, anteriorly, or posteriorly, which may decrease the volume of the supraspinatus outlet. The detection of an os acromiale is also important, as this has been associated with a tear of the rotator cuff. It is easy to detect an os acromiale if the axial MRIs include the entire acromion and acromioclavicular joint. Unfortunately, many MRI studies of the shoulder do not include a complete set of axial images; however, as long as the study contains an oblique sagittal sequence, it is still possible to diagnose an os acromiale by observing the location of the insertion of the coracoacromial ligament. If the ligament inserts on an ossicle that is separate from the remainder of the acromion, an os acromiale is present (Fig. 3).[17]

The appearance of a normal rotator cuff on MRI is similar to that of other

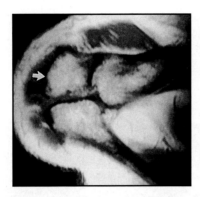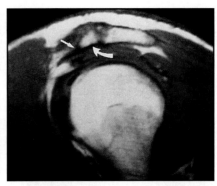

Fig. 3 Left, A proton-density-weighted axial image made through the acromioclavicular joint, showing an os acromiale (arrow). **Right,** The os acromiale (curved arrow) is also delineated on the proton-density-weighted oblique sagittal image, where a mildly thickened coracoacromial ligament (straight arrow) inserts into it.

tendons in the body. With its high collagen content, a normal cuff demonstrates little or no signal intensity on spin-echo sequences.[18] A normal cuff may demonstrate increased signal intensity, typically medial to its insertion site, because of the orientation of the collagen fibers in the cuff relative to the main magnetic field in the magnetic resonance scanner. When collagen fibers are oriented approximately 55° to the main magnetic field, increased signal intensity within the substance of the cuff may be detected on T1-weighted and proton density-weighted sequences. This area of increased signal intensity is not seen on a T2-weighted sequence. This phenomenon is referred to as the magic-angle effect and should not be mistaken for evidence of a tear or degeneration of the cuff.[19] In addition, a normal cuff does not have any morphologic changes such as attenuation, hypertrophy, or fraying.

Abnormalities of the rotator cuff are seen as altered morphology along with abnormal signal intensity. Inflammation, degeneration, or intrasubstance tears, or all three, whether elicited by extrinsic impingement or intrinsic overload, are detected on a T1-weighted or proton density-weighted sequence as a focus of increased signal intensity because of increased hydration of the tissue. In one

study, eight of ten patients who had clinically suspected impingement syndrome had abnormal signal intensity within the rotator cuff on MRI.[20] Degeneration and inflammation were demonstrated in all biopsy specimens from the cuff of five of these eight patients.

The signal intensity on a T2-weighted sequence depends on the degree of hydration because of the pathologic changes in the collagen fascicles and the type of reactive tissue in the tendon. Generally, the greater the hydration of the tissue, the higher the signal intensity on the T2-weighted sequence. The morphology of the cuff may be altered (attenuated or hypertrophied), and the margins of the cuff may be ill defined but not focally torn. If there is fluid or edema in the tissues surrounding a degenerated or inflamed cuff, it will be detected on a spin-echo T2-weighted or a STIR sequence as a focus of high signal intensity. Fluid within the subacromial or subdeltoid bursa is detected easily on fat-saturated T2-weighted sequences. Kjellin and associates,[10] in a study of cadavera, compared the abnormalities detected in the rotator cuff on MRI with the histologic findings. Areas of the cuff that demonstrated abnormally increased signal intensity on spin-echo proton density-weighted sequences but no increase in

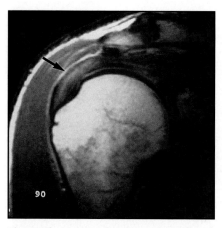 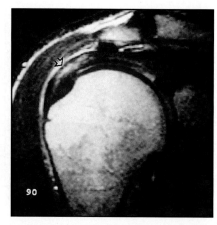

Fig. 4 Left, A proton-density-weighted oblique coronal image showing increased signal intensity within a thickened supraspinatus segment of the cuff (arrow). **Right,** A T2-weighted oblique coronal image showing persistently increased signal intensity within the substance of the supraspinatus tendon (arrow) but no tear extending to the bursal or articular surface of the cuff.

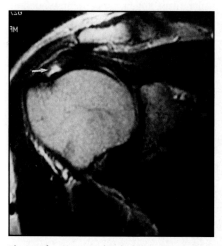 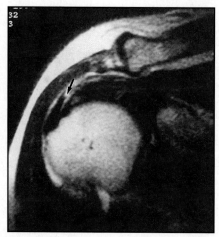

Fig 5 Left, A T2-weighted oblique coronal image showing a small, deep, partial-thickness tear (arrow) involving the articular surface of the cuff. **Right,** A T2-weighted oblique coronal image of a different shoulder, showing an irregular oblique tear (arrow) involving the bursal side of the cuff.

intensity on T2-weighted sequences corresponded to areas of eosinophilic, fibrillar, or mxyoid degeneration as well as areas of fibrosis. Areas that demonstrated increased signal intensity on a T2-weighted sequence corresponded to areas of severe degeneration and disruption of the fibers (Fig. 4). Degenerated supraspinatus tendons demonstrating increased signal intensity on T2-weighted and gradient-echo sequences have also been shown to contain interstitial tears, fibrocartilaginous metaplasia, and fatty infiltration.[21]

A partial-thickness tear of the rotator cuff is detected on spin-echo T2-weighted sequences as a focal area of disrupted fibers on the bursal or articular surface of the cuff (Fig. 5) or within the substance of the cuff. It is frequently possible to determine whether the partial tear involves more or less than 50% of the thickness of the cuff, which may help the surgeon to determine whether the cuff should be debrided or repaired. Discontinuity or detachment of the tendon, along with fluid extending from the articular to the bursal surface, appears to be the most specific finding on MRI for the diagnosis of a full-thickness tear[22] (Fig. 6). By imaging the tear in at least two planes, it is possible to measure the size and to determine the location of the tear accurately. Unfortunately, fluid is not always detected extending through a full-thickness tear, particularly when the tear is chronic and has generated a fibrous reaction in the peritendinous tissue[23] (Fig. 7). In these cases, assessment of the morphology of the cuff or detection of retraction of the cuff may provide the information needed to make an accurate diagnosis. With MRI, it is also possible to determine the degree of retraction of the cuff, the quality of the torn cuff fibers, and the degree of associated muscle atrophy (Fig. 8). The residual function of the muscles of a torn cuff may be determined by assessment of the muscle morphology.[24,25]

Isolated full-thickness tears of the subscapularis segment of the cuff may be difficult to detect clinically;[26] however, MRI provides an excellent means to detect these tears[27] (Fig. 9). On MRI, it is also possible to detect partial detachment of the deep fibers of the superior segment of the subscapularis tendon that may be associated with medial subluxation of the biceps tendon (Fig. 10). If the deep fibers are detached completely, medial intra-articular dislocation of the biceps tendon is possible. In dissection studies, Clark and Harryman[9] detected a tendinous sleeve surrounding the biceps tendon where it enters the bicipital groove, with the subscapularis fibers located under and the supraspinatus fibers located over the biceps tendon. It also appears that the superficial subscapularis fibers are continuous with a fibrous fascia that extends over the biceps tendon.[28]

Iannotti and associates[29] reported on the efficacy of MRI in the evaluation of 91 patients who had a surgical procedure

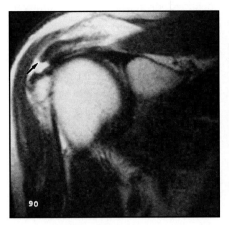
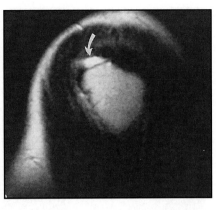
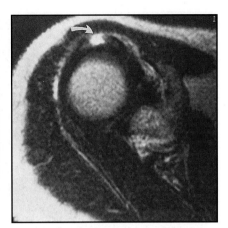

Fig. 6 A small full-thickness tear (arrow) at the insertion site of the rotator cuff, posterior to the rotator interval. **Left,** T2-weighted oblique coronal image. **Center,** T2-weighted oblique sagittal image. **Right,** T2-weighted axial image.

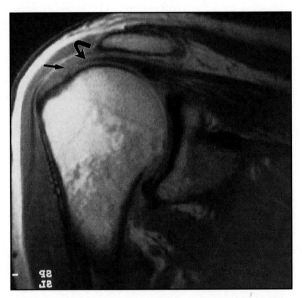
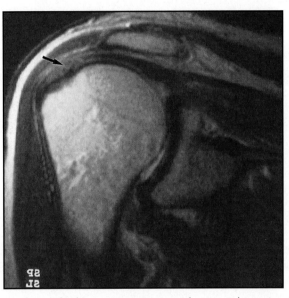

Fig. 7 Left, A proton-density-weighted oblique coronal image showing a tapered, completely torn supraspinatus tendon (curved arrow) and tissue demonstrating intermediate signal intensity (straight arrow) in the region of the gap in the tendon. **Right,** A T2-weighted oblique coronal image showing high-signal-intensity fluid within the glenohumeral joint but no fluid extending through the defect in the cuff. The reactive tissue within the defect (arrow) demonstrates intermediate signal intensity.

for dysfunction of the shoulder and in the assessment of 15 asymptomatic volunteers. With regard to the detection of a complete tear, MRI was 100% sensitive and 95% specific. Tendinitis was defined arthroscopically as an area of hyperemia on the undersurface of the cuff or as thickening of the subacromial bursa. Degeneration or a partial tear was defined arthroscopically as fraying or fibrillation of the cuff. MRI had a sensitivity of 82%

and a specificity of 85% with regard to the differentiation between tendinitis and degeneration of the cuff and a sensitivity of 93% and a specificity of 87% with regard to differentiation of a normal tendon from one showing signs of impingement. Those authors concluded that high-resolution MRI is an excellent noninvasive tool for the diagnosis of disorders of the rotator cuff mechanism. The MRI examinations in that study were

made and interpreted by musculoskeletal radiologists with extensive experience with MRI.

In addition to the study by Iannotti and associates,[29] there have been reports recently on the high accuracy of MRI made with the new fast-imaging techniques to detect full-thickness tears of the cuff.[30-32] Robertson and associates[33] recently demonstrated that full-thickness tears can be diagnosed accurately with

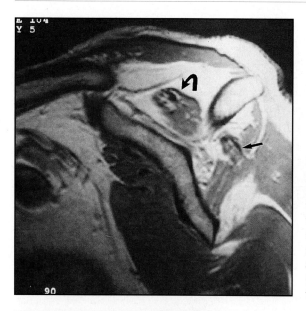

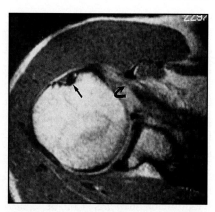

Fig. 8 A proton-density-weighted oblique sagittal image of a large, chronic, full-thickness tear involving the supraspinatus and infraspinatus segments of the cuff, showing moderate-to-severe atrophy of the supraspinatus (curved arrow) and infraspinatus (straight arrow) muscles.

Fig. 9 A proton-density-weighted axial image showing a completely detached subscapularis tendon (curved arrow). The biceps tendon (straight arrow) is still located within the bicipital groove, which is covered by an intact transverse ligament.

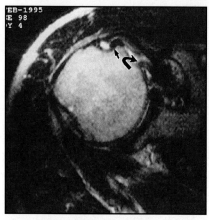

Fig. 10 A T2-weighted axial image showing the biceps tendon (straight arrow) to be medially subluxated and resting on the medial wall of the bicipital groove. The deep fibers of the subscapularis tendon (curved arrow) are detached from the lesser tuberosity, but the superficial fibers are still continuous with the fibrous fascia covering the bicipital groove.

MRI with little interobserver variation with regard to the correct diagnosis. However, interobserver variation was much greater for the diagnosis of partial-thickness tears, tendinitis, and normal cuffs.

The sensitivity and specificity of MRI in the diagnosis of a partial-thickness tear of the rotator cuff are lower than those for detection of a full-thickness tear. Traughber and Goodwin,[34] in a comparison of the results of MRI with the findings at arthroscopy in 28 patients, detected five of five full-thickness tears but only four of nine partial-thickness tears. Hodler and associates[35] compared standard MRI with MR arthrography for the diagnosis of partial-thickness tears. Whereas only one of 13 partial tears was detected on standard MRI, six of the 13 tears were detected on MR arthrograms. Both Palmer and associates[36] and Karzel and Snyder[37] reported on the improved rate of detection with MR arthrography compared with standard MRI for partial and full-thickness tears. Palmer and associates[36] performed both fat-suppressed and non-fat-suppressed oblique coronal T1-weighted sequences for 37 patients along with MR arthrography. They detected 16 of 16 full-thickness tears with both techniques but only three of eight partial-thickness tears without fat suppression; all eight were detected with fat suppression. Because MR arthrography is more invasive, costly, and time-consuming than standard MRI, its efficacy must be proved with well-designed prospective clinical studies before it can be recommended on a routine basis. It is possible that in selected patients, such as athletes who perform repetitive overhead activities, MR arthrography with special positioning of the shoulder may be efficacious.[38]

Occasionally, a patient is seen because of recurrent symptoms after repair of the rotator cuff. The same MRI studies performed preoperatively can be performed to evaluate the cuff postoperatively.[39] Gaenslen and associates[40] evaluated 29 patients (30 shoulders) postoperatively with MRI, and they correctly diagnosed 16 of 19 full-thickness and five of six partial-thickness tears detected at the time of a reoperation on the cuff. If there is any type of metallic hardware in the shoulder, fat-saturated spin-echo sequences should be avoided because of amplification of metallic artefacts. Karzel and Snyder[37] reported a higher rate of detection of postoperative full-thickness tears with MR arthrography than with conventional MRI. Whereas the size of a recurrent tear appears to be related to the degree of dysfunction of the shoulder,[41] it is important to remember that a full-thickness tear after an operation may be asymptomatic. Calvert and associates[42] performed arthrography on 20 patients after repair of the rotator cuff and demonstrated leakage of contrast material, indicating a full-thickness tear, in 18 of them. Seventeen of the 18 patients were asymptomatic at the time of the arthrography.

Although MRI is very sensitive in the detection of tendon disorders, it cannot determine their clinical importance. Knowledge of the appearance of the rotator cuff on MRIs of asymptomatic subjects is necessary before the clinical relevance of changes detected in the cuffs of symptomatic patients can be determined.[43-45] Sher and associates[45] imaged the shoulders of 96 asymptomatic individuals, the youngest of whom was 19 years old. The overall prevalence of full-thickness tears was 15% (14), and the overall prevalence of partial-thickness tears was 20% (19). However, when the different age-groups were considered, no full-thickness tear and only one partial-thickness tear (4%) was diagnosed in the 25 subjects who were 19 to 39 years old, and one full-thickness tear (4%) and six partial-thickness tears (24%) were diagnosed in the 25 subjects who were 40 to 60 years old. Of the 46 individuals who were more than 60 years old, 13 (28%) were diagnosed with a full-thickness tear and 12 (26%), with a partial-thickness tear. Miniaci and associates[43] evaluated 30 shoulders in 20 asymptomatic subjects who were 17 to 49 years old. Although they detected abnormal signal intensity within the cuffs of these subjects, none had evidence of a full-thickness tear. Needell and associates[46] evaluated the prevalence of peritendinous and bone abnormalities in the same asymptomatic cohort of 96 patients studied by Sher and associates.[45] In 75% of the subjects, they detected osteoarthrosis of the acromioclavicular joint, which correlated more closely with age than with abnormalities of the rotator cuff. Unfortunately, they did not categorize the type of osteoarthrosis; specifically they did not state whether there were osteophytes projecting off the inferior margin of the joint line. The prevalence of subacromial spurs

was 12% (three of 26) in the subjects who were 19 to 39 years old and 52% (25 of 48) in the subjects who were 61 to 88 years old, and the prevalence of cysts of the humeral head was 8% (two of 26) and 40% (19 of 48), respectively. Both of these changes correlated closely with the severity of the rotator cuff abnormalities. The presence of fluid in the subacromial or subdeltoid bursa also correlated with abnormalities of the cuff. While cysts of the humeral head, subacromial spurs, and fluid within the subacromial or subdeltoid bursa may indicate an abnormal rotator cuff, it cannot be inferred that their presence reflects a symptomatic condition.

Muscle Injury

Muscle injury is one of the most frequent causes of musculoskeletal dysfunction related to sports activities. Muscle contusions occur most frequently in the lower extremities but may also occur in the shoulder girdle. Acute disruption of muscle fibers may result in intramuscular hemorrhage or a hematoma as well as incite an inflammatory response associated with interstitial edema. Because of the acute pain associated with a muscle injury, it may be difficult to determine the precise location and severity of the injury with a physical examination. Before the availability of MRI, radiographic studies were of little value in assessing acute muscle injuries. On plain radiographs, there may be obliteration of the fat planes surrounding an injured muscle secondary to the perimuscular edema. With computed tomography, the size or contour of a muscle may be seen to be altered but the detection of intramuscular hemorrhage, edema, or hematoma is limited. Because of the excellent soft-tissue contrast resolution provided by MRI, it is now possible to determine the nature and extent of a muscle injury.

A muscle contusion is indicated by abnormal signal intensity and morphology of a muscle on MRI. On spin-echo

sequences, a normal muscle demonstrates intermediate signal intensity on T1-weighted and proton density-weighted sequences and low signal intensity on T2-weighted sequences. In a contused muscle, the interstitial edema or hemorrhage, or both, is seen as high signal intensity on T2-weighted sequences. Because hemorrhage infiltrates through a muscle and mixes with the interstitial edema, it is not possible to separate it from the edematous muscle tissue. With a grade-1 contusion (failure of microstructural fiber), the size of the muscle may be slightly increased and the margins may have a feathery appearance because of the extension of interstitial edema into the perimuscular tissue.[47] Edematous changes in the adjacent subcutaneous fat are also frequently detected. With a grade-2 muscle contusion (a partial macroscopic tear), there is a focus of disrupted muscle fibers in addition to the altered signal intensity from the interstitial edema and hemorrhage. A grade-3 muscle contusion appears similar to a grade-2 contusion, except that there is complete disruption of the muscle fibers. A muscle hematoma is depicted as a focus of intermediate or high signal intensity on a T1-weighted sequence, depending on the age and chemical composition of the hematoma, and as a focus of high signal intensity on a T2-weighted sequence. It is also possible to detect the sequelae of a muscle contusion, which include muscle atrophy, fibrosis, calcification, and ossification.[48]

Muscle strain is probably the most common type of injury of the myotendinous unit. A muscle strain is an acute, stretch-induced injury secondary to excessive indirect force generated by eccentric muscular contraction. Such strains may involve the muscles stabilizing the shoulder joint. The pain elicited by an acute muscle strain typically occurs during an athletic activity or immediately at its termination. The pathologic changes in an acutely strained muscle include microtraumatic disruption of the

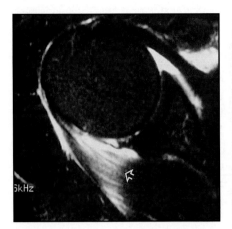

Fig. 11 A fat-saturated T2-weighted axial image showing edematous changes in the lateral segment of the teres minor muscle (arrow) due to an acute stretch-induced injury. There is no tear of the posterior aspect of the labrum or posterior capsular stripping.

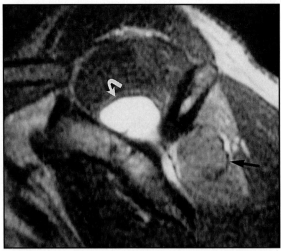

Fig. 12 A T2-weighted oblique sagittal image showing a ganglion cyst (curved arrow) located within the supraspinous fossa and extending through the spinoglenoid notch. There is increased signal intensity within the infraspinatus muscle (straight arrow) due to subacute denervation.

muscle fibers near its myotendinous junction associated with edema and hemorrhage. Because the tendon of a multipennate muscle extends into the muscle belly, the symptoms of a strain may be located anywhere within the muscle and not merely at its ends. A grade-1 muscle strain appears similar to a grade-1 contusion on MRI. The muscle may be enlarged secondary to interstitial edema or hemorrhage, or both, and there is increased signal intensity within the muscle on a spin-echo fat-saturated T2-weighted sequence (Fig. 11). Clinically, a grade-2 muscle strain presents as muscle pain associated with a loss of strength. Pathologically, there is a macroscopic partial tear of the myotendinous unit. On the MRI, there is a partial tear of the muscle fibers associated with edema or hemorrhage, or both. With a grade-3 strain, there is complete disruption of the myotendinous unit. In addition to the evaluation of muscle strains, it is also possible to detect the changes of delayed-onset muscle soreness[49,50] and to study muscle physiology with MRI.[51,52]

It should be possible to employ the same MRI techniques to evaluate the muscles of the shoulder girdle, including patterns of muscle contraction and recruitment, and to compare this information with that provided by the dynamic electromyographic studies currently employed to assess shoulder biomechanics. In athletes, such as pitchers and football quarterbacks, who present with chronic overuse syndromes, abnormalities in the dynamic stabilizers of the shoulder also may be detected with MRI. By demonstrating which muscle groups are involved, it is possible to document that an overuse condition exists and to determine the appropriate rehabilitative program.

MRI can also detect changes in a muscle after injury to its innervation. Fleckenstein and associates[53] and Uetani and associates[54] reported on the appearance of acute, subacute, and chronic muscle denervation on MRI. With acute denervation, there is no detectable difference in the appearance of normally and abnormally innervated muscles. With subacute denervation, there is an increase in the T1 and T2 relaxation values of the denervated muscles. STIR sequences or fat-suppressed spin-echo T2-weighted sequences are most sensitive for the detection of the increased signal intensity related to the prolonged T2 relaxation value of a muscle. Findings of subacute denervation caused by paralabral ganglion cysts compressing the suprascapular nerve at the level of the spinoglenoid notch have been detected in the infraspinatus muscle (Fig. 12).[55] In chronically denervated muscle, atrophy and fatty infiltration is best identified on T1-weighted sequences. The determination of exactly which muscle groups are affected by denervation may make it possible to explain functional loss and to determine treatment. Uetani and associates[54] demonstrated that the abnormal signal intensity initially identified in denervated muscle reverted to normal with the return of neural function after therapeutic intervention. To my knowledge, it is not yet known whether the abnormal signal intensity detected in the infraspinatus muscle in patients who have a ganglion cyst reverts to normal after the cyst is removed.

Whenever a patient is seen for muscular dysfunction, it is necessary to rule out a primary neuropathy or myopathy as the cause. The diagnosis of a neuropathy or a myopathy that alters the morphology or signal intensity of a muscle is possible on MRI. Direct evaluation of the brachial plexus is also possible, along with assessment of the major nerves innervating the shoulder girdle. Masses in the suprascapular and spinoglenoid notch or in the quadrilateral space that may be compressing the suprascapular or axillary nerves can be easily diagnosed with MRI as long as the study includes the appropriate anatomic regions. Direct communication between the referring physician and the radiologist is frequently needed if the maximum amount of information is to be generated for the assessment of a patient who has a suspected neuropathy or myopathy.

Although MRI is extremely sensitive to pathologic changes within a muscle, it lacks specificity. Any pathologic process that alters muscle morphology, incites an inflammatory response, or increases hydration of the muscle can be detected with MRI. The results of even a benign procedure, such as an intramuscular injection, can be detected on MRI as a focus of abnormal signal intensity in the muscle and perifascial tissue. Precise correlation of the abnormal findings on MRIs with the history and the findings of the physical examination is necessary to determine the clinical relevance of abnormal findings and to help to narrow down the differential diagnosis.

Instability

Instability of the shoulder can present in a variety of ways, and the radiographic approach should be tailored to the clinical situation. For the diagnosis of acute dislocation, the role of imaging is to confirm the presence and direction of the dislocation, to identify associated fractures or other injuries, and to evaluate the adequacy of reduction. Plain radiographs are usually adequate for the evaluation of an acute dislocation. Computed tomography helps to clarify the nature of a complex fracture-dislocation in cases of a failed reduction with intra-articular bone fragments and in cases of chronic dislocation. MRI may be helpful in evaluating patients with an irreducible dislocation caused by a dislocated biceps tendon or an avulsed rotator cuff or labrum.

MRI in the evaluation of instability is typically applicable to patients who have symptoms or signs suggestive of recurrent subluxation or dislocation of the shoulder and for whom the history and physical examination are inconclusive. Conventional MRI provides objective evidence of instability by detecting abnormalities of the capsulolabral complex, humeral head, and glenoid. MRI also provides information concerning the remainder of the shoulder girdle that may be causing the dysfunction.

In order to diagnose a torn labrum or torn glenohumeral ligaments accurately, it is necessary to know the normal range of appearance of these structures.[56,57] A normal anterior aspect of the labrum may be triangular, crescentic, cleaved, notched, or round and may be a different shape on each side of the body. Even though the labrum is composed of fibrocartilage, it may demonstrate a globular or linear focus of increased signal intensity on T1-weighted, gradient-echo, and proton-density-weighted images. As with the rotator cuff, the orientation of the collagen fibers in the labrum with respect to the main magnetic field may cause increased signal intensity that is detected in the labrum on T1-weighted and proton-density-weighted images. The posterior aspect of the labrum is normally smaller than the anterior aspect and is typically triangular. Investigators describing the appearance of a normal glenoid labrum have typically used MRIs of asymptomatic patients.[56,57] Unfortunately, this does not guarantee that the labra were normal.

An acute traumatic dislocation may damage the labrum, capsulolabral complex, supporting myotendinous structures, rim of the glenoid, or humeral head. The role of MRI is to define precisely the location and extent of the injury of these structures. In the acute situation, the presence of joint fluid helps in the evaluation of the labrum. The labrum may be torn, detached, or displaced after dislocation of the shoulder.[58] An anterior tear frequently is detected on MRI as a mass of tissue contiguous with deformed or stripped glenohumeral ligaments (Fig. 13). A torn or deformed middle or inferior glenohumeral ligament may be detected with MR arthrography,[59,60] but it may be difficult to assess with conventional MRI unless there is a large joint effusion. A strain or tear of the subscapularis muscle or tendon may be associated with an anterior dislocation. Rarely, there is stripping of the inferior aspect of the capsule from the humeral neck with an acute dislocation. This condition is difficult to diagnose clinically, but it can be diagnosed on an MRI (Fig. 14).

Additional findings indicative of previous anterior traumatic dislocation include a Hill-Sachs deformity, a Bankart lesion, and capsular stripping. A Hill-Sachs deformity is an osteochondral defect in the superior aspect of the posterolateral margin of the humeral head that results from impaction of the humeral head on the rim of the glenoid at the time of anterior dislocation of the shoulder. This deformity is detected on a MRI as an indentation in the humeral head. If there has been a recent episode of anterior instability, there may be an area of high signal intensity in the cancellous bone surrounding the deformity on a T2-weighted image. A cyst sometimes forms subjacent to a Hill-Sachs deformity in patients with a history of multiple dislocations. A Bankart lesion is a tear of the anterior capsulolabral complex that occurs with anterior dislocation of the shoulder. If there is also a fracture of the anterior part of the glenoid rim, the abnormality is referred to as an osseous Bankart lesion. The detection of a chronic osseous Bankart lesion may be subtle on MRI, but acute or subacute lesions may be associated with osseous edema in the rim of the glenoid or with anterior capsular stripping. While such stripping with associated pericapsular edema indicates an episode of anterior instability, a redundant anterior aspect of the capsule

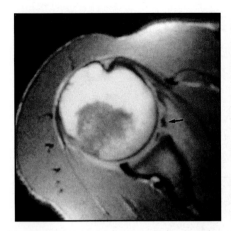
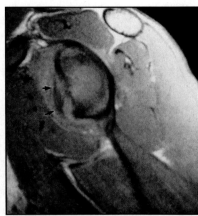

Fig. 13 Left, A proton-density-weighted axial image made after a recent anterior dislocation of the shoulder. The anterior aspect of the glenoid labrum is torn and detached (arrow). **Right,** The extent of the labral tear (arrows) is defined on the proton-density-weighted oblique sagittal image.

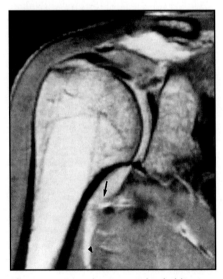

Fig. 14 A proton-density-weighted oblique coronal image showing an avulsion of the inferior aspect of the capsule from the neck of the humerus (arrow).

can be seen in asymptomatic subjects and is of uncertain clinical relevance.[57]

Signs of posterior instability include tears of the posterior aspect of the labrum and posterior capsular stripping (Fig. 15). For patients in whom instability is clinically suspected but the labrum appears normal on the initial standard imaging sequences, additional sequences made with the arm in internal and external rotation may help to demonstrate a torn labrum. Special positioning of the arm has also been used to assess the posterosuperior segment of the labrum.[61]

Several normal findings or anatomic variants depicted on a MRI may be mistaken for a torn labrum. There is a normal zone of hyaline cartilage interposed between the labrum and the rim of the glenoid that manifests increased signal intensity on T1-weighted, proton density-weighted, and gradient-echo sequences and that should not be misdiagnosed as a tear. Normal anatomic variants, such as a sublabral foramen at the level of the subscapularis recess or a Buford complex, may also be mistaken for a labral tear.[62] If there is no fluid in the shoulder joint, abutment of the glenohumeral ligaments against the anterior aspect of the labrum may simulate a deformed or torn labrum.[56]

With use of arthroscopy as the so-called gold standard, the accuracy of MRI in the detection of labral tears exceeds 90%. Legan and associates,[63] using MRI, accurately diagnosed 54 of 57 anterior labral tears, and Gusmer and associates[64] diagnosed 37 of 37 anterior labral tears detected at surgery. Legan and associates[63] diagnosed four anterior labral tears that

were not present at surgery and Gusmer and associates,[64] diagnosed three. Anterior labral tears seem to be easier to detect than posterior tears.[63] The clinical value of MRI is directly affected by factors such as the type of imaging equipment used, the completeness of the imaging sequences, the type of cohort population, and the specialization of the radiologists interpreting the studies. Garneau and associates[65] reported poor interobserver and intraobserver variability in the detection of labral abnormalities with MRI.

Other findings of instability on MRI include osseous changes in the anterior or posterior margin of the glenoid; glenoid dysplasia[66] or abnormal tilt; subluxation of the humeral head; and abnormalities of the rotator cuff, especially of the subscapularis muscle and tendon. Glenoid labral cysts are typically associated with labral tears and may indicate the direction of instability. Tirman and associates[67] reported evidence of a labral cyst on the MRIs of 20 patients; all of the cysts were associated with a labral tear. Eleven of the 20 patients had clinical evidence of instability in the direction of the labral tear and cyst. The labral tear and cyst were located superiorly in nine patients, posteriorly in nine, and anteriorly in two. The cyst extended into the spinoglenoid notch in six patients, the suprascapular notch in three, and both in four. In eight patients, the labral tear as well as a communication between the joint and the cyst was confirmed at surgery.

The shoulder joint normally contains only a small amount of fluid, making evaluation of the joint capsule and the glenohumeral ligaments difficult. MR arthrography has been used to overcome this limitation by the injection of saline solution or a dilute solution of an MR contrast agent into the joint.[68,69] Distention of the joint capsule facilitates the evaluation of the capsulolabral complex in much the same way that it does with computed tomographic arthrography. Several recent studies have demonstrated the superiority of MR arthrography compared with computed tomographic arthrography for the evaluation of instability of the shoulder.[70-72] In addition, MR arthrography is reportedly more accurate than standard MRI for the detection of capsulolabral abnormalities.[37,70] The major disadvantage of MR arthrography is that it transforms a standard noninvasive MRI study into a limited invasive study, which is more time-consuming and more expensive. In addition, MR contrast agents have not been approved by the Food and Drug Administration for intra-articular use. Although MR arthrography may be useful in a select subset of patients, such as those who have posterosuperior impingement,[61] it must be clarified whether its increased sensitivity comes at the expense of decreased specificity and, in addition, how the information affects the management of the patient and the outcome. Considering the recent report by Gusmer and associates,[64] which showed conventional unenhanced MRI to be highly accurate for the detection of labral abnormalities, it should probably remain the initial MRI screening examination for patients with symptoms of instability.

Although labral tears are typically associated with clinical or occult instability, they also may be found in patients who have a stable shoulder and pain, clicking, or locking. This has been reported in athletes who participate in overhead activities[73] as well as in nonathletes.[74] A torn labrum may appear frayed, blunted, or attenuated and may contain abnormal signal intensity extending to its articular surface. Superior labral tears involving the biceps anchor are detected both in athletes who participate in overhead sports and in nonathletes. Snyder and associates[75] reported tears of the superior aspect of the labrum that may extend anteriorly or posteriorly (SLAP lesions), and they classified these tears

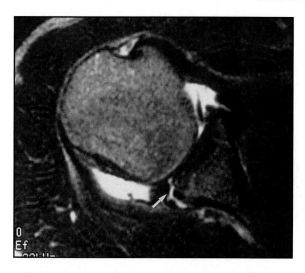

Fig. 15 A T2-weighted axial image showing a tear through the base of the posterior aspect of the glenoid labrum (arrow) along with posterior capsular stripping.

according to the type of labral deformity and the integrity of the biceps anchor. A type-I lesion represents fraying of the superior aspect of the labrum, which is attached to the rim of the glenoid; a type-II lesion, avulsion of the superior aspect of the labrum and the biceps anchor from the superior aspect of the rim; a type-III lesion, a tear of the superior aspect of the labrum, which is displaced into the shoulder joint (similar to a bucket-handle tear of the meniscus); and a type-IV lesion, a tear of the superior aspect of the labrum associated with a partially detached biceps anchor (part of the biceps inserts into the torn labrum and part into the supraglenoid tubercle). The reported accuracy of MRI in detecting these lesions has varied greatly in the literature. Some studies demonstrated the need for intra-articular contrast medium to make the diagnosis,[37] whereas in other studies routine MRI sequences successfully demonstrated the tear of the superior aspect of the labrum that extended anteriorly or posteriorly.[76,77] Both oblique coronal and axial sequences are needed for optimum detection of the presence and extent of the tear (Fig. 16).

The application of MRI for the assessment of instability of the shoulder is highly dependent on the physician managing the patient. If an orthopaedic sur-

geon uses arthroscopy to repair Bankart-type lesions and arthrotomy to repair all other types of instability, MRI may be beneficial in the preoperative planning.[78] In difficult cases, MRI may be needed to provide objective evidence of instability. While MRI appears to have contributed important information to the care of patients,[61,78] it is still necessary for each clinician to determine its appropriate role, in his or her particular medical community, in the assessment of patients who have symptoms of instability of the shoulder.

Suder and associates[79] evaluated patients after traumatic primary anterior dislocation of the shoulder and found that conventional MRI was only moderately reliable in the preoperative evaluation of labral tears and Hill-Sachs deformities and that it provided little useful information concerning capsulolabral lesions. Green and Christensen,[80] in a study of the MRIs of 33 patients who had possible anterior instability of the shoulder, detected only 21 of 28 labral tears that were present at surgery. They concluded that "magnetic resonance imaging is not useful in the surgical planning for most patients with obvious anterior shoulder instability." In a study of 41 labral tears that were detected at surgery, Liu and associates[81] accurately diagnosed

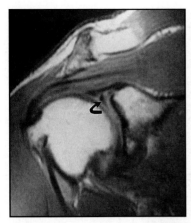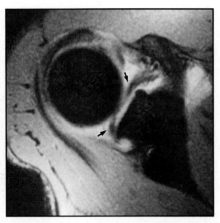

Fig. 16 Left, A proton-density-weighted oblique coronal image showing a type-III tear of the superior aspect of the labrum extending anteriorly and posteriorly (SLAP lesion) (arrow). **Right,** A gradient-echo axial image also showing a type-III tear of the superior aspect of the labrum extending anteriorly and posteriorly (arrows).

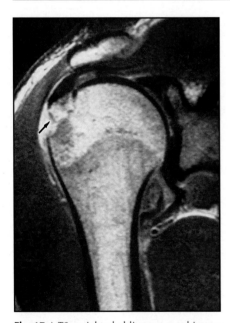

Fig. 17 A T2-weighted oblique coronal image showing a minimally displaced fracture of the greater tuberosity (arrow), which was the result of a skiing injury. The rotator cuff is intact.

37 tears on physical examination but only 24 on MRI. Two tears that were diagnosed on physical examination and with MRI were not detected at surgery. It is hoped that with the continued improvement in MRI technology, such as three-dimensional imaging of the labrum,[82] its value in the assessment of instability of the shoulder will continue to improve.

Additional Applications
Trauma
After a direct-impaction injury to an extremity, it is fairly common for an individual to have normal findings on plain radiography despite pain involving an osseous structure. Before the availability of MRI, the precise etiology of this pain was unclear; it was uncertain whether it was related to injury of soft-tissue or osseous structures, or both. With the exquisite sensitivity of MRI for the detection of bone marrow edema, it became readily apparent that many of these patients had areas of edema in the cancellous bone at the site of an osseous injury. These areas were designated bone contusions or bruises, and it was hypothesized that the osseous edema was due to trabecular microfractures. Recently, Rangger and associates[83] reported that biopsy of two foci of osseous edema in a knee demonstrated a reparative process of fractured cancellous bone. Bone contusions may occur secondary to an extrinsic impaction injury or to bones impacting against one another as a result of acute instability or malalignment. The importance of detecting a bone contusion is that it may explain the etiology of a patient's pain and eliminate the need for additional diagnostic tests.

In the shoulder, contusions in the posterior superolateral margin of the humeral head and the anterior margin of the glenoid may be detected after an episode of anterior instability. Contusions of the lesser tuberosity and the posterior margin of the glenoid are seen after a posterior dislocation. Contusions of the greater tuberosity are frequently detected after a fall while skiing. In addition, MRI can detect nondisplaced or minimally displaced fractures of the greater tuberosity in these patients (Fig. 17). These fractures are frequently difficult to detect on plain radiographs. For the evaluation of stress fractures of the humerus, MRI is as sensitive and probably more specific than a radionuclide study, because of its superior spatial resolution.

Osteonecrosis
Atraumatic osteonecrosis of the shoulder may be detected in patients who are taking steroids (Fig. 18) or those who have sickle-cell or marrow-storage disease. The appearance of the osteonecrosis depends on its stage of evolution. The diagnosis is based on detection of a well-marginated focus of abnormal subchondral cancellous bone that may be surrounded by a rim of reactive bone. Collapse of the subchondral bone plate as well as secondary degenerative changes may be detected. This problem appears to be less common in the humeral head than in the femoral head, most likely because of the nonweight-bearing function of the humeral head. Osteonecrosis of the humeral head may also be detected after a comminuted fracture that disrupts its blood supply.

Tumor
Patients who have a malignant process involving the scapula, the humeral head,

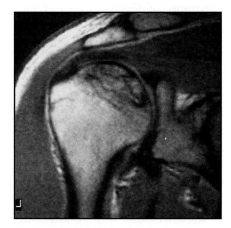

Fig. 18 A proton-density-weighted oblique coronal image showing a large osteonecrotic focus in the superomedial segment of the humeral head, without collapse of the subchondral bone plate, associated with chronic use of steroids.

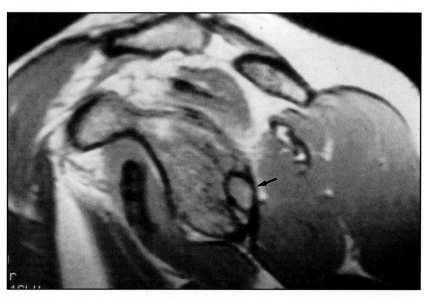

Fig. 19 A proton-density-weighted oblique sagittal image showing subchondral cysts (arrow) within the posteroinferior margin of the glenoid.

or the humeral neck may be seen for pain in the shoulder. Because of osteopenia of the shoulder girdle, which is common in older patients, it is often difficult to detect early osseous destruction on plain radiographs. As in other areas of the body, MRI provides an excellent means with which to evaluate the presence and extent of either primary or metastatic tumors of the shoulder girdle. T1-weighted sequences are used to define the interface between the tumor and the fat in the cancellous bone or at the cortical surface, and fat-suppressed T2-weighted or STIR sequences are used to define extension of the tumor into soft tissue. With MRI, it is possible to detect benign tumors, such as a scapular exostosis, that are precipitating symptoms of a snapping scapula.

MRI also provides the most comprehensive evaluation of soft-tissue tumors. Tumors that originate in synovial tissue, such as diffuse or focal pigmented villonodular synovitis and synovial chondromatosis, or tumors that are located within the muscles or perimuscular tissue of the shoulder girdle may be assessed completely with MRI. As in

other joints of the body, pigmented villonodular synovitis typically presents with foci of nodular tissue demonstrating low signal intensity on spin-echo T1-weighted and T2-weighted sequences because of its hemosiderin content. Intravenous contrast-enhanced MRI studies are frequently needed to evaluate tumor margins and to assess the degree of tumor necrosis. MR angiography is also available to evaluate the relationship of soft tissue tumors to the major vessels, as well as to determine the degree of tumor vascularity.

Arthritis and Osteoarthrosis
Patients who have a systemic arthritis, such as rheumatoid arthritis or ankylosing spondylitis, may be seen for symptoms about the shoulder. Plain radiographs are usually sufficient to evaluate these patients, unless secondary complications, such as an insufficiency fracture or infection, develop.

Osteoarthrosis of the glenohumeral joint is relatively infrequent, and it may be difficult to detect on plain radiographs. Because the articular cartilage of the humeral head and glenoid fossa is

normally 2 to 3 mm thick, it is extremely difficult to detect isolated lesions of the articular cartilage. Once subchondral edema or cystic changes are present as part of a degenerative condition, they are easily detected with the appropriate proton-density or T2-weighted sequences (Fig. 19). Small loose bodies are difficult to detect unless there is at least a little fluid within the joint. Small marginal osteophytes of the rim of the glenoid or the junction of the humeral head and neck are also difficult to detect with MRI because of the soft tissues inserting into these regions. MRI provides an excellent assessment of arthropathy of the rotator cuff by depicting the osseous alterations of the glenohumeral joint and the supporting soft-tissue structures.

Inflammation and Infection
Soft-tissue infection, septic arthritis, and osteomyelitis of the shoulder girdle are unusual causes of pain about the shoulder but they must be considered, particularly in a patient who is immunosuppressed or is receiving steroids. Any inflammatory process involving the fascia or the muscles can be detected with

MRI because of the increased tissue hydration resulting from the influx of cellular elements and the associated interstitial edema. One of the main applications of MRI in patients who have a soft-tissue infection is the determination of whether there is a focal abscess or evidence of muscle necrosis. MRI is extremely sensitive for detecting a joint effusion, osseous edema, and destruction of bone due to infection.

A common cause of pain about the shoulder is calcific bursitis. While bursitis is typically precipitated by the deposition of hydroxyapatite crystals, and is therefore readily diagnosed on plain radiographs, it can also be caused by an infectious agent such as tuberculosis. Fluid within the subacromial and subdeltoid bursa is easily detected on MRI. In addition to detection of calcification within a fluid-filled bursa, it is possible to assess the condition of the synovial tissue and the subjacent rotator cuff on MRI. It is also possible to detect so-called rice bodies within the bursa, which may be present with rheumatoid bursitis or, rarely, some infectious agents.

Overview

An imaging study should be ordered only when its results will directly affect the management of a patient. As a result of the static nature of most imaging studies, including MRI, their interpretation is predominantly focused on the detection of isolated structural abnormalities. But static images are a snapshot of the evolution of a pathologic condition, and their value is enhanced if they can elucidate the natural history of a pathologic process. MRI has greatly increased our understanding of dysfunction of the shoulder. MRI can detect not only pathologic conditions that are precipitating symptoms but also alterations in tissue resulting from chronic microtrauma or aging that do not precipitate symptoms. These subclinical abnormalities are not false-positive findings, as they

represent pathologic changes in the tissue. Although they may have no clinical relevance in the explanation of a patient's current symptoms, they may have prognostic importance if they reflect altered biomechanical properties of tissue. In the future, this information may be used to guide athletic training or to optimize patient rehabilitation.

While MRI has improved the diagnosis and treatment of musculoskeletal disorders, its efficacy can be enhanced further by a closer working relationship among physicians who care for patients who have musculoskeletal disorders. Prospective, controlled studies are still needed to compare the cost-effectiveness of the various imaging and diagnostic modalities employed to evaluate the shoulder. Redundant and unnecessary diagnostic studies must be eliminated if we hope to control the spiraling costs of health care.

References

1. Sidor ML, Zuckerman JD, Lyon T, et al: The Neer classification system for proximal humeral fractures: An assessment of interobserver reliability and intraobserver reproducibility. *J Bone Joint Surg* 1993;75A:1745–1750.
2. Davis SJ, Teresi LM, Bradley WG, et al: Effect of arm rotation on MR imaging of the rotator cuff. *Radiology* 1991;181:265–268.
3. Buckwalter JA, Woo SL, Goldberg VM, et al: Soft-tissue aging and musculoskeletal function. *J Bone Joint Surg* 1993;75A:1533–1548.
4. Crues JV III: Technical considerations, in Mink JH, Reicher MA, Crues JV III, et al (eds): *Magnetic Resonance Imaging of the Knee*, ed 2. New York, NY, Raven Press, 1993, pp 1–23.
5. Mirowitz SA: Fast scanning and fat-suppression MR imaging of musculoskeletal disorders. *Am J Roentgenol* 1993;161:1147–1157.
6. Mirowitz SA, Apicella P, Reinus WR, et al: MR imaging of bone marrow lesions: Relative conspicuousness on T1-weighted, fat-suppressed T2-weighted, and STIR images. *Am J Roentgenol* 1994;162:215–221.
7. Shellock FG: MRI biological effects, safety, and patient management, in Mink JH, Reicher MA, Crues JV III, et al (eds): *Magnetic Resonance Imaging of the Knee*, ed 2. New York, NY, Raven Press, 1993, pp 25–49.
8. Neer CS II: Impingement lesions. *Clin Orthop* 1983;173:70–77.
9. Clark JM, Harryman DT II: Tendons, ligaments, and capsule of the rotator cuff: Gross

and microscopic anatomy. *J Bone Joint Surg* 1991;74A:713–725.
10. Kjellin I, Ho CP, Cervilla V, et al: Alterations in the supraspinatus tendon at MR imaging: Correlation with histopathologic findings in cadavers. *Radiology* 1991;181:837–841.
11. Farley TE, Neumann CH, Steinbach LS, et al: The coracoacromial arch: MR evaluation and correlation with rotator cuff pathology. *Skeletal Radiol* 1994;23:641–645.
12. Fukuda H, Hamada K, Nakajima T, et al: Pathology and pathogenesis of the intratendinous tearing of the rotator cuff viewed from en bloc histologic sections. *Clin Orthop* 1994;304:60–67.
13. Solem-Bertoft E, Thuomas K-A, Westerberg C-E: The influence of scapular retraction and protraction on the width of the subacromial space: An MRI study. *Clin Orthop* 1993;296:99–103.
14. Blevins FT, Hayes WM, Warren RF: Rotator cuff injury in contact athletes. *Am J Sports Med* 1996;24:263–267.
15. Weiner DS, Macnab I: Superior migration of the humeral head: A radiological aid in the diagnosis of tears of the rotator cuff. *J Bone Joint Surg* 1970;52B:524–527.
16. Jacobson SR, Speer KP, Moor JT, et al: Reliability of radiographic assessment of acromial morphology. *J Shoulder Elbow Surg* 1995;4:449–453.
17. Uri DS, Kneeland JB, Herzog RJ: Os acromiale: Evaluation of markers for identification on sagittal and coronal oblique MR images. *Skeletal Radiol* 1997;26:31–34.
18. Zlatkin MB, Iannotti JP, Roberts MC, et al: Rotator cuff tears: Diagnostic performance of MR imaging. *Radiology* 1989;172:223–229.
19. Timins ME, Erickson SJ, Estkowski LD, et al: Increased signal in the normal supraspinatus tendon on MR imaging: Diagnostic pitfall caused by the magic-angle effect. *Am J Roentgenol* 1995;165:109–114.
20. Kieft GJ, Bloem JL, Rozing PM, et al: Rotator cuff impingement syndrome: MR imaging. *Radiology* 1988;166:211–214.
21. Nakagaki K, Ozaki J, Tomita Y, et al: Magnetic resonance imaging of rotator cuff tearing and degenerative tendon changes: Correlation with histologic pathology. *J Shoulder Elbow Surg* 1993;2:156–164.
22. Farley TE, Neumann CH, Steinbach LS, et al: Full-thickness tears of the rotator cuff of the shoulder: Diagnosis with MR imaging. *Am J Roentgenol* 1992;158:347–351.
23. Rafii M, Firooznia H, Sherman O, et al: Rotator cuff lesions: Signal patterns at MR imaging. *Radiology* 1990;177:817–823.
24. Nakagaki K, Ozaki J, Tomita Y, et al: Alterations in the supraspinatus muscle belly with rotator cuff tearing: Evaluation with MRI. *J Shoulder Elbow Surg* 1994;3:88–93.
25. Nakagaki K, Ozaki J, Tomita Y, et al: Function of supraspinatus muscle with torn cuff evalu-

ated by magnetic resonance imaging. *Clin Orthop* 1995;318:144–151.

26. Gerber C, Krushell RJ: Isolated rupture of the tendon of the subscapularis muscle: Clinical features in 16 cases. *J Bone Joint Surg* 1991;73B:389–394.

27. Patten RM: Tears of the anterior portion of the rotator cuff (the subscapularis tendon): MR imaging findings. *Am J Roentgenol* 1994;162:351–354.

28. Walch G, Nove-Josserand L, Levigne C, et al: Tears of the supraspinatus tendon associated with "hidden" lesions of the rotator interval. *J Shoulder Elbow Surg* 1994;3:353–360.

29. Iannotti JP, Zlatkin MB, Esterhai JL, et al: Magnetic resonance imaging of the shoulder: Sensitivity, specificity, and predictive value. *J Bone Joint Surg* 1991;73A:17–29.

30. Quinn SF, Sheley RC, Demlow TA, et al: Rotator cuff tendon tears: Evaluation with fat-suppressed MR imaging with arthroscopic correlation in 100 patients. *Radiology* 1995;195:497–500.

31. Singson RD, Hoang T, Dan S, et al: MR evaluation of rotator cuff pathology using T2-weighted fast spin-echo technique with and without fat suppression. *Am J Roentgenol* 1996;166:1061–1065.

32. Sonin AH, Peduto AJ, Fitzgerald SW, et al: MR imaging of the rotator cuff mechanism: Comparison of spin-echo and turbo spin-echo sequences. *Am J Roentgenol* 1996;167:333–338.

33. Robertson PL, Schweitzer ME, Mitchell DG, et al: Rotator cuff disorders: Interobserver and intraobserver variation in diagnosis with MR imaging. *Radiology* 1995;194:831–835.

34. Traughber PD, Goodwin TE: Shoulder MRI: Arthroscopic correlation with emphasis on partial tears. *J Comput Assist Tomogr* 1992;16:129–133.

35. Hodler J, Kursunoglu-Brahme S, Snyder SJ, et al: Rotator cuff disease: Assessment with MR arthrography versus standard MR imaging in 36 patients with arthroscopic confirmation. *Radiology* 1992;182:431–436.

36. Palmer WE, Brown JH, Rosenthal DI: Rotator cuff: Evaluation with fat-suppressed MR arthrography. *Radiology* 1993;188:683–687.

37. Karzel RP, Snyder SJ: Magnetic resonance arthrography of the shoulder: A new technique of shoulder imaging. *Clin Sports Med* 1993;12:123–136.

38. Tirman PF, Bost FW, Steinbach LS, et al: MR arthrographic depiction of tears of the rotator cuff: Benefit of abduction and external rotation of the arm. *Radiology* 1994;192:851–856.

39. Owen RS, Iannotti JP, Kneeland JB, et al: Shoulder after surgery: MR imaging with surgical validation. *Radiology* 1993;186:443–447.

40. Gaenslen ES, Satterlee CC, Hinson GW: Magnetic resonance imaging for evaluation of failed repairs of the rotator cuff: Relationship to operative findings. *J Bone Joint Surg* 1996;78A:1391–1396.

41. Harryman DT II, Mack LA, Wang KY, et al: Repairs of the rotator cuff: Correlation of functional results with integrity of the cuff. *J Bone Joint Surg* 1991;73A:982–989.

42. Calvert PT, Packer NP, Stoker DJ, et al: Arthrography of the shoulder after operative repair of the torn rotator cuff. *J Bone Joint Surg* 1986;68B:147–150.

43. Miniaci A, Dowdy PA, Willits KR, et al: Magnetic resonance imaging evaluation of the rotator cuff tendons in the asymptomatic shoulder. *Am J Sports Med* 1995;23:142–145.

44. Neumann CH, Holt RG, Steinbach LS, et al: MR imaging of the shoulder: Appearance of the supraspinatus tendon in asymptomatic volunteers. *Am J Roentgenol* 1992;158:1281–1287.

45. Sher JS, Uribe JW, Posada A, et al: Abnormal findings on magnetic resonance images of asymptomatic shoulders. *J Bone Joint Surg* 1995;77A:10–15.

46. Needell SD, Zlatkin MB, Sher JS, et al: MR imaging of the rotator cuff: Peritendinous and bone abnormalities in an asymptomatic population. *Am J Roentgenol* 1996;166:863–867.

47. Mink JH: Muscle injuries, in Mink JH, Reicher MA, Crues JV III, et al (eds): *Magnetic Resonance Imaging of the Knee*, ed 2. New York, NY, Raven Press, 1993, pp 401–431.

48. Greco A, McNamara MT, Escher RB, et al: Spin-echo and STIR MR imaging of sports-related muscle injuries at 1.5 T. *J Comput Assist Tomogr* 1991;15:994–999.

49. Nurenberg P, Giddings CJ, Stray-Gundersen J, et al: MR imaging-guided muscle biopsy for correlation of increased signal intensity with ultrastructural change and delayed-onset muscle soreness after exercise. *Radiology* 1992;184:865–869.

50. Shellock FG, Fukunaga T, Mink JH, et al: Exertional muscle injury: Evaluation of concentric versus eccentric actions with serial MR imaging. *Radiology* 1991;179:659–664.

51. Polak JF, Jolesz FA, Adams DF: NMR of skeletal muscle: Differences in relaxation parameters related to extracellular/intracellular fluid spaces. *Invest Radiol* 1988;23:107–112.

52. Shellock FG, Fukunaga T, Mink JH, et al: Acute effects of exercise on MR imaging of skeletal muscle: Concentric vs eccentric actions. *Am J Roentgenol* 1991;156:765–768.

53. Fleckenstein JL, Watumull D, Conner KE, et al: Denervated human skeletal muscle: MR imaging evaluation. *Radiology* 1993;187:213–218.

54. Uetani M, Hayashi K, Matsunaga N, et al: Denervated skeletal muscle: MR imaging. Work in progress. *Radiology* 1993;189:511–515.

55. Uppal GS, Uppal JA, Dwyer AP: Glenoid cysts mimicking cervical radiculopathy. *Spine* 1995;20:2257–2260.

56. Liou JT, Wilson AJ, Totty WG, et al: The normal shoulder: Common variations that simulate pathologic conditions at MR imaging. *Radiology* 1993;186:435–441.

57. Neumann CH, Petersen SA, Jahnke AH: MR imaging of the labral-capsular complex: Normal variations. *Am J Roentgenol* 1991;157:1015–1021.

58. McCauley TR, Pope CE, Jokl P: Normal and abnormal glenoid labrum: Assessment with multiplanar gradient-echo MR imaging. *Radiology* 1992;183:35–37.

59. Chandnani VP, Gagliardi JA, Murnane TG, et al: Glenohumeral ligaments and shoulder capsular mechanism: Evaluation with MR arthrography. *Radiology* 1995;196:27–32.

60. Palmer WE, Brown JH, Rosenthal DI: Labral-ligamentous complex of the shoulder: Evaluation with MR arthrography. *Radiology* 1994;190:645–651.

61. Tirman PF, Bost FW, Garvin GJ, et al: Posterosuperior glenoid impingement of the shoulder: Findings at MR imaging and MR arthrography with arthroscopic correlation. *Radiology* 1994;193:431–436.

62. Tuite MJ, Orwin JF: Anterosuperior labral variants of the shoulder: Appearance on gradient-recalled-echo and fast spin-echo MR images. *Radiology* 1996;199:537–540.

63. Legan JM, Burkhard TK, Goff WB II, et al: Tears of the glenoid labrum: MR imaging of 88 arthroscopically confirmed cases. *Radiology* 1991;179:241–246.

64. Gusmer PB, Potter HG, Schatz JA, et al: Labral injuries: Accuracy of detection with unenhanced MR imaging of the shoulder. *Radiology* 1996;200:519–524.

65. Garneau RA, Renfrew DL, Moore TE, et al: Glenoid labrum: Evaluation with MR imaging. *Radiology* 1991;179:519–522.

66. Trout TE, Resnick D: Glenoid hypoplasia and its relationship to instability. *Skeletal Radiol* 1996;25:37–40.

67. Tirman PF, Feller JF, Janzen DL, et al: Association of glenoid labral cysts with labral tears and glenohumeral instability: Radiologic findings and clinical significance. *Radiology* 1994;190:653–658.

68. Flannigan B, Kursunoglu-Brahme S, Snyder S, et al: MR arthrography of the shoulder: Comparison with conventional MR imaging. *Am J Roentgenol* 1990;155:829–832.

69. Tirman PF, Stauffer AE, Crues JV III, et al: Saline magnetic resonance arthrography in the evaluation of glenohumeral instability. *Arthroscopy* 1993;9:550–559.

70. Chandnani VP, Yeager TD, DeBerardino T, et al: Glenoid labral tears: Prospective evaluation with MR imaging, MR arthrography, and CT arthrography. *Am J Roentgenol* 1993;161:1229–1235.

71. Jahnke AH Jr, Petersen SA, Neumann C, et al: A prospective comparison of computerized arthrotomography and MRI of the glenohumeral joint. *Am J Sports Med* 1992;20:695–701.

72. Sano H, Kato Y, Haga K, et al: Magnetic resonance arthrography in the assessment of anterior instability of the shoulder: Comparison with double-contrast computed tomography arthrography. *J Shoulder Elbow Surg* 1996;5:280–285.

73. Rafii M, Firooznia H, Bonamo JJ, et al: Athlete shoulder injuries: CT arthrographic findings. *Radiology* 1987;162:559–564.

74. Neviaser TJ: The GLAD lesion: Another cause of anterior shoulder pain. *Arthroscopy* 1993;9:22–23.

75. Snyder SJ, Banas MP, Karzel RP: An analysis of 140 injuries to the superior glenoid labrum. *J Shoulder Elbow Surg* 1995;4:243–248.

76. Cartland JP, Crues JV III, Stauffer A, et al: MR imaging in the evaluation of SLAP injuries of the shoulder: Findings in 10 patients. *Am J Roentgenol* 1992;159:787–792.

77. Monu JU, Pope TL Jr, Chabon SJ, et al: MR diagnosis of superior labral anterior posterior (SLAP) injuries of the glenoid labrum: Value of routine imaging without intraarticular injec-tion of contrast material. *Am J Roentgenol* 1994;163:1425–1429.

78. Minkoff J, Cavaliere G: Glenohumeral insta-bilities and the role of MRI techniques: The orthopedic surgeon's perspective. *Magn Reson Imaging Clin North Am* 1993;1:105–123.

79. Suder PA, Frich LH, Hougaard K, et al: MRI evaluation of capsulolabral tears after traumatic primary anterior shoulder dislocation: A prospective comparison with arthroscopy of 25 cases. *J Shoulder Elbow Surg* 1995;4:419–428.

80. Green MR, Christensen KP: Magnetic reso-nance imaging of the glenoid labrum in anteri-or shoulder instability. *Am J Sports Med* 1994;22:493–498.

81. Liu SH, Henry MH, Nuccion S, et al: Diagnosis of glenoid labral tears: A compari-son between magnetic resonance imaging and clinical examinations. *Am J Sports Med* 1996;24:149–154.

82. Loehr SP, Pope, TL Jr, Martin DF, et al: Three-dimensional MRI of the glenoid labrum. *Skeletal Radiol* 1995;24:117–121.

83. Rangger C, Klestil T, Kathrein A, et al: Influence of MRI on indications for arthroscopy of the knee. *Clin Orthop* 1996;330:133–142.

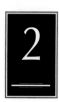

Arthroscopic Acromioplasty: Indications and Technique

David W. Altchek, MD
Eric W. Carson, MD

Introduction

Impingement syndrome of the shoulder is one of the most common causes of shoulder pain and dysfunction. Neer,[1] in 1972, was the first to coin the term "impingement syndrome." In 100 dissected shoulders, Neer observed evidence of impingement in 11, with a characteristic ridge of proliferative spurs and excrescences on the undersurface of the anterior process of the acromion. He described this condition as compression of the supraspinatus tendon against the anterior edge of the acromion, the coracoacromial ligament, and, at times, a projecting spur localized to the acromioclavicular joint. This chronic, repetitive syndrome, characterized by microtrauma, causes a progressive inflammatory process and a subsequent degenerative process within the rotator cuff, accompanied by pain and weakness of the shoulder. Neer[2] proposed three stages in the development of impingement syndrome: stage I, a reversible stage, in which edema and hemorrhage predominate; stage II, an irreversible stage, in which tendinitis and fibrosis have occurred; and stage III, characterized by significant tendon degeneration and tearing.

Stage I and most stage II lesions respond to a conservative program consisting of gentle exercise, nonsteroidal anti-inflammatory medications, and occasional corticosteroid subacromial injection. Stage II lesions refractory to conservative treatment and stage III lesions are candidates for surgical intervention.

Historically, various procedures had been used, including complete acromionectomy and lateral acromionectomy.[3-5] Neer[1] developed a new surgical procedure for impingement syndrome, an open anterior acromioplasty. This procedure has gained wide acceptance with universally excellent long-term results that ranged from 80% to 90% in most series, including Neer's original group.[2,6-10]

In 1985, Ellman[11] presented an alternative method, an arthroscopic subacromial decompression/acromioplasty technique. His preliminary data revealed results comparable to those of open acromioplasty. Subsequently, in 1987, the long-term results of this new and innovative technique were published.[12] Reports of the first 50 consecutive arthroscopic acromioplasties, with a follow-up of 1 to 3 years, revealed an 88% satisfactory rating (excellent or good) and a 12% unsatisfactory rating (fair or poor). Subsequently, other authors have documented similar results of arthroscopic acromioplasty. [10,13-16] Altchek and associates[17] reported follow-up on 40 patients who underwent arthroscopic acromioplasty. Ten of these patients had full-thickness cuff tears. Good or excellent results were noted in 73% of patients, with a 77% rate of return to sports. Speer and associates[18] reported 88% good or excellent results after arthroscopic acromioplasty for patients with an intact rotator cuff. Esch[14] reported a 78% objective success rate and an 82% patient satisfaction rate for patients without full-thickness rotator cuff tears. A follow-up study by Gartsman[19] reported 88% satisfactory results in patients without rotator cuff tears and 83% satisfactory results in patients with partial cuff tears.

After the initial introduction of an arthroscopic subacromial decompression/acromioplasty by Ellman,[11] there was great doubt and skepticism about the technical difficulties of this procedure and concern about the adequacy of arthroscopic acromial resection. In a cadaver study published by Gartsman and associates,[20] the predictability of the bone resection via the arthroscopic technique was shown to be equal to that possible with the open technique. In a related study by Devine and associates (unpublished data) intraoperative measurements were made of the acromial thickness before and after acromioplasty to compare open and arthroscopic techniques. The average thickness of bone resected at a site 1 cm posterior to the anterior aspect of the acromion in the mid-axial plane was noted to be 5 mm for the open technique and 5.1 mm for the arthroscopic technique, again confirming that adequate bone removal can be achieved arthroscopically.

A comparison of the two techniques shows there are several advantages of arthroscopic acromioplasty. First, arthroscopic acromioplasty involves significantly less surgical morbidity and allows quicker rehabilitation. Open acromioplasty requires some degree of detachment of the anterior deltoid from the acromion and protection of the deltoid repair during early rehabilitation. By preserving the deltoid origin during arthroscopic acromioplasty, an active rehabilitation regimen can be safely started immediately postoperatively. Ultimately, return to high-load overhead activity still requires establishment of overall shoulder girdle strength, as demonstrated in the study by Altchek and associates,[17] in which the overall average time to return to work was 9 days, and the average return to sports was 2.4 months.

It should not be overlooked that direct visualization of the glenohumeral joint at the time of an arthroscopic acromioplasty may prove to be invaluable in those cases in which the clinical diagnosis is not absolutely clear. Two common examples are middle-aged patients with early osteoarthritis of the shoulder and younger patients with subtle instability, which may mimic the symptoms of impingement syndrome. Abnormalities such as labral tears, biceps tears, undersurface rotator cuff tears, subscapularis tendon tears, and synovitis or adhesive capsulitis of the shoulder may go otherwise undetected during an open acromioplasty.

Pathoanatomy/Etiology

A variety of factors have been described and proposed in the development and exacerbation of the subacromial impingement. Traditionally, these have been grouped into structural factors and dynamic factors.

Structural

Acromial shape has received significant attention with respect to causation of impingement syndrome. In a review of 140 shoulders in 71 cadavers (average age, 74.4 years), Bigliani and associates[21] described three types of acromion: type I

- flat, seen in 17%; type II - curved, seen in 43%; and type III - hooked, seen in 40%. Bilateral concurrence of shape was seen in 58% of the cadavers. A third of the specimens had full thickness tears, of which 73% were seen with a type III acromion, 24% with a type II, and 3% with type I. This cadaveric study was supported in a clinical review of 200 modified lateral scapular radiographs by Morrison and Bigliani.[22] Eighty percent of the patients with full thickness rotator cuff tears had hooked acromia (type III); the remainder had curved acromia (type II). Gartsman[19] subsequently described an additional type of acromion associated with impingement syndrome, a type I acromion with an increase in the angle of inclination that narrows the supraspinatus outlet.

Other causes of decreased space within the supraspinatus outlet have been identified, including osteophytes of the acromioclavicular joint; hypertrophy and enthesopathy of the coracoacromial ligament; os acromiale; malunion of the greater tuberosity, distal clavicle, or acromion; inflammatory bursitis (rheumatoid arthritis); thickening of the rotator cuff (calcific tendinitis); or a flap of rotator cuff secondary to a partial tear on the bursal side. All of these conditions have a significant impact, because they decrease the overall volume of the subacromial space and space available for the tendons of the rotator cuff, leading to eventual degeneration and tearing.

Overuse/Dynamic Impingement

Traditionally, the pathologic changes of impingement have been attributed to mechanical causes, based on Neer's gross anatomic findings related to the anterior inferior one third of the acromion. In recent years, however, an alternative mechanism for the etiology of impingement has been put forth. Altchek and others have proposed that the initial stages of impingement syndrome are caused either by an injury to the rotator

cuff or by repetitive microtrauma of the rotator cuff.[23] Either of these injuries causes a weakened and dysfunctional rotator cuff. Imbalance of the shoulder musculature between the weakened rotator cuff and a normal deltoid causes abnormal superior migration of the humeral head during arm elevation. Because of this, the tuberosity repetitively abuts the coracoacromial arch, resulting, over a long period of time, in bony hypertrophy of the coracoacromial arch and tuberosity, as well as further injury to the rotator cuff. In a study performed by Deutsch and associates,[23] no statistically significant superior migration of the humeral head on the glenoid was noted in patients with stage II and stage III impingement when they were compared with a group of normal patients.

This dynamic imbalance supports the role of rehabilitation of the musculature of the shoulder girdle in patients with impingement syndrome. Successful strengthening of the rotator cuff and scapular musculature should restore the humeral head centering effect of the rotator cuff during arm elevation.

Clinical Evaluation

Despite diagnostic advances, such as magnetic resonance imaging (MRI), impingement syndrome remains a clinical diagnosis. In most cases, a thorough history and detailed physical examination will elucidate the diagnosis.

Patients with impingement syndrome typically present with the insidious onset of shoulder pain with overhead activities. This pain may awaken the patient at night and he or she may be unable to sleep lying on the involved side. The pain is often localized to the proximal lateral aspect of the humerus. Typically, patients with impingement syndrome do not complain of loss of shoulder motion. However, they may frequently have a painful arc of motion between 70° and 120° of elevation.

Inspection may reveal atrophy of the

shoulder girdle musculature if the condition has been chronic. Areas of tenderness may be localized to the region of the subacromial bursa, the anterior acromion, the coracoacromial ligament, or the greater tuberosity at the insertion of the supraspinatus tendon. Crepitus in the subacromial region is often palpable and is associated with hypertrophy and scarring of the subacromial bursa. This crepitus may be noted by placing a hand over the acromion and ranging a relaxed shoulder. Pain may limit the patient's active range of motion in abduction and forward flexion, especially above the horizontal plane. Active forward elevation and abduction of the upper extremity are usually more painful than passive motion because of the presence of tendon injury.

Neer[2] described the impingement sign, used to aid in the diagnosis of impingement syndrome. This sign is elicited when the examiner elevates the patient's arm in the forward plane and internally rotates the humerus while stabilizing the scapula with the opposite hand. This movement compresses the rotator cuff against the undersurface of the acromion and causes pain. A variation of the impingement sign, the "Hawkins' sign,"[24] is performed by flexing the shoulder forward to 90° and then forcibly internally rotating the shoulder. This maneuver drives the greater tuberosity again under the coracoacromial ligament, thereby reproducing impingement pain. Equivocal impingement signs should prompt the physician to search for other causes for the patient's symptoms.

Patients with impingement syndrome may also demonstrate associated posterior capsular tightness. The horizontal adduction test is performed when the arm is brought to 90° of forward flexion and is then adducted across the body, which may elicit pain in the posterior aspect of the shoulder. This test result must be differentiated from that associated with acromioclavicular arthritis, in which the same maneuver causes pain localized to the acromioclavicular joint.

Selective muscle testing about the shoulder musculature is also important in the evaluation of impingement syndrome. Weakness is often related to pain and is noted with supraspinatus and infraspinatus testing. Patients with extensive rotator cuff involvement, such as partial and full thickness tears, obviously will have more weakness than patients with an intact rotator cuff.

The impingement test, described and popularized by Neer,[2] is performed by injecting 10 ml of 1% xylocaine into the subacromial space. If shoulder pain and impingement signs are eliminated by the injection, a diagnosis of impingement syndrome can be made with confidence. It is important to remember that other conditions may mimic the pain and dysfunction of impingement syndrome (Outline 1).

Radiographic Evaluation
Plain radiographs are considered the best imaging tool for the initial evaluation of patients presenting with a shoulder that has been painful for at least 6 weeks. Standard radiographs of the shoulder include anteroposterior views in internal and external rotation and a supraspinatus outlet view for the work-up of a patient with impingement syndrome. The anteroposterior views in internal and external rotation are taken tangential to the glenoid and allow assessment of the glenohumeral joint space, acromioclavicular joint, humeral head position, and greater tuberosity. The supraspinatus outlet view consists of a transscapular view angled 15° caudal.[25] Morphology of the acromion, as described by Bigliani and associates[21] (type I, flat; type II, curved; and type III, hooked) can best be evaluated by this radiograph. Typically, there is anatomic narrowing of the subacromial space by an anterior acromial projection.

Additional views may be obtained to evaluate a painful shoulder. The axillary

Outline 1
The differential diagnoses of impingement syndrome
Biceps tendinitis
Glenohumeral instability
Cervical radiculitis
Viral brachial plexopathy
Visceral problems (ie, coronary insufficiency, choleocysitis)
Acromioclavicular arthritis
Calcific tendinitis
Thoracic outlet syndrome
Pancoast tumor
Adhesive capsulitis
Glenohumeral osteoarthritis
Rotator cuff pathology
Neoplasm of the proximal humerus/shoulder girdle

view may be helpful in looking for an unfused acromial epiphysis (os acromiale) and may more accurately demonstrate early arthrosis of the glenohumeral joint. The Zanca view,[26] an anteroposterior view with 20° of cephalic tilt, provides the most accurate view of the acromioclavicular joint.

Advanced imaging techniques such as arthrography, ultrasonography, computed tomographic (CT) scan, and MRI, commonly used in the evaluation of the painful shoulder, should not be used as a screening tool. These are ancillary testing techniques and should be reserved for those patients in whom the diagnosis is not completely clear from the history and physical examination. Although many consider arthrography to be the gold standard for detection of full-thickness rotator cuff tears, at our institution we have had excellent success using MRI in the evaluation of rotator cuff pathology, and we prefer MRI over arthrography. Ultrasonography techniques have seen increased use secondary to better technology and decreased cost. However, the accuracy of ultrasonography has not been reliable enough for widespread use.

Treatment

Nonsurgical Treatment

The majority of patients with impingement syndrome can be treated successfully within 3 months when placed in a well-structured rehabilitation program.[2,8,27] The most important aspect of the rehabilitation program is to allow injured tissue to heal by preventing overstress or reinjury, to minimize the effects of immobility, and to allow a gradual increase of strength of the rotator cuff and scapular musculature. Additionally, the protocol should include posterior capsular stretching, because contracture of the posterior capsule is not uncommon. Nonsteroidal anti-inflammatory medications, hot and cold therapy, ultrasound, and, in some cases, a steroid injection into the subacromial space are methods used to decrease the inflammation associated with impingement.

Surgical Treatment

Only after a 3- to 6-month period of rehabilitation should surgery be considered. If the patient has not improved with a rehabilitation program and the diagnosis is in question, a more extensive workup is warranted prior to considering surgery. Error in diagnosis is a common cause of failure of acromioplasty.

Surgical Technique

At our institution, we routinely use regional anesthesia (interscalene 1.5% mepivicaine block) for the vast majority of shoulder procedures, including arthroscopy. Regional anesthesia yields 3 to 4 hours of excellent anesthesia, allows swifter recovery, and makes outpatient discharge safer, when it is appropriate.

Patients are placed on the operating table in the "beach-chair" position. We prefer the beach-chair position over the lateral position because it allows greater freedom of positioning of the arm and easier conversion to open procedure. A total-body suction-fitted bean bag is used for patient support, with the trunk at an angle of 70° to 80° to the plane of the floor. The scapula is positioned laterally over the edge of the table and the bean bag is contoured to allow complete access to the anterior and posterior shoulder girdle to the medial edge of the scapula.

The shoulder is then carefully examined under anesthesia. Passive range of motion is documented. Anterior and posterior glenohumeral stability is examined using a modification of Hawkins' load-shift maneuvers, as previously reported. Inferior instability is evaluated with the sulcus sign test.

The upper extremity is prepared and draped in sterile fashion. An articulated forearm holder (McConnell Orthopaedic, Greenville, TX) is used to place the shoulder in a position of neutral rotation and minimal abduction. The subcutaneous anatomy of the scapular spine, acromion, acromioclavicular joint, clavicle, and coracoid process are drawn on the skin to aid in portal placement.

The subacromial space is distended with 20 to 30 ml of 1:300,000 epinephrine/saline solution prior to portal establishment. This has two positive effects: first, subacromial hemostasis is improved; second, it allows easier initial penetration of the bursal sac. The region of the posterior portal is infiltrated with 0.25% bupivacaine, as this area is often incompletely anesthetized by the interscalene block.

The anatomic principles and location of shoulder arthroscopic portal placement have been reported previously. For the vast majority of rotator cuff related procedures, we use posterior, anterosuperior, and lateral subacromial portals. Following establishment of the posterior portal, the arthroscope is inserted and the anterosuperior portal is established under direct vision. Complete methodical examination of the glenohumeral joint is then undertaken, beginning with inspection of the labrum (biceps/labral complex and anteroinferior) and articular surfaces of the glenoid and humeral head. In contrast to the common degenerative labral lesions found in the older patient, labral pathology in the younger patient is often associated with glenohumeral instability. Articular cartilage abnormalities, such as osteoarthritis of the shoulder, can mimic impingement syndrome. Ellman and associates[28] noted 18 patients who underwent shoulder arthroscopy for impingement syndrome and who at surgery were found to have coexisting glenohumeral degenerative joint disease that had not been apparent during preoperative clinical or radiographic evaluation.

The arm is then placed in the rotator cuff position, approximately 45° of forward flexion, 20° to 30° of abduction, and 10° of external rotation, with gentle traction in the plane of the scapula. The traction places tension on the supra- and infraspinatus portions of the rotator cuff, allowing better visualization. The cuff undersurface is carefully inspected and probed.

If a rotator cuff tear is present, the size, thickness, tissue quality, and mobility of any cuff tearing is assessed using probes and grasping instruments placed through the anterior and lateral subacromial portals. The lateral subacromial portal is established 2 cm distal to the lateral border of the acromion and roughly midway between the anterior border and midportion of the acromion. This location is optimized, provides access to the cuff tear for probing and potential "mini-open" repair, and can also be used for subacromial decompression and anterior acromioplasty. A blunt probe is passed through this portal and on to the bursal surface of the cuff. If a full-thickness tear is present, the probe will pass easily through the tear into the joint. If a partial-thickness tear is present, probing the bursal surface enables the surgeon to determine the thickness of the tear and the quality of the remaining tissue.

Full-thickness tear edges are debrided to stable tissue with a 4.5-mm motorized full-radius resector. Only then may a tear be fully assessed for retraction and mobility. A tear is considered mobile if, with the arm held in neutral rotation at the side of the trunk, the edge of the tear can be grasped with an arthroscopic forceps and reduced to the anatomic tendon insertion site.

If a partial-thickness articular surface rotator cuff tear is present, tear depth and tissue quality are assessed following debridement of any loose, frayed fragments. Tears of less than 50% thickness with good remaining tissue quality are debrided to stable tissue using the full-radius resector. In nonathletes, tears of greater than 50% but less than 100% thickness and that are less than 1 cm in width are also debrided to stable tissue. In athletes (particularly those who play throwing sports) these tears are of concern. To prevent their progression to larger, complete tears, they are repaired via arthroscopically placed sutures. Partial-thickness tears of greater than 50% thickness that are greater than 1 cm in width are repaired arthroscopically in all patients.

If the depth of a partial-thickness articular-surface cuff tear cannot be determined by probing, a monofilament marking suture is passed through the tear via the lateral subacromial portal. The intra-articular end of the suture is grasped and drawn out through the anterior portal. The two external ends are then clamped and retracted while the intra-articular work is completed. During subsequent subacromial arthroscopy, the suture marks the location of the bursal surface portion of the tear, and it can then be assessed for tissue quality and thickness.

Technique of Subacromial Decompression

Arthroscopic subacromial decompression is undertaken prior to cuff repair, or as a primary procedure in cases of isolated outlet impingement. Decompression reduces the mechanical source of attrition cuff wear and also improves arthro-

scopic visualization of the superior rotator cuff surface. The general technical principles of arthroscopic subacromial decompression have been reported earlier. These studies have emphasized the importance of careful attention to technical detail to achieve optimal results.

Arthroscopic subacromial decompression consists of extensive subacromial bursectomy, coracoacromial ligament recession or resection, anterior acromioplasty, and removal of impinging acromioclavicular osteophytes. We begin by inserting the arthroscope into the subacromial bursa from the posterior portal. A 5.5-mm motorized full-radius resector is inserted from the lateral subacromial portal. The subacromial bursa is completely debrided from the subacromial space, the acromial undersurface, and the entire rotator cuff outer surface with humeral rotation. Inadequate bursectomy can significantly compromise the surgical result secondary to poor visualization or retention of thickened bursa, which may continue to impinge the coracoacromial (CA) ligament. The CA ligament should be clearly visible as the "roof" of the space. Identification of the CA ligament helps the surgeon orient within this tight cavity.

Electrocautery is used to peel the ligament from the anterior acromial undersurface to the level of the deltoid insertion. Care is taken to preserve the deltoid fascia and to avoid violating the actual deltoid muscle fibers. The ligament is then divided into multiple fragments and resected.

Bleeding can impair visualization significantly and make it difficult for the surgeon to perform an adequate subacromial decompression. Several easy steps can be used to avoid this complication. Patients taking nonsteroidal anti-inflammatory medications should discontinue their use 1 week prior to the procedure to decrease the tendency to bleed. We routinely infiltrate the subacromial space with 20 to 30 ml of a 1:300,000 epineph-

rine/saline solution, as mentioned above, at the beginning of all shoulder procedures. Additionally, injection of 1 ml of 1:1,000 adrenaline into the 3-l bags of saline irrigation fluid is effective in controlling bleeding.

During this aspect of the procedure, meticulous use of electrocautery will control bleeding promptly. Rapid, intermittent suction may help clear an area so that the origin of bleeding may be identified and cauterized. If this step does not control the bleeding, the pressure of the arthroscopic pump may be elevated, or, if gravity is being used, the bags may be elevated. The pressure should be elevated only for short intervals and is lowered promptly once the bleeding is under control in order to avoid tissue extravasation. Hypotensive anesthesia is also very effective in controlling bleeding, but must be used with caution in older patients.

Anterior acromioplasty is then performed with the 5.5-mm full-radius resector or oval-shaped burr, depending upon the acromial bone density. The overriding technical principle behind this portion of the procedure is adequate biplanar visualization and bone resection using both the posterior and lateral subacromial portals. To achieve this, the arthroscope is initially kept in the posterior portal, with the arthroscopic camera held in a position parallel both to the plane of the subcutaneous acromial surface superiorly and to the underlying rotator cuff inferiorly. The axis of the arthroscope is rotated laterally or medially so that it lies parallel to these planes. With this visual orientation, a flat acromial undersurface will appear as a uniform, planar surface that runs directly away from the camera to the anterior deltoid fibers, and anterior subacromial spurring or hooking will appear as a caudally drooping wall of bone.

The anterior acromial spur, which has been exposed via coracoacromial ligament resection, is excised, beginning laterally at the anterolateral corner of the acromion and proceeding medially to the acromioclavicular joint capsule. Inability to identify the most anterior lateral aspect of the acromion will result in improper resection. The resector is simultaneously passed in an anterior-to-posterior sweeping motion from the anterior acromial edge to the mid-portion of the acromial body. To achieve wedge-shaped resection, more bone must be resected anteriorly than posteriorly. A rough estimate of the degree of anterior resection required can be determined from the preoperative supraspinatus outlet radiographs. This degree of anterior resection is then progressively "feathered" posteriorly so that no bone is being resected when the shaver reaches the acromial mid-portion. This transition zone in the mid-portion of the acromion must be planed to avoid creating a ridge between resected and unresected bone. If carefully followed, this technique will avoid both inadequate and excessive resection or the creation of a concave "well" between the anterior and posterior margins of resection. As a result, the entire anterior spur is removed and the acromial undersurface is uniplanar. Care is taken to carry the entire resection medially to the acromial facet of the acromioclavicular joint.

The arthroscope is then inserted into the lateral portal. The resector in the posterior portal is laid flush with the posterior acromial undersurface. If adequate decompression has been achieved, the resector tip should now also lie flush with the anterior acromial undersurface. If not, the posterior undersurface can be used as a so-called "cutting block," to continue resection along the anterior lip until the undersurface is uniplanar.

Any impinging osteophytes along the undersurface of the acromioclavicular joint may now be visualized and removed in similar fashion. The distal clavicle may be arthroscopically excised if necessary. Some authors have advocated routine distal clavicle resection. We reserve distal clavicle excision only for patients with

clinical and radiographic evidence of symptomatic acromioclavicular joint arthrosis.

Following subacromial decompression, the bursal surface of the rotator cuff is assessed. Complete cuff examination can be achieved by rotation and abduction/adduction of the humeral head. Previously placed partial-tear marking sutures are visualized, and the bursal-side cuff surface is probed in these areas to rule out occult full-thickness lesions. Partial-thickness tears may be repaired using either an arthroscopic or a "mini-open" technique. Larger tears are characterized through preoperative and arthroscopic evaluation as mobile, fixed-retraction/repairable, or fixed-retraction/irreparable. Mobility is assessed, as discussed previously, with a tissue-grasping forceps or retention sutures placed in the cuff through the lateral subacromial portal. Irreparability is associated with marked tendon retraction, poor remaining cuff-tissue quality, and MRI evidence of cuff muscle atrophy.

Following completion of the surgical procedure, the arthroscope and instruments are withdrawn, the shoulder is decompressed by draining remaining intra-articular or subacromial fluid, and the portals are closed with nylon sutures. A mixture of 10 ml of 0.25% bupivacaine, 5 mg (10 ml) of morphine, and 5 drops of a 1:1000 epinephrine solution are injected in the subacromial space and glenohumeral joint. The extremity is placed in an immobilizer and a cryotherapy dressing is applied to the shoulder.

Cause of Failure
Causes of failure following arthroscopic decompression are similar to the causes of failure following open acromioplasty.[29] In the literature, the documented failure rate of open and arthroscopic subacromial decompression ranges between 4% and 41%.[30] Numerous studies have documented error in diagnosis as the most common cause of failure.[29–31] Many

patients have shoulder instability,[32,33] acromioclavicular arthritis,[34] degenerative joint disease,[28] or extra-articular biceps tendon injury[17] concomitantly with impingement. Once again the importance of a detailed history and thorough examination cannot be overemphasized. If the diagnosis of impingement is in question, additional diagnostic testing, such as MRI, is indicated.

Inadequate bone resection can also cause surgical failure, in any of several ways. Preoperative films, particularly the supraspinatus outlet, must be reviewed critically to appreciate how much bone resection will be required. Not only should the type of acromion be characterized in the outlet, but the presence of osteophytes at the acromioclavicular joint on the anteroposterior view, prominence of the lateral acromion on the anteroposterior view, and hooked lateral acromion should also be noted preoperatively. At surgery, the adequacy of bone resection of the acromion should be viewed with the arthroscope from both lateral and posterior portals. An inadequate bursectomy or continuous bleeding will affect visualization within the subacromial space and can compromise the proper resection of bone.

A retained coracoacromial ligament attachment can increase the volume in the subacromial space and lead to recurrent impingement.[15] Complete detachment of the ligament is best documented by observing the appearance of the intact deltoid fascia across the full width of the acromion after the ligament has been completely cut. In some cases, after the coracoacromial ligament has been released, it may be significantly hypertrophied and compromise the decompression. In these cases, the released ligament should be completely excised using an aggressive full-resecting shaver blade.

Throwing Athletes
The use of subacromial decompression to treat refractory shoulder pain in young

throwing athletes is a controversial subject. Tibone and associates[35] reported unsatisfactory results using an open technique of formal bony acromioplasty. Others, however, have demonstrated good results with an arthroscopic soft-tissue decompression with a bursectomy and complete resection of the coracoacromial ligament.

We have followed a series of 50 throwing athletes presenting with anterior shoulder pain refractory to greater than 3 months of formal physiotherapy and all of whom had momentary relief of pain with a subacromial injection of lidocaine. Many of these athletes had moderate anterior laxity on examination, but none had a distinct history of instability. At arthroscopic inspection, many had moderate laxity of the anterior capsule as measured by the drive-through test, but none had tearing or detachment of the anterior inferior labrum or anterior glenohumeral ligaments. Most of these athletes (95%) had minor fraying of the undersurface of the supraspinatus or infraspinatus. Some (40%) had evidence of internal impingement and a frayed undersurface of the rotator cuff in association with fraying or tearing of the posterior labrum.

All patients underwent debridement of intra-articular cuff and labral pathology. In all patients, a subacromial bursitis was noted and extensively debrided. In some patients (25%), a thickened coracoacromial ligament was noted and thinned. In few patients (10%), bony narrowing of the subacromial space was noted radiographically or intraoperatively, and in these patients an arthroscopic acromioplasty was performed.

We have evaluated the results of this procedure and found that, when associated with a minimum of 3 months of formal rehabilitation emphasizing scapular strengthening and posterior scapular stretching, the results have been favorable in 80% of cases. In the other 20%, we feel that the capsular laxity is excessive and cannot be controlled by improved strength characteristics of the shoulder. In young throwing athletes, mini decompression usually does not require bony resection, and it relies heavily on postoperative rehabilitation to improve the dynamic stabilization effect of the scapular and rotator cuff musculature.

Conclusion

In recent years, arthroscopic subacromial decompression/acromioplasty has been gaining overall acceptance in the treatment of impingement syndrome, and it is quickly becoming the standard of orthopaedic care when conservative modalities have failed. A comparison of clinical results with arthroscopic techniques and the traditional "open" acromioplasty proposed by Neer has revealed very promising results. Arthroscopic acromioplasty also offers these benefits: better cosmesis (a smaller incision), lower morbidity, a more complete examination (includes evaluation of the glenohumeral joint), earlier return to work, and a more aggressive early rehabilitation. Taken together, these advantages account for the high patient satisfaction of this procedure. If the surgeon follows some basic principles and is meticulous, particularly with regard to controlling hemostasis and resection of bone, this procedure can be performed safely, effectively, and well.

References

1. Neer CS II: Anterior acromioplasty for the chronic impingement syndrome in the shoulder: A preliminary report. *J Bone Joint Surg* 1972;54A:41–50.

2. Neer CS II: Impingement lesions. *Clin Orthop* 1983;173:70–77.

3. Armstrong JR: Excision of the acromion in the treatment of the supraspinatus syndrome: Report of ninety-five excisions. *J Bone Joint Surg* 1949;31B:436–442.

4. Hammond G: Complete acromionectomy in the treatment of chronic tendinitis of the shoulder. *J Bone Joint Surg* 1962;44A:494–504;570.

5. Hammond G: Complete acromionectomy in the treatment of chronic tendinitis of the shoulder: A follow-up of ninety operations on eighty-seven patients. *J Bone Joint Surg* 1971;53A:173–180.

6. Bigliani LU, D'Alessandro DF, Duralde XA, McIlveen SJ: Anterior acromioplasty for subacromial impingement in patients younger than 40 years of age. *Clin Orthop* 1989;246:111–116.

7. Ha'eri GB, Wiley AM: Shoulder impingement syndrome: Results of operative release. *Clin Orthop* 1982;168:128–132.

8. Hawkins RJ, Brock RM, Abrams JS, Hobeika P: Acromioplasty for impingement with an intact rotator cuff. *J Bone Joint Surg* 1988;70B:795–797.

9. Post M, Cohen J: Impingement syndrome: A review of late stage II and early stage III lesions. *Clin Orthop* 1986;207:126–132.

10. Roye RP, Grana WA, Yates CK: Arthroscopic subacromial decompression: Two-to-seven-year follow-up. *Arthroscopy* 1995;11:301–306.

11. Ellman H: Arthroscopic subacromial decompression: A preliminary report. *Orthop Trans* 1985;9:49.

12. Ellman H: Arthroscopic subacromial decompression: Analysis of one-to three-year results. *Arthroscopy* 1987;3:173–181.

13. Esch JC, Ozerkis LR, Helgager JA, Kane N, Lillinot N: Arthroscopic subacromial decompression: Results according to the degree of rotator cuff tear. *Arthroscopy* 1988;4:241–249.

14. Esch JC: Arthroscopic subacromial decompression and postoperative management. *Orthop Clin North Am* 1993;24:161–171.

15. Paulos LE, Franklin JL: Arthroscopic shoulder decompression development and application: A five year experience. *Am J Sports Med* 1990;18:235–244.

16. Ryu RK: Arthroscopic subacromial decompression: A clinical review. *Arthroscopy* 1992;8:141–147.

17. Altchek DW, Warren RF, Wickiewicz TL, Skyhar MJ, Ortiz G, Schwartz E: Arthroscopic acromioplasty: Technique and results. *J Bone Joint Surg* 1990;72A:1198–1207.

18. Speer KP, Lohnes J, Garrett WE Jr: Arthroscopic subacromial decompression: Results in advanced impingement syndrome. *Arthroscopy* 1991;7:291–296.

19. Gartsman GM: Arthroscopic acromioplasty for lesions of the rotator cuff. *J Bone Joint Surg* 1990;72A:169–180.

20. Gartsman GM, Blair ME Jr, Noble PC, Bennett JB, Tullos HS: Arthroscopic subacromial decompression: An anatomical study. *Am J Sports Med* 1988;16:48–50.

21. Bigliani LU, Morrison DS, April EW: The morphology of the acromion and its relationship to rotator cuff tears. *Orthop Trans* 1986;10:228.

22. Morrison DS, Bigliani LU: Roentgenographic analysis of acromial morphology and its relationship to rotator cuff tears. *Orthop Trans* 1987;11:439.

23. Deutsch A, Altchek DW, Schwartz E, Otis JC, Warren RF: Radiologic measurement of superior displacement of the humeral head in the impingement syndrome. *J Shoulder Elbow Surg* 1996;5:186–193.

24. Hawkins RJ, Kennedy JC: Impingement syndrome in athletes. *Am J Sports Med* 1980;8:151–158.

25. Neer CS II, Poppen NK: Supraspinatus outlet. *Orthop Trans* 1989;711:234.

26. Zanca P: Shoulder pain: involvement of the acromioclavicular joint: Analysis of 1000 cases. *AJR Am J Roentgenol* 1971;112:493–506.

27. Morrison DS, Frogameni A, Woodworth P: Conservative management for subacromial impingement of the shoulder. *J Shoulder Elbow Surg* 1993;2:S22

28. Ellman H, Harris E, Kay SP: Early degenerative joint disease simulating impingement syndrome: Arthroscopic findings. *Arthroscopy* 1992;8:482–487.

29. Seltzer DG, Wirth MA, Rockwood CA: Complications and failures of open and arthroscopic acromioplasties. *Op Tech Sports Med* 1994;2:136–150.

30. Lirette R, Morin F, Kinnard P: The difficulties in assesment of results of anterior acromioplasty. *Clin Orthop* 1992;278:14–16.

31. Cahill BR: Understanding shoulder pain, in Stauffer ES (ed): American Academy of Orthopaedic Surgeons *Instructional Course Lectures XXXIV*. St. Louis, MO, CV Mosby, 1985, pp 332–336.

32. Jobe FW: Impingement problems in the athlete, in Barr JS Jr (ed): *Instructional Course Lectures XXXVIII*. Park Ridge, IL, American Academy of Orthopaedic Surgeons, 1989, pp 205–209.

33. Ogilve-Harris DJ, Wiley AM, Sattarian J: Failed acromioplasty for impingement syndrome. *J Bone Joint Surg* 1990;72B:1070–1072.

34. Flugstad D, Matsen FA, Larry I, Jackins SE: Failed acromioplasty: Etiology and prevention. *Orthop Trans* 1986;10:229.

35. Tibone JE, Jobe FW, Kerlan RK, et al: Shoulder impingement syndrome in athletes treated by an anterior acromioplasty. *Clin Orthop* 1985;198:134–140.

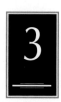

Arthroscopic Subacromial Decompression— Avoidance of Complications and Enhancement of Results

Leslie S. Matthews, MD
J. Mark Blue, MD

Introduction

Although it is technically demanding, arthroscopic subacromial decompression (ASAD) can yield results comparable to those of conventional open surgery,[1-7] with less morbidity, improved cosmesis, and lower cost. As with any difficult surgical procedure, however, results can be jeopardized by technical problems and complications. This chapter outlines pre-, intra-, and postoperative considerations that can enhance surgical results and reduce complications associated with ASAD of the shoulder.

Preoperative Planning

Once a patient is diagnosed with impingement syndrome refractory to conservative management and ASAD is under consideration, three factors are of major importance in the preoperative planning process: status of the acromioclavicular (AC) joint, acromial morphology, and status of the rotator cuff.

Status of the Acromioclavicular Joint

The surgeon cannot wait until surgery is in progress to assess what, if any, role the AC joint may play in a given patient's shoulder symptoms. Therefore, it is imperative to consider and evaluate all the various possibilities associated with the AC joint and to plan surgical management based on that evaluation.

Table 1	
Spectrum of acromioclavicular joint pathology and relevant treatment	
AC Joint Involvement	**Treatment**
AC joint normal, clinically and by radiograph	None
Primary isolated AC joint disease	Distal clavicle resection
AC joint disease (symptomatic) plus impingement	Distal clavicle resection and ASAD
Silent AC joint with inferior osteophytes/impingement	Debride osteophytes at time of ASAD

Simply stated, there are four possible clinical scenarios for which the AC joint must be scrutinized (Table 1). First is one in which the joint is both clinically and radiographically normal and asymptomatic. In this situation, it is clear that no surgical intervention directed toward the joint is necessary. The importance of making this judgment preoperatively rather than intraoperatively cannot be overemphasized. In the second scenario, the AC joint may be the sole source of the patient's symptoms, with no associated impingement or rotator cuff disease. In this setting, for patients refractory to nonsurgical treatment, AC joint resection (whether open or arthroscopic) is indicated. In turn, no subacromial decompressive surgery is necessary. Third, in certain settings, the AC joint may be involved with osteoarthritic changes that have caused the formation of inferior AC joint osteophytes that contribute to the impingement process. This impingement contribution may be evidenced by radiograph (Fig. 1) and by magnetic resonance imaging (MRI). Despite this osteophyte formation, the joint itself may be clinically "silent," ie, not otherwise contributing to symptoms. Lack of tenderness, negative AC joint stress test, and negative lidocaine injection test can all serve to confirm this situation preoperatively. Appropriate surgical management of this scenario involves debridement/resection of the offensive osteophyte at the time of ASAD. Complete resection of the distal clavicle is not indicated in this setting. Fourth, the patient with refractory subacromial impingement may also suffer from associated symptoms originating from a diseased AC joint. Possible causes of these symptoms include osteoarthritis, osteolysis, or an old fracture. In this setting, complete distal clavicle resection should be performed in conjunction with ASAD. Again, accurate preoperative assessment is essential to

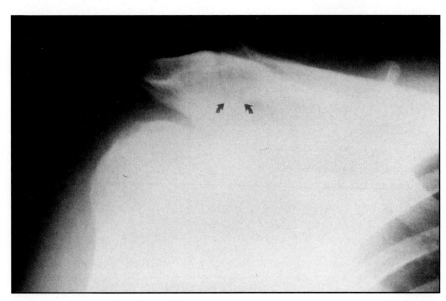

Fig. 1 Plain radiograph showing degenerative changes within the acromioclavicular joint and inferior osteophyte formation (arrows).

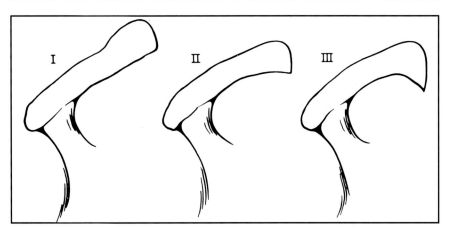

Fig. 2 Types of acromial morphology. (Reproduced with permission from Bigliani LU, Morrison DS, April EW: The morphology of the acromion and its relationship to rotator cuff tears. *Orthop Trans* 1986;10:216.)

guide the surgeon to proper judgment and execution. Aiding the orthopaedist's preoperative evaluation of the AC joint are appropriate history and physical examination techniques, radiographs, selective injection testing, and, occasionally, the use of MRI or technetium Tc99m bone scanning.

Acromial Morphology
Bigliani and associates[8] have described the variations in the morphology of the acromion process (Fig. 2) and the association of the type-III morphology with impingement and rotator cuff disease. Not all type-III acromia are comparable; some patients demonstrate dramatically larger osteophytes than others.

The goal of any subacromial decompression, whether open or arthroscopic, should be surgical creation of a flat, type-I acromion. The amount of bony resection achieved can be more difficult to quantify when arthroscopic techniques

are used, and the risks of incomplete decompression are undoubtedly greater.[1,3,9] To minimize this risk, preoperative planning should also include radiographic evaluation of acromial morphology. This can generally best be achieved by the "acromial outlet" radiograph (Fig. 3), a view obtained by adjusting the radiographic beam to the plane of the scapula while it is angled 15° caudally (Fig. 4). Once obtained, this radiograph can be used by the surgeon to measure accurately the amount of bony resection required to convert the acromial morphology to type I (Fig. 5). Preoperative knowledge of the size of the resection—whether 5, 10, or 15 mm—can greatly facilitate the surgical procedure.

Status of the Rotator Cuff
Encountering an unexpected, undiagnosed full-thickness rotator cuff tear at the time of planned ASAD can be a frustrating surgical experience. In a worst-case scenario, the surgeon must then make intraoperative decisions for treatment without adequate planning, informed consent, or patient preparation.

To avoid this pitfall, adequate preoperative rotator cuff evaluation is essential. If, at the time a subacromial decompression is planned, the surgeon cannot be assured of the rotator cuff status by history, physical examination, and radiographic evaluation, further diagnostic testing is indicated. This information will allow the surgeon to plan surgery (equipment, time allocation, resources, etc) as well as to advise the patient of risks, alternatives, time of recovery, anticipated loss of work time, and other associated considerations.

Intraoperative Factors
Proper visualization, orientation relative to subacromial landmarks, maintenance of hemostasis, and quantification of bone resection are essential intraoperative factors to consider in order to enhance surgical results and reduce the risk of complications.

Visualization

All subacromial arthroscopic surgery should be preceded by glenohumeral evaluation.[10] Evaluation of the joint can be critical in assessing partial rotator cuff tears, biceps lesions, osteoarthritis, labral pathology, and instability—all important factors that can affect results and prognosis. After thorough glenohumeral evaluation of intra-articular pathology, and treatment when possible, the arthroscope is redirected subacromially. The subacromial bursa is an anterior structure that does not fully occupy the subacromial space (Fig. 6).[11] Every attempt should be made to enter the bursa for best visualization of important subacromial structures. If only the subacromial space is entered, and not the bursa, the view achieved is poorer. The arthroscope is directed slightly medially toward the AC joint, and a slight "pop" is felt as the bursa is entered. Entrance to the bursa eliminates the need for extensive bursal debridement, thereby reducing the associated bleeding.

Orientation

The surgeon must be aware of the normal anatomic relationships within the subacromial space and create additional reference points when necessary. The coracoacromial ligament is an excellent reference point, but it is best seen only when the bursal space is entered. Placement of a reference needle marker in the AC joint is also helpful. This is best done at the start of the procedure, because soft-tissue swelling caused by fluid extravasation can make later intraoperative placement more difficult and less precise.

Once adequate orientation is achieved, bipolar, multielectrode cautery is used to debride soft tissue over the entire area of the acromion to be included in the bony resection. This exposure extends from the most anterior portion of the acromion to its midportion, as well as laterally at the deltoid origin to the AC joint medially.

Hemostasis

Bleeding can frustrate the surgeon and greatly hinder his or her ability to adequately and accurately perform this surgical procedure. A variety of methods can be used to control bleeding; not all are necessary in each case.

First, proper bursal entry and avoidance of excessive bursal debridement is helpful. Second, adequate hydrostatic pressure must be maintained throughout surgery; a pump can be used for this purpose. Third, the use of bipolar, multielectrode cautery is routine and greatly facilitates hemostasis as well as visualization. When not medically contraindicated, hypotensive anesthesia and or the use of epinephrine with an irrigation solution can also be of benefit. The fat pad beneath the AC joint is hypervascular and when AC joint resection is planned, dissection into this area is best delayed until after the ASAD has been performed.

Quantification of Bone Resection

One of the most common, if not the most common, technical errors in ASAD is resecting too little or uneven amounts of bone from the acromion.[1,12] The keys to avoiding this error are multifactorial and varied and include preoperative factors (knowledge of and planning for the appropriate amount of acromial bony resection, as previously described) and intraoperative factors (proper visualization, orientation, and control of hemostasis).

Intraoperatively, the surgeon can use a number of techniques to assess the amount of bone resection. The two techniques most commonly used are the "keyhole" and the "cutting block" methods. In the keyhole method,[1] a hole of known depth is created in the acromion and the surrounding bone is then resected to that level. When combined with preoperative radiographic assessment, very accurate quantification can then be achieved. For the less-preferred cutting block technique,[9,10] a burr is introduced

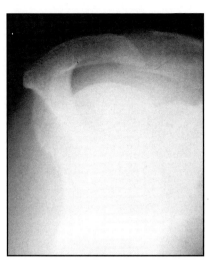

Fig. 3 Acromial outlet radiograph showing type II acromial morphology.

through a posterior portal. The posterior acromion is used to guide the amount of bony resection anteriorly, rendering the acromion flat once the burr achieves a flat orientation to the acromial undersurface.

A curved arthroscopic rasp can be very helpful in smoothing and finishing the resection of the acromion. To validate a complete and adequate bony resection, it is perfectly acceptable to extend a portal sufficiently to allow palpation of the acromion with a gloved finger. Postoperative acromial outlet radiographs also can be used to confirm adequacy of decompression.

Postoperative Considerations
Evaluation of Results

When the aforementioned approaches to patients with subacromial impingement are followed, good results can be expected in most cases. However, evaluation of the patient with a poor result after ASAD presents a challenge. The first step in evaluating such a patient is to retrace the preoperative steps and look for other problems that may have been misdiagnosed and inadequately treated. Most commonly included in this setting are AC joint disease, rotator cuff tears, biceps lesions, instability, and pain referred from

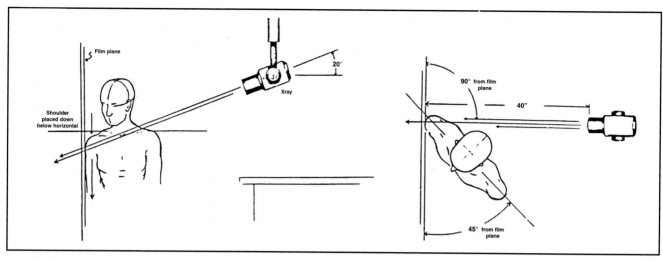

Fig. 4 Technique required to obtain the acromial outlet radiographic view. (Courtesy of Steven Snyder, MD.)

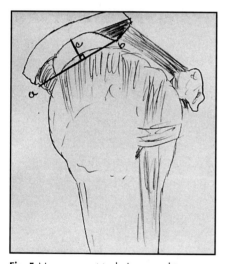

Fig. 5 Measurement technique used to preoperatively determine the extent of bony resection: a, posterior acromion; b, inferior aspect of anterior acromial spur; c, line drawn perpendicular to line a-b indicates amount of planned bony resection.

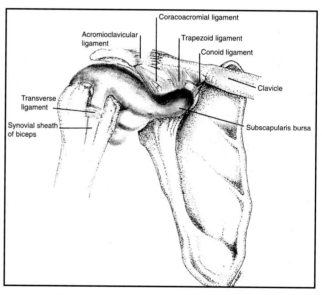

Fig. 6 Anatomic extent of the subacromial bursa. (Reproduced with permission from Anderson JE (ed): *Grant's Atlas of Anatomy,* ed 8. Baltimore, MD, Williams & Wilkins, 1983.)

other sites, such as the cervical spine, thorax, or viscera.

In the second step, the potential for technical errors (such as poor/incomplete bony resection or incomplete treatment of the AC joint), which led to the poor results, must also be considered. Most poor results can be attributed to failure of diagnosis and/or technical errors.

Complications of ASAD

Fortunately, complications from ASAD are rare and, when encountered, are usually minor, self-limited, and not deleterious to final outcomes.[3,5,6,12] This includes complications such as infection, bleeding, neurovascular injury, and fistula formation. There does not appear to be an increased incidence of any of these com-

plications associated with ASAD when compared to open surgery.[1,2,4-6]

The most potentially serious complication after ASAD is acromial fracture (Fig. 7).[13] Although problems with resection are more commonly related to too little bony resection, acromial fracture after ASAD has been attributed to too much or to poorly placed bony resection.

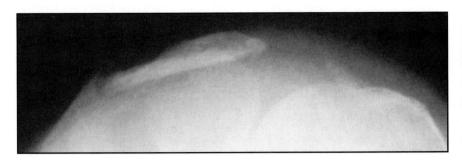
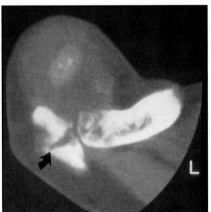

Fig. 7 Acute acromial fracture after ASAD. **Left,** Plain radiograph. **Right,** Computed tomograph (Reproduced with permission from Matthews LS, Burkhead WZ, Gordon S, et al: Acromial fracture: A complication of arthroscopic subacromial decompression. *J Shoulder Elbow Surg* 1994;3:256-261.).

Although rare, this is a devastating and permanent complication, for which prevention is the best cure.

Conclusion

ASAD has justifiably become the state-of-the-art surgical treatment for refractory subacromial impingement syndrome. Although technically demanding, this procedure offers results equal to or better than conventional open surgery while improving cost, cosmesis, and morbidity. With careful preoperative planning, intraoperative technique, and postoperative evaluation, consistently gratifying results can be achieved.

References

1. Altchek DW, Warren RF, Wickiewicz TL, et al: Arthroscopic acromioplasty. Technique and results [see comments]. *J Bone Joint Surg* 1990;72A:1198-1207.

2. Van Holsbeeck E, DeRycke J, Declercq G, et al: Subacromial impingement: open versus arthroscopic decompression. *Arthroscopy* 1992;8:173-178.

3. Paulos LE, Franklin JL: Arthroscopic shoulder decompression development and application: A five year experience. *Am J Sports Med* 1990;18:235-244.

4. Ellman H, Kay SP: Arthroscopic subacromial decompression for chronic impingement: Two- to five-year results. *J Bone Joint Surg* 1991;73B:395-398.

5. Speer KP, Lohnes J, Garrett WE Jr: Arthroscopic subacromial decompression: Results in advanced impingement syndrome. *Arthroscopy* 1991;7:291-296.

6. Esch JC, Ozerkis LR, Helgager JA, et al: Arthroscopic subacromial decompression: Results according to the degree of rotator cuff tear. *Arthroscopy* 1988;4:241-249.

7. Roye RP, Grana WA, Yates CK: Arthroscopic subacromial decompression: Two- to seven-year follow-up. *Arthroscopy* 1995;11:301-306.

8. Bigliani LU, Morrison DS, April EW: The morphology of the acromion and its relationship to rotator cuff tears. *Orthop Trans* 1986;10:216.

9. Sampson TG, Nusbet JK, Glick JM: Precision acromioplasty in arthroscopic subacromial decompression of the shoulder. *Arthroscopy* 1991;7:301-307.

10. Caspari RB, Thal R: A technique for arthroscopic subacromial decompression. *Arthroscopy* 1992;8:23-30.

11. Matthews LS, Fadale PD: Subacromial anatomy for the arthroscopist. *Arthroscopy* 1989;5:36-40.

12. Gartsman GM: Arthroscopic acromioplasty for lesions of the rotator cuff. *J Bone Joint Surg* 1990;72A:169-180.

13. Matthews LS, Burkhead WZ, Gordon S, et al: A complication of arthroscopic subacromial decompression. *J Shoulder Elbow Surg* 1994;3:256-261.

Arthroscopic Distal Clavicle Resection

Robert H. Bell, MD

Introduction

The application of arthroscopy in the shoulder began in the early 1970s, with glenohumeral inspection. In the 1980s, therapeutic applications of arthroscopy were realized, beginning with labral debridements and synovectomies. As our comfort level grew, with it came a heightened level of curiosity for other applications about the shoulder. Next, the subacromial space was explored, introducing a new set of anatomic landmarks and another learning curve for instrumentation. The arthroscopic subacromial decompression (ASAD) for chronic impingement tendinitis was developed and its efficacy demonstrated.

With the 1990s came even greater exploration arthroscopically about the shoulder. As the technology improved and surgeons gained technical competency, many orthopaedists began to delve into the area of arthroscopic rotator cuff and instability repairs. It was during this time that another area of interest, the acromioclavicular (AC) joint, gained prominence. Surgeons were quick to note that this represented a different kind of joint with very irregular contours, narrow width, and varying degrees of inclination. They also felt that many of the procedures commonly performed on the AC joint would likely be amenable to arthroscopic techniques.

Clinical Presentation (Symptoms)

The typical presentation for patients with disorders of the AC joint is an early sub-tle change in activities of daily living, specifically those requiring internal rotation and adduction, such as batting or follow-through on a golf swing. Discomfort with internal rotation posterior to the coronal plane is also seen, such as in hooking a bra or reaching for a coat sleeve. Interestingly, forward elevation is not as much of a problem for these patients unless there is a strong component of impingement tendinitis.

In most patients, the onset of pain is insidious with no well-defined traumatic event. Occasionally, a young athlete will describe an injury to the AC joint as one that causes persistent pain and "popping" afterwards. This likely represents meniscal damage with secondary arthropathy. In idiopathic osteolysis (weight lifter's shoulder), repetitive overloading of the joint and its articular cartilage has been postulated as the cause of this inflammatory, localized disorder of the AC joint.[1-3]

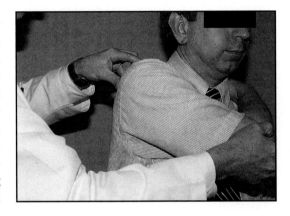

Fig. 1 The swimmer's sign or cross-arm adduction test. Gentle forward elevation with adduction and internal rotation result in compression of the painful acromioclavicular joint.

Physical Examination

Unlike many other shoulder disorders with varying locations of referred pain, AC joint disorders often present with pain readily localized by the patient to the AC joint. Typically positive is the swimmer's sign or cross-arm adduction test. This is performed by asking the patient to raise the arm in forward elevation, internally rotate, and then adduct, reaching for the contralateral shoulder (Fig. 1). This compresses the joint and stretches the posterior joint capsule. Impingement may also be a component in these patients, and in those instances forward elevation and abduction will be painful. Range of motion and strength are preserved, although more advanced AC joint disease may result in diminished internal rotation.

Diagnostic Modalities

As is the case with all shoulder problems,

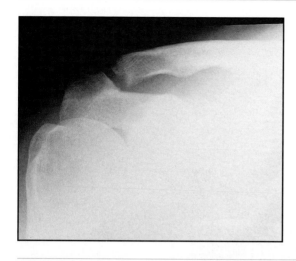

Fig. 2 The Zanca view. Obtained by tipping the tube 10° to 15° cephalad, this view allows an unobstructed look at the acromioclavicular joint without soft-tissue or bony overlay. Note the cystic changes in the distal clavicle.

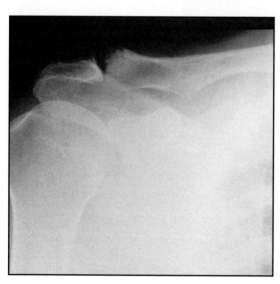

Fig. 3 Osteoarthritis of the acromioclavicular joint manifests with joint narrowing and trumpeting of the distal clavicle caused by superior and inferior osteophytic spurring.

routine radiographic studies should be ordered including scapular anteroposterior (AP), outlet, and axillary views. In the case of the AC joint, the AP view allows the orthopaedist to assess joint narrowing as well as superior and inferior osteophytic changes consistent with osteoarthritis. The outlet view will demonstrate inferior clavicular osteophytes, as well as subacromial changes, which may need to be addressed concomitantly. The axillary view helps to define anterior or posterior displacement of the clavicle or irregularities secondary to arthritis. A fourth view that is extremely helpful is the Zanca.[4,5] This view is obtained by tipping the x-ray tube 10Υ to 15° cephalad,

which allows for imaging the AC joint without as much soft-tissue and bony overlay from the scapular spine (Fig. 2). This view is helpful in early idiopathic osteolysis for demonstrating cystic changes at the distal clavicle.

Technetium bone scans can also be helpful in early cases of idiopathic osteolysis and other inflammatory arthritides when radiographic changes have yet to take place. Similarly, magnetic resonance imaging (MRI), although seldom necessary, may help demonstrate soft-tissue irregularities and early erosive changes in the distal clavicle as seen in idiopathic osteolysis.

Although not an imaging study, selec-

tive injections about the shoulder are helpful, both diagnostically and therapeutically, especially with the AC joint. These can be useful to help sort out impingement tendinitis, sternoclavicular problems, and rotator cuff pathology. The technique employs a 2-cc mixture of a long-acting anesthetic and steroid. It is imperative that the patient be examined before and after the injection in order to benefit from its diagnostic aspect.

Specific Disorders of the Acromioclavicular Joint
Osteoarthritis
In osteoarthritis of the AC joint, the onset of symptoms is fairly gradual and often accompanies other joint involvement. It is not unusual for radiographic changes to precede clinical symptoms. Typical findings include joint narrowing and trumpeting of the distal clavicle due to superior and inferior osteophytic spurring (Fig. 3). The differential diagnosis will include impingement syndrome, biceps tendinitis, rotator cuff tears, and glenohumeral arthritis. Impingement tendinitis typically results in pain on forward elevation, pain that is less common in isolated AC pathology. Biceps tendinitis will have more distal pain localized to the bicipital groove. Rotator cuff tears, either isolated or associated with AC problems, will demonstrate weakness on forward elevation and, in larger tears, on external rotation. Osteoarthritis of the glenohumeral joint will be marked by a global decrease in range of motion and radiographic evidence of glenohumeral joint narrowing. The definitive treatment in osteoarthritis of the AC joint is a distal clavicle resection, done either arthroscopically or by open technique.

Rheumatoid Arthritis
Rheumatoid arthritis seldom presents as an isolated entity in the AC joint. The more common presentation is that of a patient with polyarticular disease, often with ipsilateral glenohumeral involve-

ment and a painful AC joint. Radiographically, these patients demonstrate periarticular erosions and osteopenia, yet there is less spurring or trumpeting than in osteoarthritis (Fig. 4). Because this is seldom an isolated entity, the surgeon needs to define the level of involvement of the rotator cuff and glenohumeral joint prior to any surgical intervention.

Idiopathic Osteolysis (Weight Lifter's Shoulder)

Idiopathic osteolysis is classically seen in individuals participating in heavy overhead work or recreational activities such as weight lifting. The onset is insidious and the pain well localized to the AC joint. Radiographically, a Zanca view will demonstrate cystic changes, often on the dorsal aspect of the distal clavicle. Injections can be helpful to confirm the diagnosis, especially in those instances in which radiographic changes have yet to take place. Alternatively, a technetium bone scan will define the site of involvement.

Treatment

Historically, many individuals have put forth treatment options for disorders of the AC joint. The most widely recognized is that of Mumford[6] in his operation to address arthritides and painful separations of this joint using a simple excision of the distal clavicle. It is a proven procedure with a low level of morbidity, and it can be performed on an outpatient basis. The question then is, given the efficacy of this operation, is there really a need to consider an arthroscopic approach?

A similar argument ensued regarding arthroscopic acromioplasty. The open acromioplasty was a time-proven technique that had only moderate morbidity, and that was reproducible in the general orthopaedist's hands. The response by the arthroscopist was that the arthroscopic approach preserved the anatomy, lessened the morbidity, and shortened hospi-

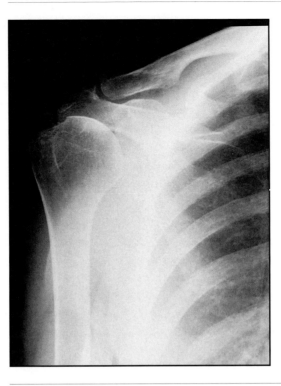

Fig. 4 Rheumatoid arthritis of the acromioclavicular joint presents with diffuse osteopenia, periarticular erosions, and joint narrowing but little osteophytic formation.

talization. Over time, the efficacy of that technique and its application were accepted.

Similarly, arthroscopic distal clavicle resection has been looked at from a scientific standpoint as well. Gartsman,[7] in 1991, performed a study on ten cadaveric shoulders. Five underwent an open excision of the distal clavicle and five were treated by an arthroscopic excision. He concluded that the arthroscopic resection was technically comparable in its resection rate to the open. Flatow and associates,[8] in 1992, looked at 12 patients; six arthroscopic and six open, and found that the resection rates were comparable in both groups. However, although overall improvement in preoperative pain was comparable, it was achieved earlier in the arthroscopic group. Additional reports by Bigliani and associates,[9] Meyers,[10] and Snyder and Tolin[11] have further demonstrated the reproducibility and clinical success of this arthroscopic application to the AC joint.

In a preliminary series of 30 patients who underwent concomitant arthroscopic Mumford and arthroscopic subacromial decompression, all patients were noted to have a conversion to a Type I acromion with an average AC joint resection of 13 mm. All patients noted a rapid return of range of motion and function with an overall 93% satisfactory result.[1] Furthermore, Cook and Tibone[12] have shown a loss of flexion and extension strength in athletes who have undergone open Mumford procedures, indicating that the open approach may result in some long-term deficits.[12] Thus, it would appear that the arthroscopic approach to the AC joint does generate less morbidity with a confirmed resection rate and quicker rehabilitation. Clearly, the arthroscopic approach affords many advantages, yet, as with all arthroscopic procedures, there are potential technical limitations and an inherent learning curve that must be overcome. There are two approaches available to the joint; a direct, or superior, approach and an indirect, or bursal, approach.

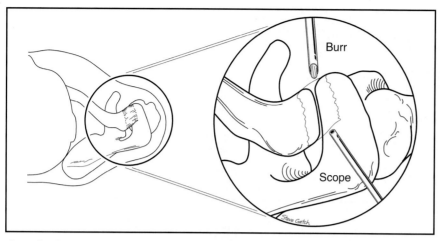

Fig. 5 The direct approach to the acromioclavicular joint employs a posterior portal for the arthroscope and an anterior one for the burr and shaver.

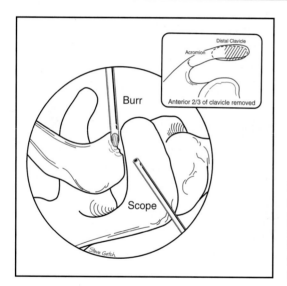

Fig. 6 The resection begins at the anterior, inferior aspect of the joint and works its way posteriorly and superiorly. In most cases, the anterior two thirds of the distal clavicle can be removed from this anterior portal.

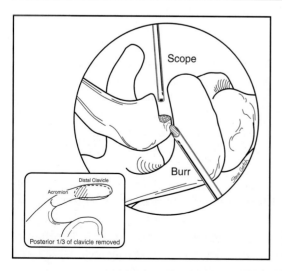

Fig. 7 In the final step the arthroscope is moved to the anterior portal, the burr to the posterior, and the residual posterior one third of the clavicle is removed.

Technique
Direct Approach

The direct approach to an AC joint resection is best suited for those patients with early idiopathic osteolysis or early osteoarthritis in which there remains at least 5 mm of joint space. Furthermore, this is to be used only in individuals with isolated AC joint problems and does not address subacromial changes. The technique begins with the patient in either the beach chair or lateral decubitus position, depending on surgeon preference. For direct AC joint resections, I prefer the beach chair position because, unlike most other arthroscopic shoulder procedures, it requires no traction and the arm may remain at the patient's side. A long-acting scalene anesthetic is used.

If there is concern about concomitant glenohumeral pathology, that joint is inspected first using the standard posterior viewing portal. All topographic landmarks are marked so as to maintain a point of reference in cases of excessive swelling. Both anterior and posterior portals are marked, each approximately 1 cm anterior and posterior to the joint. The inclination of the joint itself is confirmed with the needle to give a reference for the angle of trocar introduction.

The arthroscope is inserted in the posterior portal and an anterior working portal is created to introduce a shaver system. This portal location is best determined with needle localization while viewing intra-articularly. This method will help to avoid inaccurate portal placement. The joint is initially debrided, and any retained meniscal fragments are excised. Electrocautery and a pump irrigation system are used throughout the procedure. In most cases, a 4-mm burr may be used and the decompression is begun at the anteroinferior corner of the distal clavicle (Fig. 5). If the joint space is narrow, a 2.7-mm arthroscope and small joint instruments may be used to initially debride the joint and begin the resection. The resection progresses from anterior to posterior

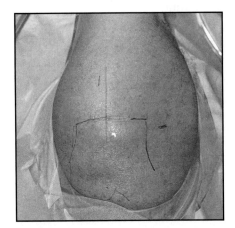

Fig. 8 The "Finish Line" is drawn as a perpendicular to the lateral border of the acromion beginning from just posterior to the acromioclavicular joint. The lateral working portal for the arthroscopic subacromial decompression and the clavicle resection is made just anterior to this line and 2 to 3 cm lateral to the acromion.

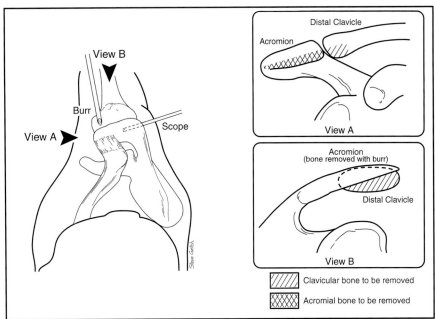

and inferior to superior (Fig. 6). On completion of resection of the anterior two thirds, using switching sticks, the arthroscope is moved to the anterior portal and the burr brought in from the posterior portal (Fig. 7). The posterior one third of the remaining distal clavicle is then excised.

Indirect or Bursal Approach

The indirect or bursal approach is applicable to situations in which the joint is markedly narrowed, such as in advanced osteoarthritis and rheumatoid arthritis. This approach also allows the surgeon to visualize the bursal side of the rotator cuff and, at the same time, to decompress the acromion.

The patient is placed in the lateral decubitus position and all potential pressure areas are identified and padded. The body is rolled posteriorly 15Υ and the arm is placed in traction at 30Υ to 40Υ of abduction with 10 to 15 lb of weight. Extreme care is taken to position the head so as to avoid traction on the brachial plexus.

All pertinent bony topographic anato-

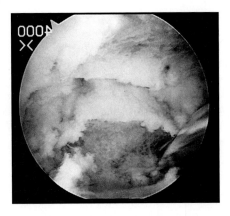

Fig. 9 Top left and **right,** Viewing from the posterior portal and working from the lateral, the inferior one half to two thirds of the exposed distal clavicle is resected. This begins at the anterior inferior corner and works posteriorly. These views demonstrate the amount of bone that should be removed in this portion of the procedure as seen from anterior and lateral. **Bottom,** This intraoperative arthroscopic view shows the resection beginning at the anterior inferior corner of the clavicle.

my is marked and portal locations confirmed. A standard posterior viewing portal is marked 1 cm medial and 2 to 3 cm inferior to the posterolateral corner of the acromion. A line is drawn from the posterior aspect of the AC joint out laterally, perpendicular to the lateral margin of the acromion. This line will mark the most posterior extent of the arthroscopic acromioplasty and is called the "finish line." This line should mark the point at which the decompression begins to taper out and is completed. The lateral portal, the portal for all subacromial work, is marked just anterior to this line and 2 to 3 cm lateral to the edge of the acromion (Fig. 8). The majority of the arthroscopic

subacromial decompression (ASAD) will be performed using these two portals.

The subacromial portion of this procedure is carried out using a standard technique. First, the subacromial bursa is resected and the coracoacromial ligament is released. The bony resection begins at the anterolateral corner of the acromion and moves medially towards the AC joint and posteriorly towards the "finish line." Upon completion of the ASAD, the inferior one half of the distal articular surface of the clavicle will be exposed. In order to properly visualize this area from the posterior portal, the arthroscope is rotated 90Υ medially. Electrocautery is used to release any residual AC joint capsule, and

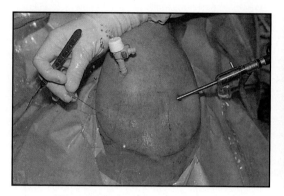
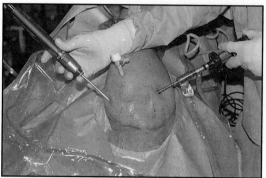

Fig. 10 Left, this shows the technique of needle localization for establishment of the anterior portal. Note the arthroscope is still in the posterior viewing portal. **Right,** With the portal location confirmed, the burr is introduced anteriorly to complete the resection.

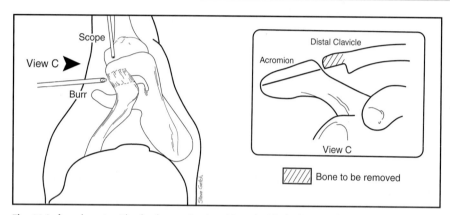
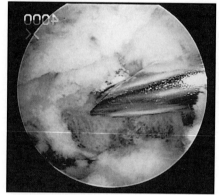

Fig. 11 Left and **center,** The final resection is achieved with the burr in the new anterior portal and the arthroscope either posterior or lateral. The righthand illustration shows the intended area of resection. **Right,** This intraoperative arthroscopic view shows the burr removing the superior half of the distal clavicle.

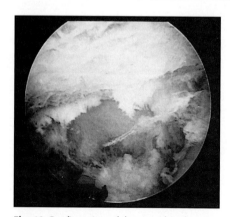

Fig. 12 Confirmation of the completed resection is shown in this view from the lateral portal.

a shaver or a basket complete the task. If need be, the remaining acromial facet of the AC joint is removed with the burr to improve visualization. Using the lateral portal, the exposed inferior half of the distal clavicle is resected to a depth of approximately 10 to 15 mm (Fig. 9). With the acromial facet removed with the acromioplasty, at least half of the articular surface of the clavicle will be seen. Care must be used to avoid injuring the supraspinatus myofibrils inferior to the clavicle and the anterior and posterior joint capsule. The window of the burr may be used as a guide to confirm the amount of bony resection.

At this point, the arthroscope may be either moved to the lateral portal for viewing or maintained posteriorly if the view is adequate. In most cases, I have found it unnecessary to change portals because all arthroscopes provide a 20° to 30° offset angle in their lens. Rarely, a very broad clavicle will have such a wide posterior expanse that the posterior portal alone is inadequate for viewing and the lateral portal must be used. Once the inferior resection is complete, attention is directed to the residual superior half. To achieve this portion of the resection, an additional anterior portal is used to gain the proper angle for the burr. Under direct visualization, a needle is introduced from a point just anterior to the AC joint, directed toward the inferior aspect of the clavicle (Fig. 10, *left*). In similar fashion, under direct visualization, a small stab wound is made with a #11 blade and the burr is introduced (Fig. 10, *right*). Working from inferior to superior and from anterior to posterior, the residual superior or dorsal half of the distal clavicle is resected (Fig. 11). Again, care is taken to preserve the dorsal capsule of the AC joint. Confirmation of the resection is achieved via direct viewing from either the posterior or lateral portals (Fig. 12).

Alternatively, a 70Υ scope may be employed from the lateral portal.

Postoperative Care

The advantage of the arthroscopic approach to AC joint resections is the decreased pain and early return of motion. After the first week, most of these patients will have regained at least 75% of their forward elevation and abduction. Many patients will have noted improved cross-arm adduction and internal rotation. These patients rarely require a course of formal physical therapy but, instead, should be instructed on home range-of-motion exercises. At approximately 3 weeks, as comfort allows, they may be started on a gentle strengthening program with an anticipated return to manual work-related activities at approximately 4 to 6 weeks and recreational activities in a similar time frame.

Acknowledgments

The author wishes to thank Steve Getch for his invaluable assistance with illustrations.

References

1. Cahill BR: Osteolysis of the distal part of the clavicle in male athletes. *J Bone Joint Surg* 1982;64A:1053–1058.

2. Cahill BR: Atraumatic osteolysis of the distal clavicle: A review. *Sports Med* 1992;13:214–222.

3. Scavenius M, Iversen BF: Nontraumatic clavicular osteolysis in weightlifters. *Am J Sports Med* 1992;20:463–467.

4. Rockwood CA Jr, Matsen FA III (eds): *The Shoulder.* Philadelphia, PA, WB Saunders, 1990, pp 42–43, 210–211.

5. Zanca P: Shoulder pain: Involvement of the acromioclavicular joint. Analysis of 1,000 cases. *Am J Roentgenol* 1971;112:493–506.

6. Mumford EB: Acromioclavicular dislocation: A new operative treatment. *J Bone Joint Surg* 1941;23:799–802.

7. Gartsman GM: Arthroscopic resection of the acromioclavicular joint. *Am J Sports Med* 1993;21:71–77.

8. Flatow EL, Cordasco FA, Bigliani LU: Arthroscopic resection of the outer end of the clavicle from a superior approach: A critical, quantitative, radiographic assessment of bone removal. *Arthroscopy* 1992;8:55–64.

9. Bigliani LU, Nicholson GP, Flatow EL: Arthroscopic resection of the distal clavicle. *Orthop Clin North Am* 1993;24:133–141.

10. Meyers JF: Arthroscopic debridement of the acromioclavicular joint and distal clavicle resection, in McGinty JB, Caspari RB, Jackson RW, et al (eds): *Operative Arthroscopy.* New York, NY, Raven Press, 1991, pp 557–560.

11. Tolin BS, Snyder SJ: Our technique for the arthroscopic Mumford procedure. *Orthop Clin North Am* 1993;24:143–151.

12. Cook FF, Tibone JE: The Mumford procedure in athletes: An objective analysis of function. *Am J Sports Med* 1988;16:97–100.

Biomechanics of Rotator Cuff Repair: Converting the Ritual to a Science

Stephen S. Burkhart, MD

Technological advancement can occur only when changes in technology and technique are based on science rather than opinion. Unfortunately, some of the longstanding tenets of rotator cuff surgery, such as the need for watertight repairs and the desirability of tendon transfers to achieve watertight repairs, were based primarily on opinion. My goal in this review is to present my perspective on the science of rotator cuff fixation to bone and to show how that relates to the optimal technique of suture anchor repair of the torn rotator cuff.

Biomechanics

Bone Tunnels Versus Suture Anchors

The superiority of transosseous rotator cuff repair through bone tunnels has recently become suspect. A recent biomechanical study suggests that distal tunnel placement into cortical bone is essential in order to avoid bone failure.[1]

My perception of rotator cuff fixation failure underwent a radical change as a result of two recent studies that we performed to investigate cyclic loading of two different repair constructs. We had previously studied bone tunnel fixation by means of a single pull to failure (ultimate load), and we had found that suture breakage was the most common failure mode.[2] Therefore, we concluded that the suture was the "weak link," and we investigated means to improve suture strength (eg, simple versus mattress suture configuration). However, when we studied the failure patterns of rotator cuff repairs

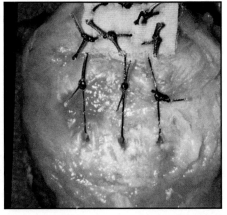 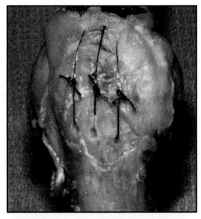

Fig. 1 Left, Specimen from cyclic loading experiment, with rotator cuff tear repaired through three bone tunnels. **Right,** After cyclic loading, this specimen demonstrates how the suture "sawed through" the bone, causing bone failure.

under cyclic loading at physiologic loads and rates, which is a much more realistic model than the single-pull model, we found that the failure mode of the repaired rotator cuff changed radically.[3] Instead of suture failure of the cuff repair, bone failure was the predominant failure mode, occurring in approximately two thirds of our specimens. The pattern of bone failure was intriguing. Under cyclic loading, the braided multifilament suture gradually but relentlessly "sawed through" the bone bridge like a wire going through butter until the cuff margin pulled away from the bone to the point that the original cuff defect (1 cm by 2 cm) was restored (Fig. 1). Our interpretation of that failure mode was that our closure of the cuff defect resulted in a "tension mismatch" of the resting ten-

sions of the muscle-tendon units of the rotator cuff, with the fibers at the central portion of the defect having the greatest "tension overload" under cyclic loading (Fig. 2). Therefore, the central sutures failed first and by the largest amount as the construct equalized the tension in its muscle-tendon units by this "controlled failure." Because of this consistent failure pattern, we concluded that cuff repairs should, inasmuch as possible, respect the crescent shape of the margin of the tear, and be repaired adjacent to the articular margin so as not to create a "tension overload."

After concluding the cyclic loading experiment for bone tunnel fixation, we repeated the experiment using suture anchor fixation of the rotator cuff tear.[4] Instead of three bone tunnels, we used

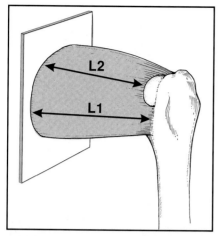

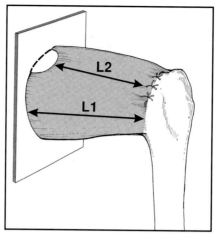

Fig. 2 Left, Muscle-tendon unit lengths (L1 and L2) are referenced to a plane through the medial scapula. The intact muscle-tendon unit (L1) is longer than the muscle-tendon unit at the apex of the defect (L2). **Right,** Repair of the rotator cuff defect can be accomplished either by releasing the origin of the muscle-tendon units that comprise the defect and repairing the defect without undue tension, or by closing the defect under tension, thereby creating a "tension mismatch" between L1 fibers and L2 fibers.

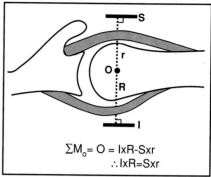

$$\sum M_o = O = IxR - Sxr$$
$$\therefore IxR = Sxr$$

Fig. 3 A balanced force couple (equipollent forces) is one in which the moments created by two forces about a center of rotation are equal and opposite, so that the object on which the forces act is in equilibrium. In the transverse plane of the shoulder, the moment created by the subscapularis (Sxr) is equal to the moment created by the posterior cuff (IxR). (©1995, University of Texas Health Science Center.)

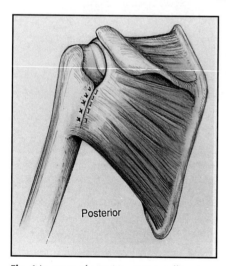

Fig. 4 In cases of massive rotator cuff tears with posterior extension, repair of the lower half of the infraspinatus is usually sufficient to restore a balanced force couple.

three Mitek-RC suture anchors (Mitek Products, Inc, Westwood, MA) for repairing the 1 cm by 2 cm cuff defect in each specimen. Surprisingly, only one of the 48 suture anchors underwent any failure within the bone. Instead, under cyclic loading, the constructs all eventu-ally failed when the suture progressively pulled through the tendon.

Comparing the results of these two cyclic loading studies, we concluded that fixation failure of the rotator cuff to bone was less likely to occur with the use of suture anchors than with the use of bone tunnels. Furthermore, using suture anchors instead of bone tunnels had shifted the "weak link" of the construct to the suture-tendon interface.

Partial Repair

Partial repair of the rotator cuff can be either end-on (tendon to bone) or side-to-side (tendon to tendon). These two techniques have different biomechanical implications and consequences, but they can be used in a complementary fashion to achieve the optimal repair of large and massive rotator cuff tears.[5]

The goal of partial repair of tendon to bone is to create a balanced force couple between the anterior cuff and the posteri-or cuff, thereby creating a stable fulcrum for glenohumeral motion (Fig. 3).[6,7] In 1994, we reported the results of partial repair (tendon to bone) in patients with massive irreparable cuff tears.[7] Most of these cases involved partial repair of at least the lower half of the infraspinatus. (Fig. 4) The improvement in function with this technique was dramatic. Active forward elevation improved from a pre-operative average of 59.6° to a postopera-tive average of 150.4°, for an average gain of 90.8°. The UCLA strength score improved from a preoperative average of 2.2 to a postoperative average of 4.4.

Margin Convergence

Despite the excellent results of partial repair of tendon to bone, there are many large U-shaped rotator cuff tears that require an additional side-to-side repair of the medial portion of the tear. Although the medial margin of the tear may appear to be retracted, it often repre-sents the apex of a lateral-to-medial split, rather than a pure retraction. Such tears can often be repaired to a large extent by side-to-side repair. This type of repair will shift (converge) the free margin of the rotator cuff closer to its anatomic

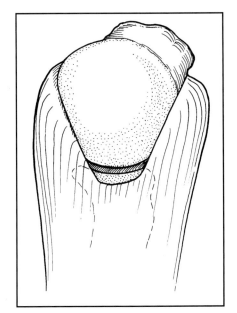
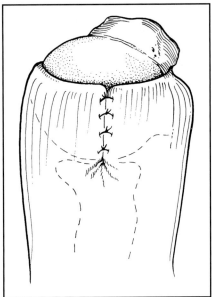

Fig. 5 Left, A U-shaped rotator cuff tear. **Right,** Partial side-to-side repair causes a "margin convergence" of the tear toward the greater tuberosity. This increases the cross-sectional area and decreases the length of the tear, thereby decreasing strain and elongation.

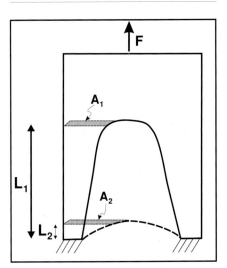

Fig. 6 Free-body diagram showing the mechanical conditions before and after partial side-to-side repair. The length of the tear has been reduced from L1 to L2, and the cross-sectional area of the cuff tissue at the apex of the margin of the tear has been increased from A1 to A2. These changes decrease the elongation of the tear and decrease the strain at the tear margin.

insertion on the greater tuberosity, so I have called this margin-shift phenomenon "margin convergence"[8] (Fig. 5).

Margin convergence by side-to-side repair effects a strain reduction at the "converged" free margin of the rotator cuff tear that can be very significant. For example, partial side-to-side repair of two thirds of the length of a U-shaped tear will reduce the elongation or strain at the margin of the tear by a factor of six. This means that the fiber elongation in the repaired configuration is only one sixth the elongation in the pre-repair configuration. Reduction in strain or elongation occurs because the repair decreases the length of the tear and increases the cross-sectional area at the margin of the tear (Fig. 6). Strain and elongation decrease because they are directly proportional to the length of the tear and inversely proportional to the cross-sectional area, according to the formula: $\Delta L = FL/AE$, where ΔL = elongation; F = rotator cuff force acting on the tear; L = length of tear; A = cross-sectional area; and E = modulus of elasticity (Young's Modulus).

Strain reduction such as that shown in the above example should be protective in two ways: (1) It should be protective against suture failure as well as propagation of the tear if the cuff is left in the crescent-shaped configuration; and (2) It should be protective of a repair of the free margin to bone, should the surgeon elect to repair the reconfigured crescent-shaped free margin to bone.

The matter of tissue fixation security can be positively influenced by this technique of strain reduction. By reducing the strain so that weaker tissue fixation will still be adequate, we enhance our safety tolerances for the strength characteristics of suture, tendon, and bone, thereby making suture breakage, tendon failure, and bone failure less likely.

Combined Techniques for Repair of Massive Rotator Cuff Tears

In order to deal adequately with a massive rotator cuff tear, the surgeon must fully understand the configuration of the tear. Very often, he or she must combine partial side-to-side repair with tendon-to-

bone repair. For a large U-shaped tear, the surgeon should begin medially with a side-to-side repair, progressing laterally until the anterior and posterior leaves of cuff tissue can no longer be approximated in a side-to-side fashion. At that point, suture anchors can be used to repair the "converged" margin to bone as much as possible, leaving a hole at the central portion of the cuff defect if the tear cannot be completely repaired (Fig. 7). By combining margin convergence (tendon-to-tendon repair) with partial repair of the margins of the tear (tendon-to-bone repair), one can obtain significant closure of many rotator cuff defects that initially appear irreparable.[5]

Suture Anchors
The Deadman Analogy: How to Insert the Anchor
Suture anchors are simply a clever means of attaching bone to soft tissue. They function in exactly the same way that a "deadman" functions to support the cor-

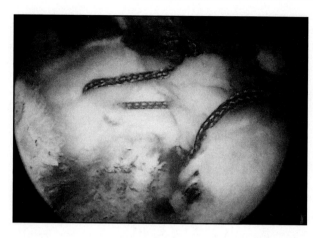

Fig. 7 Partial repair of a massive rotator cuff tear using a single suture anchor to repair the "converged" margin of the cuff to bone. Note the residual small defect in the cuff after combined tendon-to-tendon and tendon-to-bone repair.

pendicular to the anchor (θ_1, the pullout angle) and the other is the angle that the suture makes with the direction of pull of the rotator cuff (θ_2, the tension-reduction angle) (Fig. 9). These two angles are important in different ways. Mathematically, it has been shown that the tension in the suture decreases as θ_2 decreases. Therefore, a low angle of θ_2 is protective against suture breakage because it lowers the tension in the suture in comparison to a high angle of θ_2.

θ_1 is defined as the angle that the suture makes with the perpendicular to the anchor. This is the pullout angle, and, obviously, the more acute the angle θ_1, the more difficult it will be to pull out the anchor.

The clinical importance of the deadman theory is that suture anchors should be inserted at an angle toward the free margin of the rotator cuff tear (Fig. 10), and that from the anchor the suture should make an acute angle with the direction of pull of the rotator cuff.

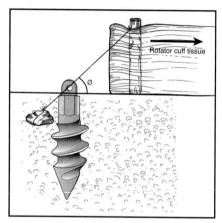

Fig. 8 Analogy of the deadman system to the suture anchor system for rotator cuff repair. The deadman is analogous to the suture anchor; the deadman wire is analogous to the suture; the pull of the fence wire on the corner post is analogous to the pull of the rotator cuff; and the fence post is analogous to the compressed rotator cuff tissue between the suture and the bone.

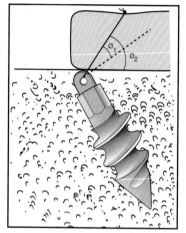

Fig. 9 Representation of θ_1 and θ_2. θ_1, the pullout angle for the anchor (angle the suture makes with the perpendicular to the anchor); θ_2, the tension-reduction angle (angle the suture makes with the direction of pull of the rotator cuff). Ideally, θ_1 and θ_2 should both be less than or equal to 45°.

Tension Overload:
Where to Insert the Anchors
In the section on *Margin Convergence*, the concept of "tension overload" was introduced. In the lab, we have demonstrated that a rotator cuff defect that is closed under tension will fail 100% of the time when it is subjected to cyclic loading.[3,4] Therefore, it seems most logical to respect the crescent-shaped free margin of the cuff and to repair it without tension, adjacent to the articular margin if possible (Fig. 11). If the free margin extends far medially, the repair should be started in a side-to-side manner from medial to lateral, and an attempt should be made to converge the margin of the cuff close enough to the junction between the articular surface and the greater tuberosity that the cuff margin can be secured (either partially or completely) to the bone bed with suture anchors.

ner fencepost on a South Texas ranch.[9] The "deadman" of a corner fencepost is a large rock buried 3 feet under the ground, and it has an attached wire that extends above ground to the top of the fence post as a guywire. This deadman system serves to support the corner fence post like a guywire. The deadman analogy to suture anchors is obvious: The deadman is analogous to the suture anchor; the guywire is analogous to the suture; and the fence post is analogous to the compressed rotator cuff tissue

beneath the suture (Fig. 8). In the case of the fence post, there is an ideal "deadman angle" (the angle that the guywire makes with the ground) of 45° or less that the ranchers must achieve, or else the fence post will lean. Extending the analogy to suture anchors, one can determine the ideal "deadman angle" for the suture anchor.

There are actually two "deadman angles" that are important in studying the properties of suture anchors. One is the angle that the suture makes with the per-

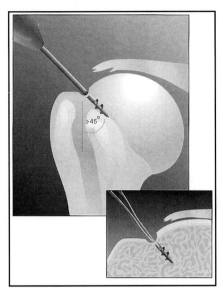

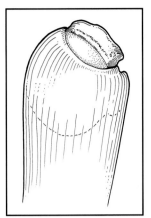 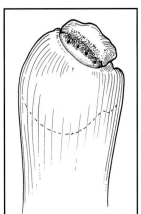 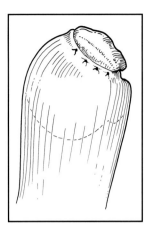

Fig. 11 Left, Crescent-shaped margin of rotator cuff tear. **Center,** Preparation of bone bed adjacent to articular surface. **Right,** Repair of crescent margin of rotator cuff adjacent to the articular margin to minimize tension on the repair.

Fig. 10 Proper angle of insertion of a suture anchor at 45° (deadman angle).

The Ideal Suture Anchor

At the present time, my opinion is that the ideal suture anchor should be made of a high-strength metal alloy such as titanium. Such an anchor will be visible radiographically, which is advantageous to the surgeon because he can identify the exact location of the anchor if a problem arises. Previous reports have pointed out the potentially catastrophic complications of metal migration from the shoulder to the lung, subclavian artery, and spinal canal.[10-14] I am concerned about the potential migration of radiographically undetectable plastic anchors. If an anchor becomes loose and has the potential to migrate, I would rather be able to see it on the radiograph, so that I can safely remove it.

Biodegradable anchors are currently under investigation for rotator cuff fixation.[15] The polyglyconate tack that has been approved for fixation of Bankart lesions is not appropriate for rotator cuff fixation under tension because of its rapid degradation and loss of strength. The polyglyconate tack retains only 60% of its strength at 2 weeks.[15] Therefore, it is not appropriate for the repair of a cuff tear

under any tension whatsoever.

I have a second concern about biodegradable suture anchors. As the anchor degrades, the smaller cross-sections will weaken first, and the eyelet will weaken before the body of the anchor weakens. My concern is that suture cut-out through the eyelet is likely to occur before the anchor becomes loose, causing loss of rotator cuff fixation at an early stage. Studies of bioabsorbable implants have so far focused on the initial pull-out strengths and degradation of the entire implant.[15,16] However, for suture anchors, animal studies need to be conducted to show the time relationship of eyelet degradation to the degradation of the body of the anchor, as well as the degradation profile of fixation ribs or screw-threads on the anchor. Once the boundary fixation (ribs, threads) is lost, the entire anchor will become loose whether the body of the anchor has degraded or not.

The ideal anchor must possess adequate pull-out strength, but what is "adequate pull-out strength"? The most obvious answer is that it must be stronger than the suture that is used with it, so that the suture would break before the anchor would pull out. In the case of the rotator cuff, most anchors will accept a #2 Ethi-

bond suture, which is a suture commonly used for cuff repair. I prefer to use nonabsorbable sutures such as #2 Ethibond. The average breaking strength (ultimate load) of #2 Ethibond is 30 lbs, so we would like the pull-out strength of our anchor to be greater than 30 lbs, as it is in all of the commercially available anchors today.[15,16]

My preference is to use an anchor that accepts two #2 Ethibond sutures through the eyelet. This accomplishes two things. First of all, it gives an added margin of safety for suture breakage, so that if one suture breaks the anchor can still be used with the remaining suture. Secondly, two sutures give an additional soft tissue fixation point per anchor, allowing greater fixation security with fewer anchors. This potentially shortens the operating time and minimizes the need (and cost) of additional anchors. Such cost issues become more important in areas where managed care predominates.

Three suture anchor configurations (with minor variations) are available commercially: (1) the press-fit plug anchor (eg, Mitek anchor); (2) the predrilled screw (eg, Linvatec Revo screw); and (3) the nonpredrilled compressing screw (eg, Arthrex corkscrew).

Of these three, the nonpredrilled compressing screw has exhibited the greatest pullout strength (FA Barber, unpublished data). The pullout strength of a screw is further enhanced when the thread diameter is large relative to the core diameter of the screw.[17] With nonpredrilled compressing screws, bone compaction with screw insertion increases the security of the anchor in bone.

Insertion of suture anchors through tendon and then into bone has been advocated. My experience with a screw-type anchor, using a trans-tendon insertion technique, is that the residual hole in the cuff is approximately the size of the core diameter of the screw-anchor rather than being the size of the thread diameter, since the threads simply appear to separate the fibers instead of cutting them. Therefore, the residual hole from the anchor insertion is an acceptable 2 mm (core diameter) rather than 5 mm (thread diameter). However, I would be reluctant to place a large-diameter plug-type anchor through the cuff, because I would be concerned about leaving a large defect where the anchor pierced the cuff.

The Approach: Open Versus Mini-Open Versus Arthroscopic
The standard open approach for rotator cuff repair has proven reliable if meticulous attention is given to repairing the deltoid securely to bone.[18-20] Paulos and Kody[21] introduced the concept of the mini-open rotator cuff repair, in which an arthroscopic acromioplasty is combined with an open repair of the cuff through a small (4 cm) split in the deltoid. This approach does not detach any deltoid from the bone, and it avoids the potentially devastating complication of deltoid retraction.[22] Other authors[23-25] have shown the mini-open approach to be a reliable means of repairing the torn rotator cuff.

The natural extension of the trend toward less invasive surgery has been the development of arthroscopic techniques of rotator cuff repair. Most of these arthroscopic techniques use suture anchors for fixation to bone.[24] I have also developed an arthroscopic technique of transosseous bone tunnel repair, using a sub-axillary nerve portal.[26] However, suture anchor techniques are easier to perform arthroscopically than bone tunnel techniques, and they have been shown to be mechanically more secure than bone tunnel techniques.[3,4] Although the mini-open technique can be routinely carried out on an outpatient basis, the arthroscopic approach has the added advantage of minimizing the risk of a "captured shoulder" from subacromial adhesions.[27] Obviously, the cost advantages of procedures that can be performed on an outpatient basis are a significant consideration now in the United States.

Author's Preferred Technique
Mini-Open Approach
Although I perform the majority of rotator cuff repairs in my patients arthroscopically, I use the mini-open approach in two situations: The patient with a massive tear that extends far posteriorly to involve all of the external rotators; and the patient with significant cardiopulmonary pathology that necessitates that the anesthesia time be minimized. For large subscapularis tears, a more extensile open approach is usually indicated, but such anterior tears are rare in comparison to tears with posterior extension.

For the mini-open repair, I place the patient in the lateral decubitus position, secured by a vacuum bean bag. Five to 10 pounds of balanced suspension is used for the arm, with the shoulder in 20° of abduction and 20° of forward flexion. An arthroscopic acromioplasty is performed by a modified cutting-block technique, similar to the procedure described by Bachner and Snyder.[24] If indicated, an arthroscopic distal clavicle excision is also performed.

The arm can be more easily manipulated during the cuff repair if it is left in traction. The patient is maintained in the lateral decubitus position during the mini-open portion of the procedure since that position affords the best access to the posterior part of the rotator cuff, simply by internally rotating the shoulder. A 4-cm muscle-splitting incision is made in the anterolateral portion of the deltoid, and the cuff tear is visualized. A traction suture is placed to assess the mobility of the tear. Elevators and dissecting scissors are used to free the bursal surface of the cuff from adhesions. If need be, the articular surface of the cuff can be dissected free from the glenoid margin in order to further mobilize the tendon. A bone bed is prepared adjacent to the articular surface of the humerus using a high-speed burr. The burr is used to develop a bleeding bone bed without decorticating the bone. Nonpredrilled compressing screw-anchors are placed at 10 mm intervals in the bone bed, just adjacent to the articular surface so as to minimize tension on the repair. The anchors are placed within the bone at a "deadman angle" of approximately 45°. Each anchor has two #2 braided sutures that are placed through the cuff as simple sutures with a free curved needle. I prefer simple sutures, rather than mattress sutures, because they produce a more stable rotator cuff margin than mattress sutures. I begin the repair at the posterior and anterior margins of the tear and progress centrally with the repair. If the tear is U-shaped, I place side-to-side sutures medially, from the posterior leaf to the anterior leaf, before repairing the converged margin to bone with suture anchors. If the central portion of the tear will not reach the bone bed without undue tension, I do not repair the central portion to bone. I would rather leave a portion of the cuff unrepaired than to overtension a portion of the repair.

Arthroscopic Approach
The patient is placed in the lateral decubitus position, and the cutting-block

technique is used for the subacromial decompression, just as in the mini-open approach. If indicated, an arthroscopic distal clavicle excision is performed. The torn rotator cuff edge is conservatively debrided to a stable margin with a power shaver, and a bone bed is then prepared adjacent to the articular surface. Adhesions are dissected from the cuff with an elevator or with a shaver. The arthroscope is placed through the posterior portal, and a tendon grasper is placed through a lateral working portal. I prefer to use an 8-mm clear cannula laterally to facilitate visualization, particularly during knot-tying. With the tendon grasper, I assess the mobility of the tear. If it is quite mobile and can be pulled over the prepared bone bed, I prefer to use a trans-tendon approach to place the suture anchor. A spinal needle is used to determine the proper location, adjacent to the lateral edge of the acromion, to make a small stab wound for placement of the screw-anchor. If the patient has hard bone, a bone punch is used through the stab wound to make a pilot hole in the bone. Then the anchor is introduced clockwise through the stab wound so that it easily screws through the deltoid muscle and into the subacromial space. The screw-anchor is then centered onto the rectangular "target" of the tendon grasper and screwed through the tendon (Fig. 12). The arthroscope is then positioned to visualize the pilot hole, and the screw-anchor is inserted into bone under direct visualization. It is critical to watch the anchor go into bone, so that the surgeon is certain that the anchor did not deflect obliquely off the bone surface without obtaining purchase. Because the trans-tendon approach eliminates the need for special instrumentation to pass braided sutures through soft tissues, those steps can be omitted from the procedure. However, if the rotator cuff lacks sufficient mobility to allow trans-tendon anchor insertion, the anchors may be inserted directly into bone, and the

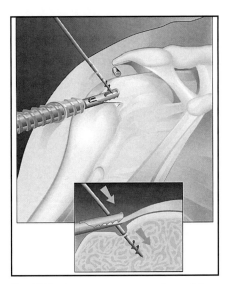

Fig. 12 Tendon grasper acts as a "target" for trans-tendon insertion of screw-anchors. The surgeon must watch the screw enter the bone to be sure there is secure osseous fixation.

sutures may then be passed through the tendon by means of arthroscopic suture passers or transporters. The anchors should be placed in the bone bed directly adjacent to the articular surface and at a 45° "deadman angle."

With the trans-tendon approach, one limb of each suture is withdrawn to the undersurface of the cuff by means of a crochet hook. This allows the surgeon to tie a simple suture, which gives a more stable edge to the cuff than a mattress suture. I prefer to use a double-diameter sliding knot pusher, which prevents slippage of the previously-placed loop as each subsequent loop is placed, providing maximum knot security. Every other half hitch is alternated in direction, and the post may be switched if desired (Figs. 13 and 14).

For large U-shaped tears, side-to-side repair of anterior and posterior leaves of the tear is done as a first stage using soft-tissue suture passers or transporters, in order to "converge" the margin of the cuff tear toward the bone bed. Screw-anchors are then used to repair the cuff margin to bone. If the central portion of

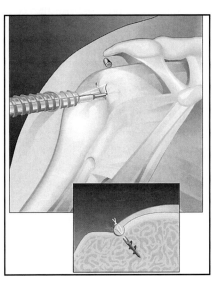

Fig. 13 Tying knots with a double-diameter knot pusher, which holds each throw tightly while subsequent throws are passed with the plastic sliding sleeve. Simple sutures give a more stable edge to the cuff than mattress sutures.

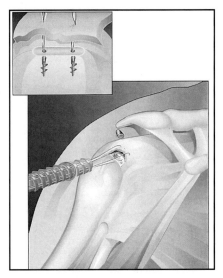

Fig. 14 All anchors must be placed prior to tying the knots, so as not to obscure visualization of the entry point of each anchor into the bone bed.

the tear cannot be completely repaired to bone, I leave a hole in the cuff centrally.

From Ritual to Science
Arthroscopic techniques of rotator cuff repair are rapidly being refined and have

the potential to revolutionize the treatment of rotator cuff tears. The combined principles of margin convergence and balanced force couples have provided us with a logical approach to achieve mechanically sound repairs of all but the most global tears. The torn rotator cuff should no longer be approached ritualistically by crude and unscientific means of simply covering the hole. Instead, each rotator cuff tear should be recognized as a unique biomechanical problem with a unique solution that is defined by its boundary conditions. By accurately defining the problem, we automatically determine the solution. In so doing, we elevate the ritual to a science.

References

1. Caldwell GL Jr, Warner JJP, Miller MD, et al: Transosseous rotator cuff fixation: The weak link? A biomechanical evaluation. *Orthop Trans* 1995;19:368.

2. Burkhart SS, Fischer SP, Nottage WM, et al: Tissue fixation security in transosseous rotator cuff repairs: A mechanical comparison of simple versus mattress sutures. *Arthroscopy* 1996;12:704-708.

3. Burkhart SS, Johnson TC, Wirth MA, et al: Cyclic loading of transosseous rotator cuff repairs: "Tension overload" as a possible cause of failure. *Arthroscopy* 1997;13:172-176.

4. Burkhart SS, Diaz-Pagàn JL, Wirth MA, et al: Cyclic loading of anchor-based rotator cuff repairs: Confirmation of the "tension overload" phenomenon and comparison of suture anchor fixation to transosseous fixation. *Arthroscopy*, in press.

5. Burkhart SS: Partial repair of massive rotator cuff tears: The evolution of a concept. *Clin Orthop* 1997;28:125–132.

6. Burkhart SS: Reconciling the paradox of rotator cuff repair versus debridement. A unified biomechanical rationale for the treatment of rotator cuff tears. *Arthroscopy* 1994;10:4-19.

7. Burkhart SS, Nottage WM, Ogilvie-Harris DJ, et al: Partial repair of irreparable rotator cuff tears. *Arthroscopy* 1994;10:363-370.

8. Burkhart SS, Athanasiou KA, Wirth MA: Margin convergence: A method of reducing strain in massive rotator cuff tears. *Arthroscopy* 1996;12:335-338.

9. Burkhart SS: The deadman theory of suture anchors: Observations along a south Texas fence line. *Arthroscopy* 1995;11:119-123.

10. McCaughan JS Jr, Miller PR: Migration of Steinmann pin from shoulder to lung. *JAMA* 1969;207:1917.

11. Mazet R Jr: Migration of a Kirschner wire from the shoulder region into the lung: Report of two cases. *J Bone Joint Surg* 1943;25:477-483.

12. Norrell H Jr, Llewellyn RC: Migration of a threaded Steinmann pin from an acromioclavicular joint into the spinal canal: A case report. *J Bone Joint Surg* 1965;47A:1024-1026.

13. Sethi GK, Scott SM: Subclavian artery laceration due to migration of a Hagie pin. *Surgery* 1976;80:644-646.

14. Lyons FA, Rockwood CA Jr: Migration of pins used in operations on the shoulder. *J Bone Joint Surg* 1990;72A:1262-1267.

15. Barber FA, Herbert MA, Click JN: Suture anchors: Update 1997. *Arthroscopy*, in press.

16. Barber FA, Herbert MA, Click JN: The ultimate strength of suture anchors. *Arthroscopy* 1995;11:21-28.

17. Asnis SE, Ernberg JJ, Bostrom MP, et al: Cancellous bone screw thread design and holding power. *J Orthop Trauma* 1996;10:462-469.

18. Ellman H, Hanker G, Bayer M: Repair of the rotator cuff: End-result study of factors influencing reconstruction. *J Bone Joint Surg* 1986;68A:1136-1144.

19. Matsen FA III, Arntz CT: Rotator cuff tendon failure, in Rockwood CA Jr, Matsen FA III (eds): *The Shoulder*. Philadelphia, PA, WB Saunders, 1990, vol 2, pp 647-677.

20. Codd TP, Flatow EL: Anterior acromioplasty, tendon mobilization, and direct repair of massive rotator cuff tears, in Burkhead WZ Jr (ed): *Rotator Cuff Disorders*. Baltimore, MD, Williams & Wilkins, 1996, pp 323-334.

21. Paulos LE, Kody MH: Abstract: Arthroscopically enhanced "mini-approach" to rotator cuff repair. *Arthroscopy* 1991;7:333.

22. Neer CS II, Marberry TA: On the disadvantages of radical acromionectomy. *J Bone Joint Surg* 1981;63A:416-419.

23. Levy HJ, Uribe JW, Delaney LG: Arthroscopic-assisted rotator cuff repair: Preliminary results. *Arthroscopy* 1990;6:55-60.

24. Bachner EJ, Snyder SJ: Arthroscopic subacromial decompression, arthroscopic-assisted (mini-open) rotator cuff repair, and arthroscopic cuff repair, in Burkhead WZ Jr (ed): *Rotator Cuff Disorders*. Baltimore, MD, Williams & Wilkins, 1996, pp 271-289.

25. Liu SH, Baker CL: Arthroscopically assisted rotator cuff repair: Correlation of functional results with integrity of the cuff. *Arthroscopy* 1994;10:54-60.

26. Burkhart SS, Nassar J, Schenck RC Jr, et al: Clinical and anatomic considerations in the use of a new anterior inferior subaxillary nerve arthroscopy portal. *Arthroscopy* 1996;12:634-637.

27. Mormino MA, Gross RM, McCarthy JA: Captured shoulder: A complication of rotator cuff surgery. *Arthroscopy* 1996;12:457-461.

Combined Arthroscopic and Open Treatment of Tears of the Rotator Cuff

Gary M. Gartsman, MD

In the last decade, arthroscopy of the shoulder has advanced from a diagnostic tool to an effective treatment option for stage-II impingement (fibrosis and thickening of the tendon), partial-thickness tears of the rotator cuff, and arthrosis of the acromioclavicular joint.[1-7] Full-thickness tears of the rotator cuff have been treated with arthroscopic decompression without repair of the tendon.[2,3,8] However, this procedure does not reliably produce good results, and it is clear that most full-thickness tears require repair.

At present, the technique for achieving shoulder decompression and tendon repair varies. Some surgeons prefer open repair; others use arthroscopic techniques exclusively. A third option combines arthroscopic and open operative methods. This chapter presents the rationale and technique of combined arthroscopic and open treatment of partial-thickness and complete tears of the rotator cuff. The treatment of stage-II impingement and massive, irreparable tears will not be covered.

Rationale of Combined Approach
Full-thickness rotator cuff tears can be treated successfully with traditional open methods. The results have been well documented.[9,10] However, this approach is not successful in all patients. In an attempt to improve the outcome, orthopaedists have investigated two areas: the detection and treatment of intra-articular

lesions of the rotator cuff and the use of limited surgical exposure. Intra-articular lesions of the glenohumeral joint are possible, and it might be beneficial to identify and treat them. These lesions are almost certainly overlooked when an open surgical technique is used, as the glenohumeral joint is not well visualized except when there is a massive tear of the rotator cuff. Arthroscopic techniques allow the surgeon to perform a subacromial decompression without detaching the deltoid. This appears to eliminate the rare but potentially devastating complication of dehiscence of the deltoid.

The theoretical advantages of combined arthroscopic and open techniques are the diagnosis of coexisting lesions and their possible treatment when the glenohumeral joint is examined, the identification of partial-thickness tears on the articular surface of the cuff, and the evaluation of the subacromial space through the use of small puncture sites. In addition, the deltoid remains attached to the acromion, smaller incisions result in less dissection and less postoperative pain, and appearance is improved. Moreover, the procedure can potentially be done on an outpatient basis and the postoperative rehabilitation may be accelerated.

Surgical Options
for the Combined Approach
When using a combined approach, the surgeon can choose one of two surgical

options, depending on the severity of the lesion and on his or her level of skill with arthroscopy of the shoulder. The first option involves arthroscopic evaluation of the glenohumeral joint. Coexisting lesions are identified and treated as appropriate. The arthroscope is then removed, and the rotator cuff is approached through a standard open incision. This technique has the advantages of arthroscopy—that is, it allows intra-articular inspection—and also permits the surgeon to repair the cuff with use of familiar methods. Surgical time is minimized with this approach, and the surgeon is able to treat the complete spectrum of rotator cuff disease. The second option involves a greater level of arthroscopic skill. The glenohumeral joint is examined arthroscopically and then the arthroscope is inserted into the subacromial space. A bursectomy is performed, if needed, to allow visualization of the lesion. If the local anatomy allows, a small open incision is made directly over the lesion and the repair is completed with the open technique. Alternatively, the surgeon can continue with arthroscopic techniques, resecting the coracoacromial ligament and performing an acromioplasty before opening the shoulder. As the surgeon becomes more skilled in arthroscopy of the shoulder, he or she may prepare the repair site on the greater tuberosity and place traction sutures in the edge of the cuff before the shoulder is opened.

The goal of the combined approach is to evaluate both the glenohumeral joint and the subacromial space completely and to allow repair of the torn rotator cuff through a small incision without detaching the deltoid.

Partial-Thickness Rotator Cuff Tears

Neer originally described three gradations of tears of the rotator cuff.[11] Stage I denotes hemorrhage and edema of the tendon; stage II, tendinitis and fibrosis; and stage III, an incomplete or full-thickness rotator cuff tear. Most orthopaedic literature has been devoted to the diagnosis and treatment of either stage-II lesions or full-thickness tears.[3,7,11] Little has been written regarding partial tears.[5,6,12-15] Two factors seem to be responsible for this. First, most partial-thickness tears occur on the articular surface and are not visualized during open acromioplasty for stage-II impingement; they may not be seen well even if the tendon is split in line with its fibers. Second, when partial tears were noted, they did not fit well into the Neer classification because they represent more damage than a stage-II lesion but cannot be categorized properly as a stage-III lesion.

With the advent and increased use of arthroscopy of the shoulder, partial articular surface tears have been described more frequently[5,6,12-16] because the surgeon is able to view the articular surface of the rotator cuff clearly and can measure the damaged area precisely. Various classification systems have been devised to categorize these lesions. The system used in this article was described by Ellman and me;[17] we classified partial-thickness tears according to the depth and anatomic site of the lesion. Tears are noted as being on the articular surface or the bursal surface. Grade-1 lesions demonstrate definite disruption of the tendon fibers but involve less than one fourth (< 3 mm) of the thickness of the tendon. Grade-2 lesions involve less than

one half of the thickness of the tendon and are 3 to 6 mm deep. Grade-3 lesions involve more than one half of the thickness of the tendon and are more than 6 mm deep.

Lesions of the rotator cuff are diagnosed as partial-thickness tears if there is disruption of the tendon fibers but no full-thickness tear is noted visually or by palpation with a probe or an arthroscopic instrument. Fraying, roughening, abrasion, or discoloration of the synovial lining or the surface of the tendon were not classified as partial-thickness tears.

Preoperative Evaluation

A complete history and a physical examination of the upper extremity and the cervical spine is vital. Elements in the history are reviewed for indications as to the etiology of the tear. Most lesions of this type are secondary to the impingement process, but partial-thickness tears can also be secondary to glenohumeral instability or an episode of trauma. The level of activity desired by the patient should also be noted.

The physical examination documents findings of impingement without regard to the etiology of the tear. Particular attention should be paid to symptomatic glenohumeral translation. The surgeon must be cautious about making definitive conclusions, because the examination for instability may be unreliable if the patient is in pain.

Radiographic evaluation is particularly critical for these patients. Anteroposterior, axillary, and scapular outlet radiographs are made and are examined for anterior acromial sclerosis, osteophytes on the anterior aspect of the acromion, and the shape of the acromion. Magnetic resonance images provide additional data on the location and extent of the partial tear.

Surgery is indicated for persistent pain that interferes with activities of daily living, work, or sports activities and is unresponsive to a 6- to 12-month course of nonsurgical care. Nonsurgical treatment

consists of modification of activity, anti-inflammatory medication, injections of cortisone, and a home rehabilitation program designed to improve or maintain the range of motion along with exercises to improve strength in the shoulder and scapular muscles.

The surgeon should understand the four essential elements that determine appropriate management of the patient: the etiology of the tear (impingement or instability), the extent of the tear, osseous abnormalities, and the patient's level of activity. A decision-making process that balances the four factors most reliably results in patient satisfaction.

In one study, Milne and I[14] found that the partial-thickness tear was attributable to impingement in 85 (77%) of 111 patients, to glenohumeral instability in 14 (13%), and to direct trauma in 12 (11%). If the tear was caused by instability, surgery that only repairs the tear will not be beneficial. The instability must also be corrected at the time of the operation.

Partial-thickness tears that are secondary to impingement require more complex analysis, and the following are general guidelines. Lower-grade lesions and smaller tears of the rotator cuff may be treated with decompression, while more advanced lesions must be repaired. Certain osseous shapes or changes are consistent with extrinsic compression of the tendon. Radiographic findings that suggest that the lesion will respond to surgical decompression are a type-III, or hooked, acromion; anterior acromial spurs; and inferior acromioclavicular joint osteophytes. Patients who have normal osseous anatomy are more likely to have intrinsic lesions and to need repair of the tendon. Less active patients may have a good result with decompression alone; more active patients may need repair of the tendon. The appropriate surgical treatment is more clearly defined at the ends of the spectrum. Decompression alone should be successful for the treatment of a grade-1 lesion in a sedentary patient who has a type-III acromion, while repair of the tendon is necessary for a grade-3 lesion in an active patient who has a type-I (flat) acromion. The decision process is more complex in the middle zone—for example, a grade-2 lesion in a weekend recreational athlete who engages in sports requiring overhead activities and who has a type-II (curved) acromion. The surgeon's ability to weigh the involved factors correctly allows for the most successful postoperative course.

Operative Setup

Anesthesia I use interscalene block anesthesia supplemented with general anesthesia. Regional anesthesia allows decreased use of anesthetic agents, which minimizes postoperative side effects and affords excellent postoperative relief of pain so that the patient can begin physical therapy comfortably. General anesthesia eliminates discomfort as well as unwarranted movement on the operating table.

Positioning of the Patient I prefer the patient to be in the sitting position, as easy access is afforded to the anterior, lateral, and posterior aspects of the shoulder without the need to turn the patient. This is also the position most commonly used for open repair; therefore, the patient does not need to be moved as the surgeon switches from the arthroscopy to the open portion of the operation. Positioning of the upper extremity is facilitated by the use of a McConnell arm-holder (McConnell, Greenville, TX). This holder allows the upper extremity to be positioned without the help of an assistant and is invaluable for maintaining proper rotation and elevation so that the site of the repair may be brought directly underneath the incision.

Some surgeons use the lateral decubitus position. This position is familiar to most shoulder surgeons who perform arthroscopy, and many are comfortable performing the open portion of the surgical procedure with the patient in this position. Either position may be used.

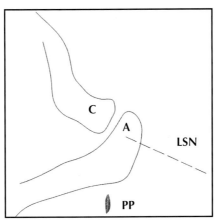

Fig. 1 The posterior portal (PP) and the lateral skin incision (LSN) in the right shoulder. C = clavicle and A = acromion.

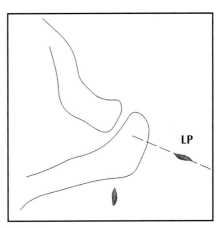

Fig. 2 The lateral portal (LP) created in line with the lateral skin incision.

Portals The acromion and the lateral portion of the clavicle are outlined with a surgical marker. The site of the proposed open incision is also drawn (Fig. 1). Three portals are used. The posterior portal is 1.5 cm medial and 1.5 cm inferior to the posterolateral acromial border. The posterior portal is made superior to the point of entry used by many surgeons (which is 2.5 cm inferior and 2.5 cm medial to the posterolateral acromial border) so that the arthroscope enters the subacromial space parallel and immediately inferior to the acromial undersurface. This places the arthroscope at the maximum distance from the greater tuberosity and improves the surgeon's perspective of the tear. The lateral portal is made along the line of the open incision, 5 mm posterior to the anterior acromial border and approximately 3 to 5 cm lateral to the acromial border (Fig. 2). The axillary nerve can be in jeopardy if the lateral portal is placed more than 5 cm lateral to the acromial border. The lateral portal should allow the cannula to enter midway between the humeral head and the acromion. The anterior portal is placed midway between the acromioclavicular joint and the lateral aspect of the acromion, approximately 2 cm from the anterior acromial margin. Additional por-

tals are rarely necessary as the upper extremity can be rotated to bring various portions of the tear underneath the lateral portal.

Glenohumeral Joint

A blunt trocar and cannula are used to penetrate the glenohumeral joint capsule through the posterior portal. A systematic inspection of all structures is necessary. The surgeon can generally view partial-thickness tears easily as they are most commonly located in the anterior aspect of the supraspinatus. Tears in other locations necessitate changes in rotation and abduction of the shoulder so that the entire tear is visualized clearly.

The surgeon should then establish the anterior portal. The arthroscope is moved anteriorly, and the posterior structures are examined. The arthroscope is then replaced in the posterior portal and a motorized shaver is inserted anteriorly. The partial tear is debrided until the surgeon can determine the dimensions and depth of the lesion. If the lesion is grade 1, the surgeon may remove the instruments, redirect them into the subacromial space, and perform an arthroscopic subacromial decompression, using previously described techniques.[6]

Grade-2 lesions in less active patients

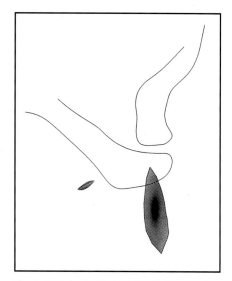

Fig. 3 The lateral skin incision is deepened.

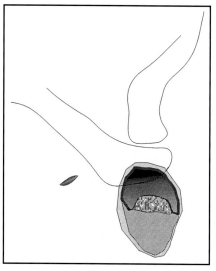

Fig. 4 The tear of the rotator cuff is exposed.

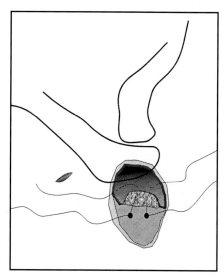

Fig. 5 Sutures are passed through the edges of the tendon.

or in those who have a type-III acromion may be treated with decompression alone. Grade-2 lesions may be repaired if the patient is active or if the acromial shape is type I or II. If the lesion is grade 3, it is necessary to repair the tendon. The partial tear is then converted into a full-thickness tear by debridement with a soft-tissue shaver. Alternatively, the surgeon may choose to mark the area of the partial tear with a spinal needle placed percutaneously. The entry point for the needle should be in line with the proposed open incision, generally 5 mm posterior to and 5 mm lateral to the anterolateral acromial border. The needle is advanced until it enters the middle of the tear. A number-1 dark blue (for easy visualization) absorbable monofilament suture is passed down the spinal needle until 4 cm of suture are in the joint. A soft-tissue grasping instrument inserted anteriorly holds the suture within the joint as the needle is removed. The arthroscope is then removed from the joint.

Surgical Repair

At this point, the surgeon may proceed directly to open repair by making a 3- to 5-cm-long lateral skin incision, incising the superficial deltoid fascia and spreading the deltoid fibers (Figs. 3 and 4). The split in the deltoid muscle fibers should begin approximately 1 cm posterior to the anterior aspect of the acromion. If the deltoid split is started at the anterior acromial border, traction applied during surgical repair may inadvertently detach the anterior aspect of the deltoid. Acromioplasty and resection of the coracoacromial ligament are performed when there is either radiographic evidence of bone that narrows the subacromial space (a type-III acromion or an anterior acromial protuberance) or arthroscopic findings consistent with impingement, such as fraying or fibrillation of the coracoacromial ligament. The surgeon should then rotate the upper extremity until the full-thickness tear or the marking suture is brought directly into the surgical field. The marking suture is removed, and the tendon is debrided until a full-thickness defect is created. The surgeon may then create a trough or a cancellous bed and repair the tendon to bone through tunnels in the bone or with suture anchors (Figs. 5 and 6). The superficial deltoid fascia is reapproximated with absorbable sutures, and the subcutaneous tissue and the skin are

closed routinely (Figs. 7 and 8).

If the surgeon wishes to perform more of the operation arthroscopically before the open repair and after the inspection of the glenohumeral joint, the arthroscope is introduced into the subacromial space through the original posterior portal. A lateral cannula is placed 5 mm posterior to the anterior aspect of the acromion and is positioned distal to the lateral aspect of the acromion so that it enters the subacromial space midway between the rotator cuff and the acromion. The marking suture is identified, and bursectomy, acromioplasty, and resection of the coracoacromial ligament are performed as necessary. The marking suture is identified and removed, and a synovial resector is used to debride the area of the partial tear until it is converted to a full-thickness tear. A traction suture may be placed in the margin of the tendon. The instruments are then withdrawn, and the open repair is performed as described.

Postoperative Rehabilitation

Tears repaired with this technique are generally small (1 to 3 cm long). Rehabilitation begins the afternoon of surgery

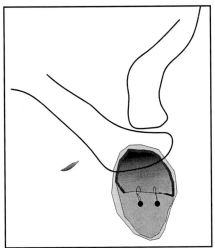

Fig. 6 The repaired tear.

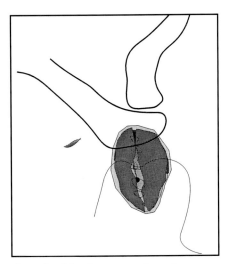

Fig. 7 The deltoid is reapproximated.

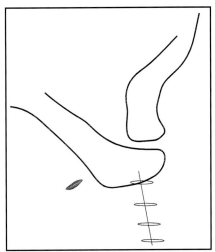

Fig. 8 The skin is closed.

with passive range-of-motion exercises in elevation and external rotation and is continued for 6 weeks. A sling is worn for protection during this period. Active range-of-motion exercises are started 6 weeks postoperatively; strengthening exercises, 3 months postoperatively. A return to full activities is allowed 6 months after surgical repair.

Results
The reported rate of good and excellent results is 88% (98 of 111) with this surgical technique.[14,15]

Complete Tears of the Rotator Cuff
Combined arthroscopic and open techniques can also be used to treat complete tears of the rotator cuff successfully. Blevins and associates[8] as well as Paulos and Kody[18] reported their experience with this technique. The theoretical advantages proposed by those authors are similar to those for partial tears, the most important being the ability of the surgeon to perform an acromioplasty and a resection of the coracoacromial ligament without deltoid detachment, to make a smaller incision, and to evaluate and treat coexisting abnormalities of the glenohumeral joint.

Preoperative Evaluation
An estimation of the size and repairability of the tear is the primary focus of the physical examination. Atrophy of the supraspinatus and infraspinatus muscles, inability to maintain the upper extremity in abduction, and weakness of resisted elevation and external rotation to manual muscle-testing of grade 3 or less are signs of a large tear. As the open approach in the combined technique employs a small incision and visualization is limited, this method is generally not suitable for larger (> 3 cm) tears or tears that need extensive mobilization. In these situations, the surgeon may elect to use conventional open repair techniques.

Operative Setup
The anesthesia, positioning of the patient, and placement of the portals are identical to those described for partial-thickness tears.

Glenohumeral Joint
Miller and Savoie[19] documented intra-articular abnormality in 74 of 100 patients who had a mini-open repair and concluded that arthroscopic examination of the glenohumeral joint is useful. However, the clinical importance of the lesions described in that report is unclear. My

experience has been that, while abnormalities of the glenohumeral joint were common (137 of 200 patients) in association with a complete tear of the rotator cuff, most of these abnormalities were minor, with only 25 (13%) of the 200 patients having findings of any importance.[20] Taverna and I used three criteria to define a major intra-articular abnormality: a lesion that required surgical treatment, one that changed the course of the postoperative rehabilitation, or one that altered the expected goals of the procedure.

Three patients were noted to have a severe partial tear of the biceps tendon that was not visible during the subacromial portion of the procedure.[20] All three tears were located within 1 to 2 cm of the attachment of the biceps to the superior portion of the glenoid. This finding delayed the biceps-strengthening exercises. No patient had a complete tear of the biceps noted during arthroscopy of the glenohumeral joint that had not been identified during examination of the subacromial space.

In our study,[20] lesions involving the cartilage included exposed bone of seven humeral heads. The lesions were all located in the medial aspect of the humeral head, were circular, and averaged

30 mm in diameter. Two patients had noticeable areas of full-thickness cartilage loss from the glenoid. No attempt was made to abrade the area of exposed bone. No loss of joint space or other findings consistent with arthrosis were detected on the preoperative radiographs.

Lesions of the labrum included separation in seven patients (anterior and posterior separation of the superior aspect of the labrum in five and a Bankart lesion in two) and a flap tear in three.[20] All of the labral separations were reattached with suture anchors and nonabsorbable suture. The patients who had anterior and posterior separation of the superior aspect of the labrum had injured the shoulder during a fall but had no history of locking or catching and no findings on physical examination indicative of glenohumeral instability or the separation. The labral flap tear was located in the anterior-superior quadrant of the glenoid in one patient and anteriorly in two patients; the tears were debrided with a motorized instrument.

Three patients had major synovitis involving the entire shoulder capsule.[20] A complete synovectomy was performed with electrocautery and a motorized shaver after a biopsy specimen was taken. The biopsies demonstrated nonspecific inflammatory changes.

Arthroscopy of the glenohumeral joint has a role in the management of patients who have a complete tear of the rotator cuff. It is possible that the identification and treatment of these lesions, previously overlooked with conventional open repair techniques, can improve results.

Surgical Repair

After the surgeon completes the glenohumeral portion of the procedure, the arthroscope is repositioned in the subacromial space through the posterior portal. The first goal is to visualize the tear of the rotator cuff accurately and to document its size and shape; therefore, bursa

is removed as necessary. If the tear is large (> 3 cm) or retracted and is not amenable to repair through a limited incision, the surgeon should halt the arthroscopy and proceed directly to traditional open repair. If the site and size of the tear allow for a repair through the proposed incision, the surgeon has two options: proceed to open repair or, if he or she has advanced arthroscopy skills, continue to perform the operation arthroscopically. The surgeon must remain aware of both the duration of surgery (so that anesthesia time is kept to a minimum) and soft-tissue swelling (so that the open repair is not technically difficult). It is not in the best interest of the patient or the surgeon to perform a combined arthroscopic and mini-open repair that doubles the duration of the operation or that involves an incision that is 90% as long (because of soft-tissue swelling), compared with traditional open methods.

The lateral portal is created in line with the proposed open incision, and an operating cannula is inserted into the subacromial space. Resection of the coracoacromial ligament, anterior partial acromionectomy, and inferior acromioplasty are performed as necessary. Osteophytes on the inferior surface of the lateral aspect of the clavicle are removed with a power burr if they impinge on the rotator cuff, as determined on preoperative radiographic imaging or as observed during the operation. The acromioclavicular joint is resected only if, on preoperative examination, the patient has pain localized to that joint. A traction suture may then be placed through the edge of the tendon. The arthroscopic instruments are removed.

The previous skin marking is used, and a 3- to 4-cm-long incision is made. The superficial deltoid fascia is incised, the deltoid fibers are spread with retractors, and the subacromial space is entered. The anterior portion of the middle of the deltoid must be retracted gen-

tly. Arthroscopic acromioplasty can weaken the deltoid attachment, and an unrecognized avulsion can substantially compromise function. The tear of the rotator cuff is identified and is repaired with nonabsorbable sutures through a bone trough or over a decorticated area of bone with suture anchors. The retractors are removed, the superficial fascia is repaired with absorbable sutures, and the subcutaneous tissue and the skin are closed.

Postoperative Rehabilitation

Tears repaired with this technique are generally small (< 3 cm). Rehabilitation begins with passive range-of-motion exercises in elevation and external rotation, starting the afternoon of the operation and continuing for 6 weeks. A sling is worn for protection during this period. Active range-of-motion exercises are started 6 weeks after surgery, and strengthening exercises, after 3 months. Full activities are allowed 6 months after surgery.

Results

Blevins and associates,[8] in a report on The Hospital for Special Surgery experience, documented an excellent or good result in 53 (83%) of 64 patients, according to the modified shoulder-rating scale of The Hospital for Special Surgery; 57 (89%) were satisfied with the result. Paulos and Kody[18] reported a good or excellent result in 16 of 18 patients according to the rating scale of the University of California at Los Angeles; 17 patients were satisfied.

Overview

Open repair of full-thickness tears of the rotator cuff has a documented history of success.[9,10] However, not all patients have a successful result after surgery. The selection of patients, the severity of the tear, the technique of repair, and the postoperative rehabilitation have a substantial influence on the end result. A technique that combines arthroscopic and open surgical repair has the theoretical advantages of identification and treatment of previously undiagnosed lesions of the glenohumeral joint, minimized soft-tissue dissection, preservation of the deltoid attachment, and improved appearance. Whether these theoretical advantages are real will be determined by studies that compare matched series of patients and torn tendons. Two other theoretical advantages do not seem valid. Rehabilitation is not accelerated by the combined approach because the limiting factor is healing of the tear to bone, and this is identical after open and arthroscopic operations. Also, the ability to treat tears of the rotator cuff surgically on an outpatient basis depends more on whether regional anesthesia can be used, education of the patient, and economic pressure than on the type of surgery used.

The combined arthroscopic and open technique may prove to be the desired method for some surgeons and may serve as a transition from conventional open repair to complete arthroscopic repair for others. It should be stressed that, at present, no ideal repair technique is applicable to all surgeons and all patients. Each

surgeon should determine, on the basis of his or her level of arthroscopic proficiency and the type of lesion identified, which technique is likely to be most effective.

References

1. Altchek DW, Warren RF, Wickiewicz TL, et al: Arthroscopic acromioplasty: Technique and results. *J Bone Joint Surg* 1990;72A:1190–1207.

2. Cofield RH: Tears of rotator cuff, in Murray DG (ed): American Academy of Orthopaedic Surgeons *Instructional Course Lectures XXX*. St. Louis, MO, CV Mosby, 1981, pp 258–273.

3. Cofield RH: Rotator cuff disease of the shoulder. *J Bone Joint Surg* 1985;67A:974–979.

4. Ellman H: Arthroscopic subacromial decompression: Analysis of one- to three-year results. *Arthroscopy* 1987;3:173–181.

5. Esch JC, Ozerkis LR, Helgager JA, et al: Arthroscopic subacromial decompression: Results according to the degree of rotator cuff tear. *Arthroscopy* 1988;4:241–249.

6. Gartsman GM: Arthroscopic acromioplasty for lesions of the rotator cuff. *J Bone Joint Surg* 1990;72A:169–180.

7. Hawkins RJ, Abrams JS: Impingement syndrome in the absence of rotator cuff tear (stages 1 and 2). *Orthop Clin North Am* 1987;18:373–382.

8. Blevins FT, Warren RF, Cavo C, et al: Arthroscopic assisted rotator cuff repair: Results using a mini-open deltoid splitting approach. *Arthroscopy* 1996;12:50–59.

9. Hawkins RJ, Misamore GW, Hobeika PR: Surgery for full-thickness rotator-cuff tears. *J Bone Joint Surg* 1985;67A:1349–1355.

10. Neer CS II, Flatow EL, Lech O: Tears of the rotator cuff: Long term results of anterior acromioplasty and repair. *Orthop Trans* 1988;12:735.

11. Neer CS II: Impingement lesions. *Clin Orthop* 1983;173:70–77.

12. Fukuda H, Hamada K, Yamanaka K: Pathology and pathogenesis of bursal-side rotator cuff tears viewed from en bloc histologic sections. *Clin Orthop* 1990;254:75–80.

13. Fukuda H, Mikasa M, Yamanaka K: Incomplete thickness rotator cuff tears diagnosed by subacromial bursography. *Clin Orthop* 1987;223:51–58.

14. Gartsman GM, Milne JC: Articular surface partial-thickness rotator cuff tears. *J Shoulder Elbow Surg* 1995;4:409–415.

15. Snyder SJ: Partial thickness rotator cuff tears: Results of arthroscopic treatment. *Arthroscopy* 1991;7:1–7.

16. Ellman H: Diagnosis and treatment of incomplete rotator cuff tears. *Clin Orthop* 1990;254:67–74.

17. Ellman H, Gartsman GM (eds): *Arthroscopic Shoulder Surgery and Related Procedures*. Philadelphia, PA, Lea & Febiger, 1993.

18. Paulos LE, Kody MH: Arthroscopically enhanced "miniapproach" to rotator cuff repair. *Am J Sports Med* 1994;22:19–25.

19. Miller C, Savoie FH: Glenohumeral abnormalities associated with full-thickness tears of the rotator cuff. *Orthop Rev* 1994;23:159–162.

20. Gartsman GM, Taverna E: The incidence of glenohumeral joint abnormalities associated with complete, reparable rotator cuff tears. *Arthroscopy* 1996;12:575–579.

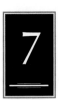

Arthroscopic Rotator Cuff Repair:
Current Indications, Limitations, Techniques, and Results

George T. Stollsteimer, MD
Felix H. Savoie III, MD

Introduction

Arthroscopic rotator cuff repair is still in its infancy, and its absolute indications, limitations, and results have yet to be truly delineated. Although data are presently being generated by multiple authors, no definitive statements can be made concerning its place within the surgeon's armamentarium. However, guidelines for basic indications and limitations can be gleaned from this research.

Levy and associates[1] and Baker and Liu[2] discussed many of the advantages of arthroscopically assisted rotator cuff repair. Advantages include inspection of the glenohumeral joint with treatment of any abnormalities at the time of surgery, the ability to perform subacromial decompression with a concomitant treatment of acromioclavicular (AC) joint lesions, preservation of the deltoid origin, decreased inpatient hospital stay, and an earlier return to full activity. These advantages, reported for arthroscopically assisted rotator cuff repairs, also exist for fully arthroscopic repair of rotator cuff injuries.

Arthroscopic repair of rotator cuff tears may be considered as an option for most patients being evaluated for surgical intervention. The size of the tear, quality of the bone and soft tissue, and the skill of the surgeon all play a role in the decision-making process.

Indications

Arthroscopic repair of the rotator cuff is indicated in small to medium tears with adequate bone and tendon quality. The ability to position the tendon over the greater tuberosity without undue tension is also important.

Currently, we consider patients with tears less than or equal to 3 cm optimal candidates for arthroscopic repair. Tears of this size are usually minimally retracted and present an "edge" amenable to arthroscopic repair using conventional techniques.

Large tears (> 3 cm) may also be repaired arthroscopically, but these require more advanced techniques. Arthroscopic sutures of horizontal and vertical splits are often necessary. Margin convergence (closure of the longitudinal component of the tear) is required to decrease repair tension. These techniques, which require advanced arthroscopic skills, should be reserved for situations in which open surgery is not an option. In most patients, complex tears should be repaired through a mini-open or open approach.

Surgical Technique
Glenohumeral Arthroscopy

Every arthroscopic rotator cuff repair begins with a standard glenohumeral arthroscopy. The arthroscopy is performed either in the standard lateral decubitus position with the patient tilted posteriorly approximately 30° or in semi-sitting position. If the patient is placed in the lateral decubitus position, the arm is placed in a traction device with 10 to 15 lbs of traction. All intra-articular pathology is addressed. The rotator cuff itself is then debrided in preparation for its eventual repair.

Debridement and Decompression

Prior to every arthroscopic rotator cuff repair, a diagnostic bursoscopy, subacromial decompression, and, if necessary, excision of the distal clavicle is performed. During our subacromial decompression, a lateral portal is created approximately 3 cm distal to the anterolateral edge of the acromion. A spinal needle is used to identify the exact area on the shoulder in which to create this portal. The spinal needle should enter perpendicular to the arthroscope, bisecting the acromion and greater tuberosity. A universal cannula is placed into this lateral portal. It is this portal that will be used to assist in repair of the rotator cuff. Completion of the arthroscopic acromioplasty occurs when the anterior edge of the acromion is noted to be posterior to the clavicle as visualized from the lateral portal. Every arthroscopic rotator cuff repair we perform is preceded by a subacromial decompression. If indicated, a distal clavicle resection is also performed. We routinely remove 1 cm of distal clavicle while preserving the superior AC joint capsule.

Rotator Cuff Repair Preparation

Once the intra-articular pathology has been identified and addressed, and the

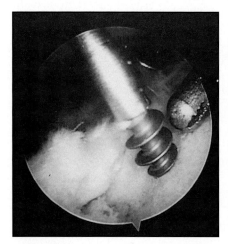

Fig. 1 With the cuff medial, the Revo screw is placed into the pilot hole for an alignment check.

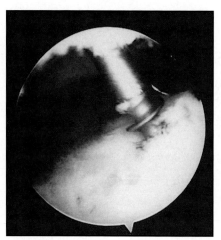

Fig. 2 Revo screw being placed through the tendon into the pilot hole.

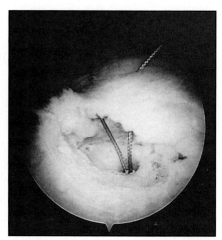

Fig. 3 View of the anchor in its cancellous bed with suture through the tendon as viewed from the lateral portal.

subacromial decompression and distal clavicle resection completed, attention is directed toward repair of the rotator cuff. The inflow portal is placed anteriorly and the arthroscope posteriorly into the subacromial space. The universal cannula is brought in through the lateral portal. Assessment of the shoulder for arthroscopic cuff repair is initiated. Three areas of concern must be evaluated: (1) tendon excursion/tension, (2) tendon quality, and (3) bone quality. Tendon excursion/tension is assessed using an arthroscopic tissue grabber brought in through this lateral portal. The supraspinatus tendon is pulled laterally to check for adequate excursion, tension, and quality. If required for adequate mobilization, capsular and coracohumeral soft-tissue attachments to the rotator cuff can be released. This may be performed with a blunt shaver or with an elevator, which is introduced through the lateral portal and used to free both the bursal and articular sides of the cuff. These maneuvers can aid in developing a tension-free repair. It is extremely important that the cuff have enough excursion to overlie the lateral bony trough without undue tension. The rotator cuff tendon will seek to return to

its normal resting length, ie, the position at which it is tension-free. If the cuff cannot be easily brought over to its insertion site, the repair is at risk of failing, and arthroscopic repair should be abandoned in favor of an open procedure.

The cuff tissue must be substantial enough to hold suture. Atrophic tissue is at risk for suture pull-out.

Finally, the cancellous bony bed must be dense enough to hold anchors. Advanced age, longstanding tears, and significantly compromised function are all factors that will negatively influence the patient's bone density. If cuff excursion, soft-tissue quality, and bone density are all satisfactory, the cuff may be repaired arthroscopically.

The greater tuberosity is lightly abraded just lateral to the articular surface of the humerus. Trough depth should be approximately 1 mm to 2 mm. Trough length will be determined by the width of the rotator cuff tear. Each anchor will need approximately 1 cm of bone between it and all adjacent anchors.

A spinal needle is inserted at the anterolateral corner of the acromion directly overlying the cancellous trough. The purpose of this is to identify the spot

to create a direct path to the cancellous bed. A small puncture wound is made in the skin at the optimal position established by the spinal needle.

Transtendon Technique With Suture Anchors

This technique involves the placement of the anchor directly through the cuff tendon into the trough. The anchor is placed in a "blind" fashion, because the cuff overlies the trough prior to insertion of the anchor. Many different anchors can be used in this fashion, including Revo, Mitek G2, Fastak, and Harpoon (Revo, Linvatec, Largo, FL; Mitek G2, Mitek Surgical Products, Inc, Norwood, MA; Fastak, Arthrex, Inc, Naples, FL; Harpoon, Arthrotek, Inc, Ontario, CA). This section describes the use of a Revo screw, but the technique is similar for all the anchors.

In hard bone, the Revo awl is brought in through the superior lateral portal. The cuff is allowed to move medially away from the cancellous bed. The awl is brought down to create a pilot hole, which will become the bed for the Revo screw itself. The awl is removed and the Revo screw is then brought in through this superior portal. With the cuff still medial to the cancellous trough, the tip of the screw is placed into the hole to allow an alignment check (Fig. 1) for eventual final setting of the screw. The screw is pulled away from the trough enough to allow the cuff to be pulled laterally to its final resting position. The anchor is then placed through the cuff into the pilot hole (Fig. 2), and the screw is set securely into bone. Both ends of the suture itself will exit out of this superior portal (Fig. 3). They are secured with a hemostat. The awl is then brought back in through the portal, and the procedure is repeated posterior to the first anchor. Using a crochet hook, one of the suture limbs from each anchor should be brought out of the lateral portal. One must secure the free superior limb of each suture with a hemostat so as not to pull the complete suture out of its eyelet in the screw. These two lateral limbs (one from the anterior anchor, one from the posterior anchor) are tied together using the knot technique of Wagner. A firm, gentle pull on the two superior suture limbs will bring the lateral knot back into the subacromial space through the lateral portal and will secure the cuff down to its cancellous trough. A mattress stitch is created between the two anchors, which holds the supraspinatus tendon down to the abraded bone trough. The crochet hook is again used to bring the remaining limbs of the suture out through the lateral portal. These are tied with a Revo knot technique and advanced with a knot pusher, firmly securing the cuff to its bony trough. The scope is placed in the lateral portal and fixation is checked with a probe. We generally use two anchors for this technique with two mattress sutures. A larger, even number of anchors can be used with this technique depending on the size of the rotator cuff tear. If the surgeon prefers, simple sutures can be used to tie the cuff down to its bony bed. One of the suture limbs of each anchor is retrieved from under the cuff and brought out through the lateral por-

tal. This leaves one remaining limb through the cuff. The stitch can be tied down with either a sliding knot or a series of alternating half-hitches.

Anchor/Suture Passing Technique

The suture passing technique is very similar to the transtendon technique: the preparation, portals used, and placement of the anchors are the same. The primary differences are that the anchors are placed into the cancellous trough under direct visualization and the sutures are passed through the tendon with a suture passing device. In this technique, the anchor is inserted directly into the bone trough without passing through the tendon. One (simple) or both (mattress) sutures are then retrieved through the tendon. There are two methods of suture passage. A suture retriever of varying angle can be placed through the tendon. The suture is placed into the wire loop and retrieved through the tendon and out the appropriate portal. The technique is repeated if a mattress suture is desired.

The second method of suture passage is to use a suture punch. In this technique, a modified Caspari punch is placed through the lateral portal after anchor placement. A significant bite can be taken and the "suture shuttle" is placed through the tendon. One limb of the suture is then placed into the shuttle and retrieved through the cuff. This procedure may be repeated for a mattress suture. A standard (nonmodified) suture punch with a double 2-0 prolene may be used in the same way if a one-portal technique is desired. Once retrieval of one limb of the suture through the cuff is accomplished, the suture may be tied if a simple stitch is preferred. Alternatively, the suture retriever may be placed through the tendon approximately 5 mm away from the first site, creating a mattress suture that can be tied arthroscopically. This process is then repeated for each subsequent

anchor. A tear of any size may be repaired in this fashion.

Screw/Staple Technique

The use of screws or staples in repair of rotator cuff tears is described here primarily for the purpose of condemnation. Zuckerman and Matsen[3] have previously described the significant complications that can be seen with the use of these devices. France and associates[4] evaluated the pull-out strength of staples in rotator cuff repair and found them to be less secure than trough-in-bone suture repair. We are unable to recommend their use in rotator cuff surgery.

Assessing the Repair

Assessment of the repair is an ongoing process occurring throughout the arthroscopic procedure. However, three main checkpoints need to be evaluated during every surgery. First, check for adequate excursion and quality of the soft tissues. As discussed, undue tension or poor tissue quality are significant risk factors for failure. Second, check the purchase of the anchor in bone. After placement, every suture anchor should be tested for adequacy of fixation. This is easily accomplished by applying a gentle pull on the suture. Under direct visualization, the anchor should be checked for stability at the bone-anchor interface. Third, once the cuff has been repaired, the overall construct should be evaluated. Under direct visualization, the cuff-bone interface should be checked for gaps or separation. The inferior aspect of the cuff should adhere securely to the cancellous trough. A probe should be used to aid in this evaluation. The bursal surface of the cuff should be visualized through the posterior and lateral portals (Figs. 4 and 5).

A poor evaluation at any one of these points indicates an inadequate repair. Suture and anchor removal and refixation must be accomplished. At this point, the surgeon may decide to convert to a mini-open repair.

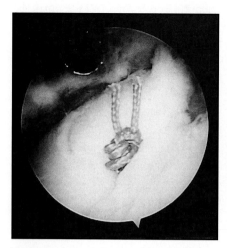

Fig. 4 Final repair as viewed through the posterior portal.

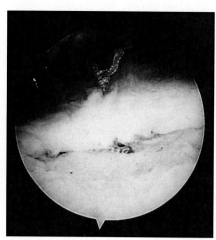

Fig. 5 Final repair as viewed through the lateral portal.

Conversion to Mini-Open Repair

Current techniques dictate that a majority of repairs be performed via open or mini-open incisions. Conditions identified intraoperatively that require conversion to a mini-open rotator cuff repair are generally related to the three factors discussed previously: (1) tendon excursion, (2) tendon quality, and (3) bone quality.

At times, the surgeon will find that it is not possible to develop a tension-free repair arthroscopically. Large or massive tears, long-standing tears, or tears with significant retraction may not be amenable to arthroscopic repair.

These same patients may also have poor tissue quality. If this is the case, simple stitches or mattress sutures may be inadequate to securely maintain the cuff in its bony trough. More involved tension-absorbing suture techniques, such as the Southern California Orthopedic Institute (SCOI) suture technique, may be required.[5] Complex suture techniques are often more easily performed via an open or mini-open repair. This procedure has been reported in detail previously.[1,5]

Briefly, our mini-open technique is performed by extending an incision along the anterior acromion distally for 1 to 3 cm. The incision should not run greater than 3 cm to 5 cm distal to the acromion, to avoid injury to the axillary nerve. The size of the tear will dictate, to a great extent, the length of the incision. Rarely do we need to extend the incision as far caudal as the lateral portal. Most repairs can be accomplished through a 3 cm to 4 cm incision. The deltoid fascia is sharply opened and the deltoid itself is bluntly separated to prevent injury to the axillary nerve. This allows direct visualization of the rotator cuff.

The cuff is debrided and the arthroscopic soft-tissue releases are evaluated for adequate excursion of the tendon. The rotator cuff is then repaired down to a decorticated bony trough via osseous tunnels or anchors, as the surgeon prefers.

Postoperative Rehabilitation

Postoperatively, the patient is placed in an abduction pillow for comfort. This is maintained for 1 week. At the first postoperative office visit, 5 days postsurgery, the patient is started on passive forward flexion. The patient is placed in an abduction sling for daytime activities and continues to wear the abduction pillow at night.

For the next 2 to 3 weeks following the surgery the patient is advanced to active-assisted external rotation and forward flexion. Full passive mobilization is begun by postoperative week 4, along with active rotator cuff exercises. Active range of motion and rotator cuff exercises are progressed as tolerated. Full rehabilitation begins at week 8 and functional activities at week 12.

Results: Our Patients

Forty-eight patients undergoing arthroscopic repair of full thickness rotator cuff tears were evaluated for this paper. The repairs were performed from May 1992 through August 1995. There were 31 males and 17 females in this study. The average age of the patients was 54 years, with a range of 38 to 88 years of age. Follow-up of these patients ranged from 12 months to 53 months with an overall average follow-up of 34 months after surgery.

All repairs were performed completely arthroscopically by the same surgeon (FHS). All arthroscopic repairs were accompanied by a full glenohumeral arthroscopic evaluation with subsequent burscoscopy and arthroscopic subacromial decompression. Distal clavicle resection was performed in patients with symptomatic acromioclavicular joints. The hardware used to perform the repairs were 21 Mitek G-2 anchors, 14 Revo screws, six Harpoon suture anchors, and seven ROC XS (Innovasive Devices, Inc, Marlborough, MA) suture anchors. Twenty-seven were transtendon techniques and 21 were suture-passing techniques.

UCLA scores for the total patient population averaged 33 out of a possible 35. The range of scores was 28 to 35. Results were also evaluated based on the size of the rotator cuff tear. Groups were divided into tears less than 1 cm (16 patients), 1 cm to 3 cm (24 patients), or greater than 3 cm in size (eight patients). In addition, the patients were looked at according to age, with groups divided up into subjects less than 45 years of age, 45 to 60 years old, and older than 60 years of age. There were nine patients in the first group, 28 patients in the second group, and 11 patients in the third group. UCLA scores for these three groups were 33 for patients under 45, 34 for the 45- to 60-year-old group, and 33 for those older than 60. Of note, among the 48 patients, there was one failure, which occurred in a 40-year-old male. The patient had a rupture of his rotator cuff repair after the initial surgery. He then underwent open revision repair and has done well since the second procedure. The most common findings for a nonperfect score in the UCLA grading system ran between occasional or slight pain to slight restrictions in overhead function and slight decreases in strength.

Of importance, all patients were carefully evaluated throughout the arthroscopic procedure at the points previously mentioned as significant for rotator cuff repair: tension, soft tissue quality, and bone-anchor stability. Only after all patients satisfactorily passed the evaluations was the full arthroscopic procedure performed. During the same period of time, 843 patients had open cuff repairs by the same surgeon.

Discussion
Indications
The indications for arthroscopic rotator cuff repair have not been delineated. As far as we are aware, no studies have been performed to answer this question.

Baker and Liu[2] state that full thickness tears less than 2 cm or tears less than 5 cm with a minimal or moderate (less than 2 cm) retraction were amenable to this technique. Our current indications for arthroscopic rotator cuff repair follow similar guidelines. However, as definitive research is yet to be performed, we evaluate these three factors in our decision-making process. (1) Size and retraction of tear: As stated previously, the cuff must be mobile enough to establish a tension-free repair. Further, although no millime-

ter cut-off limit can be quoted, a good rule of thumb is that the complete tear should be visible in a single view of the arthroscope. (2) Quality of the tissue: The cuff tendon itself must be of adequate quality to securely hold suture. If the tissue is too atrophic to be firmly held with simple or mattress sutures, a mini-open repair with placement of tension-absorbing sutures may be required. (3) Adequate bone quality: Just as the soft tissues must be adequate to hold suture, the bone must be dense enough to secure the anchor firmly. Intraoperative evaluation of the anchor-bone interface is mandatory during all arthroscopic repairs.

Technical Considerations
Osseous Tunnels Versus Anchors
Hecker and associates,[6] in 1993, evaluated the pull-out strength of suture anchors as compared to suture repair through osseous tunnels. In his study, he found no significant difference in the fixation strength of rotator cuff repairs using sutures only versus a rod or wedge polyacetyl suture anchor. There was also no significant difference in the pull-out force between the rod or the wedge anchors themselves. Several modes of failure were identified: suture breakage, suture tear-out through the tendon, and anchor pull-out. The primary mode of failure was by suture tearing through the tendon. Anchor failure was rare, but noted in two groups. Polyacetyl anchor failure occurred at the anchor/bone interface with an abrupt failure or pull-out of the anchor. Metallic anchors tended to cut out in the direction of the load prior to complete anchor failure. Hecker felt that the increased surface area and stiffness of the polyacetyl anchors closely mimicked the bone and provided improved resistance to pull-out forces.

Reed and associates[7] also evaluated full thickness rotator cuff tears comparing suture anchor techniques versus osseous tunnel repairs of rotator cuff

tears. They evaluated full thickness tears created in fresh frozen human cadavers. On one side, the repair was performed via sutures through bone tunnels. The other side was repaired with suture anchors. They found the overall mean strength of the suture repair to be 194 Newtons versus 261 Newtons for anchors, a statistically significant difference. Failures were predominantly caused by suture breakage. However, there was one anchor pull-out and one soft-tissue failure, in which the suture pulled through the tendon. Suture failures were all caused by cut-out of the sutures through the lateral cortex. Reed concluded that suture anchors provided stability superior to that of osseous tunnels. The anchor should be placed into the edge of the subchondral bone directly adjacent to the articular surface and should be countersunk below the bone surface. Finally, the anchor should be directed so that the pull of the rotator cuff is approximately 90° to the anchor with the humerus at 30° of abduction. This is essentially the position discussed by Burkhart in his "deadman's" suture anchor theory.[8] In this theory, Burkhart discusses two essential angles for suture anchor placement: the anchor pull-out angle and the tension-reduction angle. The anchor pull-out angle is the angle the suture makes with a line drawn perpendicular to the long axis of the anchor. The tension-reduction angle is the angle the suture makes with the direction of pull of the rotator cuff. Both the anchor pull-out angle and the tension-reduction angle should be kept ≤ 45°. This allows for an increase in the anchor's pull-out strength and a decrease in the tension in the suture.

Anchor Strength Goble and associates[9] developed the first suture anchor in 1985. Since that time, there has been a large increase in the number and types of anchors, as well as research concerning their overall properties.

Suture anchor choice depends primarily on surgeon preference. The limiting factors appear to be the quality of the bone and the strength of the suture. In almost all cases, the suture fails first, before the anchor. In soft bone, the expansile ROC XS appears to provide a significant advantage over nonexpansile anchors.

Histology of Absorbable Anchors Barber and Deck,[10] in a recent study, evaluated the foreign body reaction of a poly L-lactic acid suture anchor (ESP anchor by Arthrex) in ram femurs. This was evaluated over a 12-week period. They found no substantial acute, chronic, or foreign body reaction to this anchor. It seems that this poly L-lactic acid suture anchor will be very compatible with the in-vivo environment. However, more research is needed in this area, and no recommendations can be made at this time regarding their use.

Suture Anchor Insertion Technique In his paper on the deadman theory, Burkhart[8] discussed the optimal angle to place an anchor, as well as the suture itself, to increase pull-out strength of the anchor and reduce suture tension. It is hoped that these principles would decrease the risk of suture anchor construct failure.

Tippett (JW Tippett, MD, 1995, San Antonio, TX, personal communication) also gave recommendations concerning the techniques used for arthroscopic repair of rotator cuffs. He discussed the importance of the avoidance of tension on the cuff repair. Further, he also stressed the need to anchor the tendons to the bone with suture anchors using the deadman theory.

Attention to these details in anchor placement and suture fixation will lead to a secure suture anchor construct.

Suture Material Barber, in his update discussion in 1996 (FA Barber, MD, 1996, Atlanta, GA, personal communication), stated that the most suitable selections for arthroscopic rotator cuff repair are either PDS (polydioxanone) or nonabsorbable suture. He found that PDS retains approximately 80% of its strength in-vivo at 3 weeks. However, it drops to 40% at 6 weeks and was only 5% at 9 weeks.

Gerber and associates[11] also examined suture material. Gerber's study agreed with an earlier 1989 study by Trail and associates[12] that nonabsorbable, braided polyester is an extremely stiff material with excellent ultimate tensile strength, appropriate for rotator cuff repair. They found braided absorbable sutures have similar in vitro mechanical properties; but after 2 weeks of implantation, the ultimate tensile strength decreased 50%. Based on the findings of previous authors that 6 weeks are needed for secure biologic fixation of tendon to bone after repair, sutures such as Vicryl (polyglactin-910) or Dexon (polyglycolic acid) are not appropriate for rotator cuff repair.[13-15] Gerber and associates[11] felt that PDS-2 probably is an absorbable monofilament with a slow enough degradation for use in rotator cuff repair. However, the suture was felt to be extensible. Separation of the bone tendon interface occurs largely secondarily to the elongation of the suture material. They found elongation of 10.2 ± 0.6 mm for PDS versus an elongation of 2.8 ± 0.1 mm for braided polyester. Therefore, PDS probably can be used for small rotator cuff repairs without any tension. However, there is concern about failure secondary to degradation and elongation. For this reason, we recommend the use of a nonabsorbable braided suture, #2 or larger.

Suture Mechanics Burkhart found that two simple sutures were 40% stronger than one mattress suture (SS Burkhart, MD, 1996, Atlanta, GA, personal communication). He attributed this primarily to the increased load sharing that occurs with multiple simple sutures.

However, this finding is contrary to studies performed by Gerber and associates,[11] which found that simple stitches were less effective than mattress sutures. This study reported an ultimate tensile strength with two simple sutures of 184 Newtons and 208 Newtons with four simple sutures. Six simple stitches were needed to develop an ultimate tensile strength of 273 Newtons. This is in contrast to mattress sutures, each of which has an ultimate tensile strength of 269 Newtons. It was Gerber's feeling that simple sutures could only be recommended for small cuff tears with easily mobile tissues. He did not feel that simple sutures would be appropriate for larger tears or if the tendon was under tension.

Abrasion of Tuberosity St. Pierre, in 1996, discussed the process of tendon healing to cortical bone (P St. Pierre, MD, 1996, Atlanta, GA, personal communication). He questioned the need for actually developing a cancellous trough and evaluated this in a prospective, randomized study of infraspinatus tendon healing to a cancellous trough versus to a cortical bed in goats. The repair of tendons to a cancellous trough did not provide a significant mechanical advantage over direct repair to cortical bone at 6 or 12 weeks. In this study, he looked at the load-to-failure, energy-to-failure, and the overall stiffness of the repair. From this it seems that one may only be required to remove the soft tissues from the cortical bone surface prior to placing the suture anchor directly into the bone. No data are available regarding human patients.

At present, we perform an arthroscopic decortication, creating a cancellous trough in all our rotator cuff repairs.

Transtendon Versus Anchor First We currently perform our repairs using both a transtendon technique and anchor first technique. There are pros and cons to both procedures.

Placing anchors transtendon eliminates an entire step of the repair. As the sutures are already through the tendon, there is no need for a suture-passing device. However, placement of the anchor is performed in a "blind" manner, which greatly increases the technical difficulty of anchor positioning, and could result in improper anchor placement.

In the anchor-first technique, the anchor is delivered into the bone under direct visualization. The sutures are then passed through the tendon, requiring an additional step. However, this method allows more precise control of suture positioning in the tendon—a significant advantage in medium to large tears.

We recommend that the surgeon familiarize himself with both techniques. Arthroscopy is a dynamic process; the more options available to the surgeon, the greater the chance of success.

Reported Results

In 1996, Tippett reported on 36 patients who underwent arthroscopic repair of the rotator cuff (JW Tippett, MD, 1996, Atlanta, GA, personal communication). Mean age of the patients was 66 years, with a 16-month average follow-up. Of the 29 patients available for follow-up, 21 patients, based on a modified UCLA scale, had a satisfactory outcome.

Wolf, in 1995, reported on his results with arthroscopic repair (EM Wolf, MD, 1995, San Antonio, TX, personal communication). Outcome for 85% of his 66 patients was rated as good to excellent, also based on a modified UCLA scale. Ninety-two percent of all patients were satisfied with their procedure. Of note, 75% of 27 patients undergoing second-look arthroscopies had intact repairs.

The findings of Tippett and Wolf match closely with the findings in our limited study. The majority of patients undergoing arthroscopic rotator cuff repair have a satisfactory outcome with good results as far as pain relief, function, range of motion, and strength.

Future Considerations

Continued research will be of the utmost importance in determining the role of arthroscopy in rotator cuff surgery. Much has already been done in the way of evaluating technique and hardware. We are beginning to see promising research in the use of absorbable suture anchors (possibly eliminating the concerns of retained metal in the shoulder). Studies on the need for creation of a cancellous bed, as well as determinations of suture anchor strength, have advanced the development of arthroscopic technique.

Yet, the most important research will be in the area of long-term outcome for arthroscopic repairs. The true limitations of and indications for the technique have yet to be determined. Further study concerning tear size, patient age, and outcome in heavy laborers and athletes will prove invaluable in carving out the role of arthroscopic repair in the surgeon's armamentarium.

Conclusion

Early results demonstrate that arthroscopic repair of the rotator cuff may be a viable option in many patients. Criteria used to evaluate those tears amenable to arthroscopic repair include adequate excursion and quality of the avulsed tendons, and the bone's ability to securely hold a suture anchor. Anchors must be positioned using the deadman theory of suture anchor placement.

Arthroscopic rotator cuff repair is a technically demanding operation. The surgeon and operating room personnel must be familiar with the many facets of the procedure. Arthroscopic rotator cuff repair can offer the patient excellent results with advantages over open techniques in selected patients.

References

1. Levy HJ, Uribe JW, Delaney LG: Arthroscopic assisted rotator cuff repair: Preliminary results. *Arthroscopy* 1990;6:55–60.

2. Baker CL, Liu SH: Comparison of open and arthroscopically assisted rotator cuff repairs. *Am J Sports Med* 1995;23:99–104.

3. Zuckerman JD, Matsen FA III: Complications about the glenohumeral joint related to the use of screws and staples. *J Bone Joint Surg* 1984;66A:175–180.

4. France EP, Paulos LE, Harner CD, et al: Biomechanical evaluation of rotator cuff fixation methods. *Am J Sports Med* 1989;17:176–181.

5. Snyder SJ: Evaluation and treatment of the rotator cuff. *Orthop Clin North Am* 1993;24:173–192.

6. Hecker AT, Shea M, Hayhurst JO, et al: Pull-out strength of suture anchors for rotator cuff and Bankart lesion repairs. *Am J Sports Med* 1993;21:874–879.

7. Reed SC, Glossop N, Ogilvie-Harris DJ: Full-thickness rotator cuff tears: A biomechanical comparison of suture versus bone anchor techniques. *Am J Sports Med* 1996;24:46–48.

8. Burkhart SS: The deadman theory of suture anchors: Observations along a South Texas fence line. *Arthroscopy* 1995;11:119–123.

9. Goble EM, Somers WK, Clark R, et al: The development of suture anchors for use in soft tissue fixation to bone. *Am J Sports Med* 1994;22:236–239.

10. Barber FA, Deck MA: The in-vivo histology of an absorbable suture anchor: A preliminary report. *Arthroscopy* 1995;11:77–81.

11. Gerber C, Schneeberger AG, Beck M, et al: Mechanical strength of repairs of the rotator cuff. *J Bone Joint Surg* 1994;76B:371–380.

12. Trail IA, Powell ES, Noble J: An evaluation of suture materials used in tendon surgery. *J Hand Surg* 1989;14B:422–427.

13. Forward AD, Cowan RJ: Tendon suture to bone: An experimental investigation in rabbits. *J Bone Joint Surg* 1963;45A:807–823.

14. Ketchum LD, Martin NL, Kappel DA: Experimental evaluation of factors affecting the strength of tendon repairs. *Plast Reconstr Surg* 1977;59:708–719.

15. Clancy WG Jr, Narechania RG, Rosenberg TD, et al: Anterior and posterior cruciate ligament reconstruction in Rhesus monkeys. *J Bone Joint Surg* 1981;63A:1270–1284.

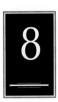

The Treatment of Stiffness of the Shoulder After Repair of the Rotator Cuff

Jon J. P. Warner, MD

Patrick E. Greis, MD

Repair of the rotator cuff usually eliminates pain and improves the overall function of the shoulder. Good shoulder function depends on the patient regaining a nearly normal passive and active range of motion with sufficient strength to perform activities of daily living, work, and sports.[1] Failure of procedures for repair of the rotator cuff usually is ascribed to disruption of the repair itself and may be associated with both pain and loss of active motion. However, loss of motion may occur with or without disruption of the repair and may be due to postoperative adhesions and actual capsular contracture.

The prevalence of loss of motion has not been clearly reported in previous studies of the results of repair of the rotator cuff. A review of series of such procedures that were performed over the previous two decades revealed that, of 500 patients, 21 (4%) had loss of motion that was believed to be due to postoperative adhesions.[2-13] Many reports have not included quantitative measurements of postoperative motion compared with preoperative motion; thus, it is difficult to arrive at an accurate appraisal of the prevalence of shoulder stiffness after repair of the rotator cuff. The senior one of us (JJPW) has found that loss of passive motion is not uncommon after repair of the rotator cuff, and although the patient may not always be symptomatic treatment may be necessary.

The purpose of the current chapter is to review the variables involved in loss of motion after repair of the rotator cuff and to describe an approach for its evaluation and treatment.

Etiology and Clinical Evaluation

Some loss of motion after repair of a large tear of the rotator cuff may be inevitable, as dissection of the subscapularis and infraspinatus tendons free from surrounding tissue and local transposition of the tendons to repair the defect of the rotator cuff may result in limitation of the overall passive excursion of portions of the cuff. For example, repair of a chronic rupture of the subscapularis often is associated with some loss of external rotation.[14] This is because of the shortening resulting from the repair of the tendon-muscle unit, as there is actual loss of tendon tissue. Furthermore, some patients may not be bothered by painless loss of motion as long as function and strength are improved.

Symptomatic loss of motion after repair of the rotator cuff can have a variety of causes. One possible etiology is failure of a motor unit of the shoulder—that is, a tear of a rotator-cuff tendon, muscle failure (avulsion of the deltoid or disuse atrophy), or injury of the axillary nerve, the brachial plexus, or the suprascapular nerve. Shoulder stiffness can also be caused by soft-tissue contracture, which can be intra-articular (capsular

contracture or tendon shortening) or extra-articular (subacromial or subdeltoid scarring or scarring of the subscapularis-conjoined tendon region). Other causes are intrinsic disease or abnormality of the glenohumeral joint, such as osteoarthrosis or an osseous deformity, and a pain complex. These factors may occur in isolation or in combination. The history given by the patient is very important, as it may provide insight into the cause or causes of the loss of motion. For example, prolonged immobilization of the shoulder without any passive motion might be expected to lead to adhesions between tissue planes and thus to stiffness after a repair of the rotator cuff. An inappropriate load on the repair, such as that caused by a fall or by the initiation of an active range of motion during the first few weeks after the procedure, might lead to disruption of the repair.

Additional patient-related factors of importance are a history of insulin-dependent diabetes mellitus and the formation of keloid scars.[15] These factors appear to be associated with a predisposition to loss of motion of the shoulder in the postoperative setting.[16]

The most important observation to make during an evaluation of stiffness after a repair of the rotator cuff is whether the loss of motion is active, passive, or both.[17] Motion must always be compared with that of the contralateral,

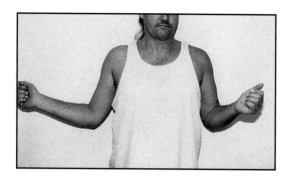

Fig. 1 Photograph of a 36-year-old man who had painful loss of external rotation of the left shoulder after a repair of the supraspinatus tendon and tight closure of the rotator interval.

asymptomatic shoulder, if possible. Elimination of pain with use of a subacromial injection of 10 ml of 1% Xylocaine (lidocaine) can allow the physician to discriminate between loss of active motion due to pain and that due to a tear or contracture of the rotator cuff.[18] Testing should include not only flexion but also abduction in the scapular plane, internal and external rotation, and horizontal flexion (cross-chest adduction).[16,19] The presence of pain with any of these motions also should be evaluated. Any differences between the arcs of active and passive motion should be noted. Careful measurements of isolated glenohumeral motion should be made with a goniometer, as patients who have shoulder stiffness often have scapulothoracic substitution (compensatory movement of the scapula on the thorax) and tilting of the trunk, which may give the appearance of more motion at the glenohumeral joint than is really present.

Active motion is measured with the patient seated, and passive motion is measured with the patient supine. When the patient is supine, scapulothoracic substitution and tilting of the trunk are reduced, allowing more accurate measurement of glenohumeral rotation.[18]

Loss of active motion but preservation of passive motion indicates failure of the repair of the rotator cuff or an injury of the axillary or suprascapular nerve, or both. In most patients, the location of the tear can be predicted on the basis of the pattern of lag between the arcs of active and passive motion.[20] For example, greater passive than active internal rotation indicates a tear of the subscapularis, while greater passive than active external rotation when the shoulder is abducted indicates a tear of the infraspinatus.

Loss of passive motion and an equivalent limitation of active motion, with good strength, after a repair may or may not indicate a repeat tear; however, such findings do indicate postoperative adhesions and, sometimes, capsular contractures that limit motion. In some patients, articular incongruity, as might occur with osteoarthrosis, also may contribute to loss of motion.

The pattern of motion loss is a particularly important indicator of the location or locations of adhesions. For example, loss of external rotation with the upper extremity at the side may be associated with contracture of the rotator-interval region of the anterosuperior portion of the glenohumeral joint, whereas limited abduction and external rotation usually indicates contracture of the inferior aspect of the capsule.[16,21-23] Loss of internal rotation is usually associated with a contracture of the posterior aspect of the capsule.[16,23]

Persistent loss of motion after a repair of the rotator cuff often can be attributed to one of three causes: a pre-existing comorbid condition, such as osteoarthrosis or shoulder stiffness, in addition to the tear of the rotator cuff; the surgical technique; or the technique used for postoperative rehabilitation. Some patients who

have loss of motion caused by osteoarthrosis may be managed, incorrectly, for a tear of the rotator cuff. Furthermore, some degree of passive motion loss may not have been recognized or treated effectively before the repair of the rotator cuff. The result will be shoulder stiffness after the repair. This situation is analogous to performing a repair of the anterior cruciate ligament in a stiff knee. The result will be a healed ligament in a stiff knee. Therefore, it is preferable to recognize and treat shoulder stiffness adequately before performing a repair of the rotator cuff.

Incorrect surgical technique can lead directly to stiffness after a repair of the rotator cuff. For example, tight closure of the rotator-interval region with the upper extremity in internal rotation leads to loss of both external rotation and flexion (Fig. 1).[24-26] In some patients, over-advancement of a tendon[16,27,28] to close a tendon defect may lead to loss of motion by capturing the shoulder. However, most failures that are due to incorrect surgical technique are caused by inadequate mobilization and repair of the torn tendon or by repair of the tendon under excessive tension.

Assuming that a technically adequate repair has been performed, the postoperative treatment has a direct bearing on the prevalence of shoulder stiffness after a repair of the rotator cuff. The aim during the initial phase of treatment (the first 6 weeks after the operation) is to protect the repair until it has healed while preserving passive motion. Thus, failure to begin a passive range of motion in the first week after the operation can lead to loss of motion. This loss of motion is usually caused by adhesions between tissue planes, but it also may be caused by capsular contracture.

Some patients have a very low tolerance for pain during early passive motion, and this places them at risk for shoulder stiffness. Also, these patients tend to have a form of shoulder stiffness that is particularly resistant to nonsurgical therapy.[16,29,30]

When a patient has loss of motion after a repair of the rotator cuff, additional important clinical observations include the presence of atrophy, which suggests a chronically torn tendon; painful flexion, which suggests residual impingement; tenderness over the acromioclavicular joint or the biceps tendon, which suggests an untreated pathologic condition; weakness, which suggests an incomplete repair of the rotator cuff or a nerve injury; decreased skin sensation, which suggests an axillary nerve injury; and a defect of the deltoid, which suggests an iatrogenic injury to the origin of the deltoid.

Standard radiographs may be helpful for determining the extent of previous surgical treatment for impingement and acromioclavicular disease. Our preference is to make a supraspinatus outlet radiograph, a 30° caudal tilt radiograph, a radiograph of the acromioclavicular joint, and an axillary radiograph.[31,32] These radiographs demonstrate the extent of the resection of the acromion and the acromioclavicular joint and provide information about the glenohumeral joint. Common problems that may be disclosed include failure to recognize and treat an os acromiale, excessive or inadequate resection of the acromion or the acromioclavicular joint, fracture of the os acromiale, and previously unrecognized osteoarthrosis of the glenohumeral joint.

Additional adjuvant imaging that may be useful includes arthrography and magnetic resonance imaging. While the former will demonstrate a repeat tear after a repair, a watertight repair is not necessary for good function. Furthermore, arthrography does not directly show the degree and location of capsular contracture and adhesions.[33]

Magnetic resonance imaging may provide additional useful information about the thickness of the tendon tissue as well as the degree of muscle atrophy and fatty degeneration.[34,35] This information can help the physician to decide on the treat-

ment for stiffness of the shoulder and a repeat tear of the tendon repair. For example, thin tendon tissue might be expected to tear with closed manipulation, and a muscle with extensive atrophy and fatty degeneration would not be expected to function normally after a repair.[34]

When all of the previously mentioned factors are taken into account, it appears that shoulder stiffness that might necessitate treatment is found in four types of patients: those who have stiffness without a tear after the repair, those who have both stiffness and a repeat tear after the repair, those who have stiffness in association with untreated osteoarthrosis of the glenohumeral joint, and those who have stiffness in combination with an injury of the deltoid or a nerve injury, or both, with or without a repeat tear after the repair. The treatment of each group of patients will be discussed.

Treatment Options
Stiffness Without a Tear of the Repaired Rotator Cuff

These patients often have a history of prolonged immobilization after the repair. Passive motion may not have been initiated following surgery, or the patient may have had too much pain to allow this motion. Both the passive and the active range of motion are limited and, although there may be pain, strength is good. The pain may be due to an inadequate acromioplasty, untreated disease of the acromioclavicular joint or the biceps, or stiffness of the shoulder. Such stiffness may cause pain by changing the biomechanics of the glenohumeral joint. For example, a patient who has lost internal rotation because of a contracture of the posterior aspect of the capsule may have increased superior translation of the humeral head on the glenoid when flexion is attempted. This can cause so-called non-outlet impingement.[16,23] Furthermore, loss of glenohumeral motion results in a compensatory increase in

scapulothoracic motion, and some of these patients have symptoms referable to the scapular area.[16]

Treatment options for these patients include intensive physical therapy, closed manipulation, and arthroscopic or open release of adhesions. All patients should be managed with stretching techniques by a physical therapist for at least 3 to 6 months after the repair, before other options for treatment are considered. During this period, the pain may subside and the patient's tolerance for stretching may improve. However, if no motion is gained during this period, it is neither clinically useful nor cost effective to continue with this course of treatment.

Closed manipulation, while appropriate for the treatment of idiopathic adhesive capsulitis, usually is not helpful for patients who have stiffness after a repair of the rotator cuff.[16,21,24,26,30] These patients usually have more extensive adhesions involving the tissue planes between the rotator cuff and the deltoid and the acromion, as well as actual capsular contractures. Furthermore, forceful manipulation after a repair of the rotator cuff may pose a risk to the integrity of the repair. Therefore, we usually do not attempt this form of treatment.

Arthroscopic release of contracted capsule and adhesions is the method that we usually employ. This technique allows precise, selective release of adhesions between tissue planes as well as division of shortened, thickened capsular tissue.[16,21,26,36] Subsequently, gentle, controlled manipulation of the shoulder can restore motion with a reduced risk to the repair of the rotator cuff. Concomitant intra-articular and subacromial disease also may be detected and treated. For example, previously untreated disease of the biceps tendon can be managed with an arthroscopic tenotomy, and acromioclavicular disease and residual subacromial impingement also may be treated. An additional advantage of this technique is that it permits an immediate active

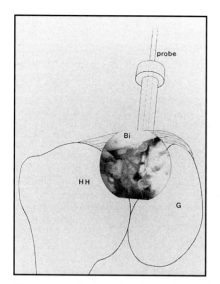
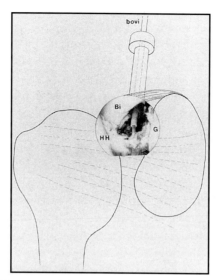
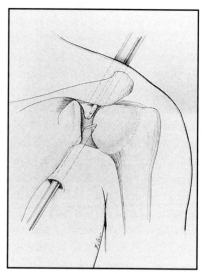

Fig. 2 Schematic drawings of the left shoulder of the patient shown in Figure 1. **Left,** Arthroscopic view of the rotator-interval region. The arthroscope is in the posterior portal. There is thick scar and synovial tissue in the rotator-interval region underneath the biceps tendon (Bi). HH = humeral head and G = glenoid. **Center,** An arthroscopic release of the rotator-interval region was performed with use of an electrocautery device (bovi). Bi = biceps tendon, HH = humeral head, and G = glenoid. **Right,** The arthroscopic release of the rotator interval has allowed the humeral head to distract away from the glenoid, permitting better access to adhesions in the anterior aspect of the joint capsule. (Adapted with permission from Warner JJP, Allen A, Marks PH, et al: Arthroscopic release for chronic, refractory adhesive capsulitis of the shoulder. *J Bone Joint Surg* 1996;78A:1808.)

range of motion without the need to await healing of repaired soft tissues. Contraindications to this technique are malunion of the tuberosity causing an osseous block to motion, articular incongruity due to osteoarthrosis, and extra-articular contractures such as entrapment or shortening of the subscapularis after a previous Putti-Platt or Bristow procedure, for example.

Arthroscopic Release The method of anesthesia and postoperative analgesia is very important to the overall success of this technique. We therefore use regional anesthesia, either by means of an interscalene block during the surgical procedure followed by additional blocks postoperatively or with the placement of an indwelling interscalene catheter and administration of anesthesia followed by a continuous slow drip of a local anesthetic.[37,38] The interscalene block is performed with use of about 30 ml of 0.5% bupivacaine with 1:200,000 epinephrine. This anesthesia effect lasts for about 6 hours, although analgesia may last for as

long as 12 hours. If a catheter is not used, then the block is repeated on the mornings of the first and second postoperative days, as our patients remain in the hospital for 48 hours after the procedure in order to have intensive physical therapy.

When an interscalene catheter is used, a continuous infusion of 0.25 % bupivacaine is administered at a rate of 6 ml per hour for 48 hours. All of our patients also use a self-administered pain-relief system (patient-controlled analgesia) through an intravenous pump set to administer 1 mg of morphine every 8 minutes as needed, to a maximum of 30 mg in 4 hours.

Anterior Capsular Release We always measure and record the passive range of motion after adequate anesthesia has been achieved. Although there may be some concern about articular injury with insertion of an arthroscope into a stiff joint, our technique enables us to avoid this problem.[16,29]

We perform shoulder arthroscopy with the patient seated in the beach-chair position, without any traction on the

arm.[39] The joint is distended with sterile saline solution through an 18-gauge spinal needle inserted into a posterior portal. The hydrostatic pressure tends to push the humeral head away from the glenoid and reduces the risk of injury to the cartilage as the arthroscope is inserted. The arthroscope is guided carefully over the humeral head. As the volume of the joint is usually small, retrograde flow of saline solution out of an open port in the arthroscopic sheath confirms the intra-articular placement of the arthroscope. Usually, only the anterosuperior region of the joint capsule can be visualized; no attempt should be made to force the arthroscope inferiorly into the joint (Fig. 2, *left*). The long head of the biceps tendon defines the region of the rotator interval, which is the area between the anterior edge of the supraspinatus tendon and the superior edge of the subscapularis tendon.[22] This region usually is contracted in individuals who lack external rotation of the adducted shoulder.[24,25]

An 18-gauge spinal needle is introduced from a superior and anterior location so that it enters the joint just underneath the long head of the biceps tendon. The needle then is withdrawn, and it is replaced with a 7-ml arthroscopic shoulder cannula (Linvatec, Concept Arthroscopy, Largo, Florida). A 4.5-mm motorized shaver (full radius resector; Linvatec, Concept Arthroscopy) is placed through the cannula, and the anterosuperior region of the joint is debrided of synovial tissue and adhesions. This allows the thick sheet of the scarred anterosuperior portion of the capsule to be clearly visualized (Fig. 2, *left*). An arthroscopic electrocautery device with a hooked tip (Linvatec, Concept Arthroscopy) is inserted through the anterior cannula, and the capsular scar is divided, beginning just anterior and inferior to the long head of the biceps and continuing inferiorly until the superior border of the subscapularis can be seen (Fig. 2, *center*). As this thick capsular tissue is divided, visualization of the joint improves, as the humeral head moves inferior and lateral to the glenoid with the release of this portion of the capsule (Fig. 2, *right*). This allows the arthroscope to be introduced farther anteriorly and inferiorly into the joint. If the anterior aspect of the capsule inferior to the superior border of the subscapularis is also thickened and contracted, it can be divided down to the inferior aspect of the glenoid. We never attempt to divide the capsule into the axillary pouch, as we believe that this creates a major risk of injury to the axillary nerve, which is in close proximity to that region of the capsule. After the anterior capsular release, the arthroscope is withdrawn and gentle closed manipulation is performed, first to restore external rotation and then to restore flexion and internal rotation.

Patients who continue to have marked limitation of internal rotation and cross-chest adduction have a posterior capsular contracture as well. In these individuals, a posterior capsular release is also necessary.

Posterior Capsular Release The

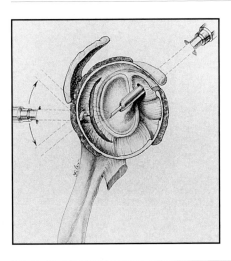

Fig. 3 The technique for posterior capsular release. The arthroscope is placed through an anterior portal, and the contracted posterior aspect of the capsule is divided along the glenoid rim through a posterior portal with use of an electrocautery device. (Adapted with permission from Warner JJP, Allen AA, Marks PH, et al: Arthroscopic release of postoperative capsular contracture of the shoulder. *J Bone Joint Surg* 1997;79A:1154.)

arthroscope is placed through the anterior cannula so that the posterior part of the joint can be visualized. A posterior cannula is used for the arthroscopic release. An electrocautery device is placed through the posterior cannula, and the thickened posterior aspect of the capsule is divided adjacent to the glenoid labrum, beginning just posterior to the biceps tendon and continuing down to the posteroinferior aspect of the glenoid rim but not into the axillary pouch (Fig. 3). The posterior aspect of the capsule is divided along the glenoid rim, as at this level the muscles of the rotator cuff are superficial to the capsule and the extent of the capsular release can be determined when muscle fibers of the infraspinatus are visualized. The arthroscope is then removed, and the arm is manipulated to regain internal rotation, cross-chest adduction, and forward elevation.

Subacromial Arthroscopy If motion has not been restored after what is believed to have been an adequate release of capsular tissue, several possible reasons should be considered, including subacromial or subdeltoid scarring and over-advancement of rotator-cuff tissue during the previous repair. The scarring can be treated with an arthroscopic technique.

Scarring in the subacromial space is common after a repair of the rotator cuff, especially if appropriate postoperative

mobilization was not instituted (Fig. 4). Subacromial bursoscopy and debridement is effective for freeing up extra-articular adhesions in the subacromial space. A lateral portal such as that used for routine subacromial decompression is made, and a motorized shaver is used to remove the tissue between the acromion and the rotator cuff. Debridement is carried out to the anterior aspect of the acromion but not into the fibers of the deltoid muscle. Additional anteroinferior acromial bone is removed arthroscopically if an incomplete or inadequate acromioplasty had been done previously. If loss of motion persists even after complete capsular release and subacromial debridement, then an open release usually is needed to address other extracapsular scarring and to permit tendon mobilization or z-plasty lengthening for the treatment of any residual loss of external rotation.

Stiffness With a Tear of the Repaired Rotator Cuff

This is a particularly challenging situation to manage. If the repair of the rotator cuff has failed within the first few months after the initial operation, then gentle closed manipulation may restore motion, after which an open repair can be performed. These patients are prone to subsequent loss of motion, so early pas-

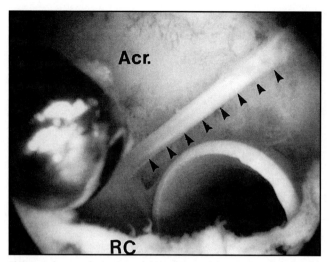 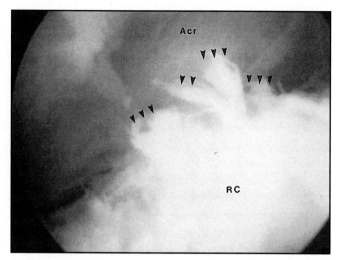

Fig. 4 Arthroscopic images of the subacromial space in a left shoulder. **Left,** Subacromial adhesions (arrowheads) are seen extending from the rotator cuff (RC) to the acromion (Acr.). **Right,** After division of subacromial adhesions (arrowheads), the rotator cuff (RC) can glide freely underneath the acromion (Acr).

sive motion is instituted and an interscalene catheter or repeated interscalene blocks are used for postoperative analgesia as described previously.

If closed manipulation does not improve motion, either an open or an arthroscopic release can be performed. If there is marked loss of passive motion and extensive scarring, it may be best to release the adhesions without revising the repaired rotator cuff at the same time, as the combination of both operations may increase the likelihood of subsequent shoulder stiffness. Instead, intensive postoperative physical therapy can be used to maintain the gains in motion, and several months later, when the shoulder is supple, a repeat repair of the tendon can be performed.

Open Release Patients who have contractures or adhesions that are resistant to an arthroscopic release, or those who have contraindications to an arthroscopic release, may need an open release to restore motion. The advantages of this procedure are that extra-articular adhesions outside of the subacromial space can be released and lengthening of the subscapularis tendon can be performed if needed. Conversion to an open procedure after an attempted arthroscopic release is accomplished easily by lowering the head of the bed so that it is positioned at a 45° angle. This changes the beach-chair position to a semiseated position, which is more suitable for an anterior approach to the shoulder. We use interscalene anesthesia and analgesia as described previously.

The open release can be accomplished through either an anterosuperior deltoid-splitting approach or a standard deltopectoral approach. Dissection and freeing up of the subscapularis muscle and tendon, however, should be performed through the latter approach so that the axillary nerve and the brachial plexus can be thoroughly visualized and protected.[16] Adhesions between the deltoid and the humerus are released first. This area may be densely scarred, and a combination of blunt and sharp dissection is needed to free up this interval. Care must be taken to avoid injury to the axillary nerve as it enters the deltoid through the quadrilateral space. If the muscle substance of the deltoid is violated as the dissection proceeds posteriorly, the axillary nerve can be injured. It is therefore important to keep the dissection on the humerus as it pro-gresses posteriorly. The axillary nerve often can be identified 3 to 5 cm distal to the acromion, coursing from posteroinferior to anterosuperior and lying directly on the subdeltoid fascia. When the interval between the deltoid and the humerus has been developed, the dissection is carried superiorly into the subacromial space. Any scar or bursal tissue between the acromion and the superior aspect of the cuff should be excised, along with the coracoacromial ligament if it is present. Completion of this part of the dissection should leave the deltoid and the subacromial space free of the humeral head and rotator-cuff muscles.

In order to free up the subscapularis, the interval between it and the conjoined tendon and coracoid must be dissected. The dissection should start at the coracoid and should proceed inferiorly along the lateral border of the conjoined tendon. The coracohumeral ligament is divided sharply, and the interval between the subscapularis and the conjoined tendon is dissected. Care is taken as the dissection proceeds medially so that the musculocutaneous nerve is not injured as it enters the muscle substance of the coracobrachialis and the biceps. If necessary, we identify the musculocutaneous nerve during this step in the dissection.

The goal of this portion of the dissection is to free the subscapularis from adhesions in order to restore external rotation. In patients who have a marked loss of external rotation, the subscapularis must be completely released, beginning on its superficial surface, continuing around its superior and inferior borders, and finally releasing its inferior adhesion to the joint capsule and the scapula. During this procedure, the axillary nerve must be identified on the superficial surface of the muscle.[16] In order to do this, we detach the tendon of the subscapularis from its humeral insertion either by performing a z-plasty or by releasing the underlying capsule with the tendon. A humeral head retractor then can be used to displace the humeral head posteriorly, to facilitate the dissection of the subscapularis and the axillary nerve. A long, thin retractor placed over the subscapularis allows the brachial plexus and the axillary nerve to be visualized. The axillary nerve then is elevated with a right-angle clamp, and a vessel loop is placed around it. Adhesions fixing the subscapularis to the inferior aspect of the capsule then can be released down to the axillary nerve. Adhesions between the subscapularis and the underlying capsule then are divided, and the interval between the subscapularis and the glenoid labrum also is developed.

This complete release and freeing of the subscapularis usually restores enough mobility to the tendon so that it can be repaired to the lesser tuberosity, resulting in improved external rotation. However, if the tendon is still not mobile enough to allow external rotation of more than 30°, a z-plasty lengthening of the subscapularis and the capsule in the coronal plane can be performed.[40-43] The subscapularis and the scarred capsule initially are dissected with some of the scarred tendon and capsule left attached to the lesser tuberosity. The subscapularis tendon

then is repaired to this limb of tissue with the shoulder in external rotation, thus completing the z-plasty repair.

Some patients who have severe loss of motion may have marked thickening and contracture of the inferior aspect of the capsule as well as contracture of the posterior aspect of the capsule. In these patients, the capsule can be released circumferentially with use of a humeral head retractor to displace the humeral head posteriorly and with the axillary nerve dissected away from the inferior aspect of the capsule. Next, a blunt retractor is placed along the inferior aspect of the capsule, which may then be sharply divided. As the inferior aspect of the capsule is divided, the humeral head can be moved farther away from the glenoid with the humeral head retractor, allowing access to the scarred posterior aspect of the capsule. This portion of the capsule can be divided by placing a small knife-blade on a long handle through the joint. The posterior aspect of the capsule should be divided along the glenoid labrum in order to avoid injury to the posterior rotator-cuff tendon, which attaches to the posterior aspect of the capsule in a more lateral location. After these releases, the subscapularis and the capsule are closed as described earlier.

Postoperative Treatment After an open or an arthroscopic release, the patient is admitted to the hospital for 48 hours of pain management. An indwelling interscalene catheter can be used to provide continuous analgesia, or repeated interscalene blocks can be performed on the mornings of the first and second postoperative days with use of bupivacaine as described earlier. Physical therapy is performed twice each day, in the morning and the afternoon. We have not found that use of a continuous passive motion machine is either cost effective or clinically useful in conjunction with this approach.

After an open release or a repeat repair of the rotator cuff, or both, passive

motion only is permitted within the safe limits defined by the soft-tissue repair. When an arthroscopic release has been performed, both active motion and passive motion are permitted. Narcotic analgesics are used during the first several days after the procedure, and physical therapy is initiated immediately on an outpatient basis. Physical therapy sessions are conducted five times a week for the first 2 weeks and three times a week for the next 2 weeks. In current managed-care insurance plans, it is important to advise the primary-care physician of this mandatory and essential aspect of postoperative treatment. Patients who have had an arthroscopic release also perform a home program using a pulley and self-assisted stretching, while those who have had an open release or a tendon repair, or both, continue with passive motion only for 6 weeks after the operation.

Stiffness With Untreated Osteoarthrosis

Consideration of the treatment of osteoarthrosis and stiffness is beyond the scope of this paper; however, recognition of articular incongruity and osteoarthrosis is important in order to avoid unnecessary and inadequate treatment of only the tear of the rotator cuff. In fact, although patients who have a tear of the rotator cuff and osteoarthrosis usually have stiffness before the surgical repair of the tendon, they are at additional risk for stiffness after the repair. Adequate treatment usually necessitates both resurfacing of the joint and repair of the rotator cuff with release of adhesions.

Stiffness With Deltoid or Nerve Injury

Occasionally, patients have a combination of complications after a repair of the rotator cuff. The combination of stiffness with an injury of the deltoid or a nerve injury, or both, is particularly difficult to treat. The ultimate prognosis is determined more by the latter two complica-

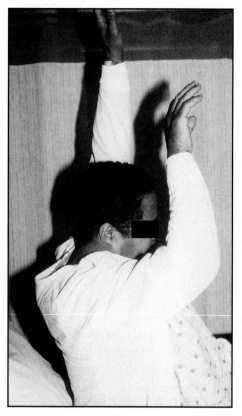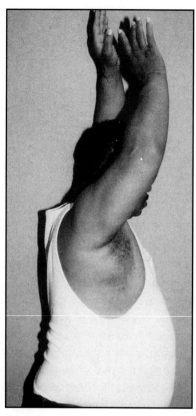

Fig. 5 Left, A 41-year-old man who had loss of motion 8 months after a repair of the rotator cuff. **Right,** Four months after an arthroscopic capsular release and subacromial debridement of adhesions, flexion is symmetrical with that of the contralateral normal shoulder.

tions than by the stiffness.

While disruption of the deltoid origin is infrequent after a repair of the rotator cuff, it is a devastating complication.[44] The senior one of us has found that, if it is recognized within the first 3 weeks after the repair of the rotator cuff, it can be repaired satisfactorily, provided that excessive acromial bone has not been removed. In this procedure, all adhesions are released and the deltoid is mobilized and repaired.

If a nerve injury has occurred, it should be determined whether it is a neurapraxic injury caused by a retractor or a direct axonotmesis caused by surgical trauma. Most of these injuries are of the former type and will resolve; therefore, shoulder stiffness and disruption of the tendon repair should be treated according to the methods described previously.

Our Experience

The senior one of us has treated five cases of shoulder stiffness after a total of 221 repairs of the rotator cuff. An additional five patients were referred to us for treatment of stiffness associated with an intact repair following a repair of the rotator cuff that had been done elsewhere. The indication for the treatment of shoulder stiffness was painful limitation of motion in all planes that affected the ability of the patient to perform activities of daily living. Although no specific loss of motion was used as an absolute indication, all patients had marked shoulder stiffness after more than 6 months of postoperative therapy.

Eight patients were managed with an arthroscopic capsular release and release of subacromial adhesions, with a satisfactory outcome (Fig. 5), whereas two need-

ed an open release because of extra-articular scarring of the subscapularis. All patients had improved motion and relief of pain.

We concluded that, although symptomatic stiffness after a repair of the rotator cuff is a relatively uncommon problem, it can be well treated with either an arthroscopic or an open technique. After the operation, intensive supervised physical therapy is essential. Occasionally, a repeat repair of the rotator cuff should be delayed until passive motion has been restored.

References

1. Constant CR, Murley AH: A clinical method of functional assessment of the shoulder. *Clin Orthop* 1987;214:160–164.

2. Baker CL, Liu SH: Comparison of open and arthroscopically assisted rotator cuff repairs. *Am J Sports Med* 1995;23:99–104.

3. Bigliani LU, Cordasco FA, McIlveen SJ, et al: Operative repairs of massive rotator cuff tears: Long-term results. *J Shoulder Elbow Surg* 1992;1:120–130.

4. Bigliani LU, McIlveen SJ, Cordasco FA, et al: Operative management of failed rotator cuff repairs. *Orthop Trans* 1988;12:674.

5. Blevins FT, Warren RF, Cavo C, et al: Arthroscopic assisted rotator cuff repair: Results using a mini-open deltoid splitting approach. *Arthroscopy* 1996;12:50–59.

6. DeOrio JK, Cofield RH: Results of a second attempt at surgical repair of a failed initial rotator-cuff tear. *J Bone Joint Surg* 1984;66A:563–567.

7. Ellman H, Hanker G, Bayer M: Repair of the rotator cuff. End-result study of factors influencing reconstruction. *J Bone Joint Surg* 1986;68A:1136–1144.

8. Grana WA, Teague B, King M, et al: An analysis of rotator cuff repair. *Am J Sports Med* 1994;22:585–588.

9. Harryman DT II, Mack LA, Wang KY, et al: Repairs of the rotator cuff: Correlation of functional results with integrity of the cuff. *J Bone Joint Surg* 1991;73A:982–989.

10. Hawkins RJ, Misamore GW, Hobeika PE: Surgery for full-thickness rotator-cuff tears. *J Bone Joint Surg* 1985;67A:1349–1355.

11. Levy HJ, Uribe JW, Delaney LG: Arthroscopic assisted rotator cuff repair: Preliminary results. *Arthroscopy* 1990;6:55–60.

12. Liu SH: Arthroscopically-assisted rotator-cuff repair. *J Bone Joint Surg* 1994;76B:592–595.

13. Paulos LE, Kody MH: Arthroscopically enhanced "miniapproach" to rotator cuff repair. *Am J Sports Med* 1994;22:19–25.

14. Warner JJP, Allen AA, Gerber C: Diagnosis and management of subscapularis tendon tears. *Tech Orthop* 1994;9:116–125.

15. Janda DH, Hawkins RJ: Shoulder manipulation in patients with adhesive capsulitis and diabetes mellitus: A clinical note. *J Shoulder Elbow Surg* 1993;2:36–38.

16. Allen AA, Warner JJP: Management of the stiff shoulder. *Op Tech Orthop* 1995;5:238–247.

17. Clarke GR, Willis LA, Fish WW, et al: Preliminary studies in measuring range of motion in normal and painful stiff shoulders. *Rheumatol Rehab* 1975;14:39–46.

18. Ben-Yishay A, Zuckerman JD, Gallagher M, et al: Pain inhibition of shoulder strength in patients with impingement syndrome. *Orthopedics* 1994;17:685–688.

19. Boone DC, Azen SP: Normal range of motion of joints in male subjects. *J Bone Joint Surg* 1979;61A:756–759.

20. Hertel R, Ballmer FT, Lambet SM, et al: Lag signs in the diagnosis of rotator cuff rupture. *J Shoulder Elbow Surg* 1996;5:307–313.

21. Harryman DT II: Shoulders: Frozen and stiff, in Heckman JD (ed): *Instructional Course Lectures 42.* Rosemont, IL, American Academy of Orthopaedic Surgeons, 1993, pp 247–257.

22. Harryman DT II, Sidles JA, Harris SL, et al: The role of the rotator interval capsule in passive motion and stability of the shoulder. *J Bone Joint Surg* 1992;74A:53–66.

23. Harryman DT II, Sidles JA, Clark JM, et al: Translation of the humeral head on the glenoid with passive glenohumeral motion. *J Bone Joint Surg* 1990;72A:1334–1343.

24. Neer CS II, Satterlee CC, Dalsey RM, et al: The anatomy and potential effects of contrac-ture of the coracohumeral ligament. *Clin Orthop* 1992;280:182–185.

25. Ozaki J, Nakagawa Y, Sakurai G, et al: Recalcitrant chronic adhesive capsulitis of the shoulder: Role of contracture of the coraco-humeral ligament and rotator interval in patho-genesis and treatment. *J Bone Joint Surg* 1989;71A:1511–1515.

26. Pollock RG, Duralde XA, Flatow EL, et al: The use of arthroscopy in the treatment of resistant frozen shoulder. *Clin Orthop* 1994;304:30–36.

27. Cofield RH: Subscapular muscle transposition for repair of chronic rotator cuff tears. *Surg Gynecol Obstet* 1982;154:667–672.

28. Neviaser RJ, Neviaser TJ: Transfer of the sub-scapularis and teres minor for massive defects of the rotator cuff, in Bayley I, Kessel L (eds): *Shoulder Surgery.* Berlin, Germany, Springer-Verlag, 1982, pp 60–63.

29. Neviaser RJ, Neviaser TJ: The frozen shoul-der: Diagnosis and management. *Clin Orthop* 1987;223:59–64.

30. Zuckerman JD, Cuomo F: Frozen shoulder, in Matsen FA III, Fu FH, Hawkins RJ (eds): *The Shoulder: A Balance of Mobility and Stability.* Rosemont, IL, American Academy of Orthopaedic Surgeons, 1993, pp 253–267.

31. Bigliani LU, Morrison DS, April EW: The morphology of the acromion and its relation-ship to rotator cuff tears. *Orthop Trans* 1986; 10:228.

32. Bigliani LU, Ticker JB, Flatow EL, et al: The relationship of acromial architecture to rotator cuff disease. *Clin Sports Med* 1991;10:823–838.

33. Itoi E, Tabata S: Range of motion and arthrog-raphy in the frozen shoulder. *J Shoulder Elbow Surg* 1992;1:106–112.

34. Goutallier D, Postel JM, Bernageau J, et al: Fatty muscle degeneration in cuff ruptures: Pre- and postoperative evaluation by CT scan. *Clin Orthop* 1994;304:78–83.

35. Iannotti JP, Zlatkin MB, Esterhai JL, et al: Magnetic resonance imaging of the shoulder: Sensitivity, specificity, and predictive value. *J Bone Joint Surg* 1991;73A:17–29.

36. Wiley AM: Arthroscopic appearance of frozen shoulder. *Arthroscopy* 1991;7:138–143.

37. Brown AR, Weiss R, Greenberg C, et al: Interscalene block for shoulder arthroscopy: Comparison with general anesthesia. *Arthroscopy* 1993;9:295–300.

38. Kinnard P, Truchon R, St-Pierre A, et al: Interscalene block for pain relief after shoulder surgery: A prospective randomized study. *Clin Orthop* 1994;304:22–24.

39. Warner JJP: Shoulder arthroscopy in the beach-chair position: Basic set-up. *Op Tech Orthop* 1991;1:147–154.

40. Hawkins RJ, Angelo RL: Glenohumeral osteoarthrosis: A late complication of the Putti-Platt repair. *J Bone Joint Surg* 1990;72A: 1193–1197.

41. Kieras DM, Matsen FA III: Open release in the management of refractory frozen shoulder. *Orthop Trans* 1991;15:801–802.

42. Lusardi DA, Wirth MA, Wurtz D, et al: Loss of external rotation following anterior capsulor-rhaphy of the shoulder. *J Bone Joint Surg* 1993;75A:1185–1192.

43. MacDonald PB, Hawkins RJ, Fowler PJ, et al: Release of the subscapularis for internal rota-tion contracture and pain after anterior repair or recurrent anterior dislocation of the shoul-der. *J Bone Joint Surg* 1992;74A:734–737.

44. Groh GI, Simoni M, Rolla P, et al: Loss of the deltoid after shoulder operations: An operative disaster. *J Shoulder Elbow Surg* 1994;3:243–253.

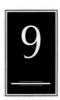

The Treatment of Failed Rotator Cuff Repairs

Frank A. Cordasco, MD
Louis U. Bigliani, MD

Introduction

Surgical treatment of a rotator cuff tear was first reported by Codman in 1911,[1] three quarters of a century after the first description of a tear by the English anatomist J.G. Smith in 1835.[2] The pathogenesis and treatment of rotator cuff tears was subsequently reviewed by McLaughlin.[3-5] Numerous techniques for reconstruction of rotator cuff tears have been described in the ensuing period.[6-35] However, several of the earlier series reported a notable percentage of unfavorable results.[10,13,14,17,22,34,36] The results of open rotator cuff repair improved significantly following Neer's report in 1972 on anterior acromioplasty in combination with cuff mobilization and repair.[24] Subsequent series have reported good to excellent results in both pain relief (85% to 100%) and function (70% to 95%) with the use of this approach.[8,16,18,21,29,30,37-46]

Notwithstanding these favorable results, complications do occur and can lead to failure of rotator cuff repairs. The causes of a failed rotator cuff repair are complex and have multifactorial etiologies. Several factors have been associated with failed repairs, including a large or massive tear, a rotator cuff tendon of poor quality, an inadequate repair, failure of graft materials, suture anchor or hardware failure, deltoid origin compromise with or without lateral or radical acromionectomy, an insufficient sub-acromial decompression, failure to treat associated acromioclavicular joint pathology, denervation of the deltoid or rotator cuff, infection, and deficient or overly aggressive physical therapy.[16,18,32,35,41,44,47-55] These factors can be evaluated in the context of the stages of rotator cuff repair, which include the approach, the decompression, the mobilization and repair, and the postoperative rehabilitation program.[56] Revision rotator cuff surgery is a technically demanding procedure, and the results are not as good as those of primary repairs.[47,49,53,54] The primary indication for reoperation in patients with failed rotator cuff repairs should be persistent pain, because improvement in function has been less predictable than pain relief.[47,49,54] Patients who have an intact deltoid, an intact lateral portion of the acromion, and good quality tissue of the rotator cuff are better candidates for the procedure.[47,54]

Clinical Presentation

Pain is the primary complaint of patients who have undergone unsuccessful rotator cuff repairs. DeOrio and Cofield[49] reported a series of 27 patients with failed initial repairs of the rotator cuff. Twenty-one patients in the group had severe pain. All 50 patients in the series reported by Neviaser and Neviaser[54] complained of nocturnal discomfort. We reviewed a group of 31 patients with failed repairs of the rotator cuff, 21 of whom described severe pain that required daily use of narcotics.[47] It is essential to obtain a comprehensive history, beginning with the patient's condition before the initial repair, and including the operative notes as well as details regarding the postoperative rehabilitation program. Determine if the patient had a period of pain-free activity following the initial repair. Twenty-six of the 31 patients in our series were never relieved of pain after the initial repair.[47] Failure of a repair of the rotator cuff should be suspected within the first 6 months postoperatively if pain and function have not improved markedly. Characterizing the pain is important, because this is the primary indication for revision surgery. If a patient can function with minimal pain, conservative management may be the preferred option.

The physical examination may demonstrate significant spinati atrophy or a long head biceps tendon disruption. Previous incisions should be carefully evaluated for such sources of pain as suture granulomas or neuromas. Warmth or erythema may represent a low-grade infection. The acromioclavicular joint should be palpated to determine if there is any underlying pathology, which may be contributing to the patients symptoms. Horizontal adduction and internal rotation maneuvers used to elicit acromioclavicular joint symptoms may be compromised by glenohumeral joint stiffness.

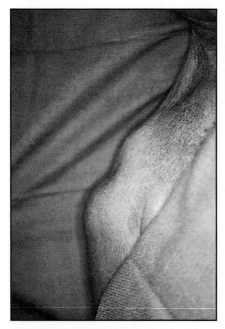

Fig. 1 This 57-year-old female developed a deltoid origin avulsion following a rotator cuff repair that included a lateral acromionectomy.

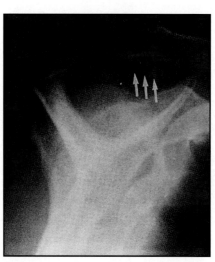

Fig. 2 Supraspinatus outlet view of a 52-year-old male, demonstrating a residual acromial spur after an insufficient subacromial decompression. (Reproduced with permission from Iannotti JP (ed): *Rotator Cuff Disorders*. Park Ridge, IL, American Academy of Orthopaedic Surgeons, 1991, pp 63–74.)

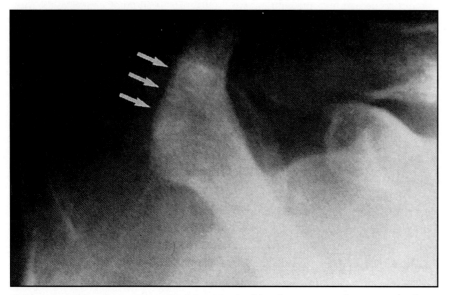

Fig. 3 A modified axillary radiograph of the right shoulder, demonstrating the acromion of a 60-year-old male who had persistent pain and weakness after a lateral acromionectomy. The deltoid was retracted distally. A true lateral radiograph could not be made because of the pain and stiffness of the shoulder. The arrows are directed towards the substantial amount of bone that was removed from the lateral portion of the acromion. (Reproduced with permission from Bigliani LU, Cordasco FA, McIlveen SJ, et al: Operative treatment of failed repairs of the rotator cuff. *J Bone Joint Surg* 1992;74A:1505–1515.)

Compromise of the origin of the deltoid muscle can result in a failure after rotator cuff surgery, either from inadequate repair of the deltoid split or because an associated lateral or radical acromionectomy was performed.[16,44,47–49,52–54] The deltoid origin should be meticulously inspected during the physical exam (Fig. 1). It is also important to assess the function of the deltoid in all three portions, particularly the anterior component, to be certain an axillary nerve injury has not occurred.

Passive and active range of motion may both be restricted to an equal extent in patients with a stiff, frozen shoulder that has developed because of inadequate rehabilitation. The impingement sign may be positive in the patient with persistent subacromial pathology. There may be a notable discrepancy between passive and active range of motion in those patients who have a residual tear or who have retorn their rotator cuff. Weakness is often present in forward elevation and external rotation. The patient with a large, persistent or recurrent rotator cuff tear cannot maintain the humerus in an externally rotated position, and this suggests a significant infraspinatus component. Hertel and associates[57] described three useful clinical signs, the external rotation lag sign, the drop sign, and the internal rotation lag sign, to assess specific components of the rotator cuff.

The cervical spine should be assessed to rule out any radicular symptoms, which may contribute to shoulder pain or stiffness. The patient who presents with little or no pain and significant weakness should be evaluated carefully for neurologic lesions, including cervical radiculopathy, Parsonage-Turner syndrome (brachial neuritis), and suprascapular nerve lesions.

Routine radiographic evaluation should include axillary, supraspinatus outlet,[58] and anteroposterior (AP) views of the scapula with the humerus in neutral, internal, and external rotation. The

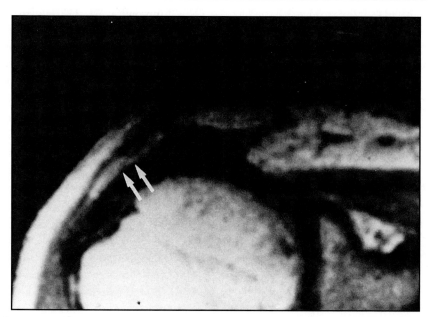

Fig. 4 MRI, revealing retraction of the deltoid from the edge of the acromion in this 48-year-old male following a rotator cuff repair, is noted by the white arrows. (Reproduced with permission from Iannotti JP (ed): *Rotator Cuff Disorders*. Park Ridge, IL, American Academy of Orthopaedic Surgeons, 1991, pp 63–74.)

acromial morphology can be determined and any source of residual impingement (Fig. 2) or lateral acromial compromise (Fig. 3) can be identified. The acromiohumeral interval can be used to assess the degree of cuff pathology,[59] however, this can be imprecise due to the inherent variability in obtaining an AP view. Radiographs should be evaluated carefully for signs of early cuff tear arthropathy.[60] In cases of long-standing impingement, large or massive rotator cuff tears may result in superior humeral migration and erosion into the acromioclavicular joint, and in this situation an arthrogram will demonstrate a so-called "geyser sign."[61]

The presence of a full thickness rotator cuff tear can be confirmed by arthrogram, ultrasonography, or magnetic resonance imaging (MRI). In most cases, MRI is preferable, because it can provide additional information regarding the rotator cuff tear size, the integrity of the deltoid origin and long head biceps tendon, the vascularity of the humeral head, the integrity of the articular cartilage, and the quality of the remaining tissue (Fig. 4). Gaenslen and associates[62] found MRI to be useful in identifying full-thickness tears of the rotator cuff, intact cuffs, ruptures of the biceps tendon, and detachments of the deltoid origin in a series of 25 shoulders following a previous rotator cuff repair.

Electrodiagnostic studies may be helpful in patients who have significant weakness or muscle atrophy after a rotator cuff repair and in cases in which cervical spine pathology is present as well. Injury to the axillary and/or suprascapular nerves as a result of previous trauma or surgery should be investigated with appropriate studies, if suspected.[44,47,55,63]

Approach

Although the skin incision does not play a major role in the functional result of a repair of the rotator cuff, a painful scar can be a persistent problem. Additionally, the appearance of the incision is a factor with many patients. The skin overlying the shoulder is fairly extensile, and ade-quate exposure can be achieved without creating excessively large, curved incisions or damaging the deltoid or acromion. We prefer a 5- to 7-cm skin incision on the anterosuperior aspect of the shoulder in the skin flexion creases (perpendicular to the fibers of the deltoid), this provides cosmesis and decreases the potential for spreading of the scar. The incision extends from the lateral aspect of the anterior third of the acromion towards the lateral tip of the coracoid.

Deltoid retraction has been a devastating problem following rotator cuff repair.[47,49,53,54] Excellent exposure can be obtained with minimal, if any, removal of the deltoid origin from the acromion.[8,56] The deltoid split is performed with the electrocautery, beginning approximately 5 mm anterior to the acromioclavicular joint and extending directly laterally past the anterolateral corner of the acromion. This method leaves a strong healthy cuff of tissue attached to the anterior aspect of the acromioclavicular joint and acromion, preserving the deltoid origin. The deltoid split is then generally extended for a distance of 3 to 5 cm lateral and slightly posterior to the anterolateral corner of the acromion, in line with the fibers of the middle deltoid. A stay suture is then placed at the distal end of the split to avoid injury to the axillary nerve. The axillary nerve generally is located 5 to 6 cm distal to the anterolateral aspect of the acromion. In smaller individuals however, Burkhead and associates[63] have shown that the nerve can approach 3 cm distal to the anterolateral corner of the acromion, particularly when the arm is in an abducted position.

Repair of the deltoid split following acromioplasty is crucial. If there is an inadequate cuff of soft tissue remaining on the acromion, the deltoid should be reattached to the acromion and distal clavicle with drill holes through bone. When a distal clavicle resection has been performed, the deltoid must be repaired

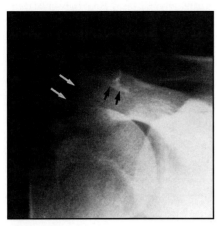

Fig. 5 This 44-year-old female had persistent impingement symptoms after a lateral acromionectomy (white arrows) was performed. Anteroposterior view of a persistent anterior acromial spur (black arrows). (Reproduced with permission from Iannotti JP (ed): *Rotator Cuff Disorders*. Park Ridge, IL, American Academy of Orthopaedic Surgeons, 1991, pp 63–74.)

to the leading edge of trapezius fascia. Deltoid origin avulsion can occur because of an inadequate repair of the split. When deltoid retraction occurs, it should be repaired as soon as possible, because the most successful deltoidplasties have been those which were repaired acutely.[44,53]

Lateral and radical acromionectomies should not be performed. Neer and Marberry[53] emphasized that, while some investigators have reported satisfactory results following lateral and radical acromionectomy,[64,65] the procedure is anatomy deforming and has many disadvantages. Radical acromionectomy weakens the deltoid by removing the fulcrum afforded by the acromion and can result in a permanent contracture of the middle deltoid. A high incidence of wound complications, including sinus tract formation, has been noted as well.[53] Additionally, revision rotator cuff repair in the presence of previously performed lateral or radical acromionectomies and transacromial approaches is technically demanding and is less likely to provide a satisfactory result.[47,49,53]

Decompression

Neer postulated that variations in acromial slope and morphology were clinically relevant[24,58] and emphasized that radical and lateral acromionectomy compromised the deltoid origin, resulting in weakness.[53] Bigliani and associates[66] demonstrated a relationship between acromial morphology and the incidence of rotator cuff tears. Using stereophotogrammetry, Flatow and associates[67] determined that shoulders with type III acromions consistently had increased contact, compared with shoulders of other acromial types, and that this contact was greatest on the distal supraspinatus tendon with the arm in elevation.

The performance of a subacromial decompression has been shown to provide significant pain relief. Two studies have demonstrated that patients who underwent anterior acromioplasty, but whose small rotator cuff tears were unrepaired, had satisfactory pain relief.[6,68] Fifty percent of the patients in the study by DeOrio and Cofield[49] did not undergo anterior acromioplasty during their first, unsuccessful repair. Twenty-eight of the 31 patients (90%) in our series of failed repairs had a persistent subacromial impingement lesion (Fig. 5) because of inadequate care of the acromion.[47] Rockwood and associates[31] also noted the importance of subacromial decompression alone as a means of pain relief.

Subacromial impingement can occur at the anterolateral aspect of the coracoacromial ligament, the anteroinferior acromion, and/or the acromioclavicular joint. An adequate subacromial decompression has generally included a coracoacromial ligament release, anterior acromioplasty, and a modified or complete acromioclavicular arthroplasty as indicated. We begin by identifying the anterolateral edge of the coracoacromial ligament. The entire coracoacromial liga-

ment is then subperiosteally elevated and tag sutures should be placed in preparation for later repair. The remaining cuff of strong deltoid origin tissue is meticulously elevated 3 to 5 mm to expose the anterior aspect of the acromion. The inferior aspect of the acromion often has adherent bursal or rotator cuff tissue which should be cleared with an elevator. It is important to check the thickness of the acromion before proceeding to the acromioplasty. A thin, sharp beveled osteotome is used to perform the procedure. The bevel is directed upward to avoid removing excessive bone or fracturing the acromion. The wedge of bone excised should consist of the full width of the acromion from the medial to lateral border. The anteroinferior aspect of the acromion should have a smooth contour for subacromial contact.

However, aggressive decompression in the presence of an unrepaired or nonfunctional rotator cuff can lead to anterosuperior humeral head subluxation or even dislocation.[69] Flatow and associates[70] reported a modified acromioplasty technique in a series of patients with massive rotator cuff tears. The coracoacromial ligament is preserved by reattaching it after a conservative acromioplasty has been performed. This may help to preserve the passive and static, buffering function of the coracoacromial arch and prevent anterosuperior humeral head subluxation in patients who have lost the dynamic, head-depressing function of the rotator cuff.[70] Flatow and associates[71] reported favorable preliminary results of coracoacromial arch reconstruction in a series of patients with anterosuperior subluxation after failed repairs of the rotator cuff.

It is important to evaluate the acromioclavicular (AC) joint as a potential source of symptoms in patients with rotator cuff tears, because this joint can contribute to the impingement process.[8,45,47,49,56] Five of the 31 patients in our series had persistent pain and AC joint tenderness, which contributed to the failure of their repair. Each of these patients had AC joint symptoms prior to the index repair.[47] Generally, the inferior portion of the acromial side of the acromioclavicular joint is removed as part of the acromioplasty, leaving the inferior aspect of the distal clavicle prominent. The coracoacromial arch should be restored by performing a modified AC arthroplasty using a double-action rongeur, rasp, or burr. This also extends the subacromial space medially. A complete AC arthroplasty or distal clavicle resection is reserved for those patients with preoperative AC joint tenderness and clinical findings such as pain with horizontal adduction or internal rotation.[8,56] Currently, this is performed from the inferior aspect of the joint, preserving the superior AC ligaments to maintain AC joint stability in the anteroposterior plane.

An unfused acromial epiphysis can occasionally cause pain and impingement, which may result in full thickness rotator cuff tears.[47,48,72,73] If a small pre-acromial fragment is encountered at the time of revision surgery, it can be excised. If a stable fibrous union is present without motion, a routine anterior acromioplasty is acceptable. Excision of the larger meso- and meta-acromial fragments can lead to weakness and retraction of the deltoid, although Mudge and associates[73] reported satisfactory results with excision. These larger fragments pose a challenge, and we no longer advocate the use of hardware because of the potential for hardware failure and concomitant damage to the rotator cuff.[47,72] We have found that removal of the inferior surface of the fragment while retaining the superior cortex with the associated deltoid origin has been successful.[47]

Rotator Cuff Repair

The factor most commonly associated with failure of a primary rotator cuff repair is the presence of a large or massive rotator cuff tear.[21,29,35,44,47,49,53,54,56] Repair of a large or massive tear is more difficult, because the tear has usually been present for a long time and the quality of the cuff tissue may be poor. Significant bursal scarring and tendon retraction may be exhibited, and several techniques have been described to aid in mobilization and reconstruction of these defects.[3,4,7,8,11,12,15,17,20,24–28,44,52,56,74–78] These techniques include the mobilization of existing tendons,[5,8,16–18,21,24,44,56] transfer of tendons,[3,8,12,15,25,26,44,50,52,56,75] and implantation of fascia,[7,77] allografts,[27] and synthetic material.[28] Results have generally been more satisfactory when the repair has been performed with mobilization and transposition of existing cuff tissue rather than implantation of fascia, allografts, or synthetic material.[8,16,40,44,47,56]

At the revision surgery, the size of the rotator cuff tear and the quality of the remaining tissue should be thoroughly assessed. The long head of biceps tendon is evaluated. Tenodesis is rarely necessary, and is reserved for those patients with a long head biceps tendon disruption and associated pain and spasm at the musculotendinous junction. The classification system suggested by Post and associates[30] is most often used and determines size before mobilization of the tendons. In this scheme, large tears are those with diameters 3 to 5 cm in size and massive tears are greater than 5 cm in diameter. Gerber and associates[19] proposed a system of classification based upon the ability of the tear to be approximated to bone after mobilization has been performed. Classifying the size of the tear by the number of tendons involved is undependable because the tendons become confluent near the insertion upon the greater tuberosity.[79] Multiple sutures are placed into the leading edge of the tendon in preparation for mobilization. The suture material used is 0 or #1 nonabsorbable multifilament and is passed in an interrupted simple fashion. An elevator is used to sweep the superficial bursa

overlying the cuff tissue, particularly in the area of the subscapularis and near the base of the coracoid. Only the superficial bursa is removed and minimal rotator cuff tissue is debrided from the leading edge of the tendon. It has been shown that the deep bursa may provide blood flow to the edge of the torn cuff tendon and that the cuff tendon tissue has a vascular supply as well.[80,81]

The stay sutures are used to sequentially mobilize the rotator cuff from anterior to posterior. Various portions of the rotator cuff can be visualized by changing the position of the humerus. Extension and internal rotation allows visualization of the infraspinatus and teres minor, while flexion and external rotation facilitates evaluation of the subscapularis. The bursal surface of the rotator cuff is carefully assessed, in revision cases there may be adhesions between the deltoid and cuff posterolaterally in the "lateral gutter." Commonly these adhesions are attached to the undersurface of the acromion and should be elevated from beneath the acromion before performing the acromioplasty to avoid inadvertent extension of the tear in the cuff. Release of these bursal adhesions is necessary in order to adequately mobilize the posterior cuff. This should be performed bluntly with an elevator or using a scissors to spread. Sharp dissection in this area may cause injury to the posterior cuff and should be performed carefully.[8,44] In addition, the location of the axillary nerve in patients who have had prior surgery is often difficult to determine. The "tug-test" can be used gently to clarify the location of the nerve in revision cases.[82] For patients with large or massive tears at revision surgery, additional posterior exposure can be gained by depressing the humeral head with a blunt retractor. The Gerber retractor may also be useful to depress the humeral head and gain posterior exposure. This device is a modified laminar spreader which has a ring to depress the humeral head. At this time a

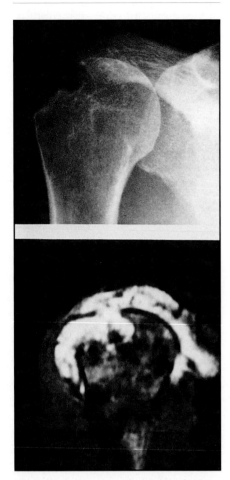

Fig. 6 Anteroposterior radiograph and MRI demonstrating humeral head destruction and the extent of articular cartilage involvement 2 years following rotator cuff repair with cadaveric graft. (Reproduced with permission from Iannotti JP (ed): *Rotator Cuff Disorders.* Park Ridge, IL, American Academy of Orthopaedic Surgeons, 1991, pp 63–74.)

complete assessment of the posterior tissues should be possible to determine the full extent of the tear. Generally, a small portion of the infraspinatus and teres minor remain attached at the insertion site, and care should be exercised to avoid injury to this area during the mobilization phase.

Patients with failed repairs often have rotator cuff tissue that is scarred down to the glenoid rim and base of the coracoid. This is particularly true when inadequate mobilization was performed for long-standing tears with chronic

retraction. The undersurface release is carried out bluntly with an elevator. Sharp dissection should be performed with care to avoid injury to the suprascapular nerve.[55,83] The posterior rotator cuff may also be cut if sharp dissection is used, as it is closely adherent to the posterior capsule.

After a systematic release of the extra-articular and intra-articular aspects of the rotator cuff has been performed, it is essential to check the excursion of the tendon edge by placing tension on the stay sutures. To assure a successful repair, the edges of the torn tendon should reach the anatomic neck of the humerus with the arm in a functional position of 10° to 15° of forward elevation and 10° of abduction. Often, in large and massive tears the tendon edge cannot be approximated to the anatomic neck. There are several maneuvers that can be employed in such cases.

The coracohumeral ligament is often retracted and scarred down to the base of the coracoid.[8,44,76] This limits the lateral and distal advancement of the supraspinatus. "The interval slide" describes a complete release of the rotator interval and coracohumeral ligament from the base of the coracoid.[8] This release has provided 1 to 1.5 cm of increased supraspinatus tendon excursion. Since this technique has been developed, we have less frequently performed other maneuvers such as a subscapularis transfer.[8] Transfer of the subscapularis tendon to repair large or massive rotator cuff defects was described by Cofield and has subsequently been used by other investigators.[8,15,26,44,46,75] However, it has been suggested that this transfer may result in superior migration of the humerus by destabilizing force couples.[11] When transfer of the subscapularis is employed, it is important to leave the underlying capsule and glenohumeral ligaments undisturbed to avoid problems with instability and to transfer the superior third of the tendon only.

In the vast majority of cases these maneuvers have been successful in achieving a satisfactory repair. When complete repair is not possible using these techniques, procedures using supraspinatus advancement,[17,20] transposition of the long head biceps tendon,[12] fascial autografts,[7] allografts,[27] and synthetic materials[28] are not currently advocated. Serious complications involving graft rejection and joint destruction have been noted (Fig. 6). When complete repair is not possible, we prefer partial repair with particular emphasis placed on establishing anterior-posterior stability[11,78] or transfer of the latissimus dorsi[19] depending on the patient in question.

Once the rotator cuff has been adequately mobilized, the repair begins with preparation of the greater tuberosity. The anatomic neck region is "scarified" with a curette. A deep trough is not necessary to facilitate healing and compromises bone (Fig. 7). Multiple drill holes are placed into the greater tuberosity depending on the size of the tear. The holes begin medially at the anatomic neck and extend laterally, through the tuberosity, for a distance of 1 to 1.5 cm. This provides a satisfactory bone bridge and 0 or #1 braided multifilament sutures are passed through the drill holes. Suture anchors may be used in the greater tuberosity as well.[50,84–86] However, bone of poor quality can preclude the use of anchors, as they tend to fail at the bone-anchor interface. Non suture-anchor metallic implants have associated complications which include impingement, loosening (Fig. 8), and failure.[48,87]

The repair is performed with the humerus in 10° to 15° of flexion and 10° of abduction. Extension of the humerus during repair is counterproductive and should be avoided.[8] Before securing the tendon-to-bone sutures, the anterior and posterior aspects of the repair should be performed first to reestablish the intratendinous relationships of the rotator cuff. Anteriorly, if an interval slide has

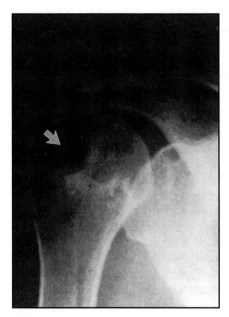

Fig. 7 Anteroposterior radiograph of the right scapula of a 63-year-old female who had a large defect in the greater tuberosity and the humeral head created as a trough for fixation of the rotator cuff tendon at the initial repair. The tear recurred at the site of repair. (Reproduced with permission from Bigliani LU, Cordasco FA, McIlveen SJ, et al: Operative treatment of failed repairs of the rotator cuff. J Bone Joint Surg 1992;74A:1505–1515.)

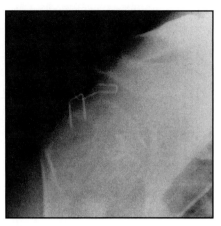

Fig. 8 Anteroposterior radiograph revealing displaced staples used during the repair of a rotator cuff tear in this 59-year-old male. The staples also created additional tears in the rotator cuff tendon. (Reproduced with permission from Iannotti JP (ed): *Rotator Cuff Disorders*. Park Ridge, IL, American Academy of Orthopaedic Surgeons, 1991, pp 63–74.)

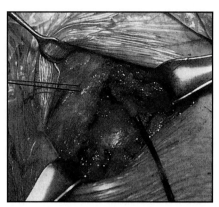

Fig. 9 The coracoacromial ligament is repaired to the acromion in a slightly medial location following the repair of large or massive rotator cuff tears. (Reproduced with permission from Cordasco FA, Bigliani LU: Large and massive tears: Technique of open repair. *Orthop Clin North Am* 1997;28:179–193.)

been performed, the rotator interval should be closed in a manner that realigns the mobilized supraspinatus edge further laterally than the corresponding subscapularis edge of the interval. Posteriorly, if there is a split between the infraspinatus and teres minor, it should be repaired. Depending upon the tear configuration, a tendon-to-tendon repair may also be appropriate for a portion of the cuff superiorly, prior to securing the tendon-to-bone sutures. The rotator cuff tendon-to-bone sutures are then repaired while the humerus is maintained in the position noted above. The sutures are tied superiorly over the bone bridge.

In large and massive rotator cuff tears, the coracoacromial ligament is repaired.[46,70,71] The preserved coracoacromial ligament is reattached to the acromion in a slightly more medial position to provide a buttress to superior migration of the humeral head (Fig. 9). The deltoid split is repaired to the cuff of strong deltoid origin using buried 0 braided multifilament suture material. If this tissue is of poor quality, the deltoid is repaired directly to bone with drill holes. The subcutaneous tissue is closed with a few absorbable sutures and the skin is closed with a subcuticular stitch. The arm is immobilized in a sling. Abduction pillows are used occasionally in cases where a deltoidplasty has been performed. When abduction devices are used it is important to avoid extension of the humerus, because to do so places tension across the repair.

Rehabilitation

Passive-assisted range-of-motion exercises should be started early in the postoperative period to avoid stiffness.[88] The physical therapy program should be modified depending on the pathology encountered at the time of revision surgery. The standard Neer Phase I rehabilitation program is modified in the care of patients with large or massive tears. During the first 6 weeks only three exercises are performed. These include pendulum exercises, passive-assisted forward elevation to 140°, and supine passive-assisted external rotation using a stick to 30°. Pulley exercise and extension of the humerus, which can stress the repair, is avoided in the first 4 to 6 weeks. Active-assisted and isometric exercise is started between 6 and 8 weeks beginning with supine external rotation and supine forward elevation. Erect forward elevation with a stick is then initiated. At first the stick is used alone, and, then, at 12 weeks 1 to 3 pound weights are added. The use of weights early in the rehabilitation program has been associated with failed repairs.[47,54] Strength and resistance exercises can be gradually progressed, and, at 6 to 9 months postoperatively, more dynamic strengthening may begin with light-weight medicine balls in appropriate patients.[89] Following primary repairs, it has been noted that many patients continue to gain improvements in strength and function during the first 12 to 18 months postoperatively.[90,91]

Results

DeOrio and Cofield[49] reported on 27 patients who underwent a second attempt at repair of a rotator cuff tear that had failed an initial repair. Pain was at least diminished in 76% of the group, particularly in patients who had symptoms of continuing subacromial impingement (86%). This result did not meet the patients' or authors' expectations, as 63% of the patients still had moderate to severe pain. There was minimal improvement in active motion and function, particularly in those patients with a coexisting deltoid problem and/or a massive tear at the second surgery. The authors concluded that a second attempt at repair of a torn rotator cuff most often resulted in incomplete relief of pain and little improvement in active abduction or active strength. Furthermore, a maximum effort was advocated to achieve success with the initial repair including an anterior acromioplasty and protection of the deltoid origin during the procedure.[49]

We reviewed a series of 31 patients who had a revision surgery following a failed initial rotator cuff repair. Overall, only 16 patients (52%) had a satisfactory result. Twenty-five (81%) of the 31 patients had good or excellent pain relief. Functional motion improved significantly in seventeen patients (55%). There were two dominant factors in the 15 patients with fair or poor results. Poor quality of existing rotator cuff tissue was noted in ten patients, and deltoid deformity secondary to deltoid detachment or lateral acromionectomy was present in nine. Nine of the 13 patients with a deltoid deformity had an unsatisfactory result. Three of six patients who had a detached deltoid origin but an intact acromion had a satisfactory result. Conversely, only one of seven patients with a lateral acromionectomy had a satisfactory result.[47]

Neviaser and Neviaser[26] reported a series of 50 patients with failed rotator cuff repairs. Forty-six patients (90%) noted improvement in pain from their preoperative status. Active elevation improved in 26 patients (52%) an average of 50°. Twenty-two patients retained the same motion as before the surgery, and two patients lost motion. The authors concluded that factors important in achieving success included an adequate subacromial decompression and the presence of an intact deltoid. A negative factor was the use of weights early in the postoperative period (3 months).

Summary

Results following surgical management of failed rotator cuff tears are clearly inferior to those obtained in the treatment of primary repairs.[47,49,53,54] Conservative management may be the treatment of choice in selected patients with failed rotator cuff repairs. The primary goal for revision rotator cuff surgery should be relief of pain, not improvement in function. If the level of pain is manageable, and the patient is functioning with respect to activities of daily living, additional surgery may not be helpful. As there are multiple etiologies associated with failure of the initial repair, each patient should be carefully evaluated on an individual basis to determine if a subsequent procedure would be appropriate. Repeat repair is more likely to succeed in patients with an intact and functioning deltoid, an intact lateral portion of the acromion, and good quality of rotator cuff tissue. Conversely, patients who have had a lateral or radical acromionectomy, a detached or nonfunctioning deltoid, or poor quality of remaining rotator cuff tissue are less likely to have a successful result after repeat repair.

It is evident that some of the factors associated with failure are avoidable. As the best chance for a successful result is at the time of the primary repair, the following points will briefly review these factors. The skin incision should be made in the flexion creases which are perpendicular to the deltoid fibers. The deltoid origin should be meticulously protected during the repair and lateral or radical acromionectomy should not be performed. Adequate anterior acromioplasty is essential for removal of the impingement lesion and to prevent subsequent wear on the repaired cuff tendon. The acromioclavicular joint should be evaluated preoperatively and treated as indicated at the time of the surgery. Adequate release of adhesions and mobilization of rotator cuff tissue should be performed using the coracohumeral ligament release and interval slide when necessary. The rotator cuff should be repaired to bone using tendon to bone sutures and/or secure suture anchors. In large and massive tears, there appears to be a role for the reattachment of the coracohumeral ligament. Early phase I range of motion should be initiated following rotator cuff repair and early resistance exercise with weights should be avoided.

References

1. Codman EA: Complete rupture of the supraspinatus tendon: Operative treatment with report of two successful cases. Boston Med Surg J 1911;164:708–710.
2. Smith JG: Pathological appearances of seven cases of injury of the shoulder-joints with remarks. Am J Med Sci 1835;16:219–224.
3. McLaughlin HL: Lesions of the musculotendinous cuff of the shoulder: I. The exposure and treatment of tears with retraction. J Bone Joint Surg 1944;26:31–51.
4. McLaughlin HL: Repair of major cuff ruptures. Surg Clin North Am 1963;43:1535–1540.
5. McLaughlin HL, Asherman EG: Lesions of the musculotendinous cuff of the shoulder: IV. Some observations based upon the results of surgical repair. J Bone Joint Surg 1951;33A:76–86.
6. Bakalim G, Pasila M: Surgical treatment of rupture of the rotator cuff tendon. Acta Orthop Scand 1975;46:751–757.
7. Bateman JE: The diagnosis and treatment of ruptures of the rotator cuff. Surg Clin North Am 1963;43:1523–1530.
8. Bigliani LU, Cordasco FA, McIlveen SJ, et al: Operative repairs of massive rotator cuff tears: Long-term results. J Shoulder Elbow Surg 1992;1:120–130.

9. Björkenheim JM, Paavolainen P, Ahovuo J, et al: Surgical repair of the rotator cuff and surrounding tissues: Factors influencing the results. *Clin Orthop* 1988;236:148–153.

10. Bosworth DM: An analysis of twenty-eight consecutive cases of incapacitating shoulder lesions, radically explored and repaired. *J Bone Joint Surg* 1940;22:369–392.

11. Burkhart SS, Nottage WM, Ogilvie-Harris DJ, et al: Partial repair of irreparable rotator cuff tears. *Arthroscopy* 1994;10:363–370.

12. Bush LF: The torn shoulder capsule. *J Bone Joint Surg* 1975;57A:256–259.

13. Codman EA: Rupture of the supraspinatus tendon and other lesions in and about the subacromial bursa, in Codman EA (ed): *The Shoulder: Rupture of the Supraspinatus Tendon and Other Lesions In or About the Subacromial Bursa.* Malabar, FL, RE Kreiger Publishing, 1984.

14. Codman EA: Rupture of the supraspinatus-1834 to 1934. *J Bone Joint Surg* 1937;19:643–652.

15. Cofield RH: Subscapular muscle transposition for repair of chronic rotator cuff tears. *Surg Gynecol Obstet* 1982;154:667–672.

16. Cofield RH: Rotator cuff disease of the shoulder. *J Bone Joint Surg* 1985;67A:974–979.

17. Debeyre J, Patte D, Elmelik E: Repair of ruptures of the rotator cuff of the shoulder: With a note on advancement of the supraspinatus muscle. *J Bone Joint Surg* 1965;47B:36–42.

18. Ellman H, Hanker G, Bayer M: Repair of the rotator cuff: End-result study of factors influencing reconstruction. *J Bone Joint Surg* 1986;68A:1136–1144.

19. Gerber C, Vinh TS, Hertel R, et al: Latissimus dorsi transfer for the treatment of massive tears of the rotator cuff: A preliminary report. *Clin Orthop* 1988;232:51–61.

20. Ha'eri GB, Wiley AM: Advancement of the supraspinatus muscle in the repair of ruptures of the rotator cuff. *J Bone Joint Surg* 1981;63A:232–238.

21. Hawkins RJ, Misamore GW, Hobeika PE: Surgery for full-thickness rotator-cuff tears. *J Bone Joint Surg* 1985;67A:1349–1355.

22. Heikel HV: Rupture of the rotator cuff of the shoulder: Experiences of surgical treatment. *Acta Orthop Scand* 1968;39:477–492.

23. Lindblom K, Palmer I: Ruptures of the tendon aponeurosis of the shoulder joint: The so-called supraspinatus ruptures. *Acta Chir Scand* 1939;82:133–142.

24. Neer CS II: Anterior acromioplasty for the chronic impingement syndrome in the shoulder: A preliminary report. *J Bone Joint Surg* 1972;54A:41–50.

25. Neviaser JS: Ruptures of the rotator cuff of the shoulder: New concepts in the diagnosis and operative treatment of chronic ruptures. *Arch Surg* 1971;102:483–485.

26. Neviaser RJ, Neviaser TJ: Transfer of subscapularis and teres minor for massive defects of the rotator cuff, in Bayley I, Kessel L (eds): *Shoulder Surgery.* Berlin, Germany, Springer-Verlag, 1982, pp 60–63.

27. Neviaser JS, Neviaser RJ, Neviaser TJ: The repair of chronic massive ruptures of the rotator cuff of the shoulder by use of a freeze-dried rotator cuff. *J Bone Joint Surg* 1978;60A:681–684.

28. Ozaki J, Fujimoto S, Masuhara K, et al: Reconstruction of chronic massive rotator cuff tears with synthetic materials. *Clin Orthop* 1986;202:173–183.

29. Packer NP, Calvert PT, Bayley JI, et al: Operative treatment of chronic ruptures of the rotator cuff of the shoulder. *J Bone Joint Surg* 1983;65B:171–175.

30. Post M, Silver R, Singh M: Rotator cuff tear: Diagnosis and treatment. *Clin Orthop* 1983;173:78–91.

31. Rockwood CA Jr, Williams GR, Burkhead WZ Jr: Debridement of degenerative, irreparable lesions of the rotator cuff. *J Bone Joint Surg* 1995;77A:857–866.

32. Samilson RL, Binder WF: Symptomatic full thickness tears of rotator cuff: An analysis of 292 shoulders in 276 patients. *Orthop Clin North Am* 1975;6:449–466.

33. Watson M: Major ruptures of the rotator cuff: The results of surgical repair in 89 patients. *J Bone Joint Surg* 1985;67B:618–624.

34. Wilson PD: Complete rupture of the supraspinatus tendon. *JAMA* 1931;96:433–438.

35. Wolfgang GL: Surgical repair of tears of the rotator cuff of the shoulder: Factors influencing the result. *J Bone Joint Surg* 1974;56A:14–26.

36. Godsil RD Jr, Linscheid RL: Intratendinous defects of the rotator cuff. *Clin Orthop* 1970;69:181–188.

37. Adamson GJ, Tibone JE: Ten-year assessment of primary rotator cuff repairs. *J Shoulder Elbow Surg* 1993;2:57–63.

38. Bassett RW, Cofield RH: Acute tears of the rotator cuff: The timing of surgical repair. *Clin Orthop* 1983;175:18–24.

39. Cofield RH, Hoffmeyer P, Lanzer WL: Surgical repair of chronic rotator cuff tears. *Orthop Trans* 1990;14:251–252.

40. Flatow EL, Fischer RA, Bigliani LU: Results of surgery, in Iannotti JP (ed): *Rotator Cuff Disorders: Evaluation and Treatment.* Park Ridge, IL, American Academy of Orthopaedic Surgeons, 1991, pp 53–63.

41. Iannotti JP, Bernot MP, Kuhlman JR, et al: Postoperative assessment of shoulder function: A prospective study of full-thickness rotator cuff tears. *J Shoulder Elbow Surg* 1996;5:449–457.

42. Misamore GW, Ziegler DW, Rushton JL II: Repair of the rotator cuff: A comparison of results in two populations of patients. *J Bone Joint Surg* 1995;77A:1335–1339.

43. Neer CS II: Impingement lesions. *Clin Orthop* 1983;173:70–77.

44. Neer CS II: Cuff tears, biceps lesions, and impingement, in Neer CS II (ed): *Shoulder Reconstruction.* Philadelphia, PA, WB Saunders, 1990, pp 41–142.

45. Neer CS II, Flatow EL, Lech O: Tears of the rotator cuff: Long term results of anterior acromioplasty and repair. *Orthop Trans* 1988;12:673–674.

46. Pollock RG, Black AD, Self EB, et al: Abstract: Surgical management of rotator cuff disease. *J Shoulder Elbow Surg* 1996;5:S37.

47. Bigliani LU, Cordasco FA, McIlveen SJ, et al: Operative treatment of failed repairs of the rotator cuff. *J Bone Joint Surg* 1992;74A:1505–1515.

48. Bigliani LU, Steinmann S, Flatow EL: Complications, in Iannotti JP (ed): *Rotator Cuff Disorders: Evaluation and Treatment.* Park Ridge, IL, American Academy of Orthopaedic Surgeons, 1991, pp 63–74.

49. DeOrio JK, Cofield RH: Results of a second attempt at surgical repair of a failed initial rotator-cuff repair. *J Bone Joint Surg* 1984;66A:563–567.

50. Gerber C, Schneeberger AG, Beck M, et al: Mechanical strength of repairs of the rotator cuff. *J Bone Joint Surg* 1994;76B:371–380.

51. Harryman DT II, Mack LA, Wang KY, et al: Repairs of the rotator cuff: Correlation of functional results with integrity of the cuff. *J Bone Joint Surg* 1991;73A:982–989.

52. Iannotti JP: Full-thickness rotator cuff tears: Factors affecting surgical outcome. *J Am Acad Orthop Surg* 1994;2:87–95.

53. Neer CS II, Marberry TA: On the disadvantages of radical acromionectomy. *J Bone Joint Surg* 1981;63A:416–419.

54. Neviaser RJ, Neviaser TJ: Reoperation for failed rotator cuff repair: Analysis of fifty cases. *J Shoulder Elbow Surg* 1992;1:283–286.

55. Warner JP, Krushell RJ, Masquelet A, et al: Anatomy and relationships of the suprascapular nerve: Anatomical constraints to mobilization of the supraspinatus and infraspinatus muscles in the management of massive rotator-cuff tears. *J Bone Joint Surg* 1992;74A:36–45.

56. Cordasco FA, Bigliani LU: Large and massive tears: Technique of open repair. *Orthop Clin North Am* 1997;28:179–193.

57. Hertel R, Ballmer FT, Lambert SM, et al: Lag signs in the diagnosis of rotator cuff rupture. *J Shoulder Elbow Surg* 1996;5:307–313.

58. Neer CS II, Poppen NK: Supraspinatus outlet. *Orthop Trans* 1987;11:234.

59. Weiner DS, Macnab I: Superior migration of the humeral head: A radiological aid in the diagnosis of tears of the rotator cuff. *J Bone Joint Surg* 1970;52B:524–527.

60. Neer CS II, Craig EV, Fukuda H: Cuff-tear arthropathy. *J Bone Joint Surg* 1983;65A:1232–1244.

61. Craig EV: The geyser sign and torn rotator cuff: Clinical significance and pathomechanics. *Clin Orthop* 1984;191:213–215.

62. Gaenslen ES, Satterlee CC, Hinson GW: Magnetic resonance imaging for evaluation of failed repairs of the rotator cuff. *J Bone Joint Surg* 1996;78A:1391–1396.

63. Burkhead WZ Jr, Scheinberg RR, Box G: Surgical anatomy of the axillary nerve. *J Shoulder Elbow Surg* 1992;1:31–36.

64. Armstrong JR: Excision of the acromion in treatment of the supraspinatus syndrome: Report of ninety-five excisions. *J Bone Joint Surg* 1949;31B:436–442.

65. Hammond G: Complete acromionectomy in the treatment of chronic tendinitis of the shoulder: A follow-up of ninety operations on eighty-seven patients. *J Bone Joint Surg* 1971;53A:173–180.

66. Bigliani LU, Morrison DS, April EW: The morphology of the acromion and its relationship to rotator cuff tears. *Orthop Trans* 1986;10:216.

67. Flatow EL, Soslowsky LJ, Ticker JB, et al: Excursion of the rotator cuff under the acromion: Patterns of subacromial contact. *Am J Sports Med* 1994;22:779–788.

68. Apoil A, Dautry P, Koechlin P, et al: The surgical treatment of rotator cuff impingement, in Bayley I, Kessel L (eds): *Shoulder Surgery*. Berlin, Germany, Springer-Verlag, 1982, pp 22–26.

69. Wiley AM: Superior humeral dislocation: A complication following decompression and debridement for rotator cuff tears. *Clin Orthop* 1991;263:135–141.

70. Flatow EL, Weinstein DM, Duralde XA, et al: Abstract: Coracoacromial ligament preservation in rotator cuff surgery. *J Shoulder Elbow Surg* 1994;3:S73.

71. Flatow EL, Connor PM, Levine WN, et al: Abstract: Coracoacromial arch reconstruction for anterosuperior subluxation after failed rotator cuff surgery: A preliminary report. *J Shoulder Elbow Surg* 1997;6:228.

72. Bigliani LU, Norris TR, Fischer J, et al: The relationship between the unfused acromial epiphysis and subacromial impingement lesions. *Orthop Trans* 1983;7:138.

73. Mudge MK, Wood VE, Frykman GK: Rotator cuff tears associated with os acromiale. *J Bone Joint Surg* 1984;66A:427–429.

74. Constant CR: Shoulder function after rotator cuff tears treated by operative and nonoperative means, in Post M, Morrey BF, Hawkins RJ (eds): *Surgery of the Shoulder*. St. Louis, MO, Mosby-Year Book, 1990, pp 231–233.

75. Karas SE, Giachello TL: Subscapularis transfer for reconstruction of massive tears of the rotator cuff. *J Bone Joint Surg* 1996;78A:239–245.

76. Neer CS II, Satterlee CC, Dalsey RM, et al: On the value of the coracohumeral ligament release. *Orthop Trans* 1989;13:235–236.

77. Bayne O, Bateman JE: Long term results of surgical repair of full thickness rotator cuff tears, in Bateman JE, Welsh RP (eds): *Surgery of the Shoulder*. Philadelphia, PA, BC Decker, 1984, pp 167–171.

78. Burkhart SS: Reconciling the paradox of rotator cuff repair versus debridement: A unified biomechanical rationale for the treatment of rotator cuff tears. *Arthroscopy* 1994;10:4–19.

79. Clark JM, Harryman DT II: Tendons, ligaments, and capsule of the rotator cuff: Gross and microscopic anatomy. *J Bone Joint Surg* 1992;74A:713–725.

80. Swiontkowski MF, Iannotti JP, Boulas HJ, et al: Intraoperative assessment of rotator cuff vascularity using Laser Doppler Flowmetry, in Post M, Morrey BF, Hawkins RJ (eds): *Surgery of the Shoulder*. St Louis, MO, Mosby-Year Book, 1990, pp 208–212.

81. Uhthoff HK, Sarkar K, Lohr J: Repair in rotator cuff tendons, in Post M, Morrey BF, Hawkins RJ (eds): *Surgery of the Shoulder*. St Louis, MO, Mosby-Year Book, 1990, pp 216–219.

82. Flatow EL, Bigliani LU: Locating and protecting the axillary nerve in shoulder surgery: The tug test. *Orthop Rev* 1992;21:503–505.

83. Bigliani LU, Dalsey RM, McCann PD, et al: An anatomical study of the suprascapular nerve. *Arthroscopy* 1990;6:301–305.

84. Barber FA, Cawley P, Prudich JF: Suture anchor failure strength: An in vivo study. *Arthroscopy* 1993;9:647–652.

85. France EP, Paulos LE, Harner CD, et al: Biomechanical evaluation of rotator cuff fixation methods. *Am J Sports Med* 1989;17:176–181.

86. Hecker AT, Shea M, Hayhurst JO, et al: Pull-out strength of suture anchors for rotator cuff and Bankart lesion repairs. *Am J Sports Med* 1993;21:874–879.

87. Zuckerman J, Matsen F: Complications about the glenohumeral joint related to the use of screws and staples. *J Bone Joint Surg* 1984;66A:175–180.

88. Neer CS II, McCann PD, Macfarlane EA, et al: Earlier passive motion following shoulder arthroplasty and rotator cuff repair: A prospective study. *Orthop Trans* 1987;11:231.

89. Cordasco FA, Wolfe IN, Wootten ME, et al: An electromyographic analysis of the shoulder during a medicine ball rehabilitation program. *Am J Sports Med* 1996;24:386–392.

90. Gore DR, Murray MP, Sepic SB, et al: Shoulder-muscle strength and range of motion following surgical repair of full-thickness rotator-cuff tears. *J Bone Joint Surg* 1986;68A:266–272.

91. Walker SW, Couch WH, Boester GA, et al: Isokinetic strength of the shoulder after repair of a torn rotator cuff. *J Bone Joint Surg* 1987;69A:1041–1044.

Failed Repair of the Rotator Cuff: Evaluation and Treatment of Complications

Evan H. Karas, MD
Joseph P. Iannotti, MD

Surgical repair of a tear of the rotator cuff usually provides relief of pain.[1-7] Restoration of strength is somewhat less predictable, but the rate of overall patient satisfaction after primary repair of the rotator cuff has been reported to be as high as 91% in a series of 340 shoulders.[2,4] Improved surgical techniques that have been developed over the last several decades have been largely responsible for this success. However, surgical repairs can fail. These failures present diagnostic and therapeutic challenges, because they may have multiple causes. Identification of the cause in a given patient requires a thorough evaluation that includes a complete history, physical examination, and review of the radiographs and the ancillary studies. Only then can an effective treatment plan be established. Although the results of repair of recurrent tears of the rotator cuff have not been as satisfactory as those of primary repair,[7,8-11] proper diagnosis and treatment can greatly increase the chance for success.

The major reasons for failure of repair of the rotator cuff are an incomplete or incorrect diagnosis; postoperative complications; errors in surgical technique; and errors in or poor performance of postoperative rehabilitation, or both. A combination of these factors may be responsible for a poor result in a given patient. The clinical evaluation of these parameters must be extremely thorough in order to avoid failure of treatment.

A careful history, including a review of the medical record, surgical notes, and preoperative and postoperative imaging studies, must be obtained. This information should allow the preoperative diagnosis to be established on the basis of both the clinical data and the anatomic abnormalities. An inaccurate or incomplete diagnosis or an error in the execution of the surgical procedure or the postoperative rehabilitation program may then be revealed. Accurate definition of all of the factors resulting in failure of the initial procedure is the first step in deciding on future treatment and improving the likelihood of a successful revision when surgery is indicated.

Errors in Diagnosis

Physical examination and injection tests help to define the patient's current problems. Care must be taken to specifically identify referred pain due to thoracic outlet syndrome and lesions of the cervical spine. Pain secondary to cervical lesions often presents in a dermatomal pattern over the posterior and lateral aspects of the shoulder; the pain may radiate to the occiput and the thoracic spine. Tenderness to palpation and a decreased range of motion of the neck are indicative of cervical disk disease. Provocative maneuvers, such as the Spurling test for diskogenic disease and the Wright[12] and Adson[13] tests for thoracic-outlet syndrome,[14,15] may be helpful if the results

are positive. The Spurling test is performed by passive lateral bending and ipsilateral rotation of the neck. A positive test reproduces radicular symptoms. With the Adson test, the arm is positioned in extension with ipsilateral rotation of the neck. With the Wright test, the arm is placed in extension and abduction. The Adson and Wright tests are positive when they reproduce the symptoms of the upper extremity and the hand. If selective injection of lidocaine into the subacromial space or the acromioclavicular joint, or both, relieves pain, the cervical spine may be eliminated from consideration.

Neuropathies of the suprascapular and axillary nerves also may mimic disease of the rotator cuff and cause misdiagnoses. The suprascapular nerve, a branch of the superior trunk of the brachial plexus, may be compressed beneath the suprascapular ligament in the suprascapular notch[16] or by a ganglion in the spinoglenoid notch.[17] In addition, if a superior capsular release was performed during the original procedure, it is possible that dissection more than 2 cm medial to the superior aspect of the glenoid rim had resulted in iatrogenic suprascapular nerve injury.

Clinical presentation of these neuropathies usually consists of pain in the posterior aspect of the shoulder with accompanying muscle weakness specific to the site of nerve compression.

Proximal compression at the suprascapular notch or iatrogenic injury at this level denervates both the supraspinatus and the infraspinatus, while more distal compression at the spinoglenoid notch causes selective weakness of the infraspinatus. Similarly, weakness of the deltoid and the teres minor secondary to postoperative neuropathy of the axillary nerve may have a presentation very similar to that of a tear of the rotator cuff. Electromyographic analysis can help to confirm these diagnoses.[16,18,19] Magnetic resonance imaging (MRI) is the only useful imaging modality for defining neuropathy of the suprascapular nerve as a cause of failed rotator cuff surgery. It may reveal space-occupying lesions such as a ganglion cyst, or it may show severe muscle atrophy without a defect of the cuff.

Acromioclavicular joint arthropathy also can complicate the clinical presentation of disorders of the rotator cuff and can lead to failures in diagnosis and treatment. Careful clinical examination of the acromioclavicular joint, including direct palpation for tenderness and cross-arm adduction maneuvers, should be performed routinely for patients who have a possible lesion of the cuff. Imaging studies may be useful for diagnosing residual abnormalities of the acromioclavicular joint, a common cause of persistent pain following rotator cuff surgery. A Zanca radiograph (an anteroposterior radiograph made with the x-ray beam centered on the acromioclavicular joint with 15° of cephalic angulation) shows the full extent of the joint and may reveal lesions that were missed on routine anteroposterior radiographs. If radiographs are inconclusive and a lesion of the acromioclavicular joint is strongly suspected, a bone scan may confirm the diagnosis and lead to appropriate treatment.

An unrecognized os acromiale can cause persistent pain after subacromial decompression and repair of the rotator cuff. This lesion is most readily identified on routine axillary radiographs of the shoulder or on axial MRIs of the acromion. If small fragments are mobile and painful, they can be excised with reattachment of the deltoid to the remaining edge of the acromion. Larger lesions may require excision of the intervening synchondrosis and fixation with a tension-band wire with use of local bone graft obtained from a simultaneous acromioplasty.

Lesions of the biceps tendon and the superior glenoid labrum often are found in patients who have impingement syndrome and rotator cuff tears.[20] Failure to recognize and treat these problems appropriately can lead to a poor surgical result. An arthroscopic mini-open repair offers the advantage of improved visualization of the biceps tendon and its attachment to the superior aspect of the labrum. A finding of tenderness of the biceps tendon to palpation on physical examination, and a positive result on the Speed or the Yergason test, are suggestive of but nonspecific for biceps tendinitis.[21] The Yergason test is performed by resisting supination and flexion of the forearm. The Speed test is performed by resisting flexion of the elbow and the shoulder with the elbow in 90° of flexion and the shoulder in approximately 30° of flexion. Both tests are performed to evaluate referred pain to the long head of the biceps tendon. Standard radiographs are not particularly helpful for assessing the status of the biceps tendon. An axial radiograph of the intertubercular sulcus may provide indirect evidence of a lesion of the biceps tendon.[22] Arthroscopy is the most useful tool for delineating severe lesions of the biceps tendon. Tendon fraying and labral detachments can be both assessed accurately and treated arthroscopically. These intra-articular structures may be difficult to visualize and treat during routine open repair of defects of the cuff that are less than 2 cm long. Additionally, arthroscopy can be helpful for distinguishing internal posterosuperior glenoid impingement or secondary subtle glenohumeral instability,[23,24] especially in athletes who have pain during the late cocking phase (marked external rotation and abduction) of throwing.

Errors in Surgical Technique

Errors in the surgical technique of acromioplasty and rotator cuff repair can undermine the results of treatment of even the most accurately diagnosed lesions of the cuff. These errors include inadequate surgery and intraoperative complications. Inadequate surgeries include those in which a lesion of the biceps tendon or the labrum, or both, is missed; those in which arthropathy of the acromioclavicular joint is missed, as discussed previously; and inadequate acromioplasty. Intraoperative complications include fracture of the acromion, detachment or denervation of the deltoid, and failure to preserve the coracoacromial arch in patients who have an irreparable tear of the cuff.

The principles of acromioplasty include removal of sufficient bursa for adequate evaluation of the underlying rotator cuff and adequate removal of anteroinferior acromial bone without excessively shortening or narrowing the acromion. Inadequate anterior acromioplasty has been reported by many investigators as a common source of failures requiring revision surgery.[8,9,25-29]

In a study by Flugstad and associates,[26] 15 of 19 patients who had failure of surgical treatment for impingement syndrome were found to have residual acromial spurs. Of 117 patients who had a failed acromioplasty in a study by Rockwood and Williams,[29] all 90 who had recurrent symptoms of impingement had a residual anterior acromion at the time of surgery. DeOrio and Cofield[9] also demonstrated the importance of adequate subacromial decompression in their study of failed rotator cuff repairs; more than 50% of their 27 patients had not had an acromioplasty during the first, unsuccessful, operation.

Removal of an excessive amount of the anterior or lateral portion of the acromion may be associated with a fracture of the acromion or with detachment of the deltoid and a poor surgical result.[30] In the early development of techniques for repair of the rotator cuff, radical acromionectomy or subtotal lateral acromionectomy was advocated for subacromial decompression.[31-34] More recently, however, it has become clear that the acromion serves a necessary function in providing a strong attachment point and fulcrum for the powerful deltoid muscle. In 1981, Neer and Marberry[35] reported on 30 patients who had had removal of 80% of the acromion with resultant adhesions of the deltoid to the rotator cuff, deltoid retraction, and loss of the acromial fulcrum. Attempted surgical correction in 20 of these patients was unsuccessful. It is now accepted that acromionectomy is fraught with complications and should be abandoned.[17,25,33]

Frank acromial fractures can occur either intraoperatively or postoperatively.[30] Careful visualization and palpation of the thickness of the acromion is necessary to avoid this complication. Meticulous surgical technique, with emphasis on the correct angle of progression of the osteotome and with great care taken not to lever on the acromion with a subacromial retractor, is mandatory. An intraoperative fracture should be identified readily at the time of surgery and corrected with open reduction and internal fixation to prevent a painful nonunion and consequent deltoid weakness. Acromial fractures also have been reported after arthroscopic subacromial decompression[29] (Fig. 1), emphasizing the need for excellent visualization of the undersurface of the acromion and careful control of bone removal. Excessive use or trauma, or both, during the postoperative period also can cause an excessively thinned acromion to fracture.

The manner in which the deltoid is handled during an acromioplasty and rotator cuff repair is critical to a successful result. Avoidance of lateral acromionectomy to prevent deltoid retraction and scarring of the rotator cuff has been discussed previously. However, deltoid detachment from an intact acromion can still occur. The technique for removing and repairing the origin of the deltoid from the acromion can help to minimize the occurrence of this complication. In 1972, Neer[36] reported a method of acromioplasty in which a limited portion of the deltoid origin is removed subperiosteally from the anterior acromion and the acromioclavicular joint. Blunt dissection between the anterior and lateral heads of the deltoid muscle then allows exposure of the rotator cuff without excessive acromial destruction or deltoid detachment.[36] The deltoid-splitting technique was modified by Bigliani and Rodosky[37] to provide better access to the posterior cuff tendons without necessitating additional deltoid origin detachment.

Arthroscopic acromioplasty and mini-open repair of the rotator cuff theoretically should decrease the prevalence of detachment of the deltoid. To our knowledge, there have been no reported cases of detachment of the deltoid after mini-open or arthroscopic techniques. However, the senior one of us (JPI) has seen such detachment after both arthroscopic mini-open repair of the cuff and arthroscopic acromioplasty alone. Therefore, it is possible for this complication to occur with both arthroscopic techniques.

Reattachment of the deltoid to the acromion after repair of a tear of the rotator cuff is crucial. If an inadequate soft-tissue cuff of fascia remains on the acromion, or if excessive deltoid detachment is necessary for repair of a massive tear, then the deltoid should be reattached to the osseous edge of the acromion and the clavicle (if necessary) through drill holes. If the lateral portion of the clavicle has been resected, the deltoid must be repaired to the leading edge

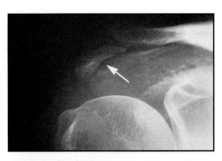

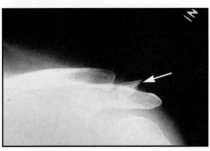

Fig. 1 Postoperative fractures of the acromion (arrows). (Top, Reproduced with permission from Naranja RJ, Iannotti JP, Gartsman GM: Complications of rotator cuff surgery, in Norris TR (ed): *Orthopaedic Knowledge Update: Shoulder and Elbow.* Rosemont, IL, American Academy of Orthopaedic Surgeons, 1997, pp 157-166.)

of the trapezius fascia. Improper reattachment may result in retraction of the deltoid and may substantially compromise the functional result. When poor-quality deltoid tissue is encountered, an extended period of protected mobilization of the shoulder may be necessary.

Examination of the shoulder of a patient who has deltoid detachment reveals a defect at the deltoid origin from the acromion and a prominence of the deltoid distal to the defect that is accentuated by active elevation of the arm (Fig. 2, *left*). An MRI may be helpful for confirming this diagnosis (Fig. 2, *right*). Surgical repair of a retracted deltoid should proceed as soon as possible. Prolonged retraction leads to scarring and subsequent stiffness, pain, and loss of shoulder function.

Sher and associates (personal communication, Sher JS, Warner JJ, Gross Y, et al, 1996.) reported on 24 patients who

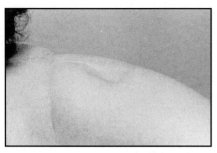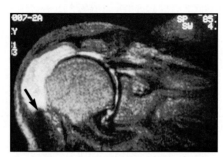

Fig. 2 Postoperative detachment of the deltoid. **Left,** Clinical evaluation reveals a defect that is accentuated by attempted active elevation of the arm. **Right,** T2-weighted magnetic resonance image demonstrates detachment and retraction of the origin of the deltoid (arrow). (Reproduced with permission from Naranja RJ, Iannotti JP, Gartsman GM: Complications of rotator cuff surgery, in Norris TR (ed): *Orthopaedic Knowledge Update: Shoulder and Elbow.* Rosemont, IL, American Academy of Orthopaedic Surgeons, 1997, pp 157-166.)

had had either deltoid repair (for an acute tear) or rotational deltoidplasty of the middle deltoid anteriorly (for a chronic tear) to reconstruct a postsurgical deltoid disruption. At an average of 39 months, 16 patients (67%) had an unsatisfactory clinical result. The poor results were associated with a previous lateral acromionectomy; involvement of the middle deltoid; duration of symptoms of more than 12 months; and a concomitant, poorly compensated for, massive rotator cuff tear. Conversely, a satisfactory result was associated with an acute disruption isolated to the anterior deltoid, an intact acromion, and preserved function of the rotator cuff.

Iatrogenic deltoid denervation is a serious complication of rotator cuff surgery. Knowledge of the anatomy of the terminal branches of the axillary nerve as they relate to the splitting of the deltoid muscle is critical. The axillary nerve arises from the posterior cord of the brachial plexus near the coracoid process and then courses through the quadrilateral space to reach the posterior aspect of the shoulder. While in the quadrilateral space, it divides into posterior and anterior terminal branches, which supply the posterior one-third and the anterior two-thirds of the deltoid muscle, respectively. The anterior branch travels approximately 5

cm inferior to the lateral and anterior margin of the acromion, and is perpendicular to the direction of the muscle fibers. The deltoid split, therefore, should not extend beyond this distance. A stay suture can be placed at the apex of this split to prevent its propagation from excessive deltoid retraction. Furthermore, Burkhead and associates[38] showed that, in some smaller patients, the nerve may be located slightly closer than 5 cm from the acromial margin.

Axillary nerve neuropathy initially presents as weakness in abduction and forward elevation of the shoulder. Chronic disorders are accompanied by deltoid atrophy. Loss of sensation in the dermatome overlying the lateral deltoid is variable, as the cutaneous nerves supplying this area often arise from the posterior terminal branches of the axillary nerve.

Electromyography should be used when denervation of the deltoid is suspected postoperatively, both to confirm the diagnosis and to establish the nature of the injury as either a neurapraxia or a neurotmesis. Neurapraxias can be managed expectantly, with institution of passive range-of-motion exercises to prevent stiffness of the shoulder. Nerve transections should be evaluated for recovery on a monthly basis; nerve repair can be considered if no improvement is evident by 3

to 4 months and if it is warranted by the degree of the functional impairment. However, these recommendations are based on results obtained after repair of axillary nerve injuries secondary to dislocation of the shoulder or surgery for anterior stabilization in which the nerve was injured at its larger, main-branch region.[39] There is little information in the literature with regard to the treatment of terminal branch lesions after cuff repair. Leffert[40] described rotational deltoidplasty with excision of the denervated portion of the muscle as a valuable alternative to nerve repair for this problem.

The importance of the coracoacromial arch in providing anterosuperior stability for the humeral head has been the subject of several recent investigations.[41,42] Lazarus and associates[41] demonstrated anterosuperior escape of the humeral head from beneath the coracoacromial arch in five of six cadaver shoulders after coracoacromial ligament release and anterior acromioplasty. In a more elaborate cadaver model, Flatow and associates (personal communication, Flatow EL, Raimondo Ra, Kelkar R, et al, 1996.) demonstrated that this superior migration is most severe in the presence of large rotator cuff tears, especially when the edges of the tear approach the equator of the humeral head. Repair of the rotator cuff tears restored nearly normal glenohumeral kinematics in their patients. Failure to recognize the role of the coracoacromial arch in shoulders with a torn rotator cuff may lead to clinically evident anterosuperior instability (Fig. 3). In an attempt to circumvent this problem, Flatow and associates[43] recently described a technique of limited subacromial decompression and reattachment of the coracoacromial ligament in patients with a massive irreparable rotator cuff tear.

Postoperative Complications

Complications of repair of the rotator cuff include infection, heterotopic ossification, frozen shoulder, and recurrent tearing. Because these complications can be related both to the surgical technique and to the postoperative rehabilitation, they will be discussed separately.

Postoperative infections may be difficult to diagnose, as they often present in a delayed and unimpressive fashion. Superficial wound infections are characterized by erythema with or without drainage, induration, warmth, and fever. These findings may be subtle initially and may be overlooked as normal postoperative inflammation. Laboratory and imaging studies are often unrevealing at this stage. If left to worsen, these infections eventually will manifest themselves as wound dehiscence, drainage, cellulitis, and lymphadenopathy. Treatment is most successful if begun early and based on positive cultures. A heightened awareness of this potential problem is critical, and aspiration of the joint or the wound should not be delayed in suspicious cases. Intravenous administration of anti-staphylococcal and antistreptococcal antibiotics (first-generation cephalosporin) should be initiated after surgical debridement and exploration of the extent of the infection. If the infection does not pass deep to an intact repair of the cuff, then the repair can be left intact if this allows for adequate debridement of necrotic tissue. If the infection extends into the shoulder joint, then it should be debrided arthroscopically. The subacromial space and the biceps tendon sheath should be debrided in an open fashion. Nonabsorbable suture and any metallic suture anchors should be removed. Closed suction drains should be left in place, and antibiotics should be given intravenously as dictated by the results of gram stains and specimens of intraoperative cultures.

Heterotopic ossification is rare after acromioplasty and repair of the rotator cuff. It occurs in approximately 3% to 5% of patients, in our experience, but not all of these patients are symptomatic. Copious irrigation to remove all bone fragments after acromioplasty reduces the chance of heterotopic bone formation. When ossification occurs in the subacromial space or in the space created by resection of the lateral portion of the clavicle, it can be a source of pain (Fig. 4). The diagnosis is best made with use of routine radiographs. Lesions that cause severe pain or that limit motion can be treated with excision. Preoperative bone scans help to delineate mature lesions when they do not display markedly increased uptake of radioisotope. In our center, low-dose irradiation (7 Gy in a single dose) given within the first 48 hours after resection, or indomethacin given orally for 6 weeks, has been successful in preventing recurrence. This regimen is based on its effectiveness in patients who have had a total hip arthroplasty; we are unaware of any scientific data that support its use specifically for heterotopic ossification of the shoulder.

Postoperative stiffness after rotator cuff repair can lead to severe functional limitations. Bigliani and associates[8,25] reported on five patients who had frozen shoulder after the procedure. Those authors attributed the failures to inadequate postoperative rehabilitation and they recommended gentle pendulum exercises and passive elevation in the scapular plane, beginning on the first or second postoperative day, as preventive measures. One must be careful to identify patients who have a severe loss of motion of the shoulder preoperatively, as they are at higher risk for frozen-shoulder syndrome during the postoperative period. Passive shoulder-stretching exercises should be initiated, and a nearly full range of motion should be achieved before the cuff is repaired. If rehabilitation fails to restore motion, then manipulation with the patient under anesthesia followed by arthroscopic capsular release for shoulders that are resistant to manipulation should be performed. The patient can be brought back to the operating room at a later date, after motion of the shoulder

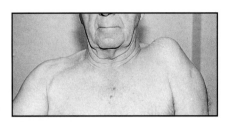

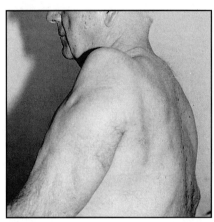

Fig. 3 Top, Coracoacromial arch insufficiency. (Reproduced with permission from Naranja RJ, Iannotti JP, Gartsman GM: Complications of rotator cuff surgery, in Norris TR (ed): *Orthopaedic Knowledge Update: Shoulder and Elbow.* Rosemont, IL, American Academy of Orthopaedic Surgeons, 1997, pp 157-166.) **Bottom,** Attempted shoulder evaluation results in superior migration of the humeral head.

has been restored, for definitive surgical treatment of the lesion of the cuff.

More recently, Mormino and associates[44] reported on 13 patients who had subdeltoid adhesions after rotator cuff repair. These patients had arthroscopic release of the adhesions, which was universally successful in alleviating pain. The average score according to the system of the University of California at Los Angeles increased from 14.8 to 30.1 points. These authors postulated that the adhesions acted as a functional tenodesis, thus altering the normal biomechanics of the shoulder by preventing rolling of the humeral head on the glenoid. This restriction of motion is distinct from that secondary to capsular contracture or to scarring in the classic frozen shoulder

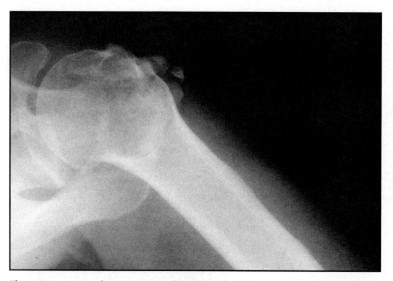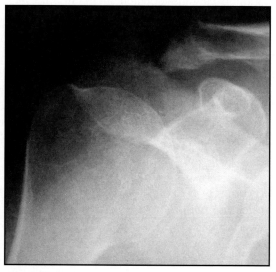

Fig. 4 Postoperative heterotopic ossification. **Left,** Axillary radiograph demonstrating heterotopic bone in the vicinity of an anterior acromioplasty. **Right,** Zanca (acromioclavicular joint) radiograph demonstrating heterotopic bone formation in the space created by resection of the lateral portion of the clavicle. ((Reproduced with permission from Naranja RJ, Iannotti JP, Gartsman GM: Complications of rotator cuff surgery, in Norris TR (ed): *Orthopaedic Knowledge Update: Shoulder and Elbow.* Rosemont, IL, American Academy of Orthopaedic Surgeons, 1997, pp 157-166.)

and has been termed the captured shoulder. Early mobilization of the shoulder postoperatively may reduce the prevalence of this complication. However, all of the patients in this series began therapy on the first postoperative day. These authors did not explore factors that may have been associated with the development of the adhesions.

Persistent Rotator Cuff Defects

Persistent defects of previously repaired rotator cuff tendons may be related to an inadequate initial repair of the cuff, poor-quality tendon or bone, persistent impingement, or improper physical therapy. The results of clinical evaluation and radiographs must be evaluated concomitantly in order to determine the presence of a persistent defect as well as its relative clinical importance.

Persistent impingement usually is related to inadequate acromioplasty. Inadequate repair of the original tear may be secondary to improper identification of thickened, hypertrophic subacromial bursal tissue as rotator cuff tendon or to inadequate mobilization of the torn tendons with consequent tension on the site of the repair. Bigliani and associates[25] identified the cause of 11 of 31 failed repairs as secondary to inadequate mobilization. Observation of the ease with which the bursal tissue pulls away from the underlying rotator cuff, as well as the differential motion of the bursa as compared with that of the rotator cuff with rotation of the humeral head, should serve as guides with which to determine the proper tissue to repair.

Overly intensive physical therapy during the early postoperative period may lead to avulsion of the tendon before healing. This mechanism was associated with five of the 31 failures in the series of Bigliani and associates.[25] In addition, Neviaser and Neviaser[10] found that early use of weights was a factor leading to failure of repair of rotator cuff tears. Rehabilitation must be tailored individually to intraoperative observations of the repair in each patient. A small tear that is repaired without detachment of the deltoid will withstand more intensive thera-py than will a large or massive tear necessitating takedown and repair of the deltoid origin. Intraoperative assessment of the quality of the tissue and the amount of tension on the site of the repair also will help to guide therapy.

The identification of persistent defects of the cuff with use of imaging modalities can be difficult. The most useful study in the postoperative setting is arthrography. Communication of contrast medium between the subacromial and glenohumeral joint spaces was reported to be 100% sensitive and 96% specific for the diagnosis of full-thickness rotator cuff tears in series ranging from 20 to 805 shoulders.[45-47] Ultrasonography also has been used successfully to delineate full-thickness defects in the shoulder postoperatively. Accurate interpretation of sonographic images requires an extremely experienced sonographer who has the frequent opportunity to correlate the readings with the intraoperative findings. The sensitivity for the diagnosis of postoperative tears of the cuff approached 95% overall, and failure to visualize a supraspinatus musculotendinous unit was virtually 100% predictive of a complete tear, in series of 50[48] and 72[49] patients. Unlike preoperative MRI scans, postoperative scans do not delineate partial rotator cuff tears accurately. Persistent full-thickness tears can be assessed accurately when there is a well-defined defect in the tendon that displays high signal intensity on T2-weighted images (Fig. 5).

The clinical importance of a persistent full-thickness tear must be integrated within the context of the growing body of literature defining the presence of asymptomatic or minimally symptomatic tears. These data come from cadaver studies, imaging studies of shoulders after repair, clinical series of shoulders that have had subacromial decompression without repair of a massive tear, and imaging studies of asymptomatic individuals.

DePalma and associates,[50] in their classic study of 108 cadavera, determined the prevalence of defects of the rotator cuff relative to aging. Although no specimens from individuals who had died before the fifth decade of life had a tear of the rotator cuff, 33% from those who had died in the fifth decade and 100% from those who had died in the seventh decade had a complete tear. Of these specimens, 44 were obtained during autopsies on patients for whom the history and the findings on physical examination had been negative for a lesion of the rotator cuff.

Calvert and associates[45] used arthrography to study 20 shoulders after repair of the rotator cuff. They found that 18 of the shoulders had a persistent defect and that 17 of the 18 had satisfactory relief of the preoperative pain. Harryman and associates,[51] in a larger, more detailed study, performed bilateral ultrasonography on 122 patients after repair of the cuff. Of 105 patients who had a postoperative defect of the cuff, 94 were satisfied with the decrease in pain. Persistent defects were related to a decreased range of motion of the shoulder and to an

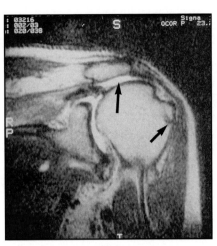

Fig. 5 T2-weighted magnetic resonance image, made in the coronal plane, of a recurrent defect of the rotator cuff. There is a full-thickness, high-signal-intensity defect in the supraspinatus tendon (large arrow). Note the bone trough and the suture through the bone tunnel (small arrow).

inability to perform activities of daily living. Additionally, the subjective results associated with intact repairs of recurrent tears were as successful as those associated with intact repairs of primary tears. The size of the tear was not related to the subjective assessment of function or pain relief at the latest follow-up evaluation if the repair had remained intact. However, a repair of a large defect is less likely to heal than is a small tear.

These results are not surprising, given the recent reports in the literature concerning the results of imaging of asymptomatic shoulders. With use of ultrasonography of the contralateral, asymptomatic shoulder of 73 patients who had a unilateral tear, Harryman and associates[51] noted rotator cuff defects in 40 (55%). Sher and associates[52] performed MRI on 96 asymptomatic shoulders and found an over-all prevalence of full-thickness and partial-thickness tears of 15% and 20%. All but one full-thickness defect was in a patient who was more than 60 years old.

Finally, the clinical importance of postoperative defects of the cuff must be

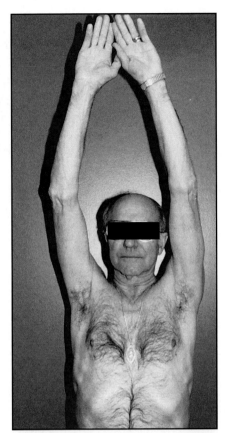

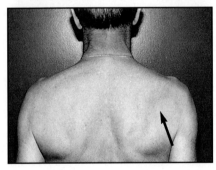

Fig. 6 This patient had an excellent result 2 years after debridement of a massive rotator cuff tear. **Top,** The range of motion is excellent. **Bottom,** There is marked atrophy of the infraspinatus (arrow).

interpreted in light of the evidence that acromioplasty and partial debridement or partial repair of a portion of the cuff is successful for the treatment of some large degenerative tears. Rockwood and associates[53,54] showed that this technique, coupled with intensive postoperative rehabilitation, can provide relief of pain and adequate function. Selection of the patients is critical, as the best results have been in patients who have had preoperative forward elevation of the shoulder above the horizontal plane, an intact long head of the biceps, and excellent function of the deltoid[53,54] (Fig. 6). Less favorable results have been noted in patients who have had a previous operation, anterior deltoid dysfunction, or a biceps tendon tear.[53,54] Although detachment of the cuff can provide favorable results in selected patients, we recommend repair of the cuff whenever possible.

To establish a treatment plan for patients in whom recurrent defects of the cuff are suspected, the results of imaging studies must be interpreted within the context of each patient's clinical presentation. Symptomatic patients who have subacromial crepitus, weakness of abduction and external rotation, and positive lag signs on external rotation as noted on physical examination are potential candidates for repeat repair. Findings at the time of the reoperation, including the size and location of the recurrent defect and the quality of the tendon and its degree of retraction and ability to be mobilized, will help to determine whether repeat repair of the torn edges of the tendon to bone is justified. A discussion of the patient's goals and expectations preoperatively is also important for guiding intraoperative decisions.

In conclusion, there are many potential causes of failure of rotator cuff repair. The categories of incomplete and incorrect diagnosis, errors of surgical technique or postoperative rehabilitation, and postoperative complications are convenient for classification, but it must be remembered that there may be several causes of failure in any given patient. Clinical evaluation is most dependent on a careful history, a review of the medical record and the preoperative imaging studies, and a physical examination with use of injection tests as indicated. On the basis of this evaluation, a definitive diagnosis or a limited differential diagnosis often can be established. The selective use of additional imaging studies and diagnostic arthroscopy will define the anatomic abnormalities. These lesions must be correlated carefully with the clinical findings in order to determine their relative importance and to choose the appropriate treatment.

References

1. Cofield RH: Rotator cuff disease of the shoulder. *J Bone Joint Surg* 1985;67A:974–979.
2. Hawkins RJ, Misamore GW, Hobeika PE: Surgery for full-thickness rotator-cuff tears. *J Bone Joint Surg* 1985;67A:1349–1355.
3. Iannotti JP: Full-thickness rotator cuff tears: Factors affecting surgical outcome. *J Am Acad Orthop Surg* 1994;2:87–95.
4. Neer CS II, Flatow EL, Lech O: Tears of the rotator cuff: Long term results of anterior acromioplasty and repair. *Orthop Trans* 1988;12:735.
5. Petersson C: Long-term results of rotator cuff repair, in Bayley I, Kessel L (eds): *Shoulder Surgery.* Berlin, Germany, Springer-Verlag, 1982, pp 64–69.
6. Samilson RL, Binder WF: Symptomatic full thickness tears of the rotator cuff: An analysis of 292 shoulders in 276 patients. *Orthop Clin North Am* 1975;6:449–466.
7. Wolfgang GL: Surgical repair of tears of the rotator cuff of the shoulder: Factors influencing the result. *J Bone Joint Surg* 1974;56A:14–26.
8. Bigliani LU, McIlveen SJ, Cordasco FA, et al: Operative management of failed rotator cuff repairs. *Orthop Trans* 1988;12:674.
9. DeOrio JK, Cofield RH: Results of a second attempt at surgical repair of a failed initial rotator-cuff repair. *J Bone Joint Surg* 1984;66A:563–567.
10. Neviaser RJ, Neviaser TJ: Reoperation for failed rotator cuff repair: Analysis of 46 cases. *Orthop Trans* 1989;13:509.
11. Sahlstrand T: Operations for impingement of the shoulder: Early results in 52 patients. *Acta Orthop Scand* 1989;60:45–48.
12. Wright IS: The neurovascular syndrome produced by hyperabduction of the arms: The immediate changes produced in 150 normal controls, and the effects on some persons of prolonged hyperabduction of the arms, as in sleeping, and in certain occupations. *Am Heart J* 1945;29:1–19.
13. Adson AW: Surgical treatment for symptoms produced by cervical ribs and the scalenus anticus muscle. *Surg Gynecol Obstet* 1947;85:687–700.
14. Leffert RD: Thoracic outlet syndrome: Orthopaedic perspective on diagnosis and treatment. *Orthop Trans* 1988;12:190.
15. Leffert RD: Thoracic outlet syndrome, in Gelberman RH (ed): *Operative Nerve Repair and Reconstruction.* Philadelphia, PA, JB Lippincott, 1991, vol 2, pp 1177–1195.
16. Rengachary SS, Burr D, Lucas S, et al: Suprascapular entrapment neuropathy: A clinical, anatomical, and comparative study. Anatomical study and comparative study. *Neurosurgery* 1979;5:447–455.
17. Neviaser TJ, Ain BR, Neviaser RJ: Suprascapular nerve denervation secondary to attenuation by a ganglionic cyst. *J Bone Joint Surg* 1986;68A:627–628.
18. Donovan WH, Kraft GH: Rotator cuff tear versus suprascapular nerve injury: A problem in differential diagnosis. *Arch Phys Med Rehabil* 1974;55:424–428.
19. Drez D Jr: Suprascapular neuropathy in the differential diagnosis of rotator cuff injuries. *Am J Sports Med* 1976;4:43–45.
20. Neer CS II, Bigliani LU, Hawkins RJ: Rupture of the long head of the biceps related to subacromial impingement. *Orthop Trans* 1977;1:111.
21. Yergason RM: Supination sign. *J Bone Joint Surg* 1931;13:160.
22. Cone RO, Danzig L, Resnick D, et al: The bicipital groove: Radiographic, anatomic, and pathologic study. *Am J Roentgenol* 1983;141:781–788.
23. Lombardo SJ, Jobe FW, Kerlan RK, et al: Posterior shoulder lesions in throwing athletes. *Am J Sports Med* 1977;5:106–110.
24. Snyder SJ, Karzel RP, Del Pizzo W, et al: SLAP lesions of the shoulder. *Arthroscopy* 1990;6:274–279.
25. Bigliani LU, Cordasco FA, McIlveen SJ, et al: Operative treatment of failed repairs of the rotator cuff. *J Bone Joint Surg* 1992;74A:1505–1515.
26. Flugstad D, Matsen FA, Larry I, et al: Failed acromioplasty: Etiology and prevention. *Orthop Trans* 1986;10:229.
27. Hawkins RJ, Chris AD, Kiefer GN: Failed anterior acromioplasties. *Orthop Trans* 1987;11:233.
28. Packer NP, Calvert PT, Bayley JI, et al: Operative treatment of chronic ruptures of the rotator cuff of the shoulder. *J Bone Joint Surg* 1983;65B:171–175.
29. Rockwood CA Jr, Williams GR: The shoulder impingement syndrome: Management of surgical treatment failures. *Orthop Trans* 1992;16:739–740.
30. Matthews LS, Burkhead WZ, Gordon S, et al: Acromial fracture complicating arthroscopic subacromial decompression. *J Shoulder Elbow Surg* 1994;3:256–261.
31. Armstrong JR: Excision of the acromion in treatment of the supraspinatus syndrome: Report of ninety-five excisions. *J Bone Joint Surg* 1949;31B:436–442.
32. Hammond G: Complete acromionectomy in the treatment of chronic tendinitis of the shoulder: A follow-up of ninety operations on

eighty-seven patients. *J Bone Joint Surg* 1971;53A:173–180.

33. McLaughlin HL: Lesions of the musculotendinous cuff of the shoulder: I. The exposure and treatment of tears with retraction. *J Bone Joint Surg* 1944;26:31–51.

34. Smith-Petersen MN, Aufranc OE, Larson CB: Useful surgical procedures for rheumatoid arthritis involving joints of the upper extremity. *Arch Surg* 1943;46:764–770.

35. Neer CS II, Marberry TA: On the disadvantages of radical acromionectomy. *J Bone Joint Surg* 1981;63A:416–419.

36. Neer CS II: Anterior acromioplasty for the chronic impingement syndrome in the shoulder: A preliminary report. *J Bone Joint Surg* 1972;54A:41–50.

37. Bigliani LU, Rodosky MW: Techniques of repair of large rotator cuff tears. *Tech Orthop* 1994;9:133–140.

38. Burkhead WZ Jr, Scheinberg RR, Box G: Surgical anatomy of the axillary nerve. *J Shoulder Elbow Surg* 1992;1:31–36.

39. Petrucci FS, Morelli A, Raimondi PL: Axillary nerve injuries: 21 cases treated by nerve graft and neurolysis. *J Hand Surg* 1982;7A:271–278.

40. Leffert RD: Neurological problems, in Rockwood CA Jr, Matsen FA III (eds): *The Shoulder.* Philadelphia, PA, WB Saunders, 1990, vol 2, pp 750–773.

41. Lazarus MD, Yung SW, Sidles JA, et al: Abstract: Anterosuperior humeral displacement: Limitation by the coracoacromial arch. *J Shoulder Elbow Surg* 1996;5:S7.

42. Moorman CT III, Deng XH, Warren RF, et al: Abstract: The coracoacromial ligament: Is it the appendix of the shoulder? *J Shoulder Elbow Surg* 1996;5(suppl):S9.

43. Flatow EL, Pollock RG, Bigliani LU: Coracoacromial ligament preservation in rotator cuff surgery. *Tech Orthop* 1994;9:97–98.

44. Mormino MA, Gross RM, McCarthy JA: Captured shoulder: A complication of rotator cuff surgery. *Arthroscopy* 1996;12:457–461.

45. Calvert PT, Packer NP, Stoker DJ, et al: Arthrography of the shoulder after operative repair of the torn rotator cuff. *J Bone Joint Surg* 1986;68B:147–150.

46. Mink JH, Harris E, Rappaport M: Rotator cuff tears: Evaluation using double-contrast shoulder arthrography. *Radiology* 1985;157:621–623.

47. Stiles RG, Otte MT: Imaging of the shoulder. *Radiology* 1993;188:603–613.

48. Drakeford MK, Quinn MJ, Simpson SL, et al: A comparative study of ultrasonography and arthrography in evaluation of the rotator cuff. *Clin Orthop* 1990;253:118–122.

49. Olive RJ Jr, Marsh HO: Ultrasonography of rotator cuff tears. *Clin Orthop* 1992;282:110–113.

50. DePalma AF, Callery G, Bennett GA: Part I: Variational anatomy and degenerative lesions of the shoulder joint, in Blount WP, Banks SW (eds): American Academy of Orthopaedic Surgeons *Instructional Course Lectures VI.* Ann Arbor, MI, JW Edwards, 1949, pp 255–281.

51. Harryman DT II, Mack LA, Wang KY, et al: Repairs of the rotator cuff: Correlation of functional results with integrity of the cuff. *J Bone Joint Surg* 1991;73A:982–989.

52. Sher JS, Uribe JW, Posada A, et al: Abnormal findings on magnetic resonance images of asymptomatic shoulders. *J Bone Joint Surg* 1995;77A:10–15.

53. Rockwood CA Jr: The management of patients with massive rotator cuff defects by acromioplasty and rotator cuff debridement. *Orthop Trans* 1986;10:622.

54. Rockwood CA, Williams GR, Burkhead WZ: Debridement of degenerative, irreparable lesions of the rotator cuff. *J Bone Joint Surg* 1995;77A:857–866.

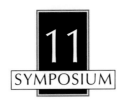

Instability of the Shoulder: Complex Problems and Failed Repairs: Part I. Relevant Biomechanics, Multidirectional Instability, and Severe Glenoid Loss

Evan L. Flatow, MD

Jon J.P. Warner, MD

Historically, much of the literature on glenohumeral instability has concerned recurrent locked anterior glenohumeral dislocation. As the standard objective of surgical intervention was the elimination of such a dislocation, many operations yielded a high proportion of successful results. However, increased attention to the special needs of active, athletic individuals has led to a higher standard for the success of surgical reconstruction: the maintenance of full motion and strength in addition to the restoration of stability. Modern repair procedures avoid over-tightening and emphasize restoration of the integrity of the capsular-ligamentous-labral complex. Although there is controversy as to whether an operation for uni-directional anterior instability should include a capsulorrhaphy in addition to repair of a Bankart lesion, most investigators agree that no more than a minor capsular tightening, with no procedure on bone, is needed for this most common type of shoulder instability.[1-4]

The situation is understandably more complex in the small number of patients in whom the instability of the shoulder is associated with more severe anatomic distortions. The recognition that symptomatic glenohumeral translations could occur in multiple directions in shoulders with global capsular laxity led to the development of more extensive capsular reconstructions. Furthermore, although capsular and ligamentous structures are usually the major sites of abnormality, in

Table 1 Anatomic factors affecting the stability of the shoulder		
Factor	**Function**	**Abnormality**
Congruity of articular surface	Concavity-compression effect	Glenoid dysplasia, fracture, Hill-Sachs lesion, and reverse Hill-Sachs lesion
Glenoid labrum	Increased depth of socket and surface area; anchoring point for ligaments and capsule	Bankart lesion
Negative intra-articular pressure	Vacuum effect	Capsular rupture, defect of the rotator interval, capsular laxity, and capsular injury
Coracohumeral ligament/superior glenohumeral ligament	Limits external rotation and inferior translation in adduction and posterior translation in flexion	Lesion of the rotator interval
Middle glenohumeral ligament	Limits external rotation and inferior translation in adduction and anterior translation in mid-abduction	Bankart lesion and capsular injury
Inferior glenohumeral ligament complex	Limits anterior, posterior, and inferior translation in abduction	Bankart lesion and capsular injury
Posterior aspect of the capsule	Limits posterior translation in the flexed, adducted, and internally rotated shoulder	Posterior capsular laxity and injury
Rotator cuff	Dynamic compression of the joint; steering effect	Overuse injury (fatigue) and rupture
Biceps (long head)	Dynamic restraint to anterior and superior translation	Lesion of the superior portion of the labrum, anterior and posterior (SLAP lesion) and rupture

(Reproduced with permission from Warner JJP, Schulte KR, Imhoff AB: Current concepts in shoulder instability. *Adv Op Orthop* 1995;3:219.)

unusual instances severe loss of glenoid bone or a large humeral impression fracture may require surgical treatment.

Little information is available to guide the clinician in the care of these difficult problems as reports in the literature and discussions at meetings have tended to

focus on recurrent anterior glenohumeral instability, especially with regard to the choice between open and arthroscopic techniques. The purpose of this chapter is to review the evaluation and management of patients who have multidirectional instability, major loss of bone from

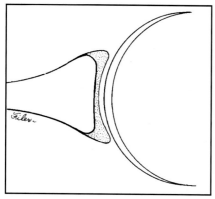

Fig. 1 The glenohumeral joint. The subchondral bone of the glenoid is less curved than the humerus, but the articular cartilage of the glenoid is thicker peripherally, so that the true articular surfaces are, in fact, highly conforming. Because the surface area of the glenoid is far smaller than that of the humerus, the articular surfaces provide less stability in the shoulder than do those in the hip, where the socket is larger and contains a large portion of the femoral head. (Reproduced with permission from Warner JJP, Caborn DNM: Overview of instability. *Crit Rev Phys Rehab Med* 1992;4:149.)

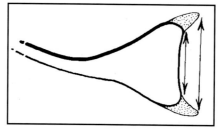

Fig. 2 The glenoid labrum extends around the perimeter of the glenoid and increases the surface area (arrows) and depth of the glenoid socket. (Reproduced with permission from Warner JJP, Caborn DNM: Overview of instability. *Crit Rev Phys Rehab Med* 1992;4:149.)

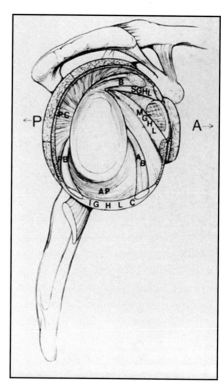

Fig. 3 The capsuloligamentous anatomy, viewed from the side with the anterior aspect (A) to the right and the posterior aspect (P) to the left. The humeral head has been removed, leaving the glenoid and the superior glenohumeral (SGHL) and middle glenohumeral (MGHL) ligaments. The inferior glenohumeral ligament complex (IGHLC) consists of an anterior band (AB), a posterior band (PB), and the interposed axillary pouch (AP). The posterior capsule (PC) is the area proximal to the posterior band. B = biceps. (Reproduced with permission from O'Brien SJ, Neves MC, Arnoczky SP, et al: The anatomy and histology of the inferior glenohumeral ligament complex of the shoulder. *Am J Sports Med* 1990;18:449–456.)

the glenoid, or a large humeral impression fracture, each of which substantially increases the level of complexity of surgical reconstruction.

Biomechanical Considerations

An effective approach to the management of glenohumeral instability, with either primary or revision surgery, depends on a clear understanding of the normal anatomy and biomechanics of the shoulder. The history of the treatment of shoulder instability is based on an evolving understanding of the unique anatomic aspects of this joint, which allow it to have a huge range of motion but also to remain stable.[5] Although some early approaches such as the Bristow-Latarjet procedure[6] were designed to constrain the motion of this joint or to distort the anatomy in order to substitute for injured structures such as the capsule and the labrum, more contemporary approaches have been directed toward the restoration of normal

anatomy and selective correction of the abnormality encountered in each patient. An increased understanding of the contribution of both static and dynamic soft-tissue and osseous factors to the stability of this joint has led to a more accurate appreciation of the spectrum of abnormality that contributes to instability (Table 1). With all approaches to the treatment of instability, the surgeon should consider which anatomic factor or factors are abnormal in each patient and should then address each factor systematically.

Static Stabilizers

Articular Anatomy Although the glenohumeral joint surfaces are congruent (Fig. 1), the surface areas of the larger humeral head and the smaller glenoid fossa do not match.[7,8] This congruent articulation allows for a very secure concavity-compression effect, which is created by the rotator cuff as it dynamically compresses the humeral head into the matched concavity of the glenoid.[9] Furthermore, the fibrocartilaginous labrum, which extends around the perimeter of the glenoid, increases the depth and surface area of the articulation[10] (Fig. 2) and enhances the stability of the joint.

These joint surfaces are related to one another by the orientation of the proximal part of the humerus and the glenoid.

Within a wide range of normal retrotorsion for the humerus and retroversion or anteversion for the glenoid, the joint surfaces maintain contact with one another during active overhead motions in both work and sports activities.[11–14]

Any injury that distorts the relationship of the joint surfaces or their congruity may manifest as instability[15–20] (Table 1). For example, a glenoid fracture that results in a loss of concavity of the glenoid leads to a loss of the normal con-

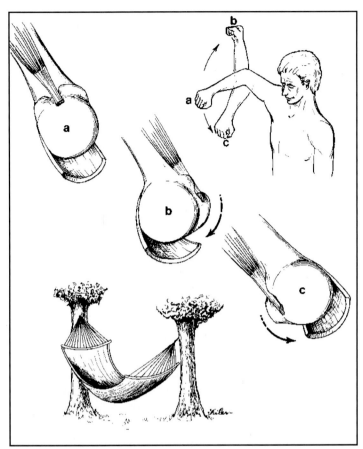
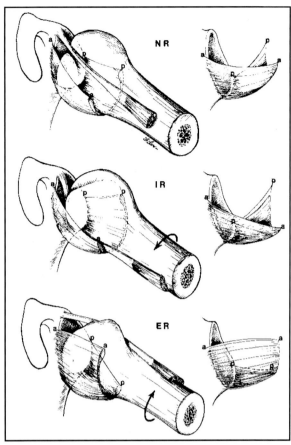

Fig 4. Left, Drawing of the hammock-like anatomy of the inferior glenohumeral ligament complex, which allows for reciprocal tightening of its anterior and posterior portions when the arm moves from neutral rotation in abduction (a) to external rotation (b) and to internal rotation (c). (Reproduced with permission from Warner JJP, Caborn DNM: Overview of instability. *Crit Rev Phys Rehab Med* 1992;4:151.) **Right,** Orientation changes of the anterior band (aa) and the posterior band (pp) during neutral (NR), internal (IR), and external rotation (ER). (Reproduced with permission from Warner JJP, Caborn DNM, Berger R, et al: Dynamic capsuloligamentous anatomy of the glenohumeral joint. *J Shoulder Elbow Surg* 1993;2:131.)

cavity-compression mechanism. A Bankart lesion[3,9] also can disrupt the normal concavity-compression relationship of the joint in addition to representing a detachment of the origin of the glenohumeral ligaments. Other osseous lesions that can affect the normal articular relationships include a large Hill-Sachs lesion[3,21–24] or congenital dysplasia[25] of the joint surfaces.

Articular and labral injuries may exist alone or in combination with other abnormalities, and all of them must be carefully identified and corrected. The goal of treatment is to reconstruct the normal relationships between the articular surfaces.

Capsuloligamentous Structures

The thin capsular tissue is reinforced by collagenous thickenings, which are termed ligaments and may have the appearance of band-like structures[26] (Fig. 3). Different regions of the capsule each play an important role in the constraint of the humeral head in the glenoid and the prevention of excessive translations and rotations of the joint.[27–33] During rotation of the arm, the glenohumeral ligaments and capsule tighten and loosen reciprocally (Fig. 4), thus limiting translations and rotations in a load-sharing fashion.[5] When the shoulder is in a mid-range of rotation, these capsuloligamentous structures are relatively lax and most stability is maintained by the rotator cuff and the biceps, which create a

concavity-compression effect across this articulation.[9,34,35] Any surgical procedure that tightens the capsule and ligaments with the arm in this mid-range of rotation, risks constraining the joint and preventing rotation.[36,37] The Putti-Platt procedure, for example, may cause loss of external rotation. Furthermore, an overly tight anterior repair can lead to posterior humeral subluxation with the joint load focused on the posterior part of the glenoid,[38,39] which may be a factor in the development of arthrosis after tight instability repairs.[40]

The capsuloligamentous structures also may provide afferent feedback that modulates contraction of the rotator cuff during active motion of the shoulder.[41]

This feedback may occur through the sensory modality of proprioception.

Although there is substantial variation in the development and robustness of portions of the capsule and ligaments, the ligamentous or band-like components can be seen consistently on arthroscopic inspection. However, it is important to remember that only the synovial surface of the capsule can be observed with the arthroscope. Thin, flimsy synovial tissue can appear robust and impressive if pleated or folded by the rotation of the arm. Conversely, a band of capsular thickening may be indistinguishable from the surrounding capsule. Only recently has information about the structural and material properties of these ligaments been gained.

The material properties of the inferior glenohumeral ligament have been investigated extensively. The strength of the inferior glenohumeral ligament in tension has been found to be far lower than that of the knee ligaments, which is to be expected as the shoulder ligaments share load with the muscles and other stabilizing mechanisms.[14] Another interesting finding is that regions of the inferior glenohumeral ligament become stronger and stiffer at higher strain rates,[42] suggesting a functional adaptation that stabilizes the humeral head during high-speed athletic activities, when the muscles may be surprised or fatigued.

When loaded in tension, the inferior glenohumeral ligament was found to fail most commonly at the glenoid insertion, which is analogous to a Bankart avulsion, and in its mid-substance, which might be expected to result in capsular stretching and laxity.[14] However, there was substantial strain in the mid-substance before failure even in the ligaments that ultimately tore at the glenoid insertion. Recently, a study of repetitive loading of the inferior glenohumeral ligament at increasing levels of subfailure strain demonstrated dramatic decreases in peak force with unrecovered elongation.[43] These findings suggest that the capsule may be subject to plastic deformation, especially after repetitive trauma.

Repetitive injuries from athletic activities often stretch out many different parts of the capsule, as each episode stresses only the portion of the capsule that was taut in the particular position in which the arm was injured. The reason that acquired laxity, such as that seen in gymnasts or in swimmers who perform the butterfly stroke, is often multidirectional may be that the cumulative effect of multiple minor injuries with the arm in various positions is a globally lax capsule. Conversely, a single violent traumatic episode would tend to focus the worst damage more to a specific region; for example, a traumatic anterior dislocation would result in a Bankart avulsion with anteroinferior capsular stretch.

Intraoperative determination of the region of injury of the capsule and ligaments is important when deciding on the best method of treatment. Labral detachment (a Bankart lesion), humeral detachment, or intraligamentous rupture can occur. Debate continues about the importance of a Bankart lesion compared with a capsular injury. Some surgeons favor isolated Bankart repair, whereas others believe an associated capsular shift is necessary to treat a concomitant capsular injury.[3,14,24,37,44–47]

Laxity Compared with Instability
Laxity is a necessary attribute of the capsule and ligaments of the shoulder and allows for the normal large range of motion of this joint. Instability, however, is abnormal symptomatic motion of the humeral head relative to the glenoid during active shoulder motion. As the parameters of normal laxity are quite variable, confusion may develop if an examiner tries to define instability only on the basis of passive movement of the humeral head relative to the glenoid with the patient under anesthesia.[34,35,48–52] The surgeon must be very careful to correlate the laxity perceived on examination with the patient under anesthesia with the symptoms and physical findings observed on examination when the patient is awake.[37,44] A shoulder that can be subluxated when the patient is under anesthesia may or may not be truly unstable. Certainly, many young athletic individuals have relatively lax shoulders, and the assumption that the pain in such an individual is due to instability that necessitates repair with a capsular shift procedure may be erroneous.

Dynamic Stabilizers
Rotator Cuff The rotator cuff is a complex of four muscles that encircle the humeral head and are conjoined to regions of the joint capsule. These muscles function primarily to stabilize the humeral head in the glenoid and secondarily to move the joint surfaces relative to one another.[53,54] The rotator cuff has two major stabilizing mechanisms: concavity-compression[9,10] and synchronous coordinated contraction of the muscle units that steer the humeral head into the glenoid during motion of the arm.[55,56]

Injury of the rotator cuff can occur from a single traumatic event or from cumulative trauma, as with repetitive overhead throwing motions. In either case, instability can result. The goal of treatment, either by physical therapy or by surgery, should be to restore the function of the rotator cuff.

Long Head of the Biceps Brachii Studies have shown that the long head of the biceps brachii has an important dynamic stabilizing role for both anterior and superior translation of the humeral head.[53,57–59] Injury of the origin of the tendon (a so-called SLAP lesion; superior portion of the labrum, anterior, and posterior) often is observed in association with instability, and it may represent the failure of a dynamic stabilizing mechanism.[60,61]

Additional Factors Affecting Stability
Glenohumeral stability also is affected by negative intra-articular pressure and by scapulothoracic motion. Negative intra-

articular pressure develops in the sealed compartment of the joint, and it is basically a vacuum effect that prevents the joint surfaces from being displaced away from one another. The magnitude of this stabilizing force is relatively small compared with the force of muscle contraction, and it functions mainly to keep the joint surfaces opposed in the relaxed dependent arm.[62–64] Any condition that vents the capsule, such as a tear or defect of the rotator interval, reduces this stabilizing effect.

Normal scapulothoracic motion is essential for normal glenohumeral function. Patients who have shoulder instability often have abnormal scapulothoracic motion, and sometimes they may have frank winging of the scapula.[65–67] Whether scapulothoracic dysfunction is primary or secondary in these patients, it has several important biomechanical consequences for the glenohumeral joint. First, failure of the scapula to rotate properly so that the glenoid remains underneath the rotating humeral head increases the tendency for instability because of loss of the stable glenoid platform on which the humeral head can rotate. Second, if the scapula wings, the coracoacromial arch will descend relative to the advancing greater tuberosity and the patient will have functional impingement.[67] Therefore, it is imperative for the orthopaedic surgeon to assess scapulothoracic function in a patient who has shoulder instability. In shoulders in which instability is treated nonsurgically, muscle rehabilitation should include the axioscapular stabilizers (the serratus anterior, trapezius, and rhomboid muscles) as well as the rotator-cuff muscles.

In conclusion, in order to treat shoulder instability successfully, the physician must consider all static and dynamic factors that stabilize the joint. Isolated lesions as well as combined conditions must be identified and treated according to sound principles of anatomy and biomechanics.

Multidirectional Instability

The most common form of shoulder instability is recurrent anterior subluxation or dislocation. When this condition is initiated by a major traumatic event, there is often detachment or stripping of the labrum and the inferior glenohumeral ligament complex from the anteroinferior aspect of the glenoid (a Bankart lesion).[68–70] Most investigators[1–4,12,47] agree on the need to repair this lesion, but there is debate about whether a concomitant capsulorrhaphy is needed. Thomas and Matsen[4] argued that most patients who have unidirectional anterior instability of traumatic onset need only a repair of the Bankart lesion. However, the translations induced by a Bankart lesion in an experiment were found to be small (inadequate to allow a complete dislocation).[46] Indeed, Jobe (personal communication, 1990) noted that, geometrically, in order for the labrum to pull away from the glenoid, both the labrum and the attached capsule must deform (for example, the way a turtleneck collar stretches while being pulled off over the head). Early arthroscopic repairs that focused only on the Bankart lesion thus may have had a high rate of failure because, as minimally invasive procedures, they did not cause scarring of the lax capsule. In contrast, open approaches either include an explicit capsulorrhaphy or at least reduce capsular laxity through scarring. In any event, a wide variety of anterior reconstructions have been found to be effective for the treatment of unidirectional anterior glenohumeral instability. Multidirectional instability is more complex. Bankart lesions are less frequent, and capsular laxity becomes the dominant abnormality.

In 1980, Neer and Foster[45] reviewed the literature on glenohumeral instability[11,71–73] and introduced a new type of capsular procedure, which they termed inferior capsular shift, for reconstruction of multidirectional instability. In that and subsequent reports,[2,45,74,75] Neer emphasized several points. (1) Shoulders may become loose not only because of trauma and inherent ligamentous laxity but also because of repetitive minor injury and stress (as occurs in swimming the butterfly stroke or performing gymnastics). These stresses are often an important factor in the development of multidirectional instability. (2) Not all loose shoulders are painful, and the surgeon must be convinced that the instability is symptomatic before considering repair. (3) Standard anterior repairs may correct multidirectional instability incompletely, resulting in persistent symptomatic inferior and posterior instability. (4) Overly tight anterior repairs may tighten the joint asymmetrically, causing a fixed subluxation to the posterior side, which can result in arthrosis. (5) Rehabilitation of the muscles that stabilize the humerus is important not only in nonsurgical management but also to protect the repair postoperatively, as "the capsule and ligaments normally function only as a check-rein."[45]

Multidirectional instability is defined as symptomatic glenohumeral instability in more than one direction: anterior, inferior, and posterior.[2,45,74–80] There has been controversy about whether multidirectional and unidirectional instability are always distinct conditions or just extreme examples from a continuing degree of joint laxity, as has been proposed by Bigliani and associates.[12] The latter approach suggests that varying degrees of capsulorrhaphy may be necessary depending on the lesion that is encountered.

Clinical Presentation
Although extremely hypermobile shoulders can become symptomatic without unusual trauma, there may be a discrete injury that initiates symptoms. Repetitive stress on the shoulder from athletic activities or work-related events, often is involved. Patients who have multidirec-

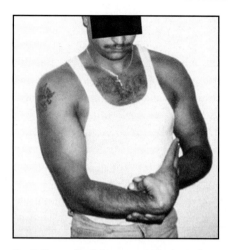 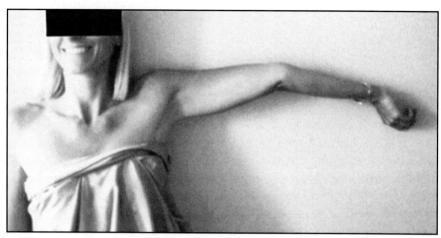

Fig. 5 Generalized ligamentous laxity. **Left,** Laxity of the thumb is demonstrated by this patient who can approximate the thumb to the forearm. **Right,** Laxity of the elbow is demonstrated by this patient who can hyperextend the elbow. (Reproduced with permission from Bigliani LU (ed): *The Unstable Shoulder.* Rosemont, IL, The American Academy of Orthopaedic Surgeons, 1996, p 81.)

tional instability report recurrent subluxation and a sense of instability more commonly than locked dislocation. When dislocations occur, they often do so without a major injury and spontaneously reduce or can be reduced by the patient. It is important to evaluate the history of each patient carefully for suggestions of voluntary instability.[73]

Symptoms may be vague, but they can suggest the directions of instability involved. Pain in the overhead, abducted, and externally rotated position is associated with anterior instability. Discomfort with the arm in forward elevation and internal rotation (for example, when pushing open heavy doors) suggests posterior instability. Patients who have inferior instability often report pain and paresthesias (traction on the brachial plexus) when carrying heavy objects.

The patient may have a history of laxity of many joints, sometimes involving ankle sprains, patellar dislocations, or other ligament problems. Family members also may have a history of these types of disorders. The role of biochemical abnormalities, generalized laxity syndromes, and defined collagen disorders (for example, Ehlers-Danlos syndrome) in multidirectional instability have been investigated but not well characterized.[49,81-85]

The physical examination may demonstrate generalized joint laxity with findings such as hyperextension at the elbows or the metacarpophalangeal joints or the ability to approximate the thumbs to the forearms (Fig. 5). Laxity of the contralateral shoulder may be a clue to the multidirectional nature of the instability. Scapulothoracic instability with scapular mistracking may coexist with glenohumeral instability, and the examiner should look for this disorder.[2]

The key part of the examination is to elicit unwanted glenohumeral translations that reliably reproduce the symptoms (Fig. 6). This is not always easy because laxity may be dramatic but asymptomatic, and symptomatic instability may be impossible to demonstrate if pain, muscle spasm, and guarding prevent subluxation. There are many maneuvers to demonstrate instability, including the anterior and posterior apprehension tests, the anterior and posterior load and shift tests, the fulcrum test, the relocation test, the Fukuda test, and the push-pull or stress test with the patient supine.[2,45,86,87] The sulcus sign (inferior sag of the humerus with the arm at the side) and inferior translation of the abducted humerus are especially helpful for elucidating inferior laxity.[45]

Plain radiographs of a shoulder with multidirectional glenohumeral instability generally demonstrate normal findings, but they should be evaluated for the presence of humeral head defects or glenoid lesions (such as osseous Bankart fragments), or both, and for reactive bone or wear. Regular or computed tomographic (CT) arthrograms may demonstrate an increased capsular volume and, less commonly, labral detachments. Magnetic resonance imaging (MRI) may demonstrate labral lesions and chondral wear. It also may reveal capsular laxity, although it does so somewhat less reliably than arthrography because of the lack of joint distention. Evaluation of multidirectional glenohumeral instability with stress radiographs and cine MRI has been described, but these studies generally are not used.[88,89]

Nonsurgical Treatment
Multidirectional instability usually can be treated nonsurgically, and this approach is tried in all patients initially. Rehabilitation is designed to strengthen

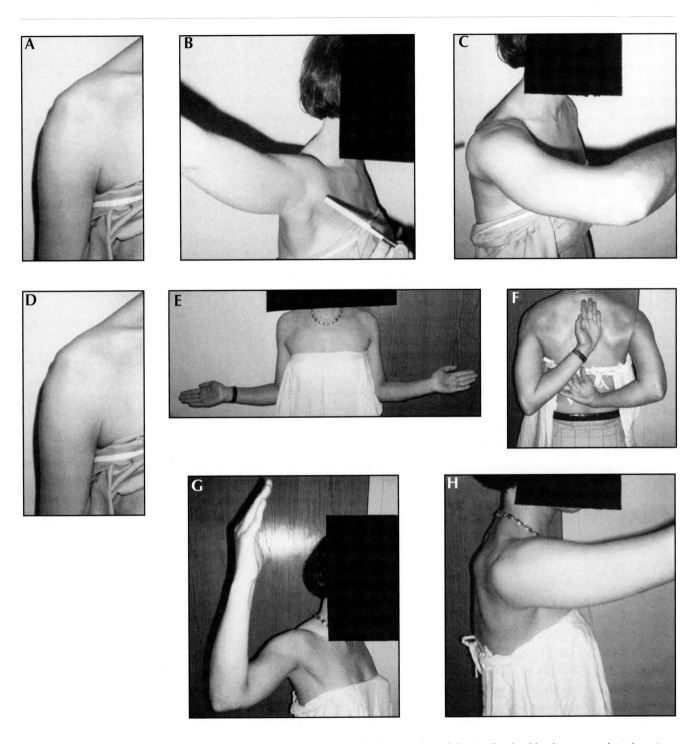

Fig. 6. Top, Preoperative photographs of a 22-year-old woman who had multidirectional instability. **A,** The shoulder demonstrated a sulcus sign of 3+ as the arm was pulled distally by the examiner (not shown). **B,** The shoulder subluxated anteriorly when the arm was extended and externally rotated. The instability was symptomatic and prevented overhead activities. **C,** The shoulder dislocated posteriorly when the arm was flexed and internally rotated. The patient was unable to reach for objects or to push open doors. **Bottom,** Photographs made 7 years after treatment with an inferior capsular shift from a posterior approach. **D,** Elevation. **E,** External rotation. **F,** Slight loss of internal rotation. **G,** The shoulder had no anterior subluxation when the arm was extended and externally rotated. The shoulder was stable and strong, and the patient was able to use the arm overhead for athletic activities. **H,** The shoulder did not dislocate posteriorly when the arm was flexed and internally rotated.

the deltoid, rotator cuff, and scapular stabilizers.[90,91] Studies of patients who had generalized laxity and instability of the shoulder have demonstrated imbalances in muscle coordination[92] and deficits in shoulder joint proprioception.[41] The aim of treatment is to improve muscle tone and coordination and generally to increase the patient's functional adaptation.

Activities are modified to avoid movements that cause symptoms in the shoulder. A brief course of non-steroidal, anti-inflammatory medication may be helpful when chronic joint discomfort results from secondary inflammation. Occasionally, secondary bursitis or rotator-cuff tendinitis may develop, causing shoulder pain that prevents the patient from performing the indicated exercises. In this rare situation, a subacromial injection of a steroid preparation may provide sufficient relief for the patient to resume the exercise regimen.

Surgical reconstruction is considered only if the patient does not respond to a lengthy program of conservative treatment (usually a minimum of 6 months). Most surgeons try to refrain from operating on a patient younger than 16 years of age, because glenohumeral instability may decrease as the normal laxity of adolescence diminishes with age and because nonsurgical treatment avoids injury to the important proximal humeral physeal plate.

It is important to avoid surgery on a patient who is voluntarily dislocating the shoulder.[73] Patients who have this syndrome may have underlying psychiatric problems and are able to use asymmetric muscle pull to dislocate the shoulder, often maintaining the position despite attempted manipulations by perplexed physicians in front of distraught parents.[93,94] However, overt psychiatric disturbance often is difficult to identify, and patients may have more subtle types of secondary gain or just may have a habitually improper pattern of muscle coordination that results in subluxation.

Whatever the cause, individuals who voluntarily dislocate the shoulder with use of their own muscles (so-called muscular dislocators) are poor candidates for stabilization procedures. These patients should be managed with skillful neglect of the shoulder in conjunction with strengthening and retraining of the muscles as well as treatment of any underlying psychological disorder.

Not all patients who can demonstrate shoulder instability to the examiner are voluntary dislocators. Even if the instability is involuntary or began after substantial trauma, many patients learn which positions to avoid (for example, forward elevation and internal rotation in a patient prone to posterior subluxation). Such individuals, described as positional dislocators, may demonstrate dislocation for the examiner, if requested, but otherwise do their best to avoid it. These patients generally are good candidates for surgical reconstruction.

Surgical Technique
The most widely used reconstruction is the one described by Neer and Foster[45] or a modification of it. The procedure is designed to reduce capsular volume on all sides of the capsule by thickening and overlapping the anterior aspect of the capsule, if the procedure is carried out through an anterior approach, after completely detaching the inferior aspect of the capsule around the neck of the humerus to reduce the capsular pouch. The inferior portion of the capsule is then shifted anteriorly to increase the tension on the posterior aspect of the capsule so that it equals the tension on the anterior aspect. Neer termed the procedure the inferior capsular shift because of the novel feature of tensioning both the anterior and the posterior aspect of the capsule through one approach by shifting the inferior aspect of the capsule. The procedure occasionally has been misinterpreted as an operation performed primarily or exclusively

on the inferior aspect of the capsule. When done through a posterior approach, the procedure on the anterior and posterior aspects of the capsule is reversed.

Examination with the patient under anesthesia can be very helpful with regard to confirming the components of instability. The shoulder is tested for anterior, inferior, and posterior translations in a variety of positions to bring different portions of the capsule and ligament system into play. Although it is rare to change the approach that was determined by preoperative clinical assessment, a surprising finding should not be ignored. Examination with the patient under anesthesia is most helpful when preoperative pain and spasm have precluded a revealing examination in the office.

The goal of treatment is to balance the capsular tension on all sides, and usually this can be accomplished through one surgical approach, anterior or posterior. Although Cooper and Brems[95] reported that they always performed an anterior approach, many surgeons use an approach on the side of the greatest instability as it is the side that will be best reinforced and strengthened by the overlap of flaps and the scar from the surgical approach.[2,13,76] Shoulders that dislocate both anteriorly and posteriorly usually are approached from the anterior side.

Anterior Approach for Inferior Capsular Shift The details of the operative technique have been previously described.[45,76,94] The patient is anesthetized with either regional (scalene block) or general anesthesia, and a concealed axillary skin incision leading to a deltopectoral approach is used. Subscapularis-splitting approaches have been helpful for discrete anterior capsular repairs of unidirectional anterior subluxation.[1] However, anatomic detachment and repair of the subscapularis is preferred as part of the approach for capsular

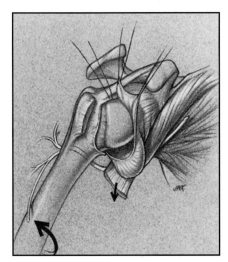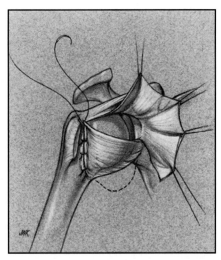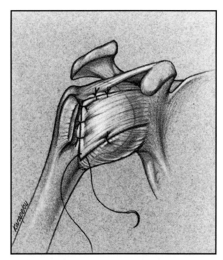

Fig. 7 An inferior capsular shift performed from an anterior approach. **Left,** The subscapularis tendon (straight arrow) is detached. Then the capsule is detached laterally, leaving a cuff for repair. As the humerus is externally rotated (curved arrow), the capsule is detached from around the humeral neck. The extent of this release—that is, how far around the neck posteriorly to detach the capsule—is tailored to the size of the pouch and the degree of instability present. **Center,** The inferior flap of the laterally-based T-capsulorrhaphy is brought anteriorly and superiorly. **Right,** The rotator interval is closed, and the superior flap is brought down and across the inferior flap. This procedure thickens and reinforces the capsule on the side of the approach, while the shift of the inferior aspect of the capsule tensions (but cannot thicken) the opposite (posterior) side. (Reproduced with permission from Bigliani LU: Anterior and posterior capsular shift for multidirectional instability, in Paulos LE, Tibone JE (eds): *Operative Techniques in Shoulder Surgery.* Gaithersburg, MD, Aspen, 1991, pp 138–139.)

shift repairs of multidirectional instability for two major reasons. First, these repairs necessitate the detachment of the capsule around the inferior part of the humeral neck, which generally requires external rotation of the humerus. However, external rotation of the humerus tends to tension the subscapularis and to close any attempted subscapularis-splitting approach. Second, a large portion of the capsule must be freed from adhesions and attachments to surrounding tendons in order to be shifted and therefore must be freed from the overlying subscapularis tendon in particular.

Neer and Foster[45] referred to the gap between the supraspinatus and subscapularis as the rotator interval and termed the deeper layer at the same location the cleft between the superior and middle glenohumeral ligaments. They believed that this cleft was generally enlarged in patients who had multidirectional instability. Neer and Foster described closing the cleft and drawing the superior flap tight to cause the middle

glenohumeral ligament (and the attached superior glenohumeral ligament) to "act as a sling against inferior subluxation."[45] Recent biomechanical studies have confirmed this view by showing the antero-superior (rotator-interval) aspect of the capsule to be important for inferior stability of the adducted arm.[33] Indeed, some surgeons have found that, in certain patients, the major lesion is in this region and isolated closure of rotator-interval defects may be all that is needed surgically.[96] However, in shoulders with multidirectional instability, closure of the rotator interval is just one part of a global capsular tensioning.

Standard anterior capsulorrhaphies may be done in a variety of fashions. When a capacious capsule in a shoulder with multidirectional instability needs reconstruction, many investigators have preferred the lateral T-capsulorrhaphy described by Neer and Foster.[45] The capsule can be shifted most effectively to reduce capsular volume where the capsular circumference is largest, which is in

the lateral aspect. Nevertheless, medial T-capsulorrhaphies or even H-capsulorrhaphies (reconstruction in which the vertical limbs of the incision are made both medially and laterally) have been used.[44]

Stay sutures are placed in the free edge of the capsule as it is detached (Fig. 7). As the humerus is externally rotated and flexed, the capsule is incised around the neck of the humerus. A finger may be placed in the inferior pouch to assess how large it is and how much redundant capsule needs to be released from the humerus before repair. The inferior portion of the capsule has been shown to be important for inferior stability of the abducted arm.[33] In an anterior approach to a shoulder with classic multidirectional instability, the capsule is detached all the way down to its posterior aspect, which then can be tensioned as the detached inferior aspect of the capsule is shifted anteriorly.

If there is detachment of the glenohumeral ligament complex (a Broca-

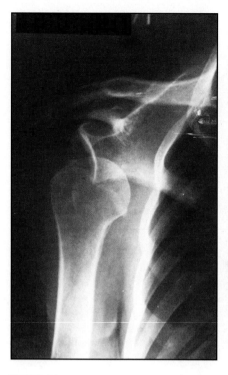 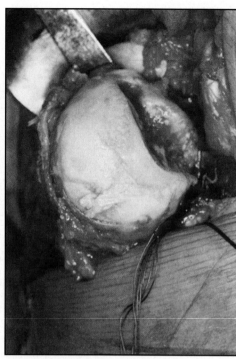

Fig. 8 Left, Chronic unreduced anterior dislocation in an elderly patient. **Right,** An enormous humeral impression fracture was seen at the open reconstruction. The fracture was treated with a humeral head replacement.

Perthes-Bankart lesion), it is repaired through an inside-out approach in conjunction with the capsular procedure. Ligament detachments occur in shoulders with multidirectional instability, although less frequently. As patients who have multidirectional instability frequently have symptoms in the midrange, where the ligaments often are lax, it has been suggested that containment of the humeral head by the glenoid and labrum may also be impaired (D Harryman, MD, personal communication, 1995). Bigliani (personal communication, 1994) has used a so-called barrel stitch (a superior-inferior imbricating stitch just lateral to the labrum) during open reconstruction, and others (D Harryman, MD, personal communication, 1995) have used arthroscopic pleating of the capsule adjacent to the labrum (sewing a fold of capsule side-to-side to the labrum) to remove capsular stretch medially and to build up the height of the glenoid rim, deepening the socket to help to contain the head.

The capsular flaps are overlapped and repaired with the arm in a balanced position of slight external rotation and slight flexion. Warner and associates[97] suggested that it might be desirable to repair the superior flap with the arm adducted and the inferior flap with the arm abducted, as these are the positions that tension those areas, according to basic science studies.

Arthroscopic capsular tensioning[98] and arthroscopic laser contraction of the capsule[99] have both been described for the treatment of multidirectional instability. However, because stiffness is a less frequent problem than recurrent instability after repairs for multidirectional instability and because most surgeons place the upper extremity in a brace or cast for 6 weeks after the operation in an attempt to achieve stability, the value of minimally invasive surgery is less obvious.

The upper extremity is immobilized in neutral rotation (to allow symmetrical healing of the anterior and posterior aspects of the capsule) for 6 weeks, and only gentle isometric exercises and

supervised motion of the elbow are permitted during that time. At 6 weeks, use of the brace is discontinued and range-of-motion exercises are gradually introduced. At 12 weeks, progressive strengthening is instituted on an individualized basis. When repetitive microtrauma is the dominant etiology and excessive generalized laxity is not present, the rehabilitation program may be accelerated. However, when there are multiple loose joints, the major mode of failure usually is recurrent instability from stretching of the repair rather than stiffness; in this situation, the aim of rehabilitation should be to regain shoulder motion slowly over a period of 6 months or more.

When a capsular shift approach is used for intermediate degrees of instability (for example, so-called bidirectional [anterior and inferior] instability), without a substantial posterior component, the upper extremity is protected in a sling for 6 weeks. However, after 10 days, the upper extremity is removed from the sling, and exercises, including

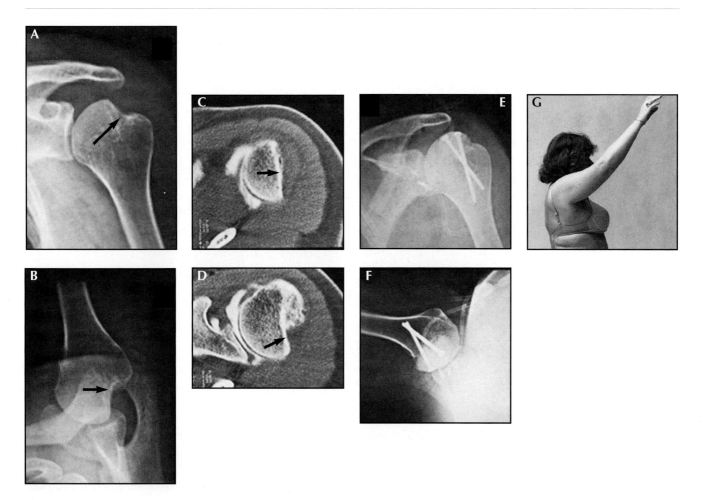

Fig. 9 An active young female patient who had recurrent anterior instability of the shoulder. **A** and **B,** Radiographs showing a large humeral impression defect (arrows). **C** and **D,** Computed tomographic scans showing the large size of the defect (arrows). **E** and **F,** Ligament reconstruction, which was accompanied by reconstruction of the humeral head defect with a segment of an allograft humeral head. **G,** The patient went on to a good functional result.

isometrics and external rotation to 10° as well as forward elevation to 90°, are begun. At 2 to 4 weeks, external rotation is increased to 30°, forward elevation is increased to 140°, and isometric strengthening is added. At 4 to 6 weeks, external rotation is increased to 40°, forward elevation is increased to approximately 160°, and resistive exercises are begun. After 6 weeks, external rotation is increased to 50° and forward elevation, to 180°. After 3 months, external rotation may be progressed. Strengthening begins with the arm in neutral below 90°. Careful and frequent postoperative follow-up is necessary, as patients who are not progressing quickly enough may

need an accelerated program and those who are regaining motion too quickly may need to be slowed down. Return to contact sports generally is restricted until 9 to 12 months have elapsed.

Posterior Approach for Inferior Capsular Shift A variety of skin incisions have been used for a posterior approach. Although oblique or vertical incisions generally leave less prominent scars than transverse incisions, an anterior axillary scar is best from a cosmetic standpoint. For isolated posterior instability, a deltoid split and an infraspinatus-splitting approach to the capsule may allow adequate exposure.[100] An approach under the deltoid also has been used.

However, for an extensive capsular mobilization, many surgeons prefer to detach a small portion of the origin of the posterior part of the deltoid and to detach the infraspinatus.[76]

Capsular mobilization and repair is performed in a manner that is similar to that used for the anterior approach. Again, several methods have been described,[2,74,76] with the classic procedure being a laterally based T-capsulorrhaphy.

After the operation, all patients wear a brace with the shoulder in neutral or slight extension and in slight external rotation for 6 weeks. Thereafter, the pace of mobilization is determined by the degree of generalized laxity, the pace of

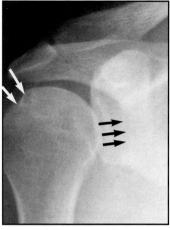
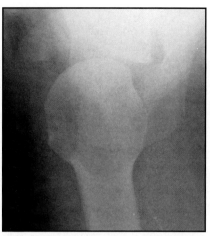
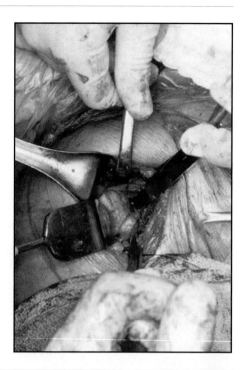

Fig. 10 A young patient who had recurrent anterior dislocation of the shoulder. **Left,** This anteroposterior radiograph shows evidence of a Hill-Sachs lesion (white arrows) and loss of the sclerotic line representing the anteroinferior aspect of the glenoid rim (black arrows). **Center,** The axillary radiograph shows loss of bone from the anteroinferior aspect of the glenoid, which was confirmed by a computed tomographic scan (not shown). **Right,** This intraoperative photograph shows loss of 30% of the anteroinferior aspect of the glenoid.

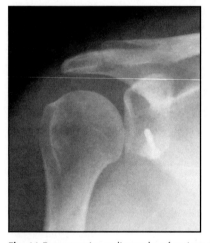
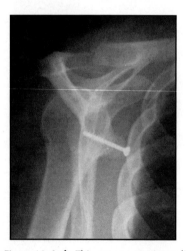
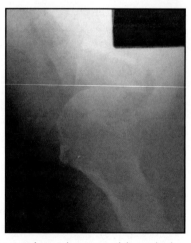

Fig. 11 Postoperative radiographs of patient shown in Figure 10. **Left,** This anteroposterior radiograph shows inferior placement of the graft. The capsule was repaired to the edge of the intact glenoid articular surface, and the coracoid was transferred behind the capsule to reinforce it. **Center,** This lateral radiograph shows anteroinferior placement of the graft. **Right,** The axillary radiograph shows placement of the graft to reconstruct the anterior aspect of the glenoid rim.

healing, and other factors as have been described for repairs from an anterior approach.

Results
Treatment of multidirectional instability with a capsular shift reconstruction has been successful in several studies.[101–103]

Altchek and associates[44] reported good results with use of a T-plasty modification of the Bankart procedure for repair of multidirectional instability. Hawkins and associates[104] reported less favorable results in a series of 31 patients who were followed for 2 to 5 years postoperatively; 12 (39°) had an unsatisfactory result.

In a study by Cooper and Brems,[95] 39 (91%) of 43 shoulders that had been followed for at least 2 years after an inferior capsular shift were rated by the patient as satisfactory with no recurrent instability. Bigliani and associates[13] reviewed a series of 52 shoulders with classic multidirectional instability that had been treated

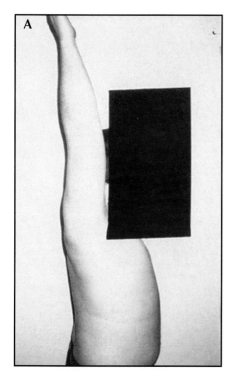

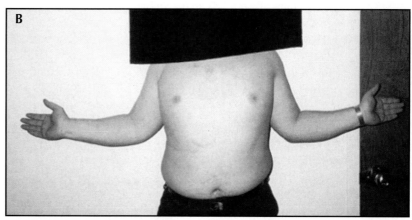

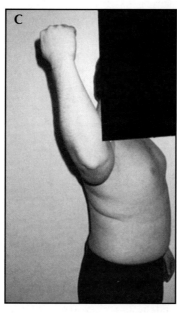

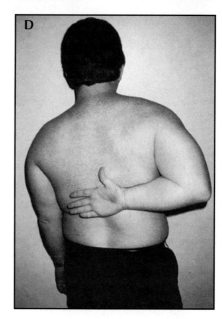

Fig. 12 Photographs of the same patient, made one year postoperatively. **A,** Elevation. **B,** External rotation. **C,** Full external rotation at 90° of elevation. **D,** Full internal rotation.

with an inferior capsular shift. An anterior approach was used in 36 shoulders and a posterior approach in 16. All were completely immobilized in a brace for 6 weeks postoperatively. Forty-six (94%) of the 49 shoulders that had been followed for an average of 5 years (range, 2 to 11 years) had a satisfactory result.

Major Loss of Humeral or Glenoid Bone

Although glenoid wear or fracture and humeral impression fractures are common in unstable shoulders, only rarely are they large enough to warrant specific treatment. When they are, the reconstruction is made much more complex.

Humeral Impression Fractures

Chronic locked anterior and posterior dislocations, especially in older patients who have soft bone, often result in large humeral impression fractures. However, the chronic dislocations are not the same as recurrent dislocations or subluxations, and their treatment has been discussed elsewhere.[105-107] Recurrent posterior instability rarely involves large humeral impression fractures, and little information is available on such cases.

When reconstruction for recurrent anterior dislocation is being done in a shoulder with an unusually large Hill-Sachs lesion, several options may be considered. A slightly tighter anterior repair

may prevent the extreme of rotation that would allow the edge of the defect to engage the glenoid rim.[2] However, given the risk of late arthrosis after an overly tight anterior repair,[37,49,108] this option is rarely advocated. A derotational humeral osteotomy[109] may shift the functional range of the arm so that it is rarely externally rotated enough to approximate the defect to the glenoid rim, but this procedure generally is not used in North America. Filling the defect with the infraspinatus tendon also has been described but has been infrequently performed.[110]

Prosthetic replacement is always an option if more than 40% of the humeral head is involved. However, the procedure is used more readily in elderly patients who have a locked unreduced dislocation than in young patients who have recurrent instability (Fig. 8).

Bone-grafting of the defect may appear to be the most logical and direct approach. Neer[2] described use of local autogenous bone graft from the surgical neck of the humerus to fill in an unusually large humeral head defect. Gerber (personal communication, 1993) used an allograft consisting of a segment of a humeral head, with some early success (Fig. 9). As far as we know, no long-term studies of the procedures are available to help the surgeon to select among these options.

Loss of Glenoid Bone

The glenoid rim may be flattened either by a fracture or by wear from repeated dislocations. Despite frequent discussion of this problem in the literature and at courses, very little information is available regarding how large a defect must be before it needs specific treatment. Steinman and associates[111] believed that if the defect involved at least 25% of the surface area of the glenoid, then some type of bone reconstruction was necessary.

Defects involving less than 20% of the surface area of the glenoid may be rendered extra-articular by repairing the detached labrum and capsule back to the edge of the remaining intact glenoid articular cartilage. If a chip of bone has been avulsed with the capsule and ligaments attached, then it is repaired with sutures as is done in a standard repair. If the fragment is large enough and can be mobilized, a screw may be used, with the surgeon taking care that the screw head does not contact the humeral articular surface.

Defects involving at least 25% of the glenoid surface usually are reconstructed. If a large single fragment is still present, then it is freshened and repaired.[112]

If no fragment is available, then the coracoid tip with attached muscle is transferred into the defect behind the repaired capsule in an extra-articular fashion (Figs. 10, 11, and 12). A screw and washer generally are used. The aim of the procedure is to deepen the socket and to support the capsule, not to act as a bone block.

Overview

Most patients who have glenohumeral instability can be managed successfully without surgery. When surgery is necessary, most patients who have post-traumatic unidirectional anterior instability do well after any of several anatomic capsular reconstructions and repair of an associated Bankart avulsion, if one is present. When a patient has severe capsular redundancy or marked loss of glenoid or humeral bone, a more complex reconstruction is needed. An understanding of the biomechanics of the shoulder, careful and appropriate surgical technique, and individualized postoperative rehabilitation usually lead to a gratifying result, even in these challenging and complex situations.

References

1. Jobe FW, Giangarra CE, Kvitne RS, et al: Anterior capsulolabral reconstruction of the shoulder in athletes in overhand sports. *Am J Sports Med* 1991;19:428–434.

2. Neer CS II (ed): *Shoulder Reconstruction.* Philadelphia, PA, WB Saunders, 1990, pp 273–362.

3. Rowe CR, Patel D, Southmayd WW: The Bankart procedure: A long-term end-result study. *J Bone Joint Surg* 1978;60A:1–16.

4. Thomas SC, Matsen FA III: An approach to the repair of avulsion of the glenohumeral ligaments in the management of traumatic anterior glenohumeral instability. *J Bone Joint Surg* 1989;71A:506–513.

5. Warner JJP, Flatow EL: Anatomy and biomechanics, in Bigliani LU (ed): *The Unstable Shoulder.* Rosemont, IL, American Academy of Orthopaedic Surgeons, 1996, pp 1–24.

6. Ferlic DC, DiGiovine NM: A long-term retrospective study of the modified Bristow procedure. *Am J Sports Med* 1988;16:469–474.

7. Saha AK: Dynamic stability of the glenohumeral joint. *Acta Orthop Scand* 1971;42:491–505.

8. Soslowsky LJ, Flatow EL, Bigliani LU, et al: Articular geometry of the glenohumeral joint. *Clin Orthop* 1992;285:181–190.

9. Lippitt SB, Vanderhooft JE, Harris SL, et al: Glenohumeral stability from concavity-compression: A quantitative analysis. *J Shoulder Elbow Surg* 1993;2:27–35.

10. Howell SM, Galinat BJ: The glenoid-labral socket: A constrained articular surface. *Clin Orthop* 1989;243:122–125.

11. Bateman JE, Fornasier VL (eds): *The Shoulder and Neck,* ed 2. Philadelphia, PA, WB Saunders, 1978, pp 475–564.

12. Bigliani LU, Kurzweil PR, Schwartzbach CC, et al: Inferior capsular shift procedure for anterior-inferior shoulder instability in athletes. *Am J Sports Med* 1994;22:578–584.

13. Bigliani LU, Pollock RG, Owens JM, et al: The inferior capsular shift procedure for multidirectional instability of the shoulder. *Orthop Trans* 1993;17:576.

14. Bigliani LU, Pollock RG, Soslowsky LJ, et al: Tensile properties of the inferior glenohumeral ligament. *J Orthop Res* 1992;10:187–197.

15. Brewer BJ, Wubben RC, Carrera GF: Excessive retroversion of the glenoid cavity: A cause of non-traumatic posterior instability of the shoulder. *J Bone Joint Surg* 1986;68A:724–731.

16. Chaudhuri GK, Sengupta A, Saha AK: Rotation osteotomy of the shaft of the humerus for recurrent dislocation of the shoulder: Anterior and posterior. *Acta Orthop Scand* 1974;45:193–198.

17. Cyprien JM, Vasey HM, Burdet A, et al: Humeral retrotorsion and glenohumeral relationship in the normal shoulder and in recurrent anterior dislocation (scapulometry). *Clin Orthop* 1983;175:8–17.

18. Kronberg M, Bronström LA: Humeral head retroversion in patients with unstable humeroscapular joints. *Clin Orthop* 1990;260:207–211.

19. Kronberg M, Broström LA, Söderlund V: Retroversion of the humeral head in the normal shoulder and its relationship to the normal range of motion. *Clin Orthop* 1990;253:113–117.

20. Randelli M, Gambrioli PL: Glenohumeral osteometry by computed tomography in normal and unstable shoulders. *Clin Orthop* 1986;208:151–156.

21. Calandra JJ, Baker CL, Uribe J: The incidence of Hill-Sachs lesions in initial anterior shoulder dislocations. *Arthroscopy* 1989;5:254–257.

22. Hermodsson I: Röntgenologische Studien über die traumatischen und habituellen Schultergelenkverrenkungen nach vorn und nach unten. *Acta Radiol* 1934;20(suppl):1–173.

23. Rowe CR, Sakellarides HT: Factors related to recurrences of anterior dislocations of the shoulder. *Clin Orthop* 1961;20:40–48.

24. Rowe CR, Zarins B, Ciullo JV: Recurrent anterior dislocation of the shoulder after surgical repair: Apparent causes of failure and treatment. *J Bone Joint Surg* 1984;66A:159–168.

25. Morrey BF, Janes JM: Recurrent anterior dislocation of the shoulder: Long-term follow-up of the Putti-Platt and Bankart procedures. *J Bone Joint Surg* 1976;58A:252–256.

26. O'Brien SJ, Neves MC, Arnoczky SP, et al: The anatomy and histology of the inferior glenohumeral ligament complex of the shoulder. *Am J Sports Med* 1990;18:449–456.

27. Gagey O, Bonfait H, Gillot C, et al: Anatomic basis of ligamentous control of elevation of the shoulder (reference position of the shoulder joint). *Surg Radiol Anat* 1987;9:19–26.

28. Jerosch J, Moersler M, Castro WH: The function of passive stabilizers of the glenohumeral joint: A biomechanical study. *Z Orthop Ihre Grenzgeb* 1990;128:206–212.

29. O'Connell PW, Nuber GW, Mileski RA, et al: The contribution of the glenohumeral ligaments to anterior stability of the shoulder joint. *Am J Sports Med* 1990;18:579–584.

30. Oversen J, Nielsen S: Stability of the shoulder joint: Cadaver study of stabilizing structures. *Acta Orthop Scand* 1985;56:149–151.

31. Terry GC, Hammon D, France P, et al: The stabilizing function of passive shoulder restraints. *Am J Sports Med* 1991;19:26–34.

32. Turkel SJ, Panio MW, Marshall JL, et al: Stabilizing mechanisms preventing anterior dislocation of the glenohumeral joint. *J Bone Joint Surg* 1981;63A;1208–1217.

33. Warner JJ, Denz XH, Warren RF, et al: Static capsuloligamentous restraints to superior-inferior translation of the glenohumeral joint. *Am J Sports Med* 1992;20:675–685.

34. Harryman DT II, Sidles JA, Harris SL, et al: Laxity of the normal glenohumeral joint: A quantitative in vivo assessment. *J Shoulder Elbow Surg* 1992;1:66–76.

35. Harryman DT II, Sidles JA, Harris SL, et al: The role of the rotator interval capsule in passive motion and stability of the shoulder. *J Bone Joint Surg* 1992;74A:53–66.

36. Lusardi DA, Wirth MA, Wurtz D, et al: Loss of external rotation following anterior capsulorrhaphy of the shoulder. *J Bone Joint Surg* 1993;75A:1185–1192.

37. Warner JJ, Johnson D, Miller M, et al: Technique for selecting capsular tightness in repair of anterior-inferior shoulder instability. *J Shoulder Elbow Surg* 1995;4:352–364.

38. Bigliani LU, Flatow EL, Kelkar R, et al: The effect of anterior capsular tightening on shoulder kinematics and contact. *J Shoulder Elbow Surg* 1994;3:S65.

39. Flatow EL, Ateshian GA, Soslowsky LJ, et al: Computer simulation of glenohumeral and patellofemoral subluxation: Estimating pathological articular contact. *Clin Orthop* 1994;306:28–33.

40. Bigliani LU, Weinstein DM, Glasgow MT, et al: Glenohumeral arthroplasty for arthritis after instability surgery. *J Shoulder Elbow Surg* 1994;3:S65.

41. Lephart SM, Warner JJP, Borsa PA, et al: Proprioception of the shoulder joint in healthy, unstable, and surgically repaired shoulders. *J Shoulder Elbow Surg* 1994;3:371–380.

42. Ticker JB, Bigliani LU, Soslowsky LJ, et al: Viscoelastic and geometric properties of the inferior glenohumeral ligament. *Orthop Trans* 1992;16:304–305.

43. Pollock RG, Bucchieri JS, Wang VM, et al: Subfailure repetitive loading of the IGHL affects its mechanical properties. *Trans Orthop Res Soc* 1997;22:164.

44. Altchek DW, Warren RF, Skyhar MJ, et al: T-plasty modification of the Bankart procedure for multidirectional instability of the anterior and inferior types. *J Bone Joint Surg* 1991;73A:105–112.

45. Neer CS II, Foster CR: Inferior capsular shift for involuntary inferior and multidirectional instability of the shoulder: A preliminary report. *J Bone Joint Surg* 1980;62A:897–908.

46. Speer KP, Deng X, Borrero S, et al: Biomechanical evaluation of a simulated Bankart lesion. *J Bone Joint Surg* 1994;76A:1819–1826.

47. Warner JJ, Miller MD, Marks P, et al: Arthroscopic Bankart repair with the Suretac device: Part I. Clinical observations. *Arthroscopy* 1995;11:2–13.

48. Dowdy PA, O'Briscoll SW: Shoulder instability: An analysis of family history. *J Bone Joint Surg* 1993;75B:782–784.

49. Emery RJ, Mullaji AB: Glenohumeral joint instability in normal adolescents: Incidence and significance. *J Bone Joint Surg* 1991;73B:406–408.

50. O'Driscoll SW, Evans DC: Contralateral shoulder instability following anterior repair: An epidemiological investigation. *J Bone Joint Surg* 1991;73B:941–946.

51. Uhthoff HK, Piscopo M: Anterior capsular redundancy of the shoulder: Congenital or traumatic? An embryological study. *J Bone Joint Surg* 1985;67B:363–366.

52. Warner JJ, Micheli LJ, Arslanian LE, et al: Patterns of flexibility, laxity, and strength in normal shoulders and shoulders with instability and impingement. *Am J Sports Med* 1990;18:366–375.

53. Flatow EL, Kelkar R, Raimondo RA, et al: Abstract: Active and passive restraints against superior humeral translation: The contributions of the rotator cuff, the biceps tendon, and the coracoacromial arch. *J Shoulder Elbow Surg* 1996;5:S111.

54. Thompson WO, Debski RE, Boardman ND III, et al: A biomechanical analysis of rotator cuff deficiency in a cadaveric model. *Am J Sports Med* 1996;24:286–292.

55. Bradley JP, Tibone JE: Electromyographic analysis of muscle action about the shoulder. *Clin Sports Med* 1991;10:789–805.

56. Cain PR, Mutschler TA, Fu FH, et al: Anterior stability of the glenohumeral joint: A

dynamic model. *Am J Sports Med* 1987;15:144–148.

57. Itoi E, Kuechle DK, Newman SR, et al: Stabilising function of the biceps in stable and unstable shoulders. *J Bone Joint Surg* 1993;75B:546–550.

58. Rodosky MW, Harner CD, Fu FH: The role of the long head of the biceps muscle and superior glenoid labrum in anterior stability of the shoulder. *Am J Sports Med* 1994;22:121–130.

59. Warner JJ, McMahon PJ: The role of the long head of the biceps brachii in superior stability of the glenohumeral joint. *J Bone Joint Surg* 1995;77A:366–372.

60. Snyder SJ, Karzel RP, Del Pizzo W, et al: SLAP lesions of the shoulder. *Arthroscopy* 1990;6:274–279.

61. Warner JJ, Kann S, Marks P: Arthroscopic repair of combined Bankart and superior labral detachment anterior and posterior lesions: Technique and preliminary results. *Arthroscopy* 1994;10:383–391.

62. Gibb TD, Sidles JA, Harryman DT III, et al: The effect of capsular venting on glenohumeral laxity. *Clin Orthop* 1991;268:120–127.

63. Kumar VP, Balasubramanium P: The role of atmospheric pressure in stabilising the shoulder: An experimental study. *J Bone Joint Surg* 1985;67B:719–721.

64. Warner JJP, Deng X, Warren RF, et al: Superoinferior translation in the intact and vented glenohumeral joint. *J Shoulder Elbow Surg* 1993;2:99–105.

65. Leffert RD, Gumley G: The relationship between dead arm syndrome and thoracic outlet syndrome. *Clin Orthop* 1987;223:20–31.

66. Ozaki J: Glenohumeral movements of the involuntary inferior and multidirectional instability. *Clin Orthop* 1989;238:107–111.

67. Warner JJ, Micheli LJ, Arslanian LE, et al: Scapulothoracic motion in normal shoulders and shoulders with glenohumeral instability and impingement syndrome: A study using Moir, topographic analysis. *Clin Orthop* 1992;285:191–199.

68. Bankart ASB: The pathology and treatment of recurrent dislocation of the shoulder-joint. *Br J Surg* 1938;26:23–29.

69. Broca A, Hartmann H: Contribution a l'etude des luxations de l'epaule (luxations dites incomletes, decollements periostiques, luxations directes et luxations indirectes). *Bull Mem Soc Anat Paris* 1890;4:312–336.

70. Perthes G: Über Operationen bei habitueller Schulterluxation. *Dtsch Ztschr Chir* 1906;85:199–227.

71. De Palma AF (ed): *Surgery of the Shoulder*, ed 2. Philadelphia, PA, JB Lippincott, 1973, pp 403–432.

72. Neer CS II, Foster CR: Inferior capsular shift for involuntary inferior and multiedirectional instability of the shoulder: A preliminary report. *J Bone Joint Surg* 1980;62A:897–908.

73. Rowe CR, Pierce DS, Clark JG: Voluntary dislocation of the shoulder: A preliminary report on a clinical, electromyographic, and psychiatric study of twenty-six patients. *J Bone Joint Surg* 1973;55A:445–460.

74. Neer CS III: Involuntary inferior and multidirectional instability of the shoulder: Etiology, recognition, and treatment, in Stauffer ES (ed): American Academy of Orthopaedic Surgeons *Instructional Course Lectures XXXIV.* St. Louis, MO, CV Mosby, 1985, pp 232–238.

75. Neer CS II: Special lecture: Recent concepts in dislocation and subluxation, in Takagishi N (ed): *The Shoulder: Proceedings of the Third International Conference on Surgery of the Shoulder.* Tokyo, Japan, Professional Postgraduate Services, 1987, pp 7–12.

76. Bigliani LU: Anterior and posterior capsular shift for multidirectional instability. *Tech Orthop* 1989;3:36–45.

77. Cordasco FA, Pollock RG, Flatow EL, et al: Management of multidirectional instability. *Oper Tech Sports Med* 1993;1:293–300.

78. Flatow EL: Multidirectional instability, in Kohn D, Wirth CJ (eds): *Die Schulter: aktuelle operative Therapie.* Stuttgart, Germany, Thieme, 1992, pp 180–187.

79. Foster CR: Multidirectional instability of the shoulder in the athlete. *Clin Sports Med* 1983;2:355–368.

80. Mallon WJ, Speer KP: Multidirectional instability: Current concepts. *J Shoulder Elbow Surg* 1995;4:54–64.

81. Belle RM: Collagen typing in multidirectional instability of the shoulder. *Orthop Trans* 1989;13:680–681.

82. Carter C, Sweetnam R: Recurrent dislocation of the patella and of the shoulder: Their association with familial joint laxity. *J Bone Joint Surg* 1960;42B:721–727.

83. Endo H, Takigawa T, Takata K, et al: A method of diagnosis and treamtent for loose shoulder. *Cent Jpn J Orthop Surg Traumat* 1971;14:630–632.

84. Finsterbush A, Pogrund H: The hypermobility syndrome: Musculoskeletal complaints in 100 consecutive cases of generalized joint hypermobility. *Clin Orthop* 1982;168:124–127.

85. Jerosch J, Castro WH: Shoulder instability in Ehlers-Danlos syndrome: An indication for surgical treatment? *Act Orthop Belg* 1990;56:451–453.

86. Hawkins RJ, Bokor DJ: Clinical evaluation of shoulder problems, in Rockwood CA Jr, Matsen FA III (eds): *The Shoulder.* Philadelphia, PA, WB Saunders, 1990, pp 149–177.

87. Silliman JF, Hawkins RJ: Classification and physical diagnosis of instability of the shoulder. *Clin Orthop* 1993;291:7–19.

88. Friedman RJ, Bonutti PM, Genez B, et al: Cine magnetic resonance imaging of the glenohumeral joint. Proceedings of the 60th Annual Meeting of the American Academy of Orthopaedic Surgeons, San Francisco, CA. Rosemont, IL, American Academy of Orthopaedic Surgeons, 1993, p 207.

89. Jalovaara P, Myllyla V, Paivansalo M: Autotraction stress roentgenography for demonstration anterior and inferior instability of the shoulder joint. *Clin Orthop* 1992;284:136–143.

90. Burkhead WZ Jr, Rockwood CA Jr: Treatment of instability of the shoulder with an exercise program. *J Bone Joint Surg* 1992;74A:890–896.

91. Rockwood CA Jr: Management of patients with multi-directional instability of the shoulder. *Orthop Trans* 1994;18:328.

92. Kronberg M, Brostrom LA, Nemeth G: Differences in shoulder muscle activity between patients with generalized joint laxity and normal controls. *Clin Orthop* 1991;269:181–192.

93. Flatow EL: Multidirectional instability, in Bigliani LU (ed): *The Unstable Shoulder.* Rosemont, IL, American Academy of Orthopaedic Surgeons, 1996, pp 79–90.

94. Yamaguchi K, Flatow EL: Management of multidirectional instability. *Clin Sports Med* 1995;14:885–902.

95. Cooper RA, Brems JJ: The inferior capsular-shift procedure for multidirectional instability of the shoulder. *J Bone Joint Surg* 1992;74A:1516–1521.

96. Field LD, Warren RF, O'Brien SJ, et al: Isolated closure of rotator interval defects for shoulder instability. *Am J Sports Med* 1995;23:557–563.

97. Warner JJP, Johnson DL, Miller MD, et al: The concept of a "selective capsular shift" for anterior-inferior instability of the shoulder. *Orthop Trans* 1994;18:1183.

98. Duncan R, Savoie FH III: Arthroscopic inferior capsular shift for multidirectional instability of the shoulder: A preliminary report. *Arthroscopy* 1993;9:24–27.

99. Thabit G III: Laser-assisted capsular shift for the treatment of glenohumeral instability. *Orthopedics* 1994;3:10–12.

100. Jobe CM: Anatomy and surgical approaches, in Jobe FW, Pink MM, Glousman RE, et al (eds): *Operative Techniques in Upper Extremity Sports Injuries.* St. Louis, MO, Mosby-Year Book, 1996, pp 124–163.

101. Lebar RD, Alexander AH: Multidirectional shoulder instability: Clinical results of inferior capsular shift in an active-duty population. *Am J Sports Med* 1992;20:193–198.

102. Mizuno K, Itakura Y, Muratsu H: Inferior capsular shift for inferior and multidirectional instability of the shoulder in young children: Report of two cases. *J Shoulder Elbow Surg* 1992;1:200–206.

103. Welsh RP, Trimmings N: Multidirectional instability of the shoulder. *Orthop Trans* 1987;11:231.

104. Hawkins RJ, Kunkel SS, Nayak NK: Inferior capsular shift for multidirectional instability of the shoulder: 2-5 year follow-up. *Orthop Trans* 1991;15:765.

105. Flatow EL, Miller SR, Neer CS II: Chronic anterior dislocation of the shoulder. *J Shoulder Elbow Surg* 1993;2:2–10.

106. Hawkins RJ: Unrecognized dislocations of the shoulder, in Stauffer ES (ed): American Academy of Orthopaedic Surgeons *Instructional Course Lectures XXXIV.* St. Louis, MO, CV Mosby, 1985, pp 250–263.

107. Hawkins RJ, Neer CS II, Pianta RM, et al: Locked posterior dislocation of the shoulder. *J Bone Joint Surg* 1987;69A:9–18.

108. Hawkins RJ, Angelo RL: Glenohumeral osteoarthrosis: A late complication of the Putti-Platt repair. *J Bone Joint Surg* 1990;72A:1193–1197.

109. Weber BG, Simpson LA, Hardegger F, et al: Rotational humeral osteotomy for recurrent anterior dislocation of the shoulder associated with a large Hill-Sachs lesion. *J Bone Joint Surg* 1984;66A:1443–1450.

110. Connolly J: Abstract: X-ray defects in recurrent shoulder dislocations. *J Bone Joint Surg* 1969;51A:1235–1236.

111. Steinmann S, Bigliani LU, McIlveen SJ: Glenoid fractures associated with recurrent anterior dislocation of the shoulder. Proceedings of the 57th Annual Meeting of the American Academy of Orthopaedic Surgeons, New Orleans, LA. Park Ridge, IL, American Academy of Orthopaedic Surgeons, 1990, p 173.

112. Boulris CM, Horwitz DS, Pollock RG, et al: Open reduction internal fixation of intra-articular glenoid fractures. *Orthop Trans* 1996;20:12.

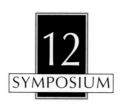

Instability of the Shoulder: Complex Problems and Failed Repairs: Part II. Failed Repairs

Evan L. Flatow, MD

Anthony Miniaci, MD

Peter J. Evans, MD, PhD, FRCSC

Peter T. Simonian, MD

Russell F. Warren, MD

Most patients who have instability of the shoulder can be well managed nonsurgically. When such treatment fails, modern anatomic repairs achieve stability and function in a high proportion of patients. When these goals are not achieved, an increasing number of patients and surgeons are considering revision surgery. A repair for instability may fail because of incorrect diagnosis, improper surgical technique, or inappropriate rehabilitation.[1] These complex situations represent both a diagnostic challenge to pinpoint the etiology of the failure of the first repair and a technical challenge to reconstruct the shoulder in the face of scarring and anatomic distortion from prior surgery. Although there is considerable overlap, it can be helpful to group these patients broadly according to the outcome of the primary procedure. These groups consist of those who have recurrent instability, those who have a stiff or overly tight shoulder, and those who have an arthrotic shoulder.[2]

The purpose of the current paper is to describe the evaluation and management of patients who have recurrent instability or stiffness of the shoulder after previous instability surgery. Reconstruction of an arthrotic shoulder with joint replacement[3] is briefly reviewed.

Recurrent Instability

We organized this complex subject by considering the factors that may be associated with the failure of a repair for the treatment of instability. These include errors in diagnosis (for example, a missed diagnosis of multidirectional instability), a patient with impaired motivation (for example, one who has voluntary instability), incomplete correction of pathologic lesions (especially Bankart lesions and capsular laxity), overcorrection (for example, an overly tight repair) leading to stiffness, improper rehabilitation or a patient who does not comply with rehabilitation, new injury, complications related to the use of hardware, aberrant healing (for example, stretching of the capsule after a repair in a patient who has a collagen disorder and generalized laxity), and arthrotic degeneration. Revision surgery should be considered only if extensive nonsurgical treatment has failed to relieve the symptoms in a motivated patient. Success is most probable if an anatomic lesion that was ignored at the first procedure (for example, an unrepaired Bankart lesion) can be identified and is amenable to correction at revision surgery. In contrast, there is an increased risk of failure if a revision repair is done in a patient with atraumatic multidirec-

tional instability who had capsular stretching despite a well–performed repair that shifted the inferior portion of the capsule superiorly. In many instances, it may be better to tell a patient that no good surgical option is available than to embark on a procedure without a clear chance of success.

Persistent or recurrent glenohumeral instability after a previous surgical stabilization is a difficult problem.[4-14] Careful evaluation of the patient's history, meticulous physical examination, and judicious use of diagnostic modalities can help to identify the reason for recurrence and to allow the formulation of a treatment plan.[4,7,15,16]

Etiology of Recurrence
Improper Previous Diagnosis Shoulder laxity may be dramatic but asymptomatic, and other diagnoses (for example, a painful lesion in the acromioclavicular joint) may have been responsible for the symptoms.[17,18] The examiner should look for other etiologies of the shoulder pain and dysfunction as well as problems in the cervical spine that may cause shoulder pain and thus simulate a lesion in the region of the shoulder.

Improper assessment of the instability, especially the failure to diagnose multidi-

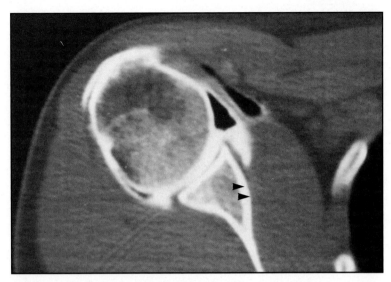 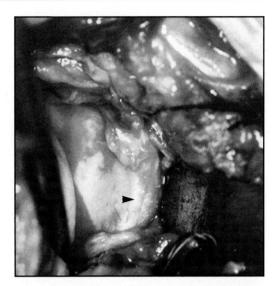

Fig. 1 A patient who had recurrent anterior glenohumeral instability after a previous repair for instability. Five years after the revision operation, which included repair of a Bankart lesion, the shoulder remained stable and had excellent motion and strength. **Left,** Arthrographic computed tomography scan showing unrepaired capsuloligamentous-labral stripping (arrowheads) from the anteroinferior aspect of the glenoid. **Right,** Intraoperative photograph showing the Bankart lesion (arrowhead).

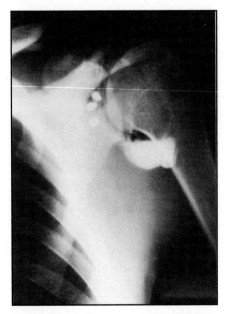

Fig. 2 Arthrographic computed tomography scan of a shoulder, showing failed correction of a large, redundant inferior capsular pouch. The patient had continued inferior instability despite previous surgical repair with multiple implants and tightening of the anterior aspect of the capsule.

rectional instability, may have led to an improper surgical procedure. All records and imaging studies from the initial eval-

uation should be reviewed. It is important to recall that a shoulder capsule may be both stiff and loose at the same time (for example, if a shoulder with multidirectional instability has been overtightened anteriorly). In these situations, in which the rotator interval and the anterosuperior aspect of the capsule as well as the inferior capsular pouch have not been addressed, the shoulder may continue to subluxate inferiorly despite being tight anteriorly to the point of restricted external rotation.

A particularly serious diagnostic error is the failure to recognize voluntary instability. These patients should be managed nonsurgically.

Incomplete Correction of Anatomic Lesions Even if the correct diagnosis was made, the pathologic lesions still may have been inadequately repaired initially. The most common unrepaired lesions are an avulsion of the capsuloligamentous-labral complex (a Bankart lesion) (Fig. 1), capsular laxity (Fig. 2), and erosion or irregularity of the glenoid rim through wear or fracture[1,2,7–9,12,16] (Fig. 3).

The high rate of failure of initial arthroscopic stabilization has been thought to be due to inadequate retensioning of the capsule and ligaments (Jobe C: Symposium on anterior shoulder instability. Presented at the Fourth Congress of the European Society for Surgery of the Shoulder and the Elbow, Milan, Italy, October 4, 1990). It also has been proposed that these approaches tended to repair the avulsed labrum too medially, on the glenoid neck rather than on the glenoid rim, thus failing to restore the socket-containment mechanism.[19]

Glenoid or humeral version is not usually a factor, but it may be one in the rare instance of a patient who has glenoid hypoplasia or rotational malunion after a humeral fracture. Although humeral impression fractures may be biomechanically important in chronic, unreduced anterior or, especially, posterior dislocations, they are rarely of consequence in recurrent instability.

New Injury Clearly, a new injury can disrupt even the best repair. Although this can occur at any time, the greatest risk is early in the postoperative period,

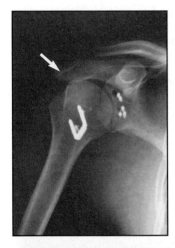
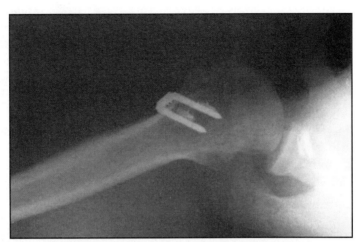
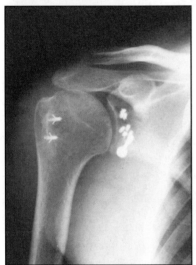
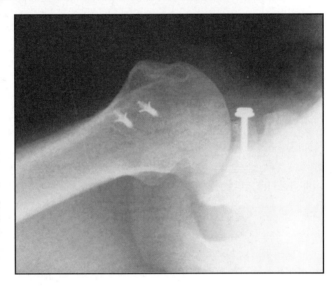

Fig. 3 An active young male patient who had recurrent dislocation after three previous failed repairs for instability. **Top left,** Anteroposterior radiograph showing a large Hill-Sachs lesion (arrow) (an impression fracture of the posterosuperior aspect of the humeral head), suture anchors and a staple from a previous operation, as well as loss of the sclerotic line of the anteroinferior aspect of the glenoid rim. **Top right,** Axillary radiograph showing loss of about one-third of the anteroinferior portion of the glenoid. **Bottom left,** Anteroposterior radiograph, made at the revision reconstruction, showing anteroinferior placement of graft. The coracoid tip was transferred as an extra-articular support to the capsule, which was repaired to the edge of the remaining intact glenoid. **Bottom right,** Axillary radiograph made after the coracoid transfer.

before the tissues have had a chance to mature. Trauma seems to be related more commonly to failures of repairs performed for unidirectional instability. In one study of recurrent instability after stabilization procedures, 12 of the 23 failures that occurred after a repair for unidirectional instability were associated with a new traumatic event compared with only two of the 20 that occurred after a repair for multidirectional instability.[12]

Improper Rehabilitation and Abnormal Healing A common cause of failure of a repair of a loose shoulder with multidirectional instability is overly intensive rehabilitation. Although stiffness is possible, it typically occurs in patients who have acquired laxity that is due to repetitive microtrauma. Patients who have inherited generalized ligamentous laxity rarely have stiff shoulders; rather, the repair tends to fail because of gradual stretching of the capsule. This type of failure can be prevented by tailoring the rehabilitation of the shoulder to regain motion slowly over a period of a full year, with avoidance of early intensive range-of-motion exercises.

Treatment of Recurrent Instability
Nonsurgical Treatment Recurrent instability should be classified with regard to the frequency of recurrence, the degree of trauma involved, and the direction and degree of instability.[20] The initial treatment should always be nonsurgical. New traumatic lesions may heal if the shoulder is protected, and laxity may be better tolerated if muscle strength and control are improved.[21,22] In a series of 39 shoulders that had recurrent instability after previous stabilization attempts, Rowe and associates[9] used specific resistive exercises to treat seven shoulders. The result was excellent in one shoulder, good in four, fair in one, and poor in one.

Revision Surgical Treatment The surgical approach varies according to the type of previous procedure and the degree of contracture associated with the instability. When the skin incision is made, generally previous scar tissue must be excised and, in some instances, the incision must be placed in a more correct position.

The anatomic planes should be identified and the cephalic vein, if it is present, should be preserved. Often there is considerable scar tissue between the clavipectoral fascia and the subscapularis. An incision lateral to the short head of the biceps up to the coracoacromial ligament, as well as rotation of the humeral head, facilitates identification of the proper plane. A periosteal elevator allows separation of the conjoined tendon and the deltoid from the cuff and the humeral head. The axillary nerve must be preserved medially and laterally. The subscapularis muscle then is released from the capsule to allow a capsular advancement and repair to be performed medially or laterally as needed. An elevator can be used to separate the muscle from the capsule; then this dissection is carried out superiorly and inferiorly. The anterosuperior portion of the capsule should be inspected. This region has been termed the cleft between the superior and middle glenohumeral ligaments,[23] and it is referred to as the rotator interval as well, although that term also is used to describe the gap between the tendons of the subscapularis and the supraspinatus. If it is enlarged, the cleft may be closed or incorporated in the capsulorrhaphy.

If there is a Bankart lesion and little or minor unidirectional capsular laxity, a variety of capsular repairs, performed either medially or laterally, can be effective. The Bankart lesion should be repaired to freshened bone at the glenoid rim. Suture anchors, if they are used, should be placed at the margin of the glenoid and not along the neck.

When substantial capsular laxity is present, especially when the inferior pouch is enlarged, an inferior capsular shift is performed. This is one of the rare situations in which anterior and posterior incisions may be necessary, because adhesions from the initial repair may make it impossible to mobilize the inferior portion of the capsule sufficiently to tension both sides from one approach. Although the ligaments and the capsule should be attached medially and laterally without slack, overtightening should be avoided, as contracture may lead to humeral subluxation in the opposite direction with subsequent arthrosis.[3,7,16]

A capsular release may be necessary in shoulders that have a capsular contracture, especially of the anterior part of the capsule and the middle glenohumeral ligament. If the contracture includes the subscapularis, that structure also has to be released or lengthened. If stiffness seems to be the dominant factor, it may be preferable to do only a release and then wait to see if renewed rehabilitation can control any remaining laxity. When anterior tightness is combined with major inferior or posterior instability, or both, a release combined with the appropriate capsulorrhaphy generally is used.

At times the subscapularis has avulsed and contracted medially, which necessitates dissection along the glenoid neck. The brachial plexus must be identified. In some patients, scarring prevents reattachment. In these instances, one of us (RFW) prefers to fill the defect with an Achilles tendon allograft attached to the glenoid and the humeral head. Alternatively, reconstruction may include the use of a hamstring or plantaris graft (Ziegler DW, Harryman DT II, Matsen FA III, Atlanta, GA, February 25, 1996) or the transfer of the pectoralis minor or the sternal head of the pectoralis major.[24]

Rehabilitation after revision surgery is the same as that after a primary repair for instability and is tailored to the ligamentous laxity and healing response of the patient. It is best to have the patient regain motion gradually, over a period of many months, and to monitor the progress and to adjust the exercises accordingly.

Results of Revision Repairs

Few reports in the literature document the outcome of revision instability surgery. Furthermore, although most of those reports concern failed repairs of traumatic unidirectional anterior instability, some do not clearly delineate the etiology or classify the type of instability. This makes comparisons difficult.

Rowe and associates[9] reported on a series of 39 shoulders that had recurrent anterior dislocation after failed initial surgical repair. The previous operations included a Bankart procedure (19 shoulders), a Putti-Platt procedure (seven), a Magnuson procedure (five), a DuToit procedure (three), a Bristow procedure (two), and a Nicola procedure (three). Thirty-two shoulders were revised surgically. The most common lesions found and corrected were Bankart lesions and excessive laxity of the capsule. Of the 32 shoulders, 24 were followed for at least 2 years; there were ten excellent results, 12 good, and two poor results. Recurrent instability developed after only two of the revision procedures.

Hawkins and Hawkins[16] reviewed a series of 46 shoulders that had failure of an initial anterior instability repair. Thirty-one shoulders were still unstable; 20 of these were revised, and about 80% of the patients were satisfied with the result.

In 1986, Walch and associates[11] reported 79 recurrences after surgery to treat recurrent dislocation. Most of the initial stabilization procedures had consisted of distal displacement or lengthening of the coracoid process. Of the 23 shoulders that had a revision repair, only 17 (74%) were stabilized.

Young and Rockwood[13] reported on 40 shoulders in 39 patients who had continuing symptoms after a failed Bristow procedure. Failure of the initial repair was related to recurrent anterior instability (primarily due to capsular laxity), posterior instability, damage of the articular cartilage, coracoid nonunion, loosening of the screw, and neurovascular injury. Multidirectional instability was identified in 23 (59%) of the 39 patients, and an untreated Bankart lesion was identified in four (20%) of 20 patients who had had a capsular shift or capsular release for treatment of chronic painful anterior instability. A revision capsulorrhaphy was performed in 15 shoulders because of recurrent instability. Of the 13 shoulders followed for at least 2 years, only eight had a good or excellent result.

Warren[12] evaluated the results of revision stabilization in 44 shoulders. Of the 44, 23 had had an initial repair for treatment of unidirectional anterior instability, and 21 shoulders had had reconstruction for treatment of multidirectional instability. At revision surgery, a Bankart lesion was identified in 19 of the 23 shoulders that had unidirectional instability and in only five of the 21 shoulders that had multidirectional instability. Major capsular laxity was present in 19 of the 23 shoulders with unidirectional instability and in all 21 shoulders with multidirectional instability. At an average of 77 months after revision surgery, eight of the 23 shoulders with unidirectional instability had an excellent result; seven, a good result; four, a fair result; and four, a poor result. The results achieved in the group that had multidirectional instability were much worse. At an average of 62 months, two shoulders had an excellent result; four, a good result; two, a fair result; and 13, a poor result. Eleven of the 13 shoulders that had a poor result had a total of 24 additional revision operations, including four glenohumeral arthrodeses.

Levine and associates (Levine WN, Connor PM, Arroyo JS, San Francisco, CA, February 16, 1997) reviewed the results in 54 shoulders in 53 patients who underwent revision stabilization surgery for failed anterior glenohumeral instability procedures. Patients requiring revision for postoperative stiffness, posterior instability, or arthrosis were

excluded. The initial procedure failed following a new traumatic event in only 17 shoulders. At revision surgery, all patients demonstrated anteroinferior instability when they were examined under anesthesia. Forty-six shoulders had excessive capsular laxity, and 25 had either a recurrent or a persistent Bankart lesion. Eleven shoulders had tight anterosuperior structures (the coracohumeral ligament, rotator interval, or superior aspect of the subscapularis) that tended to push the humeral head inferiorly into a large, redundant capsular pouch. The revision repair in 53 shoulders included an anterior-inferior capsular shift procedure; 25 also had repair of a Bankart lesion. One shoulder had a coracoid transfer for repair of a large fracture of the anterior aspect of the glenoid rim. At an average of 4.5 years, there were 40 excellent and three good results. Eleven shoulders were considered to have an unsatisfactory result because of recurrent subluxations (two shoulders) or dislocations (nine shoulders). Seven of the 11 patients were later diagnosed as voluntary dislocators. All 17 patients who had failure of the index procedure after substantial trauma had excellent results after revision surgery, compared with only 23 (62%) of the 37 patients in whom the failure after the initial repair was not associated with trauma. Interestingly, all of the patients who had a failed arthroscopic stabilization procedure had an excellent result after revision. Four of the nine shoulders that had had multiple previous stabilization attempts had recurrent instability after the revision procedure, compared with only seven of the 45 shoulders that had had only one previous stabilization procedure.

Overview
Recurrent instability of the shoulder after a stabilization procedure may be related to a missed diagnosis; a new injury; a missed anatomic lesion (especially a

Bankart lesion); or capsular laxity that was inadequately addressed at the initial procedure, was treated with improper rehabilitation postoperatively, or healed unsatisfactorily because of an underlying collagen disorder. Nonsurgical treatment options should be exhausted before surgical intervention is performed. Range of motion, function, and glenohumeral stability can be restored by a revision repair in a high percentage of patients. However, the results are not as predictable as those after a primary procedure.

The factors associated with a poor result after revision surgery include a diagnosis of multidirectional instability, failure of the initial repair without a new traumatic event, avulsion of the subscapularis, voluntary instability, and multiple previous stabilization attempts. Open revision instability repair after failed arthroscopic stabilization appears to yield good results. The reason may be that there is less scarring and soft-tissue disruption from an arthroscopic procedure or that failure of an arthroscopic procedure is related more commonly to incompletely repaired anatomic lesions (technical failure) than to poor collagen (biologic failure).

Stiffness
The major goals in the treatment of recurrent glenohumeral instability (subluxation and dislocation) are the restoration of stability and the maintenance of pain-free motion. When nonsurgical modalities fail, numerous operations to reconstruct the static (osseous and capsuloligamentous) and dynamic (rotator cuff) stabilizers of the shoulder have been used. The success rate of most procedures in the prevention of recurrent dislocation is more than 90%.[1] Although many of these procedures restore stability, they have resulted in loss of mobility and function. Furthermore, excessive loss of motion (principally external rotation) after surgical intervention has been implicated as a cause of degenerative arthropa-

Table 1
Surgical procedures for recurrent anterior and anteroinferior instability of the shoulder

Procedure	Surgical Correction
Motion-sparing	
Bankart repair	Open or arthroscopic capsuloligamentous release in both
Horizontal capsulorrhaphy	procedures
Motion-restricting	
Vertical capsulorrhaphy	Open or arthroscopic capsuloligamentous release
Putti-Platt	Open subsscapularis release or capsuloligamentous release, or both
Magnuson-Stack	Open subscapularis release or capsuloligamentous release, or both
Bristow	Open release of the subscapularis-conjoined tendon interval or subscapularis-lengthening, or both

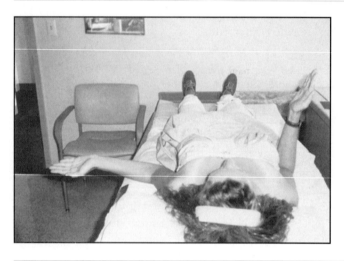

Fig. 4 Loss of external rotation after a Putti-Platt repair for recurrent instability.

thy.[3,5,7,16,25–27] Indeed, many early repairs were designed explicitly to restrict motion to avoid the positions in which the shoulder was at risk for instability. These repairs were often extra-articular and did not deal with intra-articular abnormalities such as labral detachments and capsular laxity. Reconstructions for repair of instability thus can be classified into two categories: those that restrict motion and those that spare motion (Table 1). Motion-restricting procedures reduce external rotation, thus preventing the patient from placing the arm in a vulnerable position (abduction and external rotation). This objective is achieved by means of medial-lateral tightening of either the capsuloligamentous complex (a

vertical capsulorrhaphy) or the subscapularis (a Magnuson-Stack or Bristow procedure), or both (a Putti-Platt procedure) (Fig. 4). In contrast, motion-sparing operations correct capsuloligamentous laxity, emphasizing a superior-inferior (Neer[23] or Jobe-type[28]) capsulorrhaphy. Both types of procedures have been combined with a simultaneous repair of a detached anterior capsulolabral complex (a Bankart lesion).

Loss of motion following shoulder stabilization can occur as a result of the type of procedure, technical errors in the performance of the procedure, or inadequate postoperative therapy. The management of a patient who has disabling loss of motion and pain after stabilization

requires a clear understanding of the available surgical procedures and their potential pitfalls as well as a systematic clinical and radiographic evaluation in order to implement an effective treatment protocol.

Etiology and Prevention of Stiffness After Instability Surgery
Capsulolabral Complex Procedures
The traditional Bankart repair[29] was directed solely at the capsuloligamentous and labral detachment from the anterior aspect of the glenoid rim, and tightening of the anterior aspect of the capsule was not a specific goal. The repair involves the separation of the subscapularis from the underlying capsule followed by a vertical capsulotomy 5 to 10 mm lateral to the glenoid rim. The lateral capsular flap then is advanced to the glenoid rim and repaired through drill holes in bone followed by suturing of the medial flap in a double-breasted fashion over the top.

Several technical points are relevant to the prevention of postoperative stiffness when this procedure is used. As the capsuloligamentous complex is tightened to a small degree with this procedure, care must be taken not to make the capsulotomy too far lateral from the glenoid rim in order to avoid excessive medial advancement of the lateral portion of the capsule and loss of external rotation. The site of attachment of the capsulolabral complex on the glenoid rim also is critical to anterior tensioning, which may restrict postoperative motion. The traditional Bankart repair should be performed on the edge of the articular surface of the glenoid. However, newer techniques such as suture anchors and biodegradable tacks used in either an open or an arthroscopic procedure often result in attachment of the capsulolabral complex to the anterior part of the glenoid neck. If the capsule is placed too medially, medial-lateral shortening of the anterior portion of the capsule can result, potentially with a loss of external rotation.

Table 2
Summary of reported cases of patients who had loss of motion after anterior stabilization of the shoulder

	Study					
	Samilson and Prieto[27]	Hawkins and Hawkins[16]	Hawkins and Angelo[5]	MacDonald and associates[26]	Lusardi and associates[25]	Total
Total*†	74 (45 ops)	10	11	10	20	96
Bankart repair†	2				2	4 (4%)
Capsulorrhaphy†						0
Putti-Platt procedure†	9	9	11	7	4	40 (42%)
Magnuson-Stack procedure†	6	1		1	10	18 (19%)
Bristow procedure†	17	1		2	7	27 (28%)
Other procedures†	11			2		13 (14%)
Range of motion (degrees)	0 to 30 (n = 27) 31 to 50 (n = 16) 51 to 70 (n = 12) > 70 (n = 19)		-5 (-30 to 25)‡	-8 (-30 to 5) ‡	-11 (-50 to 10) ‡	
Osteoarthrosis†		6				88
Mild	32		3	3	5	
Moderate	8		4	1	2	
Severe	5		4	6	9	

* Some shoulders had more than one procedure at a single or multiple operations. Forty-five of the shoulders in the report of Samilson and Prieto[27] had loss of motion after an operative procedure

† The values are expressed as the number of shoulders

‡ The values are expressed as the average with the range in parentheses

In a series of 20 shoulders that had loss of external rotation after various stabilization procedures, Lusardi and associates[25] found only two that had this complication after a Bankart procedure (Table 2). Thomas and Matsen[30] described a technically easier modification of the Bankart procedure, in which the subscapularis and the capsule are divided together off the humerus and reflected medially. This modification allows for an intra-articular repair of the capsulolabral complex followed by an anatomic repair of the subscapularis-capsular flap, thus avoiding the medial advancement of the lateral portion of the capsule and the potential loss of external rotation. However, others have expressed concern that this approach may not adequately correct the variable degrees of capsular laxity often seen in combination with Bankart lesions.[31]

Procedures for Capsuloligamen-tous Laxity Capsuloligamentous laxity is unidirectional (usually anterior), bidirectional (usually anterior-inferior), or multidirectional. Although a history of traumatic injury of the shoulder usually is associated with unidirectional instability and a history of atraumatic injury, with multidirectional instability, this dichotomy does not always hold true. Frequently, a patient whose laxity of the shoulder was initially caused by trauma can acquire, over time and with repeated episodes of instability, capsuloligamentous laxity. Therefore, a capsulorrhaphy alone or in combination with a modified Bankart repair often is necessary. If there is excessive capsular laxity at the time of a Bankart repair, medial advancement of the lateral portion of the capsule has been advocated by some investigators.[32] However, as has been mentioned, this may result in a restriction of external rotation. One method for avoiding a

severe loss of motion is to tension and close the capsulorrhaphy with the arm in at least 30° of external rotation.

More frequently, a repair with a horizontal capsular incision is recommended so that the superior flap may be drawn inferiorly and the inferior flap may be drawn superiorly, shortening the superior-inferior dimension of the capsule but not shortening the medial-lateral dimension. This is mandatory when inferior instability plays a role. Variations include a T-type inferior capsular shift on the humeral[23] or the glenoid side;[28] both allow for adequate exposure for repair of a Bankart lesion through an inside-out approach, if necessary, and a reduction in capsuloligamentous volume in a superior-inferior direction. T-type capsulorrhaphies also allow for more precision and individualization, as the superior-inferior and medial-lateral tension may be independently adjusted to suit the degree of capsular laxity present in each shoulder.[31] Although the risk of inadvertent tightening of the anterior aspect of the capsule is far less than that with a purely medial-lateral capsulorrhaphy, the humerus should be placed in at least 30° of external rotation and care must be taken to avoid overtightening. When performing the procedure on athletes who throw, the surgeon must allow for far more external rotation as the flaps are set.[28,31] It also has been suggested that, as different parts of the capsule are tensioned by specific positions, the inferior flap in a T-type repair should be positioned with the arm in abduction and external rotation, and the superior flap with the arm in external rotation and at the side.[33]

The arthroscopic capsular shift procedure reduces capsular volume, but it may result in decreased motion if the stabilizing sutures are placed too laterally in the capsuloligamentous complex or secured too far medially on the anterior portion of the glenoid neck. With use of suture techniques,[34,35] the ability of the surgeon to place the anchoring site for the transglenoid sutures at the junction of the articular surface may be better than that with use of suture anchors and biodegradable devices. The accurate placement of this anchoring site can be achieved only by disregarding the commercially available drill-guide placement and manually using the guide to place the drill site at the articular margin, exactly as was done in the original open Bankart procedure.

Bone Procedures The most common bone abnormalities found at shoulder surgery are Hill-Sachs lesions and, less frequently, variable erosion of the anteroinferior portion of the glenoid.[6] Reconstruction of these defects is rarely necessary to achieve stability. The Bristow procedure, as originally described by Helfet[36] (transfer of the coracoid process with the attached conjoined tendon to the anterior surface of the gle-

noid process), was designed to function, in part, as an osseous block to anterior movement of the humeral head. However, the Bristow procedure may function more as a dynamic musculotendinous sling, holding the humeral head in the joint when the arm is abducted and externally rotated. The modified Bristow procedure described by May[37] reefs the subscapularis and places the coracoid transfer through a split between the superior and inferior portions of this muscle. Thus, this modified procedure probably confers stability by tethering the distal portion of the subscapularis and by preventing it from migrating superiorly with abduction and external rotation.

Helfet[36] reported only a slight limitation in external rotation after the Bristow procedure, and May[37] found a limitation of less than 15° in most patients. Lombardo and associates[38] reported an average loss of 11° (range, 0 to 30°) of external rotation and an inability of the patients to return to sports activities involving overhead motion. Seven of the 20 shoulders that had disabling loss of external rotation in the study by Lusardi and associates[25] had had a Bristow procedure. Anatomically, the loss of rotation probably resulted from the tethering of the subscapularis and excessive scarring between the conjoined tendon and the subscapularis. Clancy suggested that the amount of internal rotation contracture related to the Bristow procedure could be minimized by positioning the humerus in 90° of abduction and maximum external rotation before closure of the defect in the subscapularis created by the coracoid graft. This would shift the site of tethering of the subscapularis more medially (WG Clancy Jr, MD, personal communication, 1997).

Motion-Restricting Procedures Although loss of external rotation is a complication of the procedures just described, it is the stated goal of the Putti-Platt and Magnuson-Stack proce-

dures. The Magnuson-Stack operation rarely is used alone and often is performed in conjunction with a capsulorrhaphy.[32] It involves the lateral and distal advancement of the subscapularis tendon, which is intended to decrease external rotation and inferior subluxation, respectively. Lusardi and associates[25] found that ten of 20 shoulders that had disabling loss of external rotation had had a Magnuson-Stack procedure. Until the current time, the most widely used surgery for repair of anterior instability was that described by Putti in 1923 and by Platt in 1925 and later termed the Putti-Platt procedure by Osmond-Clarke.[39] The procedure involves a vertical incision directly through the subscapularis and the capsuloligamentous complex into the joint followed by attachment of the lateral flap to the anterior rim of the glenoid or the periosteal tissue of the glenoid neck. The medial stump is then overlapped (double-breasted) over this repair and attached to the lesser tuberosity or to the bicipital groove.[39]

The Putti-Platt procedure has been implicated more frequently in the loss of external rotation and subsequent degenerative osteoarthrosis than has any other stabilization procedure. Hawkins and Hawkins[16] found that nine of ten patients who presented with substantial loss of motion had had a Putti-Platt repair, and six of these nine had osteoarthrosis. Hawkins and Angelo[5] described 11 shoulders that had become stiff and arthrotic after the Putti-Platt procedure. MacDonald and associates[26] reported on ten patients who had an anterior release for treatment of severe loss of motion after an anterior repair; seven had had a Putti-Platt repair originally, and five of the seven demonstrated severe osteoarthrosis. Lusardi and associates[25] found that four of 20 patients who had loss of external rotation after stabilization had been managed with a Putti-Platt operation; all of them required anterior soft-tissue release, and two required arthroplasty.

Treatment of a Stiff Shoulder

The treatment of a stiff shoulder following stabilization requires a systematic history and physical examination, followed by radiographic evaluation. It is necessary to rule out other causes of the pain in the neck, shoulder, and arm as well as the loss of motion. These possible etiologies include abnormality of the cervical cord and nerve roots, reflex sympathetic dystrophy, rotator-cuff tendinitis, primary intra-articular abnormality (adhesive capsulitis, infection, osteoarthrosis, inflammatory and crystalline arthropathy, and osteonecrosis), secondary gain, and psychological dysfunction. Details of the operation, postoperative rehabilitation, and the patient's motivation as well as whether the patient is receiving or has applied for Workers' Compensation and whether legal issues are involved, should be determined. If the patient has pain, it should be noted if it is constant or intermittent; if it occurs at night; if it is related to activity; and, if so, in what position of motion it occurs. The type and amount of analgesics used should be documented.

Physical examination should include subjective and objective measurement techniques, as described by the Society of Shoulder and Elbow Surgeons.[32] In addition, evidence of shoulder atrophy, areas of tenderness, contractures, and signs of other shoulder abnormalities should be documented. Standard shoulder radiographs should include anteroposterior, transscapular lateral outlet, and axillary lateral radiographs.

On the basis of the history as well as the physical and radiographic findings, the cause or causes of the loss of motion can be attributed to an anatomic site. Capsuloligamentous causes include generalized adhesive capsulitis or anterior contracture due to either overzealous medial-lateral capsulorrhaphy, inadequate postoperative physiotherapy, idiosyncratic scar contracture, or a combination of these conditions. Extracapsular causes can be related to specific operations (the Bristow, Magnuson-Stack, or Putti-Platt procedure), scarring along anatomic tissue planes used for exposure during reconstruction, inadequate postoperative physiotherapy, or primary or secondary rotator-cuff tendinitis. Anatomically, loss of motion can be related to scarring and contractures within any of the rotator cuff tendons and the pectoralis major, long head of the biceps, teres major, and latissimus dorsi muscles; around the coracobrachial and clavipectoral fascia as well as the coracohumeral and coracoacromial ligaments; and between the conjoined tendon and the subscapularis, subacromial space, and subdeltoid space.

Pain associated with reduced motion (principally external rotation) may be due to impingement, osteoarthrosis, capsular contracture, posterior instability, or muscle spasm. Capsuloligamentous contractures can alter the dynamic pressures within the glenohumeral joint and may be partly responsible for pain-induced spasms in the muscles surrounding the shoulder.[40] In a series of 46 shoulders in which a repair that had been performed because of instability had failed, Hawkins and Hawkins[16] found that pain was the major problem in 20 shoulders; nine shoulders had subacromial impingement syndrome, seven (six of which had had a tight anterior repair) had osteoarthrosis, and four had pain caused by the hardware.

Treatment of a shoulder that is stiff or painful, or both, should be individualized and based on the patient's lifestyle, the demands on the shoulder, and the level of pain. Treatment should begin with nonsurgical measures, including modification of activity, periodic use of analgesics, nonsteroidal anti-inflammatory medication, gentle range-of-motion exercises, and strengthening exercises for the rotator cuff. Hawkins and Angelo[5] managed seven of 11 patients who had osteoarthrosis and painful internal rotation contractures in this manner. Surgical release is warranted when pain or dysfunction, or both, do not improve after an adequate course of nonsurgical treatment. Surgical release also may be advisable for a patient who has early osteoarthrosis and reduced motion because, in addition to pain relief and increased motion, the progression of osteoarthrosis may be delayed. The value of a release before arthrosis develops in a stiff but pain-free shoulder is unclear. Many surgeons, wishing to avoid the dilemma of how to treat arthrosis of the shoulder in a young active patient, would consider a release for a shoulder with substantial loss of external rotation, even if the shoulder was not painful at that time. However, the precise guidelines for such an approach, as well as clinical data to support them, are not available. Our current approach is to consider a release when external rotation is less than 0°, to accept a loss of more than 30° of external rotation (if there is no pain or sign of osteoarthrosis) in most patients, and to individualize the decision when external rotation is between 0° and 30°. Functional considerations also are very important; in particular, throwing athletes cannot function with almost any loss of external rotation, especially at 90° of elevation. Most throwers have more than 90° of external rotation at 90° of elevation, and if external rotation is less than 90° in this position, release may need to be considered. Whatever the final decision, it is important to counsel a patient on the reasons to consider a release, with respect to both the current function and the risk of later osteoarthrotic degeneration, so that he or she may participate in the choice of treatment.

Preoperative assessment helps to direct the planning of the surgical procedure. If previous surgery involved only a capsuloligamentous or labral procedure,

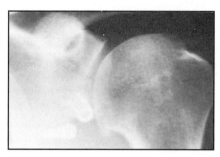

Fig. 5 Articular surface damage can result from loose or misplaced hardware.

then the shoulder release often may be performed arthroscopically, as no lengthening of the subscapularis is necessary. However, even a purely capsular procedure may lead to extra-articular adhesions, and an open release may sometimes be needed. If the previous surgery was extracapsular (a Bristow or Magnuson-Stack procedure) or capsular and extracapsular (a Putti-Platt procedure), then usually only an open procedure is effective. Although several methods of open release have been suggested,[23,24,32] all are based on release, lengthening, or medial transfer of the subscapularis musculotendinous unit and release or medial-lateral lengthening of the capsuloligamentous complex. Recurrent instability after release is rare.

As discussed already, patients may have a loss of external rotation but continue to have instability inferiorly; in these situations, a capsulorrhaphy in addition to an anterior release may be needed. The precise indications are unclear. When the stiffness predominates, it may be better to release the tight side so that asymmetric stiffness is eliminated. If this is done, the patient must be warned that a later capsular procedure may be needed if the instability cannot be treated with rehabilitation. However, once the soft tissues are balanced, mild laxity is often well tolerated. This approach avoids the difficulties of designing a postoperative rehabilitation program to follow a combined proce-

dure that includes a release, which normally is followed by early and vigorous motion, and a capsulorrhaphy, which is followed by a program of more gradual motion. When the inferior instability is extreme, however, a combined anterior release and appropriate capsular repair generally is used.

Surgical Procedure It is important to assess the shoulder for loss of motion in all planes and at various positions. In particular, external and internal rotation should be measured at 90° of elevation as well as with the arm at the side. An arthroscopic evaluation can be helpful even if an open release is planned, as the entire joint may be inspected for arthrosis or another abnormality. A capsular release may be easily performed arthroscopically. The subscapularis may be freed from the glenoid margin, and the rotator interval and the coracohumeral ligament may be released if necessary. It seems paradoxical to consider a capsular release when instability was the initial problem, but instability after a release is almost never a problem unless it was present before the release. As already discussed, when a shoulder is tight on one side and loose on another, the release is focused on the tight structures, usually the anterosuperior and anterior portions of the capsule and ligaments.

Typically, the arthroscope is placed through a standard posterior portal and a high anterior working portal is created. A transverse cut superior to the biceps with the cautery or laser releases the rotator interval. The incision then continues down the anterior portion of the capsule just lateral to the labrum in a superior-to-inferior direction. The muscular fibers of the subscapularis are exposed, and care must be taken to liberate this muscle fully. The arthroscope then is repositioned through the anterior portal, and, if internal rotation is restricted, the posterior capsule may be released through the posterior portal. If the inferior capsular pouch is tight, some sur-

geons, to avoid injury of the axillary nerve, remove the arthroscope and instruments at this point and perform a gentle manipulation. Other surgeons continue arthroscopically and carefully release the inferior aspect of the capsule, taking care to avoid the nerve, especially posteriorly where it crosses just inferior to the capsule. It may be advantageous to use the laser in this situation as the energy is less deeply transmitted (to the nerve). If there is still a loss of full external rotation, most surgeons convert to an open release, which may include a lengthening of the subscapularis if it has been previously shortened (for example, during a Putti-Platt procedure). One of us (RFW) has, on occasion, arthroscopically sectioned the internal two-thirds of the thickness of the tendon of the subscapularis obliquely and then stretched the remaining tendon thickness with manipulation to gain external rotation.

When an open release is planned or if the arthroscopic release cannot achieve full motion, the shoulder is exposed through a deltopectoral approach and the origin of the conjoined tendon and the insertions of the subscapularis, pectoralis major, and deltoid muscles are identified. First, scar tissue along interfascial planes is resected by blunt dissection if possible and by sharp dissection if necessary. The clavipectoral and coracobrachial fasciae are released. The subdeltoid and subacromial spaces are freed, and the conjoined tendon is bluntly separated from the underlying subscapularis, taking care not to injure the musculocutaneous or axillary nerve.

External rotation of the humerus allows the remaining tight anterior structures to be identified. The superior and inferior borders of the subscapularis are identified, and the axillary nerve is isolated at this point. The subscapularis may be lengthened in the coronal plane, as described by MacDonald and associates.[26] The superficial three-quarters of the subscapularis is divided vertically at a

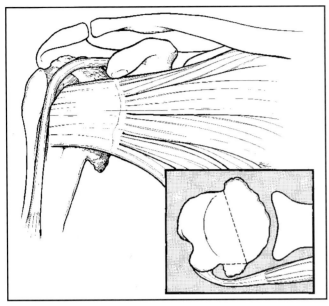 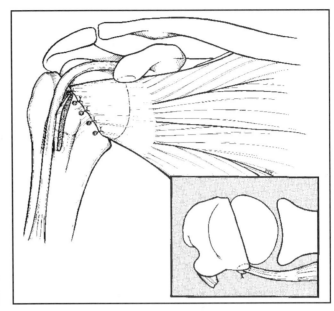

Fig. 6 Arthroplasty for treatment of arthrosis after an overly tight repair for the treatment of anterior instability. **Left,** Removal of the anterior humeral osteophytes effectively lengthens the subscapularis. **Right,** Repair of the subscapularis to the anatomic neck, medial to its original insertion, also functionally lengthens the tendon. (Reproduced with permission from Pollock RG, Bigliani LU: The management of anterior soft tissue contractures in glenohumeral arthroplasty. *Tech Orthop* 1994;9:94–95.)

point 15 mm medial to the biceps tendon, leaving a 10-mm cuff of the tendon's insertion attached to the humerus. This superficial flap is separated from the underlying one-quarter of the subscapularis and the capsule and is then reflected medially and transected deeply and medially onto the neck of the glenoid. External rotation of the humerus then is possible. Approximately 1 cm of subscapularis-lengthening equals a 20° increase in external rotation. The upper limit of lengthening that allows a stable repair is approximately 2 cm. The superficial three quarters of the subscapularis then is sutured to the underlying one quarter subscapularis-capsular flap in a double-breasted fashion with full-thickness, nonabsorbable sutures. The repair should be tensioned with the upper extremity at the side and the humerus externally rotated at least 30°. This type of formal subscapularis lengthening generally is reserved for situations in which the subscapularis has been previously shortened (as in a Putti-Platt procedure).

Otherwise, circumferential release of the subscapularis usually is adequate.

If any necessary capsular releases were not performed during an initial arthroscopic procedure, they are performed at this time. Full motion should be achieved, especially external rotation with the upper extremity at the side and at 90° of elevation. A standard closure is performed, and a drain is placed.

Passive-assisted range-of-motion exercises, including terminal stretching, are begun immediately postoperatively under the supervision of the surgeon and a physiotherapist. When the pain is severe, perioperative scalene blocks or an intermittent regional block by injection through an indwelling interscalene catheter can be used to help to relieve the pain and to facilitate early motion.[41]

The results of a release for stiffness after instability surgery have been gratifying, even when early osteoarthrotic changes are already present.[26] Whether the long-term progression of arthrosis is altered is still unknown.

Overview

Prevention is the best method of treatment for loss of motion associated with shoulder reconstruction for instability. A clear understanding of the goals and potential pitfalls of the chosen surgical procedure is essential. Operations that emphasize medial-lateral tightening of the capsule (a vertical capsulorrhaphy), the subscapularis (a Magnuson-Stack or Bristow procedure), or both (a Putti-Platt procedure), are not recommended because of the loss of motion and the subsequent dysfunction with overhead activities and the potential for degenerative osteoarthrosis. However, when a patient has loss of motion despite an appropriately chosen and executed procedure, a systematic approach to the diagnosis and treatment can provide satisfactory relief of pain and increased function.[5,16,25,26]

Arthrosis

Patients with severe arthrosis after an instability repair generally need prosthet-

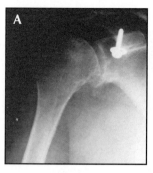 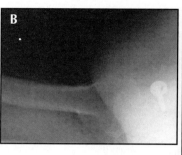 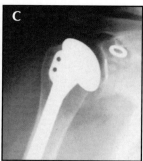 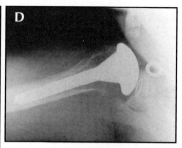

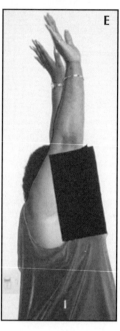 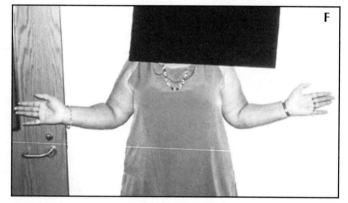 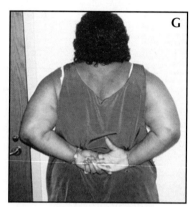

Fig. 7 A female patient with secondary arthrosis after a Bristow procedure who had a very stiff shoulder, constant pain, and very little use of the upper extremity. **A,** Anteroposterior radiograph of the shoulder. **B,** Axillary radiograph showing posterior subluxation of the humerus with eccentric posterior wear of the glenoid. **C,** Anteroposterior radiograph made after a total shoulder replacement. The washer was embedded in the bone and was not removed. **D,** Axillary radiograph, made after the total shoulder replacement, showing proper positioning of the component and partial restoration of normal glenoid version. **E,** Active elevation 1 year after the shoulder replacement and soft-tissue rebalancing. The patient had little pain and full use of the upper extremity. **F,** External rotation. **G,** Internal rotation.

ic replacement and soft-tissue rebalancing. Long-standing anterior contracture tends to drive the humeral head posteriorly, resulting in a fixed posterior subluxation, altered contact stresses, arthrotic degeneration, and posterior glenoid wear.[42,43] In addition, articular surface damage may result from loose or misplaced hardware (Fig. 5). A complete description of the technical steps of shoulder replacement is outside the scope of this chapter. However, it is helpful to review briefly the issues involved.

A release for arthrosis is performed in the same general fashion as already described. Rather than attempting to lengthen the subscapularis, the surgeon usually gains length by releasing adhesions, removing osteophytes, and repair-

ing the subscapularis more medially, at the anatomic neck (Fig. 6).

When a joint has been replaced because of arthrosis after a repair for anterior instability, recurrent anterior instability is extremely rare. If any instability occurs, it is likely to be posterior subluxation. This can occur for two major reasons. First, chronic posterior humeral subluxation (due to anterior tightness) tends to leave a posterior capsular recess. Second, posterior glenoid wear leads to a tendency to resurface the glenoid in excessive retroversion. Soft-tissue rebalancing, especially an anterior release, combined with appropriate sizing of the humeral head component, usually takes care of the posterior recess, although in rare instances imbricating

sutures may be necessary in the posterior portion of the capsule. Excessive glenoid retroversion is generally reduced by reaming down the anterior aspect of the glenoid rim, although usually not by the same amount that the posterior aspect of the glenoid has been lowered by wear. The remaining degree of increased retroversion of the glenoid component may, in most instances, be accepted and compensated for by reducing the retroversion of the humeral component. Bone grafts are almost never used.

The results of shoulder replacement and soft-tissue rebalancing are generally good[3,13] (Fig. 7). However, as many of these patients are quite young, the long-term issues with respect to the longevity of the implant are a source of concern.

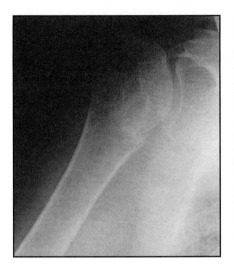

Fig. 4 Anteroposterior radiograph of a 56-year-old female who had nonsurgical treatment of a three-part proximal humerus fracture. There is varus malunion of the articular segment. The axillary lateral radiograph demonstrated flattening of the articular segment. At reconstructive surgery, the articular segment was found to be osteonecrotic. A humeral head replacement was performed.

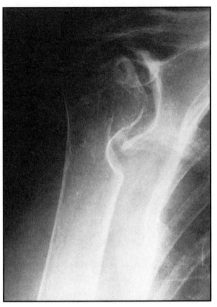

Fig. 5 Anteroposterior radiograph of a 70-year-old female with a long history of rheumatoid arthritis and shoulder pain. Note the severe glenoid erosion with medialization of the proximal humerus. The inferior aspect of the glenoid had eroded into the surgical neck of the humerus. This patient was treated with a humeral head replacement.

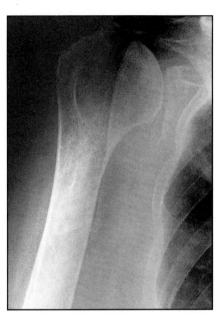

Fig. 6 Anteroposterior radiograph of a 74-year-old female with a long history of shoulder pain and weakness. Note the elevation of the humeral head relative to the glenoid, and the narrowing of the acromial humeral distance. At surgery, there was a massive irreparable rotator cuff tear and loss of the articular surface of the humeral head. She was successfully treated with a humeral head replacement.

Glenoid replacement is reserved for patients with adequate glenoid bone stock and intact or easily repairable rotator cuff.[37,39,40] Several retrospective studies have reported satisfactory results in about 90% of cases. Longer follow-up suggests that the rotator cuff deteriorates and that component loosening is a late problem.[39]

Rotator Cuff Tear Arthropathy

Neer was the first to suggest that glenohumeral arthritis in the presence of a chronic massive rotator cuff tear and primary glenohumeral osteoarthritis were distinct diagnostic entities.[41] Patients with rotator cuff tear arthropathy are older, on average in their early 70s, than patients in the other diagnostic groups discussed in this review. There is often a long history of shoulder pain and no antecedent trauma. The majority of patients are female. Active shoulder motion is usually limited; passive motion is not. Passive shoulder rotation is occasionally greater than normal because

of extensive rotator cuff and capsular tearing. Unlike primary osteoarthritis, patients with rotator cuff tear arthropathy have an external rotation lag, which signifies marked rotator cuff weakness. The radiographic features are clearly distinct from those of glenohumeral osteoarthritis. Aside from loss of glenohumeral joint space, the humeral head is usually elevated relative to the glenoid, there is narrowing of the acromial humeral space, and the normal prominence of the greater tuberosity is worn (Fig. 6).

Over the past decade there has been growing experience with shoulder arthroplasty for rotator cuff tear arthropathy. Prior to the development of shoulder arthroplasty, the surgical alternatives were limited. Arthrodesis reduces pain but has marked functional limitations, and is impractical and difficult to achieve in the typical elderly osteopenic female who has

rotator cuff tear arthropathy.[42] Early attempts at total shoulder arthroplasty included constrained implants that often led to failure.[9,10] Although unconstrained total shoulder arthroplasty predictably reduces shoulder pain, longer follow-up has led to the recognition that the altered biomechanics of rotator cuff deficiency predisposes to glenoid loosening.[43]

More recently, several reports have demonstrated that humeral head replacement is a satisfactory treatment for rotator cuff tear arthropathy. Arntz and associates[44] and Williams and Rockwood[45] reported satisfactory results in about 90% of cases when using Neer's limited goals criteria for evaluation of results. Pollock and associates[40] reported better results for humeral head replacement compared to total shoulder arthroplasty and attempted rotator cuff reconstruction.

Currently, humeral head replacement is the procedure of choice for rotator cuff tear arthropathy. The technical nuances relate to the rotator cuff deficit and the tendency toward anterior superior instability. Normal humeral retroversion must be maintained and in some instances should be increased. Some authors have recommended that an oversized humeral component be used. The appropriate humeral head size is one that articulates concentrically with the glenoid and coracoacromial arch and still permits anterior and posterior glenohumeral translation of about 50% of the humeral head diameter. The coracoacromial arch must be preserved. If there has been an acromioplasty and resection of the coracoacromial ligament, there may be uncontrollable superior subluxation of the humeral head. Postoperative rehabilitation emphasizes deltoid and external rotation strengthening.

Capsulorrhaphy Arthropathy

Capsulorrhaphy arthropathy refers to glenohumeral arthritis after anterior instability repair. It is an uncommon entity that has been recognized recently with increasing frequency. Capsulorrhaphy arthropathy is probably caused by the altered joint biomechanics that result from internal rotation contracture rather than as a sequela of glenohumeral dislocations and instability. It most commonly presents after nonanatomic instability repairs such as the Bristow, Magnusen-Stack, and Putti-Platt procedures.[46–48]

Although the joint pathology resembles primary glenohumeral osteoarthritis, patients with capsulorrhaphy arthropathy are much younger, with an average age in the mid 40s. During the early stages of joint destruction, subscapularis lengthening and anterior capsular release can significantly reduce shoulder pain and improve function.[49] However, when the articular damage is more extensive, shoulder arthroplasty is indicated.

Often, there is internal rotation contracture and posterior glenoid bone loss that require special surgical techniques.[19] Internal rotation contracture is corrected with subscapularis lengthening and anterior capsular release. Posterior glenoid bone loss can be corrected with anterior glenoid reaming and medialization of the glenoid or glenoid bone graft.[19,20] The decision to perform total shoulder arthroplasty, as opposed to humeral head replacement, is difficult. Due to the patients' young age, humeral head replacement is advantageous because it avoids the possibility of glenoid loosening. However, the results of humeral head replacement are inferior if there is eccentric glenoid wear.[30] This is a frequent finding in these patients and necessitates total shoulder arthroplasty. Overall, the results of shoulder replacement for capsulorrhaphy arthropathy are inferior when compared to the results for primary glenohumeral osteoarthritis.[50]

Osteonecrosis

The humeral head is the second most common site of nontraumatic osteonecrosis. Unlike osteonecrosis of the femoral head, the etiology of humeral head osteonecrosis is usually known. Systemic corticosteroid use is the cause of the majority of reported cases of humeral osteonecrosis.[5,33,51] On a worldwide basis, sickle cell anemia is also a common cause of humeral osteonecrosis.[52] A few cases are the result of Gaucher's disease or alcohol use.

The pathology of humeral osteonecrosis is similar to that of femoral head osteonecrosis. Ficat's classification scheme is useful for describing the pathologic involvement.[5,33] Shoulder arthroplasty is indicated once there has been collapse of the humeral articular segment. As collapse of the humeral head progresses, the glenoid becomes involved. Eventually the humeral head can engulf the glenoid.

The treatment of osteonecrosis before collapse is controversial. The role of core decompression and bone grafting is unclear.[53,54] The results of shoulder arthroplasty are excellent. Early surgical intervention, prior to glenoid involvement, consists of humeral head replacement. With more advanced disease, total shoulder arthroplasty may be necessary. This adds the possibility of late glenoid component loosening. Additionally, soft-tissue contracture complicates the situation of late treatment. The inevitable progression of humeral head osteonecrosis supports the recommendation for early humeral head replacement in symptomatic patients with humeral collapse.

Summary

Shoulder arthroplasty is an accepted treatment for certain proximal humerus fractures and for glenohumeral arthritis. The indications for shoulder arthroplasty are fairly well defined and the outcomes are predictable and highly successful. However, it is a technically demanding surgical procedure, with which few orthopaedic surgeons gain much experience. Most of the currently available implant systems are modifications of the original unconstrained components that were introduced by Neer. Current issues of controversy include implant modularity, glenohumeral mismatch, implant fixation, and the role of glenoid replacement in outcome.

References

1. Bankes MJ, Emery RJ: Pioneers of shoulder replacement: Themistocles Gluck and Jules Emile Péan. *J Shoulder Elbow Surg* 1995;4: 259–262.

2. Neer CS II: Articular replacement for the humeral head. *J Bone Joint Surg* 1955;37A: 215–228.

3. Neer CS II: Replacement arthroplasty for glenohumeral osteoarthritis. *J Bone Joint Surg* 1974;56A:1–13.

4. Neer CS II, Watson KC, Stanton FJ: Recent experience in total shoulder replacement. *J Bone Joint Surg* 1982;64A:319–337.

5. Cofield RH, Becker DA: Shoulder arthroplasty, in Morrey BF, An KN (eds): *Reconstructive Surgery of the Joints*, ed 2. New York, NY, Churchill Livingstone, 1996, pp 753–771.

6. Cofield RH: Shoulder arthrodesis and resection arthroplasty, in Stauffer ES (ed): American Academy of Orthopaedic Surgeons *Instructional Course Lectures XXXIV*. St. Louis, MO, CV Mosby, 1985, pp 268–277.

7. Cofield RH, Briggs BT: Glenohumeral arthrodesis: Operative and long-term functional results. *J Bone Joint Surg* 1979;61A:668–677.

8. Burkhead WZ Jr, Hutton KS: Biologic resurfacing of the glenoid with hemiarthroplasty of the shoulder. *J Shoulder Elbow Surg* 1995;4: 263–270.

9. Post M, Jablon M, Miller H, et al: Constrained total shoulder joint replacement: A critical review. *Clin Orthop* 1979;144:135–150.

10. Post M, Jablon M: Constrained total shoulder arthroplasty: Long-term follow-up observations. *Clin Orthop* 1983;173:109–116.

11. Cofield RH, Daly PJ: Total shoulder arthroplasty with a tissue-ingrowth glenoid component. *J Shoulder Elbow Surg* 1992;1:77–85.

12. McElwain JP, English E: The early results of porous-coated total shoulder arthroplasty. *Clin Orthop* 1987;218:217–224.

13. Roper BA, Paterson JM, Day WH: The Roper-Day total shoulder replacement. *J Bone Joint Surg* 1990;72B:694–697.

14. Gartsman GM, Russell JA, Gaenslen E: Modular shoulder arthroplasty. *J Shoulder Elbow Surg* 1997;6:333–339.

15. Collins D, Tencer A, Sidles J, et al: Edge displacement and deformation of glenoid components in response to eccentric loading: The effect of preparation of the glenoid bone. *J Bone Joint Surg* 1992;74A:501–507.

16. Conn RA, Cofield RH, Byer DE, et al: Interscalene block anesthesia for shoulder surgery. *Clin Orthop* 1987;216:94–98.

17. Neer CS II, Kirby RM: Revision of humeral head and total shoulder arthroplasties. *Clin Orthop* 1982;170:189–195.

18. Groh GI, Simoni M, Rolla P, et al: Loss of the deltoid after shoulder operations: An operative disaster. *J Shoulder Elbow Surg* 1994;3:243–253.

19. Bigliani LU, Weinstein DM, Glasgow MT, et al: Glenohumeral arthroplasty for arthritis after instability surgery. *J Shoulder Elbow Surg* 1995; 4:87–94.

20. Neer CS II, Morrison DS: Glenoid bone-grafting in total shoulder arthroplasty. *J Bone Joint Surg* 1988;70A:1154–1162.

21. Neer CS II: Displaced proximal humerus fractures: Part II. Treatment of three-part and four-part displacement. *J Bone Joint Surg* 1970; 52A:1090–1103.

22. Norris TR: Fractures of the proximal humerus and dislocations of the shoulder, in Browner BD, Jupiter JB, Levine AM, et al (eds): *Skeletal Trauma: Fractures, Dislocations, Ligamentous Injuries*. Philadelphia, PA, WB Saunders, 1992, vol 2, pp 1201–1290.

23. Hawkins RJ, Switlyk P: Acute prosthetic replacement for severe fractures of the proximal humerus. *Clin Orthop* 1993;289:156–160.

24. Green A, Barnard WL, Limbird RS: Humeral head replacement for acute, four-part proximal humerus fractures. *J Shoulder Elbow Surg* 1993; 2:249–254.

25. Stableforth PG: Four-part fractures of the neck of the humerus. *J Bone Joint Surg* 1984;66B: 104–108.

26. Leyshon RL: Closed treatment of fractures of the proximal humerus. *Acta Orthop Scand* 1984; 55:48–51.

27. Barrett WP, Franklin JL, Jackins SE, et al: Total shoulder arthroplasty. *J Bone Joint Surg* 1987; 69A:865–872.

28. Cofield RH: Total shoulder arthroplasty with the Neer prosthesis. *J Bone Joint Surg* 1984; 66A:899–906.

29. Wirth MA, Rockwood CA Jr: Complications of total shoulder-replacement arthroplasty. *J Bone Joint Surg* 1996;78A:603–616.

30. Levine WN, Djurasovic M, Glasson J-M, et al: Hemiarthroplasty for glenohumeral osteoarthritis: Results correlated to degree of glenoid wear. *J Shoulder Elbow Surg* 1997;6:449–454.

31. Green A, Norris TR: Complications of non-operative management and internal fixation of proximal humerus fractures, in Flatow EL, Ulrich C (eds): *Musculoskeletal Trauma Series: Humerus*. Oxford, England, Butterworth-Heinemann, 1996, pp 106–120.

32. Norris TR, Green A, McGuigan FX: Late prosthetic shoulder arthroplasty for displaced proximal humerus fractures. *J Shoulder Elbow Surg* 1995;4:271–280.

33. Frich LH, Sojbjerg JO, Sneppen O: Shoulder arthroplasty in complex acute and chronic proximal humeral fractures. *Orthopedics* 1991; 14:949–954.

34. Tanner MW, Cofield RH: Prosthetic arthroplasty for fractures and fracture-dislocations of the proximal humerus. *Clin Orthop* 1983; 179:116–128.

35. Neer CS II: Glenohumeral arthroplasty. in Neer CS II (ed): *Shoulder Reconstruction*. Philadelphia, PA, WB Saunders, 1990, pp 143–271.

36. Friedman RJ, Thornhill TS, Thomas WH, et al: Non-constrained total shoulder replacement in patients who have rheumatoid arthritis and class-IV function. *J Bone Joint Surg* 1989; 71A:494–498.

37. Sneppen O, Fruensgaard S, Johannsen HV, et al: Total shoulder replacement in rheumatoid arthritis: Proximal migration and loosening. *J Shoulder Elbow Surg* 1996;5:47–52.

38. Stewart MP, Kelly IG: Total shoulder replacement in rheumatoid disease: 7- to 13-year follow-up of 37 joints. *J Bone Joint Surg* 1997;79B: 68–72.

39. Boyd AD Jr, Thomas WH, Scott RD, et al: Total shoulder arthroplasty versus hemiarthroplasty: Indications for glenoid resurfacing. *J Arthroplasty* 1990;5:329–336.

40. Pollock RG, Deliz ED, McIlveen SJ, et al: Prosthetic replacement in rotator cuff deficient shoulders. *J Shoulder Elbow Surg* 1992; 1:173–186.

41. Neer CS II, Craig EV, Fukuda H: Cuff-tear arthropathy. *J Bone Joint Surg* 1983 ;65A: 1232–1244.

42. Arntz CT, Matsen FA III, Jackins S: Surgical management of complex irreparable rotator cuff deficiency. *J Arthroplasty* 1991;6:363–370.

43. Franklin JL, Barrett WP, Jackins SE, et al: Glenoid loosening in total shoulder arthroplasty: Association with rotator cuff deficiency. *J Arthroplasty* 1988;3:39–46.

44. Arntz CT, Jackins S, Matsen FA III: Prosthetic replacement of the shoulder for the treatment of defects in the rotator cuff and the surface of the glenohumeral joint. *J Bone Joint Surg* 1993;75A:485–491.

45. Williams GR Jr, Rockwood CA Jr: Hemiarthroplasty in rotator cuff-deficient shoulders. *J Shoulder Elbow Surg* 1996;5: 362–367.

46. Hawkins RJ, Angelo RL: Glenohumeral osteoarthrosis: A late complication of the Putti-Platt repair. *J Bone Joint Surg* 1990;72A: 1193–1197.

47. Norris TR, Bigliani LU: Analysis of failed repair for shoulder instability: A preliminary report, in Bateman JE, Welsh RP (eds): *Surgery of the Shoulder*. Philadelphia, PA, BC Decker, 1984, pp 111–116.

48. Young DC, Rockwood CA Jr: Complications of a failed Bristow procedure and their management. *J Bone Joint Surg* 1991;73A:969–981.

49. MacDonald PB, Hawkins RJ, Fowler PJ, et al: Release of the subscapularis for internal rotation contracture and pain after anterior repair for recurrent anterior dislocation of the shoulder. *J Bone Joint Surg* 1992;74A:734–737.

50. Green A, Norris TR: Capsulorraphy arthropathy: Glenohumeral arthrosis after anterior instability repair. Proceedings of the American Academy of Orthopaedic Surgeons 62nd Annual Meeting, Orlando, FL. Rosemont, IL, American Academy of Orthopaedic Surgeons, 1995, p 342.

51. Cruess RL: Steroid-induced avascular necrosis of the head of the humerus: Natural history and management. *J Bone Joint Surg* 1976;58B: 313–317.

52. David HG, Bridgman SA, Davies SC, et al: The shoulder in sickle-cell disease. *J Bone Joint Surg* 1993;75B:538–545.

53. Mont MA, Maar DC, Urquhart MW, et al: Avascular necrosis of the humeral head treated by core decompression: A retrospective review. *J Bone Joint Surg* 1993;75B:785–788.

54. L'Insalata JC, Pagnani MJ, Warren RF, et al: Humeral head osteonecrosis: Clinical course and radiographic predictors of outcome. *J Shoulder Elbow Surg* 1996;5:355–361.

Treatment of Proximal Humerus Fracture Malunion with Prosthetic Arthroplasty

Pedro K. Beredjiklian, MD
Joseph P. Iannotti, MD, PhD

Introduction

Patients with failed treatment of proximal humerus fractures resulting in malunion invariably present with severe pain and loss of motion and function of the affected shoulder. Disruption of the normal anatomic relationships between the tuberosities, humeral head, and shaft, as well as glenohumeral joint incongruity, can result in pain and in loss of motion and strength of the shoulder joint. Soft-tissue scarring due to posttraumatic or postsurgical changes and tears of the rotator cuff also contribute to this stiffness and loss of strength. These patients often experience significant functional impairment.

The goals of treatment are pain relief and restoration of premorbid functional status. Because nonsurgical treatment options for these patients are limited, surgical reconstruction is often necessary. Conservative management, in the form of physical therapy and anti-inflammatory medications, can be considered for patients with mild disability. Surgical options, in the form of osteotomies of the malpositioned elements of the proximal humerus (such as the greater tuberosity and surgical neck), can be effective in providing pain relief and functional improvement.[1-3] In addition, soft-tissue procedures, such as closed or open capsular release and repair of the torn rotator cuff, can relieve pain and improve function. Prosthetic arthroplasty is considered a treatment option in the management of joint incongruity.[4-8] Although it has been suggested that arthroplasty is widely regarded as a straightforward alternative if initial fracture treatment fails,[5] the truth is that the results of surgical treatment have often proven unsatisfactory.[5-7] In fact, management of malunions of proximal humerus fractures with arthroplasty represents one of the most challenging problems in shoulder surgery.

The treatment of these patients requires careful preoperative assessment of causative factors of malunion and directed surgical treatment of these issues intraoperatively. This discussion will serve to identify the etiologic factors that contribute to the pathologic processes and will establish an algorithm for treatment of these difficult fracture malunions.

Review of the Literature

Many authors have recognized the difficulty in treating patients with complications arising from proximal humerus fractures, but few reports in the literature deal with the treatment of fracture malunion with prosthetic arthroplasty.[4-8] In general, prosthetic replacement for malunions appears to have less satisfactory results than arthroplasty performed either for acute fractures or for glenohumeral arthrosis. For the late reconstruction group, most studies agree that pain relief is seen in about 75% to 85% of patients. Functional outcome, however, is generally less favorable because of persistent stiffness.

Tanner and Cofield[4] compared the results of humeral head replacement in acute and chronic fractures and fracture-dislocations in 49 shoulders. Among the patient population with chronic fractures, they included 16 patients with malunion and glenohumeral joint incongruity. They found that patients with late reconstruction had better range of motion of the affected joint on follow-up than did the acute fracture group. However, there were more complications in the chronic group, and these were ascribed to surgical difficulty, tissue scarring, and distortion of anatomy.

In a similar report, Norris and associates[5] describe late reconstruction for failed treatment of 23 three- and four-part fractures. Their series included 17 cases of malunion, which were treated with either total shoulder arthroplasty or humeral head replacement. They found that the results were inferior to those for reconstruction of acute fractures and that late reconstruction was technically demanding with more complications.

Frich and associates[6] studied a group of 42 patients with acute and chronic fractures treated with prosthetic arthro-

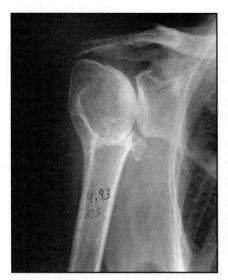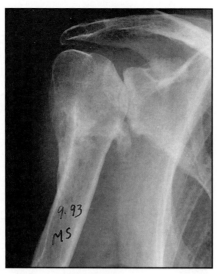

Fig. 1 Three-part fracture with a malunited greater tuberosity and secondary osteonecrosis with humeral head collapse joint incongruity. **Left,** Six months after fracture. **Right,** Eighteen months after fracture.

plasty.[6] The authors reported significantly better results in the acute fracture group, and only four of the 27 patients treated with late reconstruction had good or excellent results. The chronic fracture group had a high incidence of complications associated with instability, which the authors concluded was due to difficulty in soft-tissue balancing. The authors also found a fairly high incidence of infection, which they attributed to the multiple prior surgeries in the late reconstruction group.

Dines and associates[7] reported on a group of 11 patients treated with late reconstruction for proximal humerus malunion. Only five of the 11 had a good or excellent result on follow-up. The authors found poor results to be associated with patient age greater than 70 years and cases in which a tuberosity osteotomy was performed.

Pathology

The pathologic changes seen in shoulders with malunited fractures can be subdivided into bony and soft-tissue abnormalities. Osseous anomalies can be characterized as follows.

Osseous Anomalies

Tuberosity Displacement Malunion of the greater tuberosity in a posterior or cephalad position can cause impingement on the rotator cuff tendon in the subacromial space. This impingement can result in a chronic subacromial bursitis, and it may even lead to partial and complete tears of the rotator cuff. In addition, superior malposition of the greater tuberosity can act as a bony block against the acromion, limiting forward elevation. Similarly, a posteriorly displaced greater tuberosity will limit external rotation when the tuberosity contacts the glenoid rim or neck. Finally, the muscles of the rotator cuff lose their mechanical advantage as their point of insertion in the proximal humerus is changed, and the patient can experience weakness in elevation and external rotation.

Incongruence of the Articular Surface Lack of congruence of the glenohumeral articulation will result in painful motion of the shoulder joint. This in turn will exacerbate the stiffness that is characteristic of these patients. Frequent causes of articular incongruence in the setting of malunion include

osteonecrossis (ON) of the humeral head, humeral articular step off secondary to a head split fracture, subluxation or dislocation of the glenohumeral joint, and posttraumatic arthrosis.

Articular Segment Malalignment Fractures in which the surgical neck heals in a nonanatomic position can result in malalignment of the entire glenohumeral articular segment. Malalignment can occur in the sagittal and/or coronal planes. This malposition will also contribute to poor motion and function of the affected shoulder. Depending on the position of the malunited surgical neck, the malalignment can occur in any one (or a combination) of three directions—varus, valgus, and rotational.

Tuberosity malposition, articular incongruity, and articular segment malalignment are often present in combination. For example, a patient with a three-part greater tuberosity fracture in whom the greater tuberosity heals in a cephalad position and who concomitantly develops ON of the humeral head with collapse, is said to have a combination of criteria I and II (Fig. 1).

Soft-Tissue Pathology

In addition to the bony anomalies described above, soft-tissue pathology is quite common in these patients. These soft-tissue abnormalities are responsible, in large part, for the clinical picture seen in these patients. The three types of soft-tissue pathology are capsular contractures, rotator cuff tears, and neurologic injury.

Capsular Contracture Some degree of capsular contracture is seen in many patients with proximal humerus fracture malunions. The contracture, which can be the result of posttraumatic changes, is more pronounced in those patients whose postinjury rehabilitation protocol was inadequate. Similarly, the contracture can be the result of postsurgical scarring, and this problem is seen predominantly in patients who were treated surgically for the initial fracture. In addition, this process is exacerbated by the pain experienced from glenohumeral joint arthrosis, as well as soft-tissue and bony impingement caused by fracture malunion.

Rotator Cuff Tears Tears of the rotator cuff are seen commonly in association with malunited proximal humerus fractures. The tears may predate the fracture, or they can have occurred at the time of initial injury, as in a two-part anterior fracture-dislocation. Similarly, rotator cuff pathology can result from attritional changes caused by a malpositioned greater tuberosity. These tears contribute significantly to the poor functional capacity of the affected shoulder. Large rotator cuff tears, in the setting of advanced age or poor quality tissues, can severely compromise the postoperative results.

Neurologic Injury Nerve injury is often present in these patients. The neural deficit can occur at the time of the initial injury or during the initial surgical intervention. Commonly encountered deficits include brachial plexopathies, as well as isolated axillary, suprascapular, and musculocutaneous nerve injuries.

Finally, retained hardware from initial fracture fixation can contribute to the pathology in each case. Loose or malpositioned hardware can cause pain, impingement, and neurologic injury. Distally placed hardware (screws, plates, cerclage wires) in the middiaphyseal region can result in bone defects, which can act as stress risers. These stress risers can increase the risk of an intraoperative humeral shaft fracture, or they may require use of a long-stem humeral prosthetic component.

Evaluation
Clinical Evaluation
Preoperative planning is an essential part of the surgical treatment of these patients. Clinical evaluation must include a careful history to determine the time and mechanism of initial injury. It is of utmost

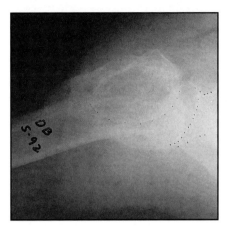
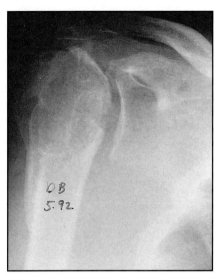

Fig. 2 Anteroposterior and axillary radiographs of a four-part fracture malunion.

importance to ascertain the exact nature of the initial fracture treatment, and it is advisable to obtain an operative report if the initial fracture treatment was surgical. Knowledge of the pathology addressed at the original surgery and the technique used for reconstruction can be helpful in planning the late reconstruction.

On physical examination, the degree of capsular contracture should be assessed. Passive range of motion measurements in forward flexion and external rotation are helpful in this regard. It must be kept in mind that bony and soft-tissue impingement may also contribute to a decrease in range of motion, and for this reason the determination of the exact etiology of stiffness should be performed intraoperatively. The influence of pain on apparent loss of motion observed in the awake patient can also be determined intraoperatively.

The integrity of the rotator cuff tendon must be established. As mentioned previously, cuff tears are often present in association with proximal humerus fracture malunion, and an attempt should be made to ascertain cuff function preoperatively. Specifically, strength of external rotation and the Gerber "lift off" test should be performed to evaluate posteri-

or cuff and subscapularis function, respectively. Again, bony abnormalities and periarticular scarring may render these tests unreliable, making intraoperative inspection of the cuff tissue a more accurate appraisal of rotator cuff integrity. Finally, preoperative imaging studies also can be helpful adjuncts in determining the integrity of the rotator cuff.

As mentioned previously, many of these patients have neurologic deficits. A careful neurovascular examination should be carried out in all patients. Specifically, assessment of axillary, suprascapular, and musculocutaneous nerve function (as well as combined brachial plexus injuries) should be carried out and accurately documented preoperatively. Electromyographic and nerve conduction studies may be helpful in establishing the pattern of nerve injury as well as the prognosis of nerve function recovery.

Imaging Studies
All patients require high quality radiographs, which should include an anteroposterior (AP) view in the plane of the scapula as well as an axillary view (Fig. 2). Each patient should be assessed individually for the need of computed tomographic (CT) or magnetic resonance

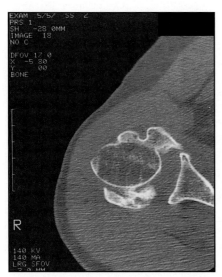

Fig. 3 CT scan of the patient shown in Figure 2. Patient has a four-part fracture malunion.

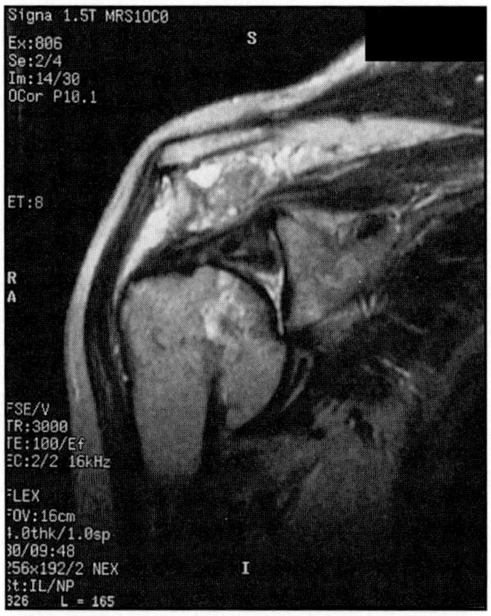

Fig. 4 MRI of a malunited four-part fracture with cuff tear and atrophy and focal ON of the humeral head.

imaging (MRI) scanning. The CT scan can be helpful in helping determine the three-dimensional spatial relationships between the malunited tuberosities, head, and shaft fragments (Fig. 3). In addition, CT scans provide a clear image of the glenohumeral articular surface, thus helping to assess the presence of articular congruity. Similarly, the MRI scan can provide information regarding the integrity of the rotator cuff tendon and degree of atrophy of the deltoid and rotator cuff musculature, as well as early ON of the humeral head (Fig. 4).

Nevertheless, as will be discussed later, intraoperative determinations regarding soft-tissue contracture, rotator cuff integrity, and spatial relationships between bony parts in the proximal humerus remain the most accurate way to assess the pathology in these patients. Intraoperative assessment is often necessary to determine the surgical techniques that will be required to correct the pathology.

Surgical Indications
The primary indications for prosthetic arthroplasty in the setting of malunion of the proximal humerus are severe pain and stiffness, with glenohumeral joint incongruity as the salient pathologic process of the criteria described above. If the bony pathology involves only tuberosity malposition or surgical neck malalignment, the patient can be treated with an osteotomy and repositioning of the malunited fragment.

Technical Considerations
Prothetic arthroplasty for the treatment of proximal humerus fracture malunion is, as mentioned previously, one of the most difficult shoulder procedures faced by the orthopaedic surgeon. Disruption of the normal anatomy and tissue planes, scarring, a weak bony framework, and muscular contracture, among other problems, can contribute to the technical difficulties encountered during surgery.

The procedure is carried out through an extended deltopectoral approach. It may be necessary to perform a coracoid osteotomy to improve exposure. A meticulous take-down of the deltoid origin may occasionally be necessary. When the take-down is performed, the surgeon should maintain the deltotrapezius fascia on the deltoid for later closure. The choices for reconstruction include hemiarthroplasty or total shoulder arthroplasty.

The surgeon must carry out a systematic evaluation of all the different aspects of bony and soft-tissue pathology present in each case. The arthroplasty itself will address the issue of articular incongruity. However, if the greater tuberosity is malpositioned or the surgical neck is malaligned, osteotomies should be performed with the arthroplasty.

Occasionally, an acromioplasty is indicated for patients who may have bony impingement under the coracoacromial arch due to slight tuberosity malposition. In this setting, an osteotomy may not be necessary, but an acromioplasty performed at the time of the reconstructive procedure may effectively decompress the subacromial space.

In addition, soft-tissue pathology in the form of capsular contracture and rotator cuff tears must be carefully evaluated. In most of these cases, the capsule either should be released circumferentially or completely excised, if it is severely contracted. Scar about the conjoint tendon and above and below the subscapularis tendon should be released to regain normal soft-tissue tension. Finally, the entire subdeltoid space should be mobilized.

At the time of initial exposure, the rotator cuff should be evaluated to determine its integrity and repairability. If the cuff tendon is not repairable, the coracoacromial ligament should be preserved for later repair in order to maintain an intact coracoacromial arch, thus minimizing the likelihood of postoperative proximal migration of the humeral component. In addition, an unrepairable large cuff tear precludes the use of total shoulder arthroplasty, even if there is loss of the articular cartilage on the glenoid surface.

The placement of the humeral component is difficult and requires a good understanding of the three-dimensional relationships between the fragments. The level and orientation of the humeral osteotomy for placement of the prosthetic component should take into account any preexisting malalignment of the surgical neck. If the greater tuberosity is malpositioned and lies below or within the confines of the articular surface of the prosthesis, it may not be necessary to perform a tuberosity osteotomy.

The height and version of the humeral component should be individualized in each case in order to maximize stability and motion. The height should be such that effective soft-tissue tension is maintained, while at the same time allowing adequate repositioning of the osteotomized tuberosities. The version should be individualized in order to improve stability of the prosthetic components. In most cases, the prosthesis is cemented.

At the time of closure, the stability of the shoulder is tested, as are the safe ranges of passive motion. The degrees of internal and external rotation that can be achieved without significant tension on either the tuberosities or the rotator cuff repair should be noted, and motion should be limited to this range for the first 6 to 8 weeks postoperatively.

University of Pennsylvania/California Pacific Medical Center Experience

We have recently reviewed our experience with a group of 39 patients treated for fracture malunion of the proximal humerus. These patients were all treated surgically and were followed up for an average of 44 months with a minimal follow-up of 12 months. Their mean age at presentation was 54 years, with an equal distribution among men and women. Initial fracture treatment for 77% of this patient group consisted of sling immobilization and early range of motion; 23% of them had surgical treatment. Malunions were categorized according to the presence of osseous abnormalities (tuberosity malalignment, articular surface incongruity, and articular segment malalignment) and soft-tissue abnormalities (capsular contracture and tears of the rotator cuff).

Most of the malunions in this series presented with a combination of tuberosity malalignment, articular incongruity, and malalignment of the articular segment. The most common type of isolated malunion was a malpositioned tuberosity fragment. Associated soft-tissue pathology included capsular contracture in 64% and full-thickness rotator cuff tears in 38% of cases. Treatment was considered complete if all bony and soft-tissue pathology was treated at the time of the surgical procedure for the treatment of malunion. The results of surgical intervention were analyzed according to successful correction of deficits, and were considered satisfactory based on pain relief, range of motion (active forward flexion equal to or greater than 90°), and ability to perform activities of daily living (ADL). A total of 27 patients (69%) had a satisfactory result based on these criteria.

Twenty-six (67%) of the patients in our group were found to have glenohumeral joint incongruity. For 23 of these 26, the joint incongruity was treated with either prosthetic arthroplasty (n = 22) or glenohumeral arthrodesis (n = 1). Of the 23 patients treated in this fashion, 17 (74%) had satisfactory results. In contrast, all three patients in whom joint incongruity was not addressed with arthroplasty or arthrodesis at the time of surgery had unsatisfactory results.

A large number of the patients in our study group had significant pain relief after surgical treatment of malunion, especially those in whom all bony and soft-tissue pathology was addressed at the time of surgical intervention. Modest gains in motion and functional capacity were also obtained. Of the patients in whom all pathology was addressed intraoperatively, forward elevation improved from 84° to 117° postoperatively, while the functional capacity to perform ADL improved from 44% to 75% of the unaffected shoulder. In the subset of patients in whom bony and soft-tissue pathology was only partially addressed, forward elevation actually declined from 83° to 75° postoperatively, while the functional capacity to perform ADL improved from 35% to 42% of the unaffected shoulder.

The large number of complications encountered in our study group attests to the technical difficulties involved in treating these patients surgically. These complications were much more common in patients treated with prosthetic replacement. A total of ten complications in nine patients were observed as a result of arthroplasty, and these complications can be divided into intraoperative, early postoperative, and late. Three intraoperative fractures of the humeral shaft occurred during preparation of the canal for insertion of a humeral prosthetic component. These fractures were treated intraoperatively, with insertion of a long-stemmed humeral prosthesis and cerclage on recognition of the fracture.

Six patients experienced complications in the early postoperative period. Two patients developed instability of the humeral head prosthesis after surgery. One case of posterior subluxation of a hemiarthroplasty was treated with revision hemiarthroplasty, with insertion of a component with a larger head. One case of anterior hemiarthoplasty subluxation was treated with revision hemiarthroplasty by placing the humeral component in increased retroversion. One patient in whom an osteotomy was performed for varus angulation of the surgical neck during total shoulder arthroplasty developed nonunion of the osteotomy site and loosening of the humeral component. One patient developed early loosening of the humeral component and was treated with revision total shoulder arthroplasty.

Long-term complications were seen in three patients who developed late attritional tears of the rotator cuff. In all cases, the tears presented with progressive loss of range of motion and strength. In all of these patients, a rotator cuff tear was present at the time of malunion treatment. Two of the three patients had an excellent result postoperatively, with significant range of motion and functional gains. Although these two patients had minimal or no pain, they had marked functional limitations at latest follow-up. The third patient had moderate symptom resolution and functional gains postoperatively. Due to progressive pain and disability, the patient underwent a procedure to repair the late cuff tear, but there had been no improvement in functional status at latest follow-up.

Treatment Algorithm

Based on this experience, we have developed a treatment algorithm for malunion of proximal humerus fractures. First, the nature of the bony pathology should be determined. In cases of glenohumeral surface incongruity, resurfacing in the form of arthroplasty (hemiarthroplasty or total shoulder arthroplasty) should be performed. If the tuberosities are malpositioned, tuberosity osteotomy and repositioning or acromioplasty should be performed. If the articular segment is malaligned, a surgical neck osteotomy should be considered. In addition, an assessment of capsular contracture and inspection of the rotator cuff tendon should be carried out, and the appropriate corrective measures performed in

order to address the pathology. All of these factors should be taken into account concomitantly, because they often coexist in these posttraumatic shoulders.

Conclusion

Preoperative physical examination of the affected shoulder is important to detect the presence and extent of capsular contracture, subacromial impingement, and rotator cuff integrity. Radiographs can be helpful in determining the position of the tuberosities, presence of articular incongruity, and alignment of the articular segment. However, it should be emphasized that intraoperative assessment of the position of the bony elements, the extent of glenohumeral articular degeneration, and rotator cuff pathology remains the most accurate method of determining the true nature of the malunion.

The periarticular bony and soft-tissues of the shoulder are intimately linked from an anatomic and mechanical standpoint. Disruption of the native osseous architecture of the proximal humerus, in combination with soft-tissue pathology in the form of capsular contracture and rotator cuff tears, can have considerable deleterious effects on shoulder joint function. Malunion of proximal humerus fractures can lead to such deficits, which can render a shoulder functionless. The symptomatology associated with proximal humerus fracture malun-

ion is multifactorial. Systematic preoperative analysis of the etiologic factors responsible for the clinical picture and complete surgical correction of these deficits are essential to achieve satisfactory results.

References

1. Flatow EL, Cuomo F, Maday MG, et al: Open reduction and internal fixation of two-part displaced fractures of the greater tuberosity of the proximal part of the humerus. *J Bone Joint Surg* 1991;73A:1213–1218.
2. Solonen KA, Vastamaki M: Osteotomy of the neck of the humerus for traumatic varus deformity. *Acta Orthop Scand* 1985;56:79–80.
3. Morris ME, Kilcoyne RF, Shuman W, et al: Humeral tuberosity fractures: Evaluation by CT scan and management of malunion. *Orthop Trans* 1987;11:242.
4. Tanner MW, Cofield RH: Prosthetic arthroplasty for fractures and fracture-dislocations of the proximal humerus. *Clin Orthop* 1983;179:116–128.
5. Norris TR, Green A, McGuigan FX: Late prosthetic shoulder arthroplasty for displaced proximal humerus fractures. *J Shoulder Elbow Surg* 1995;4:271–280.
6. Frich LH, Sojbjerg JO, Sneppen O: Shoulder arthroplasty in complex acute and chronic proximal humeral fractures. *Orthopedics* 1991;14:949–954.
7. Dines DM, Warren RF, Altcheck DW, et al: Posttraumatic changes of the proximal humerus: Malunion, nonunion, and osteonecrosis. Treatment with modular hemiarthroplasty or total shoulder arthroplasty. *J Shoulder Elbow Surg* 1993;2:11–21.
8. Muldoon MP, Cofield RH: Complications of humeral head replacement for proximal humerus fractures, in Springfield DS (ed): *Instructional Course Lectures 46*. Rosemont, IL, American Academy of Orthopaedic Surgeons, 1997, pp 15–24.

15

Management of the Unstable Prosthetic Shoulder Arthroplasty

Tom R. Norris, MD
Scott R. Lipson, MD

Introduction

Instability after shoulder arthroplasty is a multifactorial problem. When treating the unstable prosthetic implant, it is necessary to thoroughly evaluate all components of the shoulder, including the bony architecture, the position of the prosthesis, the condition of the soft tissues (ligament, capsule, muscle), and the function of the nerves of the shoulder. In addition, it is important to consider the timing of the instability (early postoperatively or later), the chronicity, the direction, and the degree. Treatment must be directed at correction of all of the factors that are contributing to instability in a given unstable shoulder arthroplasty. If any of the contributing factors is not corrected, the instability will recur after treatment, or another direction of instability may be manifested.

Review of Literature

In 1982, Neer and associates[1] reported on 194 total shoulder arthroplasties with a 4% incidence of postoperative instability. Included in their report were anterior, posterior, and inferior instability. Four patients sustained dislocations (two anterior, two posterior), all of which were treated with closed reduction and immobilization. One patient with a posterior dislocation failed closed treatment and developed recurrent posterior subluxation. The etiology of the instability was thought to be glenoid component retroversion caused by inadequate correction of posterior glenoid wear prior to implantation of the prosthesis. Two patients had

inferior instability, caused by deltoid weakness secondary to loss of humeral length and by inferior placement of the humeral component. Two patients with recurrent anterior subluxations caused by excessive humeral anteversion were treated with revision of the humeral component to correct the version.

Cofield[2] reviewed the literature for complications in shoulder arthroplasty. Instability was the most common complication reported, with an incidence of 5.2%. In the same paper, he reported on his own series of 419 total shoulder replacements (TSR). In this series he determined that the risk factors for postoperative instability were preoperative rotator cuff disease, older age, increased preoperative external rotation, and small prosthetic head size. In addition, instability was the most common indication for revision of a TSR in this series, and the third most common reason for revision of a humeral head replacement alone.

Moeckel and associates[3] retrospectively reviewed 236 shoulder arthoplasties, identifying ten with postoperative instability. Seven of the shoulders were unstable anteriorly, three posteriorly. All of the shoulders with anterior instability had a dehiscence of the subscapularis. Four could be repaired primarily. Three required reconstruction with a calcaneus-Achilles allograft, as a static anterior restraint. Each of the three shoulders with posterior instability had a different etiology of the instability. One had glenoid retroversion caused by uncorrected posterior glenoid wear. This was treated

with glenoid component revision and posterior bone grafting. One had excessive humeral retroversion, which was treated with humeral component revision. Another had excessive posterior soft-tissue laxity. This patient was treated with a soft-tissue instability repair, which failed.

Wirth and Rockwood[4,5] reviewed the literature and presented a series of their own in an effort to delineate the causes and treatments of instability after shoulder arthroplasty. Factors they discussed that contribute to anterior instability include humeral component malrotation (decreased retroversion), anterior deltoid dysfunction, and disruption of the subscapularis. In their experience, humeral component malrotation by itself was not sufficient to cause anterior instability. They found that shoulders with anterior instability and decreased humeral retroversion also had either subscapularis disruption or were lacking an intact coracoacromial arch secondary to prior surgery. However, the coracoacromial arch is truly an anterosuperior restraint. Thus, if it is absent, superior instability is more likely than anterior alone, and is usually found in conjunction with rotator cuff insufficiency. In addition, deltoid dysfunction does not usually cause instability. It is, however, a problem with significant functional consequences, which must often be dealt with in reconstruction of the multiply operated shoulder because they can compromise the results of surgery. They recommend pectoralis major transfer for irreparable subscapu-

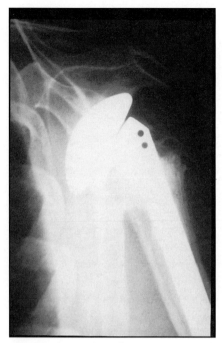

Fig. 1 This humeral prosthesis was cemented in place, 180° malrotated. Malrotation is usually not sufficient to cause instability without additional soft-tissue imbalance. However, this extreme malrotation required revision surgery.

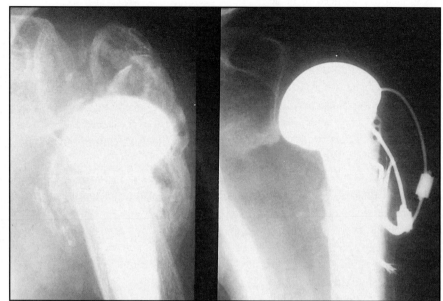

Fig. 2 This humeral head replacement was done for a proximal humerus fracture. The prosthesis was place too far distally (at the level of the surgical neck), and the tuberosities were not repaired to the humeral shaft. The prosthesis was revised, cemented at the appropriate height, and the tuberosities were osteotomized and repaired in anatomic position.

laris deficiency. In their experience, posterior instability was caused by increased humeral retroversion, glenoid component retroversion (caused by uncorrected posterior glenoid wear), and soft-tissue imbalance (posterior structures lax, anterior structures tight). They managed posterior instability with correction of humeral and glenoid component version, anterior releases and subscapularis lengthening, and posterior capsulorrhaphy.

Craig[6] divided dislocation after shoulder arthroplasty into two groups, early and late. The factors that cause dislocation differ in the two groups. Early dislocations (in the immediate postoperative period) tend to be caused by static factors: implant position, bony anatomy, inadequate postoperative protection, and soft-tissue imbalance. Late dislocations are usually caused by dynamic factors:

muscular imbalance, rotator cuff dysfunction (rotator cuff tear, suprascapular nerve injury).

Etiology of Instability

The most important aspect of treating the unstable shoulder arthroplasty is an understanding of the causative factors involved in each particular case. In order to avoid a recurrence of the instability, each factor must be addressed and corrected. The condition of the capsule must be considered; whether it is scarred and tight, or ruptured and lax. The muscular function must be assessed as well. Most importantly, the deltoid and rotator cuff must be examined to determine whether function is normal or abnormal. If the muscle function is not normal, it is necessary to determine whether the muscle is detached or denervated. Patient factors, such as potential for noncompliance and the possibility of voluntary dislocation, must be considered. The condition of the prosthesis and bone must be evaluated. The prosthesis may be loose and

malrotated, or it may have been implanted in improper rotation (Fig. 1) or height initially (Fig. 2). The position of the tuberosities should be examined to detect a tuberosity dehiscence, especially if the arthroplasty was done to treat a proximal humerus fracture.

The etiology of the arthritis that created the need for the initial arthroplasty has a bearing on the potential for postoperative instability. The shoulder with rheumatoid arthritis typically has a torn or thinned rotator cuff, central or superior glenoid erosion (Fig. 3), and inferior capsular contracture. Among the many conditions that tend to cause posterior instability are osteoarthritis, capsulorrhaphy arthropathy, and fixed posterior dislocation. All of these conditions are characterized by tight anterior structures, a stretched or torn posterior capsule, and asymmetrical posterior glenoid wear (Fig. 4). All these elements must be dealt with during the primary surgery in order to minimize the potential for superior instability. In addition, one or more of these factors may need to be addressed during revision surgery to treat postoperative instability.

Preoperative Evaluation of the Unstable Shoulder Arthroplasty

The goal of the preoperative evaluation (prior to revision surgery) is to determine the pathologic conditions present and to formulate a detailed plan based on accurate information. Deltoid function is critical for shoulder function. While deltoid dysfunction is not a significant cause of instability after arthroplasty (except inferior instability), it is a major cause of poor function after shoulder surgery. Prior to any revision shoulder surgery, the deltoid should be examined for weakness and the presence of a visible or palpable defect indicating dehiscence or denervation (Fig. 5). Electromyography (EMG) of all three divisions of the deltoid will aid in differentiating denervation from dehiscence. If deltoid dysfunction is detected preoperatively, it can be addressed during the revision with a deltoidplasty, muscle transfer, or axillary nerve exploration and repair. The condition of the rotator cuff should be determined. Magnetic resonance imaging (MRI) may be useful in determining the potential for repair of a torn rotator cuff by ascertaining the size of the tear and whether the muscles have undergone fatty degeneration. In addition, MRI is useful in the case of a chronic dislocation to evaluate the rotator cuff which cannot be examined clinically. If a large, potentially irreparable rotator cuff tear is identified prior to revision, the surgeon can plan to perform tendon transfers during the revision. EMG can be helpful in this regard as well by identifying suprascapular nerve lesions. If there is suprascapular nerve dysfunction causing rotator cuff dysfunction, it should be addressed with exploration, decompression, and repair, if warranted.

The glenoid is evaluated for the presence of uncorrected asymmetrical

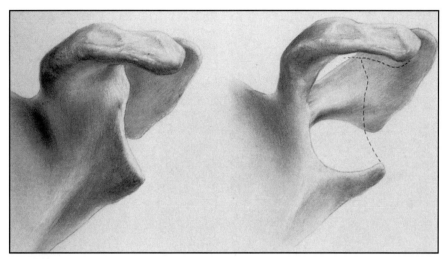

Fig. 3 Rheumatoid arthritis typically results in superior and central glenoid erosion. Often the rotator cuff is thinned or torn, as well. (Reproduced with permission from Norris TR: Unconstrained prosthetic shoulder replacement, in Watson MS (ed): *Surgical Disorders of the Shoulder.* Edinburgh, Scotland, Churchill Livingstone, 1991, p 498.)

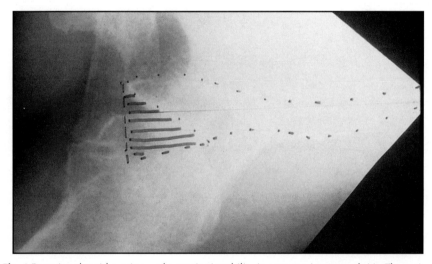

Fig. 4 Posterior glenoid erosion and posterior instability is common in osteoarthritis. The typical pathology in osteoarthritis involves increasingly scarred and shortened anterior structures, increasing internal rotation contracture, progressive posterior laxity, glenoid erosion and instability. (Reproduced with permission from Norris TR: Unconstrained prosthetic shoulder replacement, in Watson MS (ed): *Surgical Disorders of the Shoulder.* Edinburgh, Scotland, Churchill Livingstone, 1991, p 498.)

peripheral wear (Fig. 6). In a humeral head replacement the instability is the result of failure to treat the glenoid wear. In total shoulder replacement the instability is caused by glenoid component malposition, which is the result of uncorrected peripheral glenoid wear. In either situation, if asymmetrical periph-

eral wear is detected the surgeon can plan either to ream the glenoid to create a concentric glenoid that can support a prosthesis or to augment the glenoid with a bone graft. Hill and Norris[7] presented long-term follow-up data on 17 patients with glenoid bone grafts. They were able to restore glenoid version and volume in

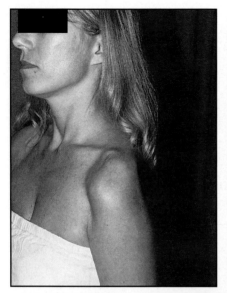
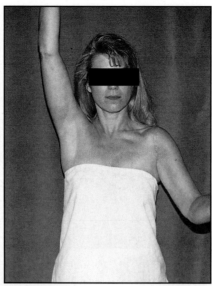

Fig. 5 Top left, This patient underwent multiple procedures for a proximal humerus fracture, including a humeral head replacement. At this point she had a fixed anterior dislocation and loss of her anterior deltoid secondary to axillary nerve injury. **Top right,** Her function was poor, with limited evaluation and strength, and she was in constant pain. **Bottom left,** An axillary view shows the fixed anterior dislocation. At the time of the revision it was found that the subscapularis had been avulsed. **Bottom right,** Revision surgery involved conversion to a total shoulder replacement, extensive posterior mobilization, retrieval of the avulsed subscapularis, and transfer of the middle deltoid to fill in for the absent anterior deltoid. This axillary view shows the humeral head centered in the glenoid component.

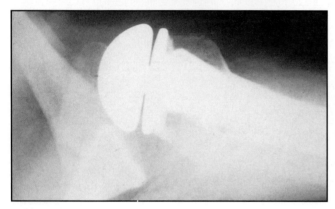
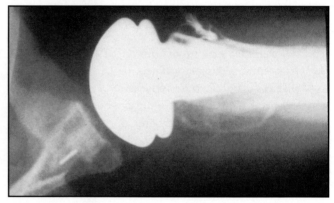

82% of the cases. Neer and Morrison[8] found that glenoid bone grafting was required in 4.3% of their total shoulder replacements.

Management of Instability After Shoulder Arthroplasty
Anterior Instability

As discussed previously, there is more than one cause of anterior instability.[3-5] The most common cause is subscapularis rupture (Fig. 5). The use of oversized humeral head components may predispose to subscapularis dehiscence by placing increased tension on the repair. Decreased humeral component retroversion does not usually cause anterior instability on its own. However, the shoulder will be anteriorly unstable if

humeral component malrotation is combined with a deficient or absent subscapularis. Glenoid component anteversion can cause anterior instability. Anterior glenoid wear or loss is most often found in arthritis of recurrent anterior dislocations (Fig. 7). If it is uncorrected (or unnoticed) at the time of arthroplasty, the glenoid component may be placed in anteversion or have insufficient anterior bony support. This can be avoided by recognizing the anterior wear on good preoperative axillary radiographs or computed tomographic (CT) scans. The anterior glenoid wear can be corrected by reaming the posterior glenoid to meet the anterior side. As long as 80% of the glenoid component is supported after reaming is completed, the prosthesis

should be stable. In severe cases, the glenoid may require bone grafting prior to insertion of a glenoid component. Revision of a malrotated glenoid may require bone grafting as well.

Subscapularis rupture can be diagnosed in the postoperative period with the lift-off test as described by Gerber and Krushell.[9] The lift-off test is performed with the arm extended and internally rotated, and the dorsum of the hand is placed on the low back. If the subscapularis is ruptured the patient will be unable to lift his hand off of his back. Once a subscapularis rupture is identified, it should be explored and repaired early. If it is not explored early, the rupture will become irreparable. Moeckel and associates[3] were able to repair only four out of seven subscapularis ruptures in their series. If the subscapularis cannot be repaired, something must be done to try to restore soft-tissue balance. A calcaneus-Achilles allograft can be used as a static anterior restraint. Active muscle power may be restored with a pectoralis major transfer or a latissimus dorsi transfer. Some combination of these reconstructive options may be used as well. The tendon transfers may help support the allograft tissue as it heals, because these grafts become quite weak during incorporation. In addition, the humeral component can be placed in increased retroversion. This alone will not correct the anterior instability, but in conjunction with an anterior reconstruction it can add some stability.

Posterior Instability

Posterior instability has more than one possible cause as well. In addition, more than one cause may be present in any particular shoulder. Vlasak and associates found that 60% of shoulders with posterior instability after arthroplasty had posterior capsular laxity. Other causes were posterior rotator cuff tears, posterior glenoid erosion (Fig. 6), increased humeral retroversion, and glenoid component retroversion (personal communication, 1995). Soft-tissue balancing is critical to restoration of stability. In posterior instability, the anterior structures are overly tight, the posterior structures are lax, or both. Thus, the anterior structures must be freed up and lengthened, and the posterior structures must be repaired, if torn, and shortened, if necessary. If external rotation is limited, the subscapularis should be lengthened, which can be accomplished by recessing the tendon medially off of the lesser tuberosity (Fig. 8). Sutures are placed in the proximal humerus prior to insertion of the humeral component to repair the subscapularis in a more medial position. Every 1 cm of lengthening increases external rotation by

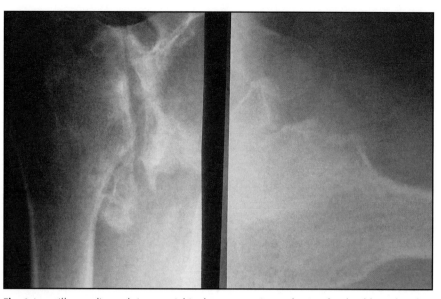

Fig. 6 An axillary radiograph is essential in the preoperative evaluation for shoulder arthroplasty. This patient with a fixed posterior dislocation has eroded the entire posterior half of the glenoid. The axillary view enables one to evaluate for asymmetrical peripheral glenoid wear. A CT scan can be used if one is unable to attain an axillary radiograph.

20°. The anterior capsule should be freed up from the anterior glenoid, and the subscapularis should be mobilized completely. If the posterior rotator cuff is torn it should be repaired. The appropriate soft-tissue tension can be determined by placing the prosthetic components and subluxating the humeral heads (Fig. 9). If the humeral head can subluxate more than 50% of the width of the glenoid, the shoulder is too loose posteriorly and a larger humeral head should be tried. If the larger head reduces the subluxation to 50% of the glenoid width, then the tension is correct. However, if this makes the anterior structures too tight to be closed or restricts motion, the smaller head should be used and the posterior capsule should be plicated. A posterior capsular plication can be performed through an anterior incision by removing the humeral head and placing a purse string suture in the capsule. After plication, the humeral head should be replaced and the trial subluxation repeated, taking care not to tear out the poste-

rior sutures.

Posterior glenoid erosion and glenoid retroversion can cause posterior instability as well. Posterior glenoid erosion can be corrected by reaming down the anterior glenoid to meet the posterior surface. Care must be taken to avoid too much medialization of the glenoid, which can make the glenoid too small to support a prosthesis. If posterior wear is severe, a bone graft may be necessary. A glenoid component that has been placed in retroversion because posterior glenoid wear has not been corrected must be revised. Revision will require reaming to equalize the anterior and posterior sides or bone graft just as described above. Decreasing humeral retroversion may also provide some stability.

Inferior Instability

Inferior instability is usually caused by placing the prosthesis too low. The most common situation occurs when a prosthesis is placed on the surgical neck when treating a four-part proximal

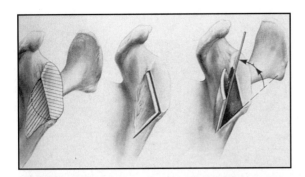
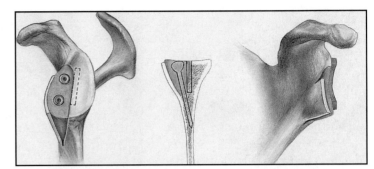
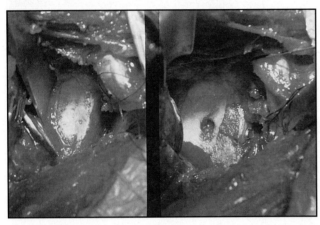
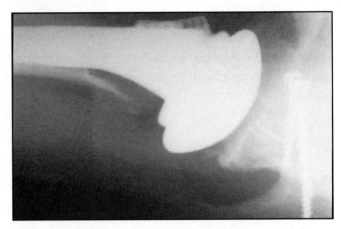

Fig. 7 Top left, Anterior glenoid wear may require the addition of an anterior glenoid bone graft prior to glenoid component insertion. A "trap-door" can be created in the anterior cortex and hinged open using an osteotome. **Top right,** The "trap-door" in the anterior cortex can then be used to sandwich in a piece of bone graft to reconstruct the glenoid. The graft is held with screws, placed to avoid interference with preparation of the glenoid. Then the glenoid is prepared as usual. **Bottom left,** Posterior glenoid wear may require bone grafting for reconstruction. The "trap-door" method does not work well posteriorly. Instead, a graft is placed posteriorly and held with screws. This operative photograph shows a piece of humeral head used as posterior bone graft. **Bottom right,** This axillary radiograph shows screws holding an anterior bone graft used in reconstruction of a glenoid with anterior wear. (Reproduced with permission from Norris TR: Unconstrained prosthetic shoulder replacement, in Watson MS (ed): *Surgical Disorders of the Shoulder.* Edinburgh, Scotland, Churchill Livingstone, 1991, p 498.)

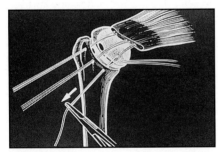

Fig. 8 Subscapularis recession is performed to lengthen the anterior structures and gain external rotation in shoulders with internal rotation contracture. Every centimeter of lengthening increases external rotation by 20°. (Reproduced with permission from Groh GI, Rockwowod CA Jr: Surgical anatomy and technique, in Friedman RJ (ed): *Arthroplasty of the Shoulder.* New York, NY, Thieme Medical Publishers, 1994, pp 80–98.)

humerus fracture (Fig. 2). Preoperative scanograms can help avoid this complication. Attention to soft-tissue tension, especially tension in the biceps tendon during implantation of the humeral component, can be helpful as well. If the prosthesis is indeed too low, it should be revised and placed at the proper height. If the prosthesis is at the correct height, the humeral head should be 3 to 5 mm above the greater tuberosity. The prosthesis can be cemented higher, or it may be necessary to use an allograft to gain humeral length.

Superior Instability
Superior instability is the most difficult form of instability to treat. Instability in this direction usually is caused by a rotator cuff tear (Fig. 10, *left*). If the coracoacromial ligament has been removed by prior surgery, the instability will be worse (Fig. 10, *right*). Rarely, superior instability can be caused by a proximally placed prosthesis. When performing an arthroplasty on a shoulder with a torn or attenuated rotator cuff, it is best either to avoid removing the coracoacromial ligament or to repair it after it is taken down. The rotator cuff should be repaired, if possible. If the rotator cuff cannot be closed directly, the subscapularis and/or the infraspinatus can be transferred superiorly, or the latissimus dorsi can be transferred. If the rotator cuff tissue is markedly attenuated or the repair is ten-

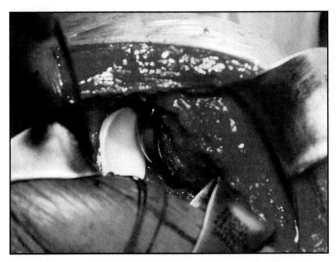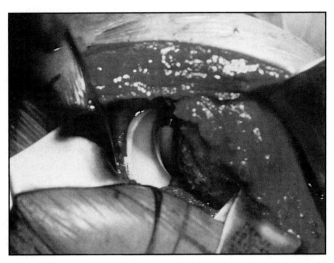

Fig. 9 Left, Proper soft-tissue balancing is the key to primary and revision shoulder arthroplasty. With a trial humeral head, the shoulder is evaluated for posterior stability. If the shoulder subluxes more than 50% of the width of the glenoid, as in this photograph, it is unstable posteriorly. If it is subluxes less than 50% it may be too tight. **Right,** The humeral head trial can be changed and the test performed again. In this photograph the humeral head subluxes the proper amount, 50%. At this point the subscapularis closure is tested. If the subscapularis is too tight to close, the smaller humeral head is replaced and the posterior capsule is tightened with a purse string suture.

uous, a glenoid component should not be used because the component will become loose if superior instability does develop.[10] The glenoid should be reamed to a more uniform shape to fit the humeral head instead. If superior instability develops in the postoperative period, an arthrogram is unnecessary to identify a rotator cuff tear. If the rotator cuff is good, a repair should be done early. All of the techniques mentioned above can be used as necessary to close the rotator cuff. If the glenoid component is loose, it should be removed and the defect packed with bone graft (autograft, allograft, or both) or reimplanted, in the few cases in which adequate bone is still available in the glenoid. It is best to try to avoid the development of superior instability by repairing rotator cuff tears early and by not taking down the coracoacromial ligament when the cuff is deficient.

The Unreconstructible Shoulder

Shoulders in which the rotator cuff and deltoid are both damaged beyond repair should be treated with an arthrodesis (Fig. 11). Usually, the unstable shoulder

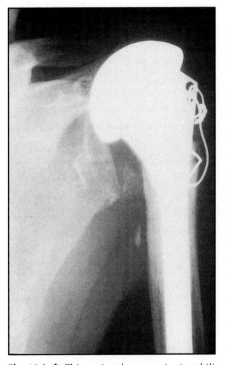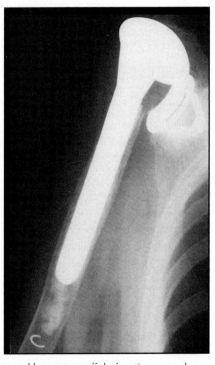

Fig. 10 Left, This patient has superior instability caused by rotator cuff dysfunction secondary to tuberosity nonunion. This is difficult to rectify with revision surgery. At times the contractures are too severe to allow mobilization of the tuberosity and attached muscle in order to replace it to its anatomic position. **Right,** This patient with superior instability is at risk for glenoid loosening, caused by eccentric loading of the glenoid component by the superiorly subluxed humeral head. Ideally, a glenoid component should not be used in a shoulder with poor quality tissue, or an irreparable rotator cuff tear. In addition, every attempt should be made to save the coracoacromial ligament or repair it.

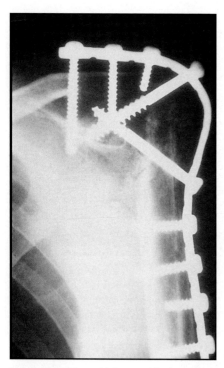

Fig. 11 Shoulders with irreparable damage to the deltoid and rotator cuff should be managed with arthrodesis.

arthroplasty does not result in an unsalvageable situation. Occasionally, soft-tissue balance is impossible to attain. The scarred, contracted tissues are too shortened to allow adequate mobilization. If the shoulder is painful and its function is unacceptable, arthrodesis should be considered. The arthrodesis can be done with allograft interposition to avoid shortening, or a humeral shortening can be done. Another situation in which arthrodesis can be considered is in the patient who has been noncompliant and

whose revision surgery is likely to fail secondary to noncompliance as well. Other options for this patient are psychiatric evaluation, nonsurgical treatment, and the use of a fiberglass shoulder spica cast.

Postoperative Measures

The postoperative care must be tailored to fit the needs of the patient and the surgical procedure performed. If an allograft soft-tissue reconstruction is performed, the patient should be protected for a prolonged period during biologic replacement of the graft, sometimes for several months. Tendon transfers and rotator cuff repairs may require the use of an abduction orthosis. Residual posterior instability after adequate soft-tissue balancing can be treated with a brace or cast, with the arm placed in neutral rotation and extension for 4 to 6 weeks.

Summary

Instability is the most common complication of shoulder arthroplasty. An understanding of the predisposing factors for developing instability is critical to the avoidance of this complication. Soft-tissue balance and proper component positioning must be attained during the index procedure to minimize the risk of developing postoperative instability. Once the shoulder does become unstable, the reason for the instability must be determined. Is the instability secondary to soft-tissue imbalance, component malposition, bony deformity, or a combination of these? Next, a decision must be

made as to how to treat the instability. Nonsurgical treatment may be tried if no obvious cause is present. However, if the instability fails to resolve or recurs, surgical intervention should be undertaken early. If the instability is not treated, it may result in loosening of the prosthesis and early wear of the components. Once surgical intervention is undertaken, all elements of the instability must be recognized and treated.

References
1. Neer CS II, Watson KC, Stanton FJ: Recent experience in total shoulder replacement. *J Bone Joint Surg* 1982;64A:319–337.
2. Cofield RH: Total shoulder arthroplasty complication and revision surgery, in *Shoulder Surgery: The Asian Perspective.* Taipai, Taiwan, Veterans General Hospital, 1995, pp 60–64.
3. Moeckel BH, Altchek DW, Warren RF, et al: Instability of the shoulder after arthroplasty. *J Bone Joint Surg* 1993;75A:492–497.
4. Wirth MA, Rockwood CA Jr: Complications of shoulder arthroplasty. *Clin Orthop* 1994;307:47–69.
5. Wirth MA, Rockwood CA Jr: Complications of total shoulder-replacement arthoplasty. *J Bone Joint Surg* 1996;78A:603–616.
6. Craig EV: Complications in shoulder arthroplasty. *Semin Arthroplasty* 1990;1:160–171.
7. Hill JM, Norris TR: Long term results of bone grafting for glenoid deficiency in total shoulder arthroplasty. *Orthop Trans* 1996;20:58.
8. Neer CS II, Morrison DS: Glenoid bone-grafting in total shoulder arthroplasty. *J Bone Joint Surg* 1988;70A:1154–1162.
9. Gerber C, Krushell RJ: Isolated rupture of the tendon of the subscapularis muscle: Clinical features in 16 cases. *J Bone Joint Surg* 1991; 73B:389–394.
10. Barrett WP, Franklin JL, Jackins SE, et al: Total shoulder arthroplasty. *J Bone Joint Surg* 1987; 69A:865–872.

SECTION

2

Elbow

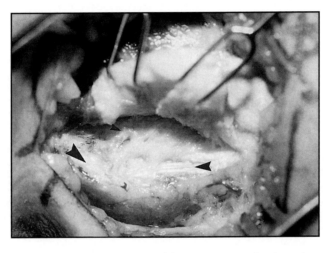

16

Surgical Management of the Extensor Mechanism of the Elbow

Gerard T. Gabel, MD
Brad Zwahlen, MD
Bernard F. Morrey, MD

The extensor mechanism of the elbow is a relatively uncommon source of clinical dysfunction but can be debilitating due to a need for forceful elbow extension with many activities of daily living. Disorders of the elbow that require surgical manipulation of the extensor mechanism are common and present a variety of diagnoses and exposures. Although the awareness and treatment of these diagnoses as well as of these surgical exposures involved have increased over the past two decades, an anatomic evaluation of the extensor mechanism of the elbow has only recently been completed. The traditional anatomic representation of the extensor mechanism of the elbow, the triceps tendon and its insertion upon the olecranon, is one of a singular, discrete insertion.[1-3] As with most anatomic assessments, a more complex system is required to accurately define the triceps mechanism.

Anatomy

The triceps tendon originates intramuscularly at a point 21 cm proximal to the olecranon. The posterior muscle coverage of the tendon terminates obliquely at a level 14 cm proximal to the olecranon. Approximately 50% of the posterior tendon is intramuscular and 50% extramuscular.

The triceps mechanism consists of two components, the triceps proper, that portion inserting on the olecranon, and the triceps expansion, which inserts distally and laterally (Fig. 1). The decrease in width and increase in thickness of the triceps mechanism, triceps proper, and triceps expansion are shown in Tables 1 and 2. The triceps proper thickens rapidly as it approaches the olecranon, while the triceps expansion remains relatively thin. The mechanism, tendon proper, and the expansion each narrow proportionately, decreasing in width by 30% to 40% from 15 cm to the level of the olecranon.

The triceps proper inserts on the posterior 40% of the olecranon (Fig. 2) with the anterior 60% covered only by capsule and fat. The triceps tendon has a maximum thickness at this level averaging 9 mm and a width of 18 mm. The tendon insertion extends to the medial margin of the olecranon; whereas, 2 to 4 mm of the lateral olecranon has no triceps insertion.

The triceps expansion, the lateral continuation of the extensor mechanism, consists of the triceps expansion tendon as well as the continuum of the medial head of the triceps and anconeus. Through this extension, the triceps expansion finds its insertion on the posterior crest of the ulna medially; the fascia of the extensor carpi ulnaris origin laterally, the antebrachial fascia distally and the anconeus insertion deep. There is no

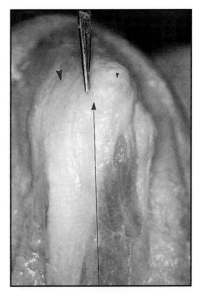

Fig 1 Posterior view of distal one-half of triceps tendon. Olecranon and triceps proper (small arrow), triceps expansion (large arrow), triceps decussation (interval between expansion and triceps proper - medium arrow). Line defines proximal extension of triceps decussation. Triceps proper tendon is mostly covered posteriorly by triceps musculature. Note the large triceps expansion laterally.

medial fascial extensor, no medial expansion (Fig. 3).

In 50% of specimens, a well-defined interval is located between the triceps expansion and triceps proper just proximal to the olecranon. This interval is the

Table 1
Triceps tendon width

Distance From Insertion (cm)	Triceps Mechanism (Total, in mm)	Triceps Proper (mm)	Triceps Expansion (mm)
15	68	23	45
10	57	20.5	36.5
5	51	20.5	30.5
0	43	17.5	25.5

Table 2
Tendon thickness

Distance From Insertion	Tendon Proper (mm)	Triceps Expansion (mm)
20 cm	0.8	N/A
15 cm	1.1	0.4
10 cm	1.8	0.6
5 cm	3.98	1.1
Insertion	9.5	0.9
5 cm Distal to Insertion	N/A	0.5

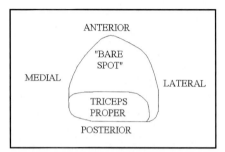

Fig. 2 Diagram of olecranon insertion of triceps proper. Note that the insertion involves the posterior 40% of the olecranon and does not extend to the lateral margin. This has surgical significance in triceps repair, triceps tendinitis, and posterior impingement.

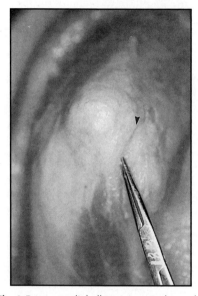

Fig. 3 Posteromedial elbow view. Probe and arrow define medial olecranon, with ulnar nerve immediately adjacent. Note the absence of medial fascial extension, ie, no medial expansion.

Outline 1
Clinical and surgical implications

CLINICAL DYSFUNCTION

Triceps Proper
   Triceps Tendinitis/Olecranon Spur
   Triceps Avulsion
   Triceps Repair in Olecranon Fractures
   Triceps Insufficiency

Osseous
   Posterior Impingement
   Type I Capitellum Fractures

SURGICAL APPROACHES

Reflecting Approaches
   Lateral-Reflecting (Bryan-Morrey)
   Medial-Reflecting
   Osteoanconeus

Transolecranon Approaches
   Anconeus Sparing
   Transolecranon-reflecting approach

Triceps-Splitting Approach

anatomic triceps decussation, with the fibers of the triceps proper coursing directly distally to its olecranon insertion, while the fibers of the triceps expansion diverge laterally to its forearm insertion. This interval in all specimens is the lateral margin of the triceps proper tendon located at the lateral one-fourth of the olecranon and lateral olecranon margin bare spot (Fig. 2).

Clinical Significance
The anatomy of the extensor mechanism of the elbow has multiple clinical and surgical implications (Outline 1), relating to the anatomy of the triceps proper and its insertion as well as the triceps expansion. Disorders of the triceps mechanism relate to compromise of the triceps proper. Deficiency of the triceps expansion, with an intact triceps proper, has not been described. Although the triceps proper appears to be able to compensate for

injury to the triceps expansion (eg, sacrificing the triceps expansion in the classic intra-articular olecranon osteotomy exposure), the triceps expansion is unable to fully compensate for injury to the triceps proper (eg, triceps avulsion injuries). Because of this it is critical that the triceps proper integrity be maintained.

Two primary processes may affect the triceps proper tendon, triceps tendinitis and triceps avulsion injuries. Triceps tendinitis is manifested by chronic posterior elbow pain with extension activities. The diagnosis is confirmed by resisted extension pain and direct tenderness at the distal triceps insertion on the olecranon. It is

seen almost exclusively in males and is caused by longstanding forceful elbow extension. Radiographically, an olecranon spur is typically seen on the posterior olecranon at the location of the triceps proper insertion (Fig. 4). Surgical management, when required, involves subperiosteal excision and exposure of the spur and the olecranon tip. Because as much as 80% of the triceps proper inserts on the spur, a formal triceps repair is required to restore the triceps proper and avoid postoperative triceps avulsion. The results of this procedure and prognosis are good for restoration of strength and motion.

Avulsion of the triceps proper is a

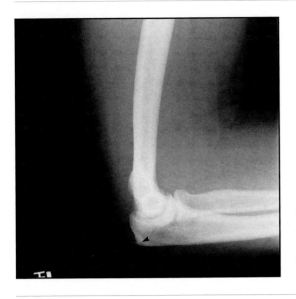

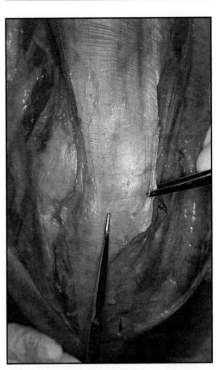

Fig. 4 Olecranon spur and triceps tendon (arrow). Mobile fragment found at surgery treated with excision of spur and olecranon tip and triceps repair.

Fig. 5 Triceps expansion transposition from lateral (left) medially to midline of olecranon (probe), recreating triceps proper axis.

result of eccentric contraction of the triceps, usually due to a fall on an outstretched arm.[4-6] Triceps tendinitis may antedate the injury. Although the triceps proper is avulsed completely, the triceps expansion is uninvolved. Elbow extension is weakened, but active extension is maintained through the triceps expansion. This may result in a failure to diagnose the avulsion and delay treatment. Since the primary extensor of the elbow is the triceps proper, repair is mandated. Debridement of any spur that is present and repair with 5 mm mersilene tape through drill holes is effective in restoring the extensor mechanism.

Secondary disorders of the triceps proper include chronic triceps insufficiency and triceps repair in olecranon fractures. Postoperative or post injury triceps insufficiency,[7,8] as with triceps avulsions, usually spares the triceps expansion. Unlike acute avulsions, direct repair of the triceps is usually not possible because of deficiency of the triceps proper tendon. Interpositional tendon grafting may be equally difficult. Reconstruction of the triceps proper, using the triceps expansion, can be performed. In this case, the triceps expansion is elevated in toto, incising the lateral margin along

the lateral intermuscular septum, extending distally along the anconeus/extensor carpi ulnaris interval to a point approximately 4 to 5 cm distal to the lateral epicondyle, leaving the distal insertion intact. The lateral expansion is translated medially to lie centrally over the olecranon (Fig. 5) and repaired with 5 mm mersilene tape to the posterior olecranon. This restores the extensor mechanism overall through the continuity of the triceps expansion, transposed to the axis of the triceps proper.

Excision of the proximal olecranon in olecranon fractures without anterior instability and less than 50% of the sigmoid notch is a well accepted method of management of nonreconstructible fractures. Repair of the triceps to the subchondral level of the proximal ulna, to support the articular surface, has been advocated as the appropriate method of repair. Placement of the tendon at a subchondral level versus repair to the posterior aspect of the remaining ulna results in a 1 cm or 40% decrease in the moment arm of the triceps proper relative to the axis of rotation of the elbow. This may result in extension weakness, especially through the last 60° of extension. Repair of the triceps should be anatomic, ie, so

that the posterior margin of the triceps is confluent with the posterior margin of the ulna.

Osseous reconstructive surgery related to the extensor mechanism includes posterior impingement of the elbow and Type II (Kocher-Lorenz) or shear fractures of the capitellum. Posterior impingement of the elbow manifests itself usually in chronic, repetitive elbow extension activities or, on occasion, an acute event. Examination demonstrates olecranon fossa level pain with both passive and active terminal extension. The pain results from impingement of the olecranon, especially its lateral margin, on the olecranon fossa and its contents. Surgical management consists of removal of a portion of the olecranon to prevent contact in full extension. As the anterior 60% of the olecranon has no tendinous insertion (Fig. 6), up to 60% of the olecranon may be removed without violation of the triceps proper (Fig. 7).

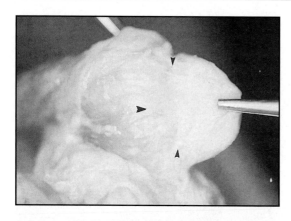

Fig. 6 Picture of proximal olecranon. Olecranon tip/bare spot (right). Triceps proper tendon (large arrow). Anterior margin of triceps proper tendon (medium arrows). Bare spot of approximately 60%.

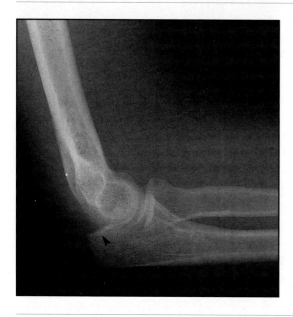

Fig. 7 Postoperative lateral radiograph showing excision of 30% of olecranon, via triceps-splitting approach.

Exposure of the olecranon through the triceps decussation (see triceps-splitting approach) also avoids triceps proper compromise and allows immediate active range of motion and early restoration of activity.

Type II (Kocher-Lorenz) or shear fractures of the capitellum consist essentially of a loss of the hyaline cartilage with a variable, but minimal, amount of the underlying bone. Due to comminution of the articular cartilage and lack of substance for fixation, these injuries may prove very difficult to reconstruct. If the subchondral shape of the capitellum has been reasonably well preserved, a resurfacing procedure with a vascularized fascial arthroplasty consisting of the tendon

and mesotendon of the triceps expansion can be performed. The triceps expansion tendon in its full width (3 to 4 cm) is elevated along with its mesotendon from the underlying triceps and anconeus. It is sectioned transversely distally to give a 5- to 6-cm pedicle based proximally (Fig. 8). The fascial pedicle is rotated 90° to cover the capitellum and is sutured into place with suture anchors. Follow-up on the cases treated in this manner is insufficient to allow for definitive recommendations, but this may prove to be a useful flap for reconstruction of the radiocapitellar joint.

Approaches to the posterior elbow have evolved in a manner to minimize injury to the extensor mechanism.[9-12]

Reflecting exposures have been described for surgical procedures of the posterior elbow. The laterally based reflecting approach (Bryan-Morrey) involves elevation of the triceps medially to preserve the triceps expansion.[9] The plane of dissection initiates at the ulnar nerve/triceps interval medially, extending laterally, elevating the triceps proper insertion. The triceps expansion and anconeus insertion on the posterior crest of the ulna is elevated to a limited degree, and the entire extensor apparatus is reflected on the anconeus/triceps expansion insertion laterally. This approach preserves the majority of the triceps expansion.

In a similar manner, the osteoanconeus flap[12] follows an essentially identical plane of dissection but involves osteotomizing a wafer of the olecranon tip rather than elevating the triceps proper off of the olecranon. The intent of this modification is to preserve the bone-tendon interface of the triceps proper insertion. In order to accomplish this, the wafer must include 9 mm of the posterior surface of the olecranon (Fig. 2), the triceps proper insertion on the posterior olecranon.

The medial-based reflecting approach, an extended Kocher approach, involves elevation of both the triceps expansion and the triceps proper. Due to the absence of a medial expansion, this reflecting approach is without an anatomic basis and has the potential to disrupt the entire extensor mechanism. Although useful as an extensile approach to the lateral elbow, it is rarely indicated for primary exposure of the posterior elbow.

The triceps-splitting approach has been described for access to the distal humerus. Proximal extension of this approach is limited by the intramuscular anatomy of the radial nerve innervation of the triceps. As usually described, with incision to the midpoint of the ulna, distal dissection extends through the triceps proper. Because the triceps proper thickens rapidly in the last 5 cm, this results in a difficult plane of dissection and the integrity of the tendon may be violated if dissection is extended fully to the level of the olecranon insertion.

The interval between the triceps proper and triceps expansion, the triceps decussation, is well defined in 50% of cases by a divergence of the superficial fibers of these tendons as they approach the olecranon. This interval, even in the absence of this divergence, occurs at the lateral margin of the triceps proper at the lateral one fourth of the olecranon. Dissection in this plane is quite easy, as it involves a pure muscle-splitting approach through the inferior aspect of the medial head. Exposure of the distal humerus is identical to a conventionally performed triceps-splitting approach, but it is facilitated by passing through an anatomically more accessible plane (Fig. 9). This triceps-splitting approach gives optimum exposure for olecranon level procedures, eg, ulnohumeral arthroplasty, partial olecranon excision for posterior impingement.

Transolecranon approaches, with an intra-articular osteotomy of the proximal ulna, allow optimum visualization of the distal humerus for comminuted intra-articular fractures of the distal humerus. This approach, as classically performed, preserves the triceps proper insertion but transects the triceps expansion, anconeus/medial head continuum and denervates the anconeus. An alternate approach, a combination of an intra-articular osteotomy and the Bryan-Morrey approaches, allows for the same distal humeral exposure but preserves the anconeus and lateral expansion. This approach involves initially a standard intra-articular osteotomy of the olecranon. The triceps expansion insertion on the posterior crest of the ulna, distal to the osteotomy, is elevated to the extent necessary to reflect the olecranon and triceps expansion laterally (Fig. 10). Elevation of the deep surface of the anconeus then allows full reflection of

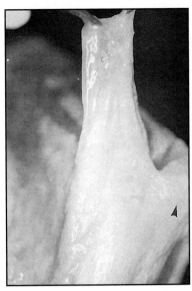

Fig. 8 Proximally based triceps expansion fascial pedicle. Note triceps proper/olecranon (arrow). This flap may be rotated 90° to resurface capitellum or radial head.

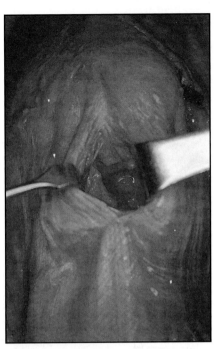

Fig. 9 Interval at lateral margin of triceps proper, the anatomic triceps splitting interval.

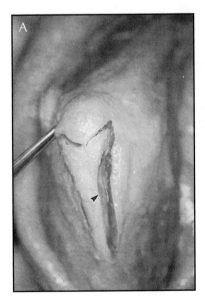

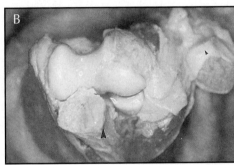

Fig. 10 A, Olecranon osteotomy with incision of triceps expansion/anconeus along lateral margin of posterior ulnar crest. The incision may stop at the level of the arrow and still allow full retraction of the extensor mechanism. B, Posterior view of flexed elbow with olecranon osteotomy reflecting approach. Olecranon/triceps proper (small arrow), lateral expansion elevation off lateral ulna (medium arrow). Note the full exposure of distal humerus with preservation of the triceps expansion.

the extensor mechanism and exposure of the entire distal humerus. This approach preserves the triceps expansion and the anconeus innervation. A second exposure, which preserves the anconeus innervation but still allows proximal retraction of the triceps, involves simply incising the borders of the anconeus and elevating it with the triceps and olecranon osteotomy.

Conclusion

The anatomy of the extensor mechanism of the elbow is more complex than the singular triceps insertion, on the olecranon. Knowledge of the triceps mechanism, triceps proper, triceps expansion and olecranon insertion of the triceps proper allows for improved management and surgical exposure of traumatic and degenerative disorders of the elbow. The triceps proper, which occupies the posterior 40% of the olecranon, must be preserved to maintain full elbow extension strength. The triceps expansion, the secondary component of the triceps mechanism, should be retained in exposures of the posterior elbow and is useful in reconstructive surgical procedures of the elbow.

References

1. Morrey BF: Anatomy of the elbow joint, in Morrey BF (ed): *The Elbow and Its Disorders*, ed 2. Philadelphia, PA, WB Saudners, 1993 pp 16–52

2. Netter FH (ed): *Musculoskeletal System*, in Netter FH: The CIBA Collection of Medical Illustrations. Summit, NJ, CIBA-GEIGY Corporation, 1987, pp 36-37.

3. Salmons S: Muscle, in Williams PL, Bannisdxter LH, Berry MM, et al (eds): *Gray's Anatomy*, ed 38. New York, NY, Churchill Livingstone, 1995, pp 737–900.

4. Anzel SH, Covey KW, Weiner AD, et al: Disruption of muscles and tendons: An analysis of 1,014 cases. *Surgery* 1959;45:406–414.

5. Conwell HE, Alldredge RH: Rutures and tears of muscles and tendons. *Am J Surg* 193735:22–33.

6. Viegas SF: Avulsion of the triceps tendon. *Orthop Rev* 1990;19:533–536.

7. Morrey BF: Complications of elbow relacement urgery, in Morrey BF (ed); *The Elbow and its Disorders,* ed 2. Philadelphia, PA, WB Saunders 1993, pp 665–675.

8. Morrey BF, Askew LJ, An KN: Strength function after total elbow arthroplasty. *Clin Orthop* 1988;234:43–50.

9. Bryan RS, Morrey BF: Extensive posterior exposure of the elbow: A triceps-sparing approach. Clin Orthop 1982;166:188–192.

10. Campbell WC: Incision for exposure of the elbow joint. *Am J Surg* 1932;16:65–67.

11. Kocher T (ed): *Text-book of Operative Surgery*, ed 3. London, England, A and C Black, 1911.

12. Wolfe SW, Ranawat CS: The osteo-anconeus flap: An approach for total elbow arthroplasty. *J Bone Joint Surg* 1990;72A:684–688.

Complex Instability of the Elbow

Bernard F. Morrey, MD

Complex instability of the elbow is the condition resulting from both the injury and the resultant loss of function due to damage to the articular surface and the ligamentous structures that stabilize the elbow. The clinical presentation may be subluxation, or it may be incongruity with malalignment in either the lateral or the anteroposterior plane. The specific goal of this report is to provide a rationale for the reliable treatment of a spectrum of these acute injuries. To accomplish this, the relative contributions of the articulation and the ligaments to normal stability, as well as their interactions, must first be defined.

Contributions to Normal Stability
Articular Elements

For the purpose of this discussion, it is assumed that the distal humerus is intact. Therefore, the elements of the articulation to be discussed include the radial head and the proximal ulna, specifically the coronoid. The ligamentous structures include the medial collateral ligament (MCL) and the ulnar part of the lateral collateral ligament (LCL). The various interactions between the soft-tissue and articular constructs are well known (Fig. 1). Some of these interrelationships have been quantified.

Radial Head

It is known clinically that the radial head may be resected without altering the normal stability of the elbow.[1] Therefore, the contribution of the radiohumeral joint to the stability of the elbow is intimately related to and dependent on the integrity of the collateral ligaments. Because the

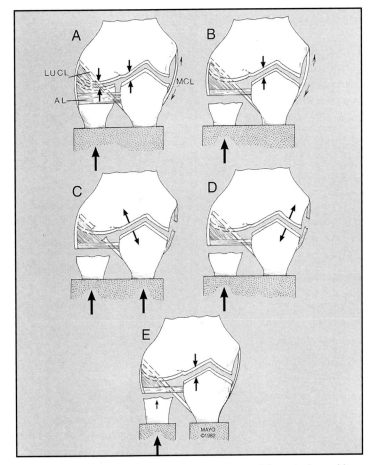

Fig. 1 Schematic drawings showing the complex interactions of the articular and ligamentous constraints at the ulnar part of the lateral collateral ligament (LUCL), annular ligament (AL), and medial collateral ligament (MCL) of the elbow. **A,** An off-center force (large arrow) demonstrates the shared compressive load (medium arrows) borne by the radial head and the coronoid, with tension (smallest arrows) being borne by the MCL. **B,** With an absent radial head, loads similar to those in A are shared by the collateral ligaments as well as the coronoid. If the soft-tissue attachments of the wrist are intact, the radius is axially stable and hence the over-all complex is stable. **C,** With an absent radial head and both collateral ligaments torn, loading of the forearm (large arrows) causes pivoting and instability at the elbow as a result of the abnormally divided load (small arrows) on the coronoid. **D,** With the radial head removed, a valgus stress (off-center load; large arrow) is inadequately resisted by the coronoid in the presence of a torn MCL, causing valgus instability as a result of the abnormally divided load (small arrows) on the coronoid. **E,** After the radial head has been removed, if there has been disruption of the triangular fibrocartilage complex at the wrist a longitudinal pattern of instability develops. (Reproduced with permission from the Mayo Foundation, Rochester, MN.)

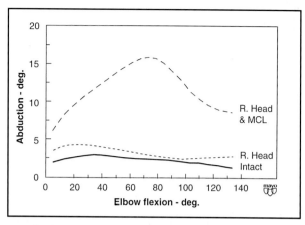 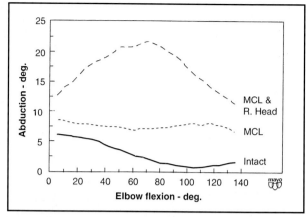

Fig. 2 Graphs showing two sequences documenting the radial (R) head as a secondary stabilizer against valgus stress at the elbow. **Left,** When the radial head has been excised and the MCL is intact, valgus stress causes little displacement (small-dotted line). However, after the MCL has been removed, the joint subluxates (large-dotted line). **Right,** In an alternative sequence, some instability occurs when the radial head is intact and the MCL is absent (small-dotted line). Removal of the radial head causes increased instability and subluxation (large-dotted line). (Reproduced with permission from the Mayo Foundation, Rochester, MN.)

radial head involves the lateral aspect of the articular complex, its particular contribution is best studied by evaluating its role in preventing valgus instability. Experimental data have clearly demonstrated that the resistance to valgus stress provided by the radial head is minimal[2] when the MCL is intact (Fig. 2). However, the radiohumeral joint offers enough resistance to valgus stress to prevent subluxation of the joint if the MCL is attenuated or torn. The major structure resisting initial valgus displacement, even with an intact radial head, is the MCL. Thus, the radial head is an important secondary stabilizer that prevents valgus instability; if the MCL is intact, the radial head offers little resistance to valgus stress, but if the MCL is attenuated or torn, the radial head assumes the role of an important stabilizer.

The relationship of the radial head to the ulnar part of the LCL has also been studied experimentally. O'Driscoll and associates[3] demonstrated the clinical manifestation of an attenuated or torn LCL; posterolateral rotatory subluxation can occur in the presence or absence of the radial head.[4] However, clinical experience suggests that elbows without a radial head do less well after reconstruction of the ulnar part of the LCL than do those in which the radial head is intact.[5] This suggests that the radial head provides some resistance to posterolateral rotatory instability but, once again, in a secondary capacity.

The Proximal Ulna
The major determinant of stability of the elbow is clearly the ulnohumeral joint. Although the stabilizing influence of this joint has not been studied to any great extent, the relative contribution of the olecranon in resisting various loading configurations has been shown to be linearly correlated with the extent of resection of the proximal ulna (Fig. 3).[6] A critical amount of articulation is required to maintain stability, but the relevance of these data is tempered by the lack of dynamic studies. At least 30% of the articular portion of the ulna appears to be needed for stability, as this is also the site of attachment of the collateral ligaments.

Coronoid
I know of no experimental data with regard to the amount of the coronoid required for stability with or without ligamentous integrity. This question is currently under investigation in our laboratory. There is a moderate amount of clinical experience suggesting that at least 50% of the coronoid must be present for the ulnohumeral joint to be functional, and this is consistent with our preliminary laboratory findings. An important clinical correlate is the ability to estimate the amount of the coronoid that no longer remains functional on the basis of the opening angle (the angle defined by a line connecting the tip of the olecranon and the tip of the coronoid and a line along the long axis of the ulna). Normally, this angle is 30°; however, fractures involving 50% of the coronoid reduce it to 0° (Fig. 4).

Ligamentous Contributions
The relative contributions of the MCL and LCL to varus-valgus stability with the elbow in flexion and extension have been studied experimentally.[7] Investigation has shown that the collateral ligaments provide approximately 50% of the stability of the joint, while the articular surfaces after an additional 50%. The only exception is with the elbow in full extension: under this condition, the ante-

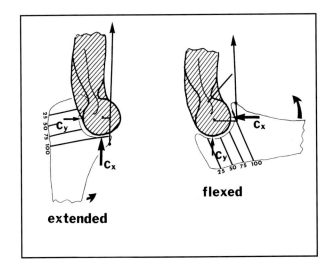

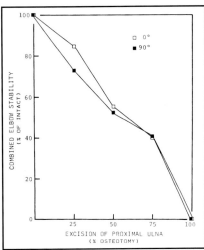

extended

flexed

Fig. 3 Left, Axial (Cx) and transverse (Cy) loading configurations of the ulna in extension and flexion after resection of 25%, 50%, 75%, and 100% of the proximal part. **Right,** The graph shows a linear correlation of the residual stability as a function of the amount of ulna resected. (Reproduced with permission from the Mayo Foundation, Rochester, MN.)

rior part of the capsule has been found to resist both varus and valgus stress. This may be important in patients who have a fracture-dislocation with disruption of both the MCL and the LCL as well as the anterior part of the capsule.

Principle

The basic principle underlying the treatment of complex instability of the elbow, which has been defined on the basis of careful evaluation of the experimental data and my clinical experience, is that it is essential that all treatment options take advantage of or restore a stable ulnohumeral joint. In this paper, complex instability is discussed on the basis of this principle. The most common conditions are classified primarily according to the articular injury.

Radial Head Fracture With Attenuation or Tear of the MCL

The presentation of an isolated fracture of the radial head can be extremely subtle. The prevalence is difficult to ascertain, but in my experience it has occurred in about 1% to 2% of patients who had a fracture of the radial head.[4] The diagnosis requires a high level of suspicion of injury of the ligament when there is a compression fracture of the radial neck. However, some comminuted fractures

may also be caused by an axial load and severe valgus stress, causing concurrent rupture of the MCL.

Treatment of this difficult problem is based first on the recognition of the pathologic features and second on the realization that the radial head is an important secondary stabilizer when the MCL has been disrupted. The primary goal of treatment is to restore the stabilizing function of the radial head by osteosynthesis if possible. If the fracture is amenable to fixation, the stable arc is determined during the procedure. If the arc is stable and within 40° of extension, unrestricted motion is allowed after 2 weeks of protection. If dislocation occurs with extension of approximately 60°, the elbow is immobilized for 2 weeks and motion in a hinged splint, with use of a 30° extension stop, is allowed for 2 weeks. The collateral ligament is not repaired in either instance.

If osteosynthesis is not possible, then restoration of the radiohumeral joint with use of a prosthesis is considered. Unfortunately, the silicone implant does not reliably offer the material characteristics necessary to achieve stability; therefore, the possibility of use of metal implants has been reintroduced,[8-10] although there is limited clinical evidence to document their efficacy. I have there-

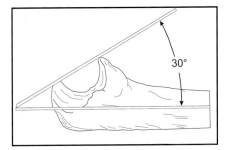

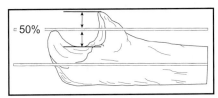

Fig. 4 Top, When the coronoid is intact, a line between the tips of the olecranon and coronoid forms an angle of approximately 30° with the long axis of the ulna. **Bottom,** When 50% of the coronoid is absent, the line from the residual coronoid through the tip of the olecranon is approximately parallel to the long axis of the ulna. This correlation assists the surgeon in anticipating instability on the basis of the radiographic appearance of the fracture. (Reproduced with permission from the Mayo Foundation, Rochester, MN.)

fore resorted, in some instances in which the MCL has been disrupted, to replacement with a cadaveric radial head in an effort to provide stabilization (Fig. 5).

If the radiohumeral joint cannot be reconstructed, it is appropriate to address the injury of the MCL directly and to

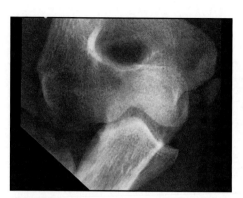 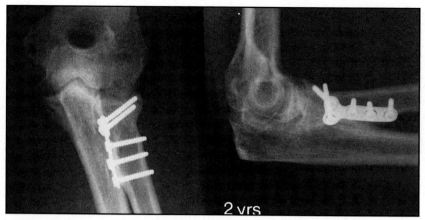

Fig. 5 Left, Radiograph showing gross valgus instability in a patient who had resection of the radial head in the presence of an unrecognized disruption of the MCL. **Right,** Two years after reconstruction with an allograft, the patient had excellent function.

repair it as soon as possible. The ligament may be avulsed from the medial epicondyle, allowing direct reattachment. Mid-substance tears are more difficult to repair, and there is less likelihood of achieving immediate stabilization.

All patients should wear a locked hinged brace for protection for 4 weeks postoperatively; the brace is then unlocked, and motion is allowed in the stable arc. The hinged brace is worn for a total of at least 6 weeks or until the joint is stable.

There is insufficient clinical experience to provide clear expectations of the results. However, treatment of the acute injury is accomplished much more readily than is reconstruction for chronic or late instability.

Radial Head Fracture With Dislocation of the Elbow

This lesion is currently described as a Mason type-IV injury, an extension of the original Mason classification of fractures.[1,11] The simple, type-I fracture is undisplaced; the type-II fracture involves 30% of the radial head and is angulated more than 30° or displaced more than 3 mm; and the type-III fracture is comminuted. There is little information in the literature to help to define the optimum treatment for fracture-dislocations.[12,13]

Assuming that the coronoid is intact, the basic principle of treatment is first to reduce the dislocation and then to determine the extent to which the ulnohumeral articulation provides stability. Additional treatment is determined according to the type of fracture.[1]

Type-I Fracture
In type-I injuries, if the arc of motion is stable to within 45° to 50° of extension then nothing more need be done except to place the elbow in a splint with a 60° extension stop, which the patient wears for 10 to 12 days. Full extension is then allowed as tolerated while the elbow is protected with a hinged splint.

Type-II Fracture
Type-II fractures are treated with open reduction and internal fixation (ORIF). These injuries are the most amenable to such treatment; a rate of success as high as eight of eight was reported by King and associates.[14] It is essential that elbows with injuries of the collateral ligaments be treated with ORIF, because these injuries result in chronic instability if the radial head is resected.[8,9,15] Because these fractures are amenable to such treatment, repair of the collateral ligaments has typically not been necessary in my practice. However, if the elbow remains unstable

on examination through the arcs of motion described earlier, then enhanced stability may be obtained by repairing or stabilizing the collateral ligaments.

Josefsson and associates[16] reviewed their experience with 19 complex injuries of the elbow and recommended ORIF of the radial head fracture as well as repair of the ligament. However, treatment of four of 19 coronoid fractures had a poor result, suggesting that this component of the lesion must be specifically addressed.

Type-III Fracture
These are the most difficult injuries to treat. Experience has suggested that the entire radial head should be excised acutely if it cannot be fixed.[12] ORIF is technically difficult and was reported to be successful in only two of six instances by King and associates.[14] During surgical excision, the elbow is tested according to the scheme described for type-I fractures. If the elbow is unstable, then direct repair of the collateral ligaments should be carried out. If this does not provide sufficient stability, then a silicone implant may be considered as a temporary spacer if it would enhance stability through an additional 20°.

Alternatively, a metal implant may be considered. A successful result was reported with use of a Vitallium implant

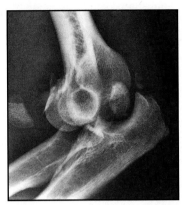 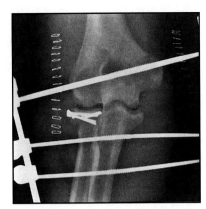 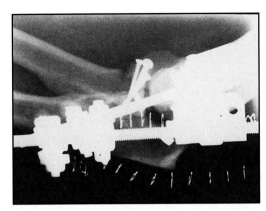

Fig. 6 Left, Radiograph showing a severe fracture-dislocation of the elbow (a Mason type-III fracture of the radial head1,11 as well as a fracture of the coronoid). **Center,** The fracture of the radial head was treated with internal fixation. **Right,** Because of the gross instability, additional stabilization was achieved with use of the Dynamic Joint Distractor.

in 24 of 31 patients after a mean duration of follow-up of 4.5 years.[10] Dislocation of the elbow was an associated injury in 21 of the 31 patients. More recently, an implant design with a so-called floating radial head was introduced; all of 12 procedures performed with this implant were associated with a successful result at a mean of 43 months.[9] Those authors particularly recommended the implant for the treatment of a type-III or complex injury. Alternatively, a cadaveric replacement may be an option; however, there has been little experience with use of such a replacement in the acute setting.

If stability remains a problem, then an external fixator allowing flexion is applied. The indication for use of the external fixator is a joint without a radial head or a healing radiohumeral joint with a torn MCL that is inherently and grossly unstable. If use of an implant or ORIF of the radial head does not restore stability, the distraction device allows a congruous alignment of the ulnohumeral joint, and motion lessens the likelihood of stiffness (Fig. 6). The device is removed in the third to fourth week, and adjustable splints are used to restore motion.

Fracture of the Proximal Ulna
Fractures of the proximal ulna, the olecranon, or the coronoid associated with

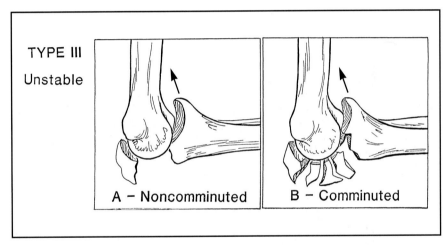

Fig. 7 A Mayo type-III ulnar fracture[4] may or may not be comminuted, but it is characterized by attenuation or disruption of the MCL or the ulnar part of the LCL, or both. This is characterized by instability of the forearm (arrows). (Reproduced with permission from the Mayo Foundation, Rochester, MN.)

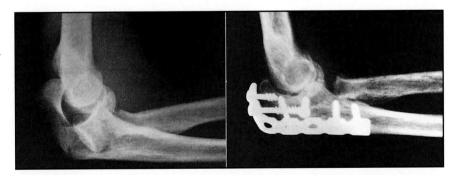

Fig 8 Left, Radiograph showing a Mayo type-III ulnar fracture[4] and a fracture of the radial head. **Right,** The fracture was treated with rigid plate fixation and resection of the radial head. Stabilization of the forearm was attained by virtue of the rigid fixation, enhanced by the 90°-angle bend in the plate.

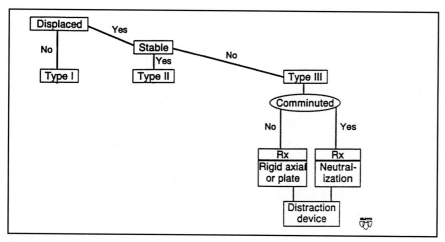

Fig. 9 Diagram for treatment of fractures of the olecranon, based on the Mayo classification.[4] For type-III unstable fractures, rigid fixation is first obtained but may need to be neutralized with a dynamic distraction device. (Reproduced with permission of the Mayo Foundation, Rochester, MN.)

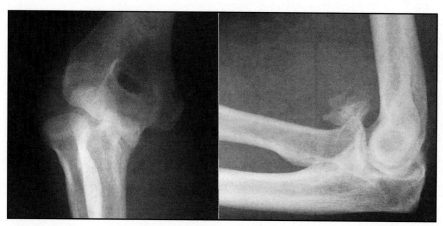

Fig. 10 Left, Radiograph showing a Regan and Morrey type-II coronoid fracture treated with reduction and controlled motion. Right, Eight months later, the joint is stable and the range of motion is from 40° to 120°.

instability fortunately are the most uncommon of these injuries, as they pose the most difficult treatment problems.[4] Treatment consists of restoring the integrity of the ulnohumeral joint, as just described. Ideally, this is accomplished by fixation of the fracture if it is amenable to osteosynthesis.

The Mayo classification scheme for fractures of the olecranon is based on displacement, comminution, and stability.[4] The injury discussed here is termed type III, meaning that the elbow is unstable

because of the injury of a collateral ligament and a displaced fracture of the olecranon (Fig. 7).

Olecranon Fractures

The type-III fracture of the olecranon is accompanied by ligamentous disruption. If there is minimum comminution of the olecranon, rigid plate fixation restores the ulnohumeral joint. If the olecranon is rigidly fixed, then the unstable injury is converted to a stable one as the ulnohumeral joint is inherently stable. Hence,

the technique for rigid fixation of the fracture is of paramount importance (Figs. 8 and 9). O'Driscoll[17] reported his experience with use of a 3.5-mm dynamic-compression plate bent at a 90° angle to attain a better position on the small, proximal fragment. Not uncommonly, one fragment may also involve the coronoid. If it does, this is the most important component of the reduction and fixation.

Coronoid Fracture

The coronoid is the most important portion of the ulnohumeral articulation. It serves as a site of attachment for the collateral ligaments and resists posterior displacement of the ulna from the pull of the biceps, brachialis, and triceps.

Type-I Fracture According to the classification of Regan and myself,[18] type-I fractures represent a small chip of the tip of the coronoid and mainly serve as an indicator that the elbow has, in all likelihood, dislocated or at least sustained an injury of the collateral ligaments. The ulnohumeral joint is stable, and rehabilitation is similar to that recommended for type-I fracture-dislocations of the radial head. Open reduction is not usually necessary.

Type-II Fracture In type-II fractures, as much as 50% of the coronoid is involved and the elbow is usually unstable. Careful examination with the patient under anesthesia reveals whether the joint is stable after reduction (Fig. 10). If posterior displacement occurs with less than 40° to 45° of flexion, the articulation is considered inadequate and the ulnohumeral joint must be stabilized. If the fracture fragment is large enough for fixation, osteosynthesis with a single screw is performed. If the fragment is too small for fixation, then a heavy number-5 suture is placed through the fragment (or fragments), which is brought to its anatomic location. In the latter situation, or even if osteosynthesis has been carried out but there is concern about stability, the system is neutralized by the applica-

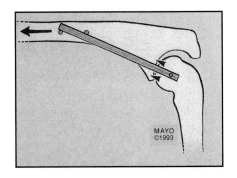

Fig. 11 Top, The pins in the ulna are placed distal to the coronoid so that the effective vector of the device displaces the ulna distally with regard to the humerus. Bottom left, The pins are placed sufficiently distal to avoid the fixation of the proximal part of the ulna. Bottom right, By introduction of distraction to the system, the ulnohumeral joint may be reduced and the forces that would ordinarily be applied to the fixation construct are neutralized. (Reproduced with permission from the Mayo Foundation, Rochester, MN.)

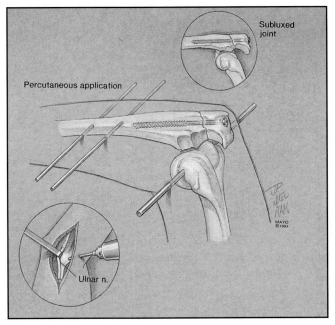

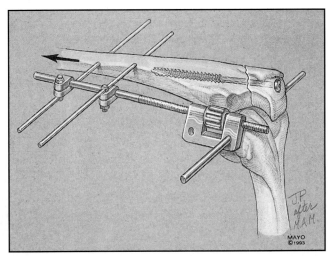

tion of a distraction device—that is, the external fixator eliminates the dynamic forces that are applied to the fracture site by the muscles that flex and extend the elbow joint. The device allows motion of the ulnohumeral joint while placing a distal distraction force on the ulna, thus protecting the articulation. The distraction device is maintained for 3 to 6 weeks, depending on the nature of the injury.[19] Cobb and I[19] reported our experience with seven such injuries and documented a successful outcome in six. In that series, the coronoid fracture was treated as described earlier, and a distraction device was applied.

Type-III Fracture These injuries are the most difficult to treat as, by definition, they render the ulnohumeral joint grossly unstable as do type-II injuries. If the coronoid is a large fragment and has not been comminuted, it may be fixed with a screw and the joint will be stable. However, because of the large forces transmitted through this relatively small surface area, as with type-II fractures these injuries should be further neutralized with the distraction device.

The severely comminuted coronoid fracture is a very uncommon injury. In this setting, I reduce the elbow and bring the fracture fragments into relative alignment with use of a heavy suture. I avoid removing any bone fragments as they may serve as a basis for substantive healing and formation of callus. The ulnohumeral relationship is maintained in a reduced position by the distraction device.

In every instance, the most important goal is to prevent posterior displacement of the ulna against the trochlea—thus, the concept of neutralization with an external fixator that permits flexion and extension while keeping the articulation aligned and eliminating the disruptive force from muscle contracture (Fig. 11).

Fracture of the Radial Head and Coronoid With Dislocation

These injuries are the most difficult in this category to treat. The principle is the same as already discussed: the radial head must be fixed or replaced. The coronoid fracture is fixed, if possible, with use of a direct or retrograde screw. In either instance, the complex is protected by the external fixator (Dynamic Joint Dis-

Elbow

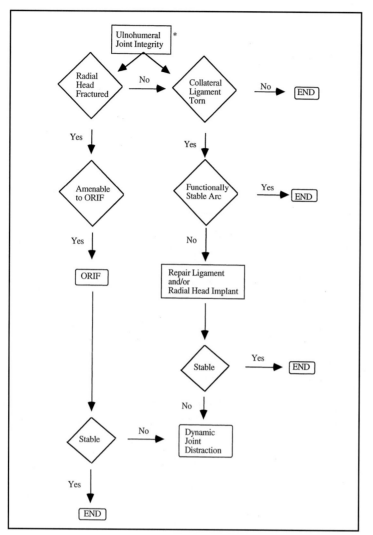

Fig. 12 Diagram for treatment of complex instability of the elbow. All decisions are predicated on restoring the integrity of the ulnohumeral joint. ORIF = open reduction and internal fixation.

tractor; Howmedica, Rutherford, New Jersey). This allows motion but eliminates force on the radial head and the coronoid.

Overview

The first principle for treating complex injuries of the elbow is to restore the essential element, the ulnohumeral joint (Fig. 12). This is done by reduction of the intact joint or, if the coronoid or the olecranon has fractured, by osteosynthesis. The second principle is that the radial head is an important secondary stabi-

lizer, so if the collateral ligaments have been injured the radial head must be restored or replaced. Finally, efforts to restore the ulnohumeral articulation are enhanced by protection with an external fixator that allows flexion. The implications for rehabilitation and the exact degree of instability are best determined after the ulnohumeral joint has been reduced and the elbow has been placed through an arc of motion. If there is any tendency for the elbow to subluxate or dislocate within 45° of extension, it should be treated appropriately.

References

1. Morrey BF: Radial head fracture, in Morrey BF (ed): *The Elbow and Its Disorders,* ed 2. Philadelphia, PA, WB Saunders, 1993, pp 383–404.
2. Morrey BF, Tanaka S, An KN: Valgus stability of the elbow: A definition of primary and secondary constraints. *Clin Orthop* 1991;265: 187–195.
3. O'Driscoll SW, Morrey BF, Korinek S, et al: Elbow subluxation and dislocation: A spectrum of instability. *Clin Orthop* 1992;280: 186–197.
4. Morrey BF: Current concepts in the treatment of fractures of the radial head, the olecranon, and the coronoid. *J Bone Joint Surg* 1995;77A: 316–327.
5. Nestor BJ, O'Driscoll SW, Morrey BF: Ligamentous reconstruction for posterolateral rotatory instability of the elbow. *J Bone Joint Surg* 1992;74A:1235–1241.
6. An KN, Morrey BF, Chao EY: The effect of partial removal of proximal ulna on elbow constraint. *Clin Orthop* 1986;209:270–279.
7. Morrey BF, An KN: Articular and ligamentous contributions to the stability of the elbow joint. *Am J Sports Med* 1983;11:315–319.
8. Harrington IJ, Tountas AA: Replacement of the radial head in the treatment of unstable elbow fractures. *Injury* 1981;12:405–412.
9. Judet T, Garreau de Loubresse C, Piriou P, et al: A floating prosthesis for radial-head fractures. *J Bone Joint Surg* 1996;78B:244–249.
10. Knight DJ, Rymaszewski LA, Amis AA, et al: Primary replacement of the fractured radial head with a metal prosthesis. *J Bone Joint Surg* 1993;75B:572–576.
11. Johnston GW: A follow-up of one hundred cases of fracture of the head of the radius with a review of the literature. *Ulster Med J* 1962; 31:51–56.
12. Broberg MA, Morrey BF: Results of treatment of fracture-dislocations of the elbow. *Clin Orthop* 1987;216:109–119.
13. Scharplatz D, Allgower M: Fracture-dislocations of the elbow. *Injury* 1975;7:143–159.
14. King GJ, Evans DC, Kellam JF: Open reduction and internal fixation of radial head fractures. *J Orthop Trauma* 1991;5:21–28.
15. Geel CW, Palmer AK, Ruedi T, et al: Internal fixation of proximal radial head fractures. *J Orthop Trauma* 1990;4:270–274.
16. Josefsson PO, Gentz CF, Johnell O, et al: Dislocations of the elbow and intraarticular fractures. *Clin Orthop* 1989;246:126–130.
17. O'Driscoll: Technique for unstable olecranon fracture-subluxations. *Op Tech Orthop* 1994; 4:49–53.
18. Regan W, Morrey B: Fractures of the coronoid process of the ulna. *J Bone Joint Surg* 1989; 71A:1348–1354.
19. Cobb TK, Morrey BF: Use of distraction arthroplasty in unstable fracture dislocations of the elbow. *Clin Orthop* 1995;312:201–210.

Tennis Elbow

Gerard T. Gabel, MD
Bernard F. Morrey, MD

Introduction

Tennis elbow is the most common clinical dysfunction of the elbow. Although it is generically applied, the term tennis elbow is most appropriately subdivided into four clinically distinct entities (Table 1). As the eponym implies, these disorders occur frequently in avocational settings; however, a more common presentation is in occupational circumstances, where it can involve either repetitive low to moderate loads or occasional high impact loads. The clinical presentation of these conditions varies as do associate diagnoses, but the one common element that exists is one of subjective complaints with little purely objective information to validate the diagnosis. This lack of objectivity means that the examiner must maintain proficiency in assessing and treating tennis elbow.

Originally described in 1873,[1] and given its current name in 1883,[2] classic tennis elbow, or lateral epicondylitis, remained an enigma until the pioneering efforts of Coonrad and Hooper,[3] Nirschl and Pettrone,[4] Froimson[5] and others in the 1970s. Although clarified over the past two decades, little fundamental change has occurred in the diagnosis or management of lateral epicondylitis. Medial epicondylitis, or golfer's elbow, which was mentioned in only one abstract prior to the 1990s, has been written about abundantly over the past 5 years, including reports by Gabel and Morrey,[6] Vangsness and Jobe,[7] and

Ollivierre and associates.[8] Triceps tendinitis, the least common of these disorders described to date, has had only limited review in the literature. Finally, the fourth condition included in this chapter, anconeus component syndrome,[9] has been identified as a separate entity.

Lateral Epicondylitis

Lateral epicondylitis, historically associated with sports injuries, now is associated to an equal or greater extent with occupational disorders. Its peak incidence is in the fourth and fifth decades with a slight male predominance. Dominant arm involvement is twice as common as nondominant. Although repetitive, indirect injury is the most common cause, direct or acute blunt trauma is implicated in 10% to 20% of cases. Concomitant or past diagnoses of similar tendinopathies, eg, rotator cuff tendinitis, deQuervain's disease, medial epicondylitis, or carpal tunnel syndrome, may be seen in up to 20% to 30% of patients, implicating a diathesis or independent response to a similar stimulus at multiple levels.[6]

Diagnosis

Physical examination at the elbow demonstrates direct tenderness over the anterior aspect of the lateral epicondyle, with occasional posterior and inferior tenderness. Resisted wrist dorsiflexion, especially with the elbow extended, is the most sensitive indirect maneuver, and its absence puts the diagnosis in question.

Table 1	
Subdivision of "tennis elbow"	
Lateral epicondylitis	85% to 95%
Medial epicondylitis	10% to 15%
Triceps tendinitis	2% to 3%
Anconeus compartment syndrome	< 1%

The radial-capitellar joint is assessed by direct palpation with pronation/supination and flexion/extension. The lateral antebrachial cutaneous nerve is evaluated as it passes the lateral margin of the biceps tendon (Tinel's sign; nerve compression test). Posterolateral rotatory instability (PLRI) is ruled out, if possible, with the PLRI test.[10] Finally, the primary local differential diagnosis (radial tunnel syndrome) is assessed by anterior local tenderness along the radial nerve in the interval between the brachioradialis and brachialis as well as at the level of the radial neck. The radial nerve, as it courses around the proximal radius, is 5 cm distal to the lateral epicondyle in full supination; pronation translates the nerve medially and distally. If direct tenderness over the radius at 5 cm distal to the lateral epicondyle in full supination is markedly greater than in pronation (the pronation/supination sign), then a presumptive diagnosis of concomitant radial tunnel syndrome is ascribed (5% coincidence). Unfortunately, even provocative electrodiagnostic studies are of no benefit in the diagnosis of radial tunnel syndrome,[11] making objective verification

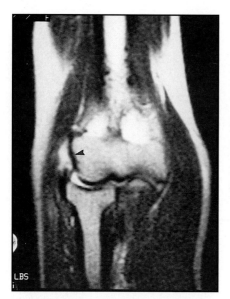

Fig. 1 Increased signal at extensor origin of extensor carpi radialis brevis (arrow), consistent with lateral epicondylitis.

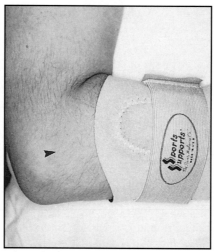

Fig. 2 Lateral counterforce brace application. Lateral pad along axis of extensor carpi radialis brevis (arrow), just distal to extensor origin, allows flexion without impingement of brace at antecubital fossa.

difficult. Proximal examination should be performed to rule out cervical radiculopathy or referred shoulder pathology, and local evaluation of the medial and posterior elbow is critical as well.

Radiographic evaluation will reveal epicondylar calcification in 5% to 20% of cases, but this is not prognostically related. Concomitant arthrosis is seen occasionally. Magnetic resonance imaging (MRI) plays an evolving role (Fig. 1), especially in today's health care cost conscious environment. MRI is useful in inconsistent cases, especially in secondary gain concerns, but its accuracy varies. Although a very consistent relationship between MRI and surgical/histopathologic findings has been reported[12] and it is considered to be in surgical planning, no specific surgical algorithm with independent verification has been offered. At present, the routine use of MRI is not recommended, and the diagnosis of lateral epicondylitis remains purely clinical. A diagnostic lidocaine injection may be useful in cases of possible concomitant intra-articular sources or radial tunnel syndrome. Intra-articular injection (6 cc

of 2% lidocaine) will help verify an intra-articular versus extra-articular source if pain is relieved with the injection. A lidocaine block (6 cc of 2% lidocaine) at the radial tunnel, just proximal to the radial-capitellar joint, may be used to substantiate radial neuropathy (J Nunley, MD, Durham, NC, personal communication, 1990).

Nonsurgical Treatment

The management of lateral epicondylitis requires a blend of patient education, anti-inflammatory measures, protective orthoses, and time. The patient should be advised of the probable duration of the disorder (3 to 9 months) and the need to avoid provocative maneuvers and to perform activities with the forearm supinated rather than pronated. For patients with a short history and mild symptoms, oral nonsteroidal anti-inflammatory drugs (NSAIDs) along with a counterforce brace[5] and wrist extension splinting are instituted. The counterforce brace pad should be centered along the extensor carpi radialis brevis (ECRB) axis distal to the radiocapitellar joint (Fig. 2). The

wrist splint should hold the wrist at approximately 30° of extension. If the symptom history exceeds 3 months duration and moderate to severe tenderness is present, a corticosteroid injection is recommended. Although still somewhat controversial, corticosteroid/local anesthetic injection is effective in decreasing pain,[13-18] especially at 2 to 6 weeks postinjection, but it is ineffective without splinting and a conditioning program. An equal volume of 2% lidocaine and triamcinolone[19] (6 mg/cc), total volume 3 cc, is injected into the point of maximum tenderness, deep to the fascia. Fatty atrophy and hypopigmentation are minimized by use of a solution (rather than suspension) and avoidance of subcutaneous deposition. The patient should be warned to expect postinjection pain for several days. Resting the extensor origin by full time use of a wrist extension splint and protection of the extensor tendon by counterforce bracing during use of the arm is critical in most cases.

Once local tenderness has resolved, a conditioning program of extensor origin stretching (gentle passive wrist flexion with the digits flexed and the elbow extended) and gradual wrist extension strengthening (1-lb increments) is instituted. The patient should be advised that, at this time, although the pain has resolved, the sense of well-being may be artificial (especially following a corticosteroid injection) and that provocative activities are to be avoided until strength and endurance equal to or greater than the preinjury state has been restored. It is at this point that most failures occur, representing not necessarily a failure of treatment, but rather a failure of completion of treatment. Repeat injection, if warranted, is preferably spaced at least 3 months from the original injection. If the patient fails to respond to two to three injections over a 6- to 12-month period, including the previously mentioned orthotics and conditioning program, surgical management is considered.

Alternate therapeutic measures, including ultrasound,[20] iontophoresis,[20] acupuncture,[21] laser,[22] dimethyl sulfoxide (DMSO),[23] electrical stimulation,[24] and shock wave therapy,[25] have generally each been supported and refuted in sequential studies, and their role is unclear, especially in the cost-conscious managed care environment. Because of the increased nonmedical costs involved, the injured worker may be an exception, especially if modified duty is unavailable.

Surgical Treatment

The surgical management of lateral epicondylitis has had varied directives, including the radial-humeral bursa,[26] synovial fringes, annular ligament,[27] denervation,[28] radial tunnel decompression,[29,30] and ECRB lengthening with release of the ECRB origin.[31] Subsequently, Coonrad and Hooper[3] (nidus excision and ECRB repair) and Nirschl and Pettrone[4] (nidus excision, lateral epicondylar decortication, and ECRB repair) have defined the central role of the ECRB and contemporary surgical management.[32-35] The recommended duration of nonsurgical management is a minimum of 6 to 9 months, although earlier intervention has been suggested.[33]

Because most patients successfully treated with conservative management require a minimum of 6 months to respond, surgical treatment before 6 months will result in overtreatment. In addition, as many patients will require more than 6 months to recover from surgery,[6] surgical intervention is not a quick fix, and it should be reserved for clearly recalcitrant cases. Concomitant radial nerve decompression can be performed if needed.

A 3-cm longitudinal incision is made just anterior to the lateral column of the distal humerus (to avoid a scar over the prominence). Dissection is carried to the investing fascia. The interval between the ECRB and the extensor digitorum communis (EDC) is identified by differential

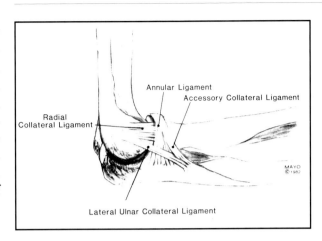

Fig. 3 Illustration demonstrating origin of the lateral ulnar collateral ligament (LUCL) at inferior margin of lateral epicondyle. Dissection of this level may compromise the ligament resulting in posterolateral rotory. (Reproduced with permission from the Mayo Foundation, Rochester, MN.)

wrist and digital passive motion. The ECRB origin is then elevated sharply off the lateral epicondyle. It is important to avoid dissection at the inferior epicondylar level to avoid the origin of the lateral ulnar collateral ligament (Fig. 3) and iatrogenic posterolateral rotatory instability.[10] A nidus, seen in approximately 50% to 75% of cases, is excised. An incidental or intentional arthrotomy typically reveals no radiocapitellar pathology. The extensor origin is decorticated with a burr, rongeur, or drill to enhance healing, and the extensor origin is repaired (side-to-side without shortening). Alternatively, the extensor origin can be released without reattachment. Because little distal translation occurs after release, especially if postoperative immobilization is used, formal repair and release may result in equivalent tendon healing length. If needed, radial nerve decompression in the ECRB-EDC interval is readily accomplished by development of this interval distally. The supinator muscle lies deep in this interval and guides localization of the radial nerve.

Postoperatively, the elbow is immobilized in a long-arm splint or Muenster cast for 1 to 3 weeks, at which time gentle active range-of-motion exercises are initiated. Counterforce bracing is resumed. A strengthening program is initiated at 4 to 6 weeks, progressing as tolerated. Impact

activities are avoided until preinjury, pain-free strength has been restored (usual minimum, 4 to 6 months).

Alternate surgical methods include manipulation under anesthesia (essentially tearing the extensor origin),[36] percutaneous release (blind extensor origin release),[37,38] the unified theory (extensive debridement/anconeus rotational flap), and endoscopic release.[39] Because the morbidity of surgery in lateral epicondylitis is the prolonged recovery and not the surgical procedure itself, closed (manipulative), blind (percutaneous) extensor origin release, or endoscopic release, although possibly less morbid in the short term, would be more morbid in the long term (due to inadequate release) and is not recommended.

The reports of the ECRB procedures demonstrate 85% to 90% good or excellent results, with the most recent findings demonstrating fewer excellent results and a longer period to attainment of the final outcome.[35,40] In addition, no correlation between surgical/histopathologic findings and outcomes has been demonstrated, with results being similar in patients with and without a surgically identifiable nidus.[35,37,41]

Medial Epicondylitis

Medial epicondylitis, or golfer's elbow, makes up approximately 10% to 15% of

Table 2
Medial epicondylitis classification

Type	Description
IA	No associated ulnar nerve symptoms/signs
IB	Minimal or mild associated ulnar nerve symptoms/signs
II	Moderate or severe associated ulnar nerve symptoms and signs

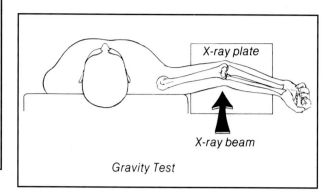

Fig. 4 Gravity valgus stress radiography to assess medial collateral ligament integrity. (Reproduced with permission from Morrey BF: Articular injuries in the athlete, in Morrey BF (ed): *The Elbow and Its Disorders*, ed 2. Philadelphia, PA, WB Saunders, 1993, p 585.)

the tendinopathies of the elbow. It represents a process similar to lateral epicondylitis, but one that involves the flexor pronator origin. The demographics, injury history, and diathesis are each comparable to that seen in lateral epicondylitis; however, unlike lateral epicondylitis, in which associated radial neuropathy is uncommon, ulnar neuropathy at the elbow is seen in 35% to 60% of medial epicondylitis cases. Although noted by Nirsch and Pettrone[42] and subsequently Vangsness and Jobe,[7] the significance of associated ulnar neuropathy at the elbow in medial epicondylitis was initially clarified by Gabel and Morrey[6] and subsequently by Kurvers and Verhaar.[43] A classification system (Table 2) provides an algorithm for surgical management and is prognostically significant.[6]

Diagnosis

The physical examination reveals direct anterior medial epicondylar tenderness in essentially all cases. The most sensitive indirect maneuver is resisted forearm pronation, seen in 90%. Resisted palmar flexion pain occurs in approximately 70% of cases. Ulnar neuropathy at the elbow is assessed with the elbow flexion test (wrist neutral, forearm supinated, elbow flexed to 135°), the nerve compression test (digital compression of the nerve at the inferior medial epicondyle) and Tinel's sign, as well as objective motor and sensory function in the hand. The anterior oblique ligament of the medial collateral complex can be palpated at the anterior inferior medial epicondyle and evaluated

with Jobe's valgus stress examination. Finally, the medial antebrachial cutaneous nerve is assessed with Tinel's sign over the nerve or hypesthesia or dysesthesia of the medial forearm.

Radiographic evaluation of medial epicondylitis is similar to that used for lateral epicondylitis, with a 10% to 20% incidence of medial epicondylar calcification and variable findings on magnetic resonance imaging. If suspected on physical examination, valgus instability may be assessed by valgus stress radiography[44] (Fig. 4). On occasion, medial epicondylar nonunion may be associated with medial epicondylitis.

If ulnar neuropathy at the elbow is suspected and if clinical examination warrants, electrodiagnostic testing is very useful. As with lateral epicondylitis, an intra-articular source of pain can be determined with an intra-articular lidocaine injection. Medial antebrachial cutaneous neuropathy can also be assessed with a diagnostic lidocaine block at the point of maximum Tinel's.

Nonsurgical Treatment

The management of medial epicondylitis mirrors that of lateral epicondylitis. A medial counterforce brace is placed over the pronator teres/flexor carpi radialis (PT/FCR) axis, distal to the elbow flexion crease. It should not be centered over the ulnar nerve or the cubital tunnel and its use should be discontinued if it exacerbates ulnar neuropathic symptoms, a

problem actually caused by improper use of the brace. A wrist splint at 0 to 10° of extension will rest the FCR; however, PT resting requires forearm immobilization, which is rarely well tolerated by the patient. Corticosteroid injections should be used cautiously and should avoid the anterior oblique ligament origin on the anterior/inferior epicondyle. The point of maximum tenderness is typically at the PT/FCR origin on the anterior epicondyle or the proximal extent of these muscles. Ulnar neuropathy is managed by avoidance of sustained elbow flexion, repetitive flexion and extension, and leaning on the elbow. Elbow extension splinting, like forearm immobilization, is poorly tolerated by patients.

Management of type IA medial epicondylitis, which has no associated ulnar neuropathy, may be based purely on the epicondylitis symptoms. Type IB medial epicondylitis, with mild associated ulnar neuropathy, is managed initially in a similar manner; however, in either type IA or type IB medial epicondylitis, if a progressive ulnar neuropathy occurs, surgical management is recommended, regardless of the status of the medial epicondylitis. Progression of a type IA or type IB medial epicondylitis to a type II medial epicondylitis, with greater ulnar neuropathy, has a poorer prognosis and should be avoided.

Surgical Treatment

If nonsurgical management fails to alleviate symptoms of either ulnar neuropathy or medial epicondylitis, surgical management is guided by relevant anatomy and clinical diagnosis. The surgical anatomy of medial epicondylitis consists of several musculotendinous neural and ligamentous concerns. The critical lesion of the PT and FCR originates off the anterior aspect of the medial epicondyle. From the proximal edge of the flexor pronator origin (the proximal edge of the PT), it extends along the anterior surface of the medial epicondyle to the accessory anterior oblique ligament. This structure, which has been recently defined, is an intramuscular septum oriented perpendicular to the flexor pronator superficial fascia. It serves as an intramuscular origin for the flexor carpi ulnaris (humeral head) and the FCR and palmaris longus. It defines the interval between the FCR and flexor carpi ulnaris (FCU) and is a very valuable landmark for medial epicondylitis surgery. Because involvement of the FCU is uncommon, medial epicondylitis surgery should usually be limited to the flexor pronator origin anterior and proximal to the accessory anterior oblique ligament. The accessory anterior oblique ligament, although a weak valgus stabilizer in extension, finds its primary function in this surgery as a landmark, not only for the FCR-FCU interval, but also for the anterior oblique ligament origin on the medial epicondyle, which is immediately posterior of the accessory anterior oblique (Fig. 5). Elevation of the flexor pronator origin posterior to the accessory anterior oblique ligament may result in iatrogenic medial elbow instability caused by injury of the anterior oblique ligament proper.

The neural anatomy of medial epicondylitis includes the medial antebrachial cutaneous nerve, which lies in the subcutaneous tissue on the anterior margin of the epicondyle. The ulnar nerve posterior to the epicondyle and beneath the cubital tunnel retinaculum and Osborne's arcade, if involved, may require surgical decompression.

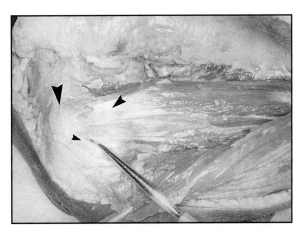

Fig. 5 Anatomy of accessory anterior oblique ligament. Medial epicondyle (large arrow), anterior oblique ligament proper (AOL) (small arrow), accessory anterior oblique ligament (AAOL) (medium arrow). Probe is in interval between AOL and AAOL. Note that the AOL is immediately posterior to AAOL at the medial epicondyle.

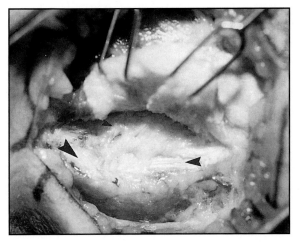

Fig. 6 Surgical anatomy of medial epicondylitis medial peicondyle (large arrow). Accessory anterior oblique ligament (AAOL) (medium arrow) and nidus (small arrow). The pronator teres/flexor carpi radialis origin is retracted anteriorly. Note that the nidus location on epicondyle is anterior to AAOL.

The surgical management of medial epicondylitis depends on the degree of involvement of the ulnar nerve. In type IA medial epicondylitis, a procedure similar to the lateral Nirschl procedure is performed. A 2 to 3 cm longitudinal incision is created just anterior to the medial epicondyle. Subcutaneous dissection with tenotomy scissors allows protection of the medial antebrachial cutaneous nerve. The flexor pronator fascia is discretely identified on the medial epicondyle. This fascia is incised, leaving a 2-mm rim of fascia on the medial epicondyle, and the underlying muscle is elevated down to the brachialis fascia/elbow capsule. Inferior dissection stops at the anterior margin of the accessory anterior oblique ligament. A nidus, if present, is almost invariably found in this interval

(Fig. 6). Dissection posterior to the accessory anterior oblique ligament, if required, must be performed with a freer elevator or tenotomy scissors to avoid injury to the anterior oblique ligament proper, which is posterior to the accessory ligament and adjacent to the capsule. Because this interval is rarely involved, this portion is generally not exposed. The anterior cortex of the medial epicondyle is roughened with a rongeur or curette. The origin of the flexor pronator is then repaired back to the retained rim of superficial fascia. Alternatively, elevation may be performed without repair.

Because the amount of retraction of the elevated flexor pronator muscle, even with full extension and supination, is small, the amount of shortening without formal repair is minimal, explaining simi-

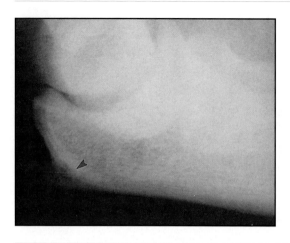

Fig. 7 Triceps tendon insertional spur (olecranon spur).

lar results with and without formal repair. In type IB medial epicondylitis, the ulnar nerve may be examined for compression with elbow flexion and forearm supination. If no indentation by Osborne's arcade occurs, the nerve is left undisturbed. If there is compression, a cubital tunnel decompression is performed. If the nerve demonstrates subluxation, adhesions, or any other alteration of its normal anatomy, it is transposed anteriorly. In type II medial epicondylitis, in which a significant associated ulnar neuropathy is present, anterior submuscular transposition, along with debridement, is performed. Postoperatively, the arm is immobilized in a single sugar-tong splint or Muenster cast for 2 to 3 weeks. An active range-of-motion program, along with splinting and counterforce utilization, is begun. Strengthening exercises are started at 6 weeks, if tolerated, and impact activities are avoided for 6 months.

The results of surgical management of medial epicondylitis depend primarily on the degree of ulnar nerve involvement. In type IA and IB patients, results similar to lateral epicondylitis (> 90% good to excellent)[6,7] are usually realized; however, in type II patients, the results are poorer (< 50% good to excellent),[6,43] primarily because of the poor recovery of the ulnar nerve in these patients. For this reason, preoperative monitoring of the ulnar nerve status is critical. In addition, the use

of cubital tunnel release exclusively[43] in these patients is frequently unsuccessful, indicating that patient-specific management of the ulnar nerve is essential. The time to recovery after medial epicondylitis procedures is 6 months or less in approximately two thirds of patients, but it is up to 2 years in the remaining third.[6]

Triceps Tendinitis

Very little has been written about triceps tendinitis, but two distinct subsets exist, those with and those without an associated olecranon traction spur. Unlike medial or lateral epicondylitis, triceps tendinitis involves a discrete tendinous insertion rather than a broad-based origin. It occurs almost exclusively in males in the fourth and fifth decades, especially weight lifers. Conservative management involves avoidance of repetitive forceful elbow extension and time. Splinting (45° elbow splint) if tolerated may be useful. Counterforce bracing proximal to the elbow is typically unsuccessful, because the cross section of the arm changes with biceps shortening. Although this intervention is limited in its scope, it is usually successful in triceps tendinitis in the absence of an olecranon spur. Corticosteroid injection into a discrete tendon insertion is contraindicated.[45] The presence of an olecranon spur is associated with a higher failure rate, and usually surgical management is required only when

such a spur exists (Fig. 7).

The surgical management of triceps tendinitis involves a posterior midline incision over the triceps proper insertion on the olecranon. The triceps tendon usually has a thin layer covering the olecranon spur and is elevated medially and laterally off the spur, preserving, as much as possible, the triceps insertion. A mobile fragment of the olecranon spur is not uncommonly found. As the triceps tendon proper inserts on the posterior 40% of the olecranon, and olecranon spurs occur posteriorly, excision of an olecranon spur usually violates the majority of the triceps proper insertion. To avoid this, a formal repair of the triceps tendon is performed and the postoperative management is similar to that following triceps avulsion repair.

Anconeus Compartment Syndrome

Anconeus compartment syndrome (ACS) is included in this chapter because it is often misdiagnosed as lateral epicondylitis.[9] ACS typically occurs in the third or fourth decade and consists of postexertional lateral elbow discomfort. Maximum tenderness is found along the anconeus muscle and is increased with resisted elbow extension. Resisted wrist extension pain and anterior lateral epicondylar tenderness are absent.

Preliminary review indicates that this is a compartment syndrome of the anconeus muscle, and increased tissue pressure has been documented. If avoiding provocative activities fails to resolve the symptoms, surgical treatment consists of an anconeus fasciotomy, incising the superficial fascia of the anconeus muscle. Unlike medial and lateral epicondylitis, no immobilization is required, and recovery is very rapid.

Failure of Tennis Elbow Surgery

An algorithm for the management of failures of surgical treatment of lateral epicondylitis has been developed by

Morrey[46] (Fig. 8). Persistent, unchanged symptoms implicate persistent extensor origin dysfunction or a misdiagnosis, eg, radial tunnel syndrome. Differential lidocaine injection may help to determine the source. Postoperative symptoms that differ from those present preoperatively indicate a possible complication of the surgery, including posterolateral rotatory instability and capsular defect with synovial sinus formation.

The management of the patient with a failed lateral epicondylar procedure requires an accurate diagnosis of the postoperative symptoms. The most common cause of persistent symptoms is persistent extensor origin dysfunction. Although lateral epicondylar procedures have a very high success rate (> 90%) on long-term follow-up, the prolonged period to attain that result has been recognized and a minimum of 6 months or possibly 1 year should pass before declaring that persistent extensor original dysfunction means that the lateral epicondylar procedure has failed.

A similar algorithm can be outlined for failed medial epicondylitis surgery. If symptoms are similar to the preoperative symptoms, persistent flexor/pronator origin dysfunction may be involved. In medial epicondylitis, as in lateral epicondylitis, a prolonged time should pass before calling the original procedure a failure. To date, the most common cause of failure has been persistent ulnar neuropathy at the elbow. The previously mentioned management algorithm of types IA, IB, and II medial epicondylitis should minimize this occurrence. If required, a revision ulnar nerve decompression is best accomplished by submuscular transposition.[47] Postoperative symptoms that differ from preoperative ones are usually caused by iatrogenic valgus instability (from anterior oblique ligament injury) or medial antebrachial cutaneous nerve injury. Valgus instability can be successfully addressed by medial collateral reconstruction as described by Jobe and associates.[48] Medial antebrachial cuta-

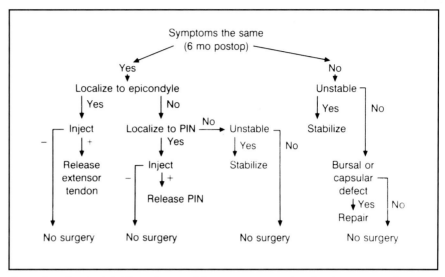

Fig. 8 Algorithm for failed lateral epicondylitis surgery. (Reproduced with permission from Morrey BF: Surgical failure of tennis elbow, in Morrey BF (ed): *The Elbow and Its Disorders*, ed 2. Philadelphia, PA, WB Saunders, 1993, p 558.)

neous neuropathy is managed by desensitization and corticosteroid injection. If symptoms persist, medial antebrachial cutaneous neurectomy and deep transposition into the brachialis muscle will alleviate the neurogenic pain but, obviously, will leave the medial forearm hypesthetic.

Conclusion

Tennis elbow is by far the most common disorder of the elbow. A detailed history, combined with comprehensive elbow examination, will usually lead to an accurate diagnosis and allow appropriate management. Each of the outlined subsets of tennis elbow described above is associated with a distinct differential diagnosis and prognosis. Patient education, activity modification, splinting, and prudent use of corticosteroid injections as indicated will resolve symptoms in the majority of cases, but the patient should be advised early on of a prolonged period of recovery. Surgical management should be undertaken only when conservative management has failed to provide relief after a diagnosis-specific period of time. The evaluation and management of the failed surgery for tennis elbow requires a com-

prehensive assessment of the elbow for appropriate treatment.

References

1. Runge F: Zur Genese und Behandlung des Schreibekrampfes. *Berl-Klin-Wochenschr* 1873;10:245–248.

2. Major HP: Letter: Lawn-tennis elbow. *Br Med J* 1883;2:557.

3. Coonrad RW, Hooper WR: Tennis-elbow: Its course, natural history, conservative and surgical management. *J Bone Joint Surg* 1973;55A:1177–1182.

4. Nirschl RP, Pettrone FA: Tennis elbow: The surgical treatment of lateral epicondylitis. *J Bone Joint Surg* 1979;61A:832–839.

5. Froimson AI: Treatment of tennis elbow with forearm support band. *J Bone Joint Surg* 1971;53A:183–184.

6. Gabel GT, Morrey BF: Operative treatment of medial epicondylitis: Influence of concomitant ulnar neuropathy of the elbow. *J Bone Joint Surg* 1995;77A:1065–1069.

7. Vangsness CT Jr, Jobe FW: Surgical treatment of medial epicondylitis: Results in 35 elbows. *J Bone Joint Surg* 1991;73B:409–411.

8. Ollivierre CO, Nirschl RP, Pettrone FA: Resection and repair for medial tennis elbow: A prospective analysis. *Am J Sports Med* 1995;23:214–221.

9. Abrahamsson SO, Sollerman C, Söderberg T, et al: Lateral elbow pain caused by anconeus compartment syndrome: A case report. *Acta Orthop Scand* 1987;58:589–591.

10. O'Driscoll SW, Bell DF, Morrey BF: Posterolateral rotatory instability of the elbow. *J Bone Joint Surg* 1991;73A:440–446.

11. Verhaar J, Spaans F: Radial tunnel syndrome: An investigation of compression neuropathy as a possible cause. *J Bone Joint Surg* 1991;73A:539–544.

12. Potter HG, Hannafin JA, Morwessel RM, et al: Lateral epicondylitis: Correlation of MR imaging, surgical, and histopathologic findings. *Radiology* 1995;196:43–46.

13. Assendelft WJ, Hay EM, Adshead R, et al: Corticosteroid injections for lateral epicondylitis: A systematic overview. *Br J Gen Pract* 1996;46:209–216.

14. Brand C: Intra-articular and soft tissue injections. *Aust Fam Physician* 1990;19:671–682.

15. Cabot A: Tennis elbow: A curable affliction. *Orthop Rev* 1987;16:322–326.

16. Coel M, Yamada CY, Ko J: MR imaging of patients with lateral epicondylitis of the elbow (tennis elbow): Importance of increased signal of the anconeus muscle. *Am J Roentgenol* 1993;161:1019–1021.

17. Day BH, Govindasamy N, Patnaik R: Corticosteroid injections in the treatment of tennis elbow. *Practitioner* 1978;220:459–462.

18. Solveborn SA, Buch F, Mallmin H, et al: Cortisone injection with anesthetic additives for radial epicondylalgia (tennis elbow). *Clin Orthop* 1995;316:99–105.

19. Price R, Sinclair H, Heinrich I, et al: Local injection treatment of tennis elbow: Hydrocortisone, triamcinolone and lignocaine compared. *Br J Rheumatol* 1991;30:39–44.

20. Ernst E: Conservative therapy for tennis elbow. *Br J Clin Pract* 1992;46:55–57.

21. Molsberger A, Hille E: The analgesic effect of acupuncture in chronic tennis elbow pain. *Br J Rheumatol* 1994;33:1162–1165.

22. Vasseljen O Jr, Hoeg N, Kjeldstad B, et al: Low level laser versus placebo in the treatment of tennis elbow. *Scand J Rehabil Med* 1992;24:37–42.

23. Percy EC, Carson JD: The use of DMSO in tennis elbow and rotator cuff tendonitis: A double-blind study. *Med Sci Sports Exerc* 1981;13:215–219.

24. Nirschl RP: Sports and overuse injuries to the elbow: Muscle and tendon trauma. "Tennis elbow," in Morrey BF (ed): *The Elbow and Its Disorders*, ed 2. Philadelphia, PA, WB Saunders, 1993, pp 537–552.

25. Rompe JD, Hope C, Kullmer K, et al: Analgesic effect of extracorporeal shock-wave therapy on chronic tennis elbow. *J Bone Joint Surg* 1996;78B:233–237.

26. Osgood RB: Radiohumeral bursitis, epicondylitis, epicondylalgia (tennis elbow): A personal experience. *Arch Surg* 1922;4:420–433.

27. Bosworth DM: The role of the orbicular ligament in tennis elbow. *J Bone Joint Surg* 1955;37A:527–533.

28. Kaplan EB: Treatment of tennis elbow (epicondylitis) by denervation. *J Bone Joint Surg* 1959;41:147–151.

29. Roles NC, Maudsley RH: Radial tunnel syndrome: Resistant tennis elbow as a nerve entrapment. *J Bone Joint Surg* 1972;54B:499–508.

30. Garden RS: Tennis elbow. *J Bone Joint Surg* 1961;43B:100–106.

31. Hohmann G: Das Wesen und die Behandlung des sogenannten Tennis ellenbogens. *Munch Med Wochenschr* 1933;80:250–252.

32. Gellman H: Tennis elbow (lateral epicondylitis). *Orthop Clin North Am* 1992;23:75–82.

33. Newey ML, Patterson MH: Pain relief following tennis elbow release. *J R Col Surg Edinb* 1994;39:60–61.

34. Nirschl RP: Lateral and medial epicondylitis, in Morrey BF (ed): *The Elbow.* New York, NY, Raven Press, 1994, pp 129–148.

35. Verhaar J, Walenkamp G, Kester A, et al: Lateral extensor release for tennis elbow: A prospective long-term follow-up study. *J Bone Joint Surg* 1993;75A:1034–1043.

36. Wadsworth TG: Lateral epicondylitis (tennis elbow). *Lancet* 1972;1:959–960.

37. Baumgard SH, Schwartz DR: Pecutaneous release of the epicondylar muscles for humeral epicondylitis. *Am J Sports Med* 1982;10:233–236.

38. Yerger B, Turner T: Percutaneous extensor tenotomy for chronic tennis elbow: An office procedure. *Orthopedics* 1985;8:1261–1263.

39. Grifka J, Boenke S, Kramer J: Endoscopic therapy in epicondylitis radialis humeri. *Arthroscopy* 1995;11:743–748.

40. Bennett JB: Lateral and medial epicondylitis. *Hand Clin* 1994;10:157–163.

41. Doran A, Gresham GA, Rushton N, et al: Tennis elbow: A clinicopathologic study of 22 cases followed for 2 years. *Acta Orthop Scand* 1990;161:535–538.

42. Nirschl RP, Pettrone F: Medial tennis elbow: Surgical treatment. *Orthop Trans* 1980;4:298–299.

43. Kurvers H, Verhaar J: The results of operative treatment of medial epicondylitis. *J Bone Joint Surg* 1995;77A:1374–1379.

44. Schwab GH, Bennett JB, Woods GW, et al: Biomechanics of elbow instability: The role of the medial collateral ligament. *Clin Orthop* 1980;146:42–52.

45. Balasubramaniam P, Prathap K: The effect of injection of hydrocortisone into rabbit calcaneal tendons. *J Bone Joint Surg* 1972;54B:729–734.

46. Morrey BF: Reoperation for failed surgical treatment of refractory lateral epicondylitis. *J Shoulder Elbow Surg* 1992;1:47–55.

47. Gabel GT, Amadio PC: Reoperation for failed decompression of the ulnar nerve in the region of the elbow. *J Bone Joint Surg* 1990;72A:213–219.

48. Jobe FW, Stark H, Lombardo SJ: Reconstruction of the ulnar collateral ligament in athletes. *J Bone Joint Surg* 1986;68A:1158–1163.

Fractures of the Radial Head and Related Instability and Contracture of the Forearm

Robert N. Hotchkiss, MD

Introduction

Fractures of the radial head and proximal forearm are often uncomplicated and heal in proper alignment, permitting adequate and near normal function. However, if the injury is of high energy or unfortunate circumstance, associated damage to the supporting ligaments of the elbow and wrist may occur. In this setting, loss of function of the wrist and forearm is due to a combination of anatomic malalignment, proximal translation of the radius relative to the ulna, and soft-tissue contracture.

The principal goal of treatment in this complex injury is to maintain the longitudinal radioulnar relationship, preserving forearm kinematics. Maintenance of the anatomy requires restoration of radial head function, either through repair or replacement, and attention to the supporting soft-tissue linkage between the radius and ulna. These structures include the posterolateral ligament complex at the elbow, the interosseous ligament (IOL) of the forearm (referred to previously as the interosseous membrane) and the triangular fibrocartilage complex (TFCC) at the distal radioulnar joint.

The Pathoanatomy of Forearm Instability and Proximal Migration of the Radius

The debate concerning the incidence of pathologic forearm instability after radial head excision has never been fully settled in the literature.[1-10] There are many reports that document both a low incidence of proximal translation of the radius and a minimal amount of displacement. In addition to patients with recognizable acute forearm dissociation (the so-called Essex-Lopresti lesion)[11] it has been suggested that other, similar injuries may be even more frequent. Whatever the epidemiology may be, once the radius rests in a position 1 cm or greater proximal to the ulna, loss of motion and pain are usually present.[10,12,13] For displacement less than 1 cm, the patient may have pain at the distal ulna, but the limitation of motion is usually not as striking.

As the radius translates proximally, the forearm gradually slips into a pronated position. The distal ulna then sits dorsally relative to the radius and carpus. The ulna impinges with the dorsal carpus and mechanically blocks supination. As a result of the mechanical block and continued scar formation, a soft-tissue pronation contracture also develops, further complicating reconstruction and salvage efforts designed to improve forearm rotation. Wrist and hand function are also notably affected in this position. Many patients experience substantial pain at the wrist and a marked loss of grip strength.[7,10,13]

The goal of treatment is therefore to recognize the injury pattern, understand the biomechanics of loadbearing in the forearm, and optimally restore the structures of import. As the first author who reported on this condition in 1930, Brockman[2] noted that this injury is complicated by both the degree of impairment and the complexity of repair and reconstruction, suggesting the best option may be surrender with the creation of a one-bone forearm. Essex-Lopresti[11] (for whom the lesion was named) later suggested that the optimal solution to acute forearm dissociation would probably be internal fixation of the radial head. His use of the subjunctive was necessitated by the lack of surgical possibilities at that time, but was, nonetheless, conceptually appropriate.

Biomechanics of the Radial Head and Forearm Stability

The elbow's unique anatomy, which combines two functionally independent articulations that share a synovial compartment, requires careful consideration after fracture of the radial head.[14] The ulnotrochlear articulation directs flexion and extension, and the radiocapitellar joint governs forearm rotation in pronation and supination. The ulnohumeral articulation is highly constrained and approximates a simple hinge with little deviation out of the frontal plane. Forearm rotation (pronation/supination) is centered at the radiocapitellar joint and distal radioulnar joint. The functional kinematics of forearm rotation are more difficult to discern because the ulna remains fixed relative to the humerus but appears to rotate at the level of the wrist. The diarthrodial joints between the radius and ulna, the proximal radioulnar joint and the distal radioulnar joint. (DRUJ), experience compressive loading during grip, lifting, and prono-supination. The coaptive joint reactive force at the two articulations creates stability and permits smooth motion. In addition to the joint reactive force and the ligamentous restraints at the DRUJ, the midforearm and proximal radioulnar joint constrain the two bones, maintaining the relative position of the forearm and the proper axis of rotation. The ligaments of the forearm axis; the triangular fibrocartilage complex, the interosseous ligament of the forearm,[15,16] the annular ligament, and the posterior lateral collateral ligament of the elbow[17] must be considered in caring for patients with these complex injuries.

Longitudinal Stability of the Forearm: Biomechanical Studies and Clinical Observations
Radial Head Function

From laboratory studies[15,16,18] and clinical observation[10,12,13] the radial head bears load at the radiocapitellar joint, undoubtedly changing with the position on the forearm and elbow.[15] The precise amount of load sharing between the radius and ulna from moment to moment can only be estimated, but it is clear that the radiocapitellar joint bears load during grip and lifting activity.[14] Morrey and associates[18] demonstrated that contact pressures increased with pronation of the forearm. Supination of the forearm was noted by Hotchkiss and associates[15] to increase the stiffness of the central ligamentous region of the interosseous membrane of the forearm, which is referred to here as the interosseous ligament of the forearm. In pronation, there is greater radiocapitellar contact, and the interosseous ligament of the forearm is less taut and less stiff.[15,18] These two independent observations support the concept that more relative load is

transferred to the ulna (from wrist to elbow) in supination in the uninjured forearm.

Once the radial head is removed, this normal, physiologic load sharing can no longer occur, and all compressive load must ultimately be transferred to the ulna. If the main soft-tissue structures that link the radius and ulna (the interosseous ligament and the TFCC) are disrupted, the radius will displace proximally relative to the ulna.[2,6,10–13,15] Detection of these associated soft-tissue injuries is not always simple. However, certain patterns should raise suspicion. Galeazzi fractures[19] or any fracture of the forearm, including isolated fractures of the radius or ulna, carry great risk of eventual pathologic displacement.[10,13] Radial head excision should be avoided if open reduction and internal fixation of the forearm is needed. The injury and surgical exposure alone is likely to compromise the interosseous ligament of the forearm, despite minimal initial displacement.

In contrast, if the radial head is intact, whether in the minimally displaced fracture or after internal fixation, proximal translation (migration) of the radius is precluded if the radiocapitellar joint remains reduced. If the radial head is not repairable, prosthetic replacement with a material of adequate stiffness is needed. In summary, a displaced radial head fracture with suspected or demonstrated forearm dissociation is treated by repair or replacement of the radial head, with repair or protection of the associated ligaments of the elbow, forearm, and wrist.

Treatment of the Displaced Radial Head Fracture: The Mason Classification and Spectrum of Associated Injuries

Because of its importance in loadbearing of the forearm, preservation of the radial head with repair, rather than excision, should be considered when technically feasible. Smaller and more suitable implants for internal fixation, combined

with an improved understanding of the anatomy, have made stable internal fixation a more reliable method of treatment for some displaced fractures.[20–28] CT scans may also improve imaging of the fracture comminution and the degree of displacement. If comminution and displacement of the fracture make internal fixation impossible, excision with replacement must be considered for support of the forearm and radius.

It is not possible to discuss management of fractures of the radial head without discussing the familiar Mason classification.[5,8,29] As with most classifications conceived by using a retrospective examination of radiographs and charts, some modification is needed for contemporary use. A modification that may be useful is based on more than the radiographs and includes features of the clinical examination and an assessment of associated injuries (Table 1).

The fractured radial head can be divided into those that are minimally displaced and do not require surgical treatment (type I), those that require surgical intervention because of displacement and can either be internally fixed or excised (type II), and, finally, those fractures that are so comminuted and displaced that internal fixation is not technically possible (type III). With type III fractures, excision is usually necessary to permit forearm rotation. Delayed radial head excision can also be considered for patients whose fractures have healed with incongruity and pain.[30]

Type II Fractures:
Internal Fixation or Excision?

The type II radial head fractures, as defined above, can be repaired using the appropriate hardware for stabilization of the head and neck. However, in an elderly, low-demand patient, internal fixation and the requisite rehabilitation effort may not be warranted. Conversely, in the higher demand, younger patient, stable internal fixation of the head and neck retains the effective load sharing at the radiocapitellar joint and precludes proximal migration of the radius.

As noted above, assessment of the possibility of proximal migration is not foolproof. A patient who presents with proximal displacement of the radius of 1 cm or more probably has suffered a tear of the IOL of the forearm and of the TFCC.[16] Imaging the IOL using MRI has been demonstrated, but in cases of significant displacement, this is probably not needed.[12] In patients with forearm or wrist pain, or associated forearm fractures, the possibility of proximal migration is high. In this setting, open reduction with internal fixation of the radial head should be strongly considered.[12,22]

The isolated head fracture can be stabilized by screw fixation.[21,22,24,25,31] Fractures that extend to the neck usually require a plate that secures the head to the shaft. Care must be taken to place the internal fixation in the "safe zone," to avoid impingement on the proximal radioulnar joint.[5,8,32] Fractures of the neck may be comminuted along the medial side. Buttress plating is not possible, because placement of the plate is limited to the non-articulating "safe zone" of the radial neck. In this setting, bone grafting should be used to support the neck, reducing the tension of the plate on the lateral side. In some patients, it is possible to use an intramedullary pin, when there is no concomitant fracture of the head.[33]

Before performing open reduction and internal fixation of the radial head, the surgeon should be comfortable with the surgical exposure, equipment, and techniques for rigid internal fixation.[5,8,32] Care must be taken to avoid any impingement of the hardware on the proximal radioulnar joint.

Type III Fracture: Excision With Instability

If the radial head cannot be repaired by stable internal fixation, excision is usually warranted. In this setting, prosthetic

Table 1
Modified Mason classification

Type I	Nondisplaced or minimally displaced fracture of head or neck	Forearm rotation (pronation/supination) is limited only by acute pain and swelling — no mechanical block Intra-articular displacement of the fracture is usually less than 2 mm or a marginal lip fracture
Type II	Displaced (usually greater than 2 mm) fracture of the head or neck (angulated)	Motion may be mechanically blocked or incongruous Technically possible to reduce and repair by open reduction with internal fixation (without severe comminution) Fracture involves more than a marginal lip of the radial head
Type III	Severely comminuted fracture of the radial head and neck	Judged not reconstructable by radiograph or during surgery Usually requires excision for movement (delayed excision should be considered)

All of these fractures may be associated injuries with elbow dislocation (usually posterior) with or without coronoid fracture, interosseous ligament injury of the forearm, and/or injury to the triangular fibrocartilage complex of the wrist

replacement is required to maintain the longitudinal relationship of the radius and ulna. Without prosthetic replacement, the radius will subside into the pronated position, with the distal ulna positioned dorsally and distally in relation to the sigmoid notch.

Prosthetic Replacement of the Radial Head

Prosthetic replacement of the radial head continues to evolve, but as of this writing no reliable material and design has yet been demonstrated. Silicone rubber seems to lack effective material properties to withstand compressive and shear forces.[5,15,32,34,35]

The use of artificial prostheses for radial head replacement dates from the 1940s, and problems of loosening and capitellar wear with synovitis have been reported.[36] Metallic radial head replacements have also been used.[37–39] Titanium is now being used to a limited extent, but no long-term studies have been reported. An articulated prosthesis, designed to reduce the toggle and loosening, has also been used, but experience with these is still preliminary.[38] There is not enough

evidence at this time to recommend the routine use of the metallic radial head implant in cases in which there is no instability. Nonetheless, when faced with a type III fracture and gross instability, a prosthesis must be used, for lack of a proven alternative, and the metallic devices may be preferable to the use of silicone rubber. Some surgeons have used allograft radial heads,[13,40] but the indications for their use are still not clear, and the number of cases is few.

If a prosthetic head is used, care must be taken to reconstruct or repair the posterolateral collateral ligaments. Metallic radial head prostheses are also more difficult to implant, because the stem is not flexible. In addition, it is necessary to protect the distal radioulnar joint, as outlined below.

Ligament Repair and Reconstruction: Proximal to Distal

The principal ligaments of the forearm include the posterolateral ulnohumeral ligament complex, the interosseous ligament (IOL) of the forearm, and the ligaments of the distal radioulnar joint, including the TFCC. Any of these structures can be injured in association with a complex radial head fracture, and each should be evaluated and, if necessary, treated.

Posterolateral Ligament Complex: Repair and Protection

Radial head function requires not only an intact head (repaired or replaced), but also effective contact with the capitellum. If there is subluxation or dislocation with associated injury to the posterolateral ligaments, proximal displacement can still occur. The posterolateral ligament complex, as described by O'Driscoll and associates,[17] has been recognized as an important component of global stability of the elbow and posterolateral instability. However, if this complex is not repaired and/or protected after radial head repair or replacement in longitudinal injury, the radial head may subluxate, losing effective contact with the capitellum. In addition, failure to recognize the importance of this structure may increase the risk of ulnohumeral dislocation. Reattachment of the posterolateral ligament may require augmentation with a palmaris tendon graft or the use of bone anchors into the isometric point at the lateral humerus.

Interosseous Ligament of the Forearm

This structure has been referred to as a membrane, although its histology (type I collagen) and function (stabilizes the position between two bones) is that of a ligament. Part of the reason for this confusion has been the broad sweep of the fibers and their varied appearance.[15,16] Nonetheless, Walker[13] surmised its function in the 1970s. Although the idea of repair is attractive, there is little to suggest that this can be done or is really helpful. Because the disruption occurs along a broad region, acute repair may be difficult or impossible.[12] It may be helpful to pin the radius out to length in combination with radial head repair or replace-

ment. The optimal position of immobilization is empirically in supination. Positioning the reduced forearm in supination for 3 to 4 weeks, and limiting pronation as motion is permitted over the subsequent weeks keeps the distal radioulnar joint reduced and maintains the distance between the radius and ulna, reducing the potential for contracture. However, theoretically, supination places the IOL under greater relative tension than pronation. Late reconstruction of the IOL using tendon graft or other materials is of theoretical value and has been performed clinically in a few cases, but its actual value is yet unproven.

Triangular Fibrocartilage Complex and the Distal Radioulnar Joint

The soft-tissue constraints at the distal forearm, specifically the TFCC, support the coronal stability of the wrist more so than the more longitudinally oriented IOL of the forearm. However, as was noted at the proximal radioulnar joint, maintaining the reduction of this joint during healing is more likely to lead to a favorable result than leaving the ulna positioned dorsally relative to the carpus and radius. Patients with Galeazzi fracture dislocations are best treated by positioning the forearm in supination and protecting this position during mobilization.[42,43] Direct repair of the TFCC, although it is of theoretical value, may not be needed if the forearm can be temporarily stabilized with a congruent reduction of the distal radioulnar joint.

Summary

Displaced fractures of the radial head that require reduction or excision are often associated with longitudinal instability. Where possible (type II), these fractures should be stabilized with rigid internal fixation. In cases in which the initial displacement reflects complete dissociation, supplemental stabilization and repair may be required. Particular attention must be paid to the posterolateral collateral liga-

ment, the interosseous ligament of the forearm, and ligaments at the distal radioulnar joint.

References

1. Adler JB, Shaftan GW: Radial head fractures: Is excision necessary? *J Trauma* 1964;4:115–136.

2. Brockman EP: Two cases of disability at the wrist-joint following excision of the head of the radius. *Proc R Soc Med* 1931;24:904–905.

3. Coleman DA, Blair WF, Shurr D: Resection of the radial head for fracture of the radial head: Long-term follow-up of seventeen cases. *J Bone Joint Surg* 1987;69A:385–392.

4. Edwards GS Jr, Jupiter JB: Radial head fractures with acute distal radioulnar dislocation: Essex-Lopresti revisited. *Clin Orthop* 1988;234:61–69.

5. Hotchkiss RN: Fractures and dislocations of the elbow, in Rockwood CA Jr, Green DP, Bucholz RW, et al (eds): *Fractures in Adults*, ed 4. Philadelphia, PA, Lippincott-Raven, 1996, pp 929–1024.

6. Johnston GW: A follow-up of one hundred cases of fracture of the head of the radius with a review of the literature. *Ulster Med J* 1962;31:51–56.

7. Lewis RW, Thibodeau AA: Deformity of the wrist following resection of the radial head. *Surg Gynecol Obstet* 1937;64:1079–1085.

8. Morrey BF: Applied anatomy and biomechanics of the elbow joint, in Anderson LD (ed): *American Academy of Orthopaedic Surgeons Instructional Course Lectures XXXV.* St. Louis, MO, CV Mosby, 1986, p 171.

9. Morrey BF, Chao EY, Hui FC: Biomechanical study of the elbow following excision of the radial head. *J Bone Joint Surg* 1979;61A:63–68.

10. Szabo RM, Hotchkiss RN, Slater RM: The use of frozen allograft radial head replacement for treatment of established symptomatic proximal translation of the radius: Preliminary experience in five cases. *J Hand Surg* 1997;22A:269–278.

11. Essex-Lopresti P: Fractures of the radial head with distal radio-ulnar dislocation: Report of two cases. *J Bone Joint Surg* 1951;33B:244–247.

12. Hotchkiss RN: Injuries to the interosseous ligament of the forearm. *Hand Clin* 1994;10:391–398.

13. Walker PS (ed): *Human Joints and Their Artificial Replacements.* Springfield, IL, Charles C Thomas, 1977, p 167.

14. An KN, Morrey BF: Biomechanics of the elbow, in Morrey BF (ed): *The Elbow and Its Disorders*, ed 2. Philadelphia, PA, WB Saunders, 1993, pp 53–72.

15. Hotchkiss RN, An KN, Sowa DT, et al: An anatomic and mechanical study of the interosseous membrane of the forearm: Pathomechanics of proximal migration of the radius. *J Hand Surg* 1989;14A:256–261.

16. Sarmiento A, Latta L (eds): *Closed Functional Treatment of Fractures.* Berlin, Germany, Springer-Verlag, 1981.

17. O'Driscoll SW, Bell DF, Morrey BF: Posterolateral rotatory instability of the elbow. *J Bone Joint Surg* 1991;73A:440–446.

18. Morrey BF, Askew L, Chao EY: Silastic prosthetic replacement for the radial head. *J Bone Joint Surg* 1981;63A:454–458.

19. Khurana JS, Kattapuram SV, Becker S, et al: Galeazzi injury with an associated fracture of the radial head. *Clin Orthop* 1988;234:70–71.

20. Bunker TD, Newman JH: The Herbert differential pitch bone screw in displaced radial head fractures. *Injury* 1985;16:621–624.

21. Esser RD, Davis S, Taavao T: Fractures of the radial head treated by internal fixation: Late results in 26 cases. *J Orthop Trauma* 1995;9:318–323.

22. Geel CW, Palmer AK: Radial head fractures and their effect on the distal radioulnar joint: A rationale for treatment. *Clin Orthop* 1992;275:79–84.

23. Geel CW, Palmer AK, Ruedi T, et al: Internal fixation of proximal radial head fractures. *J Orthop Trauma* 1990;4:270–274.

24. King GJ, Evans DC, Kellam JF: Open reduction and internal fixation of radial head fractures. *J Orthop Trauma* 1991;5:21–28.

25. Morrey BF: Radial head fracture, in Morrey BF (ed): *The Elbow and Its Disorders,* ed 2. Philadelphia, PA, WB Saunders, 1993, pp 383–404.

26. Odenheimer K, Harvey JP Jr: Internal fixation of fracture of the head of the radius: Two case reports. *J Bone Joint Surg* 1979;61A:785–787.

27. Richards RR, Corley FG Jr: Fractures of the shafts of the radius and ulna, in Rockwood CA Jr, Green DP, Bucholz RW, et al (eds): *Fractures in Adults,* ed 4. Philadelphia, PA, Lippincott-Raven, 1996, pp 869–928.

28. Sowa DT, Hotchkiss RN, Weiland AJ: Symptomatic proximal translation of the radius following radial head resection. *Clin Orthop* 1995;317:106–113.

29. Mason ML: Some observations on fracture of the head of the radius with a review of one hundred cases. *Br J Surg* 1954;42:123–132.

30. Broberg MA, Morrey BF: Results of delayed excision of the radial head after fracture. *J Bone Joint Surg* 1986;68A:669–674.

31. Khalfayan EE, Culp RW, Alexander AH: Mason type II radial head fractures: Operative versus nonoperative treatment. *J Orthop Trauma* 1992;6:283–289.

32. Speed K: Ferrule caps for the head of the radius. *Surg Gynecol Obstet* 1941;73:845–850.

33. Keller HW, Rehm KE, Helling J: Intramedullary reduction and stabilisation of adult radial neck fractures. *J Bone Joint Surg* 1994;76B:405–408.

34. Bohl WR, Brightman E: Fractures of a silastic radial-head prosthesis: Diagnosis and localization of fragments by xerography. A case report. *J Bone Joint Surg* 1981;63A:1482–1483.

35. Gordon M, Bullough PG: Synovial and osseous inflammation in failed silicone-rubber prostheses. *J Bone Joint Surg* 1982;64A:574–580.

36. Vanderwilde RS, Morrey BF, Melberg MW, et al: Inflammatory arthritis after failure of silicone rubber replacement of the radial head. *J Bone Joint Surg* 1994;76B:78–81.

37. Carr CR, Howard JW: Metallic cap replacement of radial head following fracture. *West J Surg* 1951;59:539–546.

38. Charnley G, Judet T, de Loubresse CG, et al: Articulated radial head replacement and elbow release for post head-injury heterotopic ossification. *J Orthop Trauma* 1996;10:68–71.

39. Knight DJ, Rymaszewski LA, Amis AA, et al: Primary replacement of the fractured radial head with a metal prosthesis. *J Bone Joint Surg* 1993;75B:572–576.

40. Morrey BF, An KN, Stormont TJ: Force transmission through the radial head. *J Bone Joint Surg* 1988;70A:250–256.

41. Rabinowitz RS, Light TR, Havey RM, et al: The role of the interosseous membrane and triangular fibrocartilage complex in forearm stability. *J Hand Surg* 1994;19A:385–393.

42. Sellman DC, Seitz WH Jr, Postak PD, et al: Reconstructive strategies for radioulnar dissociation: A biomechanical study. *J Orthop Trauma* 1995;9:516–522.

43. Shmueli G, Herold HZ: Compression screwing of displaced fractures of the head of the radius. *J Bone Joint Surg* 1981;63B:535–538.

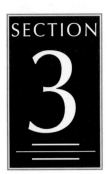

SECTION 3

Hand and Wrist

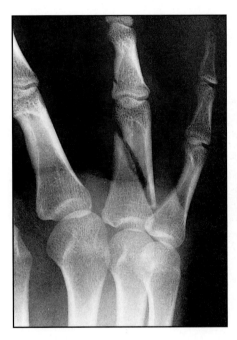
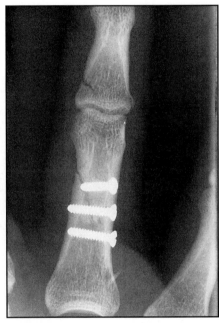

Soft-Tissue Injuries of the Hand in the Athlete

Joseph P. Leddy, MD

Soft-Tissue Injuries

Soft-tissue and tendon injuries to the athlete's hand are relatively common. A good knowledge of the pertinent anatomy and a careful physical examination are essential to the early diagnosis and treatment of these injuries. Injuries that are misdiagnosed or not treated at all may later result in disabling deformities.[1] Most of these soft-tissue injuries can be easily treated by closed means with a good end result, provided the diagnosis and treatment are rendered promptly and properly.

Tendon Injuries
Mallet Finger

This entity is also known as drop finger or baseball finger.[1,2] It normally results from a blow to the tip of the extended finger forcing the distal phalanx into flexion while disrupting the extensor mechanism over the distal interphalangeal (DIP) joint.[3,4] The joint assumes a flexed position and there is tenderness and swelling over the dorsum of the DIP joint, with no active extension. If there is generalized joint laxity, there may be an early swan neck deformity present.[5–9] The radiograph may be negative, indicating a pure tendon avulsion. There may, however, be a small fleck of bone avulsed by the tendon, or there may be a large bony fragment with a third to a half of the articular surface on it with or without palmar subluxation of the remaining distal phalanx.[9] In an adult, the preferred treatment is to splint the DIP joint in extension for 6 weeks constantly, and at night for another 4 weeks or longer.[10] When changing the splint and cleansing

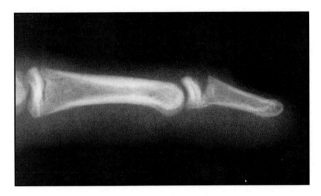

Fig. 1 Epiphyseal injury to the distal phalanx. (Reproduced with permission from Leddy JP, Dennis TR: Tendon injuries, in Strickland JW, Rettig AC (eds): *Hand Injuries in Athletes*. Philadelphia, PA, WB Saunders, 1992, pp 175–207.)

the finger during these 6 weeks, the joint should never be allowed to fall into flexion, because this may disrupt any healing which has taken place. Many of these injuries can be treated up to 2 to 3 months after the initial trauma with this splinting regimen.[2,8,11] Rarely, surgical reconstruction may be necessary in late chronic cases.

If there is a large bony fragment with palmar subluxation of the joint in a young patient, some surgeons prefer open reduction and internal fixation. Normally, the joint is reduced and transfixed with a smooth Kirschner wire (K-wire) and the fracture fragment is fixed either with small K-wire or a pull-out wire and button technique.[10] The joint is splinted as described previously. If a compound injury occurs in an athlete, the treatment is debridement and open repair with splinting as just described. In a young child, the injury is often to the epiphysis,[2,9] at the base of the distal phalanx, rather than to the tendon, and it should be treated with reduction of the fracture and splinting for approximately 3 weeks (Fig. 1).

Boutonnière Deformity (Button Hole)

The boutonnière deformity is caused by rupture of the central slip at or near its insertion into the base of the middle phalanx. The head of the proximal phalanx then "button holes" through the defect in the central slip. The triangular ligament stretches out and the lateral bands fall below the axis of motion at the proximal interphalangeal (PIP) joint, causing a flexion moment here. When the lateral bands retract, they cause an extension moment at the DIP joint. The injury is usually caused either by a blow to the dorsum of the middle phalanx, which forces the PIP joint into flexion while the athlete attempts to extend the finger, or by an unrecognized palmar dislocation of the PIP joint, which reduces spontaneously or is pulled back into place by the athlete or trainer.[12] On physical examination, there is swelling and tenderness near the central slip insertion at the base of the middle phalanx. There is weakness or inability to actively extend the PIP joint. There may be hyperextension at the DIP joint. There is full passive exten-

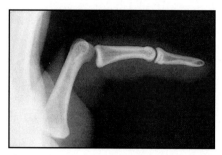 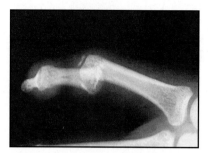 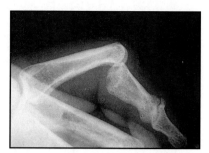

Fig. 2 Left, Palmar lateral dislocation of the proximal interphalangeal (PIP) joint. **Center,** Straight palmar dislocation of the PIP joint. Small bony flecks represent avulsion of central slip insertion. **Right,** Palmar dislocation of the PIP joint that is irreducible because of soft-tissue interposition. (Reproduced with permission from Leddy JP, Dennis TR: Tendon injuries, in Strickland JW, Rettig AC (eds): *Hand Injuries in Athletes.* Philadelphia, PA, WB Saunders, 1992, pp 175–207.)

sion of the PIP joint acutely, but in chronic cases, this deformity can become fixed. Eventually, in these unrecognized and untreated cases, passive extension is lost at the PIP joint and passive flexion is lost at the DIP joint.

There are at least three types of palmar dislocations of the PIP joint.[12] Type I, the most common type, has been described as a palmar lateral dislocation (Fig. 2, *left*). The radiograph may be normal if the athlete or trainer has pulled the finger back into place. There is tenderness over one collateral ligament and the central slip insertion. There is weak extension at the PIP joint. This injury is often missed and can later cause a boutonnière deformity. The treatment is to hold the metacarpophalangeal (MP) and PIP joints in the extended position with a safety pin type splint for 4 to 5 weeks, while encouraging active and passive flexion of the DIP joint (Fig. 3).

In type II, there is a straight palmar dislocation. On radiograph, there is an obvious deformity and the central slip has been ruptured (Fig. 2, *center*). Treatment is closed reduction and a safety pin splint again for 4 to 5 weeks holding the MP and PIP joints in the extended position and encouraging flexion at the DIP joint.

In type III, the palmar dislocation is irreducible. The radiograph shows an obvious deformity, and findings at surgery include soft-tissue interposition, such as a lateral band, collateral ligament, or central slip (Fig. 2, *right*). The central slip may or may not be torn with this injury. The treatment is open reduction with removal of the interposed tissue. If the central slip is damaged, the PIP joint can be fixed in extension with a K-wire for 3 weeks, followed by 2 more weeks in a safety pin splint. If the central slip is intact, range of motion can be started when soft-tissue healing permits.

For an acute case with a large bony avulsion from the base of the middle phalanx and joint incongruity at the PIP joint, open reduction and internal fixation are indicated. This is a rare injury. Most of these acute boutonnière injuries can be treated with closed reduction and splinting as described above. Chronic cases of boutonnière deformity usually require surgical reconstruction once full passive range of motion has been restored by splinting and/or therapy.[13,14]

Pseudo-Boutonnière Deformity
This deformity is similar in appearance to a regular boutonnière deformity, but the causes and treatment are vastly different. In a pseudo-boutonnière deformity, there is a fixed flexion deformity at the PIP joint with a mild hyperextension deformity at the DIP joint (Fig. 4, *left*). The cause is a hyperextension injury to the PIP joint with disruption of one col-

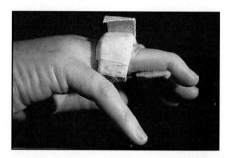

Fig. 3 Splint holding the metacarpophalangeal and proximal interphalangeal joints in extension while encouraging active and passive flexion of the distal interphalangeal joint.

lateral ligament and a portion of the volar plate.[15,16] These structures contract as they heal, causing a slowly progressive flexion deformity at the PIP joint. Over time, a telltale calcification along one side of the finger may become visible on radiograph (Fig. 4, *right*). There is no tenderness over the central slip insertion, and active and passive extension of the PIP joint are equal. Treatment of these injuries is difficult. If the deformity is less than 45° when first seen, treatment with a safety pin splint or a joint jack may help. Correction is obtained very slowly. Deformities greater than 45° when first seen often will not respond to splinting, and capsulotomy may be of benefit.[16]

Boxer's Knuckle (Soft Knuckles)
The mechanism here is a specific injury to structures on the dorsum of the MP

Soft-Tissue Injuries of the Hand in the Athlete

Chapter 20

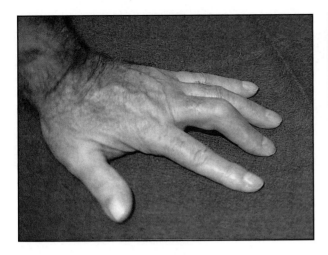

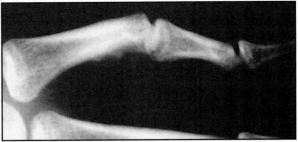

Fig. 4 Left, Pseudo-boutonnière deformity. Right, Calcification due to disruption of collateral ligament and volar plate on the injured side.

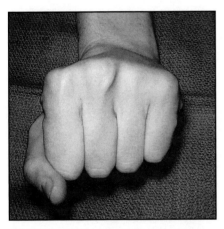

Fig. 5 Ulnar dislocation of the extensor tendon at the metacarpophalangeal joint level in the middle finger. (Reproduced with permission from Leddy JP, Dennis TR: Tendon injuries, in Strickland JW, Rettig AC (eds): Hand Injuries in Athletes. Philadelphia, PA, WB Saunders, 1992, pp 175–207.)

joint (usually the index or middle) followed by repetitive trauma reinjuring the same area.[17] The findings include swelling and tenderness over the involved MP joint. The boxer will say he just "can't punch" with that hand. The condition improves during a period of rest, but recurs as soon as the athlete begins training again. Radiographs are usually normal. Treatment may be difficult. The acute stage is seen rarely, because it is normally treated as a bruise or sprain. In the chronic case, rest or

splinting is rarely of benefit. At the time of surgical exploration, there is usually either a chronic tear in the extensor hood or the dorsal capsule of the joint.[18,19] Treatment consists of surgical repair of the damaged structures. The prognosis is good, but the recovery time may be prolonged and the athlete may not be able to return to boxing for 6 months.

Dislocation-Subluxation of the Extensor Tendons at the Metacarpophalangeal Joint

The mechanism of this injury is usually a direct blow that forces the finger into flexion or into flexion and ulnar deviation.[3,20] The extensor tendon usually dislocates or subluxes to the ulnar side. The middle finger is the most commonly affected[21] (Fig. 5). Radial subluxation is rare. Radiographs are negative. Acute cases are rarely seen, because they are usually treated as a sprain or contusion. If the injury is seen acutely, splinting the MP joint in extension for 4 to 6 weeks may be of some benefit. In chronic symptomatic cases, surgical reconstruction is often necessary. There is normally a tear in the extensor hood on the radial side. If the ulnar side is contracted, a surgical release may be necessary here.[5,21,22] If there is inadequate tissue for repair, some form of tendon transfer or reconstruction may be used.[23]

Avulsion of the Profundus Tendon Insertion (Jersey Finger)

This injury is usually caused by the finger being forcibly extended during a maximal contraction of the profundus muscle, such that the tendon insertion gives way. In more than 75% of cases, it is the ring finger that is involved. The pathognomonic finding is inability to actively flex the DIP joint. Tenderness and ecchymoses may be present, and there is normally good active flexion at the PIP joint. Radiographs are usually negative. There may be a small bony fragment opposite the PIP joint, suggesting that the tendon has retracted to this level. There may also be a large fragment of bone held up at the A4 pulley. The prognosis and treatment of this injury depends on the level to which the tendon retracts and, therefore, the remaining nutritional supply to the tendon, the time elapsed between injury and treatment, and the presence and size of a bony fragment on radiograph.[24–26] Leddy and Packer[26] have described three types of this injury.

In a type I injury, the tendon retracts to the palm so that both vinculae are ruptured, with some loss of blood supply. There is no more diffusion of synovial fluid. There is pain and tenderness in the palm at the lumbrical level. In this type, the tendon should be reinserted in 7 to

AAOS Instructional Course Lectures, Volume 47

183

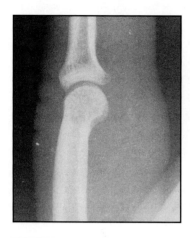
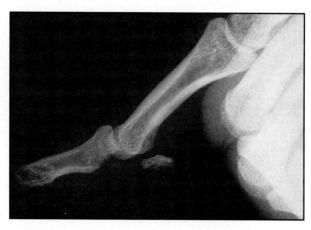

Fig. 6 Left, Small bony fragment opposite the proximal interphalangeal joint in a type II injury. (Reproduced with permission from Leddy JP, Dennis TR: Tendon injuries, in Strickland JW, Rettig AC (eds): *Hand Injuries in Athletes*. Philadelphia, PA, WB Saunders, 1992, pp 175–207.) Right, A large bony fragment held up at the A4 pulley in a type III injury.

10 days before it becomes shriveled and contracted. Radiographs are negative.

In type II, the most common type of injury, the tendon retracts to the level of the PIP joint. The long vinculum remains intact and, therefore, some blood supply is retained. Some nutrition from the synovial fluid is preserved. There may be a small bony fleck opposite the PIP joint on radiograph, marking the location of the tendon end (Fig. 6, *left*). There is pain, swelling, and tenderness at the PIP joint, with no active flexion at the DIP joint and some loss of flexion at the PIP joint. Because some length is preserved, as well as some nutritional supply, this type can often be reinserted at a later date (2 to 3 months) if necessary. Type II may convert to a type I if the long vinculum gives way and the tendon slides into the palm.

In a type III injury, there is a large bony fragment that is avulsed by the profundus insertion and held up at the A4 pulley (Fig. 6, *right*). Both vinculae are intact and, therefore, blood supply is preserved. Synovial diffusion is still present. The treatment is open reduction and internal fixation of the large fragment. This can be done as late as 2 to 3 months postinjury. The tendon may pull away from the bony fragment and become a type III B injury,[27–29] but this is unusual. Treatment in this case is open reduction and internal fixation of the large fragment, and advancement and reinsertion of the tendon into the base of the distal phalanx.

Old, untreated cases that are asymptomatic should be left alone. If the joint is unstable, consideration should be given to fusion of the DIP joint.[24–26] Flexor tendon graft through an intact superficialis may be done,[30–35] but the potential risks may outweigh the possible benefits of this procedure, particularly in the ring finger of an athlete.

Acute Rupture of the Ulnar Collateral Ligament of the Metacarpophalangeal Joint of the Thumb (Gamekeeper's Thumb, Skier's Thumb)

The mechanism of this injury is usually a fall on the outstretched thumb with a radial deviation force at the MP joint. There is pain, swelling, and weakness of pinch. There is tenderness over the ulnar aspect of the MP joint of the thumb and instability on testing of this ligament, either in extension or 30° of flexion at the MP joint or both. The radiograph may be negative. One should look for a bony fragment and also for the possibility of palmar subluxation of the base of the proximal phalanx on the metacarpal head (Fig. 7, *left*). If there is a Stener lesion[36] present, with a small avulsion of bone, this may be visualized on the radiograph (Fig. 7, *right*). If there is no bony avulsion with the Stener lesion, there is usually pain, swelling, tenderness and a feeling of a mass at the level of the metacarpal head proximal to the adductor aponeurosis. Instability, without a clear end point, is present.

Most of these injuries can be treated with 4 weeks of immobilization in a thumb spica cast. Thereafter, the thumb may be protected from 2 to 6 months with splinting during athletic endeavors, depending on the sport. Open reduction and internal fixation should be considered if there is a large displaced intra-articular fragment avulsed by the ulnar collateral ligament causing articular incongruity. If there is palmar subluxation of the base of the proximal phalanx on the metacarpal head associated with an ulnar collateral ligament injury, reduction of the joint with K-wire fixation and repair of the damaged structures is indicated. If a Stener lesion is present, with or without a bony fragment, surgical repair should be performed. If there is greater than 35° of instability when compared with the opposite normal thumb, then the surgeon should consider repair of the ligamentous injury. Postoperatively, these people are treated with 4 to 6 weeks of immobilization, depending on the surgical procedure. Protection during athletic events should be considered for 2 to 6 months following the operation.

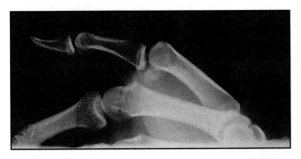

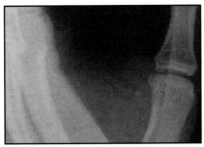

Fig. 7 Left, Palmar subluxation of the base of the proximal phalanx on the metacarpal head. **Right,** A "bony" Stener lesion, with a small fleck of bone visible proximal to the adductor aponeurosis.

Dislocation of the Carpometacarpal Joint of the Thumb

This injury is normally caused by a fall on the outstretched thumb. There is rupture of the anterior oblique ligament. Findings include pain, swelling, and deformity at the basal joint of the thumb, together with weakness of pinch. On radiograph, there is an obvious dislocation, which usually is easily reducible. In some instances, only a subluxation of the joint may be seen if there was a spontaneous reduction after the injury (Fig. 8). Treatment of these injuries is difficult. Closed reduction and cast immobilization for 6 weeks has been recommended, but careful serial radiographic evaluation must be done to make certain there is no residual or gradual subluxation. Closed reduction and percutaneous pinning may be done if there is loss of reduction or inability to maintain an anatomic reduction. If there is late instability, ligament reconstruction, such as that described by Eaton,[38] may be necessary.

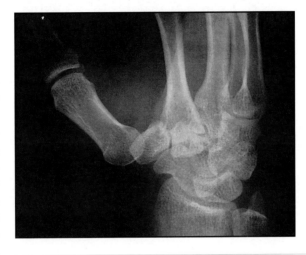

Fig. 8 Residual subluxation of the trapeziometacarpal joint after reduction of dislocation.

References

1. Posner MA: Injuries to the hand and wrist in athletes. *Orthop Clin North Am* 1977;8:593–618.

2. Abouna JM, Brown H: The treatment of mallet finger: The results in a series of 148 consecutive cases and a review of the literature. *Br J Surg* 1968;55:653–667.

3. Boyes JH (ed): *Bunnell's Surgery of the Hand*, ed 5. Philadelphia, PA, JB Lippincott, 1970.

4. Mason ML: Rupture of tendons of the hand: With a study of the extensor tendon insertions in the fingers. *Surg Gynecol Obstet* 1930;50:611–624.

5. Doyle JR: Extensor tendons: Acute injuries, in Green DP (ed): *Operative Hand Surgery*, ed 2.

New York, NY, Churchill Livingstone, 1988, vol 3, pp 2045–2072.

6. Hallberg D, Lindholm A: Subcutaneous rupture of the extensor tendon of the distal phalanx of the finger: "Mallet finger." Brief review of the literature and report on 127 cases treated conservatively. *Acta Chir Scand* 1960;119: 260–267.

7. Robb WAT: The results of treatment of mallet finger. *J Bone Joint Surg* 1959;41B:546–549.

8. Stark HH, Boyes JH, Wilson JN: Mallet finger. *J Bone Joint Surg* 1962;44A:1061–1068.

9. Wehbe MA, Schneider LH: Mallet fractures. *J Bone Joint Surg* 1984;66A:658–669.

10. Leddy JP, Dennis TR: Tendon injuries, in Strickland JW, Rettig AC (eds): *Hand Injuries in Athletes*. Philadelphia, PA, WB Saunders, 1992, pp 175–207.

11. McFarlane RM, Hampole MK: Treatment of extensor tendon injuries of the hand. *Can J Surg* 1973;16:366–375.

12. Leddy JP: Athletic injuries to the hand and wrist, in Zawadsky P (ed): *Post-Graduate Advances in Sports Medicine*. Princeton, NJ, Nassau Press, 1986, pp 3–10.

13. Peimer CA, Sullivan DJ, Wild DR: Palmar dislocation of the proximal interphalangeal joint. *J Hand Surg* 1984;9A:39–48.

14. Posner MA, Kapila D: Chronic palmar dislocation of proximal interphalangeal joints. *J Hand Surg* 1986;11A:253–258.

15. McCue FC, Andrews JR, Hakala M, et al: The coach's finger. *J Sports Med* 1974;2:270–275.

16. McCue FC, Honner R, Johnson MC, et al: Athletic injuries of the proximal interphalangeal joint requiring surgical treatment. *J Bone Joint Surg* 1970;52A:937–956.

17. Gladden JR: Boxer's knuckle: A preliminary report. *Am J Surg* 1957;83:388–397.

18. Koniuch MP, Peimer CA, VanGorder T, et al: Closed crush injury of the metacarpophalangeal joint. *J Hand Surg* 1987;12A:750–757.

19. Posner MA, Ambrose L: Boxer's knuckle: Dorsal capsular rupture of the metacarpophalangeal joint of a finger. *J Hand Surg* 1989;14A:229–236.

20. Wheeldon FT: Recurrent dislocation of extensor tendons in the hand. *J Bone Joint Surg* 1954;36B:612–617.

21. Kettelkamp DB, Flatt AE, Moulds R: Traumatic dislocation of the long-finger extensor tendon: A clinical, anatomical, and biomechanical study. *J Bone Joint Surg* 1971;53A:229–240.

22. Bin Iftikhar T, Hallmann BW, Kaminski RS, et al: Spontaneous rupture of the extensor mechanism causing ulnar dislocation of the long extensor tendon of the long finger: Two case reports. *J Bone Joint Surg* 1984;66A:1108–1109.

23. Carroll C IV, Moore JR, Weiland AJ: Posttraumatic ulnar subluxation of the extensor tendons: A reconstructive technique. *J Hand Surg* 1987;12A:227–231.

24. Leddy JP: Avulsions of the flexor digitorum profundus. *Hand Clin* 1985;1:77–83.

25. Leddy JP: Flexor tendons: Acute injuries, in Green DP (ed): *Operative Hand Surgery*, ed 2. New York, NY, Churchill Livingstone, 1988, vol 3, pp 1935–1968.

26. Leddy JP, Packer JW: Avulsion of the profundus tendon insertion in athletes. *J Hand Surg* 1977;2A:66–69.

27. Langa V, Posner MA: Unusual rupture of a flexor profundus tendon. *J Hand Surg* 1986;11A:227–229.

28. Robins PR, Dobyns JH: Avulsion of the insertion of the flexor digitorum profundus tendon associated with fracture of the distal phalanx: A brief review, in American Academy of Orthopaedic Surgeons *Symposium on Tendon Surgery in the Hand*. St. Louis, MO, CV Mosby, 1975, pp 151–156.

29. Smith JH Jr: Avulsion of a profundus tendon with simultaneous intraarticular fracture of the distal phalanx: Case report. *J Hand Surg* 1981;6A:600–601.

30. Carroll RE, Match RM: Avulsion of the flexor profundus tendon insertion. *J Trauma* 1970;10:1109–1118.

31. Chang WH, Thomas OJ, White WL: Avulsion injury of the long flexor tendons. *Plast Reconstr Surg* 1972;50:260–264.

32. Goldner JL, Coonrad RW: Tendon grafting of the flexor profundus in the presence of a completely or partially intact flexor sublimis. *J Bone Joint Surg* 1969;51A:527–532.

33. Honner R: The late management of the isolated lesion of the flexor digitorum profundus tendon. *Hand* 1975;7:171–174.

34. Jaffe S, Weckesser E: Profundus tendon grafting with the sublimis intact: An end-result study of thirty patients. *J Bone Joint Surg* 1967;49A:1298–1308.

35. McClinton MA, Curtis RM, Wilgis EF: One hundred tendon grafts for isolated flexor digitorum profundus injuries. *J Hand Surg* 1982;7A:224–229.

36. Stener B: Displacement of the ruptured ulnar collateral ligament of the metacarpo-phalangeal joint of the thumb: A clinical and anatomical study. *J Bone Joint Surg* 1962;44B:869–879.

37. Coonrad RW, Goldner JL: A study of the pathological findings and treatment in soft-tissue injury of the thumb metacarpophalangeal joint: With a clinical study of the normal range of motion in one thousand thumbs and a study of post mortem findings of ligamentous structures in relation to function. *J Bone Joint Surg* 1968;50A:439–451.

38. Eaton RG, Littler JW: Ligament reconstruction for the painful thumb carpometacarpal joint. *J Bone Joint Surg* 1973;55A:1655–1666.

Fractures in the Hand in Athletes

Arthur C. Rettig, MD

Most sports require the use of the hands for propelling a ball, defending against an opponent, or breaking a fall, and thus hand injuries are quite common. A fracture in the hand of an athlete is generally caused by torque, angular forces, compressive forces, or direct blow trauma. In most athletic hand injuries, the energy absorption level is low and the fractures are stable, with minimal soft-tissue involvement. In many cases, simple splinting or immobilization is appropriate, and may allow early return to sports. However, it is important to recognize those injuries that, if treated improperly, may result in functional impairment. The primary goal of treatment is to institute a plan that will reliably result in normal hand function.

On-the-Field Examination

The person carrying out an on-the-field examination for a possible hand fracture should answer two important questions: (1) does the injury require immediate treatment?, and (2) can the athlete continue to play? The examiner should ascertain the presence or absence of bony tenderness, crepitus, and stability. He or she should also determine the presence of any deformity, especially rotational deformity.

If there is no circulatory embarrassment, obvious deformity, or significant open wound, usually the fracture can be splinted and ice applied. Determination of whether the athlete may return to play is more difficult and depends on the per-

ceived stability of the injury, the sport involved, how much protection is consistent with participation, and finally, the comfort and desire of the athlete.

Distal Phalanx Fractures

Distal phalangeal fractures, other than the common mallet fracture, may be caused by crush forces, such as being stepped on, or a direct blow from a racquet or Lacrosse stick. Occasionally, a longitudinal fracture may result from an axially directed force secondary to contact with a ball or another player.

In general, distal phalanx fractures are stabilized by the presence of the nail plate dorsally and the pulp septa volarly. These fractures may be treated with gutter splints across the distal interphalangeal (DIP) joint for approximately 3 weeks. Return to play is allowed after approximately 7 to 10 days, depending on the athlete's level of comfort and the sport played. In racquet sports, where full DIP function is necessary, return time may be 4 to 6 weeks.

Middle Phalangeal Fractures

The middle phalanx is protected from injury in sports relatively well by its short length and by the force-absorbing adjacent interphalangeal joints. Two types of extra-articular middle phalangeal fractures occur: (1) those proximal to the insertion of the flexor digitorum sublimis (FDS), in which dorsal angulation occurs; and (2) those that occur distal to the FDS insertion, in which volar angula-

tion is the rule. Usually these fractures are caused by a direct blow or crush, which results in an oblique or transverse type fracture.

With any phalangeal fracture, it is very important to determine the stability of the fracture and the acceptability of any possible deformity that may result. In a prospective study of 284 proximal and middle phalangeal fractures, Pun and associates[1] stated that if there was less than 10° of angulation in the anteroposterior and lateral plane, no malrotation, and minimal motion at the fracture site as adjacent joints were placed through 30% of their range of motion (ROM), then treatment by free mobilization with simple buddy taping resulted in 90% good or excellent results. These criteria can be applied to many fractures in athletes with similar predictable results. Return to sport depends on the type of sport involved and the amount of protection that can be used. Periodic radiographs are recommended for confirmation of stability. If the fracture is displaced significantly or is unstable, the options of management include closed reduction and splinting, closed reduction and percutaneous fixation, or open reduction and internal fixation (ORIF).

Proximal Phalanx Fractures

Injuries of the proximal phalanx are common in many sports and can be the source of significant time loss and, if not treated properly, significant functional deficit. Direct blows or dorsally directed

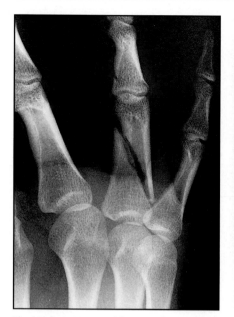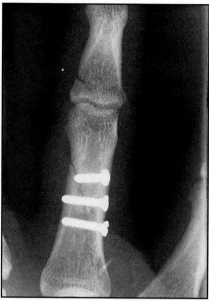

Fig 1 Left, A 20-year-old tennis player sustained an oblique rotated proximal phalanx fracture. **Right,** Treatment was by open reduction and internal fixation with an interfragmentary screw.

forces to the proximal phalanx may lead to transverse fractures, which typically angulate volarly because of the pull of the interossei on the proximal fragment. Rotational forces to the digit frequently result in spiral and oblique fractures, and these may present a problem to the clinician. The fracture pattern varies with age. In children, fractures commonly occur through the distal neck of the proximal phalanx. Physeal fractures at the base of the proximal phalanx are quite common in the adolescent. In adults, fractures occur either through the shaft or into the distal condylar area of the proximal phalanx.

In the adult, spiral oblique fractures of the shaft are commonly due to rotational stresses. When caused by athletic trauma, these fractures are usually stable because of the small amount of energy absorbed in the injury. If a spiral oblique fracture is located proximally, it may be stabilized by the A2 pulley, which is a very sturdy portion of the fibrosseous tunnel.[2] More distal fractures are less stable, because the pulley system offers less support at this level. If these fractures are

deemed stable, the position is acceptable, and rotation of the digit in full flexion is satisfactory, treatment is by splinting and buddy taping.

If the fracture pattern is unstable, closed reduction and splinting, or closed reduction and percutaneous pinning is indicated. In my experience, it is difficult to maintain closed reduction in a truly unstable fracture. I prefer, if possible, closed reduction and percutaneous pin fixation. The goals of treatment are to achieve stability with minimal soft-tissue disruption. When closed reduction is not satisfactory, ORIF with 1.5-mm or 2.0-mm interfragmentary screws may be indicated (Fig. 1). Once stability is achieved, ROM exercise is begun, and the athlete may return to sports in 2 to 6 weeks in most cases.

A common fracture that occurs in sports is the intra-articular unicondylar or bicondylar fracture. If the articular surface is anatomic, or less than 1 mm of displacement exists, management with a gutter splint for 3 weeks may be instituted. It is important to start ROM within 3 weeks of the injury or significant proxi-

mal interphalangeal (PIP) stiffness may occur. It is quite important to follow these fractures with weekly radiographs for 2 to 3 weeks to ensure maintenance of position. In the athlete, return to sport may be possible within 1 to 2 weeks, if splinting is tolerated in the sport.

If the unicondylar or bicondylar fractures are displaced more than 1 mm, internal fixation is required. Occasionally, this may be performed by means of a closed reduction and percutaneous fixation, although most cases require open reduction through a dorsal approach and internal fixation with either a K-wire or 1.5-mm or 2.0-mm screw (Fig. 2). Postoperatively, the finger is splinted in extension to protect the extensor mechanism. Early ROM may be started at 5 days.

Metacarpal Fractures
Metacarpal fractures are quite common in many sports, particularly those that involve contact, such as football or rugby. Shaft fractures are particularly common in boxing and present a special problem in management. Determination of stability of these fractures is of paramount importance. Examination should be aimed at ascertaining excessive shortening, rotation, or angulation. This is done by both physical examination and radiographic evaluation.

If the athlete has full extension, flexion, and no malrotation, the fracture is clinically acceptable and generally stable. Clinical examination should be correlated with radiographic appearance. The traditionally unacceptable clinical findings include shortening greater than 4 mm to 5 mm, angulation greater than 50° to 60° in the ring and small finger or 15° to 20° in the index and long finger, and any malrotation of the fracture. If radiographic findings are equivocal, I rely heavily on the physical examination to determine stability, acceptability, and appropriate treatment.

In a series reported in 1989 of 53

metacarpal shaft fractures that occurred in athletes (primarily football and basketball players), 82% of the fractures were stable and were treated with functional splinting, with return to sport when comfortable (Fig. 3).[3] In this series, return to football with a playing cast averaged 11 days; for basketball, return averaged 19 days. Overall, the average return to sport was 12.3 days.

In the less common, unstable metacarpal fracture where gross motion exists at the fracture site, or in cases of multiple metacarpal fractures, I recommend stabilization as quickly as possible. Closed reduction is certainly possible in certain situations, however, in my experience, reduction and percutaneous pinning or ORIF is the preferable treatment in most unstable, unacceptable metacarpal shaft fractures.

Although many methods of internal fixation have been described, Black and associates[4] pointed out that placement of a dorsal neutralization plate in a metacarpal fracture in which the volar cortices are apposed results in a construct that is essentially as strong as normal bone. Once this is achieved, the surgeon can consider the fracture to be stable and can proceed with functional treatment.

Metacarpal shaft fractures in the boxer, as reported by Melone,[5] require special consideration. Treatment attempts to restore anatomic position of the metacarpal with particular regard to angulation and length. These fractures frequently occur in the long and index finger, and if any metacarpal shortening is present it may transfer forces to the adjacent knuckles with significant problems for the boxer. Melone[5] recommends closed reduction and percutaneous pin fixation of these fractures, with either cross pinning or fixation to the adjacent metacarpal to avoid any excessive scarring on the continuously exposed dorsum of the boxer's hand. Also, in contradistinction to other sports, the metacarpal must be solidly healed in order to return to

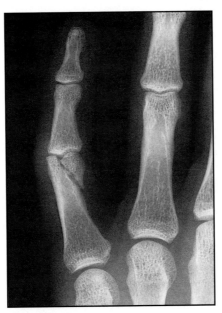 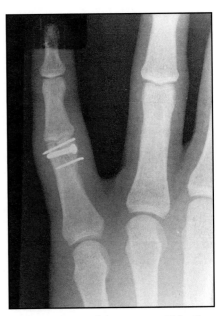

Fig. 2 Left, A 22-year-old college football player sustained a left small finger injury. **Right,** The displaced intercondylar fracture was treated by open reduction and internal fixation, using K-wire and interfragmentary screw fixation.

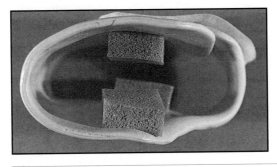

Fig. 3 Hand based othroplast splint with 3-point fixation.

boxing, healing that frequently requires a minimum of 3 months.

Metacarpal Fractures of the Thumb

Thumb metacarpal shaft fractures are quite common in sports. Caused by impact on the radial aspect of the first metacarpal, these fractures frequently occur in football as a quarterback's thumb strikes a helmet during follow through on a pass attempt. Fractures of the shaft usually occur at the proximal middle third region, with angulation occurring in adduction and volar flexion. Approximately 35° of angulation may be acceptable, and, here, too, the clinical assessment is important.

If angulation is deemed unacceptable, closed reduction and percutaneous pin fixation is indicated to prevent chronic hyperextension at the metacarpophalangeal joint. The time out of sports depends on the position and the amount of protection compatible with play, usually a minimum of 2 to 3 weeks.[6]

The Bennett's fracture-subluxation of the base of the first metacarpal occurs from a mechanism similar to that responsible for the shaft fracture. If greater than 1 mm to 2 mm of displacement or subluxation exists, reduction is indicated. Most orthopaedists prefer closed reduction with percutaneous pin fixation, although if the fragment involves greater

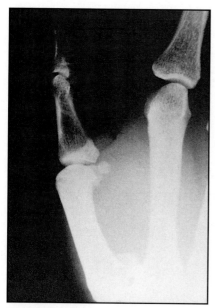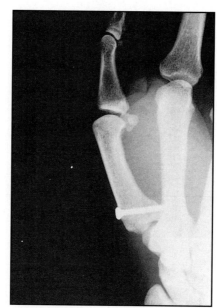

Fig. 4 Left, A professional football running back sustained Bennett's fracture. The fragment involved approximately 35% of the joint surface. **Right,** Treatment was by open reduction and internal fixation using an interfragmentary screw.

than 20% of the articular surface, ORIF with a compression screw may be performed (Fig. 4). Cancellous bone usually heals in approximately 3 weeks, and football players can frequently return to their sport within 3 weeks if they can play with cast protection and if the K-wire does not cross the carpometacarpal joint. When this injury occurs in the throwing hand of a quarterback, commonly the athlete is out for 6 to 8 weeks.

In summary, most fractures of the metacarpals and phalanges in the hand in sports activities are stable due to the lower energy absorption involved in these injuries. Therefore, in most cases the treatment is functional and involves protective splinting and return to sport when the athlete is comfortable with protective playing devices.

It should be noted, however, that many of the fractures that occur in sports are unstable, unacceptable, and require management that will assure the best possible future hand function. A thorough assessment of the injury and careful discussion of the alternatives of treatment should be undertaken with the athlete and his/her family in all situations, for all injuries.

References

1. Pun WK, Chow SP, So YC, et al: A prospective study on 284 digital fractures of the hand. *J Hand Surg* 1989;14A:474–481.

2. Hastings H II: Management of extra-articular fractures of the phalanges and metacarpals, in Strickland JW, Rettig AC (eds): *Hand Injuries in Athletes*. Philadelphia, PA, WB Saunders, 1992, pp 129–153.

3. Rettig AC, Ryan R, Shelbourne KD, et al: Metacarpal fractures in the athlete. *Am J Sports Med* 1989;17:567–572.

4. Black D, Mann RJ, Constine R, et al: Comparison of internal fixation techniques in metacarpal fractures. *J Hand Surg* 1985;10A:466–472.

5. Melone CP: Hand injuries in boxing, in *Medical Aspects of Boxing*. New York, NY, CRC Press, 1993.

6. Rettig AC, Rowdon GA: Metacarpal fractures in athletes, in Torg JS, Shephard RJ (eds): *Current Therapy in Sports Medicine*, ed 3. Philadelphia, PA, Mosby-Year Book, 1995, pp 152–155.

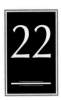

Intra-articular Fractures of the Distal Radius:
Contemporary Perspectives

Jesse B. Jupiter, MD
Diego L. Fernandez, MD
Terry L. Whipple, MD
Robin R. Richards, MD

Introduction

Fractures of the distal end of the radius are among the most common of all skeletal injuries.[1-4] Many of these injuries are relatively uncomplicated and are effectively treated by a closed manipulative reduction and plaster support. There exists, however, a subgroup of fractures that involve the articular surface of either the radiocarpal joint, the radioulnar joint, or both, and these threaten not only the integrity of the articular congruence but also the kinematics of these articulations. The varied morphology of these articular injuries, along with any associated ligamentous or other soft-tissue trauma, will require individual assessment and a treatment program tailored to the varied components of the specific intra-articular fracture.

Functional Anatomy

It is reasonable to view the distal end of the radius both as the anatomic foundation of the wrist joint and as an integral component of the forearm articulation. These units are dependent on bony and articular, as well as ligamentous, integrity both for mobility and to maintain the capacity to transmit axial load.[5] Beginning 2 cm proximal to the radiocarpal joint, at the metaphyseal flare, the distal end of the radius is uniquely designed to accomplish these functions. The distal articular surface is biconcave and triangular in shape. The apex of the triangle points toward the radial styloid process, and the base of the triangle forms the sigmoid notch, which articulates with the distal end of the ulna. The distal radial articular surface is separated into two distinct facets that are covered with hyaline cartilage. These facets articulate individually with the scaphoid and lunate carpal bones. Both facets are concave in both the anteroposterior and radioulnar directions. Because the articular end slopes in an ulnar and palmar direction, the proximal carpal row has a natural tendency to slide into an ulnar direction, a tendency that is resisted for the most part by the intracapsular and interosseous carpal ligaments.

The sigmoid notch is semicylindrical and is oriented parallel to the seat of the ulnar head. This articulation represents a trochoid joint, and rotation of the radius about the ulna is accomplished by a translation of movement, in which the ulnar head displaces anteriorly with forearm supination and dorsally with forearm pronation. The triangular fibrocartilage arises from the ulnar aspect of the lunate facet and extends onto the base of the ulnar styloid process to function as an important stabilizer of the distal radioulnar joint (DRUJ). The dorsal and volar margins of the triangular fibrocartilage are thickened and blend into what are known as the dorsal and ulnar radioulnar ligaments.

The longitudinal axis of forearm rotation passes through the articular surface of the radial head, the interosseous membrane, and the articular surface of the distal ulna at the DRUJ.[6] During pronation and supination the radius rotates around this axis. The axis of forearm rotation is parallel to neither the radius nor the ulna. Most normal activities of daily living can be accomplished with an arc of 100° of forearm rotation, with equal amounts of pronation and supination.[7] Adams and Holley[8] have demonstrated that forearm rotation, particularly pronation, produces strains in the triangular fibrocartilage. The highest strains occurred in the radial portion of the triangular fibrocartilage, particularly with axial loading when the forearm was pronated. Schuind and associates[9] performed a biomechanical study of the distal radioulnar ligaments. The palmar radioulnar ligament was taut in supination and the dorsal radioulnar ligament was taut in pronation. The length of the palmar radioulnar ligament decreased to 71% of its resting length in pronation and the dorsal radioulnar ligament decreased to an average of 90% of

Fracture types (Adults)	Fracture Equivalent in Children	Stability/ Instability*	Displacement Pattern	Number of Fragments	Associated Lesions†	Treatment
Type I Bending fracture of the metaphysis 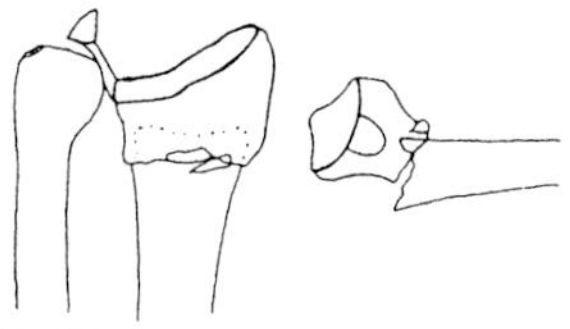	Distal forearm fracture Salter II	Stable Unstable	Nondisplaced Dorsal (Colles-Pouteau) Volar (Smith) Proximal Combined	Always two main fragments Metaphyseal comminution (Varying degree = instability)	Uncommon	Conservative (stable fractures) Percutaneous pins External fixation Bone graft, on exception
Type II Shearing fracture of the joint surface 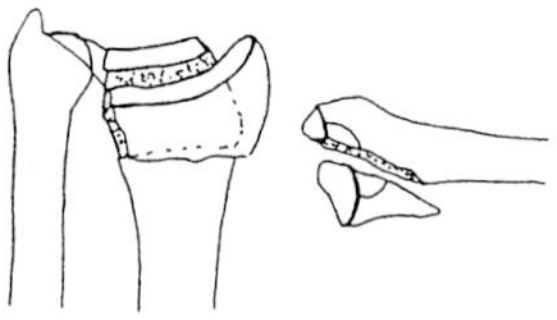	Salter IV	Unstable	Dorsal Radial Volar Proximal Combined	Two-part Three-part Comminuted	Common	Open reduction Screw-plate fixation
Type III Compression fracture of the joint surface 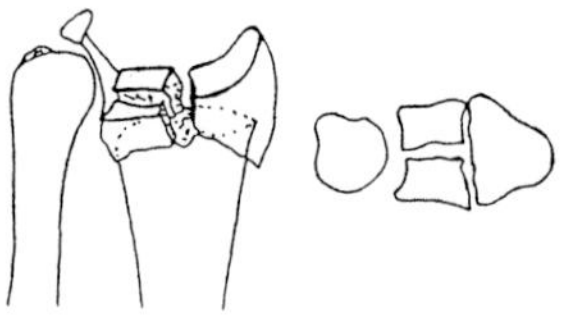	Salter III, IV, V	Stable Unstable	Nondisplaced Dorsal Radial Volar Proximal Combined	Two-part Three-part Four-part Comminuted	Frequent	Conservative Closed, limited, or extensile open reduction Percutaneous pins, combined external and internal fixation, bone graft
Type IV Avulsion fractures, radial carpal fracture dislocation 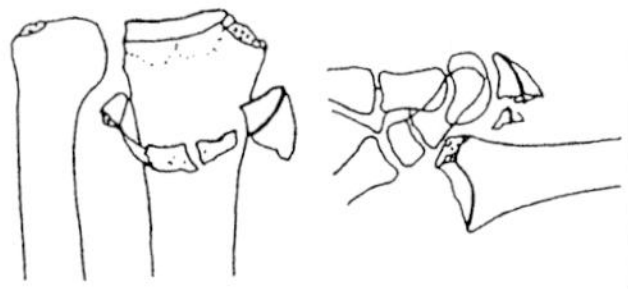	Very rare	Unstable	Dorsal Radial Volar Proximal Combined	Two-part (radial styloid, ulnar styloid) Three-part (volar, dorsal, margin) Comminuted	Very frequent	Closed or open reduction Pin or screw fixation Tension wiring
Type V Combined fractures (I, II, III IV) high velocity injury 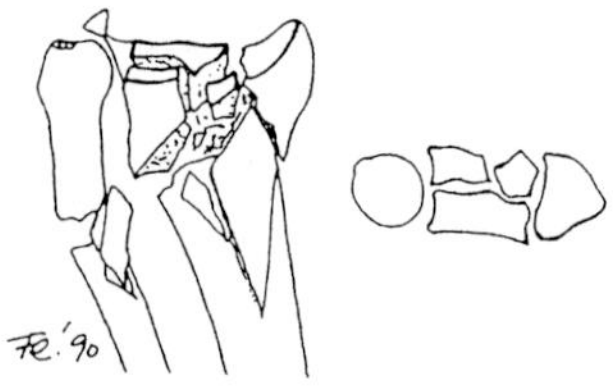	Very rare	Unstable	Dorsal Radial Volar Proximal Combined	Comminuted (frequently intra-articular, open, bone loss, seldom extra-articular)	Always present	Combined method

*High risk of secondary displacement after initial adequate reduction
†Ligaments, carpus, median, ulnar nerve tendons, ipsilateral fractures of upper extremity, compartment syndrome

Fig. 1 The classification of Fernandez of fracture types in adults based on the mechanism of injury. (Reproduced with permission from Fernandez DL: Fractures of the distal radius: Operative treatment, in Heckman JD (ed): *Instructional Course Lectures 42*. Rosemont, IL, American Academy of Orthopaedic Surgeons, 1993, pp 74–75.)

its resting length in full supination. The radioulnar ligaments were found to have material properties similar to those of the radiocarpal ligaments. King and associates[10] demonstrated, in a cadaveric study, that rotation of the radius about the ulna is accompanied by volar translation of the ulna in supination and dorsal translation of the ulna in pronation. Adams[11] has demonstrated that radial deformity alters the kinematics of the DRUJ and distorts the triangular fibrocartilage. Radial shortening, of all radial deformities, had the greatest influence on DRUJ function.

Both stability and mobility are dependent on the design and interaction of the radius with its carpal and ulnar articulations. Fractures of the distal end of the radius that disrupt these articulations can profoundly affect overall wrist and hand function.

Classification

Since Colles'[2] initial description of the fractures involving the distal end of the radius, surgeons have attempted to develop classification systems that provide clarity in defining the morphology of the injury and offer guidelines toward treatment. Saffer[12] has suggested that the various classifications can be placed into broad categories based on (1) the radiographic appearance or the fracture displacement, which would include the Comprehensive Classification of Mueller[13] and those developed by Frykman,[14] Sarmiento and associates,[15] and Lidström;[4] (2) the mechanism of injury, including the classifications of Castaing[1] and Fernandez;[16] (3) articular joint surface involvement, which would include those of Mayo,[17] McMurtry and Jupiter,[18] and Melone;[19] (4) the degree of comminution, represented by the Gartland and Werley,[20] Jenkins,[21] and Older classifications;[22] and (5) bone mineralization, as proposed by Sennwald and Segmueller.[23]

While each classification system may have inherent strengths and weaknesses,

when specifically focusing on intra-articular fractures, it has been our preference to use a classification system developed by Fernandez,[16] which is based on the mechanism of injury. Not only has this system proven to be relatively simple, but it is also particularly helpful in guiding treatment decisions (Fig. 1). The concept of a mechanistic approach is particularly relevant for fractures that involve the articular surfaces, because these often represent more complex wrist injuries, with associated ligamentous lesions, subluxations, fractures of neighboring carpal bones, and soft-tissue injury, injuries that often are directly related to the quality and extent of the causative force. At the same time, it should be emphasized that the Comprehensive Classification of Fractures provides the most detailed description of the multitude of fracture patterns that are most accurately identified by intraoperative visualization rather than radiographic interpretation[13] (Fig. 2).

Among the five major types of fracture patterns within the Fernandez classification, type II includes shearing articular fractures, which have in the past been eponymously referred to as Barton's, reverse Barton's, or Chauffeur's fractures.[24] The basic feature common to all of these is that a portion of the metaphyseal and epiphyseal area of the distal radius is intact and in continuity with the nonaffected area of the joint surface. For this reason, the overall prognosis following surgical reduction and stable fixation is favorable, because the displaced articular fragment(s) can be more exactly reduced and firmly secured to the intact distal bony column of the radius. In addition, more often than not these shearing injuries occur in young adults, whose hard cancellous bone is ideally suited for fixation with plates and screws. In a retrospective study of 49 patients with volar shearing fractures, the vast majority of the fractured bones were observed to be in at least two and, at times, three distinct fragments.[25]

Type III fractures are defined as compression fractures of the articular surface characterized by impaction of both the subchondral and metaphyseal cancellous bone. Melone[19] identified the impaction injury of the end of the radius, observing four basic components to this injury. These are the radial shaft, radial styloid process, posteromedial part of the lunate facet, and palmar medial part of the lunate facet. These compression fractures can involve both the radiocarpal and radioulnar articulations, with the component parts representing important sites of origin of the radiocarpal and radioulnar ligamentous support.

The type IV lesions are avulsion fractures of ligament attachments, which involve radiocarpal fracture-dislocations with associated ulna and radial styloid fractures. Finally, the type V lesions are high velocity injuries that involve combinations of the above lesions, often with associated soft-tissue injuries and bone loss.

One component of intra-articular fractures of the distal end of the radius that has not been the subject of extensive classification is fracture of the DRUJ. As the outcome of this component of the overall injuries depends to the large degree on residual joint stability and/or the development of posttraumatic arthrosis, the classification parameters for these injuries involve the presence of (1) DRUJ subluxation or dislocation of the ulnar head caused by concomitant rupture of the triangular fibrocartilage complex and the capsular ligaments, and (2) the extent of articular surface involvement.

Injury to the DRUJ in association with intra-articular fractures of the distal radius is classified according to the presence or absence of impingement, incongruity, or instability.[26] Impingement occurs at the DRUJ and refers to contact of the distal ulna against the ulnar aspect of the carpus (Fig. 3). When seen in the context of an acute fracture, impingement always relates to the presence of

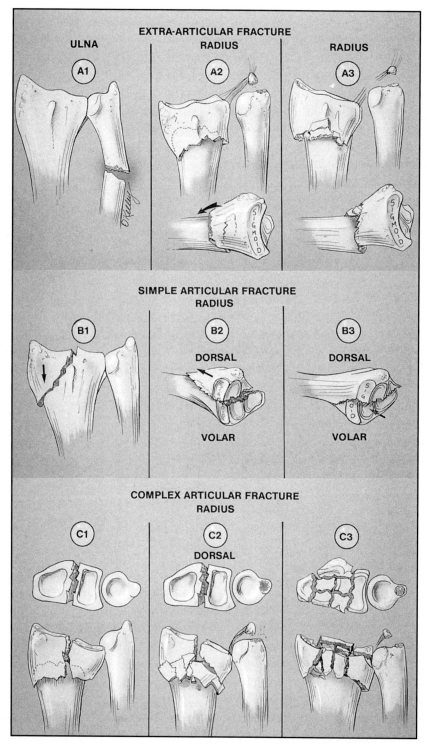

Fig. 2 The Comprehensive Classification of Fractures provides the most detailed description of the numerous extra- and intra-articular fracture patterns. (Reproduced with permission from Mueller ME: *Comprehensive Classification of Fractures: Pamphlet 1*. Berne, Switzerland, ME Mueller Foundation, 1995, pp 1–21.)

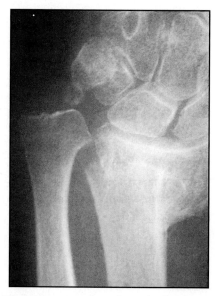

Fig. 3 Anteroposterior radiograph of an intra-articular fracture of the distal radius that has been allowed to unite in a displaced position. There is severe radial shortening, impingement of the distal ulna against the carpus, incongruity of the distal radioulnar joint, and chronic instability, as demonstrated by the radial displacement of the ununited fracture of the ulnar styloid. Reduction of the radius would probably have prevented the development of these chronic distal radioulnar joint problems.

radial shortening. Acute ulnocarpal impingement can be referred to as acute ulnocarpal abutment or acute ulnar impaction. Incongruity refers to fractures that involve either the articular surface of the distal ulna or the sigmoid notch. The resultant articular surface damage can be expected to prevent normal rotational movement of the DRUJ (Fig. 4). Because the forearm functions as an integrated unit, limitation of motion at the DRUJ affects the forearm as a whole. Instability is caused by injury to the DRUJ ligaments and/or the triangular fibrocartilage. Isolated instability of the DRUJ can occur, although the condition is most commonly seen in association with fractures of the distal radius.[27,28] The condition can also occur in association with fractures of the radial head.[29] In its most

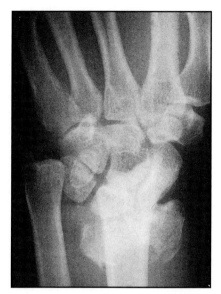

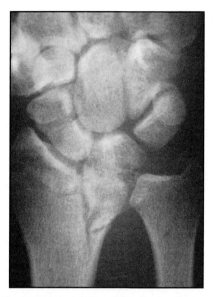

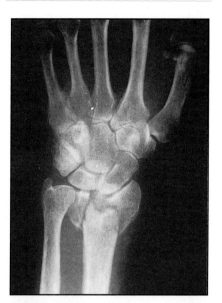

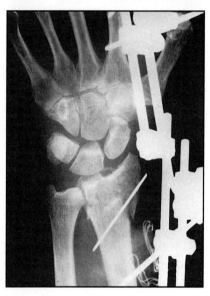

Fig. 4 Anteroposterior radiograph showing a displaced intra-articular fracture of the distal radius with involvement of the sigmoid notch. There is associated depression and dorsiflexion of the articular surface of the scaphoid facet and a fracture of the scaphoid itself.

Fig. 5 Acute instability of the distal radioulnar joint and distal forearm in association with a severely displaced intra-articular fracture of the distal radius. It is likely that there has been injury to the intraosseous membrane with this severity of displacement. The stability of the distal radioulnar joint will have to be critically assessed following reduction of the radius. If a stable position cannot be found or if the joint cannot be stabilized, surgical treatment may be required to address this facet of the injury.

Fig. 6 An anteroposterior radiograph of a three-part articular compression fracture reduced by longitudinal traction using finger traps. Note that the scaphoid is more distal than the lunate and triquetrum suggesting disruption of the scapholunate ligament.

severe form, instability can lead to dissociated movement between the radius and the ulna, affecting the forearm unit as a whole (Fig. 5). Individual patients may have various combinations and permutations of the above disorders.

Radiographic Evaluation
The basic grouping of articular injuries can most often be defined with standard anteroposterior, lateral, and oblique radiographs. The oblique radiograph is particularly helpful in identifying displacement of fractures of the dorsal aspect of the lunate facet. Special imaging studies, such as traction views following reduction, trispiral tomography, or computed tomographic scans, may provide an enhanced picture of the number of articular components as well as the extent of their displacement.

Traction views with standard posteroanterior radiographs may also provide information as to the presence of associated intracapsular carpal ligaments.

Disruption of the smooth parallel lines of the radiocarpal and midcarpal rows would suggest interosseous and/or intracapsular ligament injury[30] (Fig. 6). An additional method that can provide expanded information regarding both the nature of the articular injury and the presence of intracarpal ligament injury is the use of arthroscopic assisted reduction.

Treatment
Shearing Fractures
With shearing fractures that involve the palmar surface of the radius, shortening and palmar displacement of the fracture fragment are associated with volar subluxation of the carpus. A careful assessment of the surrounding soft tissues is important, as elevated intracompartmen-

tal pressures in the forearm or median nerve compression may coexist and mandate a more expeditious surgical intervention. In addition, the surgeon must be aware of the possibility of associated wrist ligamentous injury, in particular with displaced radial styloid involvement.

For displaced shearing fractures that

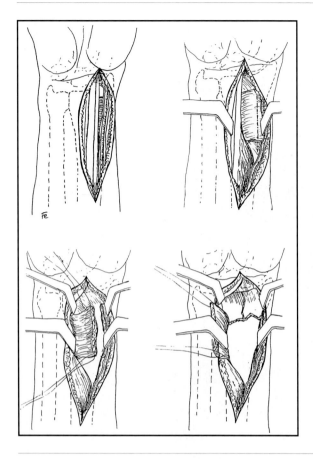

Fig. 7 A volar shearing of the distal radius requires surgical treatment. In most instances, surgical exposure can be obtained through an interval between the flexor carpi radialis tendon and radial artery. (Reproduced with permission from Jupiter JB, Fernandez DL (eds): *Management of Distal Radius Fractures.* New York, NY, Springer-Verlag, 1996, pp 76-77.)

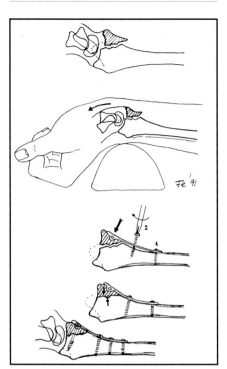

Fig. 8 Surgical reduction of volar shearing of the distal radius is facilitated by hyperextending the wrist over a rolled towel, with the forearm supinated. (Reproduced with permission from Fernandez DL: Fractures of the distal radius: Operative treatment, in Heckman JD (ed): *Instructional Course Lectures 42.* Rosemont, IL, American Academy of Orthopaedic Surgeons, 1993, pp 73–88.)

involve primarily the radial styloid (Comprehensive Classification type B1), the goals are not just to restore the articular congruence but also to realign the support for the volar capsular ligaments of the wrist. Displaced fractures may be manipulated through longitudinal traction, wrist extension, and ulnar deviation. However, these fractures are inherently unstable and require internal fixation. When using percutaneous pin or screw fixation, it is important to recognize that the radial styloid lies anterior to the mid-axis of the radius and is surrounded by a number of branches of the radial sensory nerve. Percutaneously placed wires or screws should be introduced through a drill guide and directed in a proximal, ulnarward, and dorsal direction to gain purchase in the dorsoulnar cortex of the radius.

If anatomic reduction cannot be achieved by manipulative methods, open reduction and internal fixation is recommended. Styloid fractures that involve a single fragment can be approached through a dorsoradial incision, with particular care taken to identify and protect the radial sensory nerve branches. By the same token, the surgeon should not be surprised to find the fragment in more than one piece, in which case a dorsal capsulotomy may be necessary in order to make certain that there is no impaction or rotation of any of the fragments and that the articular surfaces are realigned anatomically. In addition, this procedure will provide an opportunity to inspect the intracapsular ligaments directly.

With larger volar shearing fragments, the fractures can be exposed surgically through an interval between the flexor carpi radialis tendon and the radial artery, with detachment of the pronator quadratus from its insertion onto the radius. In the event that an associated acute median nerve compression exists, the transverse carpal ligament can be released through a separate small incision on the ulnar aspect of the palm rather than risk injury to branches of the palmar cutaneous nerve of the median nerve by extending the initial volar incision across the palmar flexion crease of the wrist (Fig. 7).

When the fracture does not involve comminution of the articular surface, the reduction can be controlled by realigning the fracture lines that extend onto the metaphysis of the volar surface of the radius. The reduction is facilitated by hyperextending the wrist over a rolled towel with the forearm in maximum supination (Fig. 8). It is imperative not to open the volar wrist capsule to visualize the articular surface, because to do so can lead to injury of the volar radiocarpal ligaments, with resultant postoperative intercarpal instability. Definitive fixation is most effectively achieved with a buttress type plate and screws (Fig. 9).

Compression Fractures

The goals of treatment of compression fractures of the articular surface involve not only the relocation of the displaced articular fragments but also restoration of the anatomic relationship of the end of the radius with the proximal carpal row and distal ulna. These goals can be more easily achieved by recognizing that many of these injuries involve distinct components that include the radial styloid and shaft and the lunate facet at the articular end of the distal radius.

Compression fractures of the end of the radius may prove to be the fracture type most amenable to arthroscopic-assisted reduction and internal fixation. The technique offers the combined advantages of joint cleansing, more accurate articular reduction, limiting the trauma from extensive surgical exposure, and rapid postoperative mobilization. It is important, however, to point out that, even in the hands of experienced surgeons, the technique is time consuming and requires a full array of arthroscopic equipment.

The optimal time to consider arthroscopic-assisted reduction is between 2 and 4 days post injury, in part to avoid excessive bleeding or thick fibrin precipitate. The technique is facilitated by mounting the wrist in a traction tower using 15 to 18 lb of finger trap traction on the index and long fingers. With the arthroscope introduced into the 3-4 portal, the joint is lavaged in order to remove clots, small fragments of cartilage debris, and small loose bony fragments via outflow through either the fifth or 1-2 portals.

Under arthroscopic guidance, the major fracture fragments can be disimpacted and, using a Kirschner wire drilled into the mid portion of each fragment parallel to the articular surface, the frac-

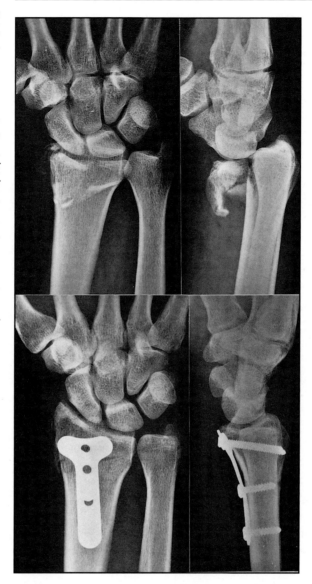

Fig. 9 Definitive fixation of the fracture shown in Figures 7 and 8 is effectively obtained by a volarly placed buttress plate. (Reproduced ith permission from Fernandez DL: Fractures of the distal radius: Operative treatment, in Heckman JD (ed): *Instructional Course Lectures 42*. Rosemont, IL, American Academy of Orthopaedic Surgeons, 1993, pp 73–88.)

ture reduction can be achieved by manipulating the fragments with these pins. A tenaculum clamp can be applied through external puncture wounds to aid in compression of the fragments. Under arthroscopic guidance, the articular fracture lines are aligned, and the pins are then advanced across the fracture lines into adjacent subchondral metaphyseal bone (Fig. 10).

Additional internal fixation, which may be required to maintain the normal palmar tilt, includes such techniques as a pin directed into the radial styloid and extending proximally into the radial meta-

physis, an external fixation frame to help prevent metaphyseal collapse, or a volar buttress plate in volar displaced fractures with metaphyseal comminution.

The pins are bent and cut short just external to the skin. Plaster splints are used, with digital mobility encouraged. After the first postoperative week, the splints can be removed on a daily basis for wrist mobility if stable fixation has been achieved. The hand and wrist should be supported, however, for approximately 5 to 6 weeks, at which time the fracture should be united. The pins should be left in place an additional 1 to 2 weeks.

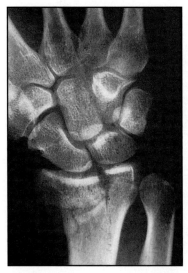 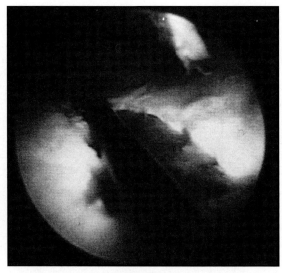 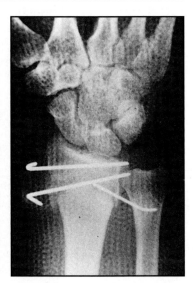

Fig. 10 A 26-year-old carpenter fell from a roof, sustaining an intra-articular fracture of his dominant distal radius. **Left,** the articular injury seen on the anteroposterior radiograph. **Center,** an arthroscopic view demonstrates the probe in a major articular displacement. **Right,** the postoperative anteroposterior radiograph shows restoration of the articular surface using three 0.045-inch smooth Kirschner wires.

Alternatively, the use of image intensification has been shown to be reasonably accurate in controlling manipulative or limited open reduction of compression type fractures. Those fractures without comminution of the underlying metaphyseal bone are often successfully reduced, either with longitudinal traction alone or with percutaneous fracture manipulation and pinning of the fracture fragments.

When one of the components of the fracture involves the displaced radial styloid, the fracture can be reduced using longitudinal traction and ulnar deviation and pronation of the hand and wrist. The styloid component can then be secured to the radial shaft using a smooth 0.045- or 0.062-in Kirschner wire directed obliquely into the radius in a more proximal and ulnar direction.

An associated lunate facet fragment may be reduced by combining longitudinal traction with radial deviation of the hand and wrist. If this proves successful, a 0.062-in smooth Kirschner wire that is directed transversely from the radial styloid and aimed directly towards the sigmoid notch. The wire is directed to lie just beneath the subchondral bone to, in effect, buttress the reduced lunate facet fragment. Oblique images or radiographs are necessary to confirm the fact that the wire has not penetrated the sigmoid notch lying in the DRUJ.

In the event that a satisfactory reduction of the "die-punch" fragment cannot be achieved by closed manipulative techniques, the fragment may be manipulated into position using a pointed awl or small elevator placed through a small (1 to 2 cm) incision. The position of the awl as well as the fracture reduction should be confirmed under image intensification. When the impacted fragment is elevated, it is useful to place a small amount of autogenous bone graft into the defect within the metaphyseal bone. The use of trephine biopsy needles will minimize the morbidity of obtaining such graft from the iliac crest.

The articular fracture morphology of these compression fractures, as defined by Melone,[19] may also involve a sagittal split of the two major fragments. In these instances, interfragmentary compression of the two fracture fragments can be achieved using a large pointed reduction clamp. One point of the clamp is placed through a dorsomedial incision into the lunate facet; the other point percutaneously grasps the radial styloid. The fragments are gently compressed together, followed by the placement of one or two transverse smooth Kirschner wires.

The fracture reduction of these two- and three-part compression fractures can be supported in above-elbow plaster for approximately 3 weeks followed by a short-arm plaster for an additional 3 weeks. When these fractures are associated with concomitant soft-tissue swelling or impaction of the articular fracture fragments, elevation and bone grafting are required. As a general rule, we prefer to apply an external skeletal fixation frame rather than plaster. This frame is especially useful when the metaphyseal support of the fracture fragment is further compromised by impaction or comminution.

When the articular fracture pattern involves a split of the lunate facet in a coronal plane, characteristic of the four-part Melone type fracture, a reduction by either manipulation alone or percutaneous manipulation with a pin or elevator will prove less successful in realigning the volarly displaced component. This difficulty occurs because the volarly displaced part of the "medial complex," as described by Melone, tends to rotate as longitudinal traction is applied. In such cases, surgical reduction through an anterior approach is necessary. A small buttress or small Kirschner wires will be necessary to support this component of the compression fracture. It is preferable, however, to reduce and support, with pins, the radial styloid component first, because this then provides a template on which the anteriorly displaced lunate facet fragment can be anatomically restored.

As a final component of the four-part fracture, the dorsal lunate facet fragment must also be anatomically repositioned. Unless this entire "medial complex" can be restored to within 1 to 2 mm of anatomic repositioning, DRUJ function cannot be assured. The dorsal component can often be remanipulated successfully through a small dorsal incision, using a pointed awl or small elevator, and pinned in place. The four-part fracture fixed with a combination of pins and/or buttress plate will require an external fixation frame for a minimum of 6 weeks in order to prevent collapse of the articular components. The Kirschner wires themselves are best left in an additional 2 weeks. Because of the association of metaphyseal impaction with a subchondral defect in many of these compression-type fractures, the placement of autogenous bone graft will not only facilitate union but will also limit the possibility of collapse of the articular restoration after removal of the fixation devices (Fig. 11).

Complications that can accompany these intra-articular fractures include loss of fixation, inadequate reduction, loss of wrist or forearm mobility, and problems related to overlying tendons or nerves. Residual articular incongruence, carpal instability, and posttraumatic arthrosis are

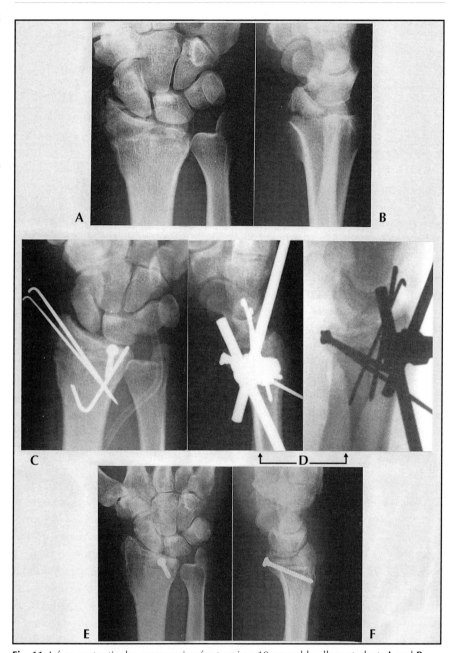

Fig. 11 A four-part articular compression fracture in a 19-year-old college student. **A** and **B,** the anteroposterior and lateral radiograph of the fracture. **C,** following manipulative reduction and percutaneous pinning of the radial styloid, the displaced volar lunate facet fragment is surgically reduced and fixed with a screw. **D,** additional pins and an external fixation device are applied. **E** and **F,** anteroposterior and lateral radiographs 12 weeks posttreatment.

among the more problematic late complications.

Distal Radioulnar Joint Disorders

The initial treatment should focus on reduction of the radius as described above. After satisfactory restoration of radial length, tilt, inclination, and articular congruity, imaging should be performed. Intraoperatively this is most easily accomplished using an image intensifier. The wrist should be imaged in the anteroposterior, oblique, and lateral planes to be certain that the relationship at the DRUJ is anatomic. DRUJ stability is assessed by ballottement of the distal ulna relative to the distal radius. Several possible scenarios exist following reduction of the radius, each of which demands a different course of action. They are as follows:[31]

DRUJ Reduced and Stable This is the most common situation. In this situation no specific treatment is required. The forearm is immobilized as dictated by the treatment method selected for management of the distal radial fracture. The wrist and forearm are mobilized according to the treatment method selected for management of the distal radial fracture. Radiographs are taken on a regular basis until fracture union occurs, and the DRUJ is reassessed clinically and radiographically at each clinic visit.

DRUJ Reducible but Unstable In this situation, it is usually possible to find a point of forearm rotation where the DRUJ is stable. Usually this position is full supination. If this is the case, the forearm is splinted in full supination and splintage is continued with a thermoplastic splint after the postoperative dressing is removed. Supination splinting is maintained for 4 weeks after the injury, after which mobilization of the forearm to neutral rotation is allowed. Six weeks after injury, full rotation is allowed, although supination splinting at night is continued until 3 months after injury.

If no stable position can be found, the DRUJ is stabilized with a radioulnar pin. The radioulnar pin is passed just proximal to the radioulnar joint and is left in place for 3 weeks. The author (JJ) uses a 2-mm pin and leaves the pin long so that it can easily be removed in the clinic. Alternatively, a "diastasis" screw can be used, using neutralization technique, a method similar to that used in the ankle. The advantage of the "diastasis" screw is that it provides more stable fixation than

can be achieved with a smooth pin. On the other hand, a screw is more difficult to remove a few weeks later.

DRUJ Not Reducible This is an uncommon scenario. The usual cause of an irreducible DRUJ is either malreduction of the radius or soft-tissue interposition within the joint. Assuming the reduction of the radius is acceptable, open reduction of the DRUJ is required.

Exposure of the Distal Radioulnar Joint

The patient is positioned supine on the operating table. The hand is placed on a hand table and the tourniquet inflated following exsanguination of the limb. A dorsal incision is made beginning 3 cm distal to the ulnar styloid. The incision is carried proximally at 45° to the long axis of the arm in a radial direction until it meets the dorsal aspect of the distal radius at its junction with the sigmoid notch. At this point the incision angles sharply (90°) towards the ulna, and as it reaches the ulnar border of the forearm it is angled sharply (45°) in a proximal direction.

The subcutaneous tissues are spread, with care taken to preserve the dorsal sensory branch of the ulnar nerve. The dorsal sensory branch of the ulnar nerve passes onto the dorsum of the hand about 1 to 2 cm distal to the ulnar styloid and branches in the same area. When dissecting the subcutaneous tissues, it is important to avoid injury to this sensory nerve because, if transection does occur, it will leave the patient with a painful neuroma. After the skin flaps have been raised, the subcutaneous tissues are elevated from the extensor retinaculum. The key to identifying the important soft-tissue structures is the extensor digiti minimi (EDM) tendon.

The supratendinous extensor retinaculum is elevated from the dorsum of the DRUJ. The retinaculum is elevated by first creating a transverse incision at the junction of the retinaculum proximally,

with the fascia over the extensor aspect of the forearm. This transverse incision is made at the proximal border of the DRUJ over the fourth extensor compartment. The transverse incision extends to the supratendinous portion of the extensor carpi ulnaris (ECU). The incision then runs longitudinally to a point just short of the distal extent of the retinaculum. It is best to preserve a small portion of the distal retinaculum to prevent bowstringing of the extensor tendons. The distal transverse limb lies just proximal to the distal border of the extensor retinaculum. As the extensor retinaculum is elevated, the tendon of the EDM is visualized. An umbilical tape is placed around this tendon and it is retracted in a radial direction.

Exposure of the DRUJ is completed by making a dorsal capsulotomy. The limbs of the dorsal capsulotomy are similar to those created in the extensor retinaculum. The base of the dorsal capsulotomy lies along the ECU tendon. The transverse limbs of the capsular flap lie along the proximal margin of the DRUJ and the dorsal surface of the triangular fibrocartilage respectively. A vertical incision is used to create the capsular flap that lies over the dorsum of the sigmoid notch, leaving a small cuff of dorsal DRUJ capsule to repair at the conclusion of the procedure.

Indications for Osseous Fixation

Displaced intra-articular fractures that involve the DRUJ require fixation. Such fractures can involve either the dorsal or volar lips of the sigmoid notch, the articular or periarticular distal ulna, or the ulnar styloid (Fig. 12). Isolated fractures of the ulnar styloid do not require internal fixation. Displaced fractures of the ulnar styloid that involve the base of the styloid should be fixed, because they are commonly associated with ulnar instability. Similarly, isolated fractures of the ulnar styloid should be fixed if there is associated translation of the carpus in relation to the distal radius. This instability pattern is often associated with a coexistent fracture of the radial styloid.

Methods of Osseous Fixation

Smooth pin fixation can be used to treat most periarticular fractures of the DRUJ (Fig. 12). Fractures of the dorsal or volar lips of the sigmoid notch can sometimes be buttressed with a volar or dorsal plate. Larger fragments can be fixed with lag screws. Tension band wires or sutures can be used to fix displaced fractures of the ulnar styloid. Juxta-articular fractures of the distal ulna can sometimes be fixed with plates. Internal fixation, particularly with pins, should avoid fixation of the periarticular tendons. Intraoperative planning should be precise in this regard in order to avoid impairing the postoperative rehabilitation program.

Soft-Tissue Repair

Careful closure of the soft tissues following open reduction of the DRUJ is required to restore stability to the joint and to prevent the development of iatrogenic instability. The dorsal capsule is repaired with interrupted horizontal mattress sutures of 3-0 braided polyester suture on a tapered needle. It is usually possible to place three or four sutures. It is important to supinate the forearm when tying these sutures and to maintain the forearm in supination as closure proceeds. Supination approximates the dorsal soft-tissue structures and allows them to be repaired in a shortened position. Forceful pronation of the forearm prior to healing of the soft tissues can disrupt their repair. The repair of the dorsal capsule is reinforced with the flap of extensor retinaculum created during exposure of the joint. The flap of extensor retinaculum is passed beneath the EDM.

Aftercare

Supination splinting is the mainstay of postoperative management. The vast majority of patients with DRUJ instability have dorsal instability, which is evident on provocative testing. In the operating room, the wrist and forearm are placed in a padded dressing with the forearm in full supination and the elbow at 90°. This position is maintained over the first 10 to 14 days until the patient returns for suture removal and check radiographs. Following removal of the sutures, a thermoplastic splint is constructed. The splint holds the elbow at 90° and the forearm in full supination. Velcro straps are used to maintain the position of the forearm. The forearm is kept in full supination for 4 weeks. During this time the splint can be removed for bathing.

After 4 weeks, the splint is removed for short periods of time. Night splinting is maintained and the patient wears the splint when outside the home. At 4 weeks, a program of active forearm rotation is begun. Passive assisted motion is begun 6 weeks following surgery. Night splinting is maintained for 3 months. The object of the rehabilitation program is

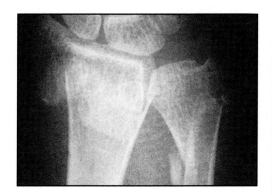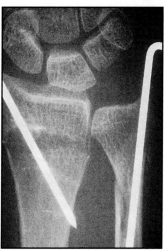

Fig. 12 Left, Anteroposterior radiograph of a displaced intra-articular fracture of the distal radius in association with a comminuted, displaced fracture of the base of the ulna. **Right,** Result following application of an external skeletal fixator and pinning of both the radial and the ulnar fractures with 2-mm pins. An excellent reduction and good fixation has been achieved. The pins were removed 6 weeks postinjury. Distal radioulnar joint function was preserved by the integrated treatment of the distal radioulnar joint injury with that of the distal radius.

progressive recovery of the range of forearm rotation while maintaining the strength of the dorsal capsular repair. During the splinting program, active finger and thumb motion is encouraged. Resistive exercises are avoided until a near-normal range of active motion is recovered. The program of rehabilitation is discontinued when the patient's progress plateaus.

Inadequate treatment of injuries of the DRUJ in association with intra-articular fractures of the distal radius can compromise treatment outcome. DRUJ instability, painful impingement, and joint incongruity can occur, either in isolation or together, leading to substantial limitation of wrist and forearm function, and compromising the function of the upper extremity as a whole. Careful clinical and radiographic assessment and the integration of treatment of the DRUJ with the treatment of the radial fracture can lead to a satisfactory outcome in these difficult injuries.

References

1. Castaing J: Les fractures récentes de l'extrémité inférieure du radius chez l'adulte. *Rev Chir Orthop* 1964;50:581–696.

2. Colles A: On fractures of the carpal extremity. *Edinburgh Med Surg J* 1814;10:182–186.

3. Jupiter JB: Fractures of the distal end of the radius. *J Bone Joint Surg* 1991;73A:461–469.

4. Lidström A: Fractures of the distal end of the radius: A clinical and statistical study of end results. *Acta Orthop Scand* 1959;41(suppl):1–118.

5. Fernandez DL, Jupiter JB (eds): Epidemiology, mechanism, classification, in *Fractures of the Distal Radius: A Practical Approach to Management*. New York, NY, Springer-Verlag, 1996, pp 23–52.

6. Mori K: Experimental study on rotation of the forearm: Functional anatomy of the interosseous membrane. *Nippon Seikeigeka Gakkai Zasshi* 1985;59:611–622.

7. Morrey BF, Askew LJ, An KN, et al: A biomechanical study of normal functional elbow motion. *J Bone Joint Surg* 1981;63A:872–877.

8. Adams BD, Holley KA: Strains in the articular disk of the triangular fibrocartilage complex: A biomechanical study. *J Hand Surg* 1993;18A:919–925.

9. Schuind F, An K-N, Berglund L, et al: The distal radioulnar ligaments: A biomechanical study. *J Hand Surg* 1991;16A:1106–1114.

10. King GJ, McMurtry RY, Rubenstein JD, et al: Kinematics of the distal radioulnar joint. *J Hand Surg* 1986;11A:798–804.

11. Adams BD: Effects of radial deformity on distal radioulnar joint mechanics. *J Hand Surg* 1993;18A:492–498.

12. Saffer P: Current trends in treatment and classification of distal radius fractures, in Saffer P, Cooney WP (eds): *Fractures of the Distal Radius*. London, England, Martin Dunitz, 1995, pp 12–18.

13. Mueller ME: Comprehensive Classification of Fractures: Pamphlet 1. Berne, Switzerland, ME Mueller Foundation, 1995, pp 1–21.

14. Frykman G: Fracture of the distal radius including sequelae: Shoulder-hand-finger syndrome, disturbance in the distal radio-ulnar joint and impairment of nerve function: A clinical and experimental study. *Acta Orthop Scand* 1967;108(suppl):3–153.

15. Sarmiento A, Pratt G, Berry N, et al: Colles' fracture: Functional bracing in supination. *J Bone Joint Surg* 1962;44A:337–351.

16. Fernandez DL: Fractures of the distal radius: Operative treatment, in Heckman JD (ed): *Instructional Course Lectures 42*. Rosemont, IL, American Academy of Orthopaedic Surgeons, 1993, pp 73–88.

17. Cooney WP: Fractures of the distal radius: A modern treatment-based classification. *Orthop Clin North Am* 1993;24:211–216.

18. McMurtry RY, Jupiter JB: Fractures of the distal radius, in Browner BD, Jupiter JB, Levine AM, et al (eds): *Skeletal Trauma: Fractures, Dislocations, Ligamentous Injuries*. Philadelphia, PA, WB Saunders, 1992, vol 2, pp 1063–1094.

19. Melone CP Jr: Distal radius fractures: Patterns of articular fragmentation. *Orthop Clin North Am* 1993;24:239–253.

20. Gartland JJ Jr, Werley CW: Evaluation of healed Colles' fractures. *J Bone Joint Surg* 1951;33A:895–907.

21. Jenkins NH: The unstable Colles' fracture. *J Hand Surg* 1989;14B:149–154.

22. Older TM, Stabler EV, Cassebaum WH: Colles fracture: Evaluation and selection of therapy. *J Trauma* 1965;5:469–476.

23. Sennwald G (ed): Fractures of the distal radius, in *The Wrist: Anatomical and Pathophysiological Approach to Diagnosis and Treatment*. Berlin, Germany, Springer-Verlag, 1987, pp 115–154.

24. Barton JR: Views and treatment of an important injury of the wrist. *Med Examiner* 1838;1:365–368.

25. Jupiter JB, Fernandez DL, Toh CL, et al: The operative treatment of volar intra-articular fractures of the distal end of the radius. *J Bone Joint Surg* 1996;78A:1817–1828.

26. Richards RR (ed): Disorders of the distal radioulnar joint, in *Soft Tissue Reconstruction in the Upper Extremity*. New York, NY, Churchill Livingstone, 1995, pp 207–222.

27. Mikic ZD: Galeazzi fracture-dislocations. *J Bone Joint Surg* 1975;57A:1071–1080.

28. Strehle J, Gerber C: Distal radioulnar joint function after Galeazzi fracture-dislocations treated by open reduction and internal plate fixation. *Clin Orthop* 1993;283:240–245.

29. Essex-Lopresti PA: Fractures of the radial head with distal radio-ulnar dislocation: Report of two cases. *J Bone Joint Surg* 1951;33B:244–247.

30. Gilula LA (ed): *The Traumatized Hand and Wrist: Radiographic and Anatomic Correlation*. Philadelphia, PA, WB Saunders, 1992.

31. Richards RR: Chronic disorders of the forearm. *J Bone Joint Surg* 1996;78A:916–930.

Wrist Instability

Walter H. Short, MD

Introduction

Carpal instability is a complicated problem that arises when there is a disturbance in the normal kinematics of the wrist. Because of the number of carpal bones and the variety of ligamentous structures that support the wrist, there is a great diversity in the types of instability patterns in the wrist. In an attempt to understand this intricate issue, many researchers have tried to organize the problem and develop classification schemes. There are several advantages to a standardized scheme for problems related to instability patterns about the wrist. The treatment and underlying cause of the problem could be more easily decided, and studies could be performed to determine the most appropriate treatment. If the classification scheme is thorough, the physician will ultimately be able to make a more accurate diagnosis and to prescribe the most effective therapy.

One of the first attempts to classify carpal instability was by Linscheid and associates[1] in their classic article on traumatic instabilities of the wrist. In this study, the basic concepts of intercalated segment instability were introduced. Based on their review, many of the patients with carpal instability could be divided either into those who had a dorsal intercalated segment instability (DISI) or those who had a volar intercalated segment instability (VISI) pattern. When the angle between the scaphoid and lunate is increased and the lunate is dorsiflexed, the instability pattern is termed DISI. When the angle between the scaphoid and lunate is decreased and the lunate is volarflexed, the pattern is termed VISI.

Dobyns and Linscheid later introduced the two terms carpal instability dissociative (CID) and carpal instability nondissociative (CIND).[2] This classification refers to whether an intrinsic or extrinsic wrist ligament is damaged. Other terms that are employed as part of this classification scheme are carpal instability complex (CIC) and carpal instability adaptive (CIA).

Most recently, a comprehensive classification scheme was developed that seeks to include all types of carpal instability.[3,4] The purpose of the scheme is to categorize all types of wrist instability. In this classification, wrist instability is divided into six categories: chronicity, constancy, etiology, location, direction, and pattern (Table 1).

Chronicity, which refers to the length of time from the beginning of the symptoms to the initiation of treatment, allows the physician to give an estimate of the potential for primary healing. It was the opinion of the authors that injuries treated less than 1 week from the time of injury offered the best opportunity for successful healing. Chronic injuries (those more than 6 weeks old) had less potential for primary healing.

Constancy refers to whether the instability is static or dynamic. Static deformities can be seen on routine radiographs; dynamic instabilities require stress views or fluoroscopy to detect any pathologic change in the position of the carpal bones.

The etiology of the wrist instability is the third category of this classification scheme. Instability can be congenital, traumatic, inflammatory, arthritic, neoplastic, iatrogenic, miscellaneous, or a combination thereof.

The segment of the classification that describes the location of the instability refers to which carpal bone or area of the wrist is involved in the pathology. Location includes specific bones and ligaments as well as the radiocarpal, intercarpal, midcarpal, and carpometacarpal regions.

Direction of the instability is also considered in this scheme. Direction refers to the change in position of the carpus relative to the radius. The terms DISI and VISI would be included in this category. DISI refers to abnormal dorsiflexion of the lunate or proximal carpal row relative to the scaphoid or radius. VISI refers to abnormal volarflexion of the lunate or proximal carpal row relative to the scaphoid or radius. Other deformities include translational changes that shift the carpus in a dorsal, volar, radial or ulnar direction. Also included in direction is rotatory subluxation of the scaphoid, as well as combinations of two or more translational instabilities.

The final category refers to the pattern of the instability. Dobyns was the first to popularize these injury patterns. They are CID, CIND, CIC, and CIA. CID (carpal

Table 1
Analysis of carpal instability

Category I Chronicity	Category II Constancy*	Category III Etiology	Category IV Location	Category V Direction	Category VI Pattern
Acute < 1 week (ie, maximum primary healing potential)	Static†	Congenital	Radiocarpal	VISI	Carpal instability dissociative (CID)
Subacute 1 to 6 weeks (ie, some primary healing potential)	Dynamic‡	Traumatic	Intercarpal	DISI	Carpal instability nondissociative (CIND)
Chronic > 6 weeks (ie, little primary healing potential; surgical repair or reconstruction needed)		Inflammatory	Midcarpal	Ulnar	Combinations (CIC)§
		Arthritis	Carpometacarpal	Radial	Carpal instability adaptive (CIA)‖
		Neoplastic Iatrogenic	Specific bone(s) Specific ligament(s)	Ventral Dorsal	
		Miscellaneous		Proximal	
		Combinations		Distal	
				Rotary	
				Combinations	

* This category also includes the concept of severity.

† Irreducible or reducible, ease of reducibility and degree of displacement may also be considered.

‡ Degree of load required to cause displacement may also be considered.

§ CIC. Combination of CID and CIND. Example: perilunate and axial injuries include both capsular (CIND) and intercarpal (CID) components.

‖ CIA, apparent carpal instability; a carpal instability pattern that exists because the carpal bones have adapted to an extended deformity (eg, a distal radius malunion).

VISI, volar flexion intercalated segment instability (palmar flexion instability); DISI, dorsiflexion intercalated segment instability. (Reproduced with permission from Larsen CF, Amadio PC, Gilula LA, et al: Analysis of carpal instability: I. Description of the scheme. *J Hand Surg* 1995;20A:757–764.)

instability dissociative) refers to instability between two carpal bones in the same row. Usually this indicates that an intrinsic ligament such as the scapholunate interosseous ligament (SLIL) is injured. CIND (carpal instability nondissociative) refers to instability between the carpal rows. Midcarpal instability may be an example of this. Many researchers have suggested that CIND implies that an extrinsic ligament is deficient. An extrinsic ligament connects the radius to the proximal carpal row or the proximal to the distal carpal row. CIC (carpal instability complex) is a combination of both CID and CIND. A perilunate dislocation is an example of this instability. CIA (carpal instability adaptive) occurs as a result of an adjustment of the carpus to some other malalignment. Examples of CIA include midcarpal instability caused by a malunion of the distal radius and ulnocarpal abutment.

This classification scheme makes it possible to separate all instabilities into unique categories and to determine the underlying pathology. The biggest advantage of this classification model is that a rational treatment protocol can be devised based on the pathology and on the experience of others who have treated the same lesion.

Midcarpal Instability

Midcarpal instability (MCI) is probably the least understood of the carpal insta-

bility patterns. It was initially reported in the literature in 1934 by Mouchet and Belot.[5] In 1981, Lichtman and asociates[6] reported on a series of ten patients who had a painful click on ulnar deviation of the wrist. It was revealed that there was instability between the proximal and distal carpal rows. Subsequently, many articles have further described and tried to explain this difficult and confusing topic.

The patient with the suspected diagnosis of midcarpal instability usually complains of a painful clunk when the wrist is used. In their series, Wright and associates[2] stated that 91% of their patients had this as their presenting symptom. Patients frequently cannot give a history of one traumatic event. Most state that they have loaded their wrist in a repetitive way either through work or sporting activities. If the history of an injury is elicited, it is usually a fall on an outstretched hand. Many of these patients give a history of being lax jointed. Physical examination of these patients can also be somewhat nonspecific. Most patients have a full range of motion of the wrist and a painful clunk that is associated with radial and ulnar deviation. In some patients there is a fullness in the ulnar aspect of the wrist associated with the synovitis that can occur in the midcarpal joint. The most important part of the physical examination involves a provocative maneuver[6] that tries to reproduce the clunk that the patient experiences. In this test, the patient assumes a grip position and is then asked to move the wrist in the plane of radial to ulnar deviation. In the normal patient, when the wrist moves from radial deviation to ulnar deviation there is a smooth, synchronous motion of the carpus. In patients with midcarpal instability, the proximal carpal row remains flexed until extreme ulnar deviation, at which time the proximal row snaps into its normal position. This spontaneous motion is accompanied by an audible or palpable clunk. Thus, in neutral or radial deviation the wrist is subluxed in VISI, and the clunk represents the spontaneous reduction of the proximal/distal row subluxation in ulnar deviation.

In another provocative maneuver,[2,7] the examiner stabilizes the forearm with one hand and applies a palmar-directed force to the wrist. In MCI, this action produces a VISI deformity of the proximal carpal row. The examiner then applies a dorsally directed force to the carpus. If the test is positive, there is a subluxation of the capitate from lunate or an exaggerated DISI deformity of the proximal carpal row.

The differential diagnosis of midcarpal instability includes any condition that produces a painful click in the wrist or pain on the ulnar side of the wrist. Many conditions on the ulnar side of the wrist can produce painful symptoms. These include tears of the triangular fibrocartilage complex (TFCC), lunotriquetral ligament (LTL) tears, ulnocarpal abutment syndrome, instability of the distal radioulnar joint, subluxation of the extensor carpi ulnaris tendon, and instability or degenerative changes of the pisiform. Some of these conditions can be seen in association with MCI.

After completing the physical examination, several diagnostic studies can be considered to further evaluate the problem. Plain radiographs may be normal. In many centers, wrist motion studies are available. Some patients with midcarpal instability may have a VISI deformity of the proximal carpal row on the lateral radiograph. Arthrograms are also usually normal. An arthrogram is sensitive to intrinsic ligament perforations. Thus, such abnormalities as injuries to the SLIL, LTL, and TFCC are usually diagnosed by this test. However, MCI does not usually involve a deficiency of these intrinsic ligaments. The pathology in this instability pattern usually involves the extrinsic ligaments of the wrist that connect one carpal row to the next or the radius or ulna to the carpus. Therefore, a

normal arthrogram does not rule out the diagnosis of MCI.

Bone scans are used with some frequency in the evaluation of wrist pain. In the case of MCI, the bone scan is not usually diagnostic. In some cases, there may be a generalized or nonspecific increased intake in the carpus. Computed tomography (CT) scans are also being used with increasing frequency in the evaluation of wrist problems. Although they can give very important information about the wrist, they are generally not very helpful to the clinician in trying to make the diagnosis of MCI. In the future, when real time CT scanning is developed, I am sure that this modality will play a bigger role in the diagnosis of this problem.

Magnetic resonance imaging (MRI) is sensitive to both soft-tissue and bone problems. Unfortunately, the ligamentous structures that contribute to the problem are small and may be incompletely imaged. In the future, as physicians gain more experience in the interpretation of this problem and dedicated wrist coils are refined, MRI will play a bigger role in the diagnostic work-up of this problem.

Fluoroscopy[8-10] is the most helpful study in making the diagnosis of midcarpal instability. By continually observing the wrist fluoroscopically, the orthopaedist is able to document the sudden shifts in carpal bone position seen during the provocative maneuvers. As the wrist is moved from radial to ulnar deviation there is normally a smooth transition as the proximal carpal row gradually moves from flexion to extension. In MCI, the proximal carpal row is in a flexed or VISI position when the wrist is in radial deviation. Instead of the smooth transition from flexion to extension of the proximal carpal row, these carpal bones remain flexed as the wrist moves into ulnar deviation. There is a sudden "catch up clunk" in ulnar deviation and the proximal carpal row suddenly dorsi-

flexes and reduces. This clunk is associated with pain and either an audible or palpable snap in the wrist. When the wrist is moved from ulnar to radial deviation, this movement is much less dramatic.

Fluoroscopy can also document the changes seen during stress testing of the wrist. When the wrist is held in the lateral projection, fluoroscopy can show the VISI of the proximal carpal row when a palmar force is applied to the wrist. When a dorsally directed force is applied to the wrist, fluoroscopy is able to detect the subluxation of the capitolunate joint and the DISI deformity that accompanies it. The term radiocapitate subluxation index, introduced by Dobyns,[2] is the distance that the capitate subluxes dorsally or palmarly from the longitudinal axis of the radius, divided by the length of the capitate. Normally this ratio averages 0.09; in patients who have midcarpal CIND this ratio is 0.25. It is recommended that the treating physician be at the examination both to stress the patient's wrist and to observe the abnormalities visible fluoroscopically.

The etiology of midcarpal instability is not completely understood. Both Lichtman and associates[6] and Wright and associates,[2] in their respective articles, have suggested multiple causative agents. Lichtman and associates[11] have developed a classification of MCI based on the suspected source of the pathology and the direction of maximum instability of the midcarpal joint. The classification is divided into palmar MCI, dorsal MCI, midcarpal CIND, and extrinsic MCI.

Palmar MCI was first investigated by Lichtman and associates,[6] who studied ten patients and did anatomic and biomechanical evaluations of 23 cadaver specimens. In the anatomic portion of this study, it was found that sectioning the volar arcuate ligament could reproduce the abnormal carpal kinematics seen in this form of MCI. Trumble and associates[12] also evaluated this form of instability biomechanically in cadaver speci-

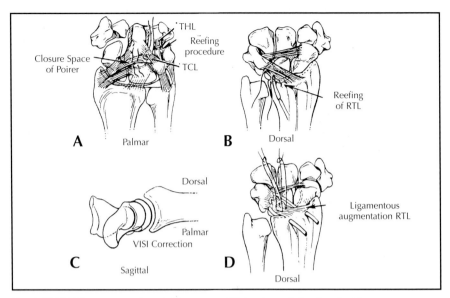

Fig. 1 CIND VISI reconstruction. **A,** The space of Poirer is partially closed with sutures between the radiolunate and radioscapho-capitate ligaments. The triquetro-hamate and tri-quetro-capitate ligaments (THL and TCL) are reefed using strong, nonabsorbable sutures with the midcarpal joint in a slightly over-corrected position. **B,** The dorsal radiotriquetral ligament (RTL) is tightened by imbrication. **C,** Correction of the VISI deformity. **D,** Ligamentous augmentation may be achieved by using a free strip of tendon to augment the tension in the radiotri-quetral ligament. (Reproduced with permission from the Mayo Foundation, Rochester, MN.)

mens. They found that, after the ulnar half of the volar arcuate ligament and the LTL were sectioned, the proximal carpal row did not rotate into dorsiflexion when the wrist was ulnarly deviated. This abnormality seems to mimic the pattern seen clinically with one form of MCI. Viegas and associates[13] also did biomechanical studies related to this problem. By serial sectioning of various intercarpal ligaments, a classification of ulnar-sided instability was developed. They found that sectioning the LTL, the ulnar portion of the palmar radiolunotriquetral ligament, and the dorsal radiocarpal ligament created a static VISI deformity with palmar subluxation of the capitate that reduced with ulnar deviation and extension. This result again resembles the circumstances found clinically. Garth and associates[14] also reported their experience with MCI. They suggested that laxity of the capitotriquetral ligament produced MCI. The capitotriquetral ligament is

presumably a portion of the ulnar limb of the arcuate ligament.

Thus, based on biomechanical and anatomic studies, palmar MCI refers to an instability pattern that consists of a VISI pattern of the proximal carpal row, which reduces in ulnar deviation and has an associated palmar subluxation of the capitate on the lunate articulation. These same studies suggest that at least the ulnar half of the arcuate ligament and probably also the LTL and possibly the dorsal radiocarpal ligament must be damaged to cause this instability pattern.

Dorsal MCI is that instability pattern that was described by both White and associates[8] and Johnson and Carrera.[15] Johnson and Carrera reported on a series of 12 patients who had symptomatic wrist pain. Under fluoroscopy it was found that the capitate could be subluxed dorsally relative to the lunate. At surgery, the authors commented that the site of pathology seemed to be the radioscapho-

capitate ligament. Clinically, the diagnosis is made by stressing the carpus, at which point radiographs reveal that the capitate subluxes dorsally to the lunate. Hankin and associates,[16] in a report of two patients, suggested that one cause of dorsal MCI is an injury to the scapho-trapezial ligament.

Midcarpal CIND is the third category in Lichtman's classification of MCI. Wright and associates[2] recently published their experience with this group of patients. Diagnosis was based on history and the reproduction of a clunk on physical examination. This clunk presumably represents the sudden reduction of the midcarpal joint when the wrist is moved into ulnar deviation. Stress radiographs also played an important role in the diagnosis. In this group of patients it was found that the midcarpal joint can sublux both dorsally and volarly. Dobyns, one of the authors, felt that when the primary subluxation is volar, the triquetral-hamate (TH) and triquetral-capitate (TC) ligaments may be elongated. When the subluxation is dorsal, the short radiolunate ligament is lax. Subluxation of the capitate-lunate joint or abnormal movement of the proximal carpal row during ulnar deviation will help to confirm the diagnosis.

The fourth category in this midcarpal instability classification is extrinsic MCI, first described by Taleisnik and Watson[17] in patients who had malunions of the distal radius. They reviewed 13 patients who had loss of normal palmar tilt of the distal radius and concluded that this deformity leads to secondary stretching of the midcarpal ligamentous structures, which in turn results in the midcarpal instability. Extrinsic MCI is a CIA type deformity.

In summary, palmar MCI is a VISI deformity that reduces abruptly with ulnar deviation. It is believed, based on anatomic and biomechanical studies, that it involves an injury to the arcuate ligament and possibly the lunotriquetral and dorsal radiocarpal ligaments. Patients with dorsal MCI have the finding of the capitate subluxing dorsally to the lunate on stress views. The injury is probably in the area of the radioscaphocapitate. Midcarpal CIND implies that there is both dorsal and volar subluxation of the joint. The area of pathology is possibly a combination of dorsal and palmar CIND. Extrinsic MCI is a secondary adaptive phenomenon that most commonly occurs after malunions of the distal radius.

The treatment of this problem is quite variable, and the results in some cases are discouraging. Many physicians recommend that these patients not be treated surgically, if at all possible. Several recommend trials of splinting, anti-inflammatories, and alteration of the use of the wrist to see if this will decrease the symptoms to a tolerable level.

Surgical treatment of MCI is not entirely satisfactory, and results depend on the location of the instability. Multiple procedures are available. Palmar MCI is thought to be caused in part by a defect in the ulnar limb of the arcuate ligament. Soft-tissue procedures include reefing the ulnar limb of the arcuate ligament, triquetral-hamate (TH) ligament reconstruction, and suturing the radioscaphocapitate to the radiolunotriquetral ligament to close the space of Poirer. In six of nine patients, this procedure[11] was considered to be a failure. In the majority of the six, the clunk observed preoperatively recurred. Another group of patients in this study[11] underwent either a TH or a triquetral-hamate-capitate-lunate (THCL) fusion. All of the THCL fusions were considered successes. Rao and Culver[18] reported on their experience with TH fusion for MCI. This fusion failed to control the symptoms of MCI in 50% of the cases. There was also an associated decrease in the range of motion compared to preoperative values.

Johnson and Carrera,[15] who published one of the first series on dorsal MCI instability, described their surgical

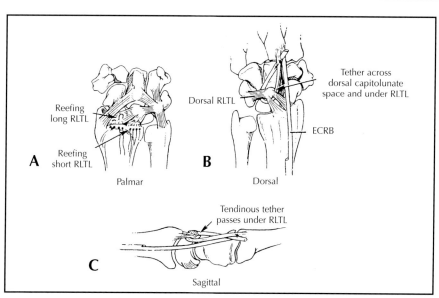

Fig. 2 CIND DISI reconstruction and ligamentous repair. **A,** The long radiolunate-triquetral ligament (long RLTL) and the short radiolunate ligament (RLL) are reefed through drill holes in the volar radial rim to prevent excessive extension of the PCR. **B,** A dorsal tether to flex the lunate on the capitate can be obtained by using a strip of the extensor carpi radialis brevis (ECRB) or longus, looping it beneath the dorsoradial triquetral ligament (dorsal RLTL) and suturing it back to itself at the insertion. **C,** The dorsal tether as seen on the sagittal view. (Reproduced with permission from the Mayo Foundation, Rochester, MN.)

approach to this problem and also reported on the results of the procedure. Surgery involves suturing the deficient radioscaphocapitate to the radiolunotriquetral ligament, thus partially closing the space of Poirer. Nine of the 11 patients in this series were considered to have a good or excellent result.

Wright and associates[2] have the most published experience with nondissociative MCI. A retrospective review of 45 patients was presented. In this study there were overall 56% good or excellent results. The best results were in those patients who underwent a joint leveling procedure or closing wedge osteotomy of the radius for MCI with an ulnar minus variant. The rationale was that on physical examination, when the triquetrum is stabilized there is no clunk. Radial shortening increases the load on the ulna, thereby stabilizing the triquetrum so that the click cannot occur. This group of patients had an overall 83% good or

excellent result. If the patient has a CIND-VISI, the proximal carpal row is flexed. Surgical treatment consists of suturing the radioscaphocapitate to the radiolunate (RL), thus closing the space of Poirer. The TH and TC ligaments are reefed and the dorsal radiotriquetral ligament is tightened by imbrication. In some cases this is augmented by a strip of free tendon graft (Fig. 1).

In CIND-DISI the short radiolunate ligament is lax and the proximal carpal row is dorsiflexed. Surgery involves tightening the long and short RL ligaments, and tethering the lunate dorsally using a slip of the radial wrist extensor (Fig. 2).

The difficulty in treating these patients is that location of the pathology is not completely known. There are several hypotheses but none have been specifically proven. This has led to a multitude of surgical procedures but the overall results are somewhat discouraging.

Treatment of MCI secondary to malunited fractures seems to have better results. Treatment should be directed at the malunion rather than the adaptive instability of the midcarpal joint. In Taleisnik and Watson's[17] series of 13 patients, nine patients had resolution of their symptoms and the MCI following a corrective osteotomy.

In summary, MCI is a problem that is not completely understood. On physical examination, the majority of patients complain of a clunk or click in their wrist with ulnar deviation of the wrist. Radiographs and arthrograms are often normal. In many cases, fluoroscopy of the wrist reveals that the motion between the proximal and distal carpal row when the wrist is moved from radial to ulnar deviation is not synchronous. A variety of ligamentous structures have been implicated in the pathologic process. Review of the published literature details a variety of different treatments. Although all authors suggest that conservative care be tried first, published reports suggest that it is effective in only about half of the cases. Surgical results are only slightly better. Based on the published results of surgical reviews, some form of midcarpal fusion seems to have slightly better results than soft-tissue procedures. Joint-leveling procedures may be helpful in selected patients. If the MCI has an extrinsic cause, such as a malunion of the

radius, corrective osteotomy is indicated. In the future, biomechanical and anatomic studies may help to further our understanding of this very confusing topic and lead to treatment protocols with a higher success rate.

In summary, the diagnosis and treatment of wrist instability is complex and can be confusing. Evaluation of these patients using a classification scheme may be of some help. Treatment of the problem depends on the location of the pathology. A variety of different soft-tissue and bony procedures have been advocated. In the future, further research may provide a more complete understanding of this problem.

References

1. Linscheid RL, Dobyns JH, Beabout JW, et al: Traumatic instability of the wrist: Diagnosis, classification, and pathomechanics. *J Bone Joint Surg* 1972;54A:1612–1632.
2. Wright TW, Dobyns JH, Linscheid RL, et al: Carpal instability non-dissociative. *J Hand Surg* 1994;19B:763–773.
3. Larsen CF, Amadio PC, Gilula LA, et al: Analysis of carpal instability: I. Description of the scheme. *J Hand Surg* 1995;20A:757–764.
4. Hodge JC, Gilula LA, Larsen CF, et al: Analysis of carpal instability: II. Clinical applications. *J Hand Surg* 1995;20A:765–776.
5. Mouchet A, Belot J: Poignet a ressaut (subluxation médiocarpienne en avant). *Bull et Mem Soc nat de Chir* 1934;60:1243.
6. Lichtman DM, Schneider JR, Swafford AR, et al: Ulnar midcarpal instability: Clinical and laboratory analysis. *J Hand Surg* 1981;6A:515–523.
7. Ono H, Gilula LA, Evanoff BA, et al: Midcarpal instability: Is capitolunate instability pattern a clinical condition? *J Hand Surg* 1996;21B:197–201.
8. White SJ, Louis DS, Braunstein EM, et al: Capito-lunate instability: Recognition by manipulation under fluoroscopy. *Am J Roentgenol* 1984;143:361–364.
9. Braunstein EM, Louis DS, Greene TL, et al: Fluoroscopic and arthrographic evaluation of carpal instability. *Am J Roentgenol* 1985;144:1259–1262.
10. Protas JM, Jackson WT: Evaluating carpal instabilities with fluoroscopy. *Am J Roentgenol* 1980;135:137–140.
11. Lichtman DM, Bruckner JD, Culp RW, et al: Palmar midcarpal instability: Results of surgical reconstruction. *J Hand Surg* 1993;18A:307–315.
12. Trumble TE, Bour CJ, Smith RJ, et al: Kinematics of the ulnar carpus related to the volar intercalated segment instability pattern. *J Hand Surg* 1990;15A:384–392.
13. Viegas SF, Patterson RM, Peterson PD, et al: Ulnar-sided perilunate instability: An anatomic and biomechanic study. *J Hand Surg* 1990;15A:268–278.
14. Garth WP Jr, Hofammann DY, Rooks MD: Volar intercalated segment instability secondary to medial carpal ligamental laxity. *Clin Orthop* 1985;201:94–105.
15. Johnson RP, Carrera GF: Chronic capitolunate instability. *J Bone Joint Surg* 1986;68A:1164–1176.
16. Hankin FM, Amadio PC, Wojtys EM, et al: Carpal instability with volar flexion of the proximal row associated with injury to the scaphotrapezial ligament: Report of two cases. *J Hand Surg* 1988;13B:298–302.
17. Taleisnik J, Watson HK: Midcarpal instability caused by malunited fractures of the distal radius. *J Hand Surg* 1984;9A:350–357.
18. Rao SB, Culver JE: Triquetrohamate arthrodesis for midcarpal instability. *J Hand Surg* 1995;20A:583–589.

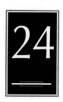

Distal Radioulnar Joint Instability

Brian D. Adams, MD

Anatomy and Mechanics

The distal radioulnar joint (DRUJ) provides the distal pivot for forearm pronation–supination, with the axis of rotation passing through the ulnar head. The ulnocarpal joint transmits approximately 20% of the axial load through the wrist.[1] This loading generates forces that tend to splay the DRUJ, and these forces must be resisted by the soft tissues.[2] Articular cartilage covers a 90° to 135° arc of the ulnar head, while the arc of the sigmoid notch of the radius is only 47° to 80°. The radius of curvature of the sigmoid notch averages 15 mm, compared to 10 mm for the ulnar head. The combination of a relatively shallow sigmoid notch and a distinct difference in the radii of curvatures of the articular surfaces results in both rotational and translational joint motions and provides minimal stability for the joint. Because of this architecture, the ligaments are essential for palmar-dorsal joint stability. The primary stabilizers of the DRUJ are the palmar and dorsal radioulnar ligaments, which are components of the triangular fibrocartilage complex (TFCC).[3] Although the articular disk of the TFCC transmits axial loads across the ulnocarpal joint and undergoes significant strains during forearm rotation,[4] it does not contribute significantly to joint stability.[5] The pronator quadratus, interosseous membrane (IOM), and DRUJ capsule, as well as other components of the TFCC, including the ulnocarpal ligaments and extensor carpi ulnaris tendon sheath, usually provide sufficient support to maintain joint alignment during healing of the radioulnar ligaments if the joint is protected from excessive forces.[6]

Physical Examination and Imaging

An acute dislocation usually produces an obvious deformity. Similarly, a chronic dislocation commonly causes a reproducible clunk that is visible or palpable during active or passive forearm rotation. The clunk usually occurs spontaneously at the extreme of pronation or supination, although occasionally additional anterior-posterior manipulation of the joint is necessary to complete the dislocation. A subluxating joint is much more subtle and difficult to detect. It is essential to compare the extremities because the normal range of motion and laxity of the DRUJ varies considerably among individuals.

A lateral radiograph of the wrist should be obtained with the arm at the patient's side and the elbow flexed 90°. However, even this standard view is unreliable for detecting instability. A posteroanterior view will identify DRUJ widening, arthritis and incongruity, ulnar styloid fractures, and bony deformity. Two orthogonal views of the forearm should be obtained when forearm deformity is suspected. Computed tomography is useful for delineating sigmoid notch incompetence, assessing arthritis, and identifying instability. However, the detection of subtle instability is often very difficult. Magnetic resonance imaging, arthrography, and scintigraphy have limited roles. These studies are useful when the diagnosis of instability is in question or there are suspected concurrent problems, such as ulnar impaction syndrome or a TFCC tear. The role of arthroscopy is evolving. Peripheral TFCC tears can be diagnosed and treated arthroscopically; however, the indications for this technique for the treatment of instability are not well defined.[7]

Principles of Treatment

The anatomic derangements responsible for instability must be identified to effect reliable treatment. The cause can be bony deformity, ligament injury, or a combination. Soft-tissue repair or reconstruction in the presence of bony malalignment will fail. The condition of the articular surfaces is a key factor in selecting among the treatment alternatives. The surfaces may be normal, incongruous, or arthritic. Unrecognized joint incongruity or arthritis will degrade the surgical outcome. Although the duration of instability may have some impact on the condition of the joint, the assumption should not be made that the articular surfaces and soft-tissues have deteriorated because of the chronicity of the instability. It may be possible to achieve a good outcome by restoring the normal anatomy with TFCC repair or corrective osteotomy even in the presence of long-standing instability. The direction of instability may be dorsal, volar, or bidirectional, with the direction defined by the position of the ulna relative to the radius.

Acute Instability

In most instances of acute instability without a fracture of the distal radius or forearm, the TFCC has been disrupted from its ulnar attachments.[8] As the severity of injury increases, other structures about the ulnar side of the wrist are torn, including the extensor carpi ulnaris (ECU) tendon sheath, the ulnocarpal ligaments, the lunotriquetral interosseous ligament, and, finally, the triquetral-capitate and triquetral-hamate ligaments. The secondary stabilizers of the joint sustain variable degrees of the injury. Dorsal dislocations are the most common. When recognized acutely, reduction is straightforward unless there is interposed soft tissue, most commonly the ECU tendon. The position of maximum stability following reduction is opposite to the position of instability; however, the joint should be tested to determine the stable arc of forearm rotation. If a stable position is found, the injury is treated by long arm casting in this position. If mild instability persists, the radius can be pinned to the ulna proximal to the joint. In severe or bidirectional instability, open repair of the TFCC should be considered.[9]

Although an ulnar styloid fracture may be associated with instability, most styloid fractures do not cause instability. A fracture through the base of the styloid is more predictive of a TFCC tear than is a fracture through the tip or shaft of the styloid.[10] The styloid tip is devoid of soft-tissue attachments. Thus, tip fractures are probably caused by compression or shear from impaction by the carpus. The styloid shaft provides an attachment for a portion of the ulnocarpal ligaments, the ECU tendon sheath, and the radioulnar ligaments. Because the primary attachment of the radioulnar ligaments is at the fovea of the ulnar head, a basilar fracture may occur without complete disruption of these ligaments. Conversely, a complete avulsion of the radioulnar ligaments and gross instability can occur without any type of styloid fracture.[8,11] Occasionally, a small fleck of bone is avulsed with the radioulnar ligaments and is seen on a radiograph in the region of the fovea. These variations must be recognized in treating instability, because ulnar styloid fixation alone will not be sufficient if the integrity of the radioulnar ligaments is not restored.

Acute instability occurs most commonly in association with distal radius fractures. Dorsal angulation of the radius causes volar dislocation of the ulna, however, radial shortening contributes to the instability. Angulation greater than 20° to 30° creates significant incongruity of the joint, distorts the TFCC, and alters DRUJ kinematics.[12,13] The radioulnar ligaments can tolerate no more than 5 mm of radial shortening before tearing occurs;[12] severe shortening indicates complete disruption. Near anatomic fracture reduction, including the sigmoid notch, is key to restoring DRUJ stability. Persistent instability following accurate reduction is uncommon even though TFCC disruption probably occurs frequently. Primary repair of the TFCC and fixation of the ulnar styloid does not produce a better result than closed reduction and long-arm casting unless there is gross instability of the joint following reduction.[14] In most cases, the secondary stabilizers of the joint will maintain sufficient stability during healing, resulting in a stable joint.

The Galleazzi fracture-dislocation should be approached similarly to the distal radius fracture complicated by DRUJ instability. Anatomic reduction and rigid fixation of the radius is essential, while TFCC repair is unnecessary unless gross or bidirectional instability persists following fracture fixation.[15,16] Because the typical Galleazzi injury produces volar dislocation of the DRUJ, positioning the forearm in some degree of supination will enhance postoperative stability.

Chronic Instability

The evaluation and treatment of chronic DRUJ instability is more challenging than that of acute instability. Chronic instability without a bony deformity is caused by inadequate healing of an acute injury or chronic inflammatory arthritis. The instability is typically dorsal subluxation of the ulna. In addition to TFCC incompetence, other soft-tissue stabilizers are usually attenuated. The condition of the articular surfaces is central to choosing the appropriate treatment alternative. Articular damage is common in long-standing cases and especially in rheumatoid arthritis.

If the articular surfaces are in good condition, TFCC repair can be attempted even in late cases of posttraumatic instability.[9] Ligament reconstruction is used when TFCC repair is not possible. Numerous extra-articular reconstructions have been described. There are three basic concepts of reconstruction: (1) tenodesis of the distal ulna using the ECU and/or the flexor carpi ulnaris (FCU) tendons, (2) an ulnocarpal tether, and (3) a radioul-

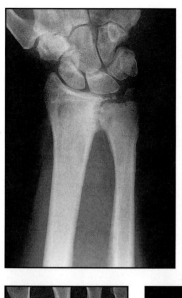
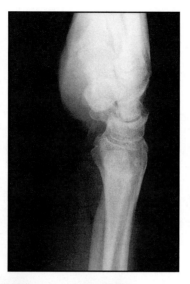
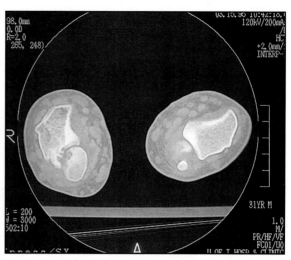
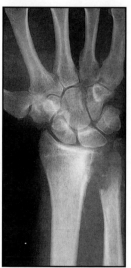
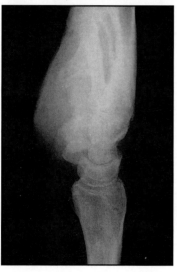

Fig. 1 Posttraumatic arthritis of the distal radioulnar joint caused severe limitation of motion and pain. Computed tomography demonstrated severe arthritis and volar subluxation of the ulna. A hemiresection arthroplasty with pronator quadratus interposition resulted in a stable distal ulna and full, painless pronation and supination.

nar tether. Although none of these approaches restores normal DRUJ stability,[17] an ulnocarpal tether also creates some support for the ulnocarpal joint.[18] A radioulnar tether provides the greatest stability, but it may result in significant loss of forearm rotation. An intra-articular reconstruction is more anatomic and can potentially restore stability with less loss of rotation. The concept is to recreate the palmar and/or the dorsal radioulnar ligaments.[19,20] In this technique, a tendon graft is routed between the margins of the sigmoid notch and the fovea. If arthritis is present, partial or complete resection of the distal ulna is indicated.

Complete resection of the head of the ulna, the Darrach procedure, is effective in the low-demand patient. The procedure should be combined with soft-tissue stabilization, and excessive resection must be avoided.[21] Partial subperiosteal bone reformation of the resected portion is common but does not adversely affect the outcome. In fact, stability may be improved by this bone growth. Hemiresection arthroplasty is indicated for the younger, high-demand patient to help preserve grip strength and stability of the wrist (Fig. 1). Several variations of this technique have been described.[22,23] Some type of soft-tissue interposition between

the distal radius and ulna is necessary to prevent abutment of the bones. Capsular flaps, an anchovy of tendon graft, and the pronator quadratus have been used successfully. Although the procedure is effective, the results are less predictable when instability is present than when it is performed for arthritis alone.

The Sauvé-Kapandji procedure is an effective alternative to resectional arthroplasty.[24,25] In this operation, the DRUJ is fused and a pseudarthrosis is created just proximal to the joint by resecting a segment of the ulnar shaft. The procedure is designed to retain support for the ulnar side of the carpus. These procedures can

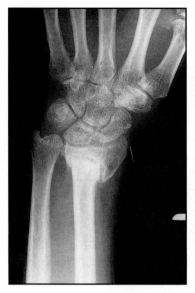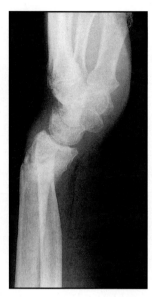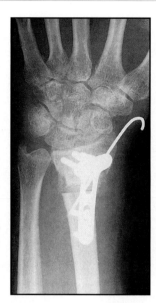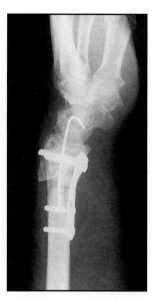

Fig. 2 A volarly angulated distal radius malunion caused dorsal dislocation of the ulna. The angular deformity and shortening were corrected by radial osteotomy and bone grafting. No soft-tissue procedure was required to restore distal radioulnar joint stability.

also be used for the rheumatoid patient. In these patients, however, the extensor tendons, especially the ECU tendon, and the retinaculum require additional care.[26]

Instability of the distal ulna after resectional arthroplasty is a difficult problem. Severe instability is most commonly associated with the Darrach procedure, but instability can occur after hemiresection or the Sauvé-Kapandji procedure. Several of the ligament reconstructions described above have been used with varying success,[27] but the techniques must be modified to include a mechanism to prevent contact between the ulnar stump and the radius. If the ulna is significantly shorter than the radius, an ulnar shaft-lengthening osteotomy may need to be combined with soft-tissue stabilization.

DRUJ instability associated with a distal radius malunion is common. In evaluating the patient, both the radiocarpal joint and DRUJ must be considered. If weakness of grip, radiocarpal joint pain, or midcarpal instability are present, a corrective osteotomy of the radius is indicated. In a low-demand patient with moderate deformity and complaints limited to

the DRUJ, a Darrach resection may be satisfactory.[28] Angulation and shortening of the radius are more problematic than displacement or loss of radial inclination. Although malunion with dorsal angulation is the most common deformity causing instability, volar angulation deformity can also cause instability (Fig. 2). Soft-tissue reconstruction alone will fail when there is significant radial deformity.

An osteotomy to correct the angular deformity of the radius will often restore DRUJ stability; however, radioulnar length discrepancy must also be addressed to improve ulnar deviation and to prevent late occurrence of an ulnar impaction syndrome. Correction of angulation and length discrepancy can be done simultaneously by a trapezoidal graft to the radius. In malunions with severe length discrepancy, this approach can be difficult because the distal radius fragment becomes harder to control with increasing distraction. An alternative is to correct the angular deformity in the radius and the length discrepancy by an ulnar shaft shortening osteotomy. A TFCC repair or soft-tissue stabilization procedure will be necessary if bony realignment does not

restore stability. If DRUJ arthritis is present, one of the arthroplasty procedures described above can be performed; however, radioulnar length discrepancy must still be addressed to prevent impingement between the ulnar styloid and the carpus.[22]

Forearm malunion can cause DRUJ instability in addition to loss of rotation.[29-31] In children, instability may not develop until years after the fracture. Fracture remodeling makes it difficult to accurately characterize a malunion in children. A rotational deformity can dominate by the time instability presents because the angular deformity corrects with growth. In adults, the deformity may initially manifest as limited forearm rotation, with instability developing later as the soft tissues stretch. Soft-tissue stabilizing procedures alone will fail in the presence of a forearm malunion. Corrective osteotomy with plate fixation will often be sufficient to restore stability;[31] TFCC repair or a reconstructive procedure is usually unnecessary. Unless there is DRUJ arthritis, a resectional arthroplasty should be avoided. The deformity may involve both the radius and ulna and require osteotomy of both bones. To achieve optimum stability and forearm rotation, different bony corrections can be tested intraoperatively by temporary fixation of the osteotomies.

Conclusion

Wrist instability is a complex problem in which there are few definitive answers. Organization of the problem is an important part of trying to diagnose and treat it. Subsequent to diagnosis, there are several treatment options available for the hand surgeon. In many cases, there is no best treatment and good results can be elusive. It is hoped that more research and clinical experience will make wrist instability easier to diagnose and address.

References

1. Palmer AK, Werner FW: Biomechanics of the distal radioulnar joint. *Clin Orthop* 1984; 187:26–35.

2. Schuind FA, Linscheid RL, An KN, et al: Changes in wrist and forearm configuration with grasp and isometric contraction of elbow flexors. *J Hand Surg* 1992;17A:698–703.

3. Palmer AK, Werner FW: The triangular fibrocartilage complex of the wrist: Anatomy and function. *J Hand Surg* 1981;6A:153–162.

4. Adams BD, Holley KA: Strains in the articular disk of the triangular fibrocartilage complex: A biomechanical study. *J Hand Surg* 1993;18A:919–925.

5. Adams BD: Partial excision of the triangular fibrocartilage complex articular disk: A biomechanical study. *J Hand Surg* 1993;18A:334–340.

6. Kihara H, Short WH, Werner FW, et al: The stabilizing mechanism of the distal radioulnar joint during pronation and supination. *J Hand Surg* 1995;20A:930–936.

7. Trumble TE, Gilbert M, Vedder N: Isolated tears of the triangular fibrocartilage: Management by early arthroscopic repair. *J Hand Surg* 1997;22A:57–65.

8. Melone CP Jr, Nathan R: Traumatic disruption of the triangular fibrocartilage complex: Pathoanatomy. *Clin Orthop* 1992;275:65–73.

9. Hermansdorfer JD, Kleinman WB: Management of chronic peripheral tears of the triangular fibrocartilage complex. *J Hand Surg* 1991;16A:340–346.

10. Hauck RM, Skahen J III, Palmer AK: Classification and treatment of ulnar styloid nonunion. *J Hand Surg* 1996;21A:418–422.

11. Adams BD, Samani JE, Holley KA: Triangular fibrocartilage injury: A laboratory model. *J Hand Surg* 1996;21A:189–193.

12. Adams BA: Effects of radial deformity on distal radioulnar joint mechanics. *J Hand Surg* 1993;18A:492–498.

13. Kihara H, Palmer AK, Werner FW, et al: The effect of dorsally angulated distal radius fractures on distal radioulnar joint congruency and forearm rotation. *J Hand Surg* 1996;21A:40–47.

14. af Ekenstam F, Jakobsson OP, Wadin K: Repair of the triangular ligament in Colles' fracture: No effect in a prospective randomized study. *Acta Orthop Scand* 1989;60:393–396.

15. Strehle J, Gerber C: Distal radioulnar joint function after Galeazzi fracture-dislocations treated by open reduction and internal plate fixation. *Clin Orthop* 1993;293:240–245.

16. Reckling FW: Unstable fracture-dislocations of the forearm (Monteggia and Galeazzi lesions). *J Bone Joint Surg* 1982;64A:857–863.

17. Petersen MS, Adams BD: Biomechanical evaluation of distal radioulnar reconstructions. *J Hand Surg* 1993;18A:328–334.

18. Hui FC, Linscheid RL: Ulnotriquetral augmentation tenodesis: A reconstructive procedure for dorsal subluxation of the distal radioulnar joint. *J Hand Surg* 1982;7A:230–236.

19. Jones KJ, Sanders WE: Posttraumatic radioulnar instability: Treatment by anatomic reconstruction of the volar and dorsal radioulnar ligaments. *Orthop Trans* 1995;19:832.

20. Scheker LR, Belliappa PP, Acosta R, et al: Reconstruction of the dorsal ligament of the triangular fibrocartilage complex. *J Hand Surg* 1994;19B:310–318.

21. Ruby LK, Ferenz CC, Dell PC: The pronator quadratus interposition transfer: An adjunct to resection arthroplasty of the distal radioulnar joint. *J Hand Surg* 1996;21A:60–65.

22. Bowers WH: Distal radioulnar joint arthroplasty: The hemiresection-interposition technique. *J Hand Surg* 1985;10A:169–178.

23. Watson HK, Gabuzda GM: Matched distal ulna resection for posttraumatic disorders of the distal radioulnar joint. *J Hand Surg* 1992;17A:724–730.

24. Minami A, Suzuki K, Suenaga N, et al: The Sauvé-Kapandji procedure for osteoarthritis of the distal radioulnar joint. *J Hand Surg* 1995;20A:602–608.

25. Sanders RA, Frederick HA, Hontas RB: The Sauvé-Kapandji procedure: A salvage operation for the distal radioulnar joint. *J Hand Surg* 1991;16A:1125–1129.

26. Leslie BM, Carlson G, Ruby LK: Results of extensor carpi ulnaris tenodesis in the rheumatoid wrist undergoing a distal ulnar excision. *J Hand Surg* 1990;15A:547–551.

27. Breen TF, Jupiter JB: Extensor carpi ulnaris and flexor carpi ulnaris tenodesis of the unstable distal ulna. *J Hand Surg* 1989;14A:612–617.

28. Hartz CR, Beckenbaugh RD: Long-term results of resection of the distal ulna for posttraumatic conditions. *J Trauma* 1979;19:219–226.

29. Matthews LS, Kaufer H, Garver DF, et al: The effect on supination-pronation of angular malalignment of fractures of both bones of the forearm: An experimental study. *J Bone Joint Surg* 1982;64A:14–17.

30. Tarr RR, Garfinkel AI, Sarmiento A: The effects of angular and rotational deformities of both bones of the forearm: An in vitro study. *J Bone Joint Surg* 1984;66A:65–70.

31. Trousdale RT, Linscheid RL: Operative treatment of malunited fractures of the forearm. *J Bone Joint Surg* 1995;77A:894–902.

Ulnar-Sided Wrist Pain and Instability

Steven F. Viegas, MD

There is a great deal of confusion over carpal instabilities, particularly in the ulnar aspect of the wrist. This confusion may arise in part from the lack of uniformity in the use of such terms as dynamic and static, and in the use of the various classifications, such as carpal instability dissociative (CID), carpal instability nondissociative (CIND), dorsal intercalated segment instability (DISI), volar intercalated segment instability (VISI), and midcarpal instability, which are not always used in the way their originators intended.

Gilford and associates[1] are credited with the first reference to carpal instability. Linscheid and associates[2] and Adelaar[3] have described common posttraumatic intercarpal instability collapse deformities. Their classification of the deformities is based primarily on the capitolunate angle. Two of the basic patterns that they describe are DISI and VISI.

A number of different lesions have been reported to result in a VISI deformity. Garth and associates[4] described laxity of the capitotriquetral ligament, which resulted in failure of the triquetral-hamate joint, which, in turn, they believe allows a VISI deformity to occur. Trumble and associates[5] also list triquetral-hamate disruption as well as capitate-lunate laxity as causes of VISI deformity. These kinds of VISI deformities are what Dobyns and associates[6] would classify as CIND lesions. The etiology most commonly attributed to the development of a VISI deformity is linked to lunate-triquetrum laxity,[3,4,7–14] which would be cat-

egorized as a CID. Different authors[10,14] have speculated that a progressive sequence of ligament disruption can occur on the ulnar side of the carpus, similar to what Mayfield and associates[15] have described on the radial side of the carpus.

There is a relative paucity of cases in the literature describing deformities that could be classified as VISI.[2,5,9,10,12,16–19] Despite scattered reports in the literature, there had not been a consensus of opinion regarding the pathology required to result in dynamic and static VISI deformities arising from the area of the lunotriquetral joint. However, clinical cases that involve documented disruptions of the lunotriquetral interosseous ligament without any VISI pattern of deformity are not uncommon.

Early cadaver experiments demonstrated increased divergent motion between the lunate and triquetrum following sectioning of the lunotriquetral interosseous and the palmar and dorsal radiotriquetral ligaments.[8,10] Some studies had also been able to reproduce dynamic VISI patterns with the application of a dorsal force on the capitate and/or hamate.[8,10] Other cadaver studies that attempted to reproduce this instability pattern had been unsuccessful.[14] A static VISI deformity in the cadaver model had not been simulated until Viegas and associates,[20] in a series of dissections, reported increased motion between the lunate and the triquetrum with a tear of the lunotriquetral interosseous ligament.

However, with disruption of this ligament alone, no appreciable dynamic or static VISI deformity was evident and none could be induced. This experiment was compatible with the findings of load studies, which, overall, demonstrated no significant differences in load distribution between the scaphoid and lunate fossa in normal wrists and in cases in which the lunotriquetral joint alone was disrupted. It is also consistent with clinical findings in which patients with incongruity between the lunate and the triquetrum generally had satisfactory clinical results.[21]

A staging system for ulnar-sided perilunate instability was developed based on a series of cadaver dissections and load studies.[20] The stages are as follows. In stage I there is partial or complete disruption of the lunotriquetral interosseous ligament and no clinical and/or radiographic evidence of dynamic or static VISI deformity. In stage II there is complete disruption of the lunotriquetral interosseous ligament, disruption of the palmar lunotriquetral ligaments, and clinical and/or radiographic evidence of dynamic VISI deformity. In stage III there is complete disruption of the lunotriquetral interosseous and the palmar lunotriquetral ligaments, attenuation or disruption of the dorsal radiocarpal ligament, and clinical and/or radiographic evidence of static VISI deformity (Fig. 1).

In a stage II ulnar-sided perilunate instability, a definite VISI deformity was evident during the application of a trans-

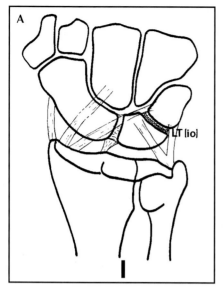
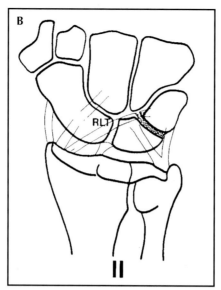
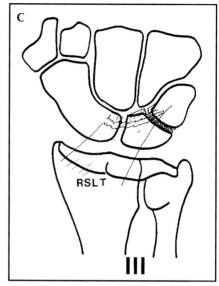

Fig. 1 A diagram depicting **(A)** the disruption of the lunotriquetral interosseous ligament (LT[io]) in a stage I ulnar-sided perilunate instability, **(B)** the additional disruption of the palmar radiolunotriquetral ligament (RLT), between the lunate and the triquetrum, in a stage II ulnar-sided perilunate instability, and **(C)** the additional disruption of the dorsal radioscapholunotriquetral ligament, also called the dorsal radiocarpal ligament, in a stage III ulnar-sided perilunate instability. (Reproduced with permission from Viegas SF, Patterson RM, Peterson PD, et al: Ulnar sided perilunate instability: An anatomic and biomechanic study. *J Hand Surg* 1990;15A:268–278.)

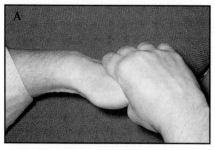
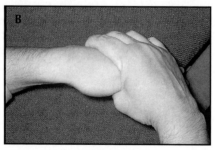

Fig. 2 The examination of a midcarpal clunk is performed by **(A)** exerting a palmarly directed translational force over the dorsal aspect of the distal carpal row with the wrist in neutral flexion/extension and slight radial deviation. The hand can be seen to be volarly translated in relation to the forearm. While maintaining the palmarly directed translational force, **(B)** the wrist is deviated in an ulnar direction, which will result in a sudden clunk as the wrist relocates into a more anatomic position. (Reproduced with permission from Viegas SF: Arthroscopic assessment of carpal instabilities and ligament injuries, in Jackson DW (ed): *Instructional Course Lectures 44.* Rosemont, IL, American Academy of Orthopaedic Surgeons, 1995, pp 151–154.)

lational force on the dorsal aspect of the capitate and/or hamate, when the wrist was in neutral or flexion and radial, neutral, or limited ulnar deviation. Sectioning the dorsal radiocarpal ligament and capsule at their attachment to the scaphoid and lunate, classified as a stage III ulnar-sided perilunate instability, allowed a static VISI deformity to arise in the wrist. This static VISI deformity could only be demonstrated, however, in those same positions in which the dynamic VISI deformity could be attained. Whenever the wrist was brought into greater than 25° of ulnar deviation or into extension, the VISI position changed to a position of normal carpal alignment. Reduction of the VISI deformity by ulnar deviation of the wrist has been described clinically. The symptomatic "clunk," often described by patients, can be reproduced by this maneuver.[22]

Arthroscopic examination of the proximal wrist joint can help to assess the integrity of the lunotriquetral interosseous ligament complex, as well as the ulnocarpal ligaments. Additionally, the laxity and diastasis of the lunotriquetral joint often can be assessed by means of midcarpal arthroscopy. The midcarpal clunk test is positive if a static or dynamic VISI instability is present. This test is performed by applying a palmarly directed translational force over the dorsum of the capitate, with the wrist in neutral flexion/extension and brought from a position of radial deviation to a position of ulnar deviation[23] (Fig. 2). During this maneuver, if there is sufficient laxity, the capitate subluxes volarly out of the lunate concavity while the wrist is in radial deviation. As the wrist is brought into ulnar deviation, the lunate is forced into a more neutral and slightly extended posture.

The capitate remains transiently perched at the volar lip of the lunate and then abruptly shifts or "clunks" dorsally to suddenly seat in a reduced position in the lunate. This maneuver can also be performed, to a limited extent, while viewing the midcarpal joint arthroscopically (Fig. 3).

Berger and associates[24] have studied the various components of the lunotriquetral interosseous ligament and found that the most substantial portion of this complex, both histologically and mechanically, is its volar component, with the dorsal component being next, and the least substantial being the proximal membranous portion of this complex. If arthroscopy reveals the proximal membranous portion of the lunotriquetral interosseous ligament complex to be disrupted and this disruption is felt to be the cause of symptoms, a local debridement of the disrupted portion of the membranous portion of the ligament is advised. If there is more significant disruption and instability, these injuries may be treated by arthroscopically assisted reduction and percutaneous pin fixation. My preference, however, is to approach the injury through an open procedure and, depending on the patient's wishes, either attempt a ligament reconstruction and repair or, alternatively, proceed to a lunate-triquetrum-capitate-hamate fusion. It is particularly important in the VISI instabilities to examine the contralateral wrist. It is not uncommon to identify physiologic laxity and a physiologic midcarpal clunk in the contralateral wrist; and, while this does not preclude the option of ligament repair and reconstruction, it raises the concern of subsequent stretching or compromise of the ligament repair due to inherent physiologic laxity. In these individuals, one might give stronger consideration to a limited arthrodesis.

In evaluating ulnar-sided wrist pain, it is important to determine whether or not there is a lunotriquetral interosseous ligament complex disruption. In previous

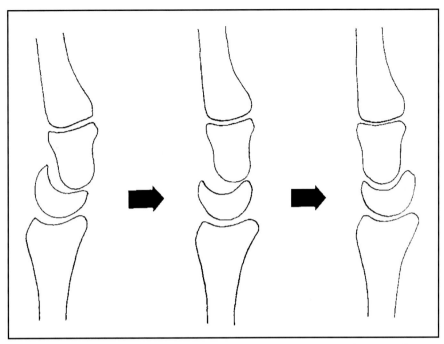

Fig. 3 This series of diagrams illustrates the alignment of the third metacarpal, capitate, lunate, and radius. The diagram on the left illustrates the VISI alignment when the palmar translational force is exerted over the dorsal aspect of the capitate with the wrist in neutral flexion/extension and slight radial deviation. In the center, as the wrist is deviated in an ulnar direction, the scaphoid and then lunate are forced into a more neutral position. Transiently, the capitate remains perched on the volar lip of the lunate and then suddenly relocates with a "clunk" into the distal lunate articulation, as illustrated on the right. (Reproduced with permission from Viegas SF: Arthroscopic assessment of carpal instabilities and ligament injuries, in Jackson DW (ed): *Instructional Course Lectures 44.* Rosemont, IL, American Academy of Orthopaedic Surgeons, 1995, pp 151–154.)

studies by Viegas and associates[25] the lunotriquetral interosseous ligament was found to be disrupted in 36% of 393 cadaver wrists dissected. Additionally, in those cadavers in which the contralateral wrist could be dissected, if there was a lunotriquetral interosseous ligament disruption on one side, there was a 53% incidence of disruption of the lunotriquetral interosseous ligament on the contralateral side. The presence of a ligament disruption alone, as demonstrated by arthroscopy and/or arthrogram, is not necessarily significant unless it correlates with the patient's symptoms.

Several interesting correlations between different anatomic features and/or pathology were revealed by statistical analysis of anatomy study results.[24]

Analysis showed a statistically significant correlation between the presence of a type II lunate and arthrosis at the proximal pole of the hamate.[25] The incidence, in fact, of arthrosis at the proximal pole of the hamate was 38.2% in the cadaver population that has a type II lunate. This compares to an incidence of only 1.8% in the population of those with type I lunates, which do not have a medial lunate facet. Arthrosis at the proximal pole of the hamate has been reported to be difficult to see on radiographs.[26] The presence of a type II lunate with a medial facet radiographically and/or arthroscopically in conjunction with ulnar-sided wrist pain should raise the question of arthrosis at the proximal pole of the hamate. This lesion is probably caused by forced ulnar deviation of the wrist, during which the hamate jumps the ridge between the lunate facets.

A previous report of the incidence and location of arthrosis in the wrist reported on a review of radiographs.[27] In this report, the radioscapholunate joint and the scaphoid-trapezium-trapezoid (STT) joint were common sites of arthrosis, and the proximal pole of the hamate was not even mentioned as a site of arthritis. In a study of a large number of cadaver wrists, the proximal pole of the hamate was the most common site of degenerative joint disease, followed by the STT joint. In 68.6% of the cases in which there was arthritis in one wrist, there was also arthritis in the opposite wrist.[25]

Another area of anatomy that is a possible site of ulnar-sided pathology and pain is the pisotriquetral joint. Relatively little information is available on the anatomy of the pisiform and its associated ligamentous attachments. Degenerative changes of the pisotriquetral joint are believed to be one of the causes of ulnar-sided wrist pain, yet the incidence and pattern of degenerative changes in the pisotriquetral joint have not been well documented. Recent anatomy studies showed that degenerative changes on the articular surface of the pisiform were present in 73.8% of the wrists and were present on the triquetrum in 75.0% of the wrists dissected. Degenerative changes were most commonly in the distal, distal radial, and radial aspects of the pisiform and triquetrum and also in the distal ulnar aspect of the triquetrum.

Summary

A variety of lesions have been associated with ulnar-sided wrist pain and/or VISI instability. A staging system for ulnar-sided perilunate instability describes progressive disruptions associated with lunotriquetral dissociation that can lead to VISI instability and emphasizes the importance of the dorsal radiocarpal ligament in preventing VISI instability. Previous studies have emphasized association between type II carpal morphology and arthrosis at the proximal pole of the hamate, which was identified as the most common location of arthrosis in the wrist. The pisotriquetral joint is another common site of degenerative changes. A better understanding of the normal anatomy and kinematics of the ulnar side of the wrist will better enable physicians to identify and treat problems in the ulnar aspect of the wrist.

References

1. Gilford WW, Bolton RH, Lambrinudi C: The mechanism of the wrist joint: With special reference to fractures of the scaphoid. *Guy Hosp Rep* 1943;92:52–59.

2. Linscheid RL, Dobyns JH, Beabout JW, Bryan RS: Traumatic instability of the wrist: Diagnosis, classification, and pathomechanics. *J Bone Joint Surg* 1972;54A:1612–1632.

3. Adelaar RS: Traumatic wrist instabilities. *Contemp Orthop* 1982;4:309–324.

4. Garth WP Jr, Hofammann DY, Rooks MD: Volar intercalated segment instability secondary to medial carpal ligamental laxity. *Clin Orthop* 1985;201:94–105.

5. Trumble T, Bour CJ, Smith RJ, Edwards GS: Intercarpal arthrodesis for static and dynamic volar intercalated segment instability. *J Hand Surg* 1988;13A:384–390.

6. Dobyns JH, Linscheid RL, Macksoud WS, Siegert JJ: Carpal instability, nondissociative. Proceedings of the American Academy of Orthopaedic Surgeons 54th Annual Meeting, San Francisco, CA. Park Ridge, IL, American Academy of Orthopaedic Surgeons, 1987, p 108.

7. Dobyns JH, Linscheid RL, Chao EY, Weber ER, Swanson GE: Traumatic instability of the wrist, in Evans EB (ed): American Academy of Orthopaedic Surgeons *Instructional Course Lectures XXIV*. St. Louis, MO, CV Mosby, 1975, pp 182–199.

8. Alexander CE, Lichtman DM: Ulnar carpal instabilities. *Orthop Clin North Am* 1984;15:307–320.

9. Lichtman DM, Noble WH III, Alexander CE: Dynamic triquetrolunate instability: Case report. *J Hand Surg* 1984;9A:185–188.

10. Reagan DS, Linscheid RL, Dobyns JH: Lunotriquetral sprains. *J Hand Surg* 1984;9A:502–514.

11. Taleisnik J: Post-traumatic carpal instability. *Clin Orthop* 1980;149:73–82.

12. Taleisnik J, Malerich M, Prietto M: Palmar carpal instability secondary to dislocation of scaphoid and lunate: Report of case and review of the literature. *J Hand Surg* 1982;7A:606–612.

13. Lichtman DM (ed): *The Wrist and Its Disorders*. Philadelphia, PA, WB Saunders, 1988, pp 53–275.

14. Taleisnik J (ed): *The Wrist*. New York, NY, Churchill Livingstone, 1985, pp 281–303.

15. Mayfield JK, Johnson RP, Kilcoyne RK: Carpal dislocations: Pathomechanics and progressive perilunar instability. *J Hand Surg* 1980;5A:226–241.

16. Chaput Vaillant: Etude radiographique sur les traumatismes du carpe. *Rev Orthop* 1913;4:227–241.

17. von Mayersbach L: Ein seltener Fall von Luxatio Intercarpea. *Dtsch Z Chir* 1913;123:179–189.

18. Navarro A: Luxaciones del carpo. *An Facultad Med* (Montevideo, Uruguay) 1921;6:113–141.

19. Sutro CJ: Bilateral recurrent intercarpal subluxation. *Am J Surg* 1946;72:110–113.

20. Viegas SF, Patterson RM, Peterson PD, et al: Ulnar-sided perilunate instability: An anatomic and biomechanic study. *J Hand Surg* 1990;15A:268–278.

21. Minami A, Ogino T, Ohshio I, Minami M: Correlation between clinical results and carpal instabilities in patients after reduction of lunate and perilunar dislocations. *J Hand Surg* 1986;11B:213–220.

22. Lichtman DM, Schneider JR, Swafford AR, Mack GR: Ulnar midcarpal instability: Clinical and laboratory analysis. *J Hand Surg* 1981;6A:515–523.

23. Viegas SF: Arthroscopic assessment of carpal instabilities and ligament injuries, in Jackson DW (ed): *Instructional Course Lectures 44*. Rosemont, IL, American Academy of Orthopaedic Surgeons, 1995, pp 151–154.

24. Berger RA, Imaeda T, Berglund L, et al: the anatomic, constraint and material properties of the scapholunate interosseous ligament: A preliminary study, in Schuind F, An KN, Cooney WP III, Garcia-Elias M (eds): *Advances in the Biomechanics of the Hand and Wrist*. New York, NY, Plenum Press, 1994, pp 9–16.

25. Viegas SF, Patterson RM, Hokanson JA, Davis J: Wrist anatomy: Incidence, distribution, and correlation of anatomic variations, tears, and arthrosis. *J Hand Surg* 1993;18A:463–475.

26. Viegas SF, Wagner K, Patterson R, Peterson P: Medial (hamate) facet of the lunate. *J Hand Surg* 1990;15A:564–571.

27. Watson HK, Brenner LH: Degenerative disorders of the wrist. *J Hand Surg* 1985;10A:1002–1006.

Radial-Sided Carpal Instability

Richard A. Berger, MD, PhD

Introduction

Radial-sided carpal instability, in particular scapholunate instability, represents the most recognized group of carpal instabilities. Although many etiologies have been postulated, traumatic ligamentous disruption is the most common cause of symptomatic instability. Although substantial knowledge has been gained over the past 2 decades about the normal motion and forces of the joints and the mechanical factors that lead to ligament disruption, many questions remain about the most effective treatment options and the ultimate outcome of those treatments.

Basic Science
Bony Anatomy

The eight bones making up the carpus are bounded proximally by the radius and ulna-triangular fibrocartilage complex (TFCC) and distally by the metacarpal bases. The carpal bones are divided anatomically into proximal and distal rows, each composed of four bones. The bones of the proximal row, from radial to ulnar, are the scaphoid, the lunate, and the triquetrum, with the pisiform located palmar to the triquetrum. The distal row is composed of the trapezium, trapezoid, capitate, and hamate. The rows are arched in both the transverse and coronal planes. In the proximal row, the lunate forms a keystone in both planes, and the capitate forms the keystone of the distal row.

Between the radius and the proximal carpal row is the radiocarpal joint, and between the proximal and distal carpal rows is the midcarpal joint. Between the bony elements of each row are individual intercarpal joints, each named according the to the bones forming the joint. The radiocarpal joint is concave distally. The midcarpal joint can be divided artificially into a concave proximal radial half and a concave distal ulnar half.

The bony elements that are of concern in radial-sided carpal instability are the radius, scaphoid, lunate, trapezium, trapezoid, and capitate. Relevant anatomic details of these bones include the distal articular surface of the radius, which is divided into a triangular-shaped scaphoid fossa and a quadrangular lunate fossa, separated by a fibrocartilaginous sagittal ridge called the interfacet prominence. The scaphoid has a complex geometry; it is shaped somewhat like a kidney bean, and can be divided into a proximal pole, the waist, and a distal pole, or tubercle. There is an offset between the proximal and distal articular surfaces, such that the distal pole normally rests palmar to the proximal pole. The lunate is wedge shaped, tapering dorsally, and is divisible into a dorsal horn and palmar horn. The capitate is composed of a semispherical head, a neck, and a body.

Ligamentous Anatomy

The palmar radiocarpal ligaments connect the radius with the proximal carpal row.[1-3] From the radial styloid process emerges the radioscaphocapitate ligament, which attaches to the lateral surface of the waist and proximal half of the distal pole of the scaphoid before passing under the waist of the scaphoid to contribute to the palmar midcarpal joint capsule. The long radiolunate ligament originates from the palmar rim of the scaphoid fossa just ulnar to the origin of the radioscaphocapitate ligament. It passes anterior to the proximal pole of the scaphoid and the scapholunate joint to attach to the radial edge of the lunate palmar horn. It is separated from the radioscaphocapitate ligament by a deep division called the interligamentous sulcus. The radioscapholunate "ligament" is essentially a mesocapsule composed of arborizing branches of vessels formed from the radial artery and the anterior interosseous artery and the anterior interosseous nerve, and surrounded by a thick layer of poorly organized connective tissue and synoviocytes.[4-6] It emerges into the radiocarpal joint space in an interval between the long and short radiolunate ligaments to merge with the scapholunate interosseous ligament. The short radiolunate ligament originates from the palmar rim of the lunate fossa of the radius and courses distally to attach to the proximal edge of the lunate palmar horn.

The dorsal radiocarpal ligament originates from the dorsal rim of the distal radius from Lister's tubercle to the sigmoid notch, attaches firmly to the dorsal horn of the lunate and terminates into the dorsal cortex of the triquetrum. The dorsal intercarpal ligament originates proximally from the triquetrum, where it passes radially across the midcarpal joint to attach firmly to the dorsal edge of the scaphoid waist and the trapezoid. The interval between these ligaments is essentially devoid of organized connective tissue.

The scapholunate ligament is a "C-shaped" structure leaving only the distal edges of the joint normally free from ligamentous connections. The ligament is divided into dorsal, proximal, and palmar regions.[7] Examination of the gross and histologic anatomy of the ligament demonstrates that the dorsal region is composed of transversely oriented collagen fascicles, the palmar region is composed of a relatively thin sheet of obliquely oriented collagen fascicles, and the proximal region is composed of fibrocartilage. The radioscapholunate "ligament" separates the proximal and palmar regions.

The radial half of the midcarpal joint is reinforced by two ligaments: the scaphotrapezium and scaphocapitate ligaments. The scaphotrapezium ligament is composed of longitudinally oriented collagen fascicles that connect the palmar cortices of the scaphoid distal pole and the trapezium.[8] The scaphocapitate ligament consists of obliquely oriented collagen fascicles that connect the palmar cortices of the scaphoid distal pole and the body of the capitate, paralleling the course of the radioscaphocapitate ligament.

Mechanics
Kinematics
The kinematics of the carpus are complex and three-dimensional. It is capable of flexion, extension, radial deviation (abduction), ulnar deviation (adduction), and limited pronation and supination. It has been determined that the centers of rotation of the wrist pass through the head of the capitate.[9] Overall, the distal row bones can be considered as a fixed unit, with essentially no clinically relevant intercarpal motion. Because of the strong ligamentous connections and articular interdigitations between the trapezoid, the capitate, and the bases of the second and third metacarpals, the motions of the distal carpal row bones

can be considered those of the hand.

The proximal row bones demonstrate a much more complex motion, both as a row and individually.[10-15] During flexion/extension motion of the wrist, the principal motion of the proximal row is also flexion and extension. The scapholunate ligament allows mutual rotation between the two bones such that the scaphoid rotates through a greater arc of motion than the lunate. Additionally, the scaphoid undergoes supination and the lunate pronates during extension of the wrist.[10,12,14] The combination of this mutual divergent rotation with the different ranges of extension arcs effectively separates the palmar edges of the two bones during wrist extension. The opposite phenomenon occurs during wrist flexion, effectively coapting the palmar edges of the joint. Because of the offset articular surfaces of the proximal and distal poles of the scaphoid, any longitudinally applied load will tend to produce flexion of the scaphoid. As the wrist deviates radially, the trapezium approximates the radial styloid process, effectively pushing the scaphoid into flexion. The scapholunate ligament, if intact, pulls the lunate into palmarflexion as well, although to a lesser degree than the scaphoid. As in flexion of the wrist, the palmar edges of the scapholunate joint approximate during wrist radial deviation. During ulnar deviation, the interaction between the triquetrum and hamate produces extension of the triquetrum, which will drag the lunate and scaphoid into extension through the connections of the lunotriquetral and scapholunate ligaments, respectively. Additionally, the scaphocapitate ligament is felt to pull the distal pole of the scaphoid dorsally, augmented by the presence of the flexor carpi radialis tendon, which passes immediately palmar to the scaphoid distal pole. Thus, the proximal carpal row behaves in a reciprocal fashion relative to the distal carpal row during wrist radial and ulnar deviation. It is important to

recognize that the proximal row represents an intercalated segment, with no direct musculotendinous control. The motions of the proximal row depend entirely on the geometry of the articular surfaces, the ligamentous constraints between the bones, and the resultant proximally directed forces of the muscles attaching distally.

Kinetics
In order to understand the principals of carpal mechanics, it must be understood that all active forces across the carpus are directed proximally by the actions of the extrinsic tendons, which uniformly insert distal to the carpus, or by weightbearing. In a stable situation, these proximally directed loads are balanced by reactive forces focused at the articular surfaces of the distal radius and ulna and the distal articular surfaces of the proximal carpal row bones. In an unstable situation, these proximally directed loads will continually attempt to drive distal bony elements into the more proximal elements. This fundamental concept will be used to explain the patterns of carpal collapse and subsequent degenerative changes that occur as a result of radial-sided carpal instability.

Using a variety of laboratory testing methods, a substantial amount of information has been gained in the last 2 decades about the magnitude and distribution patterns of loads transmitted across the carpus. As a generalization, 80% of the loads across the carpus are directed through the radiocarpal joint and 20% across the ulnocarpal joint, including the triangular fibrocartilage.[16,17] The percentage of ulnocarpal loading increases with forearm pronation (due to the relative proximal migration of the radius), ulnar deviation of the wrist, and with any conditions that effectively shorten the radius relative to the ulna, such as a distal radius fracture with subsidence or radial head resection in an Essex-Lopresti injury pattern. Although developmental minus variance of the ulna is compensated for by a proportionately greater thickness of the triangular fibrocartilage, there is a statistically greater incidence of radial-sided carpal instability associated with this condition.

Load distributions within each joint have also been characterized.[16,17] Relevant to radial-sided carpal instability, the radiocarpal load distribution averages 60% through the radioscaphoid joint space and 40% through the radiolunate joint space. Through the midcarpal joint, again with relevance to radial-sided carpal instability, the scaphoid-trapezium-trapezoid (STT) joint space averages 17% of the midcarpal load, the scaphocapitate joint, 22%, and the lunocapitate joint, 39%. A surprising characteristic of midcarpal mechanics is the very limited joint surface area that is in contact, relative to the total area available for contact: STT = 1.3%, scaphocapitate = 1.8%, and lunocapitate = 3.1%. The values are expected to change with variation in positioning of the wrist or in pathologic malpositioning of individual carpal bones, which will be explained below.

Material/Constraint Properties

Material properties of the scapholunate ligament have been studied in comparison with those of other carpal ligaments. Mayfield and associates[18] determined that the scapholunate ligament failed at an average of 359 N during tensile load application, compared to approximately 160 N for the radioscaphocapitate ligament, 210 N for the volar radiotriquetral ligament (now referred to as the long radiolunate ligament), and 60 N for the radioscapholunate ligament. They also characterized the failure modes, noting that 56% of scapholunate ligament preparations failed within the substance of the ligament, while the remaining 44% failed by avulsion fracture. Nowak[19] reevaluated the material properties of the majority of carpal ligaments, and confirmed the substantial strength of the scapholunate ligament relative to the other carpal ligaments. Only the lunotriquetral ligament

and the palmar region of the capitohamate ligaments failed at higher load applications than the scapholunate ligament.

Recently, the material and constraint properties of the dorsal, proximal, and palmar regions of the scapholunate ligament were studied using isolated bone-ligament-bone preparations from 24 adult intact cadaver wrists. (Berger RA, Imeada T, Berglund L, et al, unpublished data.) Determinations of constraint to mutual rotation and translation as well as of failure strength were made. The dorsal region of the scapholunate ligament was found to offer the greatest constraint to mutual translation, while both the dorsal and palmar regions demonstrated statistically significant constraint to mutual rotation between the scaphoid and lunate. The greatest ultimate failure strength was found in the dorsal region (260.3 ± 118.1 N), followed by the palmar region (117.9 ± 21.3 N), followed by the proximal region (62.7 ± 32.2 N).

Clinical Application
Differential Diagnosis

The differential diagnosis for radial-sided carpal instability is broad, but through the combined efforts of a detailed history, thorough physical examination, and appropriate imaging, the differential list should become substantially narrowed. Included in the differential list should be distal radius fracture, scaphoid fracture, osteonecrosis of either the scaphoid or lunate, dorsal wrist ganglion, inflammatory synovitis or arthritis, dorsal or palmar wrist ganglion, and degenerative arthritis involving the radiocarpal, radial midcarpal, or first carpometacarpal joints. Finally, other forms of carpal instability should be ruled out, including lunotriquetral dissociation and ulnar-sided carpal instability.

Examination of the Wrist

When encountering a patient with suspected radial-sided carpal instability,

information must be sought in terms of the history of the presenting problem. Typically, the patient will complain of pain in the radial aspect of the wrist, often intermittent or constant with an aching quality with sharp pain exacerbations with activities. The patient may complain of feeling a "click" or a "clunk" with wrist motion. There may be intermittent swelling, but this is not a reliable feature of radial-sided carpal instability. Depending on the source of the instability, the patient may be able to define a precise location or zone of discomfort: dorsal-radial wrist in scapholunate dissociation and generally palmar-radial wrist in radial-sided midcarpal wrist instability. There may be a definite history of injury, particularly in an acute presentation, but this recollection is not reliable in a more chronic presentation. The physician should also search out sources of pathology other than radial-sided instability when working through the differential diagnosis. Additionally, during the interview, the physician can gain a tremendous amount of information by simply observing the patient and noting how the upper extremities are being used during gesturing, writing, etc.

Generalized examination of the upper extremities is useful to be certain that more proximal pathology exists. It is always advisable to examine the contralateral extremity. Range of motion of all upper extremity joints forms the foundation of the physical examination, noting if there is pain, stiffness, crepitance, clicks, clunks, or signs of subluxation with motion. Grip strength is measured with a standard, calibrated dynomometer, as are appositional and oppositional pinch strength.

Signs of effusion or tenosynovitis are detected during palpation. At this point, a systematic examination of the wrist is begun, looking for sources of tenderness. With careful orientation, it is possible to palpate virtually every carpal bone and every intercarpal joint. For example, to locate the dorsal region of the scapholunate joint, palpate in the dorsal recess found just distal to Lister's tubercle. To palpate the scaphotrapezium joint, palpate on the palmar surface of the wrist just distal to the entrance of the tendon of flexor carpi radialis into its tendon sheath. The same joint can be palpated deep to the radial artery in the anatomic snuffbox.

Provocative maneuvers have been developed for specific joint pathology, and are quite useful in narrowing the differential diagnosis possibilities. First described by Watson and associates,[20] the "scaphoid shift" test takes advantage of the normal flexion and extension motion of the proximal carpal row during wrist radial and ulnar deviation, respectively. With the wrist in neutral flexion-extension and in maximum ulnar deviation, the examiner places a thumb directly on the palmar skin overlying the distal pole of the scaphoid, found just distal to the point where the tendon of flexor carpi radialis can no longer be palpated. The patient's wrist is then passively radially deviated, while direct pressure is applied to the distal pole of the scaphoid. As noted in the kinematic section above, the scaphoid will palmarflex during this wrist motion. If the scapholunate ligament is intact, the scaphoid palmarflexion will occur in spite of the counter-pressure applied by the examiner. If the scapholunate ligament is ruptured, it will be possible for the proximal pole of the scaphoid, unable to overcome the pressure of the examiner's thumb, to translate dorsally against the minimal constraint of the dorsal radiocarpal joint capsule. A positive test is indicated by dorsal pain in the region of the scapholunate joint and is further augmented with a sense of a "shift" of the scaphoid, which reduces when the wrist is again deviated ulnarly. Pain at the point of pressure application at the distal pole of the scaphoid does not constitute a positive test.

Because of the rarity of the condition, confidence in provocative maneuvers for radial-sided midcarpal instability is marginal, but it may be possible to sense a "reverse catch-up clunk." This is created by applying a longitudinal load across the carpus while passively moving from ulnar to radial deviation. A sudden sense of a shift or clunk through the midcarpal joint as terminal radial deviation is reached may indicate the presence of midcarpal instability.[21]

Imaging of the Wrist

Plain Radiography Standard posteroanterior (PA) and lateral radiographs are required for initial radiographic evaluation of any patient suspected of carpal instability. The position of the shoulder, elbow and forearm can dramatically affect parameters measured in the wrist. The standardized upper extremity positioning for PA radiographs is 90° of lateral shoulder abduction, 90° elbow flexion, neutral forearm rotation, neutral wrist flexion and deviation, and fingers extended. The x-ray source is positioned directly above the wrist. Proper positioning for a true PA radiograph can be confirmed by determining that the ulnar styloid process is located on the most posterior edge of the ulna, little overlap is present at the distal radioulnar joint, and there is no metacarpal overlap. Lateral wrist radiographs can be made with the arm adducted, the elbow flexed 90°, the wrist in neutral flexion and deviation, and the fingers extended. The x-ray source is positioned directly above the wrist. Proper positioning for a true lateral radiograph can be confirmed by identifying the image of the palmar cortex of the pisiform. It should be found at a level between the palmar cortices of the body of the capitate and the distal pole of the scaphoid.

When evaluating the carpal bones on standardized PA radiographs, the following points should be noted. The radiographic geometry of the scaphoid should show somewhat of a kidney-bean shape. Foreshortening of the scaphoid, especial-

ly with the distal cortical ring sign (created by the image of radiodensity of the distal pole cortices) suggests abnormal palmarflexion. The geometry of the lunate can be used to evaluate abnormal palmarflexion (triangular profile) or dorsiflexion (quadrangular profile). Under normal circumstances, the space of the scapholunate joint should not exceed that of the lunotriquetral joint, typically 2 mm or less. Contralateral comparisons are often helpful if an excessive diastasis is discovered. The carpal height ratio of Youm and associates[9] is useful to judge collapse of the carpus. It is defined as the quotient of the length of the carpus measured from the distal cortex of the capitate to the subchondral cortex of the distal radius (through the lunate) divided by the length of the third metacarpal. The normal range for the carpal height ratio is 0.054 ± 0.03.

The lateral radiograph is helpful in evaluating the angular displacement between the radius and carpal bones as well as between the carpal bones themselves. In a true lateral radiograph of a wrist, the cortical profiles of the scaphoid, lunate, and capitate should be identifiable. As such, landmarks on each bone can be identified for the purpose of determining intercarpal angles. The longitudinal axis of the scaphoid normally rests in approximately 40° of flexion relative to the longitudinal axis of the radius. The perpendicular to the longitudinal axis of the lunate normally rests within ± 10° of colinearity of the longitudinal axes of the capitate and radius. Finally, the longitudinal axis of the scaphoid normally rests in between 30° to 70° of flexion relative to the lunate. With the wrist in neutral extension, any dorsiflexion of the lunate > 10° is referred to as dorsiflexion intercalated segment instability (DISI) and palmarflexion of the lunate > 10° is referred to as volarflexion intercalated segment instability (VISI).[22]

Motion Series Although advanced carpal instability may demonstrate changes in the normal radiographic profile of the wrist, there may be a dynamic aspect to the instability pattern that cannot be verified using standard radiographs. To this end, a series of radiographs called a "motion series" has been developed. Included are PA radiographs with the wrist positioned in maximum radial and ulnar deviation and lateral radiographs with the wrist in maximum palmarflexion and dorsiflexion. Some surgeons include a PA "grip" view, which may demonstrate an increase in carpal malalignment resulting from maximized longitudinal loading. The radiographs are inspected to demonstrate any apparent profile abnormality of the carpal bones, unexpected diastases, and signs of subluxation in the various positions of the wrist. Angular measurements from these motion series radiographs are currently not possible.

Fluoroscopy Static motion series radiographs define the end position of the carpal bones at the extremes of wrist motion, but provide no information about the routes that the carpal bones took to get to these terminal positions. It is often helpful to obtain fluoroscopic images of the wrist during all phases of motion, in multiple planes, including oblique views. Subtle shifts in the relative positions of the proximal row bones, for example, may demonstrate dynamic dissociative instability. It is also helpful to videotape the fluoroscopy for in-depth analysis of the images after the radiographic session has been completed. Additionally, a widening in the scapholunate or scaphotrapezium joint with ulnar deviation is highly suggestive of a scapholunate or radial midcarpal instability pattern, respectively.

Tomography Polytomography may be useful if superimposed images of carpal elements, particularly in the lateral views, preclude clear identification of landmarks necessary for determination of intercarpal angles. Computed axial tomography can also be useful in this

manner, as well as to note the interrelationships between the carpal bones within a row in transverse views. Tomography is also useful in staging arthritis.

Arthrography Arthrography has been considered the "gold standard" for carpal instability diagnostic work-ups, especially dissociative instability patterns of the distal radioulnar and midcarpal joints. Even these measures, however, do not guarantee sufficient specificity. Studies have demonstrated abnormal joint contours and even leakage of contrast material between joint compartments in asymptomatic contralateral controls, so caution is advised in interpreting arthrograms. In terms of radial sided-carpal instability, passage of contrast material between the radiocarpal and midcarpal joints through the scapholunate interval is indicative of a tear in the scapholunate interosseous ligament. It is often helpful to videotape the fluoroscopic images for repeat viewing to be certain of the dye flow pattern. With STT dissociation, contrast material may extravasate from the midcarpal joint, and may even provide a tenogram of the flexor carpi radialis tendon sheath.

Arthrotomography Arthrotomography simply implies the application of a tomographic process after injection of a joint with contrast material. This can be accomplished either with linear tomography, trispiral (poly-) tomography or computed axial tomography. It is generally most advantageous to obtain the images in the PA projection. Using arthrotomography, it may be possible to estimate the size of the defect in the scapholunate ligament that is allowing the communication of contrast material between the radiocarpal and midcarpal joints. Unfortunately, it still does not allow determination of the state of integrity of the palmar and dorsal regions of the ligament. Lateral views may be helpful in detailing the angular relationship of the scaphoid and lunate if they are difficult to visualize using standard radiographs.

Computed Axial Tomography Computed axial tomography has limited applications in evaluating radial-sided carpal instability, other than defining bony relationships that might be difficult to visualize from standard wrist radiographs.

MRI Magnetic resonance imaging (MRI) has been reported to be a useful tool in evaluating scapholunate dissociation. Indeed, it is possible to visualize the membranous region of the scapholunate interosseous ligament in paracoronal images. It is, however, nearly impossible to predictably visualize the dorsal and palmar regions of the ligament, let alone determine if they are intact or compromised. This is due to the size of these regions and the obliquity of their fiber orientation relative to the coronal and sagittal planes imaged during MRI examinations. Therefore, MRI is felt to be no more useful than standard arthrography at the current time.

Arthroscopy Arthroscopy represents the best modality currently available for evaluating the status of the scapholunate joint in a minimally invasive fashion. The membranous region of the scapholunate ligament can easily be visualized during radiocarpal joint arthroscopy. The dorsal region is generally obscured from view by a reflection of the synovial lining of the dorsal radiocarpal joint capsule. The palmar region is completely obscured from view from the radiocarpal joint, because it lies deep to the long radiolunate ligament. Although it is generally easy to detect a tear in the proximal, or membranous, region of the scapholunate ligament, the matched curvature of the proximal articular surfaces of the scaphoid and lunate make it is difficult to determine if malrotation is present. However, from the midcarpal joint, it is indeed possible to determine not only angular displacements between the scaphoid and lunate, but also the degree of diastasis between the bones. Geissler and associates[23] have devised a grading

Table 1

Grading of scapholunate dissociation based on midcarpal arthroscopy

Grade	Radiocarpal Arthroscopy	Midcarpal Arthroscopy
I	Hemorrhage or tear in ligament	Little or no angulation, probe not admitted into joint cleft
II	Tear in ligament	Mild angulation between scaphoid and lunate, probe admitted into joint cleft, but cannot be twisted
III	Tear in ligament	Moderate angulation/separation between scaphoid and lunate, probe may be twisted in joint cleft
IV	Tear in ligament	Marked angulation and separation between scaphoid and lunate, 2.7-mm arthroscope passes between radiocarpal and midcarpal joints through scapholunate joint cleft

scale for scapholunate dissociation severity based largely upon the midcarpal arthroscopic examination (Table 1). The midcarpal arthroscopic assessment allows visualization of the distal edges of the scapholunate joint cleft, as compared to the rounded proximal articular surfaces of the scaphoid and lunate, thereby allowing a more accurate assessment of displacement between the two bones. Arthroscopy also allows the surgeon to assess other components of the carpus well beyond the capability of other imaging modalities, including the status of capsular ligaments and articular surfaces of carpal bones.

Scapholunate Instability
Pathomechanics

Scapholunate instability is probably the most recognized of all carpal instability patterns. It was formally recognized by Linscheid and associates[22] in 1972, and was noted to lead to a particular pattern of radiographic abnormalities. Scapholunate dissociation can occur insidiously or suddenly, and may be the result of traumatic disruption or inflammatory conditions such as rheumatoid arthritis. Mayfield and associates[24] have shown that scapholunate dissociation may be a part of an overall progression to perilunate instability. It is generally agreed that the fundamental pathology is disruption of the scapholunate interosseous ligament.[25-27] It is felt that this ligament typically fails traumatically in a wrist positioned in dor-

siflexion and ulnar deviation, possibly with intercarpal supination.[2] Due to the kinematics of the scaphoid and lunate, this position would likely stress the palmar region of the ligament initially, with propagation dorsally. There may be additional secondary changes in surrounding soft-tissue constraints as well, either acutely or chronically with cyclic loading.

Loss of the scapholunate interosseous ligament is believed to allow a chain of events that lead to collapse of the carpus. First, the scaphoid tends to palmarflex, because the dorsiflexing balance of the triquetrum is no longer influencing the scaphoid. This also allows the lunate to dorsiflex with the triquetrum, as the palmarflexion influence of the scaphoid is lost. Radiographically, this creates the DISI (dorsiflexed intercalated segment instability) pattern of carpal instability. Proximally directed forces transmitted through the distal carpal row from the extrinsic tendons of the hand and wrist drive the distal row into the proximal row. The capitate tends to settle between the scaphoid and lunate, often forcing them apart, with ulnar translation of the lunate and further palmarflexion of the scaphoid. The exaggeration of palmarflexion of the scaphoid and dorsiflexion of the lunate leads to abnormal loading patterns across the radiocarpal and midcarpal joints, which is felt to be responsible for the degenerative changes associated with scapholunate dissociation, termed scapho-lunate advanced col-

lapse (SLAC). These loading abnormalities have been verified in the laboratory as well.[28-30] This degenerative process typically begins at the tip of the radial styloid process (Grade I) and progresses along the dorsal half of the radioscaphoid articulation (Grade II). As the capitate articulates with a smaller portion of the lunate, due to its abnormally dorsiflexed attitude, the lunocapitate joint undergoes degenerative changes (Grade III).

Classification

Differentiation must be made between simple tears in the proximal region of the scapholunate interosseous ligament and true scapholunate dissociation. Because the proximal region of the scapholunate ligament is composed of fibrocartilage, age-related degenerative changes may occur. These changes can lead to perforations, which can, in turn, produce an abnormal arthrogram. This does not imply instability, because the important dorsal and palmar regions are likely to still be intact.

Currently, true scapholunate instability should be classified by the scheme proposed by Larsen and associates,[31] which categorizes all carpal instabilities into six parameters: chronicity, constancy, etiology, location, direction, and pattern. It is important to follow and implement this scheme, because currently little information is available that defines which parameters are the most critical, either alone or in combination, for determining the best treatment options and providing a prognosis.

Treatment

The goal of treatment for scapholunate dissociation is to provide pain relief and strength to the affected wrist and to prevent the development of degenerative changes in the articular surfaces of the radiocarpal and midcarpal joints, referred to as SLAC.[32] Treatment options for scapholunate dissociation are varied and depend on a number of factors, including the classification stratification noted above, the patient's general medical condition and age, and the treating physician's skill level and preference. Few data are available that critically analyze the outcomes of the various treatment options, and few guidelines have been published regarding specific points

Closed Reduction

Mayfield and associates[18] have described a mechanical paradox that occurs when closed reduction of a bona fide scapholunate dissociation is attempted. In order to reduce the scapholunate angle, the wrist must be dorsiflexed, which has the inadvertent effect of increasing the diastasis between the volar edges of the scaphoid and lunate. In order to reduce the diastasis between the scaphoid and lunate, the wrist must be palmarflexed, which increases the scapholunate angle. In the acute setting, with normal angles and no appreciable scapholunate diastasis, closed reduction may be attempted, and it is generally believed that a neutral position of the wrist should be maintained in a long arm thumb spica cast for 6 weeks in order to reduce the effects of the aforementioned paradox. It must also be mentioned that substantial motion and loading can occur through the carpus even with a very well conformed cast, which can reduce the effectiveness of closed reduction.

Percutaneous Pinning

Percutaneous pinning, either with closed or arthroscopically assisted reduction, offers a minimally invasive means of enhancing stability through the scapholunate joint while allowing primary healing of the scapholunate ligament to occur. Whipple advocates the use of multiple pins passed across the scapholunate interval, achieving essentially a "chondrodesis" effect. In general, the pins should be left in place 6 to 8 weeks. This procedure may be combined with a simple arthroscopic debridement of the torn membranous region of the scapholunate ligament.[33]

Capsulodesis

A dorsal capsulodesis may be used alone or in combination with any other open technique. Although variations of technique exist, the goal of the capsulodesis is to "suspend" the distal pole of the scaphoid from the radius, thus preventing excessive palmarflexion of the scaphoid. The capsulodesis may also be designed to augment the dorsal region of the scapholunate ligament and/or buttress the proximal pole of the scaphoid against excessive dorsal translation. As originally described by Blatt,[34] a section of dorsal capsule may be advanced into the distal pole of the scaphoid and secured with a pull-through suture. Alternatives include the use of a section of dorsal intercarpal ligament left attached at the scaphoid insertion and detached from the triquetrum.[35] The free end is the passed dorsally and proximally where it is anchored to the dorsal rim of the radius or to the free edge of the dorsal radiocarpal joint capsule. Most surgeons advise that, in the operating room, the scaphoid should not be allowed to flex beyond 30° to 40° following the capsulodesis.

Direct Repair

When a complete scapholunate ligament disruption is present, the remnant of the scapholunate ligament is generally avulsed from the scaphoid. Therefore, an attempt is made to draw the remnant of the ligament on the lunate toward the scaphoid. It may be secured via transosseous sutures passed through the scaphoid or it can be anchored directly into the scaphoid using a suture anchor.[36,37] Two caveats should be stressed here. First, only the dorsal and proximal regions of the scapholunate ligament are approachable from a dorsal perspective. Second, it may be difficult to properly "tension" the repair using a suture anchor technique. In either circumstance, it is strongly recommended that a dorsal capsulodesis be combined with the direct repair, because rotational control of the scaphoid is not reestablished by direct repair alone. Conyers[38] has suggested adding a palmar capsuloligamentous imbrication to direct repair, but this concept has largely fallen into disfavor.

Tenodesis

Recently, the use of the flexor carpi radialis tendon in a tenodesis technique has been advocated. A distally based strip of the tendon is passed through a drill hole in the distal pole of the scaphoid and passed proximally, where it is anchored in the distal radius.[39] This theoretically supports the distal pole of the scaphoid dynamically and statically behaves much as a dorsal capsulodesis.

Ligament Reconstruction

If insufficient ligament remnants are present for direct repair, a ligament reconstruction may be attempted. Several techniques have been advocated, including the use of bone-retinaculum-bone constructs for the wrist or ankle extensor retinaculum, proximal interphalangeal joint collateral ligaments from a central toe, and a loop of a strip of flexor carpi radialis or one of the radial wrist extensor tendons passed through drill holes in the scaphoid and lunate.[40-44] A more elaborate tendon-weave reconstruction has been advocated, which includes a pass across the midcarpal joint.[40] The tendon reconstructions offer the advantage of restoring both the dorsal and palmar functions of the scapholunate ligament. It would be advisable to add a capsulodesis to the procedural protocol if a dorsal reconstruction alone is attempted.

Limited Arthrodesis

Although there are theoretic advantages to soft-tissue stabilization of the carpus, if the carpus is to be stabilized by means other than soft-tissue reconstruction, intercarpal arthrodesis may be used.[45] The most common technique involves arthrodesis of the scaphoid-trapezium-trapezoid joint, or the so-called "tri-scaphoid" fusion.[46] This technique stabilizes the scaphoid to the distal carpal row, thus preventing abnormal palmarflexion of the scaphoid and ultimate collapse of the carpus. Although it is recognized that the scaphoid will not exhibit normal motion if arthrodesed to the distal carpal row, the untoward effect of this seems to be minimal. As an alternative, arthrodesing the scaphoid to the capitate may be technically easier and offers the same radioscaphoid contact load distribution as the scaphoid-trapezium-trapezoid arthrodesis.[47] Other arthrodeses have been attempted, including scapholunate arthrodesis.[48,49] Although this would seem to be ideal theoretically, the nonunion rate is substantial, probably due to the limited surface area of contact and the substantial deforming forces across the scapholunate joint, which will continue to tend to displace the joint. It may be sufficient to place a screw across the scapholunate articulation to act as a tether, regardless of completion of union, but no large series has been completed to validate this concept.[50]

Outcomes of Treatment
Closed Reduction
Few data are available in the literature that evaluate the efficacy of closed treatment. It is difficult to know how many patients with scapholunate dissociation have historically undergone successful closed reduction. Cast or splint immobilization is probably the most commonly employed treatment in the acute setting, for cases in which the radiographic presentation of the wrist is normal. If established radiographic changes consistent with scapholunate dissociation are present, it is currently unusual to find examples of closed treatment. The most comprehensive analysis published to date is from Palmer and associates,[43] who

reviewed five patients with acute scapholunate dissociation. At follow-up, 20% had no pain, 60% had slight pain, and 20% had moderate pain. Wrist range of motion did not differ in this series from that achieved by open repair and reconstruction techniques, averaging 46° dorsiflexion and 44° palmarflexion. Strength averaged 80% of that of the uninjured extremity, and overall patient satisfaction was rated as good in 60% and poor in 40%.

Direct Repair
In the series by Palmer and associates,[43] three patients underwent open reduction and direct repair of the torn scapholunate ligament. Postoperative pain levels were rated as none in 67% and moderate in 33%. Grip strength averaged 53% of that of the uninjured extremity and patient satisfaction rated good in 67% and poor in 33%. More recently, Lavernia and associates[36] reported their series of direct repair with capsulodesis in 24 patients treated an average of 17 months postinjury. The patients had an average loss of palmarflexion of 11°, but all had improved grip strength and pain relief and maintained improved radiographic appearance. Only one patient required occupational changes, and there were no complications.

Capsulodesis
Dorsal capsulodesis may be used alone or in combination with either ligament repair or reconstruction techniques. When used alone for the treatment of dynamic scapholunate instability in one recent series, the capsulodesis resulted in a definite improvement in stability and resulted in an average loss of palmarflexion of 12°.[21]

Ligament Reconstruction
In the acute setting, a strip of extensor carpi radialis longus or brevis, flexor carpi radialis, palmaris longus, or even abductor pollicis longus has been used to reconstruct the scapholunate ligament in

both acute and chronic settings. Palmer and associates[43] identified five patients with ligament reconstruction in the acute setting and 30 patients with ligament reconstruction in the chronic setting without evidence of arthrosis. All of the acute patients experienced pain relief following the reconstruction, with 80% reporting no pain and 20%, slight pain. The range of motion was the same as for the closed reduction and direct repair groups. Grip strength averaged 65% of the contralateral extremity, and overall satisfaction was good in 40% and fair in 60%.

Of the 30 patients treated more than 1 month following injury, all had decreased pain relative to their preoperative status, with no pain in 66%, slight pain in 30%, and moderate pain in 4%. Average wrist motion decreased to 46° of dorsiflexion and 41° of palmarflexion compared with preoperative averages of 52° and 51°, respectively. Grip strength improved in 63%, while 37% felt that their grip strength either stayed the same or diminished postoperatively. Patient satisfaction was rated as good in 73%, fair in 24%, and poor in 3%. Radiographic reviews revealed a persistent DISI deformity of at least 10° in 62% of cases, and the scapholunate gap was noted to be improved in 15 cases, unchanged in six cases, and enlarged in three cases. There was no correlation between radiographic changes and clinical status.

Arthrodesis
Tri-Scaphoid (STT) Arthrodesis
In the original series, Watson and Hempton[46] followed four patients with scapholunate dissociation treated with scaphoid-trapezium-trapezoid arthrodesis and noted marked improvement in pain, 81% of normal range of wrist flexion and extension, and 66% of normal range of wrist radial-ulnar deviation. More recently, a group of patients with rotatory subluxation of the scaphoid treated with triscaphoid arthrodesis were

followed up for an average of 3 years postoperatively.[51] Of the 30 patients studied, none changed occupations, and only four patients had mild pain with use. The average grip strength was 92% of the contralateral side, and the average dorsiflexion was 55° (75% of contralateral) and average palmarflexion was 68° (84% of contralateral). No evidence of degenerative changes was noted radiographically, and no complications were noted postoperatively. Others, however, have reported complications (up to 52%), including nonunion, pin tract infections, and dystrophic changes.[47,52]

Scaphocapitate Arthrodesis

Pisano and associates[47] reported their results of scaphocapitate arthrodesis for the treatment of scapholunate dissociation in 16 patients. Two patients experienced nonunion and seven had pain with mild use. Grip strength averaged 71% of the contralateral side. Range of motion was decreased in dorsiflexion by 28°, palmarflexion by 40°, and radial and ulnar deviation by 14° each, all relative to the nonoperated extremity. Overall, they felt that the scaphocapitate arthrodesis was technically easier than the triscaphoid arthrodesis.

Scapholunate Arthrodesis

Two series have reported results of attempted scapholunate arthrodesis. Hastings and Silver[48] reported the results of scapholunate arthrodesis attempted in five patients, with between 3 and 5 years follow-up.[48] Overall, they noted good results, with painless function and satisfactory preservation of grip, but fibrous union was noted in 66% of patients. Hom and Ruby[49] reported their results for seven patients treated with attempted scapholunate arthrodesis and followed up for an average of 9 months postoperatively.[49] Union was achieved in only one patient. Of the remaining six patients, three had no pain, and three required subsequent surgical procedures.

References

1. Berger RA, Landsmeer JM: The palmar radiocarpal ligaments: A study of adult and fetal human wrist joints. *J Hand Surg* 1990;15A: 847–854.

2. Mayfield JK, Johnson RP, Kilcoyne RF: The ligaments of the human wrist and their functional significance. *Anat Rec* 1976;186:417–428.

3. Taleisnik J: The ligaments of the wrist. *J Hand Surg* 1976;1A:110–118.

4. Berger RA, Blair WF: The radioscapholunate ligament: A gross and histologic description. *Anat Rec* 1984;210:393–405.

5. Berger RA, Kauer JM, Landsmeer JM: Radioscapholunate ligament: A gross anatomic and histologic study of fetal and adult wrists. *J Hand Surg* 1991;16A:350–355.

6. Hixson ML, Stewart C: Microvascular anatomy of the radioscapholunate ligament of the wrist. *J Hand Surg* 1990;15A:279–282.

7. Berger RA: The gross and histologic anatomy of the scapholunate interosseous ligament. *J Hand Surg* 1996;21A:170–178.

8. Drewniany JJ, Palmer AK, Flatt AE: The scaphotrapezial ligament complex: An anatomic and biomechanical study. *J Hand Surg* 1985; 10A:492–498.

9. Youm Y, McMurthy RY, Flatt AE, et al: Kinematics of the wrist: I. An experimental study of radial-ulnar deviation and flexion-extension. *J Bone Joint Surg* 1978;60A:423–431.

10. Berger RA, Crowninshield RD, Flatt AE: The three-dimensional rotational behaviors of the carpal bones. *Clin Orthop* 1982;167:303–310.

11. de Lange A, Kauer JM, Huiskes R: Kinematic behavior of the human wrist joint: A roentgen-stereophotogrammetric analysis. *J Orthop Res* 1985;3:56–64.

12. Kauer JM: The interdependence of carpal articulation chains. *Acta Anat (Basel)* 1974;88: 481–501.

13. Kobayashi M, Berger RA, Nagy L, et al: Normal kinematics of the carpal bones: A three-dimensional analysis of carpal bone motion relative to the radius. *J Biomech* 1997;30:787–793.

14. Kobayashi M, Berger RA, Linscheid RL, et al: Intercarpal kinematics during wrist motion. *Hand Clin* 1997;13:143–149.

15. Ruby LK, Cooney WP III, An KN, et al: Relative motion of selected carpal bones: A kinematic analysis of the normal wrist. *J Hand Surg* 1988;13A:1–10.

16. Viegas SF, Patterson R, Peterson P, et al: The effects of various load paths and different loads on the load transfer characteristics of the wrist. *J Hand Surg* 1989;14A:458–465.

17. Viegas SF, Tencer AF, Cantrell J, et al: Load transfer characteristics of the wrist: Part I. The normal joint. *J Hand Surg* 1987;12A:971–978.

18. Mayfield JK, Williams WJ, Erdman AG, et al: Biomechanical properties of human carpal ligaments. *Orthop Trans* 1979;3:143–144.

19. Nowak MD: Material properties of ligaments, in An K–N, Berger RA, Cooney WP III (eds): *Biomechanics of the Wrist Joint.* New York, NY, Springer-Verlag, 1991, pp 139–156.

20. Watson HK, Ashmead D IV, Makhlouf MV: Examination of the scaphoid. *J Hand Surg* 1988;13A:657–660.

21. Wintman BI, Gelberman RH, Katz JN: Dynamic scapholunate instability: Results of operative treatment with dorsal capsulodesis. *J Hand Surg* 1995;20A:971–979.

22. Linscheid RL, Dobyns JH, Beabout JW, et al: Traumatic instability of the wrist: Diagnosis, classification, and pathomechanics. *J Bone Joint Surg* 1972;54A:1612–1632.

23. Geissler WB, Freeland AE, Savoie FH, et al: Intracarpal soft-tissue lesions associated with an intra-articular fracture of the distal end of the radius. *J Bone Joint Surg* 1996;78A:357–365.

24. Mayfield JK, Johnson RP, Kilcoyne RK: Carpal dislocations: Pathomechanics and progressive perilunar instability. *J Hand Surg* 1980;5A: 226–241.

25. Ruby LK, An KN, Linscheid RL, et al: The effect of scapholunate ligament sectioning on scapholunate motion. *J Hand Surg* 1987;12A: 767–771.

26. Short WH, Werner FW, Fortino MD, et al: A dynamic biomechanical study of scapholunate ligament sectioning. *J Hand Surg* 1995;20A: 986–999.

27. Meade TD, Schneider LH, Cherry K: Radiographic analysis of selective ligament sectioning at the carpal scaphoid: A cadaver study. *J Hand Surg* 1990;15A:855–862.

28. Blevens AD, Light TR, Jablonsky WS, et al: Radiocarpal articular contact characteristics with scaphoid instability. *J Hand Surg* 1989;14A:781–790.

29. Burgess RC: The effect of rotatory subluxation of the scaphoid on radio-scaphoid contact. *J Hand Surg* 1987;12A:771–774.

30. Viegas SF, Tencer AF, Cantrell J, et al: Load transfer characteristics of the wrist: Part II. Perilunate instability. *J Hand Surg* 1987;12A: 978–985.

31. Larsen CF, Amadio PC, Gilula LA, et al: Analysis of carpal instability: I. Description of the scheme. *J Hand Surg* 1995;20A:757–764.

32. Watson HK, Ballet FL: The SLAC wrist: Scapholunate advanced collapse pattern of degenerative arthritis. *J Hand Surg* 1984;9A: 358–365.

33. Ruch DS, Poehling GG: Arthroscopic management of partial scapholunate and lunotriquetral injuries of the wrist. *J Hand Surg* 1996;21A: 412–417.

34. Blatt G: Capsulodesis in reconstructive hand surgery: Dorsal capsulodesis for the unstable scaphoid and volar capsulodesis following excision of the distal ulna. *Hand Clin* 1987;3:81–102.

35. Dobyns JH, Berger RA: Dislocations of the carpus, in Chapman MW, Madison M (eds): *Operative Orthopaedics,* ed 2. Philadelphia, PA, JB Lippincott, 1993, vol 2, pp 1289–1305.

36. Lavernia CJ, Cohen MS, Taleisnik J: Treatment of scapholunate dissociation by ligamentous repair and capsulodesis. *J Hand Surg* 1992; 17A:354–359.

37. Packer GJ, Gill PJ, Stirrat AN: Repair of acute scapho-lunate dissociation facilitated by the "TAG" suture anchor. *J Hand Surg* 1994;19B: 563–564.

38. Conyers DJ: Scapholunate interosseous reconstruction and imbrication of palmar ligaments. *J Hand Surg* 1990;15A:690–700.

39. Brunelli GA, Brunelli GR: A new surgical technique for carpal instability with scapho-lunar dislocation. *Ann Chir Main Memb Super* 1995;14:207–213.

40. Almquist EE, Bach AW, Sack JT, et al: Four-bone ligament reconstruction for treatment of chronic complete scapholunate separation. *J Hand Surg* 1991;16A:322–327.

41. Coe M, Spitellie P, Trumble TE, et al: The scapholunate allograft: A biomechanical feasibility study. *J Hand Surg* 1995;20A:590–596.

42. Minami A, Kaneda K: Repair and/or reconstruction of scapholunate interosseous ligament in lunate and perilunate dislocations. *J Hand Surg* 1993;18A:1099–1106.

43. Palmer AK, Dobyns JH, Linscheid RL: Management of post-traumatic instability of the wrist secondary to ligament rupture. *J Hand Surg* 1978;3A:507–532.

44. Svoboda SJ, Eglseder WA Jr, Belkoff SM: Autografts from the foot for reconstruction of the scapholunate interosseous ligament. *J Hand Surg* 1995;20A:980–985.

45. Augsburger S, Necking L, Horton J, et al: A comparison of scaphoid-trapezium-trapezoid fusion and four-bone tendon weave for scapholunate dissociation. *J Hand Surg* 1992;17A:360–369.

46. Watson HK, Hempton RF: Limited wrist arthrodeses: I. The triscaphoid joint. *J Hand Surg* 1980;5A:320–327.

47. Pisano SM, Peimer CA, Wheeler DR, et al: Scaphocapitate intercarpal arthrodesis. *J Hand Surg* 1991;16A:328–333.

48. Hastings DE, Silver RL: Intercarpal arthrodesis in the management of chronic carpal instability after trauma. *J Hand Surg* 1984;9A:834–840.

49. Hom S, Ruby LK: Attempted scapholunate arthrodesis for chronic scapholunate dissociation. *J Hand Surg* 1991;16A:334–339.

50. Herbert TJ: Acute rotary dislocation of the scaphoid: A new technique of repair using Herbert screw fixation across the scapho-lunate joint. *World J Surg* 1991;15:463–469.

51. Watson HK, Ryu J, Akelman E: Limited triscaphoid intercarpal arthrodesis for rotatory subluxation of the scaphoid. *J Bone Joint Surg* 1986;68A:345–349.

52. Kleinman WB, Carroll C IV: Scapho-trapezio-trapezoid arthrodesis for treatment of chronic static and dynamic scapho-lunate instability: A 10-year perspective on pitfalls and complications. *J Hand Surg* 1990;15A:408–414.

SECTION 4

Hip

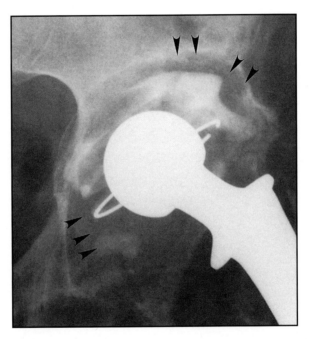

Periprosthetic Fractures of the Acetabulum During and Following Total Hip Arthroplasty

John J. Callaghan, MD

The occurrence of fractures around the femoral component of a total hip prosthesis has been well described, and the treatment options have been studied extensively. However, few reports concerning the occurrence and treatment of periprosthetic fractures of the acetabulum during and following total hip arthroplasty are available.[1-4] In this paper, I will review the literature concerning periprosthetic fractures of the acetabulum and outline measures to prevent and treat the problem.

Historical Review

In 1972, Miller[2] described ischiopubic fractures following the insertion of a Ring component without cement in five hips and following the insertion of a McKee component with cement in four. The fractures failed to unite with nonsurgical treatment, and resection arthroplasty was performed in all of the hips. McElfresh and Coventry[1] documented only one periprosthetic acetabular fracture among 5,400 total hip arthroplasties performed with cement at the Mayo Clinic. Silvello and associates[4] reported the successful treatment of a periprosthetic acetabular fracture (associated with loosening of the component) with revision of the component and bone grafting. More recently, in a study of periprosthetic acetabular fractures following total hip arthroplasty, Peterson and Lewallen[3] reported that long-term survival of the components was poor (eight of ten were revised) unless additional surgical inter-

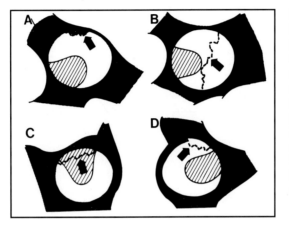

Fig. 1 Patterns of acetabular fractures observed during the insertion of oversized acetabular components. They include anterior wall (**A**), transverse (**B**), inferior lip (**C**), and posterior wall (**D**) fractures. (Reproduced with permission from Callaghan JJ, Kim A, Pederson L, et al: Acetabular preparation and insertion of cementless acetabular components. *Oper Tech Orthop* 1995;5:325-330.)

vention was performed. The occurrence and recognition of periprosthetic fractures of the acetabulum, as well as those of the femur, may be on the rise, especially during the intraoperative and early postoperative periods, because of the need for so-called press-fit stability of total hip prostheses inserted without cement.[5-7]

In Vitro Studies

As fixation of the acetabular component without cement has become the standard construct in total hip arthroplasties, problems associated with this approach are now being recognized. In vitro studies have demonstrated minimum bone-prosthesis micromotion when screws have been used to augment fixation of acetabular components without cement.[5,7,8] Clinical studies have demonstrated durability of 5 to 10 years with this form of fixation.[9-11] However, actual

and potential complications, including inadvertent perforation of vessels,[12-14] screw-fretting,[15] and channels[16] (along screw tracks or through unfilled screw holes) for the access of debris[3,10] have been concerns. These concerns have led to the use of so-called press-fit techniques (underreaming of the acetabulum in relationship to the size of the acetabular component that is to be inserted). In vitro and in vivo studies have demonstrated stability of components inserted with this approach.[5,6,11] In an in vitro study of acetabular components inserted in cadaveric human bone, performed by Kim, myself, Ahn, and Brown, a fracture occurred in four of 15 acetabula that had been underreamed by 2 mm and in four of 15 that had been underreamed by 4 mm.[17] Although most fractures were peripheral, column and transverse fractures also occurred (Fig. 1). Multiple projections were required to demonstrate

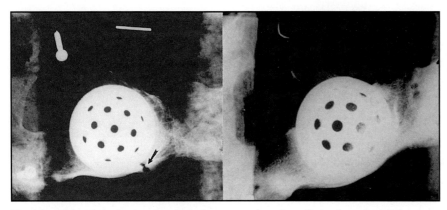

Fig. 2 A peripheral rim fracture (arrow) is demonstrated on the radiograph on the left, but not on the other. (Reproduced with permission from Callaghan JJ, Kim A, Pederson L, et al: Acetabular preparation and insertion of cementless acetabular components. *Oper Tech Orthop* 1995;5:325-330.)

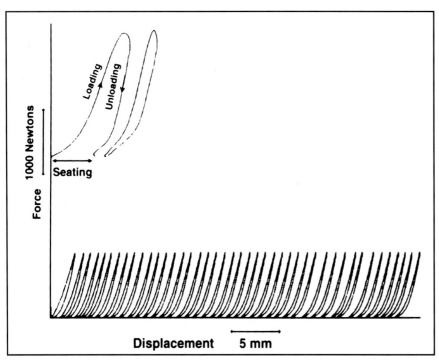

Fig. 3 Load-deflection curves. In both of these recordings, tracings of the individual loading cycles are deliberately offset for clarity. **Top,** The curve on the left shows the advancement of a cup that was oversized by 2 mm; a 2000-N pulse was used. The advancement of the cup is indicated by irrecoverable deformation (that is, the open load-deflection loop) after the unloading-curve segment. However, the curve on the right shows that a subsequent 2000-N pulse failed to advance the cup farther. **Bottom,** Multiple pulses of 1000 N failed to advance the cup. There is no net offset between loading and unloading curves (that is, the load-deflection loops are closed.) (Reproduced with permission from Kim YS, Callaghan JJ, Ahn PB, et al: Fracture of the acetabulum during insertion of an oversized hemispherical component. *J Bone Joint Surg* 1995;77A:111–117.)

many of the fractures on plain radiographs (Fig. 2). In addition, substantial impaction (approximately 2,000 N) was necessary to advance the acetabular component into the underreamed acetabulum (Fig. 3). Even with large impaction blows, gaps between the dome of the prosthesis and the bone were unavoidable (Fig. 4), as demonstrated with studies involving injection of epoxy to make molds and those employing Pressensor contact film.[17-19] When screws are used to secure the acetabular implant to bone, the posterosuperior and posteroinferior regions of the acetabulum provide optimum purchase, especially when bicortical fixation is achieved[20] (Fig. 5).

Clinical Recognition and Treatment
Intraoperative Fractures
I recently collaborated in a multicenter study of intraoperative acetabular fractures following component insertion in underreamed acetabula (Sharkey P, Hozack W, Callaghan J, et al, personal communication, 1997). Eleven of 13 fractures occurred in women who had osteopenic bone. Evaluation of these patients led me to manage this population in the following manner.

Prevention is always better than treatment. Excessive underreaming (greater than 1 mm) is strongly discouraged, especially in patients who have osteopenic bone. In my practice, patients who have osteopenic bone are managed with so-called on-line reaming (reaming of the acetabulum to the size of the acetabular component that is to be inserted), gentle insertion of the component, and augmentation of the fixation with screws through the dome of the component. In other patients, only 1 mm of underreaming is performed. I recommend that surgeons refrain from underreaming by more than 2 mm because of the potential for acetabular fracture and for leaving gaps in the prosthesis-bone interval in the polar portion of the acetabulum.

If a fracture is recognized at the time of surgery and the fracture is nondisplaced and the component is stable, the component is further stabilized by as many posterosuperior and posteroinferior bicortical screws as possible (usually two, three, or four). Only toe-touch weightbearing is allowed for 8 to 12 weeks. If a displaced intraoperative fracture is found, the component is removed and cancellous-bone screws are used to fix the displaced fragment. If the posterior column is involved, a buttress plate is used. On-line reaming is performed, and the component is gently positioned in the reconstructed acetabulum. Fixation of the component to the acetabulum is then augmented with screws through the dome of the implant. Only toe-touch weightbearing is allowed for 12 weeks. If a nondisplaced or minimally displaced intraoperative fracture is recognized during the initial hospitalization and adequate supplemental screw fixation was used at the time of the operation, a spica cast or a brace is used for 6 to 8 weeks with toe-touch weightbearing. If an intraoperative fracture is recognized later than the immediate postoperative period (Fig. 6) and the component-bone construct appears secure, the treatment consists of toe-touch weightbearing with crutches for 12 to 16 weeks. If a displaced fracture with loosening of the component occurs or is recognized late, the fracture should be fixed and the fixation of the component should be augmented with screws. If a patient has pain in the groin in the early period after the insertion of an acetabular component without cement, radiographs in multiple projections (including Judet or fluoroscopic spot radiographs) should be made to rule out an unrecognized fracture. If the fracture is displaced and adequate fixation was used, 12 weeks of toe-touch weightbearing is considered. If fixation is inadequate, I consider application of a spica cast, to be worn for 8 weeks, or a reoperation to augment the fixation with screws.

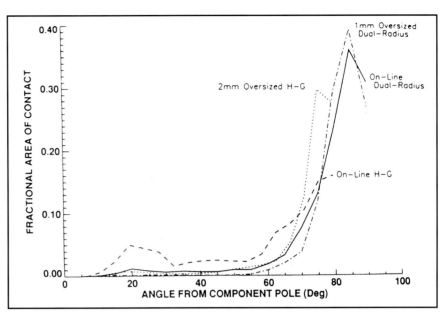

Fig. 4 Graph representing the area of contact between the acetabular prosthesis and the bone, starting from the dome and proceeding to the periphery. A change in the geometry that enlarges the periphery (the outer 1.3 cm of the dual-radius component [PSL; Osteonics, Allendale, NJ] provided better peripheral contact and similar polar contact compared with those provided by the 2-mm-oversized Harris-Galante (H-G) spherical component (Zimmer, Warsaw, IN). The spherical (H-G) component inserted after on-line reaming also provided better contact between the dome and the bone compared with that in the other conditions. (Reproduced with permission from Kim YS, Callaghan JJ, Ahn PB, et al: Reamed surface topography and component seating in press-fit cementless acetabular fixation. *J Arthroplasty* 1995;10(suppl):S14–S21.)

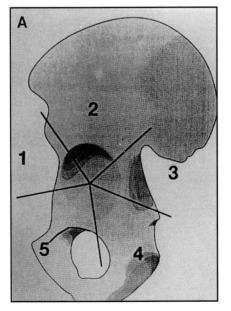

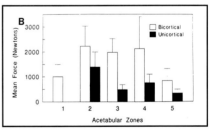

Fig. 5 Left, Schematic of the acetabular zones on the left side of a pelvis. **Right,** Graphic representation of the screw pull-out data recorded in the zones shown in the schematic. The posterosuperior quadrant provides the best screw purchase, followed by the posteroinferior quadrant. Bicortical screw purchase is better than unicortical purchase. (Reproduced with permission from Stranne SK, Callaghan JJ, Elder SH, et al: Screw-augmented fixation of acetabular components: A mechanical model to determine optimal screw placement. *J Arthroplasty* 1991;6:304.)

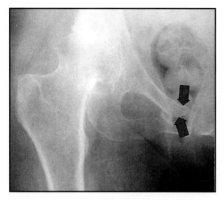
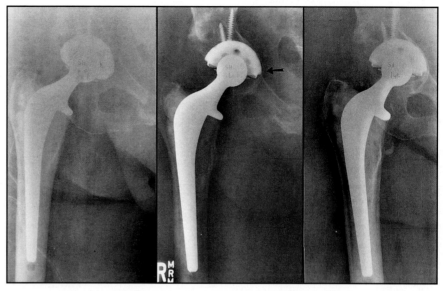

Fig 6 A woman in whom an acetabular component was inserted without cement, with 1 mm of underreaming and screw augmentation, in osteopenic bone. **Left,** Preoperative radiograph showing an insufficiency fracture (arrows) of the pubic ramus. The osteopenia is evident on the basis of this finding. **Left center,** The immediate postoperative radiograph did not show a periprosthetic fracture. **Right center,** At 6 weeks, the radiograph demonstrated a displaced healing periprosthetic fracture (arrow) and a displaced acetabular component. **Right,** At 1 year, the radiograph demonstrated no further change in the position of the acetabular component.

Postoperative Fractures

Peterson and Lewallen[3] recently classified periprosthetic fractures of the acetabulum into two types: type 1 indicates that the acetabular component is clinically and radiographically stable, and type 2 indicates that the acetabular component is unstable. Nine of the 11 fractures in their study occurred around a cemented component. The eight type-1 fractures were treated nonsurgically with toe-touch weightbearing with or without immobilization of the hip with a brace or a spica cast. Although six of these fractures healed, four of the six were associated with eventual loosening of the acetabular component that necessitated revision. I continue to treat acetabular fractures associated with a radiographically stable component nonsurgically, but I explain to the patient that the component may later have to be revised after the fracture has healed. When acute pain in the groin occurs following a total hip replacement, the diagnosis of a periprosthetic acetabular fracture should be considered, as should an insufficiency fracture of the pubic ramus. (I am regularly consulted after a workup for infection, done for acute pain that developed months or years after a total hip arthroplasty, was found to be negative. Some of these patients are found to have evidence of an insufficiency fracture of the pubic ramus on plain radiographs.)

Type-2 fractures associated with loosening of the acetabular component require surgical intervention. In the study by Peterson and Lewallen,[3] one patient was initially seen with an acute injury and migration, into the pelvis, of an acetabular component that had been fixed with screws and without cement. The patient died from vascular injury. Vascular continuity should be assessed in these patients, and preoperative vascular studies are appropriate when the component has migrated into the pelvis. If the fracture involves only the medial wall, and the anterior and posterior walls and columns are intact, a large acetabular component with bone grafting of the medial wall and augmentation of the fixation with screws may provide adequate fixation without cement, especially if at least 1 cm of the peripheral rim is intact. Patients are allowed only toe-touch weightbearing for 3 to 4 months. Elderly patients can be managed with a protrusio ring or cage with medial morcellized allograft and fixation of the acetabular component with cement.

In patients who have a transverse acetabular fracture or a posterior-column fracture, fixation of the posterior column with a plate, filling of the fracture site with morcellized bone graft, and insertion of the component without cement and with screws through the dome usually provide secure fixation. In elderly patients who have discontinuity of the posterior wall or column, or both, I use an acetabular reconstruction cage to secure the superior aspect of the hemipelvis to the ischium, morcellized

Periprosthetic Fractures of the Acetabulum During and Following Total Hip Arthroplasty   Chapter 27

graft at the fracture site, and cementing of the acetabular component.

Discussion

Periprosthetic fractures of the acetabulum are uncommon when the acetabular components are fixed with cement, but they may be more common in association with fixation without cement. Techniques for the insertion of acetabular components without cement, along with the potential for long-term factors such as medial-wall stress-shielding and pelvic osteolysis, may contribute to the potential increase in the prevalence of fractures in association with acetabular fixation without cement. Limiting the amount of underreaming of the acetabulum for the insertion of a press-fit component may prevent an intraoperative fracture. If a stable intraoperative fracture is recognized, supplemental fixation with bicortical screws and a prolonged period of toe-touch weightbearing may be adequate treatment. Stable postoperative fractures may heal with nonsurgical treatment, but the component may still have to be revised. Unstable intraoperative or postoperative fractures must be fixed securely, and the component must be fixed securely to bone. This may require plate fixation of the fracture and supplemental screw fixation of the acetabular component when cement has not been used. When cement is used, a reconstructive acetabular cage may be needed.

References

1. McElfresh EC, Coventry MB: Femoral and pelvic fractures after total hip arthroplasty. *J Bone Joint Surg* 1974;56A:483–492.

2. Miller AJ: Late fracture of the acetabulum after total hip replacement. *J Bone Joint Surg* 1972;54B:600–606.

3. Peterson CA, Lewallen DG: Periprosthetic fracture of the acetabulum after total hip arthroplasty. *J Bone Joint Surg* 1996;78A:1206–1213.

4. Silvello L, Scarponi R, Lucia G, et al: Traumatic loosening of a prosthetic acetabular cup in a young patient. *Ital J Orthop Traumatol* 1985;11:237–239.

5. Adler E, Stuchin SA, Kummer FJ: Stability of press-fit acetabular cups. *J Arthroplasty* 1992;7:295–301.

6. Curtis MJ, Jinnah RH, Wilson VD, et al: The initial stability of uncemented acetabular components. *J Bone Joint Surg* 1992;74B:372–376.

7. Stiehl JB, MacMillan E, Skrade DA: Mechanical stability of porous-coated acetabular components in total hip arthroplasty. *J Arthroplasty* 1991;6:295–300.

8. Lachiewicz PF, Suh PB, Gilbert JA: In vitro initial fixation of porous-coated acetabular total hip components: A biomechanical comparative study. *J Arthroplasty* 1989;4:201–205.

9. Latimer HA, Lachiewicz PF: Porous-coated acetabular components with screw fixation: Five to ten-year results. *J Bone Joint Surg* 1996;78A:975–981.

10. Schmalzried TP, Harris WH: The Harris-Galante porous-coated acetabular component with screw fixation: Radiographic analysis of eighty-three primary hip replacements at a minimum of five years. *J Bone Joint Surg* 1992;74A:1130–1139.

11. Schmalzried TP, Wessinger SJ, Hill GE, et al: The Harris-Galante porous acetabular component press-fit without screw fixation: Five-year radiographic analysis of primary cases. *J Arthroplasty* 1994;9:235–242.

12. Keating EM, Ritter MA, Faris PM: Structures at risk from medially placed acetabular screws. *J Bone Joint Surg* 1990;72A:509–511.

13. Kirkpatrick JS, Callaghan JJ, Vandemark RM, et al: The relationship of the intrapelvic vasculature to the acetabulum: Implications in screw-fixation acetabular components. *Clin Orthop* 1990;258:183–190.

14. Wasielewski RC, Cooperstein LA, Kruger MP, et al: Acetabular anatomy and the transacetabular fixation of screws in total hip arthroplasty. *J Bone Joint Surg* 1990;72A:501–508.

15. Huk OL, Bansal M, Betts F, et al: Polyethylene and metal debris generated by non-articulating surfaces of modular acetabular components. *J Bone Joint Surg* 1994;76B:568–574.

16. Peters PC Jr, Engh GA, Dwyer KA, et al: Osteolysis after total knee arthroplasty without cement. *J Bone Joint Surg* 1992;74A;864–876.

17. Kim YS, Callaghan JJ, Ahn PB, et al: Fracture of the acetabulum during insertion of an over-sized hemispherical component. *J Bone Joint Surg* 1995;77A:111–117.

18. Kim YS, Callaghan JJ, Ahn PB, et al: Reamed surface topography and component seating in press-fit cementless acetabular fixation. *J Arthroplasty* 1995;10(suppl):S14–S21.

19. MacKenzie JR, Callaghan JJ, Pedersen DR, et al: Areas of contact and extent of gaps with implantation of oversized acetabular components in total hip arthroplasty. *Clin Orthop* 1994;298:127–136.

20. Stranne SK, Callaghan JJ, Elder SH, et al: Screw-augmented fixation of acetabular components: A mechanical model to determine optimal screw placement. *J Arthroplasty* 1991;6:301–305.

AAOS Instructional Course Lectures, Volume 47   235

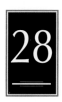

Periprosthetic Fractures of the Femur: Principles of Prevention and Management

Donald S. Garbuz, MD, FRCSC
Bassam A. Masri, MD, FRCSC
Clive P. Duncan, MD, MSc, FRCSC

Peiprosthetic fracture of the femur after hip replacement is a serious complication that can be difficult to treat. Although this complication has generally been considered uncommon,[1,2] in recent years the incidence of these serious complications has increased. This increase is due in part to the greater number of hip arthroplasties being done, especially revision procedures, in which loss of bone stock can lead to a periprosthetic fracture.[3,4] Periprosthetic fractures can occur intraoperatively and postoperatively. Prevention of such fractures is becoming increasingly important because their incidence is rising. Intimate knowledge of the risk factors, etiology, and outcome are needed to prevent or treat these injuries. When these fractures do occur, many factors are involved in the treatment decision.

Intraoperative and postoperative fractures differ with respect to etiology, risk factors, prevention, and management. For this reason this chapter will be divided in two sections, the first will address intraoperative fractures and the second postoperative fracture.

Intraoperative Fractures
Incidence, Etiology, and Prevention
In recent years the incidence of intraoperative fractures has been increasing, largely because of the increase in the use of cementless stems and the increase in

the number of revision arthroplasties being done. With the use of cemented stems, the incidence of intraoperative fracture in primary arthroplasty has been reported to be less than 1%.[4,5] With cementless implants intraoperative fracture has been reported to occur from 3% to 20% of the time.[6-8] Regardless of whether the implant is cemented or cementless, there is a markedly increased incidence of fracture in revision arthroplasty, with rates as high as 6.3% in cemented revisions[9] and 17.6% with cementless implants.

To prevent intraoperative fractures it is important to know the factors that increase the risk of this complication. Two factors already mentioned are the use of cementless implants and revision surgery.[8,10-12] Deceased bone strength resulting from osteoporosis or rheumatoid arthritis[3,13] also puts the femur at risk. Deformities of the proximal femur, as seen in patients with developmental dysplasia of the hip,[14] and previous surgery on the proximal femur other than arthroplasty[5] have also been associated with increased risk of intraoperative fracture. It is important to recognize these factors preoperatively, because careful preoperative planning and attention to specific aspects of the operation itself help prevent intraoperative fracture in the at-risk femur.

Intraoperative fractures occur at spe-

cific times during the procedure and the times differ for primary procedures and revisions. As mentioned, in primary hip arthroplasty intraoperative fracture is most often seen with cementless implants. These fractures typically occur during preparation of the femoral canal or during the final insertion of the prosthesis.[7,8,15] During preparation, fracture can occur while reaming or broaching. Eccentric reaming, in particular, can weaken the femur and predispose it to fracture during reduction or dislocation of trial components.[7] Insertion of the final prosthesis or broaching can result in a fracture caused by the wedging effect proximally as the surgeon attempts to achieve a press fit.[3,7,8] Underreaming distally or the insertion of a straight stem into the normal femoral bow can lead to fracture during final insertion of the prosthesis. To reduce the incidence of intraoperative fracture in cementless arthroplasty, careful preoperative templating is recommended to select an appropriate size implant.[7,8,16] It is important not to undersize the broach because this can lead to a proximal fracture secondary to wedging of the final prosthesis. Care has to be taken to avoid varus reaming, particularly if the greater trochanter overhangs the medullary canal. If there is doubt as to the direction of reaming, an intraoperative radiograph should be obtained to ensure adequate centering of the reamer in the canal. Lastly, during final insertion of the prosthesis, if significant resistance is met the surgeon should check to be certain the level of the rasp and prosthesis are the same. Attempting to insert the final prosthesis further than the rasp can cause a fracture.[11]

If the surgeon believes that the femur is at risk of fracture, cerclage wire, which has been shown to increase the force required to fracture the proximal femur,[17] can be used as prophylaxis before broaching or reaming. Cerclage fixation has also been shown to be effective in preventing crack propagation.[18] This is clinically very useful because a small crack caused by a femoral broach can be prevented from propagating by the use of cerclage wires proximally prior to insertion of the definitive femoral component. Preventing propagation of this crack will reduce the chance of implant-interface instability.

In revision hip surgery or in patients who have had previous surgery on the proximal femur, the risk of intraoperative fracture is increased. In these cases, fracture usually occurs during hip dislocation, cement removal, reaming of the femur, final insertion of the prosthesis.[5,9-11] During dislocation there is increased incidence of fracture in revision surgery as well as in cases where the femur is at risk as a result of local stress risers, such as old screw holes, focal weakening of the femur due to osteolysis, or stem tip impingements. To avoid this complication, any hip that has a plate on the femur should be dislocated first, before the plate is removed. In other cases in which the femur is at high risk of fracture, trochanteric osteotomy and proximal femur skeletonization should be considered prior to dislocation. To prevent fracture during cement removal and reaming, adequate visualization of the femoral canal is required. The use of an extended trochanteric osteotomy[19] will help facilitate cement removal and reaming. Other techniques for cement removal include

the use of cortical windows, but these always should be bypassed by the femoral stem to avoid the risk of postoperative fractures.

Prevention of intraoperative fracture should always be a part of preoperative planning. This planning should include clear documentation of the direction of the old stem as well as any focal areas of osteolysis. During cement removal, the surgeon should point all instruments away from these weak areas to avoid perforating or fracturing the weakened bone. Moreover, if power instruments are used for cement removal, it must be done with great care to avoid perforation.

Knowing which femurs are at risk and paying close attention to surgical technique should help avoid this complication. However, there are cases where intraoperative fractures still will occur, and, when this happens, the surgeon must treat them accordingly.

Treatment
Intraoperative fractures are not always recognized at the time of surgery.[7] When recognized, their treatment depends on their location, configuration, and the stability of the femoral component. With cementless implants, most fractures occur proximal to the lesser trochanter.[7,15,20] These usually occur as a result of aggressive rasping and broaching or during final insertion of the femoral component. Various treatment options have been suggested including cerclage wiring[7,15,20] or the use of a collared component[6,11] to prevent subsidence. In all series, if the prosthesis was stable, a good final result was obtained. Fractures that occur around the stem tip and are recognized intraoperatively present a greater challenge. The surgeon must define the extent of the fracture. These fractures can range from small fissures to perforations to spiral fractures. Whenever possible, perforations and fractures should be treated by the use of a longer stem to bypass the

weakened area.[3,8] Supplemental bone grafting should be considered. Fractures not recognized intraoperatively are often stable and may be managed conservatively with restricted weightbearing. If the fracture is not stable, or is at risk for propagating, internal fixation with cerclage wires and cortical onlay allografting should be considered. The final goals of treatment—to achieve long-term stability of the prosthesis and to allow the fracture to heal—should always be kept in mind.

Postoperative Fractures
Incidence, Etiology, and Prevention
With an increasing number of revision arthroplasties being performed, the rate of periprosthetic fractures in the postoperative period is increasing. It has been estimated by Kavanagh[11] that, while less than 1% of primary hip arthroplasties will be complicated by postoperative fracture, the rate increases to over 4% in revision cases. The true incidence of this complication for an individual hip arthroplasty is not known. Löwenhielm and associates[21] have estimated an accumulated risk of 25.3 fractures per 1,000 hip replacements over 15 years while Beals and Tower[4] estimated that the incidence over the lifetime of a prosthesis is less than 1%.

Risk factors for postoperative fractures can be anything that decreases bone strength.[5] Causes can be general, such as osteoporosis,[5,22] or more localized. Localized problems include cortical perforations, osteolysis, screw holes, or stress risers from a plate or the tip of the prosthesis. In many cases stem loosening is associated with one of these other factors, and this combination can lead to a fracture with minimal trauma.

Cortical defects have long been recognized as a major risk factor for postoperative periprosthetic fracture.[4,5,23-25] These defects can be inadvertent perforations at the time of surgery during cement removal, reaming, or insertion of the femoral prosthesis. Cortical windows

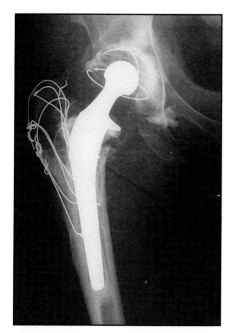 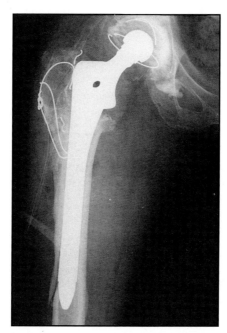 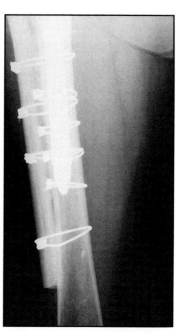

Fig. 1 Left, A 58-year-old female with a loose femoral stem. **Center,** Intraoperative radiograph demonstrating a perforation in the lateral femoral cortex due to eccentric reaming. This femur is at risk of postoperative fracture. **Right,** A cortical strut allograft is used as prophylaxis against the stress-riser in this case.

made for cement removal[4,21,22] can also put the femur at risk.

Cortical perforation is an increasingly frequent problem. Early reports estimated the incidence to be between 0.4% and 4%.[25,26] However, with the increases in revision surgery, this complication has also increased and is estimated to occur in between 13% and 18% of cases.[11,27] Prevention of cortical perforation involves careful surgical technique during the removal of cement at the time of revision. If the surgeon anticipates that the cement mantle is well fixed and that it may be difficult to remove, an extended trochanteric osteotomy will facilitate exposure and cement removal and the avoidance of inadvertent penetration.[19] Another technique used to improve the ease of cement removal is controlled perforation of the anterior femoral cortex.[28] This type of perforation is always recognized at surgery, and is bypassed with a long femoral stem, thus, eliminating the stress riser effect and decreasing the risk of fracture.

Cortical defects, whether perforations, windows, or screw holes, should be anticipated or recognized at surgery. When recognized, they should be bypassed with a long femoral stem.[11,24,29] Experimental work has shown[30] that bypassing the defect by two cortical diameters increases bone strength to 80% of normal, and this is the current recommendation for treatment of cortical defects. In addition to the use of longer stems, cortical strut grafts have been suggested as a prophylactic measure against stress risers (Fig. 1). These struts have been shown to be effective in increasing cortical strength in animal fracture models.[31] At present it is generally agreed that all defects should be grafted in addition to bypassing them with longer femoral stems.

Osteolysis has only recently been recognized as a risk factor for fracture.[3,32] These fractures usually occur in association with a loose prosthesis. Recognition of this impending pathologic fracture and early intervention will make revision eas-

ier than in the setting where a fracture is associated with a loose prosthesis.

Treatment

Although prevention is clearly the best treatment, periprosthetic fractures still occur, even in some cases in which no risk factor is evident.[4] The goals of treatment of these fractures should include a united fracture in near anatomic alignment, a stable prosthesis, return to prefracture function, and early mobilization. Numerous case series have been reported in the literature and there is little agreement on the optimum management. Early series favored nonsurgical treatment,[5,24] but recently there has been a trend toward surgical management.[4,20] Numerous treatment options have been described. These include nonsurgical management, open reduction and internal fixation, revision arthroplasty with a long stem component, or proximal femoral replacement. The choice of treatment depends on the location of the fracture, the stability of the prosthesis, available bone stock, and the age and medical status of the patient.

Early reports in the literature favored nonsurgical treatment, including traction or a hip spica cast.[4,24] The authors stated that the risk of surgery may be too high. However, conservative treatment is fraught with complications for the patient, the fracture, and the construct. Most nonsurgical regimens involve a period of traction. In elderly patients, bedrest can be complicated by such problems as skin ulcers, pneumonia, and fat embolism syndrome. It is advantageous to avoid recumbency in these patients, and this is one of the goals of modern fracture treatment. In addition to medical risks to the patient, nonsurgical treatment has been associated with an incidence of subsequent revision for femoral loosening of between 19% to 100%.[4,12,29] Nonunion rates of 25% to 42% and malunion rates of 45% have been reported with nonsurgical treatment. While nonsurgical treatment should be avoided in most cases there are certain situations in which it may be effective. In a recent series, Beals and Tower[4] showed equally good results with nonsurgical treatment in fractures that were proximal to the stem tip and that had a stable prosthesis. In their series, this accounted for only 15% of the total number of periprosthetic fractures.

As is true for femoral fractures, it is becoming increasingly clear that periprosthetic fractures in general do better with surgical stabilization. This can take the form of intramedullary fixation, extramedullary fixation, or a combination of the two. In extreme cases, proximal femoral replacement may be indicated when bone loss is severe.

Intramedullary fixation can be either prosthetic or nonprosthetic. As has been mentioned previously, periprosthetic fractures are often associated with loose femoral components. In cases in which the femoral prosthesis is loose, most authors would recommend revision with a long-stem prosthesis, which not only addresses the prosthetic stability but also provides the optimum management of femoral shaft fractures with intramedullary fixation. With the use of this technique, the combined nonunion, refracture, and revision rates have been reported to be 12% to 20%.[3] Although most reports in the literature have dealt with long-stem cemented revisions, more recent literature[4] favors uncemented revision in the fracture situation.[3,4,20] In their recent report, Beals and Tower[4] noted a significantly improved outcome ($p = 0.01$) with the use of ingrowth prosthesis versus cemented revisions for the treatment of periprosthetic fractures. In addition to the use of long-stem revisions, many authors advocate the addition of bone grafting to stimulate fracture healing.[11] In cases in which the long-stem prosthesis does not provide sufficient stability, supplementary fixation can be achieved with cerclage wires, plates, or cortical strut allografting. Nonprosthetic intramedullary fixation involves the use of devices such as Ender nails or Zickel nails,[33] but these should be used only in cases in which the implant is stable and does not completely fill the canal. These cases are rare, occurring primarily in fractures associated with Austin Moore prostheses.

Open reduction and internal fixation (ORIF) may be an attractive alternative in cases in which the prosthesis is well-fixed and the fracture is distal. Using standard AO techniques, Serocki and associates[34] and Stern and associates[35] have reported good to excellent results. If the fracture is distal to the stem tip, it is possible to achieve rigid fixation with standard plates and screws. However, in periprosthetic fractures proximal to the stem tip, the screws may violate the cement mantle or may not gain sufficient purchase if a canal-filling cementless device is in place. With cementless devices, there may not be adequate bone into which the screws may be placed. For this reason, plates were introduced that allow proximal fixation with cerclage techniques.[36] Such devices are fixed distally with screws and proximally with cerclage wires, bands, or cables. Union rate has been excellent with this device, approaching 100% in many series.[36-39] While these results with plating are encouraging, others[12] have reported that up to 50% of cases treated by ORIF required revision. Most authors would agree that ORIF should be reserved for cases in which the femoral stem is solidly fixed.[3,4,11] Cerclage wire alone has been shown to be a poor technique.[40] In postoperative fractures its use should be limited to supplemental fixation.

An attractive technique for fixation of fractures with a stable femoral component is the use of cortical onlay allograft.[11] This technique is attractive as it requires no screw fixation and has the ability to restore bone stock and bone strength. Emerson and associates[31] have shown in animal models that strut grafting is an effective technique to restore cortical strength in the presence of a fracture. In a finite element analysis, this technique was found to be as effective as Ogden plates in restoring strength to the femur. Although it is attractive theoretically, there is limited clinical experience in the use of this technique for the treatment of periprosthetic fractures. In our hands, this technique has been very effective, but in a limited number of patients.

Authors' Preferred Method

As the above review indicates, many treatment options exist for postoperative periprosthetic fractures. The goals of treatment should be a healed fracture in near anatomic position, a stable prosthesis, a return to prefracture functional status, and early mobilization. Many factors must be considered in achieving these goals. These include stability of the fracture and the prosthesis, location of the fracture, and quality of the bone stock. Additional factors that must be considered are the patient's medical status and the surgeon's experience. There are numerous classification systems in the literature but few, if any, look at these multiple factors. For this reason, the Vancouver classification was introduced.[41] This classification includes location of the fracture, implant stability, and assessment of the bone stock. The three major types are based on the location of the fracture. Type A involves fractures of the trochanteric region. Type B are fractures either around the stem tip or just distal to it. Type C fractures are so distal to the stem that they may be treated as conventional femoral fractures. The type A are divided into those fractures that involve the lesser trochanter or the greater trochanter. The B fractures that are the most common in most series are subclassified on the basis of implant stability and available bone stock. In type B1 the implant is stable. In type B2 the implant is loose, and in B3 the implant is loose and the bone stock is inadequate because of fracture comminution, severe osteolysis, or osteopenia. Since this classification was originally published, the authors have assessed its intra- and interobserver reliability and its validity (C Duncan, MD, FRCSC, Vancouver, British Columbia, unpublished data, 1997). They found this classification system to be both reliable and valid. In addition, it addresses the major issues of periprosthetic fractures, and this combination of features should make it very useful in planning treatment.

Type A proximal fractures are generally stable, and most series would support nonsurgical treatment with protected weightbearing.[3,4] In most large series, the type B fractures represent the highest proportion of cases. In two large series[4,40] they comprised between 75% and 87% of cases. In the type B fracture, the first decision to be made is if the implant is stable. To aid in determining this, prefracture radiographs and prefracture clinical status may help categorize a patient as a B1 (prosthesis stable) or not (B2 or B3). For patients with B1 fractures, the literature would support ORIF as the best treatment. As previously stated, the authors believe that cortical onlay allograft has several theoretical advantages over standard ORIF, and they advocate this as the treatment for B1 fractures. For B2 fractures, revision and a mid- or long-stem component, with or without cortical strut supplementation, is recommended. The method of stem fixation depends on the preference of the surgical team. B3 fractures are the most difficult to treat and often require replacement of the proximal femur with structural allograft or custom prosthesis. Type C fractures can be treated with standard plates or plates and cerclage, providing the prosthesis is not loose prior to the fracture.

In summary, careful preoperative planning should look at multiple factors when deciding how to treat postoperative periprosthetic fractures. Using the classification scheme we have proposed can allow a logical approach to this difficult problem.

References

1. Olerud S, Karlström G: Hip arthroplasty with an extended femoral stem for salvage procedures. *Clin Orthop* 1984;191:64-81

2. Parrish TF, Jones JR: Fracture of the femur following prosthetic arthroplasty of the hip: Report of nine cases. *J Bone Joint Surg* 1964;46A:241-248.

3. Kelley SS: Periprosthetic femoral fractures. *J Am Acad Orthop Surg* 1994;2:164-172.

4. Beals RK, Tower SS: Periprosthetic fractures of the femur: An analysis of 93 fractures. *Clin Orthop* 1996;327:238-246.

5. Scott RD, Turner RH, Leitzes SM, et al: Femoral fractures in conjunction with total hip replacement. *J Bone Joint Surg* 1975;57A:494-501.

6. Stuchin SA: Femoral shaft fracture in porous and press-fit total hip arthroplasty. *Orthop Rev* 1990;19:153-159.

7. Schwartz JT Jr, Mayer JG, Engh CA: Femoral fracture during non-cemented total hip arthroplasty. *J Bone Joint Surg* 1989;71A:1135-1142.

8. Fitzgerald RH Jr, Brindley GW, Kavanagh BF: The uncemented total hip arthroplasty: Intraoperative femoral fractures. *Clin Orthop* 1988;235:61-66.

9. Christensen CM, Seger BM, Schultz RB: Management of intraoperative femur fractures associated with revision hip arthroplasty. *Clin Orthop* 1989;248:177-180.

10. Taylor MM, Meyers MH, Harvey JP Jr: Intraoperative femur fractures during total hip replacement. *Clin Orthop* 1978;137:96-103.

11. Kavanagh BF: Femoral fractures associated with total hip arthroplasty. *Orthop Clin North Am* 1992;23:249-257.

12. Johansson JE, McBroom R, Barrington TW, et al: Fracture of the ipsilateral femur in patients with total hip replacement. *J Bone Joint Surg* 1981;63A:1435-1442.

13. Poss R, Ewald FC, Thomas WH, et al: Complications of total hip-replacement arthroplasty in patients with rheumatoid arthritis. *J Bone Joint Surg* 1976;58A;1130-1133.

14. Dunn HK, Hess WE: Total hip reconstruction in chronically dislocated hips. *J Bone Joint Surg* 1976;58A:838-845.

15. Mallory TH, Kraus TJ, Vaughn BK: Intraoperative femoral fractures associated with cementless total hip arthroplasty. *Orthopedics* 1989;12:231-239.

16. Reuben JD, Thomas M, Charnov J, et al: Femoral fracture during cementless total hip arthroplasty. *Trans Orthop Res Soc* 1991;16:219.

17. Herzwurm PJ, Walsh J, Pettine KA, et al: Prophylactic cerclage: A method of preventing femur fracture in an uncemented total hip arthroplasty. *Orthopedics* 1992;15:143-146.

18. Incavo SJ, DiFazio F, Wilder D, et al: Longitudinal crack propagation in bone around femoral prosthesis. *Clin Orthop* 1991;272:175-180.

19. Younger TI, Bradford MS, Magnus RE, et al: Extended proximal femoral osteotomy: A new technique for femoral revision arthroplasty. *J Arthroplasty* 1995;10:329-338.

20. Mont MA, Maar DC: Fractures of the ipsilateral femur after hip arthroplasty: A statistical analysis of outcome based on 487 patients. *J Arthroplasty* 1994;9:511-519.

21. Löwenhielm G, Hansson LI, Kärrholm J: Fracture of the lower extremity after total hip replacement. *Arch Orthop Trauma Surg* 1989;108:141-143.

22. Garcia-Cimbrelo E, Munuera L, Gil-Garay E: Femoral shaft fractures after cemented total hip arthroplasty. *Int Orthop* 1992;16:97-100.

23. Missakian ML, Rand JA: Fractures of the femoral shaft adjacent to long-stem femoral components of total hip arthroplasty: Report of seven cases. *Orthopedics* 1993;16:149-152.

24. McElfresh EC, Conventry MB: Femoral and pelvic fractures after total hip arthroplasty. *J Bone Joint Surg* 1974;56A:483-492.

25. Talab YA, States JD, Evarts CM: Femoral shaft perforation: A complication of total hip reconstruction. *Clin Orthop* 1979;141:158-165.

26. Pellicci PM, Inglis AE, Salvati EA: Perforation of the femoral shaft during total hip replacement: Report of twelve cases. *J Bone Joint Surg* 1980;62A:234-240.

27. Callaghan JJ, Salvati EA, Pellicci PM, et al: Results of revision for mechanical failure after cemented total hip replacement 1979 to 1982: A two to five-year follow-up. *J Bone Joint Surg* 1985;67A:1074-1085.

28. Sydney SV, Mallory TH: Controlled perforation: A safe method of cement removal from the femoral canal. *Clin Orthop* 1990;253:168-172.

29. Bethea JS III, DeAndrade JR, Fleming LL, et al: Proximal femoral fractures following total hip arthroplasty. *Clin Orthop* 1982;170:95-106.

30. Larson JE, Chao EY, Fitzgerald RH: Bypassing femoral cortical defects with cemented intramedullary stems. *J Orthop Res* 1991;9:414-421.

31. Emerson RH Jr, Malinin TI, Cuellar AD, et al: Cortical strut allografts in the reconstruction of the femur in revision total hip arthroplasty: A basic science and clinical study. *Clin Orthop* 1992;285:35-44.

32. Pazzaglia U, Byers PD: Fractured femoral shaft through an osteolytic lesion resulting from the reaction to a prosthesis: A case report. *J Bone Joint Surg* 1984;66B:337-339.

33. Pankovich AM, Tarabishy I, Barmada R: Fractures below non-cemented femoral implants: Treatment with Ender nailing. *J Bone Joint Surg* 1981;63A:1024-1025.

34. Serocki JH, Chandler RW, Dorr LD: Treatment of fractures about hip prostheses with compression plating. *J Arthroplasty* 1992;7:129-135.

35. Stern RE, Harwin SF, Kulick RG: Management of ipsilateral femoral shaft fractures following hip arthroplasty. *Orthop Rev* 1991;20:779-784.

36. Ogden WS, Rendall J: Fractures beneath hip prosthesis: A special indication for parham bands and plating. *Orthop Trans* 1978;2:70.

37. Zenni EJ Jr, Pomeroy DL, Caudle RJ: Ogden plate and other fixations for fractures compli-cating femoral endoprostheses. *Clin Orthop* 1988;231:83-90.

38. Wang G-J, Miller TO, Stamp WG: Femoral fracture following hip arthroplasty: Brief note on treatment. *J Bone Joint Surg* 1985;67A:956-958.

39. Montijo H, Ebert FR, Lennox DA: Treatment of proximal femur fractures associated with total hip arthroplasty. *J Arthroplasty* 1989;4:115-123.

40. Partridge AJ, Evans PE: The treatment of fractures of the shaft of the femur using nylon cerclage. *J Bone Joint Surg* 1982;64B:210-214.

41. Duncan CP, Masri BA: Fractures of the femur after hip replacement, in Jackson DW (ed): *Instructional Course Lectures 44*. Rosemont, IL, American Academy of Orthopaedic Surgeons, 1995, pp 293-304.

Periprosthetic Fracture of the Femur After Total Hip Arthroplasty: Treatment and Results to Date

David G. Lewallen, MD
Daniel J. Berry, MD

Postoperative periprosthetic femoral fractures have become increasingly common during the last decade. A wide range of problems, such as comminution and bone loss, are seen in association with these fractures, and the additional challenge of a loose femoral component is commonly encountered. When a femoral fracture occurs in a patient in whom the femoral component is in place, reconstruction may be reasonably straightforward or it may be nearly impossible. Options for treatment have included the use of traction, casts, and external braces; surgical reduction with internal fixation; numerous revision procedures involving insertion of a long-stem femoral component for stabilization of the fracture; and bone-grafting with use of either autogenous grafts or allografts.[1–30] These fractures must be treated according to their individual characteristics, the status of the implant, associated medical conditions, and the patient's level of physical activity.[2,10,16,18] Knowledge of the results in previously reported series and information regarding the range of treatment options can facilitate optimum decision-making with regard to these injuries.

Prevalence of Postoperative Periprosthetic Femoral Fractures

The number of patients who are seen with a postoperative periprosthetic fracture of the femur has increased steadily at our institution during the last 25 years (Fig. 1). Between 1989 and 1993, fracture

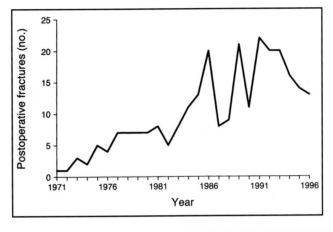

Fig. 1 Number of postoperative fractures of the femur after ipsilateral total hip arthroplasty at the Mayo Clinic during a 25-year period beginning in 1971. (Reproduced with permission of the Mayo Foundation, Rochester, MN.)

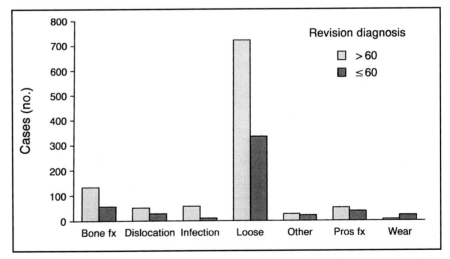

Fig. 2 Diagnoses that led to revision total hip arthroplasty at the Mayo Clinic between 1989 and 1993. Fracture was second only to loosening as a cause for revision, surpassing dislocation and infection. (Reproduced with permission of the Mayo Foundation, Rochester, MN.)

was the second leading cause of revision hip arthroplasty at the Mayo Clinic, ranking after loosening of the implant and

before dislocation and infection (Fig. 2). Reports have suggested an overall prevalence of between 0.1% and 1.1%, with ten

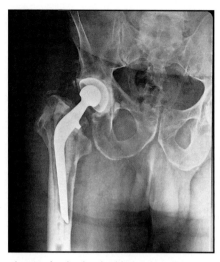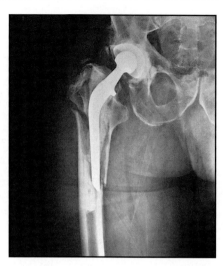

Fig. 3 Left, This hip had loosening of the implant, osteolysis, and pain 7 years after a total hip arthroplasty. The patient was advised to have a revision but refused. **Right,** Three months later, after a misstep, the patient sustained a periprosthetic fracture through an osteolytic defect.

postoperative periprosthetic fractures (0.2%) found in 5,400 patients in one of the largest series. However, these estimates apply to patients who had a femoral component that was inserted with cement and include both primary and revision total hip arthroplasties.[1,26,31–33] The time from the arthroplasty to the fracture ranged from 6 weeks to 10 years in these reports. Löwenhielm and associates,[32] reporting on a series of 1,442 primary hip arthroplasties performed with use of cement, calculated the cumulative postoperative risk of fracture to be 25.3 per 1,000 at 15 years. A survey of all records on total hip arthroplasties performed at the Mayo Clinic between 1969 and 1990, conducted with use of a computerized database from the Total Joint Registry, revealed a rate of femoral fracture of 0.6% after 17,579 primary procedures performed with cement and a rate of 0.4% after 2,078 such procedures performed without cement during the same time-period. The rates were higher after revision procedures (2.8% after 3,265 procedures performed with cement compared with 1.5% after 1,132 procedures performed without cement).

One factor that has contributed to the

increased prevalence of periprosthetic femoral fractures is the greater proportion of the population that is at risk. It has been 28 years since total hip arthroplasty was introduced in the United States; more than 120,000 primary procedures are carried out each year, and this number is growing steadily.[20] In contrast to patterns of practice in the 1970s and the early 1980s, the indications for the procedure now include younger patients, heavier patients, and those who have severe bone loss.[20] Other factors that have contributed to the greater prevalence of these fractures include an increase in the number of patients having revision hip arthroplasty and an increase in the number having more than one such procedure. Many of these revisions are related to the cumulative effects of particles of debris in the joint, as periprosthetic osteolysis increases the risk of fracture[16,24,34] (Fig. 3).

Treatment

Prevention of fractures of the femur following total hip arthroplasty is preferable to even the most successful treatment options. Preventive measures that have been recommended for use during the initial arthroplasty include avoiding the

creation of cracks, defects, or windows in the bone intraoperatively and, if these stress-risers are present, bypassing them with a stem of sufficient length that they end two to three cortical diameters distal to the defect.[35–40] Extravasation of cement out of the bone defects should be avoided as this can facilitate subsequent fracture through the unhealed stress-riser[35] (Fig. 4, *left*). The use of cerclage wires for the fixation of periprosthetic cracks produced intraoperatively has been recommended to prevent propagation and a complete fracture.[7,41–43] Bone-grafting of defects also is recommended to allow resolution of the stress-riser effect over time.

Regular radiographic follow-up of all patients who have had a total hip arthroplasty is essential for the detection of major osteolytic defects that may lead to a periprosthetic fracture as well as to failure and loosening of the implant.[20,24] At our institution, all patients who have had an arthroplasty are followed with anteroposterior, lateral, and oblique radiographs at 1, 2, 5, 7, and 10 years postoperatively and every 2 to 3 years thereafter. Radiographs should be made more often if lysis develops or if other radiographic changes warrant increased surveillance. Many of the more challenging problems associated with periprosthetic fractures are due as much to inadequate radiographic follow-up as to the type of implant and the materials that were used. Revision is recommended before extensive bone loss and a resultant periprosthetic fracture have occurred, thereby obviating the need for more extensive surgical treatment, which is associated with a greater risk of residual functional impairment. Periprosthetic fractures can be avoided only if regular radiographic follow-up is performed as recommended by the 1994 National Institutes of Health Consensus Conference on total hip replacement.[20]

Options for the treatment of postoperative periprosthetic femoral fractures have included protection of the frac-

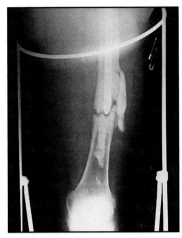
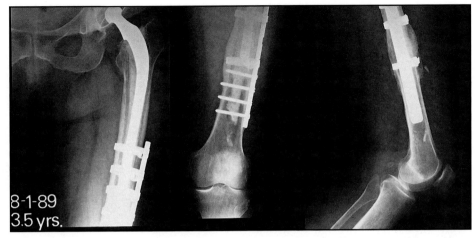

Fig. 4 Left, Periprosthetic fracture through an area of cortical perforation and extravasation of cement at the time of a revision total hip arthroplasty. Bone-grafting of any defects and avoidance of extravasation of cement can reduce the risk of fracture across this type of stress-riser. **Right,** Treatment in the presence of a well-fixed stem consisted of insertion of a plate with screws distally and cerclage bands proximally, with bone-grafting of the fracture line and the defect. The patient eventually had a solid union.

ture;[11] traction;[1,2,15,18,44] use of casts and braces;[18] and internal fixation with use of cerclage wires or cables,[2,18] screws with and without plates,[2,18,27] and special plates that have claws, bands, or cerclage wires to allow fixation in the region of the intramedullary stem[9,14,21,23,30,45] (Fig. 4, *right*). Another option for treatment is revision of the femoral component, which is frequently necessary if the fracture occurs adjacent to a loose implant. These revisions have been performed with a stem inserted with cement; a long stem with proximal or extensive porous coating, inserted without cement; a composite consisting of an allograft and a prosthesis; a proximal femoral replacement stem; and a custom implant, stem sleeve, or extension.[1,2,10,13,16,17,25,34,46] Each of these options for revision can be combined with cancellous bone-grafting or with strut allograft in the region of the fracture[47] (Fig. 5). A construct consisting of an allograft and a prosthesis should be reserved for patients who have massive proximal femoral bone loss severe enough to preclude standard reconstruction[10] (Fig. 6). In patients who have massive bone loss and a fracture, are more than 70 years of age, and place low demands on the hip, a modular proximal

femoral replacement stem may be used (Fig. 7). The appropriate treatment for a patient must be determined on the basis of the availability of the materials needed for a particular method of reconstruction; the familiarity of the surgeon with the technique in question; patient-related factors such as age, level of activity, bone quality, and configuration of the fracture; and the results that have been reported for the method under consideration.[2,10,18,48–54]

Results of Treatment

Johansson and associates,[15] in 1981, reported on a series of 23 intraoperative and 14 postoperative periprosthetic femoral fractures. The fractures had been treated with various methods, including traction, internal fixation with cerclage wires and plates, revision with a long-stem implant, and resection arthroplasty. Of the 14 postoperative fractures, eight were associated with complications. Only five of the arthroplasties that were followed by a postoperative fracture eventually yielded a satisfactory result.[15] Bethea and associates,[4] in a subsequent report, noted an association between postoperative fracture and previous procedures on the hip or a loose implant. Of 31 hips

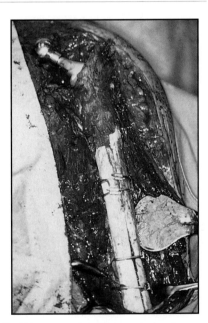

Fig. 5 Intraoperative photograph showing onlay cortical strut allograft held with cerclage cables spanning a periprosthetic fracture.

that had a fracture 4 weeks to 10 years after the arthroplasty, 18 (58%) had had at least two previous operations and 23 (74%) had had loosening of the implant or osteolysis before the fracture. A number of methods were used for treatment; nonsurgical treatment yielded the poorest results, whereas a revision with use of a

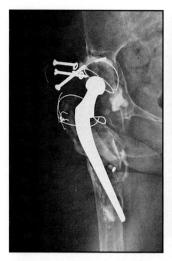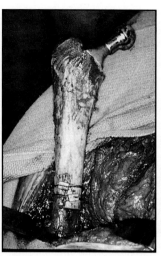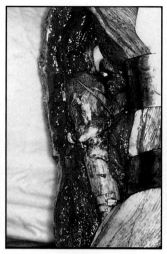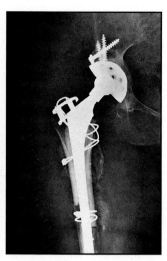

Fig 6 Left, Radiograph of a hip with loosening, osteolysis, and a periprosthetic fracture that was neglected because of inadequate medical and radiographic follow-up. **Center left,** Intraoperative photograph showing replacement of the damaged proximal aspect of the femur with a composite consisting of an allograft and a prosthesis. The procedure involved a step-cut osteotomy and cerclage wiring. The long stem of the femoral component spanned the site of the osteotomy. **Center right,** The proximal femoral remnants and the trochanter were preserved and secured to the allograft to improve function and stability of the hip. **Right,** Radiograph showing the final construct.

long-stem prosthesis yielded the best results.

Adolphson and associates[1] reported the results of treatment of postoperative fracture in 29 patients, 21 of whom had been managed with traction and eight of whom had been managed surgically. This report is important because it emphasizes the high rate of complications associated with traction. Of the 21 patients who had been managed with traction, six needed a subsequent operation because of malunion or malalignment, although all had healing of the original fracture. In contrast, three of the eight patients who had been managed surgically had a nonunion.[1]

Mont and Maar,[18] in an effort to analyze the results in a larger number of patients, reviewed 26 articles published between 1964 and 1991. The 487 patients described in those articles were stratified according to the location of the periprosthetic fracture and the type of treatment. These authors did not distinguish between patients according to the status of the fixation before the fracture, according to whether a revision had been done with or without cement, according

to whether or not bone-grafting had been done, or according to the type of graft. The fractures were categorized into five types on the basis of location, with supracondylar fractures constituting a sixth type. The rates of satisfactory results varied among the different types of fractures and the different methods of treatment. The result of traction was satisfactory for 57% of the 46 fractures that were located along the length of the stem, 43% of the 58 that were at the tip of the stem, and 77% of the 77 that were just distal to the tip of the stem. Treatment with cerclage wires alone was less successful when it was used for fractures distal to the tip of the stem than when it was used for more proximal fractures around the stem. The use of plates and screws was satisfactory treatment for seven of 15 fractures occurring along the length of the stem, 12 (48%) of 25 at the tip of the stem, and 28 (49%) of 57 distal to the tip of the stem.[18]

Beals and Tower[2] reported the results of treatment of 93 fractures in 86 patients who had had an arthroplasty performed by one of 30 different orthopaedic surgeons. Nine fractures failed to heal; therefore, the results of 102 interventions

were reported. (One fracture needed to be treated three times.) The average time to the fracture post-arthroplasty was 4.7 years; 38% of the patients had had a previous fracture of a type commonly associated with osteoporosis. The etiology could be determined for 82 fractures. Eighty-four percent were due to a fall; 8%, trauma; and 8%, spontaneous fracture. Before the fracture, the original implant had been a well-fixed cemented stem (45%), a loose cemented stem (23%), an ingrowth implant (25%), or an Austin-Moore-type stem (7%). Of the 102 surgical interventions elected by the operating surgeon, 34% consisted of implantation of an ingrowth femoral stem; 15%, revision to a stem inserted with cement; and 23%, internal fixation with use of plates, screws, or lag screws. The remaining 28% of the interventions were nonsurgical. Despite the extremely small number of interventions that were nonsurgical, complications were common, with traction resulting in a 45% rate of malunion or marked shortening of the femur and an 11% rate of nonunion. The use of lag screws alone resulted in a new fracture at the site of the screw or a nonunion after a few procedures. Of the 102 procedures involving plate fixation, 15% resulted in a new fracture and another two procedures resulted in failure of the fixation. A prosthesis, inserted with cement for revision in an additional 15% of the 102 procedures, was associated with a 31% rate of nonunion and a 15% rate of refracture. A prosthesis, inserted without cement for revision in 34% of the procedures, was associated with the best results in the series; shortening was noted after 7% of the procedures and a new fracture, after 7%, but the implant subsided after 18% of the procedures. To analyze the results of treatment, Beals and Tower[2] used a system based on the fixation of the stem and the healing status of the fracture. An excellent result was defined as a stable implant and a healed fracture; a good result, as a stable stem with some subsidence and a healed fracture with mild or moderate deformity; and a poor result, as a loose stem, nonunion, deep infection, a new fracture, or severe deformity. In this cumulative series, 32% of the interventions led to an excellent result; 16%, a good result; and 52%, a poor result.

A recent review presented the results of revision total hip arthroplasty for the treatment of 97 postoperative periprosthetic femoral fractures in 94 patients who had been managed from 1971 to 1993 at our institution. The average duration of follow-up was nearly 5 years (range, 2 to 14 years); within 2 years, three implants had failed, three patients had died, and one patient had been lost to follow-up. The fractures were categorized with use of the Vancouver classification system,[10] which defines trochanteric fractures as type A, fractures about the stem or the tip of the stem as type B, and fractures well distal to the tip as type C. Type-B fractures are further subdivided into those adjacent to a well-fixed stem (type B1), those adjacent to a loose stem (type B2), and those associated with marked osseous deficiency or destruction around the implant (type B3).[10] Approximately 60% of the fractures were type B2, and 25% were type B3. Approximately 85% of the fractures united; 15% did not. Stable long-term fixation of the stem was achieved in less than 50% of the hips. Although more than 50% of the hips had a loose femoral implant at the latest follow-up evaluation, more than 20% had no pain or only minimum symptoms despite radiographic signs of subsidence or loosening. However, approximately 33% had loosening and severe pain. Long-stem femoral components inserted with cement, proximally porous-coated long-stem components inserted without cement, and extensively porous-coated components inserted without cement all were used during the revision procedures. Insertion of a proximally porous-coated implant without cement was associated with the poorest results. An important observation was the development of a spontaneous fracture, in the absence of a fall or another inciting traumatic event, in more than 50% of the patients who had a type-B3 fracture, in which bone loss and comminution are most severe; several of these patients had had no symptoms before the spontaneous fracture occurred. This finding reinforces the importance of regular radiographic follow-up after hip arthroplasty, in order to look for the massive bone loss characteristic of type-B3 fractures, which may be asymptomatic before catastrophic failure occurs.

Treatment Recommendations

Of the available classification systems, we currently prefer the Vancouver system, because it helps to guide treatment choices.[10] The treatment of type-A fractures involving the greater or lesser trochanter depends on the underlying cause of the avulsion fracture. If the cause is severe periprosthetic osteolysis, then a revision is indicated to debride the osteolytic defects and to replace the component that

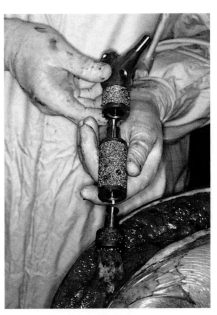

Fig. 7 A modular proximal femoral replacement stem, which can be useful for the treatment of massive bone loss and a fracture of the proximal part of the femur. This implant is an alternative to the construct consisting of an allograft and a prosthesis, especially in an older patient.

is the source of the particles of debris, whereas simple avulsion of fragments of the greater or lesser trochanter in patients who have osteoporosis may be treated nonsurgically in the presence of a well-fixed stem. Type-B1 fractures, which, by definition, are associated with a well-fixed stem, often can be treated with internal fixation. However, in patients who have a so-called first-generation implant and other problems related to the bearing surface or the position of the stem, revision may be preferable if it can be done without excessive bone damage. Type-C fractures (those well distal to a solidly fixed stem) are best treated with internal fixation unless they are minimally displaced and the position can be maintained with nonsurgical measures that do not require the patient to be recumbent for prolonged periods. All types of fractures associated with a loose femoral component are best treated with a revision, with possible rare exceptions

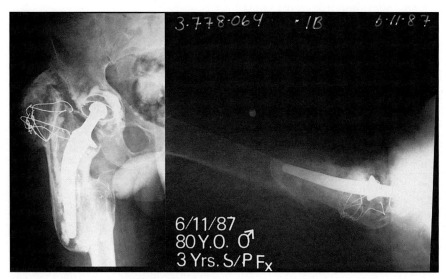

Fig. 8 Radiographs made after ill advised closed treatment, with traction, of a periprosthetic fracture associated with a loose stem. Malunion and painful loosening mandated an extensive revision procedure despite what was considered to be a successful union by the treating physician after prolonged immobilization.

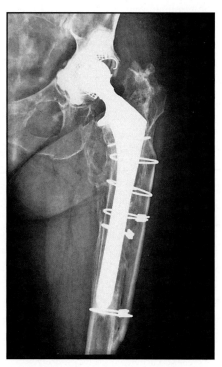

Fig. 9 Onlay strut-grafting and use of an extensively porous-coated stem resulted in fracture-healing and a stable implant.

dictated by unusual medical problems or advanced age. For all but the most debilitated patients, revision offers the best chance of achieving not only stable fixation and union of the fracture but also a functional hip and the highest over-all level of function for the patient (Fig. 8).

Several principles should be observed when a revision is performed for the treatment of a periprosthetic fracture. These include preservation of the bone stock whenever possible and achievement of stable fixation of the stem into intact host bone. This often necessitates distal fixation of the stem, which can be accomplished reliably with use of cement, with use of an extensively porous-coated stem, or with use of a stem that has grooves or slots if the diaphyseal bone segment is relatively intact. When cement is used, care should be taken to prevent it from interdigitating into the fracture fragments, as this can inhibit union. We have found that monobloc, proximally porous-coated, distally smooth femoral stems have performed poorly in routine revision situations.[55,56] This disappointing experience has also

been borne out in association with fractures. However, it is important to note that none of these situations involved stems with trochanteric bolts or distal slots and grooves, which have been designed for the enhanced stability of proximally coated implants.

After a revision, cancellous bone-grafting of all fracture lines is recommended. Strut-grafting with cerclage wires is a reliable method for restoring osseous stability at the fracture site and for promoting union (Fig. 9). The use of a construct consisting of an allograft and a prosthesis or the use of a proximal femoral replacement stem should be reserved for hips with the most severe bone loss that cannot be reconstructed with standard methods. When either of these implants is used, it is helpful to preserve the proximal bone fragments and to wrap them around the component or the allograft, employing cerclage wires or cables in order to preserve the soft-tissue attachments, improve stability of the hip, and promote union. The use of a constrained acetabular insert or a bipolar articulation is reasonable when a proxi-

mal femoral replacement stem and a large allograft is used or when the presence of poor abductor and soft-tissue attachments proximally lead to concerns about stability.

In conclusion, periprosthetic femoral fractures can present a major reconstructive challenge, but a wide variety of treatment options are available. Classification of the fracture, with assessment not only of its location but also of the fixation of the stem and the quality of the bone, allows a rational choice of reconstructive options for the management of these patients.

References
1. Adolphson P, Jonsson U, Kalen R: Fractures of the ipsilateral femur after total hip arthroplasty. *Arch Orthop Trauma Surg* 1987;106:353–357.

2. Beals RK, Tower SS: Periprosthetic fractures of the femur: An analysis of 93 fractures. *Clin Orthop* 1996;327:238–246.

3. Berman AT, Levenberg RJ: Femur fractures associated with total hip arthroplasty. *Orthopedics* 1992;15:751–753.

4. Bethea JS III, DeAndrade JR, Fleming LL, et al: Proximal femoral fractures following total hip arthroplasty. *Clin Orthop* 1982;170:95–106.

5. Booth RE Jr: Management of periprosthetic fractures. *Orthopedics* 1994;17:845–847.

6. Charnley J: The healing of human fractures in contact with self-curing acrylic cement. *Clin Orthop* 1966;47:157–163.

7. Christensen CM, Seger BM, Schultz RB: Management of intraoperative femur fractures associated with revision hip arthroplasty. *Clin Orthop* 1989;248:177–180.

8. Cooke PH, Newman JH: Fractures of the femur in relation to cemented hip prostheses. *J Bone Joint Surg* 1988;70B:386–389.

9. Dave DJ, Koka SR, James SE: Mennen plate fixation for fracture of the femoral shaft with ipsilateral total hip and knee arthroplasties. *J Arthroplasty* 1995;10:113–115.

10. Duncan CP, Masri BA: Fractures of the femur after hip replacement, in Jackson DW (ed): *Instructional Course Lectures 44*. Rosemont, IL, American Academy of Orthopaedic Surgeons, 1995, pp 293–304.

11. Dysart SH, Savory CG, Callaghan JJ: Non-operative treatment of a postoperative fracture around an uncemented porous-coated femoral component. *J Arthroplasty* 1989;4:187–190.

12. Garcia-Cuimbrelo E, Munuera L, Gil-Garay E: Femoral shaft fractures after cemented total hip arthroplasty. *Int Orthop* 1992;16:97–100.

13. Huo MH, Keggi KJ: Periprosthetic femoral fracture treatment with an intramedullary extension sleeve. *J Orthop Tech* 1994;2:191–195.

14. Jensen TT, Overgaard S, Mossing NB: Partridge Cerclene system for femoral fractures in osteoporotic bones with ipsilateral hemi/total arthroplasty. *J Arthroplasty* 1990;5:123–126.

15. Johansson JE, McBroom R, Barrington TW, et al: Fracture of the ipsilateral femur in patients with total hip replacement. *J Bone Joint Surg* 1981;63A:1435–1442.

16. Kelley SS: Periprosthetic femoral fractures. *J Am Acad Orthop Surg* 1994;2:164–172.

17. Kolstad K: Revision THR after periprosthetic femoral fractures: An analysis of 23 cases. *Acta Orthop Scand* 1994;65:505–508.

18. Mont MA, Maar DC: Fractures of the ipsilateral femur after hip arthroplasty: A statistical analysis of outcome based on 487 patients. *J Arthroplasty* 1994;9:511–519.

19. Montijo H, Ebert FR, Lennox DA: Treatment of proximal femur fractures associated with total hip arthroplasty. *J Arthroplasty* 1989;4:115–123.

20. National Institutes of Health: National Institutes of Health Consensus Conference: Total hip replacement. *JAMA* 1995;273:1950–1956.

21. Ogden WS, Rendall J: Fractures beneath hip prostheses: A special indication for Parham bands and plating. *Orthop Trans* 1978;2:70.

22. Pankovich AM, Tarabishy I, Barmada R: Fractures below non-cemented femoral implants: Treatment with Ender nailing. *J Bone Joint Surg* 1981;63A:1024–1025.

23. Partridge AJ, Evans PE: The treatment of fractures of the shaft of the femur using nylon cerclage. *J Bone Joint Surg* 1982;64B:210–214.

24. Pazzaglia U, Byers PD: Fractured femoral shaft through an osteolytic lesion resulting from the reaction to a prosthesis: A case report. *J Bone Joint Surg* 1984;66B:337–339.

25. Ries MD: Intraoperative modular stem lengthening to treat periprosthetic femur fracture. *J Arthroplasty* 1996;11:204–205.

26. Scott RD, Turner RH, Leitzes SM, et al: Femoral fractures in conjunction with total hip replacement. *J Bone Joint Surg* 1975;57A:494–501.

27. Serocki JH, Chandler RW, Dorr LD: Treatment of fractures about hip prostheses with compression plating. *J Arthroplasty* 1992;7:129–135.

28. Stern RE, Harwin SF, Kulick RG: Management of ipsilateral femoral shaft fractures following hip arthroplasty. *Orthop Rev* 1991;20:779–784.

29. Whittaker RP, Sotos LN, Ralston EL: Fractures of the femur about femoral endoprostheses. *J Trauma* 1974;14:675–694.

30. Zenni EJ Jr, Pomeroy DL, Caudle RJ: Ogden plate and other fixations for fractures complicating femoral endoprostheses. *Clin Orthop* 1988;231:83–90.

31. Fredin HO, Lindberg H, Carlsson AS: Femoral fracture following hip arthroplasty. *Acta Orthop Scand* 1987;58:20–22.

32. Löwenhielm G, Hansson LI, Kärrholm J: Fracture of the lower extremity after total hip replacement. *Arch Orthop Trauma Surg* 1989;108:141–143.

33. McElfresh EC, Coventry MB: Femoral and pelvic fractures after total hip arthroplasty. *J Bone Joint Surg* 1974;56A:483–492.

34. Reich SM, Jaffe WL: Femoral fractures associated with loose cemented total hip arthroplasty. *Orthopedics* 1994;17:185–189.

35. Eschenroeder HC Jr, Krackow KA: Late onset femoral stress fracture associated with extruded cement following hip arthroplasty: A case report. *Clin Orthop* 1988;236:210–213.

36. Fredin H: Late fracture of the femur following perforation during hip arthroplasty: A report of 2 cases. *Acta Orthop Scand* 1988;59:331–332.

37. Larson JE, Chao EYS, Fitzgerald RH: Bypassing femoral cortical defects with cemented intramedullary stems. *J Orthop Res* 1991;9:414–421.

38. Lotke PA, Wong RY, Ecker ML: Stress fracture as a cause of chronic pain following revision total hip arthroplasty: Report of two cases. *Clin Orthop* 1986;206:147–150.

39. Morrey BF, Kavanagh BF: Complications with revision of the femoral component of total hip arthroplasty: Comparison between cemented and uncemented techniques. *J Arthroplasty* 1992;7:71–79.

40. Stuchin S: Femoral shaft fracture in porous and press-fit total hip arthroplasty. *Orthop Rev* 1990;19:153–159.

41. Federici A, Carbone M, Sanguineti F: Intraoperative fractures of the femoral diaphysis in hip arthroprosthesis surgery. *Ital J Orthop Traumatol* 1988;14:311–321.

42. Fitzgerald RH Jr, Brindley GW, Kavanagh BF: The uncemented total hip arthroplasty: Intraoperative femoral fractures. *Clin Orthop* 1988;235:61–66.

43. Taylor MM, Meyers MH, Harvey JP Jr: Intraoperative femur fractures during total hip replacement. *Clin Orthop* 1978;137:96–103.

44. Missakian ML, Rand JA: Fractures of the femoral shaft adjacent to long stem femoral components of total hip arthroplasty: Report of seven cases. *Orthopedics* 1993;16:149–152.

45. Radcliffe SN, Smith DN: The Mennen plate in periprosthetic hip fractures. *Injury* 1996;27:27–30.

46. Mihalko WM, Beaudoin AJ, Cardea JA, et al: Finite-element modelling of femoral shaft fracture fixation techniques post total hip arthroplasty. *J Biomech* 1992;25:469–476.

47. Emerson RH Jr, Malinin TI, Cuellar AD, et al: Cortical strut allografts in the reconstruction of the femur in revision total hip arthroplasty: A basic science and clinical study. *Clin Orthop* 1992;285:35–44.

48. Kraay MJ, Goldberg VM, Figgie HE III: Use of an antibiotic impregnated polymethyl methacrylate intramedullary spacer for complicated revision total hip arthroplasty. *J Arthroplasty* 1992;7(suppl):397–402.

49. Levenberg R, Iorio R, Gingrich K, et al: Femur fractures associated with total hip arthroplasty. *Orthopedics* 1990;13:1188–1189.

50. Lewallen DG, Berry DJ: Femoral fractures associated with hip arthroplasty, in Morrey BF, An KN (eds): *Reconstructive Surgery of the Joints*, ed 2. New York, NY, Churchill Livingstone, 1996, vol 2, pp 1273–1288.

51. Roffman M, Mendes DG: Fractures of the femur after total hip arthroplasty. *Orthopedics* 1989;12:1067–1070.

52. Scher MA: Fractures of the femoral shaft following total hip replacement. *J Bone Joint Surg* 1981;63B:472.

53. Schwartz JT Jr, Mayer JG, Engh CA: Femoral fracture during non-cemented total hip arthroplasty. *J Bone Joint Surg* 1989;71A:1135–1142.

54. Wang GJ, Miller TO, Stamp WG: Femoral fracture following hip arthroplasty: Brief note on treatment. *J Bone Joint Surg* 1985;67A:956–958.

55. Berry DJ, Harmsen WS, Ilstrup D, et al: Survivorship of uncemented proximally porous-coated femoral components. *Clin Orthop* 1995;319:168–177.

56. Malkani AL, Lewallen DG, Cabanela ME, et al: Femoral component revision using an uncemented, proximally coated, long-stem prosthesis. *J Arthroplasty* 1996;11:411–418.

Periprosthetic Hip and Knee Fractures: The Scope of the Problem

Alastair S.E. Younger, MB, MSc, FRCSC
James Dunwoody, MD
Clive P. Duncan, MD, MSc, FRCSC

Introduction

Periprosthetic fractures after hip and knee replacement are increasingly prevalent and complex. The number of primary joint replacements performed will continue to rise as the population ages, and this will result in an increase in the prevalence of complications.

The incidence of fracture at revision arthroplasty is certain to increase. As older implants reach the end of their life span, osteolysis associated with wear debris around the hip and the knee will lead to periprosthetic fracture.

Periprosthetic fractures can occur intraoperatively, in the immediate postoperative period, or as a late complication after loosening of the component and osteolysis of the surrounding bone. Intraoperative fractures recognized and treated during the procedure are associated with a good long-term outcome. Early postoperative fractures are usually associated with intraoperative errors, such as notching of the anterior femoral cortex in total knee arthroplasty. In discussing the scope of periprosthetic fractures, the site, incidence, and outcome of periprosthetic fractures of the hip and knee will be outlined.

Perioperative Fractures Around the Hip

Incidence of Fracture After Primary Total Hip Arthroplasty

Perioperative fractures around the hip occur in approximately 1% of primary cemented replacements,[1,2] and in 3% to 18% of cementless primary procedures.[3–6] In some cases, the incidence of periprosthetic fracture may be hard to define, because the fracture may not be visible on radiographs.[7] Some designs are more prone to intraoperative fracture. Conical shaped cementless prostheses can fracture the weaker femoral metaphysis during insertion in a manner similar to the way a wedge splits wood. The stability of a conical component depends on hoop stresses around the proximal femur. Some early designs used a component that was oversized compared with the broach, which increased the incidence of fracture in these designs.[8] Fully coated cementless prostheses using line-to-line fit within the stronger cortical bone of the medullary canal may be less likely to cause an intraoperative fracture. Perioperative fractures are more likely to occur with weak bone. Conditions such as rheumatoid arthritis, Paget's disease, and osteomalacia decrease bone strength and increase the risk for fracture in both primary and revision settings.[9–10]

Intraoperative Fractures During Primary Total Hip Arthroplasty

Perioperative fractures sometimes occur during the procedure and are recognized. The surgeon should expose the proximal end of the femur if there is any question about its integrity.[8] One author recommended conversion to a cemented component if fracture occured, because cerclage wires may fail to restore rotational stability.[11] Other authors did not feel that these fractures had a significant effect on outcome, but all recognized the need for identification and management of the fracture at the time of surgery. For example, Sharkey and associates[12] followed ten patients with intraoperative femoral fractures and compared them with controls. Scores for outcome were the same for both groups. The outcome of fractures that are recognized and treated intraoperatively remains good.[4] Treatments include advancing the stem, placement of cerclage wires, and changing the component to a distally coated cementless design or use of a cemented stem.[12]

Kavanagh[8] recommended the use of bone graft. One cadaver study demonstrated that cerclage wire fixation can prevent crack propagation.[13] If the fracture line remains proximal to the tip of the stem the outcome should be favorable.[14] Unrecognized periprosthetic fractures have a very significant effect on outcome because the component may subside, causing the fracture to propagate. One solution is to use a prophylactic cerclage wire around the proximal femur to brace the femur and prevent propagation of the fracture.[15] A trial of nonweightbearing may be appropriate if the fracture is diagnosed on the postoperative film.

Careful preoperative templating can prevent fractures during cementless primary arthroplasty. The isthmus of the femur may have to be reamed to shape it to the component because the shape of the femur varies from patient to patient.[8] The fit of the prosthesis must be reassessed during the procedure, because templating is not 100% accurate.[16] Careful surgical technique can reduce the incidence of intraoperative fracture.

Postoperative Fractures After Primary Total Hip Arthroplasty

Some fractures occur in the immediate postoperative period. The femur may be weakened by overreaming of the femoral canal. Alternatively a stress riser is created at the tip of the stem by penetration of the anterior femoral cortex by reamers. A spiral fracture may propagate distal to the solidly fixed stem through the stress riser.[17] In cemented replacements, cement within the soft tissues of the thigh suggests perforation of the femur.

Acetabular Fractures During Primary Total Hip Arthroplasty

Perioperative fractures of the acetabulum decrease the strength of fixation of the acetabular component.[18] If the fracture is minimally displaced and only a small area of the rim is involved, screw fixation of the cup and a period of nonweightbear-

ing may be all that is required. No specific rates of fracture are quoted in review series, and these fractures are rare in cementless acetabular components with line-to-line fit.[19]

On occasion, an intraoperative acetabular fracture is diagnosed postoperatively. The diagnosis is suggested by a break in the ilioinguinal line, or by change of component orientation during the postoperative period. A period of nonweightbearing may allow the cup to stabilize and bone to ingrow. If further migration occurs, an acetabular revision may be required.

Perioperative Fractures and Revision Total Hip Arthroplasty

Incidence Revision procedures are at particular risk for fracture, with a rate almost double that of primary procedures.[20] In the Mayo clinic series, the rate of fracture of the femur for revision procedures was around 7%.[21] This increased risk is related to the decreased amount of bone stock, the presence of osteolysis,[22] and difficulties in removing retained cement or cementless components. Perforation of the femoral cortex increases the risk of fracture propagation.[17,23] The use of various revision techniques, such as the use of impaction allografting or cementless revision implants, can increase the risk of fracture.[24,25] Fractures occur during dislocation of the hip, during reaming, and during insertion of the broach or the prosthesis.[9,26] Fractures may develop through a cortical window, through screw holes after removal of a plate, and through areas of severe cortical erosion. Fractures can be prevented by careful exposure of the ingrowth surface during removal of a cementless stem using techniques as described by Glassman and Eng.[27] An extended trochanteric osteotomy will allow access to the femur to remove cement or, for cementless prostheses, will access the ingrowth surface.[28] Onlay segmental allograft should be used to bypass deficient

areas of the femur or to augment the femur when osteopenia is present.[29]

Fractures of the Greater Trochanter The greater trochanter is at particular risk for intraoperative or early postoperative fracture. A fracture can occur during cemented stem extraction if cement remains bonded to the femoral component.[6,8] Long-stem revision components can lever the greater trochanter and cause fracture. Finally, leverage on an osteolytic trochanter, or removal of bone to allow stem removal, can lead to fracture of the trochanter either intraoperatively or during the early postoperative period.

Outcome Missakian and Rand[30] demonstrated that complication rates were higher for those fractures managed nonsurgically. Loose components and poor fixation are associated with poor outcome.[9,26] Stable fixation after open reduction is associated with a better outcome.[31,32]

Stress Fractures

Stress fractures may occur after total hip arthroplasty. McElfresh and Coventry[33] reported that two patients from a series of 5,400 hip arthroplasties developed stress fractures of the pubic ramus. Fractures of the ipsilateral femur have been described. Fractures of the sacrum or opposite femoral neck may occur in osteopenic patients being mobilized after the procedure. Cement extrusion may be associated with a late stress fracture of the femur.[34] Osteolysis of the greater trochanter can also lead to a stress fracture.

Late Periprosthetic Fractures Around the Hip

Periprosthetic fractures around the hip can occur after the component loosens and osteolysis occurs.[26] An assessment of the bone stock will allow appropriate management of the case.[10] In some cases, osteolysis around the femur is so severe as to require complex reconstruction, including substitution of the proximal femur. In other cases, the periprosthetic fracture and bone loss is associated with infection. The surgical management of these cases is complex, and the outcome may be less than ideal.

Polyethylene wear debris cysts behind cementless acetabular components have been recently described.[35,36] These cysts can be large enough to destabilize the cup and cause fracture of the acetabulum. They have the potential to create a pelvic dissociation. This problem is especially serious because surgical management is complex, and the problem is likely to be seen more often as the patients who have these components grow older.

Classification of Periprosthetic Femoral Fractures

The most commonly quoted fracture classification system for periprosthetic fractures is the Johansson classification. In this classification system, perioperative and postoperative fractures are classified together. Type I fractures are proximal to the tip of the prosthesis, type II are at the tip of the prosthesis, and type III are distal to the tip.[26] In cementless arthroplasty, type I fractures are most common; and type II are the most common following revision surgery.[37]

The Johansson classification does not consider fixation of the component or quality of bone stock, which are both important factors in the management of periprosthetic fractures. We therefore developed a new classification system. Type A fractures involve the trochanteric region, type B are fractures around the tip of the stem, and type C fractures are distal to the stem. The B type are subgrouped into those with a solidly fixed stem (B_1), those with a loose stem and good bone stock (B_2), and those that are loose and have poor bone stock (B_3). Type B_1 fractures often occur in the perioperative period through a stress riser at the distal end of the prosthesis. Types B_2 and B_3 occur as a late complication of loosening.[10] Type A fractures are subdi-

vided depending on the trochanter involved.

Intraoperative fractures around cementless femoral components have been classified by Mallory and associates.[14] Type I fractures involve the proximal femur to the level of the greater trochanter. Type II fractures extend distal to the lesser trochanter and are no closer than 4 cm from the tip of the prosthesis. Type III fractures extend to within 4 cm of the tip of the prosthesis. Stuchin[5] classified fractures around cementless hips into four groups. Type I fractures involved the medial neck, type II were spiral fractures of the stem tip, type III originated in stress risers in the femoral shaft, and type IV were unclassified. His classification does not indicate outcome because, in his series, they all did well after the femur healed.

Bethea and associates[38] divide fractures into those below the tip of the implant (type A), spiral fractures around the tip of the implant (type B), and comminuted fractures around the stem (type C).[36] This is similar to the Johansson classification system. A number of methods of treatment were used, making it hard to interpret outcome within these groups.

Periprosthetic Fractures in Total Knee Arthroplasty
Femur

Incidence A periprosthetic fracture above a total knee arthroplasty occurs in 0.3% to 5.5% of arthroplasties.[39-45] These fractures will likely become more common as the population ages.[46] Women in their seventh decade are at particular risk.[41,42,44,46] Periprosthetic fractures have been defined as those occurring within 15 cm of the joint line,[40,47] although other authors have suggested that the limit be closer to the joint line.[47] Fractures close to the joint line are hardest to treat.[40] Osteoporosis, neuropathy, rheumatoid arthritis, anterior notching of the femur,

osteolysis, and revision arthroplasty are risk factors for periprosthetic fractures.[40,42,46,48,49] Regional osteopenia occurs around the implant and prevents secure fixation. Poor local vascularity increases the risk of nonunion. Malunion close to an implant increases the loosening rate. Cast treatment leads to prolonged stiffness. Booth[40] reports a 40% incidence of complications with closed treatment versus a 20% incidence of complications with surgery.

Causes of generalized osteoporosis include old age, hormonal changes, and use of drugs, such as corticosteroids.[46] Rheumatoid arthritis, particularly if the patient is on chronic steroid therapy, can lead to severe osteoporosis and is a major risk factor for fracture.[39,40,42,44] Aaron and Scott[39] reported on five fractures out of a series of 250 arthroplasties in rheumatoid patients.

Neurologic disorders associated with fracture of the femur include Parkinsonism, neuropathic arthropathy, polio, cerebral palsy, myasthenia gravis, cerebral ataxia, and seizures.[44,46] Culp and associates[44] found that 17 out of 61 patients with fractures had one of these diseases. Gait ataxia and seizures may have led to the fracture.

Notching of the Femur The rate of fracture after notching of the femur is variable.[39,41,44,46,50] Out of 61 supracondylar femur fractures, Culp and associates[44] found that 27 had a notched femur. When notching was present, the fracture line propagated through the notched area in 90% of cases. Their report predicted that 3 mm of notching would decrease the torsional strength of the femur by 29%. Aaron and Scott[39] reported that, of 250 knee replacements, 12 had notched femurs. Five patients with rheumatoid arthritis suffered a fracture through the notch. No unnotched femurs fractured. Notching was associated with a 40% fracture rate in another review.[41] Ritter and associates[50] reported that 180 of 670 knee replacements were notched, but only two supracondylar fractures occurred in the series. Although the relationship to fracture is not clear, notching of the anterior femoral cortex is best avoided.[40,46]

Osteolysis and Fracture Fractures have occurred through osteolytic defects.[49] One case report describes fractures that occurred 9 years after implantation of an uncemented knee. A distal femoral allograft was required to reconstruct the deficient bone. In a series of 267 cementless arthroplasties, 12 knees had to be revised because of excessive wear of the polyethylene tibial insert. Osteolytic defects were found in three patients. When thin, nonconforming designs of polyethylene are used, careful follow-up is indicated.[49,51,52] Risk factors include screw holes in the tibial baseplate, heat pressed polyethylene, thin polyethylene inserts, and nonconforming polyethylene surfaces.[53] Femoral osteolysis follows 11.1% of uncemented arthroplasties, with an average time to diagnosis of 31 months.[54] Risk factors include male sex, younger age, increased weight, osteoarthritis, and length of time prosthesis in situ.[54] Excessive polyethylene wear has been reported with increasing frequency.[49]

Periprosthetic supracondylar fracture may occur up to 10 years following surgery.[39,41,44,46,48,50,55] The average time to fracture ranges from 2 to 4 years.[46] Treatment alternatives include immobilization, open reduction and internal fixation, antegrade and retrograde intramedullary nailing, closed reduction with Rush rod fixation, and revision knee replacement with or without an allograft.[45,46,56–59] Closed treatment has been reported to have a complication rate of 40%.[40,45] Treatment by immobilization should be considered only for undisplaced fractures,[58] because open reduction and internal fixation results in better outcome.[45] Rush rod fixation results in high union rates but does not control the fracture as well.[59,60] Newer techniques include supracondylar nail fixation.[56,61–63]

Stress fracture Ipsilateral stress fracture of the femoral neck can occasionally occur. Of 12 cases reported in the literature, six patients had rheumatoid arthritis and six had osteoarthritis.[64–69] In patients who have disuse osteoporosis, forces around the hip can change after knee joint replacement.[66,67,70]

Tibia

This is a rare complication. Rand and Coventry[71] reported on 15 patients with medial plateau stress fractures associated with geometric and polycentric arthroplasties. Axial malalignment and improper component orientation increases the risk of fracture. All the tibial components were loose, and revision was required for a satisfactory result.[46,71] Tibial osteolytic defects occur in up to 16% of knees following uncemented knee replacement.[52] The configuration of porous coating on cementless implants may increase the amount of osteolysis.[72] Fractures around a knee replacement caused by high-energy trauma often result in a poor outcome.

Patella

Periprosthetic fractures of the patella occur in 3.6% to 21% of cases.[73,74] Tria and associates[74] stated that patellar fractures have become the most common complication of the extensor mechanism, but most are of mild consequence. These fractures have been reported to occur as early as 9.8 months following arthroplasty, with most occurring in the first 2 years.[74–76] Osteonecrosis of the patella, component malalignment, and inappropriate component design contribute to the risk of fracture. Increased stress at the patellofemoral articulation caused by underresection of the patella or anterior displacement of the femoral component can increase the fracture rate.[77–79] Lateral release can increase the late fracture rate.[74,80] Fat pad resection may also compromise patellar blood supply.

Component alignment was reviewed by Figgie and associates,[75] who analyzed

36 fractures and critically reviewed the radiographs. All of the fractures were associated with component malalignment. Poor alignment can also lead to poor outcome. Component design may well play a role in the 11% incidence of patellar stress fractures that occur in posterior cruciate sacrificing arthroplasty.[81] Goldberg and associates[82] contended that patellar resection thickness does not correlate with the incidence of fracture. The patella should be evenly resected to 1 to 1.5 cm of bone.[79]

If the extensor mechanism is intact, the outcome is usually good.[82] Surgery is recommended for quadriceps mechanism disruption, implant loosening, and fracture dislocations. If a major component malalignment is present, revision should be performed.[75,82] Extensor lag leads to poor outcome regardless of treatment.[76] Patellectomy may have a role in treatment in some cases.[57,83]

Summary

This review covers the present incidence, site, and outcome of periprosthetic fractures of the hip and the knee. Fractures can occur intraoperatively or postoperatively as an early or a late complication. Late postoperative fractures are related to osteolysis secondary to wear debris. These late fractures will become more prevalent with time. Intraoperative fractures can be avoided by careful technique and improved instrument design. Fractures can affect the acetabulum, femur, and trochanter of hip replacements; and the femur, tibia, and patella of knee replacements. The femur is most commonly involved for both joints. Stress fractures have been described as a rare complication of both sites of arthroplasty.

If the fracture is recognized and the bone stock is good, a good outcome can be achieved if rigid fixation is obtained. Unfortunately, poor bone stock is often present, leading to late periprosthetic fractures, which compromise the outcome.

References

1. Garcia-Cimbrelo E, Munuera L, Gil-Garay E: Femoral shaft fractures after cemented total hip arthroplasty. *Int Orthop* 1992;16:97–100.

2. Löwenhielm G, Hansson LI, Kärrholm J: Fracture of the lower extremity after total hip replacement. *Arch Orthop Trauma Surg* 1989;108:141–143.

3. Christensen CM, Seger BM, Schultz RB: Management of intraoperative femur fractures associated with revision hip arthroplasty. *Clin Orthop* 1989;248:177–180.

4. Mont MA, Maar DC, Krackow KA, et al: Hoop-stress fractures of the proximal femur during hip arthroplasty: Management and results in 19 cases. *J Bone Joint Surg* 1992;74B:257–260.

5. Stuchin SA: Femoral shaft fracture in porous and press-fit total hip arthroplasty. *Orthop Rev* 1990;19:153–159.

6. Vaughn BK: Other complications of total hip arthroplasty, in Callaghan JJ, Dennis DA, Paprosky WG, et al (eds): *Orthopaedic Knowledge Update: Hip and Knee Reconstruction.* Rosemont, IL, American Academy of Orthopaedic Surgery, 1995, pp 163–170.

7. Jantsch S, Leixnering M, Schwägerl W, et al: Shaft fissures due to implantation of cement-less total endoprostheses of the hip joint: An experimental study. *Arch Orthop Trauma Surg* 1988;107:236–241.

8. Kavanagh BF: Femoral fractures associated with total hip arthroplasty. *Orthop Clin North Am* 1992;23:249–257.

9. Scott RD, Turner RH, Leitzes SM, et al: Femoral fractures in conjunction with total hip replacement. *J Bone Joint Surg* 1975;57A:494–501.

10. Duncan CP, Masri BA: Fractures of the femur after hip replacement, in Jackson DW (ed): *Instructional Course Lectures 44.* Rosemont, IL, American Academy of Orthopaedic Surgeons 1995, pp 293–304.

11. Schutzer SF, Grady-Benson J, Jasty M, et al: Influence of intraoperative femoral fractures and cerclage wiring on bone ingrowth into canine porous-coated femoral components. *J Arthroplasty* 1995;10:823–829.

12. Sharkey PF, Hozack WJ, Booth RE Jr, et al: Intraoperative femoral fractures in cementless total hip arthroplasty. *Orthop Rev* 1992;21:337–342.

13. Incavo SJ, DiFazio F, Wilder D, et al: Longitudinal crack propagation in bone around femoral prosthesis. *Clin Orthop* 1991;272:175–180.

14. Mallory TH, Kraus TJ, Vaughn BK: Intraoperative femoral fractures associated with cementless total hip arthroplasty. *Orthopedics* 1989;12:231–239.

15. Herzwurm PJ, Walsh J, Pettine KA, et al: Prophylactic cerclage: A method of preventing femur fracture in uncemented total hip arthroplasty. *Orthopedics* 1992;15:143–146.

16. Knight JL, Atwater RD: Preoperative planning for total hip arthroplasty: Quantitating its utility and precision. *J Arthroplasty* 1992;7(suppl):403–409.

17. Fredin H: Late fracture of the femur following perforation during hip arthroplasty: A report of two cases. *Acta Orthop Scand* 1988;59:331–332.

18. Kim YS, Callaghan JJ, Ahn PB, et al: Fracture of the acetabulum during insertion of an over-sized hemispherical component. *J Bone Joint Surg* 1995;77A:111–117.

19. Schmalzried TP, Wessinger SJ, Hill GE, et al: The Harris-Galante porous acetabular component press-fit without screw fixation: Five-year radiographic analysis of primary cases. *J Arthroplasty* 1994;9:235–242.

20. Khan MA, O'Driscoll M: Fractures of the femur during total hip replacement and their management. *J Bone Joint Surg* 1977;59B:36–41.

21. Fitzgerald RH Jr, Brindley GW, Kavanagh BF: The uncemented total hip arthroplasty: Intraoperative femoral fractures. *Clin Orthop* 1988;235:61–66.

22. Pazzaglia U, Byers PD: Fractured femoral shaft through an osteolytic lesion resulting from the reaction to a prosthesis: A case report. *J Bone Joint Surg* 1984;66B:337–339.

23. Talab YA, States JD, Evarts CM: Femoral shaft perforation: A complication of total hip reconstruction. *Clin Orthop* 1979;141:158–165.

24. Elting JJ, Mikhail WE, Zicat BA, et al: Preliminary report of impaction grafting for exchange femoral arthroplasty. *Clin Orthop* 1995;319:159–167.

25. Morrey BF, Kavanagh BF: Complications with revision of the femoral component of total hip arthroplasty: Comparison between cemented and uncemented techniques. *J Arthroplasty* 1992;7:71–79.

26. Johannsson JE, McBroom R, Barrington TW, et al: Fracture of the ipsilateral femur in patients with total hip replacement. *J Bone Joint Surg* 1981;63A:1435–1442.

27. Glassman AH, Engh CA: The removal of porous-coated femoral hip stems. *Clin Orthop* 1992;285:164–180.

28. Younger TI, Bradford MS, Magnus RE, et al: Extended proximal femoral osteotomy: A new technique for femoral revision arthroplasty. *J Arthroplasty* 1995;10:329–338.

29. Head WC, Wagner RA, Emerson RH Jr, et al: Restoration of femoral bone stock in revision total hip arthroplasty. *Orthop Clin North Am* 1993;24:697–703.

30. Missakian ML, Rand JA: Fractures of the femoral shaft adjacent to long stem femoral components of total hip arthroplasty: Report of seven cases. *Orthopedics* 1993;16:149–152.

31. Stern RE, Harwin SF, Kulick RG: Management of ipsilateral femoral shaft fractures following hip arthroplasty. *Orthop Rev* 1991;20:779–784.

32. Zenni EJ Jr, Pomeroy DL, Caudle RJ: Ogden plate and other fixations for fractures complicating femoral endoprostheses. *Clin Orthop* 1988;231:83–90.

33. McElfresh EC, Coventry MB: Femoral and pelvic fractures after total hip arthroplasty. *J Bone Joint Surg* 1974;56A:483–492.

34. Eschenroeder HC Jr, Krackow KA: Late onset femoral stress fracture associated with extruded cement following hip arthroplasty: A case report. *Clin Orthop* 1988;236:210–213.

35. Astion DJ, Saluan P, Stulberg BN, et al: The porous-coated anatomic total hip prosthesis: Failure of the metal-backed acetabular component. *J Bone Joint Surg* 1996;78A:755–766.

36. Maloney WJ, Peters P, Engh CA, et al: Severe osteolysis of the pelvis in association with acetabular replacement without cement. *J Bone Joint Surg* 1993;75A:1627–1635.

37. Grigoris P, Roberts P, McMinn DJ: Failure of uncemented polyethylene acetabular components. *J Arthroplasty* 1993;8:433–437.

38. Bethea JS III, DeAndrade JR, Fleming LL, et al: Proximal femoral fractures following total hip arthroplasty. *Clin Orthop* 1982;170:95–106.

39. Aaron RK, Scott R: Supracondylar fracture of the femur after total knee arthroplasty. *Clin Orthop* 1987;219:136–139.

40. Booth RE Jr: Supracondylar fractures: All or nothing. *Orthopedics* 1995;18:921–922.

41. Figgie MP, Goldberg VM, Figgie HE III, et al: The results of treatment of supracondylar fracture above total knee arthroplasty. *J Arthroplasty* 1990;5:267–276.

42. Merkel KD, Johnson EW Jr: Supracondylar fracture of the femur after total knee arthroplasty. *J Bone Joint Surg* 1986;68A:29–43.

43. Sisto DJ, Lachiewicz PF, Insall JN: Treatment of supracondylar fractures following prosthetic arthroplasty of the knee. *Clin Orthop* 1985;196:265–272.

44. Culp RW, Schmidt RG, Hanks G, et al: Supracondylar fracture of the femur following prosthetic knee arthroplasty. *Clin Orthop* 1987;222:212–222.

45. McLaren AC, Dupont JA, Schroeber DC: Open reduction internal fixation of supracondylar fractures above total knee arthroplasties using the intramedullary supracondylar rod. *Clin Orthop* 1994;302:194–198.

46. Chmell MJ, Moran MC, Scott RD: Periarticular fractures after total knee arthroplasty: Principles of management. *J Am Acad Orthop Surg* 1996;4:109–116.

47. Zehntner MK, Ganz R: Internal fixation of supracondylar fractures after condylar total knee arthroplasty. *Clin Orthop* 1993;293:219–224.

48. Cain PR, Rubash HE, Wissinger HA, et al: Periprosthetic femoral fractures following total knee arthroplasty. *Clin Orthop* 1986;208:205–214.

49. Rand JA: Supracondylar fracture of the femur associated with polyethylene wear after total knee arthroplasty: A case report. *J Bone Joint Surg* 1994;76A:1389–1393.

50. Ritter MA, Faris PM, Keating EM: Anterior femoral notching and ipsilateral supracondylar femur fracture in total knee arthroplasty. *J Arthroplasty* 1988;3:185–187.

51. Gross TP, Lennox DW: Osteolytic cyst-like area associated with polyethylene and metallic debris after total knee replacement with an uncemented vitallium prosthesis: A case report. *J Bone Joint Surg* 1992;74A:1096–1101.

52. Peters PC Jr, Engh GA, Dwyer KA, et al: Osteolysis after total knee arthroplasty without cement. *J Bone Joint Surg* 1992;74A:864–876.

53. Engh GA, Dwyer KA, Hanes CK: Polyethylene wear of metal-backed tibial components in total and unicompartmental knee prostheses. *J Bone Joint Surg* 1992;74B:9–17.

54. Cadambi A, Engh GA, Dwyer KA, et al: Osteolysis of the distal femur after total knee arthroplasty. *J Arthroplasty* 1994;9:579–594.

55. Roffman M, Hirsh DM, Mendes DG: Fracture of the resurfaced patella in total knee replacement. *Clin Orthop* 1980;148:112–116.

56. Hanks GA, Mathews HH, Routson GW, et al: Supracondylar fracture of the femur following total knee arthroplasty. *J Arthroplasty* 1989;4:289–292.

57. Kraay MJ, Goldberg VM, Figgie MP, et al: Distal femoral replacement with allograft/prosthetic reconstruction for treatment of supracondylar fractures in patients with total knee arthroplasty. *J Arthroplasty* 1992;7:7–16.

58. Moran MC, Brick GW, Sledge CB, et al: Supracondylar femoral fracture following total knee arthroplasty. *Clin Orthop* 1996;324:196–209.

59. Ritter MA, Keating EM, Faris PM, et al: Rush rod fixation of supracondylar fractures above total knee arthroplasties. *J Arthroplasty* 1995;10:213–216.

60. Ritter MA, Stiver P: Supracondylar fracture in a patient with total knee arthroplasty: A case report. *Clin Orthop* 1985;193:168–170.

61. Jabczenski FF, Crawford M: Retrograde intramedullary nailing of supracondylar femur fractures above total knee arthroplasty: A preliminary report of four cases. *J Arthroplasty* 1995;10:95–101.

62. Murrell GA, Nunley JA: Interlocked supracondylar intramedullary nails for supracondylar fractures after total knee arthroplasty: A new treatment method. *J Arthroplasty* 1995;10:37–42.

63. Smith WJ, Martin SL, Mabrey JD: Use of a supracondylar nail for treatment of a supracondylar fracture of the femur following total knee arthroplasty. *J Arthroplasty* 1996;11:210–213.

64. Cameron HU: Femoral neck stress fracture after total knee replacement: A case report. *Am J Knee Surg* 1992;5:41–43.

65. Fipp G: Stress fractures of the femoral neck following total knee arthroplasty. *J Arthroplasty* 1988;3:347–350.

66. Hardy DC, Delince PE, Yasik E, et al: Stress fracture of the hip: An unusual complication of total knee arthroplasty. *Clin Orthop* 1992;281:140–144.

67. Lesniewski PJ, Testa NN: Stress fracture of the hip as a complication of total knee replacement: Case report. *J Bone Joint Surg* 1982;64A:304–306.

68. Palance Martin D, Albareda J, Seral F: Subcapital stress fracture of the femoral neck after total knee arthroplasty. *Int Orthop* 1994;18:308–309.

69. Devas MB: Stress fractures of the femoral neck. *J Bone Joint Surg* 1965;47B:728–738.

70. McElwaine JP, Sheehan JM: Spontaneous fractures of the femoral neck after total replacement of the knee. *J Bone Joint Surg* 1982;64B:323–325.

71. Rand JA, Coventry MB: Stress fractures after total knee arthroplasty. *J Bone Joint Surg* 1980;62A:226–233.

72. Whiteside LA: Effect of porous-coating configuration on tibial osteolysis after total knee arthroplasty. *Clin Orthop* 1995;321:92–97.

73. Cameron HU, Fedorkow DM: The patella in total knee arthroplasty. *Clin Orthop* 1982;165:197–199.

74. Tria AJ Jr, Harwood DA, Alicea JA, et al: Patellar fractures in posterior stabilized knee arthroplasties. *Clin Orthop* 1994;299:131–138.

75. Figgie HE III, Goldberg VM, Figgie MP, et al: The effect of alignment of the implant on fractures of the patella after condylar total knee arthroplasty. *J Bone Joint Surg* 1989;71A:1031–1039.

76. Hozack WJ, Goll SR, Lotke PA, et al: The treatment of patellar fractures after total knee arthroplasty. *Clin Orthop* 1988;236:123–127.

77. Reuben JD, McDonald CL, Woodard PL, et al: Effect of patella thickness on patella strain following total knee arthroplasty. *J Arthroplasty* 1991;6:251–258.

78. Scuderi G, Scharf SC, Meltzer LP, et al: The relationship of lateral releases to patella viability in total knee arthroplasty. *J Arthroplasty* 1987;2:209–214.

79. Windsor RE, Scuderi GR, Insall JN: Patellar fractures in total knee arthroplasty. *J Arthroplasty* 1989;4(suppl):S63–S67.

80. Ritter MA, Campbell ED: Postoperative patellar complications with or without lateral release during total knee arthroplasty. *Clin Orthop* 1987;219:163–168.

81. Insall JN, Lachiewicz PF, Burstein AH: The posterior stabilized condylar prosthesis: A modification of the total condylar design: Two to four-year clinical experience. *J Bone Joint Surg* 1982;64A:1317–1323.

82. Goldberg VM, Figgie HE III, Inglis AE, et al: Patellar fracture type and prognosis in condylar total knee arthroplasty. *Clin Orthop* 1988;236:115–122.

83. Clayton ML, Thirupathi R: Patellar complications after total condylar arthroplasty. *Clin Orthop* 1982;170:152–155.

The Role of Allografts
in the Treatment of Periprosthetic Femoral Fractures

Hugh P. Chandler, MD
Russell G. Tigges, MD

Fracture of the femoral shaft occurring after total hip or total knee replacement is a rare but serious complication.[1-50] If the prosthesis is loose, the logical treatment is revision surgery, with insertion of a femoral component with a longer stem to stabilize the fracture. If the stem is firmly fixed, the best method of treatment is more difficult to determine. The options available include closed treatment (traction or application of a spica cast or a cast-brace), exchange of the stem for a longer one that stabilizes the fracture, supracondylar nailing for a fracture proximal to a total knee prosthesis, and open reduction and internal fixation of the fracture.

Closed treatment of a fracture of the femoral shaft is associated with many problems,[3,5,11,14,15,20,25,29,30,34,46] including medical complications secondary to prolonged bed rest, potential loss of motion of the hip or knee, and nonunion or malunion. Malunion is particularly troubling when it is associated with a total hip or knee prosthesis. Malalignment of the femur can accelerate loosening of the implant. Also, revision of a femoral component in the presence of a deformed femur is much more difficult.

Exchange of a component that is well fixed (with either cement or bone ingrowth) for a component with a longer stem to stabilize the fracture not only is arduous but also can severely damage the surrounding bone. Anatomic alignment, union of the fracture, and a short recovery time are more likely if the stem is left intact and the fracture is treated with open reduction and internal fixation.

Technique for Treatment
Proximal Femoral Fractures Distal to a Well-Fixed Femoral Stem or Proximal to a Well-Fixed Knee Replacement

The patient is positioned on his or her side on a conventional operating table. The fracture is exposed, reduced, and temporarily stabilized with cerclage wires or cables (Fig. 1, A&B). An ipsilateral allograft femur, split into two equal pieces at the linea aspera, is used to provide biologic bone plates (Fig. 1, C). A tibia, split into two equal pieces, can be used instead, but it will not fit the host femur as well. Our experience is with fresh-frozen allografts; however, it is possible that freeze-dried allografts would also work. It is important that the femur or tibia be split into two equal parts. Three smaller struts from a single bone have not proven to be rigid enough to provide fixation.[8] The inside surfaces of the grafts should be contoured to match the outside dimensions of the recipient femur (Fig. 1, D). The two grafts are placed medial and lateral to the linea aspera, without disrupting it, in an effort to preserve its blood supply to the host bone (Fig. 1, E). The struts should extend at least 10 cm proximal and distal to the fracture to allow fixation on each side of the fracture with at least four wires.

Fixation of the grafts to the femur can be achieved with number-16 cerclage wires or with 2.0-mm cables placed at 2- to 4-cm intervals. Our current preference is to use hose clamps (from a hardware store), after they are sterilized, to compress the struts to the host bone initially and then to use double number-16 stainless-steel wires that are tightened and twisted with a Harris wire-tightener (Johnson and Johnson, Raynham, MA); the hose clamps are removed once the wires are secure (Fig. 1, F-I). Autogenous graft from the iliac crest should be added to the site of the fracture.

Postoperatively, the decision as to when a patient is allowed out of bed is made on the basis of the status of the wound and the muscular control of the lower limb, not on the basis of the fracture. Immediate protected weightbearing (60 lb) is encouraged as soon as the patient is capable of it and is continued for at least 12 weeks. After 12 weeks, the use of support can be discontinued once the patient is able to walk without pain or a limp. This technique can be used to treat a fracture distal to a well-fixed femoral stem (Fig. 2) or proximal to a well-fixed total knee replacement (Fig. 3).

Distal Femoral Fractures Distal to a Well-Fixed Femoral Stem or Proximal to a Well-Fixed Knee Replacement

With very distal femoral fractures, two allograft struts alone do not provide ade-

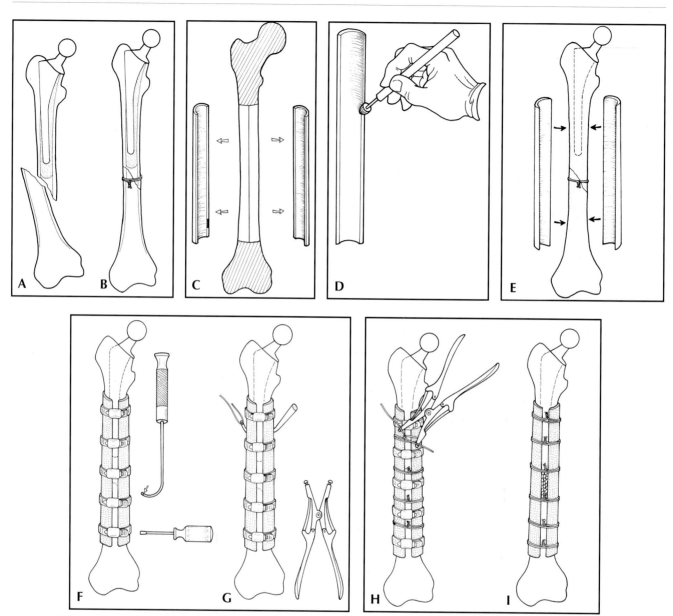

Fig. 1 A-I illustrate the technique for treatment of a proximal femoral fracture. **A** and **B,** An open reduction of the fracture is performed, and the fracture is temporarily held with cerclage wires or cables. **C,** The allograft femoral (or tibial) shaft is split into two equal parts. **D,** The inside surface of the graft is machined with a high-speed burr to conform to the outside of the host femur. **E,** The two grafts are placed medial and lateral to the linea aspera, without disrupting it, in an effort to preserve its blood supply to the host bone. These struts should extend at least 10 cm proximal and distal to the fracture. **F,** Hose clamps are used to compress the struts to the host bone initially. **G,** A bone hook with a hole in the tip is used to pass double number-16 wires around the struts. **H,** The wires are tightened and twisted with a Harris wire-tightener (Johnson and Johnson, Raynham, MA). **I,** When the wires are secure, the hose clamps are removed and bone graft is added to the site of the fracture. (Figures 1A-1E are reproduced with permission from Chandler HP, King D, Limbrid R, et al: The use of cortical allograft struts for fixation of fractures associated with well-fixed total joint prostheses. *Semin Arthroplasty* 1993;4:99–107.)

quate fixation, because they cannot extend 10 cm distal to the fracture. The optimum treatment for these fractures is probably a distal intramedullary rod with interlocking screws.[18,23,33,40,43,47] However, with a proximal total hip-replacement stem and a distal rod, there is a risk of secondary fracture at the junction of the two rigid intramedullary devices. A distal intramedullary rod works with a well-fixed femoral component of a total knee replacement only if the intercondylar notch is not occluded by a cruciate-sacrificing design and if the fracture is not so comminuted as to prevent distal fixation

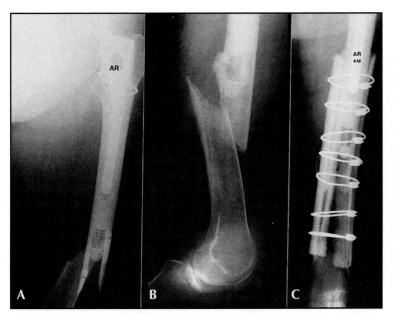
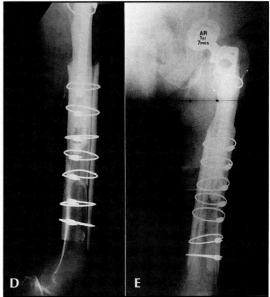

Fig. 2 An 80-year-old woman who had a total hip replacement on the right for post-traumatic osteoarthrosis following a fracture of the femoral neck. **A** and **B,** Radiographs made after the patient fell, 6 months after the total hip replacement, and sustained a Johansson type-II fracture[25] distal to a well-cemented femoral stem. She was managed with traction for 2 days. **C** and **D,** Radiographs demonstrating a healed fracture, with the struts beginning to unite with the host bone, 4 months after an open reduction and internal fixation with onlay femoral allograft struts secured with Dall-Miles cables (Howmedica, Rutherford, New Jersey). The patient began to use a walker by the second postoperative day and a cane by 3 months postoperatively. By 3.5 months, she was able to walk without support and without a limp or pain. **E,** Radiograph made 1 year and 7 months postoperatively. The patient continued to do well, and the struts had united with the femur. (Reproduced with permission from Chandler HP, King D, Limbrid R, et al: The use of cortical allograft struts for fixation of fractures associated with well-fixed total joint prostheses. *Semin Arthroplasty* 1993;4:99–107.)

with interlocking screws. If a distal intramedullary rod cannot be used, supracondylar or condylar plates are the best treatment. Unfortunately, fixation of a plate can often be tenuous because osteopenic bone cannot provide firm fixation for the screws. One solution for treatment of these difficult fractures is to use a plate on one cortex and an allograft strut on the other (Fig. 4). When a plate and strut are used together, the strut should be obtained from the corresponding portion of an ipsilateral allograft femur so that it will fit the host femur accurately. This strut can be narrower (a width of 2 cm is adequate) than those used for more proximal fractures because its function is only to provide fixation for the screw; stability is provided by the more rigid plate.

As with the proximal allograft struts, the inside of the strut is contoured to match the outside diameter of the host femur. The knee is approached through an extended medial parapatellar incision. The fracture is reduced and is held temporarily with a cerclage or Kirschner wire while the plate is placed on one cortex and the strut is placed on the other. The plate and strut are stabilized with cables or wires in the area of an intramedullary stem and with screws between the plate and the graft elsewhere (Figs. 4 and 5).

Postoperatively, a patient who has had a fracture fixed with a supracondylar plate combined with a strut is allowed motion of the knee as comfort allows and is encouraged to walk bearing 60 lb of weight for 12 weeks. If there is radiographic evidence of early union at that time, the patient is allowed weightbearing as tolerated. A combination of a metal plate on one cortex and a biologic bone plate on the other provides excellent fixa-

tion, even in the presence of poor-quality host bone (Fig. 6).

Very distal comminuted fractures, fixed with a condylar plate and screws, are less stable and should be immobilized for 4 weeks with the limb in extension or in a hinged brace that allows full extension and 30° of flexion (Fig. 7). Full motion of the knee can then be allowed. These patients can immediately walk bearing 60 lb of weight as soon as comfort allows and, at 12 weeks, can bear weight as tolerated if there is radiographic evidence of healing.

Discussion

The treatment of periprosthetic fractures of the femur with open reduction and internal fixation has the advantages of anatomic alignment, union of the fracture, and a short recovery time. However, the choice of fixation methods is of great

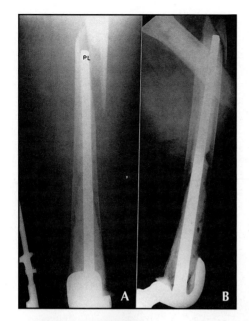
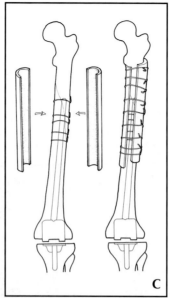
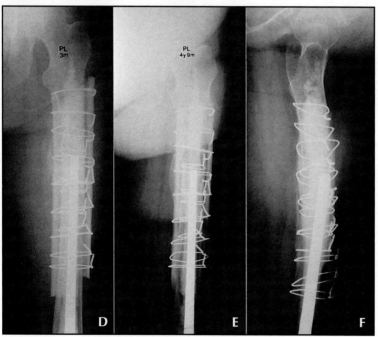

Fig. 3 A 58-year-old woman who had a customized long-stem hinged total knee prosthesis. A and B, Radiographs made after the patient sustained a proximal femoral fracture proximal to the tip of a well-fixed femoral stem. The fracture was treated unsuccessfully with traction for 6 days. C, An allograft tibia was split into two equal pieces and was secured to the femur with number-16 stainless-steel wires. The patient was kept in bed for 7 days postoperatively and walked with crutches for 3 months. D, Radiograph, made 3 months postoperatively, demonstrating union, which was evident clinically as well. The patient used a cane for 5 months. E and F, Radiographs, made 4 years and 9 months postoperatively, showing union of the grafts with the femur. (Reproduced with permission from Chandler HP, King D, Limbrid R, et al: The use of cortical allograft struts for fixation of fractures associated with well-fixed total joint prostheses. *Semin Arthroplasty* 1993;4:99–107.)

importance. Screws, cerclage wires, cables, or bands by themselves are not adequate. Conventional plates can fail because it is difficult to obtain good fixation of proximal screws around the stem and because proximal screw-holes create stress-risers that can result in fracture of the cement and loosening of the component or a new proximal fracture of the femur.

There have been many case reports and reviews in the literature regarding the results of open reduction and internal fixation of these fractures with different plates. Several authors have reported excellent results with compression plates.[2,3,9,11,12,19,21,25,31,41,44-46,48-51] Others have discouraged the use of compression plates because they had poor results.[5,10,14,15,20,22,30,34] Several specialty plates have also been designed. The Ogden plate (Zimmer, Warsaw, IN) allows proximal fixation of the plate with cerclage wires in the area of the stem. Distal fixation is obtained with screws.[50] The Howmedica (Rutherford, NJ) and Zimmer plates allow fixation with cerclage devices or screws. Partridge introduced a nylon plate used with nylon bands.[4,13,24,36] Theoretically, this more flexible plate should not cause stress-shielding. However, as the plate has not been approved for use in the United States, we have had no experience with it.

The first report in the literature, of which we are aware, on the use of massive cortical onlay grafts to immobilize femoral fractures associated with a femoral stem was published in 1989 by Chandler and Penenberg.[7] Chandler and associates,[8] in 1993, reported on a series of 19 patients who had a periprosthetic femoral fracture treated with a massive cortical onlay graft. At an average of 4.5 months postoperatively, 16 of the 19 patients had anatomic union of the fracture and had returned to their prefracture status. There was one malunion (in 8° of varus and 15° of posterior angulation), in a patient in whom a tibia split into three

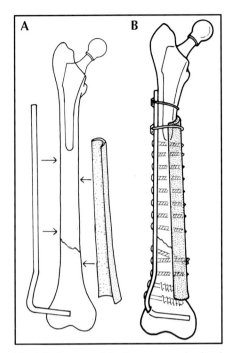

Fig. 4 A, Supracondylar fractures can be fixed with a lateral blade-plate and a medial allograft strut. **B,** Cables or number-16 wires are used in the area of the stem, and screws are used elsewhere.

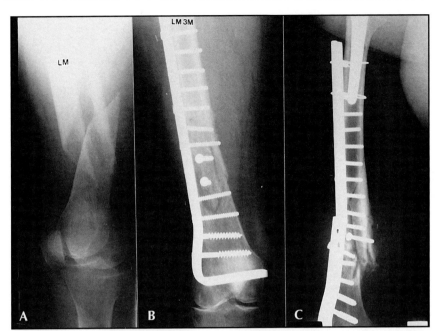

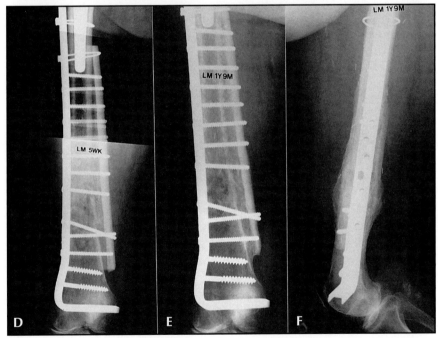

Fig. 5 A 76-year-old woman who had a total hip replacement on the right for degenerative arthritis. **A,** Radiograph made after the patient fell, 8 years after the hip replacement, and sustained a supracondylar fracture. The stem of the femoral component, which had been inserted without cement, was well fixed. **B,** Radiograph made 3 months after open reduction and fixation with a supracondylar plate. The patient walked with a walker for 3 months and then used a cane. **C,** Radiograph, made 5 months postoperatively, showing a fracture of the plate. **D,** Radiograph made 5 weeks after a repeat open reduction and fixation with a medial femoral allograft strut and a new supracondylar plate. The patient walked with a walker for 2 months and then with crutches for 1 month. **E** and **F,** Radiographs, made 1 year and 9 months after the repeat operation, showing that the fracture had healed and the medial strut had united with the femur.

equal struts had been used. A nonunion developed in two patients, who then had a reoperation. In both patients, the femoral shaft had been stripped during a previous revision procedure. The remaining 17 patients had not had a previous operation that necessitated subperiosteal dissection in the area of the fracture. All of the fractures had united, and the allograft struts had united with the host femur in all patients who were followed for more than a year. The average time in bed was slightly more than 3 days (range, 1 to 10 days), and the average stay in the hospital was 12 days (range, 9 to 19 days). The two patients who had a nonunion used support when walking until the second operation. One patient, who had used a walker before the fracture, continued to use one postoperatively (for balance only) despite union of the fracture. She died 1 year after the fracture as a result of medical problems unrelated

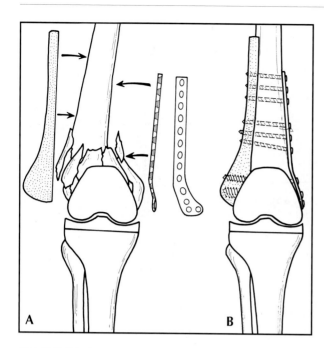

Fig. 6 A, Comminuted, very distal fractures can be stabilized with a distal allograft strut and a condylar plate. **B,** Screws have little fixation in the weak host bone but good fixation in the graft. Cancellous bone from the graft can be used to fill defects at the fracture site.

to the fracture. The average time until the other 16 patients discontinued the use of all support was 4 months (range, 6 weeks to 12 months). There were no infections and no major problems related to the wound.[8]

The use of a metal plate on one cortex and an allograft strut on the other was described by Chandler and Danylchuk[6] in 1996. Anatomic union occurred in 21 (95%) of 22 patients. The one failure was related to a technical error. The graft united with the host bone in all of the patients in whom the fracture united.

There are several advantages to the use of allografts in these situations. The struts can be customized to fit any femur; the modulus of elasticity of the struts is similar to that of the host bone and, thus, they are less likely to cause stress-shielding; the struts routinely unite with the host bone and eventually make the bone stronger than it was originally; and the graft may stimulate healing of the fracture.[52]

There are also several disadvantages to the use of allografts as biologic fixation plates. These grafts are expensive: at our institution, a femoral shaft allograft costs

about $2,400 and a tibial allograft costs about $1,950. However, these costs need to be compared with the high hospital cost of skeletal traction and the cost of various metal implants. Allograft has the potential to transmit disease.[53] Also, although these struts are initially very strong, they become weaker by 4 to 6 months as incorporation progresses.[54] Fortunately, the site of the fracture becomes stronger as the grafts weaken and, as with all fixation methods, there is a race between union of the fracture and failure of the fixation device. If healing of the fracture is delayed, the struts can fracture. Another disadvantage is that the host femur must be extensively exposed to place the struts on either side of the linea aspera. Although this theoretically compromises the blood supply of the host femur, it has not been a clinical problem in patients who have not had the shaft exposed previously. Perhaps a metal fracture plate on the lateral cortex, held with cerclage wires, is a better choice in patients who have had previous stripping of the periosteum in the area of the new fracture.

Periprosthetic femoral fractures pre-

sent a difficult treatment challenge. Open reduction and internal fixation of displaced femoral fractures with allograft femoral struts or a combination of a compression plate and an allograft strut is a proved treatment option.

References

1. Aaron RK, Scott R: Supracondylar fracture of the femur after total knee arthroplasty. *Clin Orthop* 1987;219:136–139.

2. Bethea JS III, DeAndrade JR, Fleming LL, et al: Proximal femoral fractures following total hip arthroplasty. *Clin Orthop* 1982;170:95–106.

3. Bogoch E, Hastings D, Gross A, et al: Supracondylar fractures of the femur adjacent to resurfacing and Macintosh arthroplasties of the knee in patients with rheumatoid arthritis. *Clin Orthop* 1988;229:213–220.

4. Buxton RA, Kinninmonth AW, Döhler JR: Second femur fracture after hemiarthroplasty of the hip: Salvage procedure by Partridge bands and long-stemmed prosthesis. *Arch Orthop Trauma Surg* 1986;105:375–376.

5. Cain PR, Rubash HE, Wissinger HA, et al: Periprosthetic femoral fractures following knee arthroplasty. *Clin Orthop* 1986;208: 205–214.

6. Chandler HP, Danylchuk K: Treatment of distal femoral fractures proximal to a total knee replacement or distal to the stem of a total hip replacement in osteopenic patients. Proceedings of the American Academy of Orthopaedic Surgeons 63rd Annual Meeting, Atlanta, GA, 1996. Rosemont, IL, American Academy of Orthopaedic Surgeons, p 421.

7. Chandler HP, Penenberg BL (eds): Femoral reconstruction, in *Bone Stock Deficiency in Total Hip Replacement: Classificaiton and Management.* Thorofare, NJ, Slack Inc, 1989, pp 103–164.

8. Chandler HP, King D, Limbird R, et al: The use of cortical allograft struts for fixation of fractures associated with well-fixed total joint prostheses. *Semin Arthroplasty* 1993;4:99–107.

9. Chen F, Mont MA, Bachner RS: Management of ipsilateral supracondylar femur fractures following total knee arthroplasty. *J Arthroplasty* 1994;9:521–526.

10. Cordeiro EN, Costa RC, Carazzato JG, et al: Periprosthetic fractures in patients with total knee arthroplasties. *Clin Orthop* 1990;252: 182–189.

11. Culp RW, Schmidt RG, Hanks G, et al: Supracondylar fracture of the femur following prosthetic knee arthroplasty. *Clin Orthop* 1987;222:212–222.

12. Dave DJ, Koka SR, James SE: Mennen plate fixation for fracture of the femoral shaft with ipsilateral total hip and knee arthroplasties. *J Arthroplasty* 1995;10:113–115.

13. de Ritter VA, Klopper PJ, Koomen AR: Abstract: The Partridge osteosynthesis: A prospective clinical study on the use of nylon cerclage bands and plates in the treatment of

subprosthetic femoral shaft fractures. *J Bone Joint Surg* 1990;72B:1085.

14. DiGioia AM III, Rubash HE: Periprosthetic fractures of the femur after total knee arthroplasty: A literature review and treatment algorithm. *Clin Orthop* 1991;271:135–142.

15. Dysart SH, Savory CG, Callaghan JJ: Nonoperative treatment of a postoperative fracture around an uncemented porous-coated femoral component. *J Arthroplasty* 1989;4:187–190.

16. Figgie MP, Goldberg VM, Figgie HE III, et al: The results of treatment of supracondylar fracture above total knee arthroplasty. *J Arthroplasty* 1990;5:267–276.

17. Fredin H: Late fracture of the femur following perforation during hip arthroplasty: A report of two cases. *Acta Orthop Scand* 1988;59:331–332.

18. Goodman SB: Supracondylar fractures above a total knee arthroplasty: A novel use of the Huckstepp nail. *J Arthroplasty* 1995;10:255.

19. Hanks GA, Mathews HH, Routson GW, et al: Supracondylar fracture of the femur following total knee arthroplasty. *J Arthroplasty* 1989;4:289–292.

20. Harrington IJ, Tountas AA, Cameron HU: Femoral fractures associated with Moore's prosthesis. *Injury* 1979;11:23–32.

21. Healy WL, Siliski JM, Incavo SJ: Operative treatment of distal femoral fractures proximal to total knee replacements. *J Bone Joint Surg* 1993;75A:27–34.

22. Hirsh DM, Bhalla S, Roffman M: Supracondylar fracture of the femur following total knee replacement: Report of four cases. *J Bone Joint Surg* 1981;63A:162–163.

23. Jabczenski FF, Crawford M: Retrograde intramedullary nailing of supracondylar femur fractures above total knee arthroplasty: A preliminary report of four cases. *J Arthroplasty* 1995;10:95–101.

24. Jensen TT, Overgaard S, Mossing NB: Partridge Cerclene system for femoral fractures in osteoporotic bones with ipsilateral hemi/total arthroplasty. *J Arthroplasty* 1990;5:123–126.

25. Johansson JE, McBroom R, Barrington TW, et al: Fracture of the ipsilateral femur in patients with total hip replacement. *J Bone Joint Surg* 1981;63A:1435–1442.

26. Kraay MJ, Goldberg VM, Figgie MP, et al: Distal femoral replacement with allograft/prosthetic reconstruction for treatment of supracondylar fractures in patients with total knee arthroplasty. *J Arthroplasty* 1992;7:7–16.

27. Kress KJ, Scuderi GR, Windsor RE, et al: Treatment of nonunions about the knee utilizing custom total knee arthroplasty with press-fit intramedullary stems. *J Arthroplasty* 1993;8:49–55.

28. Löwenhielm G, Hansson LI, Kärrholm J: Fracture of the lower extremity after total hip replacement. *Arch Orthop Trauma Surg* 1989;108:141–143.

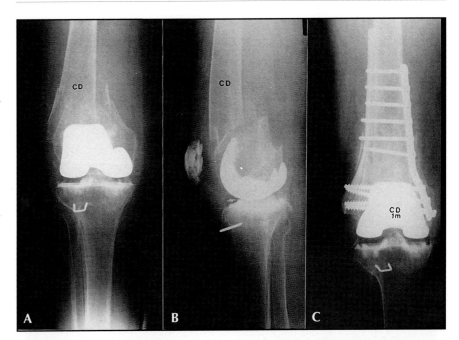

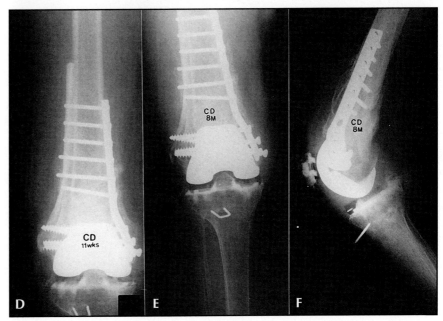

Fig. 7 An 80-year-old woman who had a well-functioning total knee replacement. **A** and **B,** Radiographs made after the patient fell, 7 years after the knee replacement, and sustained a comminuted supracondylar fracture. An attempt at closed reduction was unsuccessful. **C,** Radiograph made 1 month after an open reduction and fixation with a lateral tibial buttress plate medially and an allograft strut laterally. Postoperatively, the patient used a hinged knee-brace that limited flexion to 30° for 4 weeks, after which full motion was allowed. She was allowed partial weightbearing for 10 weeks, and she then used a cane for 4 weeks. **D,** Radiograph, made 11 weeks postoperatively, showing that the reduction has been maintained. There is early evidence of healing. **E** and **F,** Radiographs, made at 8 months, show that the fracture had united and the graft had united with the femur. The patient was able to bear full weight and had clinical evidence of union. She died from a heart attack 1 year after the fracture. At the time of death, she had been functioning at the same level as before the fracture.

29. McElfresh EC, Coventry MB: Femoral and pelvic fractures after total hip arthroplasty. *J Bone Joint Surg* 1974;56A:483–492.

30. Merkel KD, Johnson EW Jr: Supracondylar fracture of the femur after total knee arthroplasty. *J Bone Joint Surg* 1986;68A:29–43.

31. Mont MA, Maar DC: Fractures of the ipsilateral femur after hip arthroplasty: A statistical analysis of outcome based on 487 patients. *J Arthroplasty* 1994;9:511–519.

32. Montijo H, Ebert FR, Lennox DA: Treatment of proximal femur fractures associated with total hip arthroplasty. *J Arthroplasty* 1989;4:115–123.

33. Murrell GA, Nunley JA: Interlocked supracondylar intramedullary nails for supracondylar fractures after total knee arthroplasty: A new treatment method. *J Arthroplasty* 1995;10:37–42.

34. Nielsen BF, Petersen VS, Varmarken JE: Fracture of the femur after knee arthroplasty. *Acta Orthop Scand* 1988;59:155–157.

35. Parrish TF, Jones JR: Fracture of the femur following prosthetic arthroplasty of the hip: Report of nine cases. *J Bone Joint Surg* 1964;46A:241–248.

36. Partridge AJ, Evans PE: The treatment of fractures of the shaft of the femur using nylon cerclage. *J Bone Joint Surg* 1982;64B:210–214.

37. Ries MD: Intraoperative modular stem lengthening to treat periprosthetic femur fracture. *J Arthroplasty* 1996;11:204–205.

38. Ritter MA, Stiver P: Supracondylar fracture in a patient with total knee arthroplasty: A case report. *Clin Orthop* 1985;193:168–170.

39. Ritter MA, Faris PM, Keating EM: Anterior femoral notching and ipsilateral supracondylar femur fracture in total knee arthroplasty. *J Arthroplasty* 1988;3:185–187.

40. Ritter MA, Keating EM, Faris PM, et al: Rush rod fixation of supracondylar fractures above total knee arthroplasties. *J Arthroplasty* 1995;10:213–216.

41. Roscoe MW, Goodman SB, Schatzker J: Supracondylar fracture of the femur after GUEPAR total knee arthroplasty: A new treatment method. *Clin Orthop* 1989;241:221–223.

42. Schwartz JT Jr, Mayer JG, Engh CA: Femoral fracture during non-cemented total hip arthroplasty. *J Bone Joint Surg* 1989;71A:1135–1142.

43. Sekel R, Newman AS: Supracondylar fractures above a total knee arthroplasty: A novel use of the Huckstepp nail. *J Arthroplasty* 1994;9:445–447.

44. Serocki JH, Chandler RW, Dorr LD: Treatment of fractures about hip prostheses with compression plating. *J Arthroplasty* 1992;7:129–135.

45. Short WH, Hootnick DR, Murray DG: Ipsilateral supracondylar femur fractures following knee arthroplasty. *Clin Orthop* 1981;158:111–116.

46. Sisto DJ, Lachiewicz PF, Insall JN: Treatment of supracondylar fractures following prosthetic arthroplasty of the knee. *Clin Orthop* 1985;196:265–272.

47. Smith WJ, Martin SL, Mabrey JD: Use of a supracondylar nail for treatment of a supracondylar fracture of the femur following total knee arthroplasty. *J Arthroplasty* 1996;11:210–213.

48. Wang GJ, Miller TO, Stamp WG: Femoral fracture following hip arthroplasty: Brief note on treatment. *J Bone Joint Surg* 1985;67A:956–958.

49. Wittaker RP, Sotos LN, Ralston EL: Fractures of the femur about femoral endoprostheses. *J Trauma* 1974;14:675–694.

50. Zenni EJ Jr, Pomeroy DL, Caudle RJ: Ogden plate and other fixations for fractures complicating femoral endoprostheses. *Clin Orthop* 1988;231:83–90.

51. Riemer BL, Foglesong ME, Miranda MA: Femoral plating. *Orthop Clin North Am* 1994;25:625–633.

52. Mankin HJ, Friedlaender GE: Biology of bone grafts, in Chandler HP, Penenberg BL (eds): *Bone Stock Deficiency in Total Hip Replacement: Classification and Management.* Thorofare, NJ, Slack Inc, 1989, pp 1–12.

53. Tomford WW, Thongphasuk J, Mankin HJ, et al: Frozen musculoskeletal allografts: A study of the clinical incidence and causes of infection associated with their use. *J Bone Joint Surg* 1990;72A:1137–1143.

54. Springfield DS: Massive autogenous bone grafts. *Orthop Clin North Am* 1987;18:249–256.

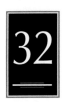

32

Impaction Morcellized Allografting and Cement

Tom J. J. H. Slooff, MD, PhD
B. Willem Schreurs, MD, PhD
Pieter Buma, PhD
Jean W. M. Gardeniers, MD, PhD

Introduction

Most total hip arthroplasties, cemented and cementless, fail because of aseptic loosening, a slow but progressive process that often results in loss of bone stock. The stability of the implant becomes compromised and the components may migrate. The key problems in revision surgery are how to manage the periprosthetic bone loss, how to achieve long-lasting stability, and how to restore hip mechanics. Although controversy still exists about the treatment of choice for the reconstruction of the failed total hip arthroplasty acetabular component, we prefer a biologic method, using impaction allografting with cement.

This chapter describes the essential general issues of bone grafting, particularly the use of morcellized grafts with cement and the rationale of the reconstruction method in acetabular revision arthroplasty. Subsequently, it describes the surgical technique, the supportive scientific studies, and the clinical and radiographic results of the reconstruction. Finally, current recommendations are presented and discussed.

General Issues
History
Bone grafting has a long history in medical science. According to folklore, it goes back to ancient times. The miracle of the saints, the twins Cosmas and Damianus, represents the first alleged bone and tissue transplant. The legend tells the histo- ry of a pious sexton, who was lying in the Roman Forum, exhausted from the pain of bone cancer in his leg. In a dream, the twin brothers came to help him, removed his diseased leg and transplanted the leg of a Moor who had just died. Because the Moor had darker skin than the sexton did, this miraculous event has been recorded as "The miracle of the black leg." Owing to the success of the operation, the twin brothers were canonized, inspiring artists over the years to create masterpieces portraying the event on canvas.

Back to reality! The early literature records that the Dutchmen Anthonie van Leeuwenhoek[1] and Job van Meekeren[2] performed excellent scientific work in the field of bone grafting and bone physiology. Anthonie van Leeuwenhoek, a contemporary of Jan van Swammerdam and Reinier de Graaf, gained international recognition through his research into microscopy and his production of the first thorough description of the histologic structure of bone. In a well-documented study published in 1668, Van Meekeren, a surgeon from Amsterdam, described the first bone graft. The graft, taken from the skull of a dog, was used successfully to restore a traumatic defect in a soldier's skull. In this case, the graft material is known as a xenograft, which indicates bone donation from one species to another. An autograft refers to bone that is transplanted from one location to another within the same individual. In the tale of the Moor, the bone graft received by the sexton represents an allograft, because another member of the same species donated the bone.

Through the centuries, the use of autografts and allografts in surgical practice has varied widely. In the 18th and 19th centuries, bone grafting was not an accepted surgical procedure; it was considered to be experimental, with an unpredictable outcome. However, the technique was developed out of sheer necessity in clinical practice, and even today clinical expertise runs ahead of science. At the end of the 19th century and the beginning of the 20th, famous surgeons such as Ollier[3] from France, Macewen[4] from Scotland, Curtis[5] from the United States, and Barth[6], Lexer[7] and Axhausen[8] from Germany stimulated the use of bone grafting. On the basis of animal experiments and clinical observations, they observed that the graft, whether it was an autograft or an allograft, largely lost its vitality and then became revitalized from the host bone. Major components in this process were considered to be the periosteum transplanted with the graft and the vascular network of the host.

The Present
Current knowledge about the histologic fate of a bone graft differs very little from the original ideas expressed in the past. It is generally accepted that to be incorporated, a graft, whether it is an autograft or

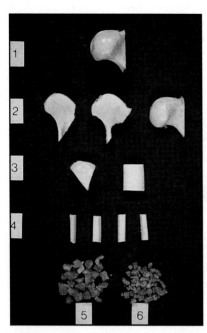

Fig. 1 Overview of the various types of bone graft: 1 to 3, solid, structural cortico-cancellous structural grafts; 4 to 6, cancellous morcellized grafts, from strips (4) to chips (5,6).

an allograft, goes through a series of processes in which the donor bone and host become closely interconnected. The host supplies the blood vessels and viable bone cells, elements that are of vital importance to the incorporation and remodeling of the dead graft material. The graft stimulates the host's cellular activity, ultimately leading to new bone formation in and around the graft, which acts as a frame-like structure for bone apposition. Important factors that influence the success of incorporation are firm fixation of the bone graft to the bone bed of the host, extent of the surface area between the graft and host bone, the vascularity of the surrounding host tissue, and the load pattern in the graft. From our clinical experience it was established that the size and architecture of the bone graft also influence the incorporation process. The distinction between structural and morcellized allografts is based on this experience (Fig. 1).

Compact structural bone grafts are very dense, which strongly compromises the ingrowth of the blood vessels essential for revitalization of the graft. In the early stages of the incorporation process, only the contact surface of the graft undergoes partial and superficial breakdown to create space for revascularization. Consequently, there is only superficial union of the graft with the host bone. Subsequently the inner part of the graft remains dead bone. It weakens due to fatigue fractures and graft resorption. We have also observed that during this incomplete and slow incorporation process it is not always possible to maintain sufficient stability of a structural bone graft after surgical fixation in a weightbearing part of the hip that is subject to considerable stress. This can also lead to movement and, thus, resorption of the graft. In contrast, impacted morcellized allografts are incorporated more uniformly and completely. Blood vessels can easily penetrate the open structure, which means rapid new bone apposition of the dead trabeculae without any loss of mechanical strength. It is well known that an individual's own bone, an autograft, incorporates better as compared to allograft due to the high osteogenic capacity and the absence of immunogenic reactions. However, it is not always possible to harvest sufficient quantities of an individual's own bone, and in elderly patients it is often of poor quality. Furthermore, the extra incision necessary to harvest the bone causes additional morbidity. For these reasons, in most cases it is necessary to use donor bone from a bone bank.

Impacted Morcellized Grafts and the Rationale for the Nijmegen Technique

The types of bone grafts used by different surgeons for acetabular reconstruction vary widely. Currently some surgeons[9,10] use morcellized allografts as routine.

Others[11–13] advocate the use of structural cancellous or corticocancellous grafts, with or without cement. This chapter deals only with morcellized allografts used with polymethylmethacrylate (PMMA) bone cement.

In the past, various surgical revision techniques have been developed to compensate for bone loss and to restore the stability of the implant. Sotelo-Garza and Charnley[14] used large quantities of bone cement to close the defect and fill the acetabular cavity. However, it is evident that in revisions where only cement is used, the bone defects still remain. Also the thin, sclerotic and smooth acetabular bone bed provides an inadequate surface for successful mechanical bone-cement interlock. The literature reports poor clinical track records. Berry and Müller[15] recommended the use of rigid metal supporting rings to bridge acetabular defects. In our opinion, the addition of these rigid metal reinforcements to bone grafting will fail because of the mismatch between the more elastic pelvic bone and the rigid metal implants and the stress shielding of the graft. Other surgeons[16] used large diameter cementless acetabular implants that were supported only by the remaining host bone. They expected spontaneous new bone formation in and around the defect.

In the 1970s, a new application for bone grafting was introduced for the reconstruction of acetabular defects in primary and revision total hip arthroplasty. In primary total hip replacement, an acetabular defect was often a congenital peripheral, segmental acetabular rim defect (Fig. 2, *top left*). A primary cavitary defect was seen fairly commonly in the advanced stages of rheumatoid arthritis. This defect has also been described as "protrusio acetabuli" (Fig. 2, *top right*). In revision total hip replacement, the defects originated mostly from the damage to the bone by the loosening process and caused cavitary, segmental, or combined defects of the acetabulum (Fig. 2, *bottom left* and *right*).

In 1975, Hastings and Parker[17] described the use of a combination of cemented total hip replacement and autogenous morcellized cancellous grafting in intrapelvic protrusio acetabuli. The graft was not impacted and was subsequently totally covered with a coarse mesh cup with a small rim.

In 1978, McCollum and Nunley[18] reported their first experience with autogenous wafers of corticocancellous bone used to augment acetabular bone stock in 25 patients with protrusio acetabuli after failed total hip arthroplasty. A fine metal mesh was subsequently tucked into acetabular anchoring holes to distribute the forces across the acetabulum. To prevent the cement from penetrating into the graft, gelfoam was used to avoid direct contact between the cement and the graft. A cemented cup was combined with an ring when the medial wall was absent.

In 1983, Marti and Besselaar[19] introduced a technique for treating protruded and dysplastic acetabuli. Medial segmental defects were closed with a corticocancellous graft supplemented with autogenous chips. Intact acetabular host bone was compressed to anchor the cement. Additionally, an Eichler ring was used. Peripheral segmental defects were repaired with segmental plugs taken from the pelvic crista and fixed with screws to the iliac wall.

In 1983, Roffman and associates,[20] in an animal model with intrapelvic protrusio, investigated the fate of autogenous chips under a layer of polymethylmethacrylate bone cement. Their model comprised a medial segmental defect. Histologic evaluation revealed the formation of bone from the acetabular wall toward the graft. The graft appeared viable, and new bone formation was induced along the surface adjoining the bone cement. Based on these experimental results in dogs, Mendes and associ-

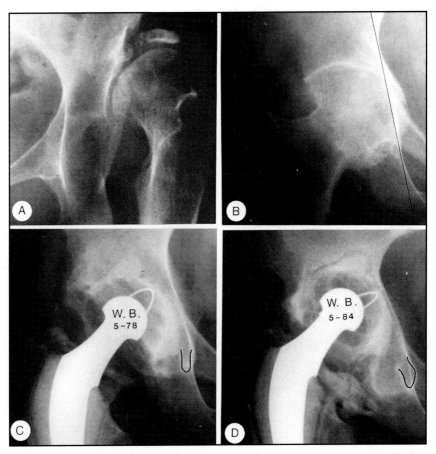

Fig. 2 Radiographs of various acetabular defects. **Top left,** View of the left hip with a dysplastic acetabulum, so-called dysplasia, which gave rise to secondary arthrosis. The femoral head has migrated in a cranial direction because of insufficient coverage. This is a case of a primary peripheral segmental rim defect. **Top right,** Preoperative radiograph of a woman with protrusio of the right acetabulum. The femoral head has migrated inwards and threatens to break through the medial wall of the acetabulum. The consequential bone loss is referred as a cavitary defect. **Bottom left,** Status after primary total hip arthroplasty that was performed in 1974. After some time both prosthetic components developed mechanical loosening. **Bottom right,** Clear signs of changes in position of the component and migration of the cup in a cranial and medial direction that resulted in bone loss and peripheral segmental rim defect. This is an example of a combined peripheral segmental and cavitary defect.

ates[21] published the results of a clinical study on primary cemented arthroplasties combined with autogenous bone chips supported with a metal mesh for intrapelvic protrusio. Follow-up studies, the longest of which were 6 years, showed clinical success in all patients.

In 1984, Slooff and associates[22] published their experience with a modified method using impacted morcellized allografts. Acetabular segmental defects were closed with corticocancellous slices or

with flexible metal wire meshes. The contained acetabulum was tightly packed with allograft chips (sized 1 cm³). The cup was inserted after pressurizing the cement directly onto the graft. To correct structural acetabular integrity loss and impairment of implant mechanical support and hip joint mechanics, our treatment strategy sought to do the following: (1) repair hip mechanics by positioning the cup at the level of the anatomic acetabulum (teardrop); (2) close segmen-

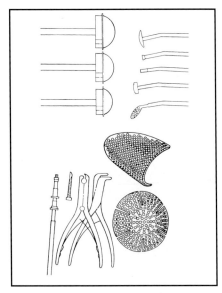

Fig. 3 Top, The instrumentation used for acetabular impaction; **bottom,** Examples of the preformed metal reconstruction mesh and the special tools used to trim, cut, and fix the mesh.

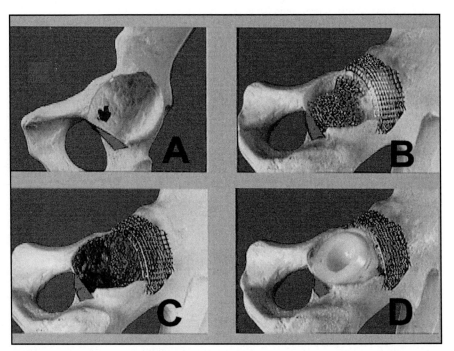

Fig. 4 The reconstruction technique. **Top left,** A combined segmental and cavitary defect. The medial wall defect is combined with a large rim defect and bone loss in the cranial part of the acetabulum. **Top right,** A preformed metal wire mesh closes the medial wall defect and a second wire mesh is used to reconstruct the acetabular rim. A confined cavitary defect remains. **Bottom left,** Solidly impacted morcellized allograft is molded in the defect and the new acetabulum is reconstructed at the level of the transverse ligament. **Bottom right,** Finally the new acetabular component is cemented directly on the impacted allograft, again at the level of the transverse ligament.

tal defects with metal wire mesh to achieve containment (a cavitary defect remains); (3) replace the periprosthetic bone loss by augmenting the cavitary defect with morcellized allograft; and (4) restore stability by impacting the chips and using bone cement.

The X-Change Acetabular Revision Instrumentation System, developed in cooperation with Howmedica International, Staines, UK, was designed to achieve these goals (Fig. 3). In use since 1978, this surgical technique has been standardized and basically has not been changed.

Surgical Technique

The posterolateral approach was used in all cases. This enabled extensive exposure of all aspects of the acetabulum and proximal femur. Trochanteric osteotomy was seldom necessary. Identification of major landmarks was helpful for orientation if scarring and distortion disturbed the anatomy. These landmarks were the tip of the greater trochanter, the tendinous part

of the gluteus maximus, the lower border of the gluteus medius and minimus, and the sciatic nerve. Aspiration of the hip was performed at this stage to obtain fluid for Gram staining and frozen sectioning to examine for possible infection.

The proximal part of the femur was exposed extensively and mobilized before the hip was dislocated. Exposure of the entire socket was achieved by removing all scar tissue, by performing circumferential capsulotomy, and by dividing the iliopsoas tendon. After removing the components and all the cement, the fibrous interface was freed completely from the irregular acetabular wall using sharp spoons and curettes. Special care was taken to locate the transverse ligament at the inferior side of the acetabulum. The socket was reconstructed from this level upwards. At least three specimens were

taken from the interfacial fibrous membrane for frozen sectioning and bacterial culture. After taking these samples, systemic antibiotic therapy was started.

The acetabular floor and walls were examined meticulously for any hidden medial and/or peripheral segmental defects (Fig. 4, *top left*). Using a pair of scissors, a flexible stainless steel mesh was trimmed and adapted to fit any of the defects and was rigidly fixed to the iliac wall with at least three screws. Any medial segmental defect was closed in a similar manner with a metal mesh. In this way, the acetabulum was contained and had become a cavitary defect (Fig. 4, *top right*). Many small drill holes (2 mm) were made in the sclerotic acetabular wall to enhance surface contact and promote vascular invasion into the graft.

Deep frozen femoral heads from the

hospital bone bank were divided into four equal parts. Substantial chips were cut with a rongeur or scissors. After cleaning the acetabulum, any existing small cavities were packed tightly with chips; then the entire socket was filled layer by layer. Impactors hammered the chips in situ, starting with the largest possible size impactor and ending with the most suitable size cup. Care was taken to reconstruct the anatomy of the hip with the new socket at the level of the transverse ligament. The acetabulum was reconstructed with a substantial layer of graft around the new cup, because the thickness of this graft layer must at least be 5 mm. After impaction, the whole acetabular hemisphere was covered with a layer of impacted allograft chips. However, it was evident that this layer was not of a uniform thickness, because the thickness depended locally on the depth of the acetabular defect. After impaction, the preexistent enlarged acetabular diameter had been reduced to a normal size (Fig. 4, *bottom left*).

While the antibiotic-loaded cement was being prepared, pressure on the graft was maintained using a trial socket. After inserting and pressurizing the cement, the cup was placed and held in position with the pusher until the cement had polymerized (Fig. 4, *bottom right*). Postoperative management included anticoagulation therapy for 3 months and systemic antibiotics for 24 hours. Indomethacin was administered for 7 days to prevent the development of heterotopic ossification. Mobilization of the patient was individualized according to the different circumstances of the revision arthroplasty. A period of 3 to 6 weeks of bed rest was required after major acetabular reconstruction.

Scientific Studies

The scientific bases for bone impaction grafting and cement are the results of the animal experiments and laboratory examinations.

Animal Experiments

To obtain more insight into the mechanical stability of reconstructions using impacted morcellized allografts with cement, and to study the incorporation process of the graft, we performed two separate animal experiments using Dutch milk goats. For the femur, follow-up was relatively brief, so this study will concentrate primarily on the mechanical stability.[23] The longer follow-up periods available for the acetabulum made this study very useful as a detailed description of the histologic incorporation process.[24] Surgical techniques used to reconstruct acetabular and femoral deficiencies were similar to those used in humans.

Mechanical Study

The medullary cavity of the femur was prepared with hand-reamers. A concentric intramedullary graft could be impacted in a retrograde fashion, using a specially developed set of instruments.[25] Cement was inserted into this construction, followed by the insertion of the femoral stem. Tantalum pellets were fixed to the implant and the bone prior to insertion in order to allow Röntgen-Stereophotogrammatic Analysis (RSA).[26] The initial stability was analyzed in four specimens; the postoperative changes were evaluated in eight goats sacrificed after 6 and 12 weeks. The prosthesis-bone construct was then loaded physiologically with a maximal load of 144% of body weight (Fig. 5). The loading mode applied resulted in bending and rotational forces, which are important for testing the stability of hip prostheses.[25] Load was applied stepwise from zero to 200, 500, and 800 N and again unloaded. Each loading period lasted 10 minutes. Stereoradiographs were taken before loading, after each loading step, and 10 minutes after the final unloading. Relative rotations and translations around and along the coordinate axes were calculated.

Six and 12 weeks after implantation the stability had clearly increased when

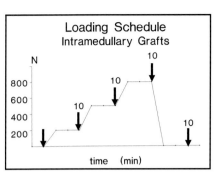

Fig. 5 The loading schedule of the femoral intramedullary grafts. Stereoradiographs were made 10 minutes after each step in load (arrows). (Reproduced with permission from Sloof TJ: Impaction grafting and cemented acetabular revision, in Villar (ed): *Revision Hip Arthroplasty*. Oxford, England, Butterworth Heinemann, 1997, pp 116-130.)

compared to the initial stability of the stems immediately after insertion (Fig. 6). In the 6- and 12-week specimens, most of the motion was axial rotation and subsidence, both of which increased with increasing load. The maximum rotation was 0.24° under 800 N, but after unloading there was significant elastic recovery, which resulted in a maximum permanent rotation of 0.14°. There were no differences between the 6- and 12-week groups. Maximum subsidence under a load of 800 N was 0.164 mm and after unloading the maximum permanent subsidence was 0.078 mm.

Although there were no significant differences between the results of the 6- and 12-week specimens, there was a trend towards greater permanent displacement in the 12-week group. The standard deviations for translations and rotations observed during biomechanical testing were estimated to be 0.036 mm and 0.07°, respectively. The results of the mechanical testing showed an increased stability postoperatively as the graft became integrated into a new bony structure. This process could indeed be confirmed by histologic analysis.

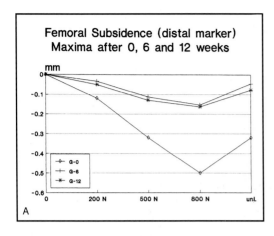

A

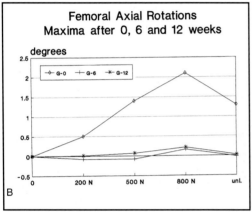

B

Fig. 6 Top, Maximal femoral subsidence after 0, 6, and 12 weeks. Note increasing stability after incorporation of the graft. **Bottom,** Maximal rotations of the graft after 0, 6, and 12 weeks show the same trend. (Reproduced with permission from Sloof TJ: Impaction grafting and cemented acetabular revision, in Villar (ed): *Revision Hip Arthroplasty.* Oxford, England, Butterworth Heinemann, 1997, pp 116-130.)

Histologic Analysis

In another animal experiment, hand reamers were used to make a cavitary defect in the anterior-superior segment of the acetabulum. Impaction grafting of the resulting defect was performed in the same way as during clinical application to patients. The acetabular component was cemented.

In each time period, three goats were sacrificed, at intervals of 6, 12, 24, and 48 weeks. Different histologic techniques were applied, including fluorochrome labeling of new bone. Directly after the operation, the impacted graft consisted of fairly large pieces of trabecular bone, which displayed small microfractures at all levels (Fig. 7). The medullary fat had been squeezed out during impaction and had been replaced by a fibrin clot. After 6 weeks, a front of vascular sprouts accompanied by loose connective tissue, with many leukocytes, penetrated into the graft at a speed of about 70 mm per day. A very high dynamic bone turnover was observed in the graft in association with this fibrovascular tissue, comprising bone graft resorption by osteoclasts and bone apposition by osteoblasts. After 6 weeks, this process resulted in a new trabecular structure in the revascularized areas. This structure consisted primarily of newly formed mainly woven bone with remnants of the graft. After 12 weeks, the percentage of graft in the new trabecular structure decreased further by bone remodeling, which produced lamellar bone. Radiographic and histologic evaluation demonstrated that the orientation of the newly formed trabecular bone was such that load transfer was possible from the cement layer to the host bone bed. At the graft-cement interface, a mixture was found of local areas where vital bone was in intimate contact with the cement layer, and other areas where fibrous tissue predominated. Between 24 and 48 weeks after surgery, the graft in the defect of the acetabulum had been completely remodeled into lamellar bone.

From our histologic and mechanical results we conclude that the reconstruction technique provides sufficient initial stability to allow incorporation of the impacted acetabular and femoral grafts.

Human Data

Histologic analysis evaluation of graft incorporation is an alternative for radiographic techniques to assess the extent of incorporation into a new trabecular structure. We were able to collect nine biopsies taken from eight grafted acetabuli, 1 to 72 months after revision.[27] Revision in all these patients was done using the technique described by Slooff and associates.[22] In one patient, who developed persistent sciatic nerve problems after a huge reconstruction in which the center of rotation was created about 5 cm more distally, the whole reconstruction had to be removed after 28 months. Histologic inspection of almost the whole previous graft, including the graft-cement interface, was then possible.

At 1 month postrevision, no signs of graft incorporation were found. In two out of the three biopsies taken at 4 months, a front of new bone was now penetrating the avascular graft. At the revascularization front, which could be recognized on the basis of vital soft tissue, osteoid and woven bone formed on the original graft trabeculae and in the interstitial space (Fig. 8). Also, local osteoclastic resorption of the graft was found.

All of the specimens taken 8 to 28 months after revision showed different stages of graft incorporation. At 8 and 9 months, various amounts of graft remnants were embedded in a new trabecular structure. Initially, the newly formed bone was woven bone, and this was later remodeled into lamellar bone in the

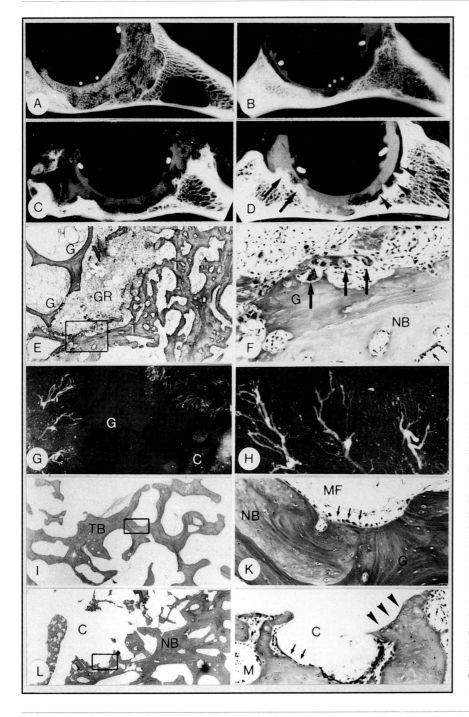

Fig. 7 A-D, Radiographs of thick sections through the acetabulum of the goat taken at 0 (**A**), 12 (**B**), 24 (**C**), and 48 weeks (**D**) after surgery. **A,** Note large pieces of graft and the clear transition zone to the host bone-bed. **B,** Complete consolidation of the graft with the host bone. The incorporation of the graft is almost completed. **C,** A radiolucent zone is present between the cement layer and the bone, indicating that a soft-tissue interface has been formed. **D,** Note local contact areas between bone and cement (arrows) and a radiolucent zone (arrow heads). Note also the dense bone adjacent the cement layer. **E,** Granulation tissue (GR) in the transition zone between a vital graft (G) and newly formed trabecular bone (T) 3 weeks after surgery. **F,** Enlargement of rectangular area outlined in **E**. Many osteoclastic bone cells (large arrows) resorb the graft (G) and osteoblasts (small arrows) synthesize new bone (NB). **G,** A vascularization front penetrates into the graft (G) 12 weeks after the surgery. Cement (C) had penetrated into the graft. **H,** Enlargement of left part of **G**. **I,** Structure of new trabecular bone after 12 weeks. **K,** Enlargement of rectangular area outlined in **I** showing active osteoblasts (arrows) and new bone (NB). Remnants of the graft (G) can be recognized by the empty osteocyte lacunae. **L,** Interface between new bone (NB) and the cement 48 weeks after surgery. Cement (C) that was removed during processing of the tissues, had penetrated deeply into the graft. **M,** Locally at higher magnification a very thin layer, one cell thick (arrows), of soft-tissue interface is present, while at other locations the new bone is in direct contact with the cement layer (arrowheads). **E, G, I, L** ×12.5; **F, H, K, M** ×125. (Reproduced with permission from Slooff TJ, Schimmel JW, Buma P: Cemented fixation with bone grafts. *Orthop Clin North Am* 1993;24:667–677.)

specimens with a longer follow-up period. The interface with the cement layer was histologically similar to that seen in earlier animal studies. Locally vital bone was in direct contact with the cement, but most locations showed a thin soft-tissue layer interfaced with the cement. The bone in the specimens with a fol-low-up of 15 months or longer closely resembled normal trabecular bone, with only a very few remnants of graft. Similar clinical results were reported after impaction grafting in the proximal femur.[28,29] The sequence of events was comparable to that which had previously been observed in animal experi-ments.[24,30–34]

From these scientific data, we conclude that impacted morcellized allograft with cement completely incorporates into a new trabecular structure and that the histologic pattern of graft incorporation is consistent in both the animal model and human biopsies.

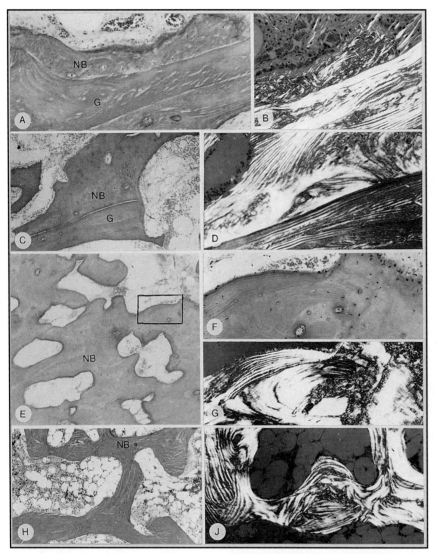

Fig. 8. A and **B,** Human core biopsy 4 months after impaction grafting in the acetabulum. Note new bone formation (NB) on remnant of graft (G). **B,** Same as **A** but with polarized light. Note woven bone formation (×140). **C** and **D,** Eight months after impaction grafting. Graft (G) has been partially resorbed. New bone formation in the form of lamellar bone. (×60 and ×140, respectively). **E-G,** Fifteen months after impaction grafting. Graft remnants are extremely scarce. Detail of boxed area shows vital (F) lamellar (G) bone. ×35 and ×140, respectively. **H** and **J,** Normal lamellar (J) bony structure with vital cell rich hemopoetic tissue (H) in specimen 28 months after impaction grafting. ×60. (Figures A and B reproduced with permission from Buma P, Lamerigts N, Schreurs BW, et al: Impacted graft incorporation after cemented acetabular revision: Histological evaluation in 8 patients. *Acta Orthop Scand* 1996;67:536-540.)

Clinical Results

In 1984 we first reported the short-term results of bone impaction grafting in total hip replacement for acetabular protrusion.[22] In 40 patients, 43 acetabular reconstructions were performed. Of these, 21 arthroplasties were primary procedures in cases with protrusion and 22 were revisions after failed total hip arthroplasties with acetabular bone stock loss. Diagnosis of the cases was osteoarthritis (15), rheumatoid arthritis (15) or trauma. The defects were mainly contained. Autografts were used in all primary total hip arthroplasties, but allografts were used in all revisions. After a short-term follow-up of 2 years (range, 0.5 to 5.5 years) there were no revisions, but radiolucent lines were seen in five cases.

Our mid-term results were presented in 1993 in a study of 88 acetabular hip revisions in 80 patients.[31] All hips were reconstructed with impacted morcellized bone grafts, and the average follow-up was 5.7 years (range, 2 to 11 years). The group consisted of 58 women and 22 men. The patients required surgery because of primary osteoarthritis (49), secondary osteoarthritis (22), or rheumatoid arthritis (nine). Defects were classified according to the AAOS classification system as cavitary (42 cases) or combined segmental-cavitary (38 cases). At this mid-term 5.7-year follow-up, four acetabular re-revisions had been performed, two for septic loosening and two for aseptic loosening. The postoperative Harris Hip Scores (HHS) averaged 87; the preoperative HHS was estimated at 44. Six cases were defined as radiologic failures, one case because of progressive radiologic loosening in all three zones, according to DeLee and Charnley.[35] Using a computer-digitizing program, in the other five cases radiologic loosening was suspected because of progressive migration.

However, only long-term follow-up can prove the true clinical value of a surgical technique. The most reliable criterion in long-term follow-up of primary hip arthroplasties and revision hip arthroplasties is the survival rate of the prosthesis using the moment of re-revision as the endpoint.[36] All patients who underwent acetabular reconstruction and revision surgery with impacted morcellized bone grafts at our department with a follow-up of at least 10 years were enrolled in our study (to be published).

In this long-term study, 62 acetabular

revisions were performed with impacted morcellized bone grafts and a cemented cup for failed acetabular components in 58 patients.[37] Two cases (2 hips) were lost to follow-up. Ten cases (ten hips) died within 10 years after the operation. None had a re-revision. Forty-six patients (50 hips) had a follow-up of 10 years or more (range, 10 to 15 years; average, 11.8 years). The defects were classified as cavitary in 37 and combined in 23 cases. There were no solitary segmental defects in this group of patients. Five acetabular re-revisions had been performed. These were due to septic loosening in two cases (3 and 6 years postoperative) and aseptic loosening in three cases (6, 9, and 12 years postoperative).

The overall survival rate was 90% when all loosenings were taken into account. But excluding the two infections, the survival rate for aseptic loosening only was 94% at an average of 11.8 years follow-up. Using the same criteria as mentioned above, there were four radiographic failures without clinical symptons of loosening.

Current Recommendations

Before attempting acetabular reconstruction with bone impaction grafting and cement, a surgeon should be informed as thoroughly as possible about the clinical, scientific, and technical details of this reconstruction method, developed at the hospitals in Nijmegen and Exeter. Experimental studies and clinical observations have clearly shown that impacted morcellized allografts lead to a predictable result: complete and rapid incorporation without impairing the strength of the graft during the process (Fig. 9). This is in contrast with the use of structural bone grafts, which incorporate incompletely, with unpredictable results.[38,39] The structural grafts that are generally used are parts of degenerative femoral heads, and this may be the cause of the incomplete incorporation. Furthermore, because of the existing

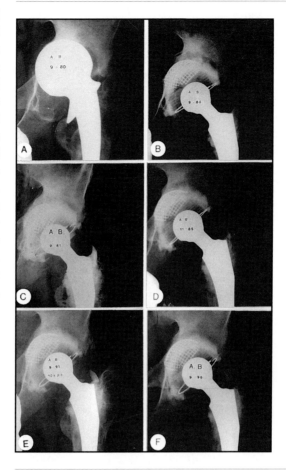

Fig. 9 A, Radiograph of a 36-year-old patient with a hemiprosthesis of the right hip that had been implanted 6 years following failed osteosynthesis of a femoral neck fracture. The metal head of the prosthesis is protruding through the acetabulum, causing central segmental defect of the acetabulum. **B-F,** Serial radiographs directly after (**B**), 1 year after (**C**), 5 years after (**D**), 10 years after (**E**), and 16 years (**F**), after reconstruction with impacted allograft bone chips. No migration, no signs of loosening, and a homogeneous structure of the graft are visible.

mismatch of the contact surfaces, it is very difficult to achieve permanent fixation of structural cancellous grafts to host bone. This lack of fixation can lead to instability of the graft and eventual resorption.

If segmental acetabular defects are present, it is mandatory to close them in order to achieve adequate impaction. We advocate the use of flexible wire meshes, which are adapted and fixed to the pelvis by screw fixation. Impaction of the morcellized grafts results in a stable and rough surface that improves the mechanical cement-bone interlock and the adaptation of the chip closely to the irregular surface of the host bone bed. Rigid impaction reduces gap formation between the host and graft, promoting the union process. The stability of the reconstruction is further improved by pressurizing the cement onto the graft.

As previously mentioned, the use of substantially sized morcellized allografts approximately 1 cm in each dimension is recommended for the acetabulum. Reduction of the chip size can cause early migration of the acetabular cup during the incorporation process because of the lack of initial stability.

In 1988, Hungerford and Jones[40] expressed their concern about allowing cement to be in direct contact with a morcellized allograft. Positive results with this combination have been reported by Roffman and associates,[20] and have been confirmed by the results of histologic studies performed by Schimmel[24] and Schreurs[34] in animal models.

As reported by other investigators, no difference was observed between the radiologic evaluation of autogenous grafts and that of allografts. However, in our view radiographic evaluation of bone incorporation is difficult. Because allograft bone can be available in sufficient quantities, there is no limit to the quantity of graft used. The economics of revision hip surgery, in general, make this procedure very unpopular for hospital administration and orthopaedic surgeons. The resource issues of these reconstruction techniques of the hip are significant and are mainly defined by the type of implant, the fixation method (with or without cement), and the use of banked bone. However, the cost aspects of special and custom-made prostheses must not be underestimated.

References

1. Leeuwenhoek van A: Microscopical observations about blood, milk bones, the brain, spittle, cuticula, sweat, fat and tears. *Philos Trans R Soc Lond* 1674;9:121–131.

2. van Meekeren J: *Heel-en Geneeskundige Aanmerkingen.* Amsterdam, The Netherlands, L Commelijn, 1668.

3. Ollier L: *Traité Experimental et Clinique de la Regeneration des os et de la Production Artificielle du Tissu Osseux.* Paris, France, Victor Masson, 1867.

4. Macewen W: Observations concerning transplantation of bones. *Proc Roy Soc Lond* 1881;32:232–247.

5. Curtis BF: Cases of bone implantation and transplantation for cyst of tibia, osteomyelitic cavities, and ununited fractures. *Am J Med Sci* 1893;106:30–37.

6. Barth A: Ueber histologische Befunde nach Knochenimplantationen. *Arch Klin Chir* 1893;46:409–417.

7. Lexer E: Die Verwendung der freien Knochenplastik nebst Versuchen über Gelenkversteifung und Gelenktransplantation. *Arch Klin Chir* 1908;86:939–954.

8. Axhausen G: Arbeiten aus dem Gebiet de Knochenpathologie und Knochenchirurgie 1: kritische bemerkungen und neue Beiträge zur freien Knochentransplantation. *Arch Klin Chir* 1911;94:241–281.

9. Hirst P, Esser M, Murphy JC, et al: Bone grafting for protrusio acetabuli during total hip replacement: A review of the Wrightington method in 61 hips. *J Bone Joint Surg* 1987;69B:229–233.

10. Olivier H, Sanouiller JL: Acetabular reconstruction using spongious grafts in reoperation of hip arthroplasties. *Rev Chir Orthop Repar Appar Mot* 1991;77:232–240.

11. Gross AE, Lavoie MV, McDermott P, et al: The use of allograft bone in revision of total hip arthroplasty. *Clin Orthop* 1985;197:115–122.

12. Harris WH, Crothers O, Oh I: Total hip replacement and femoral-head bone-grafting for severe acetabular deficiency in adults. *J Bone Joint Surg* 1977;59A:752–759.

13. Harris WH: Allografting in total hip arthroplasty: In adults with severe acetabular deficiency including a surgical technique for bolting the graft to the ilium. *Clin Orthop* 1982;162:150–164.

14. Sotelo-Garza A, Charnley J: The results of Charnley arthroplasty of the hip performed for protrusio acetabuli. *Clin Orthop* 1978;132:12–18.

15. Berry DJ, Müller ME: Revision arthroplasty using an anti-protrusio cage for massive acetabular bone deficiency. *J Bone Joint Surg* 1992;74B:711–715.

16. Harris WH: Management of the deficient acetabulum using cementless fixation without bone grafting. *Orthop Clin North Am* 1993;24:663–665.

17. Hastings DE, Parker SM: Protrusio acetabuli in rheumatoid arthritis. *Clin Orthop* 1975;108:76–83.

18. McCollum DE, Nunley JA: Bone grafting in acetabular protrusio: A biologic buttress, in Nelson CL (ed): *The Hip: Proceedings of the Sixth Open Scientific Meeting of the Hip Society, 1978.* St Louis, MO, CV Mosby, 1978, pp 124–146.

19. Marti RK, Besselaar PP: Bone grafts in primary and secondary total hip replacement, in Marti RK (ed): *Progress in Cemented Total Hip Surgery and Revision.* Amsterdam, The Netherlands, Excerpta Medica, 1983, pp 107–129.

20. Roffman M, Silbermann M, Mendes DG: Incorporation of bone graft covered with methylmethacrylate onto the acetabular wall: An experimental study. *Acta Orthop Scand* 1983;54:580–583.

21. Mendes DG, Roffman M, Silbermann M: Reconstruction of the acetabular wall with bone graft in arthroplasty of the hip. *Clin Orthop* 1984;186:29–37.

22. Slooff TJ, Huiskes R, van Horn J, et al: Bone grafting in total hip replacement for acetabular protrusion. *Acta Orthop Scand* 1984;55:593–596.

23. Schreurs BW, Huiskes R, Slooff TJJH: The initial stability of hip prosthesis in combination with femoral intramedullary bonegraft, in Odgaard A, Kjaersgaard-Andersen P, Sojbjerg JO (eds): *European Biomechanics: Proceedings of the 7th Meeting of the European Society of Biomechanics.* Aarhus, Denmark, European Society of Biomechanics, 1990, p A14.

24. Schimmel JW, Buma P, Versleyen D, et al: Acetabular reconstruction with impacted morcellized cancellous allografts in cemented hip arthroplasty: A histologic and biomechanical study on the goat. *J Arthroplasty,* in press.

25. Schreurs BW, Buma P, Huiskes R, et al: Morsellized allografts for fixation of the hip prosthesis femoral component: A mechanical and histological study in the goat. *Acta Orthop Scand* 1994;65:267–275.

26. Selvik G: *A Roentgen Stereophotogrammetric Method for the Study of the Kinematics of the Skeletal System.* Lund, Sweden, University of Lund, 1974. Thesis.

27. Buma P, Lamerigts N, Schreurs BW, et al: Impacted graft incorporation after cemented acetabular revision: Histological evaluation in 8 patients. *Acta Orthop Scand* 1996;67:536–540.

28. Ling RS, Timperley AJ, Linder L: Histology of cancellous impaction grafting in the femur: A case report. *J Bone Joint Surg* 1993;75B:693–696

29. Nelissen RG, Bauer TW, Weidenhielm LR, et al: Revision hip arthroplasty with the use of cement and impaction grafting: Histological analysis of four cases. *J Bone Joint Surg* 1995;77A:412–422.

30. Buma P, Schreurs BW, Versleyen D, et al: Histological evaluation of allograft incorporation after cemented and non-cemented hip arthroplasty in the goat, in Older J (ed): *Bone Implant Grafting.* London, England, Springer Verlag, 1992, pp 13–17.

31. Slooff TJ, Schimmel JW, Buma P: Cemented fixation with bone grafts. *Orthop Clin North Am* 1993;24:667–677.

32. Slooff TJ , Buma P, Schreurs BW, et al: Acetabular and femoral reconstruction with impacted grafts and cement. *Clin Orthop* 1996;324:108–115.

33. Slooff TJ, Buma P, Schimmel JW, et al: Impaction grafting and cement in acetabular revision arthroplasty, in Czitrom AA, Winkler H (eds): *Orthopaedic Allograft Surgery.* Wien, Germany, Springer-Verlag, 1996, pp 125–134.

34. Schreurs BW: *Reconstructive Options in Revision Surgery of Failed Total Hip Arthroplasties.* Nijmegen, The Netherlands, University of Ku Nijmegen, 1994. Thesis.

35. DeLee JG, Charnley J: Radiological demarcation of cemented sockets in total hip replacement. *Clin Orthop* 1976;121:20–32.

36. Malchau H, Herberts P: Surgical and cemented technique in total hip replacement: A revision-risk study of 136,000 primary operations. Proceedings of the American Academy of Orthopaedic Surgeons 63rd Annual Meeting, Atlanta, GA. Rosemont, IL, American Academy of Orthopaedic Surgeons, 1996.

37. Schreurs BW, Buma P, Gardeniers JW, et al: Acetabular reconstruction with impacted morcellized cancellous bone grafts in cemented revision hip arthroplasty: A ten- to 15-year follow-up study. Proceedings of the American Academy of Orthopaedic Surgeons 65th Annual Meeting, New Orleans, LA. Rosemont, IL, American Academy of Orthopaedic Surgeons, 1998.

38. Enneking WF, Mindell ER: Observations on massive retrieved human allografts. *J Bone Joint Surg* 1991;73A:1123–1142.

39. Stevenson S, Xiao Qing Li, Martin B: The fate of cancellous and cortical bone after transplantation of fresh and frozen tissue-antigen-matched and mismatched osteochondral allografts in dogs. *J Bone Joint Surg* 1991;73A:1143–1156.

40. Hungerford DS, Jones LC: The rationale of cementless revision of cemented arthroplasty failures. *Clin Orthop* 1988;235:12–24.

Neurovascular Injury Associated with Hip Arthroplasty

David G. Lewallen, MD

Neurologic and vascular complications following hip arthroplasty are uncommon, and their impact ranges from transient and trivial to permanent and devastating. The proximity of neurologic and vascular structures to the hip makes any hip surgery potentially hazardous. Direct and indirect injury of these structures can occur during surgical exposure and the subsequent procedure. The important features of the neurologic and vascular structures that are at risk during a hip arthroplasty, especially the pertinent anatomy, etiology of injuries, and treatment options, provide a foundation of information that can assist the physician who encounters neurologic or vascular complications clinically.

Neurologic Complications

Neurologic dysfunction following hip arthroplasty can be due to central neurologic injury or to a peripheral-nerve lesion. Peripheral-nerve lesions during hip arthroplasty may be categorized according to severity, location, and onset of symptoms relative to the index procedure. Central neurologic injury may occur as a result of prolonged hypoxia, a cerebrovascular accident, or fat embolism resulting from the surgery. Careful treatment by the anesthesiology team during procedures on the hip is necessary to avoid hypoxia or anoxia, to reduce major fluctuations in blood pressure that can contribute to the risk of a cerebrovascular accident, and to assist in careful position-

ing of the patient in order to prevent a peripheral-nerve lesion (such as brachial plexus stretch). Embolization of fat and marrow elements is one factor directly related to the surgical procedure that can have an important central neurologic effect and is somewhat under the control of the operating surgeon.

Neurologic Sequelae of Fat Embolism

Embolization of fat and marrow elements from the femur and, to a lesser degree, the acetabulum has been shown to occur during all primary total hip arthroplasties and to peak during portions of the procedure that involve maximum manipulation of bone, such as reaming and particularly cementing of a component.[1-5] Most patients seem to tolerate the passage of this embolic material through the right side of the heart and into the pulmonary vessels without apparent signs or sequelae.[1] Rarely, marked intraoperative hypotension, hypoxia, and even cardiac arrest and death occur as a result of those emboli, usually immediately after cementing of an implant.[6-10] A patent foramen ovale, which was documented in approximately 25% of 965 hearts of normal adults in an autopsy study, allows for the potential of paradoxical embolization of this material with passage from the right side of the heart to the left side and subsequent widespread systemic delivery.[1,11,12] Paradoxical embolization has been estimated to be possible in 10%

of normal patients.[11] The passage of this material into the left-sided circulation may cause focal neurologic deficits, perioperative delirium, and even death during the postoperative period. In individuals who do not have the potential for right-to-left shunting, the pulmonary vessels function as a filter, entrapping the material and limiting the risk that it poses to the central nervous system (Fig. 1). The use of transesophageal echocardiography intraoperatively has allowed documentation of the passage of fat and marrow elements through the right atrium and the right ventricle and has also allowed direct observation of paradoxical embolization in individuals who have right-to-left shunting at the atrial level[1] (Fig. 2). Focal cerebral infarcts can be observed on computed tomography (CT) scans (Fig. 3), and they can be seen directly in pathologic specimens when perioperative death results from paradoxical embolization.

It is not possible to prevent embolization of fat and marrow elements completely during the course of hip arthroplasty, but some measures may minimize the amount of material that is delivered. Pulsatile lavage of the osseous bed before placement of the implant, particularly in arthroplasties performed with cement, should reduce the amount of material present for potential embolization to the venous circulation.[13,14] The quantity of material embolized has been directly related to the amount of pressurization

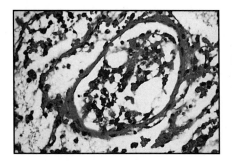

Fig. 1 Histologic autopsy specimen of a pulmonary vessel from a patient who died intraoperatively immediately after cementing of a component. Intravascular fat and marrow elements are visible (hematoxylin and eosin, approximate magnification ×100).

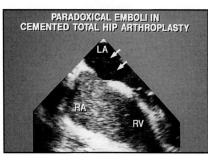

Fig. 2 Intraoperative transesophageal echocardiogram of the heart, made just after insertion of a femoral component with cement. The right atrium (RA), left atrium (LA), and right ventricle (RV) are visible. Bright-speckled echogenic material is present in the right atrium and paradoxical emboli (arrows) are visible in the left atrium.

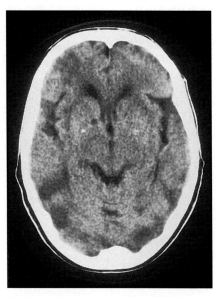

Fig. 3 Computed tomography scan of the head, showing dark areas of focal cerebral infarction (arrowheads) in a patient who went into a coma immediately after a bipolar arthroplasty with cement and subsequently died. The presence of a previously undiagnosed major right-to-left shunt at the atrial level on an echocardiogram led to the diagnosis of intraoperative paradoxical embolization. (Reproduced with permission from Lewallen DG, Ereth MH: Intraoperative mortality, in Morrey BF (ed): *Reconstructive Surgery of the Joints*, ed 2. New York, NY, Churchill Livingstone, 1996, pp 197–205.)

that occurs within the bone.[3,4,15] Thus, excessive pressurization of the cement, particularly on the femoral side, is not warranted, especially in elderly debilitated patients or in those in whom a preexisting right-to-left shunt has been recognized. Use of a vent hole in the femur allows extravasation of fat, blood, and marrow elements during placement of the femoral component and should also reduce the amount of material delivered to the right-sided circulation.[16] It is possible to switch from a femoral implant designed to be inserted with cement to one designed to be inserted without cement if indications during the surgical procedure suggest that a patient's condition is unstable or if the patient is particularly sensitive to earlier steps of the procedure known to be associated with major amounts of embolic material, such as osseous reaming, cementing of the acetabular component, or placement of an intramedullary plug.[1,9] A drop in blood pressure of at least 20% to 30% of the baseline mean arterial pressure directly associated with those particular steps should prompt consideration of a change in technique if a stem was intended to be inserted with cement. While the risk of catastrophic injury of the central nervous system or death due to paradoxi-

cal embolization is exceedingly rare, it is not known how often the commonly observed perioperative state of confusion after hip arthroplasty is caused by more subtle manifestations of this same problem. Echocardiography may be of benefit preoperatively when the medical and cardiac evaluation suggests a possible structural cardiac abnormality.

Peripheral-Nerve Complications

Injuries of peripheral nerves can be categorized according to location, severity, and etiology. The prevalence of neurologic injuries in the upper extremity following hip arthroplasty is approximately 0.15%, as documented in a review of more than 7,000 replacements.[17] Such injuries are usually caused by problems with positioning of the patient, and they are much more likely to occur in patients who have rheumatoid arthritis.[17,18] Neurologic injuries involving the contralateral lower extremity are also rare, occurring in five of 919 arthroplasties in one review, and these also are caused mainly by problems with positioning. These injuries most frequently manifest as a transient hypoesthesia or less often as motor dysfunction.[18] Most peripheral-nerve lesions associated with hip arthro-

plasty involve the treated limb and can be caused by direct injury, positioning problems, or excessive retraction.

The severity of peripheral-nerve lesions was categorized by Seddon[19] according to the degree of anatomic disruption. Neurapraxia involves an intact neurologic structure with decreased function caused by local pressure producing ischemia and contusion of the nerve. Axonotmesis involves axonal disruption with distal degeneration of the myelin but with no disruption of the endoneural tube. A return of nerve function is possible with neurapraxia or axonotmesis. Neurotmesis involves complete disruption of the nerve, such as is seen in complete transection, and results in a permanent loss of nerve function unless surgical repair is performed.[19] Clinical discrimination between neurapraxia and neurotmesis is difficult, especially initially.

Prevalence
Peripheral-nerve lesions have been clinically evident after 0.6% to 1.3% of primary total hip arthroplasties, according to reports of series involving 600 to more than 2,000 patients.[20-24] Neural injury has been observed after as many as 7.5% of revision arthroplasties, according to series ranging in size from 88 to more than 3,000 patients.[25-27] However, subclinical neural injury demonstrable on electromyographic or nerve-conduction studies is actually quite common after hip arthroplasty. In one prospective study, it was detected in 70% of 30 hips.[24] In two series, of 614 and 7,133 hips, more than 90% of the observed nerve palsies involved the sciatic nerve, with half of these involving only the peroneal division.[17,20] The femoral nerve is the next most commonly injured nerve, but such injury is rarely noted clinically and even more rarely involves prolonged dysfunction or disability.[28] Injury of the obturator nerve, at least by clinical criteria, is infrequent but can be caused by intrapelvic extrusion of cement.[29] The prevalence of injury of the superior gluteal nerve, especially that associated with the Hardinge or transgluteal approach, is not clear. While they are thought to be uncommon, these injuries may occur more often than is recognized, because weakness of the abductors is common at least temporarily after most hip surgeries and may be attributed to a variety of causes other than intraoperative neural injury. Splitting of the gluteus medius more than 6 cm proximal to the tip of the greater trochanter (or 4 cm proximal to the acetabular rim) places the superior gluteal nerve at risk.[30,31] Lateral femoral cutaneous nerve palsies are also observed occasionally and may be caused by pressure from hip rests or supports used to position the patient during the procedure. This problem is often transient, and the etiology usually is not clearly defined.

Risk factors for peripheral-nerve lesions have been examined by several authors. Female gender has repeatedly emerged as an important variable, with 80% or more of the nerve palsies in three different studies of 825 to 2,012 patients occurring in women.[21,24,32] It has been postulated that this increased prevalence in women is due to the fact that, compared with men, they have reduced muscle bulk, smaller size, shorter limbs, and possible differences in local vascular anatomy.[24,32] Experimental models have shown that neural injury will occur if the nerve is elongated more than 6% of its length. Given this 6% stretch limit, smaller individuals with shorter limbs, and thus much shorter nerves, have less of a potential for absolute neural retraction than do much larger individuals.[21,32] This factor may help to explain partially the difference in prevalence between the genders.

Etiology
In general, neural injury can occur as a result of traction, compression, or ischemia.[33] The cause of nerve injury associated with an arthroplasty may be direct damage occurring acutely during the procedure or indirect effects occurring in a delayed fashion, as may be seen with problems with positioning postoperatively or the formation of deep hematomas. However, several specific factors have been associated with an increased risk of neural injury. Prior surgery to the hip is one such factor.[20] Revision of a failed implant is associated with a 1.4% to 7.5% rate of postoperative nerve palsy according to reviews of series including 88 to 3,126 patients.[25-27] This increased risk may be caused by the more extensive and difficult dissection required with revision procedures and perhaps, in some patients, by uncertainty regarding the location of major neurologic and vascular structures when a previous surgical exposure has been performed. In addition, tethering by scar tissue may predispose the nerve to stretch with retraction, dislocation of the hip, or limb-lengthening. During isolated acetabular component revision through a posterior approach, retraction of the intact femoral component anteriorly may increase the risk of compression of the femoral nerve.

Acute limb-lengthening of more than 2 to 4 cm during arthroplasty has been associated with an increased risk of neural injury.[20,21,34] In a study of 100 patients who had a total hip replacement for the treatment of dysplasia of the hip, nerve palsy occurred in 13 (28%) of the 46 patients who had more than 4 cm of limb-lengthening, and no nerve palsy occurred in the 54 who had less than 4 cm of lengthening.[21] The peroneal division of the sciatic nerve may be particularly at risk during limb-lengthening maneuvers, because tethering at both the sciatic notch and the fibular head makes the effective length of the nerve less than that of the overall limb.

Altered anatomy in the region of the hip has been considered a factor that increases the potential for neural injuries[26] (Fig. 4). Congenital dysplasia of the hip, for example, results in abnormal anatomy because not only is lengthening sometimes attempted, but also the severity of the dysplasia inherently alters the relationship of the nearby neurologic structures. This may help to explain rates of nerve palsy ranging from 5.2% to 13% in series of 100 to 172 patients who had dysplasia of the hip treated with arthroplasty.[21,27,34]

The type of surgical approach used on the hip has not been shown to influence the observed rates of nerve palsy.[3,21] However, some neural injuries are clearly the result of direct injury of the nerve by surgical instruments during either the exposure or the subsequent arthroplasty. Thus, the femoral nerve is more at risk for direct injury during the anterolateral approach, whereas the sciatic nerve is

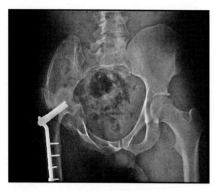 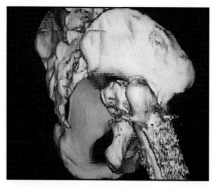 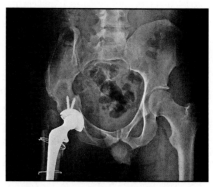

Fig. 4 A patient who had severe dysplasia and intermittent sciatic nerve sensory symptoms preoperatively as well as pain in the hip. The patient had had a previous femoral osteotomy. **Left,** Preoperative radiograph. **Center,** Preoperative computed tomography scan. **Right,** Despite derotation and shortening, anterior translation of the hip to allow articulation with a cup placed in the anatomic location resulted in a transient motor loss in the peroneal distribution. Persistent sensory symptoms and causalgia-like pain in the leg were still present 1 year after surgery.

more at risk during the posterior approach. Neural injury can also occur indirectly during exposure of the hip as a result of prolonged or excessive retraction efforts.[28] Cerclage with wire, suture, or cable may entrap the nerve, causing nerve palsy.[35] Extrusion of cement with direct contact with, or even complete entrapment of, the sciatic, femoral, or obturator nerve has been reported.[29,36,37] Extrusion of cement during placement of an acetabular component is much less a concern now that acetabular components are often inserted without cement. However, concerns regarding entrapment of nerves by cement have been replaced by potential neurovascular problems related to the screws used, instead of cement, to fix acetabular cups.[23,38,39] This concern resulted in the development of a four-quadrant system for guiding placement of the screws on the acetabular side.[39] Screws should be restricted to the posterior-superior and posterior-inferior quadrants, and care must still be taken to avoid posterior placement of the screw into the region of the sciatic notch.[23,39]

The formation of a hematoma can produce delayed-onset nerve palsy subsequent to hip arthroplasty and has been associated with excessive anticoagulation for prophylaxis against venous thrombosis.[40,41] When the hematoma involves the

gluteal compartment, the sciatic nerve is at risk.[41,42] A hematoma involving the iliacus muscle can produce femoral nerve palsy and may result from perforation of the medial wall of the acetabulum during the arthroplasty.[43] Iliacus hematoma has been noted on postoperative CT scans, and CT may sometimes facilitate the diagnosis and treatment if the exact etiology and timing of onset of the nerve palsy are unclear. Symptoms associated with the formation of a hematoma and secondary nerve palsy include not only neurologic dysfunction but also excessive pain exacerbated by passive stretch of the involved compartment.[42] Other causes of delayed-onset nerve palsy that are not directly related to the initial surgery include dislocation, late ischemia from stretch neurapraxia after lengthening, positional effects as seen with direct compression of the peroneal division at the fibular head,[44] and late migration of hardware such as trochanteric wires.[45] Prominence of an implant or associated cement spurs can also produce irritation of adjacent neurologic structures and the delayed onset of neural symptoms.[46]

Causalgia-like pain or reflex sympathetic dystrophy may complicate recovery from a neural injury and can compromise the end result even if the final motor and sensory deficits are minimum (Fig. 4).

This problem was seen in as many as 29% of 28 patients following an arthroplasty,[21] and it can be the main cause of a poor result in some instances.

Prevention

Prevention of a nerve palsy is clearly preferable to treatment of an already established neurologic problem. Careful surgical technique and avoidance of direct injury of the nerve during exposure, retraction, and placement of the implant are important. Surgical techniques that emphasize the use of instruments and sharp dissection away from rather than toward important neurologic or vascular structures are suggested. Such techniques make it possible to avoid neural injury when (not if) those instruments slip. Limiting one-stage limb-lengthening efforts to 4 cm or 6% of the calculated length of the nerve, whichever is less, should help to reduce the risk of associated nerve palsy. Identification and protection of the sciatic nerve in some high-risk situations, such as when there are major alterations in local anatomy, is probably indicated. Maintenance of the knee in flexion during retraction for exposure about the acetabulum through a posterior approach can reduce tension on the sciatic nerve and reduce the risk of nerve palsy. It is recommended that screw placement on the acetabular side into the anterior-superior and anterior-inferior quadrants be avoided. Careful subperiosteal circumferential exposure of the femoral shaft during placement of the cerclage wires, with protection of the sciatic nerve if it is immediately adjacent, is also recommended.

Intraoperative neural monitoring has been explored as a potential means to reduce the risk of neural injury.[47-50] It is possible to document intraoperative irritation of the nerves and, if necessary, to alter the surgical technique or the position of the limb. Such monitoring has been recommended as a surveillance method during revision total hip arthroplasty or when major limb-lengthening efforts are planned.[50] Simultaneous changes in amplitude and latency appear to be predictive of a postoperative alteration in the function of the sciatic nerve.[50] However, the actual reduction in the risk of nerve palsy due to intraoperative neural monitoring has not been well established, and thus the ability of this method to actually prevent neural injury remains controversial.[47-50] While routine use of this method for primary or even revision total hip arthroplasties may be difficult to support on the basis of current data, judicious use in situations that involve increased risk due to distorted anatomy or anticipated major limb-lengthening seems reasonable.

Treatment

While prevention is better than treatment, it is critically important to assess the neurologic and vascular status of all patients carefully in the postoperative period, with good written documentation that this has been done. Observation with serial examinations and sequential electromyographic and nerve-conduction studies are helpful for the follow-up of individuals in whom neurologic dysfunction is detected. Direct surgical intervention is clearly indicated in patients in

whom a postoperative hematoma has produced nerve palsy. The clinical hallmark of this problem is delayed onset or late progression of a neurologic deficit associated with evidence of local hematoma about the hip on examination. Decompression of the hematoma reduces the risk of long-term neurologic sequelae.[32,40,41] When an immediate postoperative nerve palsy is discovered, exploration of the nerve is indicated only when there is reason to believe that a major direct injury, such as complete transection or encirclement of the nerve with cerclage wires, has occurred, because these problems are associated with a poor prognosis unless exploration and appropriate repair are carried out. Routine surgical exploration of nerve palsies after an arthroplasty is not indicated. Late exploration has been suggested when there has been no sign of nerve regeneration,[51] but, at present, exploration is rarely performed unless complete disruption is strongly suspected.

Prognosis

Neurologic recovery is variable and is related to the severity of the initial injury. The prognosis is better for femoral nerve palsy than for sciatic palsy and is better for isolated peroneal palsy than for complete sciatic palsy.[20] A satisfactory functional outcome, with some residual neurologic loss, is achieved in many patients. Johanson and associates[21] reported that 79% of 34 patients who had nerve palsy had incomplete recovery, and 15 of the 28 patients who had sufficient follow-up had both motor and sensory deficits at the most recent examination. Good prognostic signs include retention of motor function with isolated sensory loss or recovery of motor function during the initial days following surgery. Both of these situations are associated with a high rate of good results and overall recovery.[27] It is important, when counseling patients, to state that improvement may continue

for at least 1 year after the injury, but the status is unlikely to change after 18 months.

Vascular Complications

Vascular injuries associated with hip arthroplasty may present either with acute hemorrhage during the procedure or with delayed, postoperative bleeding problems. Other potential sequelae include thrombosis of arterial or venous structures, formation of an arteriovenous fistula or false aneurysm, and embolic events (both venous and arterial).[52,53] Symptoms that may be noted days or years after the index arthroplasty include pain from pressure by a pseudoaneurysm, ischemia due to occlusion or embolization, and bleeding at the time of subsequent revision procedures.[54] Structures at risk include the femoral artery and vein; the obturator artery and venous branches; the external iliac, common iliac, and profunda femoris vessels; and the superior gluteal artery and vein.

Prevalence

The overall risk of vascular complications associated with hip arthroplasty is small, with an estimated prevalence of approximately 0.25%.[55] The external iliac artery and the common femoral artery are the structures most often injured.[56] One review of the literature revealed that 36 of 68 reported vascular complications involved the external iliac artery and 17, the common femoral artery; two thirds of the injuries were observed on the left side.[56] Vascular injury is more common in previously treated hips or after revision hip arthroplasty than during primary hip replacement.[56,57] The exact prevalence depends somewhat on how the investigator defines an important vascular problem. For example, excessive bleeding was reported in association with 1% (19) of 2,012 arthroplasties, with six of the 19 patients requiring reoperation; however, not all of them were thought to have had

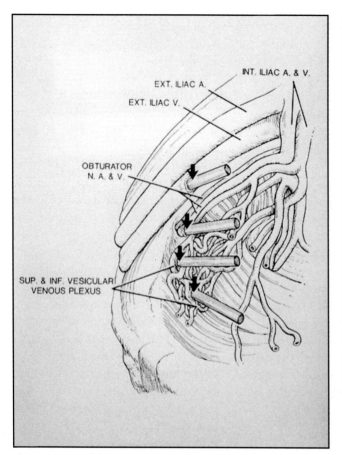

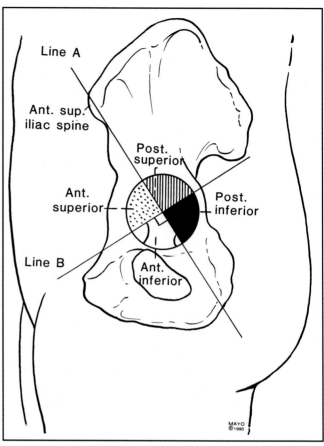

Fig. 5 Diagram of the intrapelvic vascular structures adjacent to the inner surface of the anterior column and medial wall of the acetabulum. The arrows indicate long rods extending from the anterior screwholes of an acetabular component and marking the intrapelvic trajectory of any screws placed in those positions. (Reproduced with permission from Keating EM, Ritter MA, Faris PM: Structures at risk from medially placed acetabular screws. *J Bone Joint Surg* 1990;72A:510.)

Fig. 6 Diagram of the four acetabular quadrants created by two intersecting lines from the anterior and posterior superior iliac spines. Placement of the screw in the anterior-superior or anterior-inferior quadrant should be avoided because of the risk of vascular injury. (Reproduced with permission of the Mayo Foundation, Rochester, MN.)

an injury of a major named vascular structure.[58] Shoenfeld and associates,[56] in a review of the results of 68 arthroplasties complicated by vascular injury that required surgical treatment, found a 7% mortality rate and a 15% rate of subsequent amputation.

Etiology

The etiology of vascular injuries may be either direct damage to the vessel or indirect injury from stretch, tearing, or compression. Direct injury can occur from sharp instruments, such as scalpels or osteotomes, and can involve any of the adjacent vascular structures, depending on the area and the direction of the dissection. Direct injury of the common iliac vein from excessive acetabular reaming with violation of the medial wall has been reported.[59] Damage caused by Hohmann or other sharp-tipped retractors, one of the more common mechanisms of vascular injury, tends to occur in two locations: over the anterior aspect of the acetabular rim and medial to the femoral neck. The common femoral artery and the medial and lateral circumflex femoral vessels are involved, with presentation in the form of bleeding, ischemia due to occlusion, or the late formation of a pseudoaneurysm requiring surgical repair.[55,60–62] Nachbur and associates[55] reported six such cases related to use of a Hohmann retractor, with injury of the external iliac, common femoral artery, or circumflex vessels. One of those cases resulted in amputation.

Vascular injury due to placement of a screw during fixation, without cement, of an acetabular component has received attention recently because of reports of major hemorrhage and even death.[38] Anatomic studies by Keating and associates[38] and by Wasielewski and associates[39] clearly demonstrated the close proximity of the external iliac vessels, obturator nerve and vessels, and superior and inferior vesicular venous plexus to the medial aspect of the acetabulum (Fig. 5). Wasielewski and associates[39] described a four-quadrant system for the safe placement of acetabular screws (Fig. 6). The anterior-superior and anterior-inferior quadrants are the zones in which there is a major risk of vascular injury by screws. Because the mechanical strength or quality of screw fixation in these anterior zones is inferior anyway, there is little reason to subject a patient to the risk of an attempted placement in those regions during primary arthroplasty. In revision arthroplasties in which anterior bone fixation may be desired because of bone loss elsewhere, palpation of drill-bits and screws after dissection of the anterior column can facilitate safe placement of the screw. The potential risk associated with such screws does not end after successful placement, however. In one report, a death occurred as a result of bleeding from a vascular injury associated with a traumatic acetabular fracture adjacent to a cup inserted without cement and fixed with screws; the cup and screws displaced medially, injuring the external iliac vessels.[63]

A vessel may be injured directly during extraction of components; such an injury has been reported after removal of loose acetabular components with associated intrapelvic cement.[54,64] Vascular injury may also occur because of compression or kinking of atherosclerotic vessels, with resulting arterial thrombosis or arterial emboli in the leg.[22,60,65] In one series, two of 15 vascular complications involved postoperative ischemia that was thought to be caused by late thrombosis.[55] It is also possible that some cases of postoperative ischemia without frank occlusion or direct injury are caused by disruption of the collateral blood supply by the dissection and limb-lengthening associated with hip arthroplasty in a limb in which atherosclerosis had been marginally compensated for preoperatively.[57] Vascular occlusion from compression

may also occur because of extravasation of the cement and encasement of vascular structures.[60]

Prevention
Careful surgical exposure and technique are important to avoid damage of adjacent vascular structures. The technique of sharp dissection and the use of sharp instruments away from, rather than toward, adjacent vascular structures should be encouraged. Careful placement of the retractor intraoperatively is important especially over the anterior aspect of the acetabular rim. Preoperative vascular evaluation is reasonable for patients who have severe pre-existing peripheral vascular disease. Preoperative arteriography may be indicated for high-risk situations, such as those that involve intrapelvic migration of a failed acetabular component or intrapelvic extravasation of cement.[52,53,64,66-68] Planned intrapelvic, medial exposure with mobilization or repair of the iliac vessel may be indicated in such patients to avoid injury during cup removal.[66] A thorough knowledge of the vascular anatomy in the region of the hip helps the surgeon to avoid vascular injuries. In particular, it is essential that acetabular screws not be placed into hazardous zones, as determined by the adjacent vascular anatomy medial to the acetabulum.[23,38,39]

Treatment
Contingency planning for the treatment of a potentially catastrophic vascular injury can facilitate an effective and rapid response. Prompt recognition of vascular injury is important. When such an injury is identified intraoperatively, the initial essential step is to control the bleeding. Standard measures of coagulation or ligation may be effective. Wound packing may provide temporary control or, in some instances, result in hemostasis as a result of thrombosis. However, injury of a major vessel can require surgical repair. The operating orthopaedic surgeon must

have a thorough knowledge of pertinent regional vascular anatomy, and familiarity with adjunctive surgical approaches, such as the ilioinguinal approach or the McBurney incision for retroperitoneal or intrapelvic exposure, facilitates emergent proximal vascular control and may be life-saving. The immediate availability of a vascular surgeon or a surgeon who has comparable expertise is essential in the event of a major injury necessitating vascular repair. Preoperative consultation with a vascular surgeon and intraoperative assistance may be considered when there is a risk of an intraoperative vascular injury, as in patients who have a markedly distorted anatomy, a history of previous vascular injury or repair, or intrapelvic migration of the components and cement.

Overview
Neurovascular injuries associated with hip arthroplasty are uncommon but may be catastrophic. A thorough knowledge of local anatomy, careful consideration of the structures at risk, and avoidance of maneuvers that increase the risk of these injuries can help to reduce the chance of these problems.[69] Should neurologic or vascular injury occur, prompt recognition is essential to allow appropriate treatment in order to minimize the chance of permanent sequelae.

References
1. Ereth MH, Weber JG, Abel MD, et al: Cemented versus noncemented total hip arthroplasty: Embolism, hemodynamics, and intrapulmonary shunting. *Mayo Clin Proc* 1992;67:1066–1074.

2. Herndon JH, Bechtol CO, Crickenberger DP: Fat embolism during total hip replacement: A prospective study. *J Bone Joint Surg* 1974;56A:1350–1362.

3. Kallos T, Enis JE, Gollan F, et al: Intramedullary pressure and pulmonary embolism of femoral medullary contents in dogs during insertion of bone cement and a prosthesis. *J Bone Joint Surg* 1974;56A:1363–1367.

4. Orsini EC, Byrick RJ, Mullen JB, et al: Cardiopulmonary function and pulmonary microemboli during arthroplasty using cemented or non-cemented components: The role of

intramedullary pressure. *J Bone Joint Surg* 1987;69A:822–832.

5. Rinecker H: New clinico-pathophysiological studies on the bone cement implantation syndrome. *Arch Orthop Trauma Surg* 1980;97: 263–274.

6. Dandy DJ: Fat embolism following prosthetic replacement of the femoral head. *Injury* 1971;3:85–88.

7. Duncan JA: Intra-operative collapse or death related to the use of acrylic cement in hip surgery. *Anaesthesia* 1989;44:149–153.

8. Kallos T: Impaired arterial oxygenation associated with use of bone cement in the femoral shaft. *Anesthesiology* 1975;42:210–215.

9. Lewallen DG, Ereth MH: Intraoperative mortality, in Morrey BF, An KN (eds): *Reconstructive Surgery of the Joints*, ed 2. New York, NY, Churchill Livingstone, 1996, pp 197–206.

10. Patterson BM, Healey JH, Cornell CN, et al: Cardiac arrest during hip arthroplasty with a cemented long-stem component: A report of seven cases. *J Bone Joint Surg* 1991;73A: 271–277.

11. Black S, Cucchiara RF, Nishimura RA, et al: Parameters affecting occurrence of paradoxical air embolism. *Anesthesiology* 1989;71:235–241.

12. Hagen PT, Scholz DG, Edwards WD: Incidence and size of patent foramen ovale during the first 10 decades of life: An autopsy study of 965 normal hearts. *Mayo Clin Proc* 1984;59:17–20.

13. Byrick RJ, Bell RS, Kay JC, et al: High-volume, high-pressure pulsatile lavage during cemented arthroplasty. *J Bone Joint Surg* 1989; 71A:1331–1336.

14. Sherman RM, Byrick RJ, Kay JC, et al: The role of lavage in preventing hemodynamic and blood-gas changes during cemented arthroplasty. *J Bone Joint Surg* 1983;65A:500–506.

15. Tronzo RG, Kallos T, Wyche MQ: Elevation of intramedullary pressure when methylmethacrylate is inserted in total hip arthroplasty. *J Bone Joint Surg* 1974;56A:714–718.

16. Engesaeter LB, Strand T, Raugstad TS, et al: Effects of a distal venting hole in the femur during total hip replacement. *Arch Orthop Trauma Surg* 1984;103:328–331.

17. Nercessian OA, Macaulay W, Stinchfield FE: Peripheral neuropathies following total hip arthroplasty. *J Arthroplasty* 1994;9:645–651.

18. Smith JW, Pellicci PM, Sharrock N, et al: Complications after total hip replacement: The contralateral limb. *J Bone Joint Surg* 1989;71A: 528–535.

19. Seddon HJ: Three types of nerve injury. *Brain* 1943;66:237–288.

20. Edwards BN, Tullos HS, Noble PC: Contributory factors and etiology of sciatic nerve palsy in total hip arthroplasty. *Clin Orthop* 1987;218:136–141.

21. Johanson NA, Pellicci PM, Tsairis P, et al: Nerve injury in total hip arthroplasty. *Clin Orthop* 1983;179:214–222.

22. Stubbs DH, Dorner DB, Johnston RC: Thrombosis of the iliofemoral artery during revision of a total hip replacement: A case report. *J Bone Joint Surg* 1986;68A:454–455.

23. Wasielewski RC, Crossett LS, Rubash HE: Neural and vascular injury in total hip arthroplasty. *Orthop Clin North Am* 1992;23:219–235.

24. Weber ER, Daube JR, Coventry MB: Peripheral neuropathies associated with total hip arthroplasty. *J Bone Joint Surg* 1976;58A: 66–69.

25. Amstutz HC, Ma SM, Jinnah RH, et al: Revision of aseptic loose total hip arthroplasties. *Clin Orthop* 1982;170:21–33.

26. Navarro RA, Schmalzried TP, Amstutz HC, et al: Surgical approach and nerve palsy in total hip arthroplasty. *J Arthroplasty* 1995;10:1–5.

27. Schmalzried TP, Amstutz HC, Dorey FJ: Nerve palsy associated with total hip replacement: Risk factors and prognosis. *J Bone Joint Surg* 1991;73A:1074–1080.

28. Simmons C Jr, Izant TH, Rothman RH, et al: Femoral neuropathy following total hip arthroplasty: Anatomic study, case reports, and literature review. *J Arthroplasty* 1991;(suppl 6): S57–S66.

29. Siliski JM, Scott RD: Obturator-nerve palsy resulting from intrapelvic extrusion of cement during total hip replacement: Report of four cases. *J Bone Joint Surg* 1985;67A:1225–1228.

30. Hardinge K: The direct lateral approach to the hip. *J Bone Joint Surg* 1982;64B:17–19.

31. Jacobs LG, Buxton RA: The course of the superior gluteal nerve in the lateral approach to the hip. *J Bone Joint Surg* 1989;71A:1239–1243.

32. Solheim LF, Hagen R: Femoral and sciatic neuropathies after total hip arthroplasty. *Acta Orthop Scand* 1980;51:531–534.

33. Sunderland S (ed): *Nerves and Nerve Injuries*, ed 2. Edinburgh, Scotland, Churchill Livingstone, 1978.

34. Shaughnessy WJ, Kavanagh B, Fitzgerald RH Jr: Long-term results of total hip arthroplasty in patients with high congenital dislocation of the hip. *Orthop Trans* 1989;13:510.

35. Mallory TH: Sciatic nerve entrapment secondary to trochanteric wiring following total hip arthroplasty: A case report. *Clin Orthop* 1983;180:198–200.

36. Oleksak M, Edge AJ: Compression of the sciatic nerve by methylmethacrylate cement after total hip replacement. *J Bone Joint Surg* 1992;74B:729–730.

37. Pess GM, Lusskin R, Waugh TR, et al: Femoral neuropathy secondary to pressurized cement in total hip replacement: Treatment by decompression and neurolysis. Report of a case. *J Bone Joint Surg* 1987;69A:623–625.

38. Keating EM, Ritter MA, Faris PM: Structures at risk from medially placed acetabular screws. *J Bone Joint Surg* 1990;72A:509–511.

39. Wasielewski RC, Cooperstein LA, Kruger MP, et al: Acetabular anatomy and the transacetabular fixation of screws in total hip arthroplasty. *J Bone Joint Surg* 1990;72A:501–508.

40. Brantigan JW, Owens ML, Moody FG: Femoral neuropathy complicating anticoagulant therapy. *Am J Surg* 1976;132:108–109.

41. Fleming RE Jr, Michelsen CB, Stinchfield FE: Sciatic paralysis: A complication of bleeding following hip surgery. *J Bone Joint Surg* 1979; 61A:37–39.

42. Cohen B, Bhamra M, Ferris BD: Delayed sciatic nerve palsy following total hip arthroplasty. *Br J Clin Pract* 1991;45:292–293.

43. Wooten SL, McLaughlin RE: Iliacus hematoma and subsequent femoral nerve palsy after penetration of the medial acetabular wall during total hip arthroplasty: Report of a case. *Clin Orthop* 1984;191:221–223.

44. Dhillon MS, Nagi ON: Sciatic nerve palsy associated with total hip arthroplasty. *Ital J Orthop Traumatol* 1992;18:521–526.

45. Asnis SE, Hanley S, Shelton PD: Sciatic neuropathy secondary to migration of trochanteric wire following total hip arthroplasty. *Clin Orthop* 1985;196:226–228.

46. Edwards MS, Barbaro NM, Asher SW, et al: Delayed sciatic palsy after total hip replacement: Case report. *Neurosurgery* 1981;9:61–63.

47. Black DL, Reckling FW, Porter SS: Somatosensory-evoked potential monitored during total hip arthroplasty. *Clin Orthop* 1991;262:170–177.

48. Kennedy WF, Byrne TF, Majid HA, et al: Sciatic nerve monitoring during revision total hip arthroplasty. *Clin Orthop* 1991;264:237.

49. Nercessian OA, Gonzalez EG, Stinchfield FE: The use of somatosensory evoked potential during revision or reoperation for total hip arthroplasty. *Clin Orthop* 1989;243:138–142.

50. Porter SS, Black DL, Reckling FW, et al: Intraoperative cortical somatosensory evoked potentials for detection of sciatic neuropathy during total hip arthroplasty. *J Clin Anesth* 1989;1:170–176.

51. Hagen R: Perifere nerveskader. *Tidssk Nor Laegeforen* 1970;90:945–950.

52. Heyes FL, Aukland A: Occlusion of the common femoral artery complicating total hip arthroplasty. *J Bone Joint Surg* 1985;67B: 533–535.

53. Hopkins NF, Vanhegan JA, Jamieson CW: Iliac aneurysm after total hip arthroplasty: Surgical management. *J Bone Joint Surg* 1983;65B: 359–361.

54. Bergqvist D, Carlsson AS, Ericsson BF: Vascular complications after total hip arthroplasty. *Acta Orthop Scand* 1983;54:157–163.

55. Nachbur B, Meyer RP, Verkkala K, et al: The mechanisms of severe arterial injury in surgery of the hip joint. *Clin Orthop* 1979;141:122–133.

56. Shoenfeld NA, Stuchin SA, Pearl R, et al: The management of vascular injuries associated with total hip arthroplasty. *J Vasc Surg* 1990; 11:549–555.

57. Matos MH, Amstutz HC, Machleder HI: Ischemia of the lower extremity after total hip replacement. *J Bone Joint Surg* 1979;61A:24–27.

58. Coventry MB, Beckenbaugh RD, Nolan DR, et al: 2,012 total hip arthroplasties: A study of postoperative course and early complications. *J Bone Joint Surg* 1974;56A:273–284.

59. Mallory TH: Rupture of the common iliac vein from reaming the acetabulum during total hip replacement: A case report. *J Bone Joint Surg* 1972;54A:276–277.

60. Aust JC, Bredenberg CE, Murray DG: Mechanisms of arterial injuries associated with total hip replacement. *Arch Surg* 1981;116: 345–349.

61. Kroese A, Mollerud A: Traumatic aneurysm of the common femoral artery after hip endoprosthesis. *Acta Orthop Scand* 1975;46:119–122.

62. Salama R, Stavorovsky MM, Iellin A, et al: Femoral artery injury complicating total hip replacement. *Clin Orthop* 1972;89:143–144.

63. Peterson CA, Lewallen DG: Periprosthetic fracture of the acetabulum after total hip arthroplasty. *J Bone Joint Surg* 1996;78A: 1206–1213.

64. Brentlinger A, Hunter JR: Perforation of the external iliac artery and ureter presenting as acute hemorrhagic cystitis after total hip replacement: Report of a case. *J Bone Joint Surg* 1987;69A:620–622.

65. Parfenchuck TA, Young TR: Intraoperative arterial occlusion in total joint arthroplasty. *J Arthroplasty* 1994;9:217–220.

66. al-Salman M, Taylor DC, Beauchamp CP, et al: Prevention of vascular injuries in revision total hip replacement. *Can J Surg* 1992;35: 261–264.

67. Reiley MA, Bond D, Branick RI, et al: Vascular complications following total hip arthroplasty: A review of the literature and a report of two cases. *Clin Orthop* 1984;186: 23–28.

68. Scullin JP, Nelson CL, Beven EG: False aneurysm of the left external iliac artery following total hip arthroplasty. *Clin Orthop* 1975;113:145–149.

69. Ratcliff AH: Editorial: Arterial injuries after total hip replacement. *J Bone Joint Surg* 1985;67B:517–518.

Diagnosis of Infection Following Total Hip Arthroplasty

Mark J. Spangehl, MD, FRCSC
Alastair S.E. Younger, MB, MSc, FRCSC
Bassam A. Masri, MD, FRCSC
Clive P. Duncan, MB, MSc, FRCSC

High rates of infection complicated the early experience with total hip arthroplasty (THA) and, although the rates have decreased substantially over the last several decades, infection still is a source of considerable morbidity. In the 1960s, Charnley reported a rate of infection of 9.5% (19 infections after 199 total hip arthroplasties).[1] More recently, authors have reported that infection causes failure after 1% (71 of 5,081 and 27 of 2,084) to 2% (94 of 5,500 and 36 of 1,798) of primary total hip arthroplasties,[2–10] and the rate is higher after revision procedures. Although these percentages are small, the large number of hip arthroplasties performed each year has resulted in a major burden on the health-care system.[11] Infection following THA is costly to treat because of the subsequent need for reoperation and the prolonged hospitalization often required to eradicate the infection. In the United States, the cost per year to treat the 3,500 to 4,000 infections following THA is between 150 and 200 million dollars.[11] Because of an aging population that will need an increasing number of arthroplasties, methods to prevent, diagnose, and treat infection must be perfected in order to reduce the cost of THA to society.

Infection following THA can present a diagnostic challenge. No test is 100% sensitive and 100% specific; thus, the diagnosis of infection relies on the sur-

geon's judgment of the clinical presentation, the findings on physical examination, and the interpretation of the results of previous investigations. The consequences of misdiagnosis are considerable. Reimplantation of a prosthesis into an infected tissue bed, without appropriate debridement, is likely to result in persistent infection.[12] Numerous investigations are available for the workup and diagnosis of failed total hip replacements. These investigations, as well as an algorithm to rule out the presence of infection as a cause of failure, will be presented.

Clinical Presentation

A thorough history and physical examination are of paramount importance in the diagnosis of infection. Although a conclusive diagnosis can be made in many instances, there are no data, to our knowledge, with regard to the efficacy of clinical assessment alone. Even when a conclusive diagnosis cannot be established, a careful history and physical examination can help to guide the appropriate investigations.

Coventry,[13] and later Fitzgerald and associates,[14] described what is perhaps the most common system for the classification of infection after THA. This three-stage classification system is based on the mode or timing of the presentation of infection.

Type-I infections occur in the imme-

diate postoperative period. The patient usually is seen during the first postoperative month, and the diagnosis is evident on the basis of the medical history and the physical examination. Systemic signs of infection, such as fever, chills, and sweating, may be present. Pain is usually continuous. On examination, the wound may be erythematous, swollen, fluctuant, and tender. Wound drainage, if present, is usually purulent. Type-I infections are caused by infected hematomas or superficial wound infections spreading contiguously to the periprosthetic space. The diagnostic challenge is to determine whether or not a superficial infection has penetrated deep to the fascia.

Type-II infections also are believed to originate at the time of surgery, but because of a small inoculum or the low virulence of the organism, the onset of symptoms is delayed. The patient usually is seen between 6 and 24 months after the index procedure. The hallmark of this type of infection is a gradual deterioration in function and an increase in pain. Pain is often present from the time of the original procedure; it may be activity related or it may occur at night and during rest. Often, the only clue to infection is early loosening of the components. Systemic symptoms are not part of the presentation; however, there may be a history of prolonged wound drainage at the time of the index procedure. Specific questions about a delay in the patient's discharge from the hospital, a prolonged course of antibiotics, or ongoing wound drainage should be asked while the history is being obtained. The findings on examination of the hip in a patient who has a type-II infection usually are nonspecific and are similar to those associated with aseptic loosening. Increased warmth or a draining sinus may be present. Careful examination for an old closed sinus or evidence of poor wound healing may suggest the presence of deep infection. A type-II infection represents a diagnostic challenge.

Type-III infections are the least common and are caused by a hematogenous spread to a previously asymptomatic hip, usually 2 years or more after the arthroplasty. Generally, there is an acute febrile episode accompanied by sudden, rapid deterioration in the function of the hip. The acute onset of such an infection in a hip with a previously well-functioning prosthesis is of far more importance than the temporal relationship between the onset of the infection and the insertion of the prosthesis. The diagnosis usually can be made on the basis of the history and the physical examination. The patient may recall a systemic or febrile illness that was followed by symptoms in the hip. Seeding can occur at the site of a loose prosthesis, a solidly osseointegrated prosthesis, or a solidly fixed cemented prosthesis. A type-III infection is likely to occur in patients who are immunosuppressed, such as those who have had a renal transplant or who have been managed with immunosuppressive medications for inflammatory arthropathy; those who have recurrent episodes of bacteremia, such as intravenous drug abusers; and those who need repeat urinary catheterization.[15,16] Other factors that may be associated with type-III infection are dental manipulation,[15,17–19] respiratory infection,[17] remote periprosthetic infection,[17] open skin lesions,[20] endoscopy,[21] and contamination of the operative site.[15] Early diagnosis may allow salvage of the joint by means of thorough debridement, whereas a delay in the diagnosis may necessitate a one or two-stage exchange procedure in order to eradicate the infection.

Recently, Estrada and associates[22] expanded the classification to include patients for whom intraoperative cultures are positive despite a presumed preoperative diagnosis of aseptic loosening. Tsukayama and associates[23] reported the results of treatment of 106 infections. Thirty-one patients who initially were thought to have aseptic failure were diagnosed as having an infection on the basis of positive intraoperative cultures. In that study, a minimum of two of five cultures had to be positive in order for the joint to be considered infected. Sixteen of these patients also had an elevated erythrocyte sedimentation rate (ESR) (more than 30 mm per hour), whereas just one of the 25 patients who had had a histologic examination had acute inflammation. Only the white blood-cell count and the ESR were used routinely in the preoperative workup. These results lead to the question of whether some of the patients had a preexisting chronic infection or false-positive intraoperative cultures. It is debatable whether positive intraoperative cultures represent true infection if there is no other evidence of that diagnosis.

Preoperative Investigations
White Blood-Cell Count
The white count is rarely abnormal in patients who have an infection following a THA, and it is not helpful for ruling infection in or out as a cause of failure of the procedure. Canner and associates[24] found that, of 52 patients who had an infection following a joint arthroplasty, only eight (15%) had leukocytosis. It has been our experience,[25] as well as that of others,[26] that the white blood-cell count is normal in most patients who have an infection following a THA. When a patient does have an abnormal count, the systemic infection is usually clinically obvious and is either type I or type III.

Erythrocyte Sedimentation Rate and C-Reactive Protein Level
The ESR and the C-reactive protein (CRP) level are the most useful laboratory screening investigations for the diagnosis of a potential infection following THA. The ESR is a nonspecific hematologic test that measures the distance, in millimeters, that a column of red blood cells settles in 1 hour. This is a reflection of the formation of erythrocyte rouleaux. The formation of rouleaux generally is discouraged because of the normal negative charge on the erythrocytes; however, if there is an excess of positively charged macromolecules in the serum, the erythrocyte negative charge becomes diluted. Dilution decreases the repulsion between erythrocytes, thereby allowing the formation of rouleaux, which increases both the mass of settling red blood-cell units and the sedimentation rate.[27]

Acute-phase reactants are one type of the positively charged macromolecules just mentioned. These macromolecules are manufactured in the liver in response to a number of inflammatory, infectious, and neoplastic processes. An elevated ESR is an indirect indicator of an abundance of acute-phase reactants.[27] Because acute-phase reactants are produced under a variety of conditions, the specificity of an elevated ESR is decreased; the sensitivity, however, remains high. Patients who have a chronic infection at the site of a total joint prosthesis generally have an increased ESR without systemic illness or an increased white blood-cell count. Values of more than 30 or 35 mm per hour generally are considered to be abnormal and indicative of infection unless proved otherwise. Raising or lowering the chosen value for the ESR in order to differentiate between septic and aseptic failure will inversely affect the sensitivity and directly affect the speci-

Table 1
Sensitivity and specificity of the erythrocyte sedimentation rate and the C-reactive protein level

Laboratory Screening Test	No. of Patients	No. Who Had An Infection	Value for Erythrocyte Sedimentation Rate(mm/hr)	Value for C-Reactive Protein Level (mg/l)	Sensitivity	Specificity
Erythrocyte sedimentation rate						
Sanzen and Carlsson[29]	56	23	> 30		0.61	1.00
Thoren and Wigren[30]	79	51	> 35		0.88	0.96
Roberts and associates[28]	69	14	> 30		0.84	0.79
Spangehl and associates[25]	171	34	> 30		0.82	0.85
C-reactive protein level						
Sanzen and Carlsson[29]	56	23		> 10	0.91	0.88
Spangehl and associates[25]	142	26		> 10	0.96	0.92

ficity of the test for a given sample population. As the usefulness of a test is determined by its ability to both rule in and rule out the presence of infection, the value chosen to differentiate between septic and aseptic conditions should result in sensitivities and specificities that approach each other. This value generally has been reported to be between 30 and 35 mm per hour (Table 1).[25,28–30]

C-reactive protein is an acute-phase reactant that is synthesized in the liver and is found in only trace amounts under normal conditions.[29] As is the case for the other acute-phase reactants, the CRP level increases in a nonspecific manner as a result of infectious, inflammatory, or neoplastic disorders. The CRP level increases from trace amounts (the normal state) to reach maximum values within 48 hours after surgery and then returns to trace amounts in approximately 2 to 3 weeks.[31–33] The ESR may remain elevated for months after an uncomplicated total hip replacement.[33] Therefore, the ability of the CRP to return to normal much faster than the ESR enables it to be a more sensitive indicator of infection, particularly in the early postoperative period.

In a study of 79 patients who had had a revision hip replacement and had no known factors that would have elevated the ESR, 27 of the 28 patients who did not have an infection had an ESR that

was 35 mm/hr or less.[30] The 51 patients who had an infection had a mean ESR of 59 mm/hr, and six of these patients had an ESR of 35 mm/hr or less. With use of an ESR of more than 35 mm/hr as an indication of infection, the sensitivity was 0.88 and the specificity was 0.96. In a similar study of 56 patients who had had a revision (23 of whom had an infection and 33 of whom did not),[29] the use of an ESR of more than 30 mm/hr as an indication of infection yielded a sensitivity of 0.61 and a specificity of 1.00. In that study, the CRP level also was analyzed. With use of a CRP level of more than 10 mg/l as an indication of infection, the sensitivity and the specificity were 0.91 and 0.88, respectively. In our own series, in which an ESR of more than 30 mm/hr and a CRP level of more than 10 mg/l were considered to be indicative of infection, we found a sensitivity and specificity of 0.82 and 0.85 for the ESR and of 0.96 and 0.92 for the CRP level[25] (Table 1). Combining the tests should improve the accuracy of diagnosis.

Some care must be taken in interpreting the ESR or the CRP level before a revision hip arthroplasty. The physician must determine whether any other factors, such as rheumatoid arthritis, a recent operation, neoplasia, collagen vascular disease, infection, or an inflammatory condition, are present. If no such conditions are applicable, an ESR of

more than 30 or 35 mm/hr and a CRP level of more than 10 mg/l should be considered abnormal and should warrant additional investigation to rule out infection.

Plain Radiography
Plain radiographs should be made for all patients who have a failed arthroplasty, even though radiographs are of limited value as an investigative tool for the diagnosis of infection. Many radiographic findings, such as loosening, osteolysis, and endosteal scalloping, are common to both septic and aseptic failure. Occasionally, the patient will have diagnostic changes, such as periostitis, rapidly progressive and diffuse osteolysis, or endosteal scalloping.[34–37] Periosteal new-bone formation, with or without loosening of a component, has been considered by some to be pathognomonic of deep infection.[35]

Endosteal scalloping has been shown to be suggestive of infection.[37] In a retrospective review of 50 revision total hip replacements, 29 (91%) of 32 hips in which the prosthesis failed because of infection had evidence of endosteal scalloping on radiographs.[37] Other investigators have reported endosteal scalloping in as many as 62 (24%) of 260 hips that were not infected.[36,38]

Early loosening and rapidly progressive radiolucent lines also are suggestive of infection.[34,36] This may be particularly true if obvious causes of osteolysis, such as severe polyethylene wear, are not present. In recent years, the radiographic diagnosis of loosening has evolved.[39,40] Previously, possible loosening was defined as a radiolucent line, occupying 50% to 100% of the bone-cement interface, that had not been present on the radiographs made immediately postoperatively; probable loosening, as a continuous radiolucent line surrounding the entire mantle at the bone-cement interface; and definite loosening, as a radiolucent line at the stem-cement interface, fracture of the cement mantle or the stem, or migration of the prosthesis.[41] The clinical relevance of a radiolucent line at the bone-cement interface recently has been brought into question.[39,40] Retrieval studies of asymptomatic patients have shown circumferential remodeling of trabecular bone adjacent to cement and resultant endosteal cortical-bone resorption causing what appears as a radiolucent line on radiographs.[39,40] On the acetabular side, definite loosening is indicated by migration of the socket or the cement mantle, protrusio acetabuli, or acetabular fracture.[37]

The addition of arthrography can improve the accuracy of radiographs in the diagnosis of loosening.[42,43] Arthrography may show penetration of the contrast medium between the bone and the cement. Arthrography does not have notable advantages compared with plain radiography when used for the diagnosis of loosening of the femoral component, but it is of benefit when used for the assessment of loosening of a cemented socket.[43] Loosening is often subtle, and the diagnosis is easier to make if old radiographs are reviewed in order to document fracture of the cement, migration of a component, or progression of radiolucent lines at the component-cement interface.

Although some patients initially are seen with septic loosening of a total hip replacement, loosening is not necessarily a feature of infection following THA. Most patients who have a postoperative or an acute hematogenous infection have solidly fixed components. In our series of 84 patients who had an infection following THA, 34 (40%) had solid fixation of the femoral component at the time of revision. Occasionally, plain radiographs provide clues to infection; however, they are neither sensitive nor specific for its detection.

Radionuclide Imaging

Scintigraphy continues to receive attention with regard to its potential for the diagnosis of infection following joint replacement. Scintigraphy is limited by the cost of the scans; the time required for the patient to have the procedure; and, in some situations, the inability of the scans to yield consistently acceptable levels of sensitivity and specificity. Often, scans are no more accurate than serologic investigations, which are much less expensive.

Technetium-99m (^{99m}Tc) bone scans, the first scans that were used for the diagnosis of infection following hip arthroplasty, are sensitive but not specific. Some investigators have found that a negative bone scan rules out infection;[44] however, others have reported that a ^{99m}Tc scan occasionally can be negative in a patient who has an infection if there is an inadequate blood supply to the bone.[45] The causes of photopenic defects include subperiosteal pus, soft-tissue swelling, and vasospasm. Difficulties associated with ^{99m}Tc bone scans include the fact that multiple conditions, such as fractures, tumors, heterotopic ossification, and inflammatory disorders, can result in increased uptake in the periprosthetic tissue; the fact that the scans can remain positive for as long as 1 year after an uncomplicated hip replacement and for more than 2 years after insertion of a prosthesis without cement;[46] and, most importantly, the fact that the scans cannot be used to differentiate between infection and aseptic loosening.

Gallium-67 citrate is a radioisotope that accumulates in areas of inflammation. Like technetium, it is non-specific, as any process resulting in reactive bone formation may cause increased uptake.[45] Although more accurate than individual scans, sequential technetium-gallium scans still lack sufficient accuracy to be clinically useful for the diagnosis of a potential infection following hip arthroplasty.[47,48] Merkel and associates,[48] in a prospective study comparing sequential technetium-gallium scans with indium-labeled-leukocyte scans for the diagnosis of a variety of low-grade musculoskeletal infections, found a sensitivity of only 0.50 (12 of 24) and a specificity of 0.78 (14 of 18) for the sequential technetium-gallium scans.

Indium-111-labeled white blood cells (^{111}In-WBC) are useful for the diagnosis of conditions of increased vascularity and white blood-cell uptake; however, their usefulness for the diagnosis of infection following hip arthroplasty continues to be debated.[48–51] Glithero and associates[49] reported a poor sensitivity (0.38; three of eight) but a high specificity (1.00; 17 of 17) in an analysis of 25 failed arthroplasties, eight of which were believed to be associated with an infection. Merkel and associates,[48] in their previously mentioned study of mixed infections, found a sensitivity of 0.83 (20 of 24) and a specificity of 0.94 (17 of 18) with use of indium-labeled leukocytes. In an attempt to increase its ability to aid in the diagnosis of infection, ^{111}In-WBC scanning was combined, into a sequential protocol, with scanning with various preparations of technetium.[52,53] When a zonal analysis of the prosthesis was performed, Palestro and associates[53] found greater accuracy (greater uptake) in the region of the prosthetic femoral head in infected hips. The combined scans generally had higher sensitivities and specificities (Table 2); however, cost and time constraints still

Table 2
Sensitivity and specificity of nuclear imaging

Imaging Modality	No. of Sites Tested	No. of Proved Infections	Sensitivity	Specificity
Technetium/gallium scanning				
Kraemer and associates [47]	43	13	0.38 (5/13)	1.00 (30/30)
Merkel and associates [48]	42	24	0.59 (12/24)	0.78 (14/18)
Indium-111-labeled white blood-cell scanning				
Merkel and associates [48*]	42	24	0.83 (20/24)	0.94 (17/18)
Glithero and associates [49]	25	8	0.38 (3/8)	1.00 (17/17)
Wukich and associates [51]	24	7	1.00 (7/7)	0.41 (7/17)
Johnson and associates [52]	29	9	1.00 (9/9)	0.50 (10/20)
Technetium/indium-111-labeled white blood-cell scanning				
Johnson and associates [52]	29	9	0.89 (8/9)	0.95 (19/20)
Palestro and associates [53]	50	10	1.00 (10/10)	0.98 (39/40)
Indium-111-labeled immunoglobulin-G scanning				
Oyen and associates [55*]				
Entire study	120	72	0.97 (70/72)	0.85 (41/48)
Failed arthroplasties only	37	12	0.92 (11/12)	0.88 (22/25)
Wegener and associates [57*]	15	11	0.91 (10/11)	1.00 (4/4)

*The study included various types of infections; not all were related to the prosthetics

allow these scans only a limited role.

Other radiolabeled markers have been investigated in an attempt to improve the accuracy of nuclear imaging. Radiolabeled immunoglobulin-G (IgG) has been used for the investigation of musculoskeletal infections.[54–57] Radiolabeled IgG scans are similar to ^{111}In-WBC scans in that the radiopharmaceutical agent is labeled to a carrier that targets areas of acute inflammation. However, the advantage of IgG-labeling is that the patient does not need to have a phlebotomy before the scan is made and the lengthy laboratory preparation and subsequent reinjection of white blood cells can be avoided. Oyen and associates[54] prospectively compared the results of ^{111}In-WBC scans with those of ^{111}In-IgG scans. They reported superior results with the ^{111}In-IgG scans (a sensitivity and a specificity of 0.80 [20 of 25] and 1.00 [24 of 24] compared with 0.56 [14 of 25] and 0.79 [19 of 24] for the ^{111}In-WBC scans). Unfortunately, the study population included patients who had a variety of bone and soft-tissue infections, including infections outside of the musculoskeletal system. When patients who had musculoskeletal infections were separated from

the rest of the series, the sensitivity and specificity for the ^{111}In-IgG scans were 1.00 (15 of 15 and eight of eight, respectively) whereas those for the ^{111}In-WBC scans were 0.73 (11 of 15) and 0.88 (seven of eight). In a subsequent, noncomparative study from the same institution, the sensitivity of the ^{111}In-IgG scans was 0.92 (11 of 12) and the specificity was 0.88 (22 of 25) when only scans made after failed arthroplasties were analyzed[55] (Table 2). Until additional comparative studies specifically addressing failed total joint arthroplasties are available, the routine use of ^{111}In-IgG scans cannot be recommended.

Although costly and time-consuming, radionuclide scans can be of benefit in equivocal situations in which the results of screening serologic investigations may be falsely elevated and cultures of specimens aspirated from the joint may be unreliable because of the administration of antibiotics. The use of sequential ^{99m}Tc and ^{111}In-WBC scans currently is recommended; however, for the convenience of the patient, the use of radiolabeled IgG scans may supersede the use of sequential scans, provided that they are proved to be equivalent or superior to sequential scans

for the diagnosis of infection following hip arthroplasty.

Other Imaging Modalities

Magnetic resonance imaging (MRI) can be of value after an infection has been diagnosed in a patient in whom a THA was performed with use of radiolucent cement. MRI can be used to determine the extent of the cement mantle within the femur and the pelvis so that the revision procedure can be planned appropriately.[58] Ultrasound has a limited role in the diagnosis of infection. It can be used to measure the thickness of the joint capsule, with a thick capsule being indicative of infection.[59] Soft-tissue abscesses also may be evaluated with ultrasound.

Although these imaging modalities may assist in preoperative planning, they are not currently recommended as a means of excluding infection in patients who have a failed or painful total hip replacement.

Hip Joint Aspiration

Aspiration of the hip is perhaps the most useful investigative tool for definitive confirmation of the presence or absence of infection. Recently, however, the role

Table 3
Sensitivity and specificity of preoperative aspiration

Study	No. of Sites Tested	No. of Proved Infections	Sensitivity	Specificity
Phillips and Kattapuram [64]	141	33	0.91 (30/33)	0.82 (89/108)
Tigges and associates [63]	147	14	0.93 (13/14)	0.92 (122/133)
Kraemer and associates [47]	45	14	0.57 (8/14)	0.97 (30/31)
Roberts and associates [28]	78	15	0.87 (13/15)	0.95 (60/63)
Barrack and Harris [34]	260	4	0.50 (2/4)	0.88 (224/256)
Lachiewicz and associates [61]	156	25	0.92 (23/25)	0.97 (127/131)
Mulcahy and associates [62]	71	16	0.69 (11/16)	0.91 (50/55)
Fehring and Cohen [60]	166	6	0.50 (3/6)	0.88 (141/160)
Spangehl and associates [25]	180	21	0.86 (18/21)	0.94 (149/159)

of aspiration has generated considerable debate. In the past, aspiration was advocated for all patients who had a failed hip replacement.[14,28,43] Currently, most authors favor a more limited role,[34,60-63] with aspiration being used to confirm a clinical suspicion of infection or to support or negate the findings of other preoperative investigations, such as determination of the ESR and the CRP level, which may be falsely elevated because of connective-tissue disease. An additional benefit of aspiration in instances of suspected infection is the ability to identify the organism and its antibiotic-sensitivity profile, which may influence preoperative planning as well as the type of antibiotic that is chosen if use of an antibiotic depot is planned.

As in other investigations, the usefulness of aspiration is determined by its accuracy (the sum of the numbers of true-positive and true-negative results divided by the total number of tests). The reported rates of sensitivity and specificity have varied widely, with the sensitivity of preoperative aspiration ranging from 0.50 to 0.93 and the specificity ranging from 0.82 to 0.97 (Table 3).[25,28,34,47,60-64] These results suggest that aspiration is better for ruling infection in than for ruling it out.

The wide variation in the number of positive results that are observed when aspiration is used to ascertain the presence of infection is partly a function of the different methods used to calculate the results. One such variation in methodology involves the type of sample that is obtained at the time of aspiration. If only joint fluid is aspirated, a so-called dry tap may be interpreted as a negative result. However, it is possible to obtain synovial tissue by means of a needle biopsy, and cultures of this tissue may result in a diagnosis of infection despite the dry tap. Other variations include the number of samples obtained at the time of aspiration; the performance of repeat aspirations after the initial aspiration; the lack of a so-called gold standard for comparison (in many studies, the results of aspiration are compared with those of intraoperative cultures alone, which also are associated with a certain prevalence of false results); and the unrecognized or unreported use of antibiotics before aspiration, which is an inherent problem in many retrospective studies. In a prospective review of the results of diagnostic procedures performed for the evaluation of failed total hip replacements, we found that 13 of 193 patients had been receiving antibiotics before aspiration.[25] Twelve of the 13 patients had an infection, but only six had a positive result on aspiration.

Additionally, the wide variation in positive results may be due in part to the technique of aspiration. To reduce the number of false-positive results and thereby improve accuracy, a standard protocol should be established either by the radiology department or by the surgeon performing the aspiration. Strict aseptic technique must be observed not only to reduce the rate of false-positive results but also to prevent the unlikely but definite possibility of joint contamination and subsequent infection in a painful yet uninfected hip. To reduce the rate of false-negative results, all antibiotics must be discontinued for 2 to 3 weeks before the aspiration. The intracapsular position of the needle should be confirmed with arthrography. Local anesthetics should be used only in the skin and not in the joint as they are bacteriostatic.[65] Provided that sufficient fluid is obtained, the specimen should be separated into three samples for culture; however, if insufficient fluid is obtained, the joint can be irrigated with non-bacteriostatic saline solution and then reaspirated. A needle biopsy of synovial tissue also should be performed at the time of the aspiration.

In our aspiration protocol, a diagnosis of infection is made if all three specimens are positive for the same organism and if this result coincides with the clinical profile. If only one sample is positive, the aspiration is repeated. If the result on any of the repeat aspirations is positive for the same organism and the antibiotic-sensitivity profile also is identical, then the presence of infection is confirmed. If two of the three initial samples are positive, the result is interpreted in accordance with those of other investigations. For example, if hematologic parameters are elevated and there is no other apparent cause apart from the suspected infection,

Table 4
Sensitivity and specificity of intraoperative frozen sections

Study	No. of Sites Tested	No. of Proved Infections	Sensitivity	Specificity
Fehring and McAlister[68]	97	11	0.18 (2/11)	0.90 (77/86)
Feldman and associates[69]	33	9	1.00 (9/9)	0.96 (23/24)
Athanasou and associates[67]	106	22	0.91 (20/22)	0.96 (81/84)
Lonner and associates[70]	175	19	0.84 (16/19)	0.99 (154/156)
Fehring and Cohen[60]	130	4	0.50 (2/4)	0.90 (114/126)
Spangehl and associates[25]	202	35	0.80 (28/35)	0.94 (157/167)

then infection is likely and the aspiration need not be repeated. However, if the results of the laboratory investigations are normal or the parameters are elevated for other reasons, then the aspiration should be repeated.

Intraoperative Investigations
Intraoperative Frozen Sections
Mirra and associates[66] reported on the value of intraoperative frozen sections in 1976, stating that more than five polymorphonuclear (PMN) leukocytes per high-power field is evidence of probable infection and that a lack of PMN leukocytes is evidence of an absence of infection.

Intraoperative frozen sections have become a valuable tool for the diagnosis of infection. They are most useful in equivocal situations, when preoperative investigations are confounded by false elevations in the ESR or the CRP level, or both, or when the intraoperative appearance of the joint raises a suspicion of infection. Most investigators have reported favorable results (a sensitivity of 0.80 or more and a specificity of 0.90 or more),[25,60,67-70] although the authors of two studies[60,68] reported very poor sensitivities (Table 4). As with aspiration, some of the variation in results may be due in part to the low prevalence of infection in some series as well as the various criteria used to define a positive result. Fehring and McAlister[68] used the overall histologic picture rather than a specific number of PMN cells per high-power field as the criterion. Lonner and associates[70] recommended the use of ten PMN cells per

high-power field to improve specificity without reducing sensitivity. In their prospective analysis of the results of 175 revision arthroplasties, specificity improved from 0.96 to 0.99 when ten instead of five PMN leukocytes per high-power field was used as an index of infection. The sensitivity remained the same, at 0.84, for both indices. An important observation from that study, as well as from our own analysis of frozen sections, is that tissue should be obtained from areas that appear to be most inflamed. In addition, the pathologist should be experienced in the preparation and interpretation of specimens; we have found substantial interobserver variations among pathologists who were less experienced in the interpretation of tissue obtained from patients who had a failed total hip replacement.

Gram Stain
The gram stain is used as a simple intraoperative investigation to confirm the presence or absence of bacteria and thereby the presence or absence of an infection of the joint. In equivocal situations, when intraoperative investigations are the most useful, an investigation must be both sensitive (able to detect infection) and specific (able to rule out infection). While the gram stain may be specific, it lacks any acceptable level of sensitivity (range, 0 to 0.23).[25,47,69,71] The gram stain is not reliable for determining the presence of infection in patients who are having a revision hip arthroplasty, and it should not be used as a basis for determining treatment. In equivocal situations that

call for intraoperative investigation, we have abandoned its use in favor of the frozen section.

Opinion of the Surgeon
Despite normal findings on preoperative investigation, some hips may appear infected to the surgeon during the procedure. Frank pus and the formation of an abscess are the most obvious signs of infection. Features such as diffuse synovitis, turbid joint fluid, and formation of slime are all suspicious features.

The appearance of the joint is occasionally so overwhelmingly suspicious for infection that the surgeon cannot proceed with a single-stage exchange procedure. However, false impressions do occur, and we have delayed definitive management, because an infection initially was suspected, for a number of patients who did not have an infection. In two instances, the definitive operation was delayed because purulent material was found in the joint despite normal findings on preoperative aspiration. Intraoperative cultures subsequently were negative, and severe erosion of the polyethylene liner and wear debris were thought to be responsible for the tissue reaction. Severe accumulations of wear debris can incite a reaction that is similar in appearance to that of an infection.

Unfortunately, the true value of the surgeon's intraoperative opinion may never be known because the preoperative findings inevitably will influence that opinion. Feldman and associates[69] studied the association between the surgeon's intraoperative opinion and the pathologic diagnosis and found a sensitivity of 0.70 (seven of ten) and a specificity of 0.87 (20 of 23). There are a number of treatment options for patients in whom the macroscopic appearance of the joint is suspicious, the cultures of specimens obtained from preoperative aspiration are negative, the ESR or the CRP level is equivocal, and an intraoperative frozen section is not available. One option is to leave the prosthesis in place, obtain multiple specimens for culture, and reoperate at a later date after the final results of culture are available. Another option is to perform a single-stage exchange with a thorough debridement in a patient who may not tolerate repeated procedures. Finally, the surgeon may elect to perform a Girdlestone arthroplasty on the basis of the macroscopic appearance of the joint. This procedure is preferable to implantation of a new prosthesis into an infected tissue bed without performing a full debridement or a two-stage exchange. Despite the potential for a false interpretation of the appearance of the joint, this appearance should not be disregarded because the consequences of misdiagnosis can be devastating, and it should be kept in mind that other preoperative and intraoperative investigations are not 100% accurate.

Intraoperative Cultures

Intraoperative cultures often are used as the standard for the diagnosis of infection following an arthroplasty; however, the results of these cultures are not 100% accurate. Fitzgerald and associates[4] noted positive cultures in association with 111 (25%) of 437 hips that had not been operated on previously, and others[72,73] have reported rates of false-positive cultures of as high as 29% (188 of 658) in association with THA. In more recent studies, the rate of intraoperative false-positive cultures was between 6% (ten of 159) and 13% (32 of 254) for patients who had had a revision hip replacement.[25,34,60]

As with joint aspiration, careful tech-

nique must be followed in order to avoid false results. Preoperative antibiotics should be withheld until specimens have been obtained. Clean instruments that have not been used on the skin should be employed to obtain the specimens. The specimens should be taken from an area that has not been previously cauterized, before any irrigation fluid is used and immediately after the pseudocapsule has been opened, to decrease the chance of colonization and to allow for subsequent administration of antibiotics. Samples should be obtained from close to the surface of the prosthesis and, if applicable, from inflamed tissue.

A minimum of three tissue specimens should be sent fresh to the laboratory for immediate processing. Cultures should not be considered negative until the final results of the broth subcultures are available. Although late growth of bacteria or growth in liquid medium alone often is considered a contaminant, the final results of culture should be interpreted in the context of all of the preoperative and intraoperative findings. We have detected late growth of bacteria on solid medium or growth in liquid medium alone in some cases of infection, although this finding is not common in our experience.

Molecular Analysis

Molecular technology may be used to diagnose the presence of bacterial DNA and RNA. Specific bacteria can be identified by their DNA structure. Polymerase chain reaction (PCR) enables the production of large amounts of specific sequences of target DNA from small quantities of starting material. In essence, large volumes of identical copies of the original starting material are produced. The specimen then is heat-cycled in an amino-acid broth to allow exposure and polymerization of the DNA chains. After 25 to 40 cycles, small quantities of bacterial DNA are amplified to create sufficient volumes of DNA for analysis.[74] The DNA then can be identified by sequenc-

ing, blot analysis, or enzyme digestion. Bacterial RNA, which is produced in large volumes by a single DNA gene segment, also can be sequenced with use of reverse transcriptase enzyme.[5,74,75] These techniques are currently under development and may hold promise for improved diagnostic accuracy. However, the inherent advantage of PCR—namely, the ability to identify bacteria from small quantities of DNA—makes these techniques susceptible to contamination.[74] Whether PCR is too sensitive to any bacterial particles that are encountered, thereby leading to a high rate of false-positive results, remains to be determined.

Protocol for the Diagnosis of Infection following Arthroplasty

To exclude infection as a cause of failure of an arthroplasty, certain key investigations should be performed. This should help to keep the overall number of investigations to a minimum, thereby being cost effective, yet still confirming the diagnosis of infection.

After a careful history is obtained and a physical examination is performed, with special attention being paid to the details of the index procedure and the chronology of the pain, both the ESR and the CRP level should be determined for every patient who is to have a revision. If both results are normal—that is, the ESR is less than 30 mm/hr and the CRP level is 10 mg/l or less—and there is no suggestion of infection on clinical presentation, no additional investigations are needed. If the ESR or the CRP level is elevated for any reason or if there is a clinical suspicion of infection, then an aspiration of the hip joint should be performed. A diagnosis of infection is made if the clinical suspicion is high; the ESR or the CRP level, or both, are elevated for no other known reason; and the cultures of the aspirated fluid are positive. If the ESR or the CRP level, or both, are falsely elevated, an intraoperative frozen section may be used to confirm the diagnosis, particularly if the cultures of the aspirated fluid are negative and the clinical suspicion remains high or if the clinical suspicion is low but the cultures of the aspirated fluid are positive. However, in these situations, the determination of the ESR and the CRP level, as well as the aspiration, should be repeated before the procedure. A sequential indium bone scan also may be used preoperatively to assist the physician in making the diagnosis if it is expected that an intraoperative frozen section will not be available or that it may be unreliable because of lack of local expertise (Fig. 1).

The single most important factor in determining the treatment options for a patient in whom a THA has failed is the exclusion of a diagnosis of infection. In most patients, the diagnosis can be successfully confirmed preoperatively on the basis of the clinical presentation, the results of serologic tests, or positive cultures of aspirated joint fluid. In other patients, the diagnosis can be established according to intraoperative findings at the time of the revision procedure and confirmed with frozen section. The diagnosis may be confirmed in the postoperative period by the final results of the intraoperative cultures.

References

1. Charnley J: A clean-air operating enclosure. *Br J Surg* 1964;51:202–205.

2. Charnley J: Postoperative infection after total hip replacement with special reference to air contamination in the operating room. *Clin Orthop* 1972;87:167–187.

3. Eftekhar NS, Tzitzikalakis GI: Failures and reoperations following low-friction arthroplasty of the hip: A five- to fifteen-year follow-up study. *Clin Orthop* 1986;211:65–78.

4. Fitzgerald RH Jr, Peterson LF, Washington JA II, et al: Bacterial colonization of wounds and sepsis in total hip arthroplasty. *J Bone Joint Surg* 1973;55A:1241–1250.

5. Garvin KL, Hanssen AD: Infection after total hip arthroplasty: Past, present, and future. *J Bone Joint Surg* 1995;77A:1576–1588.

6. Lidwell OM: Clean air at operation and subsequent sepsis in the joint. *Clin Orthop* 1986;211:91–102.

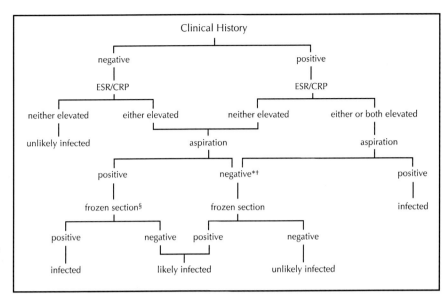

Fig. 1 Protocol for the diagnosis of infection following total hip arthroplasty.
*Repeat aspiration should be performed before the procedure if clinical suspicion of an infection is high or if the erythrocyte sedimentation rate (ESR) or the C-reactive protein (CRP) level, or both, are elevated for another reason.
†Consider performing sequential technetium-99m and indium-labeled white blood-cell scanning.
§Frozen sections should be obtained if the ESR and the CRP level are not elevated.

7. Lidwell OM, Elson RA, Lowbury EJ, et al: Ultraclean air and antibiotics for prevention of postoperative infection: A multicenter study of 8,052 joint replacement operations. *Acta Orthop Scand* 1987;58:4–13.

8. Maderazo EG, Judson S, Pasternak H: Late infections of total joint prostheses: A review and recommendations for prevention. *Clin Orthop* 1988;229:131–142.

9. Salvati EA, Robinson RP, Zeno SM, et al: Infection rates after 3,175 total hip and total knee replacements performed with and without a horizontal unidirectional filtered air-flow system. *J Bone Joint Surg* 1982;64A:525–535.

10. Schutzer SF, Harris WH: Deep-wound infection after total hip replacement under contemporary aseptic conditions. *J Bone Joint Surg* 1988;70A:724–727.

11. Sculco TP: The economic impact of infected total joint arthroplasty, in Heckman JD (ed): *Instructional Course Lectures 42*. Rosemont, IL, American Academy of Orthopaedic Surgeons, 1993, pp 349–351.

12. McDonald DJ, Fitzgerald RH Jr, Ilstrup DM: Two-stage reconstruction of a total hip arthroplasty because of infection. *J Bone Joint Surg* 1989;71A:828–834.

13. Coventry MB: Treatment of infections occurring in total hip surgery. *Orthop Clin North Am* 1975;6:991–1003.

14. Fitzgerald RH Jr, Nolan DR, Ilstrup DM, et al: Deep wound sepsis following total hip arthroplasty. *J Bone Joint Surg* 1977;59A:847–855.

15. Hughes PW, Salvati EA, Wilson PD Jr, et al: Treatment of subacute sepsis of the hip by antibiotics and joint replacement: Criteria for diagnosis with evaluation of twenty-six cases. *Clin Orthop* 1979;141:143–157.

16. Irvine R, Johnson BL Jr, Amstutz HC: The relationship of genitourinary tract procedures and deep sepsis after total hip replacements. *Surg Gynecol Obstet* 1974;139:701–706.

17. Hunter G, Dandy D: The natural history of the patient with an infected total hip replacement. *J Bone Joint Surg* 1977;59B:293–297.

18. Rubin R, Salvati EA, Lewis R: Infected total hip replacement after dental procedures. *Oral Surg* 1976;41:18–23.

19. Stinchfield FE, Bigliani LU, Neu HC, et al: Late hematogenous infection of total joint replacement. *J Bone Joint Surg* 1980;62A:1345–1350.

20. Deacon JM, Pagliaro AJ, Zelicof SB, et al: Prophylactic use of antibiotics for procedures after total joint replacement. *J Bone Joint Surg* 1996;78A:1755–1770.

21. Vanderhooft JE, Robinson RP: Late infection of a bipolar prosthesis following endoscopy: A case report. *J Bone Joint Surg* 1994;76A:744–746.

22. Estrada R, Tsukayama D, Gustilo RB: Management of THA infections: A prospective study of 108 cases. *Orthop Trans* 1993;17:1114–1115.

23. Tsukayama DT, Estrada R, Gustilo RB: Infection after total hip arthroplasty: A study of

the treatment of one hundred and six infections. *J Bone Joint Surg* 1996;78A:512–523.

24. Canner GC, Steinberg ME, Heppenstall RB, et al: The infected hip after total hip arthroplasty. *J Bone Joint Surg* 1984;66A:1393–1399.

25. Spangehl MJ, Duncan CP, O'Connell JX, et al: Prospective analysis of preoperative and intraoperative studies for the diagnosis of infection in 210 consecutive revision total hip arthroplasties. Proceedings of the American Academy of Orthopaedic Surgeons 64th Annual Meeting, San Francisco, CA. Rosemont, IL, American Academy of Orthopaedic Surgeons, 1997, p 197.

26. Eftekhar NS (ed): Diagnosis of infection in joint replacement surgery, in *Infection in Joint Replacement Surgery: Prevention and Management.* St. Louis, MO, CV Mosby, 1984, pp 115–130.

27. Covey DC, Albright JA: Clinical significance of the erythrocyte sedimentation rate in orthopaedic surgery. *J Bone Joint Surg* 1987;69A:148–151.

28. Roberts P, Walter AJ, McMinn DJ: Diagnosing infection in hip replacements: The use of fine-needle aspiration and radiometric culture. *J Bone Joint Surg* 1992;74B:265–269.

29. Sanzen L, Carlsson AS: The diagnostic value of C-reactive protein in infected total hip arthroplasties. *J Bone Joint Surg* 1989;71B:638–641.

30. Thoren B, Wigren A: Erythrocyte sedimentation rate in infection of total hip replacements. *Orthopedics* 1991;14:495–497.

31. Aalto K, Osterman K, Peltola H, et al: Changes in erythrocyte sedimentation rate and C-reactive protein after total hip arthroplasty. *Clin Orthop* 1984;184:118–120.

32. Niskanen RO, Korkala O, Pammo H: Serum C-reactive protein levels after total hip and knee arthroplasty. *J Bone Joint Surg* 1996;78B:431–433.

33. Shih LY, Wu JJ, Yang DJ: Erythrocyte sedimentation rate and C-reactive protein values in patients with total hip arthroplasty. *Clin Orthop* 1987;225:238–246.

34. Barrack RL, Harris WH: The value of aspiration of the hip joint before revision total hip arthroplasty. *J Bone Joint Surg* 1993;75A:66–76.

35. Fitzgerald RH Jr: Total hip arthroplasty sepsis: Prevention and diagnosis. *Orthop Clin North Am* 1992;23:259–264.

36. Huddleston HD: Femoral lysis after cemented hip arthroplasty. *J Arthroplasty* 1988;3:285–297.

37. Lyons CW, Berquist H, Lyons JC, et al: Evaluation of radiographic findings in painful hip arthroplasties. *Clin Orthop* 1985;195:239–251.

38. Jasty MJ, Floyd WE III, Schiller AL, et al: Localized osteolysis in stable, non-septic total hip replacement. *J Bone Joint Surg* 1986;68A:912–919.

39. Jasty M, Maloney WJ, Bragdon CR, et al: The initiation of failure in cemented femoral components of hip arthroplasties. *J Bone Joint Surg* 1991;73B:551–558.

40. Kwong LM, Jasty M, Mulroy RD, et al: The histology of the radiolucent line. *J Bone Joint Surg* 1992;74B:67–73.

41. Harris WH, McCarthy JC Jr, O'Neill DA: Femoral component loosening using contemporary techniques of femoral cement fixation. *J Bone Joint Surg* 1982;64A:1063–1067.

42. Harris WH, McGann WA: Loosening of the femoral component after use of the medullary-plug cementing technique: Follow-up note with a minimum five-year follow-up. *J Bone Joint Surg* 1986;68A:1064–1066.

43. O'Neill DA, Harris WH: Failed total hip replacement: Assessment by plain radiographs, arthrograms, and aspiration of the hip joint. *J Bone Joint Surg* 1984;66A:540–546.

44. Tehranzadeh J, Gubernick I, Blaha D: Prospective study of sequential technetium-99m phosphate and gallium imaging in painful hip prostheses (comparison of diagnostic modalities). *Clin Nucl Med* 1988;13:229–236.

45. Wegener WA, Alavi A: Diagnostic imaging of musculoskeletal infection: Roentgenography; gallium, indium-labeled white blood cell, gammaglobulin, bone scintigraphy and MRI. *Orthop Clin North Am* 1991;22:401–418.

46. Oswald SG, Van Nostrand D, Savory CG, et al: Three-phase bone scan and indium white blood cell scintigraphy following porous coated hip arthroplasty: A prospective study of the prosthetic tip. *J Nucl Med* 1989;30:1321–1331.

47. Kraemer AWJ, Saplys R, Waddel JP, et al: Bone scan, gallium scan, and hip aspiration in the diagnosis of infected total hip arthroplasty. *J Arthroplasty* 1993;8:611–616.

48. Merkel KD, Brown ML, Dewanjee MK, et al: Comparison of indium-labeled-leukocyte imaging with sequential technetium-gallium scanning in the diagnosis of low-grade musculoskeletal sepsis: A prospective study. *J Bone Joint Surg* 1985;67A:465–476

49. Glithero PR, Grigoris P, Harding LK, et al: White cell scans and infected joint replacements: Failure to detect chronic infection. *J Bone Joint Surg* 1993;75B:371–374.

50. Pring DJ, Henderson RG, Rivett AG, et al: Autologous granulocyte scanning of painful prosthetic joints. *J Bone Joint Surg* 1986;68B:647–652.

51. Wukich DK, Abreu SH, Callaghan JJ, et al: Diagnosis of infection by preoperative scintigraphy with indium-labeled white blood cells. *J Bone Joint Surg* 1987;69A:1353–1360.

52. Johnson JA, Christie MJ, Sandler MP, et al: Detection of occult infection following total joint arthroplasty using sequential technetium-99m HDP bone scintigraphy and indium-111 WBC imaging. *J Nucl Med* 1988;29:1347–1353.

53. Palestro CJ, Kim CK, Swyer AJ, et al: Total-hip arthroplasty: Periprosthetic indium-111-labeled leukocyte activity and complementary technetium-99-m-sulfur colloid imaging in suspected infection. *J Nucl Med* 1990;31:1950–1955.

54. Oyen WJ, Claessens RA, van der Meer JW, et al: Detection of subacute infectious foci with indium-111-labeled autologous leukocytes and indium-111-labeled human nonspecific immunoglobulin G: A prospective comparative study. *J Nucl Med* 1991;32:1854–1860.

55. Oyen WJ, van Horn JR, Claessens RA, et al: Diagnosis of bone, joint, and joint prosthesis infections with In-111-labeled nonspecific human immunoglobulin G scintigraphy. *Radiology* 1992;182:195–199.

56. Serafini AN, Garty I, Vargas-Cuba R, et al: Clinical evaluation of a scintigraphic method for diagnosing inflammations/infections using indium-111-labeled nonspecific human IgG. *J Nucl Med* 1991;32:2227–2232.

57. Wegener WA, Velchik MG, Weiss D, et al: Infectious imaging with indium-111-labeled nonspecific polyclonal human immunoglobulin. *J Nucl Med* 1991;32:2079–2085.

58. Fehrman DA, McBeath AA, DeSmet AA, et al: Imaging barium-free bone cement. *Am J Orthop* 1996;25:172–174.

59. Graif M, Schwartz E, Strauss S, et al: Occult infection of hip prosthesis: Sonographic evaluation. *J Am Geriatr Soc* 1991;39:203–204.

60. Fehring TK, Cohen: Aspiration as a guide to sepsis in revision total hip arthroplasty. *J Arthroplasty* 1996;11:543–547.

61. Lachiewicz PF, Rogers GD, Thomason HC: Aspiration of the hip joint before revision total hip arthroplasty: Clinical and laboratory factors influencing attainment of a positive culture. *J Bone Joint Surg* 1996;78A:749–754.

62. Mulcahy DM, Fenelon GC, McInerney DP: Aspiration arthrography of the hip joint: Its uses and limitations in revision hip surgery. *J Arthroplasty* 1996;11:64–68.

63. Tigges S, Stiles RG, Meli RJ, et al: Hip aspiration: A cost-effective and accurate method of evaluating the potentially infected hip prosthesis. *Radiology* 1993;189:485–488.

64. Phillips WC, Kattapuram SV: Efficacy of preoperative hip aspiration performed in the radiology department. *Clin Orthop* 1983;179:141–146.

65. Schmidt RM, Rosenkranz HS: Antimicrobial activity of local anesthetics: Lidocaine and procaine. *J Infect Dis* 1970;121:597–607.

66. Mirra JM, Amstutz HC, Matos M, et al: The pathology of the joint tissues and its clinical relevance in prosthesis failure. *Clin Orthop* 1976;117:221–240.

67. Athanasou NA, Pandey R, de Steiger R, et al: Diagnosis of infection by frozen section during revision arthroplasty. *J Bone Joint Surg* 1995;77B:28–33.

68. Fehring TK, McAlister JA Jr: Frozen histologic section as a guide to sepsis in revision joint arthroplasty. *Clin Orthop* 1994;304:229–237.

69. Feldman DS, Lonner JH, Desai P, et al: The role of intraoperative frozen sections in revision total joint arthroplasty. *J Bone Joint Surg* 1995;77A:1807–1813.

70. Lonner JH, Desai P, Dicesare PE, et al: The reliability of analysis of intraoperative frozen sections for identifying active infection during revision hip or knee arthroplasty. *J Bone Joint Surg* 1996;78A:1553–1558.

71. Chimento GF, Finger S, Barrack RL: Gram stain detection of infection during revision arthroplasty. *J Bone Joint Surg* 1996;78B:838–839.

72. Murray WR: Results in patients with total hip replacement arthroplasty. *Clin Orthop* 1973;95:80–90.

73. Tietjen R, Stinchfield FE, Michelsen CB: The significance of intracapsular cultures in total hip operations. *Surg Gynecol Obstet* 1977;144:699–702.

74. Rapley R, Theophilus BD, Bevan IS, et al: Fundamentals of the polymerase chain reaction: A future in clinical diagnostics? *Med Lab Sci* 1992;49:119–128.

75. Clarke AM, Mapstone NP, Quirke P: Molecular biology made easy: The polymerase chain reaction. *Histochem J* 1992;24:913–926.

Treatment of Infection at the Site of Total Hip Replacement

Eric L. Masterson, BSc, MCh, FRCS (Orth)
Bassam A. Masri, MD, FRCSC
Clive P. Duncan, MD, MSc, FRCSC

The modern era of total hip arthroplasty is little more than 30 years old, and during that time the procedure has proved to be highly effective in improving the physical function, social interaction, and overall health of millions of patients.[1] Initially, the procedure was associated with notable rates of infection,[2] but these have since been reduced considerably by measures such as prophylactic antibiotics, ultraclean-air operating rooms, and careful selection of patients.[3] However, this reduction in the prevalence of postoperative deep infection has been accompanied by a steady increase in the frequency with which the operation is performed.

It has been estimated that the prevalence of infection after all total hip replacements performed on Medicare patients in the United States, between 1986 and 1989, was approximately 2.3% (5,370 of 236,140).[4] Extrapolation of these figures to the estimated 200,000 such procedures that are performed annually in the United States suggests that more than 4,000 new cases of periprosthetic hip infection need treatment annually. These figures do not distinguish between infections that originated in the operating room and those of hematogenous origin. The total represents a sizable number of dissatisfied patients for whom the success or failure of treatment to eradicate the infection will have major implications for their quality of life.

In addition to the obvious human cost of an infection at the site of a total hip prosthesis are the considerable financial implications for the individual or the institution that must pay for the treatment. Revision hip operations necessitate a longer stay in the hospital than do primary procedures.[5] In addition, the operating time is longer, the blood loss is greater, and the rate of complications as well as the cost of implants are higher.[6] A number of factors increase the cost of revision of infected joints. These include the necessity for more than one surgical procedure for most patients, prolonged courses of parenteral antimicrobial chemotherapy, and the frequent need for periods of hospitalization between staged surgical procedures and after the completion of treatment. It has been estimated that the cost of treating an infected total hip prosthesis was at least $50,000 in 1990,[4] and current figures may well be higher. It is important that the additional costs of care be recognized by funding bodies such as Medicare and by other third-party payers.

Progress in the development of the optimum treatment of infection at the site of a total hip replacement has been slow. Such infections are sufficiently uncommon that only large tertiary referral centers can accumulate sufficient numbers of patients for study. In addition, the large number of variables in these complex cases makes it difficult to plan well-controlled prospective trials of different treatment modalities.

One of the difficulties in comparing the results of different treatment modalities is the variability in the durations of follow-up among reported series. There is evidence that the risk of recurrent infection remains increased even after several years and that the rate of recurrence increases as the duration of follow-up increases.[7,8] Whether these delayed infections are due to recurrence of the original infection or represent a new infection remains uncertain, but both mechanisms are probably important. Treatment should therefore be aimed at reducing the rate of recurrence of infection regardless of the mechanism.

Possible surgical treatment options for the infected total hip prosthesis include debridement with retention of the prosthesis; immediate one-stage exchange arthroplasty; and excision arthroplasty, either as a definitive, permanent procedure or as the first of a two or even three-stage reconstructive procedure. The use of a temporary prosthesis between the first and second stages of a two-stage exchange also has been advocated.

Antibiotics may be used as an adjunct

to surgery either systemically or locally (with use of bone cement as a vehicle), or both. Antibiotics may be used either to eradicate the infection or as a means of chronically suppressing a periprosthetic infection without concomitant surgical intervention. Occasionally, an infection at the site of a hip replacement is treated with debridement, retention of the prosthesis, and long-term administration of suppressive antibiotics. This method is particularly useful for elderly or medically unwell patients who cannot tolerate a two-stage exchange arthroplasty.

The choice of a particular treatment is influenced by a number of factors, including the acuteness or chronicity of the infection; the infecting organism, its sensitivity profile to antibiotics, and its ability to manufacture glycocalyx; the health of the patient; the fixation of the prosthesis; the available bone stock; and the particular philosophy and training of the surgeon.

Microbiologic Considerations

In most reports of periprosthetic infection, *Staphylococcus aureus* and *Staphylococcus epidermidis* are the most common infecting organisms, followed by a wide range of gram-positive and gram-negative bacteria. The importance of *S epidermidis* as a pathogen is well accepted and that organism should not be regarded as a contaminant from the skin, especially if it grows on culture on more than one occasion or in more than one broth.

Most staphylococci, with the exception of the strains designated as methicillin or oxacillin-resistant, are susceptible to cephalosporin. More than 95% of the *S aureus* organisms encountered in our hospital are sensitive to oxacillin (and therefore to cephalosporin). However, at least 30% of the *S epidermidis* isolates identified at our hospital are currently oxacillin resistant. There is substantial regional variation in the sensitivity profile of *S epidermidis*. Methicillin-resistant *S epidermidis* has been identified as an

important pathogen in patients who have an infection at the site of a total hip replacement.[9] Resistance to gentamicin has been associated with previous use of gentamicin-impregnated bone cement.[10]

Staphylococcus species with resistance to vancomycin have not yet been encountered as a clinical problem, to our knowledge. There are concerns that chronic elution of vancomycin from antibiotic-impregnated bone cement could predispose to the emergence of a vancomycin-resistant *Enterococcus* in the bowel. However, the levels of vancomycin in serum following the use of vancomycin-loaded cement have been shown to be negligible (Masri BA, Kendall RW, Duncan CP, Beauchamp CP, Bora B: The PROSTALAC system: A microbiological analysis. Read at the Combined Annual Meeting of the Canadian Orthopaedic Association and the Canadian Orthopaedic Research Society. Winnipeg, Manitoba, Canada, June 13, 1994.), and an association between the use of vancomycin in cement and the isolation of vancomycin-resistant enterococci has not been demonstrated, to our knowledge. Vancomycin should not be used for the treatment of infections that can be treated adequately with alternative antibiotics.

Much interest recently has been focused on the ability of an infecting organism to produce a slime layer, or glycocalyx. This layer is made up of a variety of polysaccharides synthesized by the bacteria as well as a range of host molecules. The ability of the organism to produce a slime layer permits it to be divided into planktonic forms, which exist as individual free-floating cells, and sessile forms, which exist within a biofilm of glycocalyx. The production of a biofilm allows the organism to adhere to and survive on synthetic surfaces. Bacteria that exist within a biofilm are at least 500 times more resistant to antibiotics than the planktonic forms.[11] They also are relatively resistant to complement activation

and ingestion by neutrophils. Biofilms require a certain minimum time to form after the inoculation of the infecting organism. In vitro evidence has suggested that infections can be eradicated with antibiotics while the inoculated organism is still in a planktonic phase but not after a biofilm has formed.[12] This finding lends support to the use of debridement, administration of antibiotics, and retention of the prosthesis for the treatment of acute-onset infections in joints with solidly fixed components. Recent research has suggested that the efficacy of antibiotics in killing biofilm bacteria is greatly enhanced by the addition of a low electrical current.[13,14] Possible therapeutic applications of electricity have yet to be explored.

Many species of *S aureus* and *S epidermidis* are slime producers. Most gram-negative organisms, with the notable exception of the *Pseudomonas* species, are poor slime producers. The eradication of pseudomonal infections also is complicated by slow rates of replication and a natural resistance to many antibiotics. There is little microbiological evidence to support contentions that other gram-negative organisms are especially difficult to eradicate, despite some clinical reports suggesting inferior results when the infecting organism was a gram-negative *Bacillus*.[15-17] Lieberman and associates,[18] in a review of the results of a two-stage treatment protocol, were unable to find any association between infection with a gram-negative organism and the risk of recurrence of infection after treatment. Tsukayama and associates[19] recently reported the results of treatment of 106 periprosthetic hip infections in 97 patients. In 13 hips the infecting organism was a gram-negative *Bacillus*, and in all 13 the infection was eradicated.

There is evidence that the material from which a component is made and the surface finish of the component may influence the ease with which infection may occur within the interstices of the prosthesis. Cordero and associates,[20] using an animal model, found that cobalt-chromium surfaces were more conducive to infection with S aureus than were titanium surfaces and that porous surfaces were more conducive to infection than were polished surfaces. The lower prevalence of infection associated with titanium surfaces may be related to superior properties of osseointegration that allow the host tissues to adhere to the surface of the implant before any microorganisms are able to adhere, elaborate glycocalyx, and cause a clinical yet indolent infection (this has been referred to as the "race for the surface").[21] The lower prevalence of infection associated with polished surfaces is probably a function of the smaller surface area for bacteria to adhere to and the shorter distances that host cells must travel in order to reach the surface of the component. In a series of in vitro experiments, Oga and associates[22] found an increased prevalence of infection with coagulase-negative Staphylococcus in association with polymethylmethacrylate and sintered hydroxyapatite surfaces,[23] although impregnation of the polymethylmethacrylate with antibiotics appeared to inhibit bacterial adhesion.[24]

A number of tests are available to determine the production of glycocalyx in laboratory cultures. However, the association between the production of glycocalyx by an organism and the development of an infection at the site of a total hip prosthesis is not sufficiently strong for the tests to have clear clinical relevance. Choosing between one and two-stage exchange procedures on the basis of production of a slime layer by the organism requires validation.

Classification of Periprosthetic Infections

Coventry,[25] in 1975, described the natural history of infections associated with total hip arthroplasty. Infection can be caused by contamination at the time of the operation. This type of infection can

present acutely, usually within 3 weeks following surgery. It also can present in the form of an indolent, chronic, low-grade infection, which usually occurs at least 8 weeks following surgery. The other mechanism of infection is hematogenous spread from a distant focus. This can happen at any time after surgery, and the presentation is similar to that of an acute infection.

Estrada and associates[26] refined the classification of periprosthetic infections by the addition of a category to describe patients who had positive intraoperative cultures without other features of obvious infection. Those authors described postoperative infections as occurring either early (within 1 month of surgery) or late (more than 1 month postoperatively). In addition, acute hematogenous infection may present at any stage in a hip joint that has been asymptomatic. Tsukayama and associates[19] recently reported the results of treatment of 106 infections that were associated with total hip arthroplasty. The infections were treated with various protocols according to four clinical settings: positive intraoperative cultures, early postoperative infection, late chronic infection, and acute hematogenous infection. Infections that were diagnosed on the basis of positive cultures of specimens that had been obtained during a revision hip arthroplasty were treated with intravenous administration of antibiotics for 6 weeks without surgical intervention, and a success rate of 90% (28 of 31) was reported. Early postoperative infections were treated with debridement, retention of the prosthesis, and administration of antibiotics; this protocol had a success rate of 71% (25 of 35). Of the remaining ten infections in that group, eight were treated successfully with a subsequent exchange procedure. Late chronic infections were treated with use of a two-stage exchange protocol, and a success rate of 85% (29 of 34) was reported. Finally, acute hematogenous infections were treated with

debridement, retention of the prosthesis, and intravenous administration of antibiotics; three of six infections were treated successfully with this protocol.

Surgical Considerations in Revisions Performed Because of Infection

The initial surgical approach for the treatment of an infection at the site of a total hip prosthesis is identical regardless of whether the surgeon plans a definitive excision arthroplasty, a single-stage exchange, or a delayed exchange. In this regard, it is appropriate to emphasize a number of points of surgical technique.

1. Old healed incisions should be used to gain access to the hip provided that the surgical exposure is not compromised. This avoids the creation of unsightly and unnecessary so-called railway-track incisions, with the attendant risk of wound-edge necrosis. Closure of the wound at the end of the procedure is facilitated if active sinus tracts can be excised readily as part of the incision. Otherwise, sinus tracts should be irrigated thoroughly and cleared of debris and loose granulation tissue.

2. Antibiotics should be withheld until the hip-joint capsule has been incised and specimens of synovial tissue have been obtained for culture, even when the probable infecting organism has been identified by means of preoperative aspiration of the hip or culture of specimens from a draining sinus. This allows for confirmation of the infecting organism and helps to rule out the presence of a polyclonal infection. If the identity of the infecting organism is in doubt or is unusual, specimens also should be sent for Ziehl-Nielsen stains and mycobacterial cultures, as well as for fungal studies. Patients who have clinical and radiographic evidence of chronic infection and who have received antibiotics orally or intravenously before referral are less likely to have a positive preoperative or intraoperative culture. In these instances, it is

useful to perform a repeat aspiration of the hip after all antibiotics have been discontinued for a minimum of 4 weeks, provided that the patient's condition permits a delay in the definitive treatment. There may, however, be some patients for whom the cultures remain negative despite other features that are strongly suggestive of infection. It is our practice to manage these patients as if the hip were infected and to obtain intraoperative specimens of the periprosthetic tissue for culture and frozen-section analysis.

3. The choice of surgical approach should be based on the need to remove all foreign material and dead tissue, including bone, while at the same time avoiding devascularization of the tissues and creation of a new potential focus of infection. The importance of removing all particles of cement has been stressed,[16,27] although some authors have found that retention of small quantities of cement did not adversely affect the clinical outcome.[18,28] If the cement around the femoral component is loose, it may be possible to remove the cement from above without damaging the femur. However, if the cement remains solidly bonded to bone, extensive damage to the femur may result from attempts to remove the cement in a retrograde fashion and consideration should be given to exposing the femoral canal directly. This can be achieved readily with use of the extended trochanteric osteotomy as described by Younger and associates.[29] We have been impressed by the ease with which solidly bonded cement can be removed using this technique and by the predictability of subsequent osseous union. If a so-called cortical window is used to gain access to distal cement, great care should be taken to ensure that the vastus lateralis muscle is not stripped from the window fragment and that the periosteal blood supply is maintained.

4. When all necrotic tissue and foreign material have been removed, the wound should be irrigated vigorously with copi- ous amounts of saline solution in order to remove as much particulate matter as possible. Pulsed-lavage systems are very effective and should be used if available. In contrast to Weber and Lautenbach,[30] we have not been impressed by the value of continuous irrigation in the postoperative period other than as a recipe for an uncomfortable patient and a medical and nursing staff that is frustrated in its attempts to prevent the system from becoming blocked.

Treatment Protocols
Antibiotics Without Surgery
Antibiotics without surgical intervention are most commonly used in the form of chronic suppressive therapy for periprosthetic infections when an operation is refused by the patient or is believed to be associated with an unacceptable risk.[31] The infection is not eradicated but is controlled so that symptoms are minimized. Certain criteria must be fulfilled in order for a patient to be considered a suitable candidate for chronic suppressive therapy. Generally, these patients are considered medically unfit to undergo major surgery or, less commonly, they have refused this option. In addition, the infecting organism must be known and must be sensitive to the chosen antibiotic. Finally, the antibiotic should be effective orally and should be well tolerated by the patient if reasonable compliance is to be expected. Side effects such as diarrhea or recurrent candidiasis usually result in the failure of treatment. The emergence of resistant strains as a result of prolonged single-agent therapy is another cause of failure of this form of treatment.

The newer fluoroquinolones have been shown to be effective in the treatment of implant-related infection caused by methicillin-susceptible Staphylococcus species.[32] The addition of rifampicin to antibiotic regimens also appears to be helpful.[33] Drancourt and associates[34] reported the results of a study on the use of oral ofloxacin with rifampicin for the treatment of infection with Staphylococcus associated with orthopaedic implants. Twenty-two hips that had a periprosthetic infection were included in the study population. Sensitivity to both antibiotics was a requirement for inclusion in the study, and antibiotics were continued orally for 6 months. The infection was eradicated in eight of the 12 joints that had a retained prosthesis after a follow-up of 12 to 57 months. One failure of treatment was due to the patient's inability to tolerate the antibiotics, and another was due to the emergence of a resistant organism. Additional reports on this treatment protocol are necessary in order to determine if these results are maintained as the duration of follow-up increases.

Debridement With Retention of the Prosthesis
There is little argument about the necessity to remove a loose total hip prosthesis from a chronically infected joint. However, removal of a well-fixed total hip implant that is associated with infection carries the risk of causing major damage to the remaining bone stock. It is therefore understandable that attempts have been made to define the circumstances in which the infection may be eradicated by debridement combined with systemic administration of antibiotics without removal of the prosthesis.

It is generally accepted that the results of debridement with retention of the prosthesis in patients who have a chronic infection are poor.[35] This is in keeping with what we understand about the ability of infecting organisms to adhere to the surfaces of the implant and to survive within a slime layer that isolates the organism from host defense mechanisms and the effects of systemic antibiotics. However, we also know that the slime layer takes some time to form after inoculation and that there is a potential so-called window of opportunity while the infecting organism is still in its planktonic form. If the infection is treated intensively with adequate debridement and appropriate systemic antibiotics, eradication should be possible. Both postoperative and late hematogenous infections can present acutely, and it appears reasonable to treat both types of infection in this manner shortly after onset.

Difficulties with this approach revolve around the determination of the time of onset of the infection and the establishment of a cutoff time beyond which it is no longer reasonable to attempt to retain the implant. Additional difficulty arises from the inability to recognize dead infected tissues that will act as an ongoing nidus of infection.

Tsukayama and associates[19] reported a 71% rate of success using a protocol of surgical debridement and intravenous administration of antibiotics to treat 35 early postoperative infections. They emphasized the importance of limiting this treatment method to infections that had developed less than 1 month postoperatively. Poor results were associated with implants that had been inserted without cement, leading those authors to suggest that such implants should be removed at the time of the debridement. The same authors reported success in eradicating three of six acute hematogenous infections.[19] However, the small numbers of patients in that group precluded extensive analysis.

There are scant prospective data in the literature to guide the surgeon as to when an attempt should be made to retain the prosthesis. The primary difficulty appears to be the lack of accuracy with which acute infections can be distinguished from chronic ones. It is our practice to limit attempts at retention of the prosthesis to patients who have a solidly fixed implant and a very clear, short history of symptomatic infection, preferably with an identifiable cause such as a bacteremia resulting from a recent dental procedure. Patients in whom the distinction between acute and chronic infection cannot be made with confidence are managed as if they have a chronic infection.

Girdlestone Arthroplasty

A number of authors have reported the use of excision arthroplasty as a definitive procedure for the control of a periprosthetic infection rather than as the first stage in a staged reconstruction.[27,28,36-39] The general consensus is that the procedure is highly effective in controlling infection and reducing pain; however, it usually is associated with a considerable loss of function. Patients who have had an excision arthroplasty walk poorly and almost always need walking aids. The absence of a fixed fulcrum for the abductor muscles results in a prominent lurching gait. Velocity and cadence are reduced, and energy expenditure is increased.[40] Limb-shortening may range from 3 to 11 cm but most typically ranges from 4 to 6 cm. This necessitates the use of external shoe-lifts that frequently are cosmetically unacceptable, especially to female patients.

Despite these drawbacks, excision arthroplasty may be the most appropriate definitive treatment for some patients, including those who are considered medically unfit to have an additional reconstructive procedure and those who are mentally impaired and may be unable to cooperate with the postoperative restrictions and the rehabilitation protocol after a complex reconstruction. A severe deficiency of bone stock also has been considered a contraindication to reimplantation.[18] However, initial encouraging results associated with the use of massive allografts suggest that a reconstruction can be performed successfully despite the poor bone stock.[41,42] Furthermore, there is evidence to suggest that postoperative function is related to the level of resection of the proximal aspect of the femur, with worse results being seen in patients who have an extensive deficiency of femoral bone stock.[38]

Excision arthroplasty is our treatment of choice for patients who have an infection at the site of a total hip prosthesis and an active history of intravenous drug abuse, because such patients have a tendency toward poor compliance with postoperative instructions and a high risk of reinfection. Another group of patients for whom we consider excision arthroplasty to be the most appropriate treatment includes those who have major immunosuppression, especially after solid organ transplantation.

Single-Stage Exchange Arthroplasty

Interest in single-stage exchange arthroplasty was perhaps first aroused by the work of Buchholz and Engelbrecht,[43] who used gentamicin-impregnated bone cement. Buchholz and associates[15] later reported a successful result in 77% of 583 patients who were managed with a single-stage exchange for the treatment of infection; this rate increased to 90% after subsequent exchange procedures. During the course of that study, the amount of gentamicin in the cement was increased, erythromycin was temporarily added, and, toward the end of the study period, antibiotics were chosen on the basis of the sensitivity of the infecting organism. Systemic antibiotics were not used routinely. The duration of follow-up ranged from 1 to 131 months. The results after a longer duration of follow-up of patients from the same unit were later reported by Nelson.[44] The prosthesis had been retained in 21 of 38 patients after a minimum follow-up of 10 years.

Carlsson and associates,[45] in 1978, reported on the use of gentamicin-impregnated bone cement in one and two-stage exchange arthroplasties performed because of infection. Their protocol included the addition of 0.5 g of gentamicin to each 40 g of bone cement and the use of systemic antibiotics. The exchange was completed during a single surgical procedure in 59 patients, and it was performed as a two-stage procedure in 18. The overall rate of success was 78%, and no significant difference was detected between the patients who had had a one-stage procedure and those who had had a two-stage procedure. It should be noted that 20 patients who had had a single-stage exchange were followed for less than 1 year and that antibiotics were administered for 6 months postoperatively.

The results after a longer duration of follow-up were later reported by Sanzén and associates[46] in a study from the same center. The rate of success after the one-stage exchanges, at a minimum of 2 years, was 76% (55 of 72 procedures). However, aseptic loosening was noted in 30 (61%) of 49 hips at 5 years.

The reported results of single-stage exchange arthroplasty were well summarized by Garvin and Hanssen.[47] They found that the cumulative success rate from 16 reports of single-stage exchange arthroplasty performed with use of antibiotic-impregnated cement was 82% (976 of 1,189 hips). The cumulative success rate from four reports of single-stage exchange arthroplasty performed without local delivery of antibiotics was 58% (35 of 60 hips). These data support the need for antibiotic-impregnated cement if a single-stage exchange is chosen. This recommendation also was supported by the results of single-stage exchange with antibiotic-impregnated cement as reported recently by Raut and associates.[7] In that study, 154 (84%) of 183 patients were infection-free after a mean duration of follow-up of more than 7 years. Almost one third of the patients had an actively discharging sinus at the time of the revision, but this did not adversely affect the outcome. The protocol included the use of oral antibiotics for 6 weeks to 3 months.

The major advantage of a single-stage exchange procedure is self-evident. The avoidance of additional surgical procedures is highly desirable for both the patient and society and is particularly important for patients who have several major medical problems, for whom the

risks of additional procedures are cumulative. However, the potential benefits must be weighed against the slightly lower rates of eradication of infection that are observed after one-stage compared with two-stage procedures as well as against the difficulty of removing a solidly fixed cemented long or mid-length stem without destroying the remaining proximal femoral bone stock should the procedure fail to eradicate the infection. Furthermore, the insertion of an implant with cement is not appropriate in many revision procedures, particularly when bone stock in the proximal portion of the femur is deficient. Because one-stage exchange techniques require that the implant be inserted with antibiotic-impregnated cement, many patients cannot be managed with this technique. The need to insert the prosthesis with cement may be responsible for the high rates of aseptic loosening that have been reported for such patients.[46]

Two-Stage Exchange Arthroplasty
In North America, periprosthetic infections of the hip are most commonly treated with a two-stage exchange arthroplasty, although the single-stage techniques remain popular in Europe. The principles of a two-stage exchange procedure include removal of the implant along with all cement containing infectious organisms and all dead or necrotic tissue, prolonged administration of antibiotics postoperatively, and eventual implantation of a new prosthesis. The popularity of this approach stems largely from reports of somewhat higher rates of eradication of infection compared with those associated with immediate-exchange protocols.[47] In a review of 12 reports of two-stage exchange procedures in which antibiotic-impregnated cement was used, Garvin and Hanssen[47] found the cumulative rate of eradication of infection to be 91% (385 of 423 hips). The rate for the nine studies in which antibiotic-impregnated cement was not

used was 82% (130 of 158 hips). These rates were somewhat higher than those in the reports of single-stage procedures.

There are many variables even within two-stage exchange protocols. These include the type and duration of postoperative systemic antibiotic therapy, the timing of the reimplantation, the use of allograft bone in the reconstruction, and the choice of fixation (with or without cement). Additional variables include the use of antibiotic-loaded cement in the form of beads and the use of a temporary spacer device in the interim between the first and second stages.

The ideal duration and route of administration of antibiotic therapy have not been determined. Most protocols have included 6 weeks of intravenous administration of antibiotics.[17,19] At least part of the advantage of the parenteral route probably stems from the more reliable administration of the antibiotic, usually by health-care workers. Adequate serum levels of many antibiotics can be achieved with use of the oral route, but compliance is always an issue when patients administer drugs to themselves. The appropriate dosage of antibiotics can be determined by measuring either bactericidal titers in serum[18] or minimum inhibitory concentrations in culture media.[47] There is some evidence that the use of parenteral therapy for less than 4 weeks is associated with a higher rate of recurrence when the infection is caused by a more virulent organism.[16]

The interval between the first and second stages of a two-stage exchange procedure has varied widely, both between different reports and within individual reports. This interval has ranged from 6 days to more than 6 years.[16] Lieberman and associates[18] reported the results of a protocol in which reimplantation was performed 6 weeks after an excision arthroplasty. Their findings did not differ importantly from the results for patients in whom reimplantation was delayed for more than 1 year.[16] Our own protocol with use of the prosthesis of antibiotic-loaded acrylic cement (PROSTALAC) includes 4 to 6 weeks of antibiotic therapy followed by repeat aspiration of the joint at a minimum of 4 weeks after discontinuation of the antibiotics.[48] We proceed with reimplantation if the culture of the aspirate is negative and the clinical appearance, erythrocyte sedimentation rate, and C-reactive protein level are indicative of resolution of the infection. This approach minimizes the possibility of attempting a reconstruction in the presence of an unresolved infection.

There has been concern that the use of bone allograft for reconstruction after infection might be associated with a higher rate of recurrent infection because the allograft might act as a sequestrum. This concern is particularly pertinent given the frequency of major cavitary and segmental bone defects in patients who have an infection at the site of a total hip arthroplasty. Such major bone loss has been regarded by some authors as a contraindication to reimplantation after infection.[17]

We are aware of only two reports that have dealt specifically with the use of allograft bone for reconstruction after infection. Berry and associates[42] retrospectively reported on 18 patients in whom various combinations of morcellized and bulk allografts were used in the second stage of a two-stage exchange that was performed because of infection. There were only two recurrent infections after a mean duration of follow-up of 4.2 years. Alexeeff and associates[41] reported on 11 patients who had a revision with use of a massive structural allograft in the second stage of a two-stage exchange protocol. There were no recurrent infections after a mean duration of follow-up of 4 years. All allografts united to host bone, and there was no major resorption of the graft apart from one small calcar graft that resorbed completely.

Most reports of exchange arthroplasty have described the results of reimplanta-

tion with use of components inserted with cement. To our knowledge, authors from only two centers have reported on large series of patients who had a revision total hip arthroplasty without cement after an infection. Nestor and associates,[49] in a report from the Mayo Clinic, described the results for 34 patients who had been managed with a two-stage exchange procedure with use of one of a variety of prostheses inserted without cement. Infection recurred in six patients (18%) after a mean duration of follow-up of almost 4 years. Of the patients who did not have a recurrence of infection, six of 28 had definite radiographic evidence of loosening and only 14 of 25 were considered to have a satisfactory functional outcome. Those authors concluded that avoidance of the use of bone cement did not improve the rate of success.

A higher rate of success was reported recently by Lai and associates,[50] who described the results of two-stage exchange procedures that were performed with use of a variety of prostheses inserted without cement. They noted recurrent infection in five (13%) of 39 patients after a mean duration of follow-up of 4 years and reported a mean Harris hip score[51] of 91 points for the 34 remaining patients who did not have an infection.

Other Surgical Options

Kostuik and Alexander[52] reported on a series of 14 patients who had had an arthrodesis of the hip, with use of a modified technique of the Association for the Study of Internal Fixation, for salvage of a failed total hip arthroplasty. Seven patients had a periprosthetic infection. The indications for the procedure were a young age, male gender, and strenuous functional demands. All hips eventually fused, and all patients were able to walk although they had a mean limb-length discrepancy of 4.6 cm. Ablation of the limb also has been reported,[53] but fortunately it is indicated only rarely.

Antibiotic-Loaded Cement and the Results With Use of the PROSTALAC System

The ability of thermostable antibiotics to elute from a bone-cement carrier has been widely documented in the literature.[54-69] Therapeutic levels of tobramycin and vancomycin have been found in drainage fluid after they were used with cement between stages in the management of patients who had an infection at the site of a total hip arthroplasty.[70] Tetracycline and chloramphenicol are not appropriate for use with bone cement because they are degraded by the exothermic curing reaction. The elution characteristics of Palacos bone cement (Merck, Darmstadt, Germany) are superior to those of other bone cements because Palacos cement has a higher surface porosity.[59] The mechanical strength of cement is substantially weakened if large volumes of antibiotic powder[63] or antibiotics dissolved in liquid[64] are added. This is a concern only when the cement is being used for fixation of a prosthesis; it is not a problem when the cement is used solely as a vehicle for antibiotics between stages in an exchange procedure.

The use of acrylic cement as an antibiotic depot is associated with improved rates of eradication of infection after both one-stage and two-stage exchange arthroplasties.[47] In a two-stage exchange arthroplasty, the cement may be used both for the definitive reconstruction[18,71] and in the form of strings of beads inserted between stages.[72,73]

Since 1986, we have been using an antibiotic-loaded implant between stages in a modified two-stage exchange protocol. This implant is known as the prosthesis of antibiotic-loaded acrylic cement; hence, the acronym PROSTALAC. The implant was designed to improve the patient's function between the first and second stages and to facilitate the definitive reconstruction by maintaining the soft tissues at their normal tension while providing the benefits of a local antibiotic depot.

The PROSTALAC includes a constrained acetabular component that is inserted with cement and a modular femoral component that consists of a stainless-steel endoskeleton surrounded by antibiotic-loaded cement. The femoral component is made intraoperatively with use of a series of molds. After thorough debridement and removal of all dead tissue and foreign material, the acetabular component is loosely cemented and fixation of the femoral component is achieved by means of a press-fit so that both components can be removed easily during the second stage without damaging the bone stock. A range of stem sizes and lengths is available to allow for the stabilization of hips with severe bone-stock deficiency. We most commonly use a combination of antibiotics consisting of 2.4 to 3.6 g of tobramycin and 1.0 to 1.5 g of vancomycin per package of bone cement. We avoid the use of wound-suction drains in order to encourage high levels of antibiotic within the infected tissues. Parenteral administration of antibiotics is continued postoperatively for 4 to 6 weeks. We proceed with definitive reconstruction if a culture of the hip aspirate, performed 4 weeks after the discontinuation of antibiotics, is negative and other indices suggest resolution of the infection. In our recent series of 61 patients, there was only one patient for whom the second stage of the exchange was delayed because of a positive culture of the hip aspirate. We believe that these organisms were contaminants because, in both cases, the organism that grew on culture was different from the initial infecting organism and the intraoperative cultures were negative. We have been impressed by the ease of exposure during the second stage as a result of appropriate soft-tissue tensioning by the temporary implant. Using this technique, we were able to eradicate infection in 45 (94%) of

48 patients at a minimum duration of follow-up of 2 years.[74]

Treatment of Tuberculous Infections

Tuberculosis is a rare cause of periprosthetic infection; the reports that we are aware of consist only of isolated cases.[75] A tuberculous infection may be diagnosed in the early postoperative period by means of a mycobacterial culture or histologic examination of specimens obtained at the time of a primary arthroplasty. Alternatively, the infection may present years after a primary arthroplasty as an unexpected pathogen in association with a loose prosthesis. There is some evidence, in case reports, that a solidly fixed prosthesis may be retained and that treatment can be successful with use of antituberculous chemotherapy alone.[76] However, such treatment is unlikely to be successful in a patient who has a loose prosthesis; in such a situation, the prosthesis should be removed. There is little information in the literature to guide the surgeon as to the timing or advisability of reimplantation, although it seems reasonable to perform the procedure after completion of a full course of antituberculous chemotherapy, provided that the clinical, radiographic, and hematological indices suggest full resolution of the infection.

Acknowledgement
The authors thank Mike Noble, MD, FRCP(C), for his assistance in the preparation of this manuscript.

References
1. Laupacis A, Bourne R, Rorabeck C, et al: The effect of elective total hip replacement on health-related quality of life. *J Bone Joint Surg* 1993;75A:1619–1626.

2. Charnley J: Postoperative infection after total hip replacement with special reference to air contamination in the operating room. *Clin Orthop* 1972;87:167–187.

3. Hanssen AD, Osmon DR, Nelson CL: Prevention of deep periprosthetic joint infection. *J Bone Joint Surg* 1996;78A:458–471.

4. Sculco TP: The economic impact of infected total joint arthroplasty, in Heckman JD (ed): *Instructional Course Lectures 42.* Rosemont, IL, American Academy of Orthopaedic Surgeons, 1993, pp 349–351.

5. Dreghorn CR, Hamblen DL: Revision arthroplasty: A high price to pay. *Br Med J* 1989;298:648–649.

6. Barrack RL: Economics of revision total hip arthroplasty. *Clin Orthop* 1995;319:209–214.

7. Raut VV, Siney PD, Wroblewski BM: One-stage revision of total hip arthroplasty for deep infection: Long-term follow up. *Clin Orthop* 1995;321:202–207.

8. Went P, Krismer M, Frischhut B: Recurrence of infection after revision of infected hip arthroplasties. *J Bone Joint Surg* 1995;77B:307–309.

9. James PJ, Butcher IA, Gardner ER, et al: Methicillin-resistant Staphylococcus epidermidis in infection of hip arthroplasties. *J Bone Joint Surg* 1994;76B:725–727.

10. Hope PG, Kristinsson KG, Norman P, et al: Deep infection of cemented total hip arthroplasties caused by coagulase-negative Staphylococci. *J Bone Joint Surg* 1989;71B:851–855.

11. Costerton JW, Lewandowski Z, Caldwell DE, et al: Microbial biofilms. *Annu Rev Microbiol* 1995;49:711–745.

12. Anwar H, Strap JL, Costerton JW: Kinetic interaction of biofilm cells of Staphylococcus aureus with cephalexin and tobramycin in a chemostat system. *Antimicrob Agents Chemother* 1992;36:890–893.

13. Costerton JW, Ellis B, Lam K, et al: Mechanism of electrical enhancement of efficacy of antibiotics in killing biofilm bacteria. *Antimicrob Agents Chemother* 1994;38:2803–2809.

14. Wellman N, Fortun SM, LcLeod BR: Bacterial biofilms and the bioelectric effect. *Antimicrob Agents Chemother* 1996;40:2012–2014.

15. Buchholz HW, Elson RA, Engelbrecht E, et al: Management of deep infection of total hip replacement. *J Bone Joint Surg* 1981;63B:342–353.

16. McDonald DJ, Fitzgerald RH Jr, Ilstrup DM: Two-stage reconstruction of a total hip arthroplasty because of infection. *J Bone Joint Surg* 1989;71A:828–834.

17. Salvati EA, Chekofsky KM, Brause BD, et al: Reimplantation in infection: A 12-year experience. *Clin Orthop* 1982;170:62–75.

18. Lieberman JR, Callaway GH, Salvati EA, et al: Treatment of the infected total hip arthroplasty with a two-stage reimplantation protocol. *Clin Orthop* 1994;301:205–212.

19. Tsukayama DT, Estrada R, Gustilo RB: Infection after total hip arthroplasty: A study of the treatment of one hundred and six infections. *J Bone Joint Surg* 1996;78A:512–523.

20. Cordero J, Munuera L, Folgueira MD: Influence of metal implants on infection: An experimental study in rabbits. *J Bone Joint Surg* 1994;76B:717–720.

21. Gristina AG, Barth E, Webb LX: Microbial adhesion and the pathogenesis of biomaterial-centered infections, in Gustilo RB, Gruninger

RP, Tsukayama DT (eds): *Orthopaedic Infection: Diagnosis and Treatment.* Philadelphia, PA, WB Saunders, 1989, pp 3–25.

22. Oga M, Sugioka Y, Hobgood CD, et al: Surgical biomaterials and differential colonization by Staphylococcus epidermidis. *Biomaterials* 1988;9:285–289.

23. Oga M, Arizono T, Sugioka Y: Bacterial adherence to bioinert and bioactive materials studied in vitro. *Acta Orthop Scand* 1993;64:273–276.

24. Oga M, Arizono T, Sugioka Y: Inhibition of bacterial adhesion by tobramycin-impregnated PMMA bone cement. *Acta Orthop Scand* 1992;63:301–304.

25. Coventry MB: Treatment of infections occurring in total hip surgery. *Orthop Clin North Am* 1975;6:991–1003.

26. Estrada R, Tsukayama D, Gustilo R: Management of THA infections: A prospective study of 108 cases. *Orthop Trans* 1993;17:1114–1115.

27. Clegg J: The results of the pseudarthrosis after removal of an infected total hip prosthesis. *J Bone Joint Surg* 1977;59B:298–301.

28. Ahlgren SA, Gudmundsson G, Bartholdsson E: Function after removal of a septic total hip prosthesis: A survey of 27 Girdlestone hips. *Acta Orthop Scand* 1980;51:541–545.

29. Younger TI, Bradford MS, Magnus RE, et al: Extended proximal femoral osteotomy: A new technique for femoral revision arthroplasty. *J Arthroplasty* 1995;10:329–338.

30. Weber FA, Lautenbach EE: Revision of infected total hip arthroplasty. *Clin Orthop* 1986;211:108–115.

31. Goulet JA, Pellicci PM, Brause BD, et al: Prolonged suppression of infection in total hip arthroplasty. *J Arthroplasty* 1988;3:109–116.

32. Desplaces N, Acar JF: New quinolones in the treatment of joint and bone infections. *Rev Infect Dis* 1988;10(suppl 1):S179–S183.

33. Widmer AF, Gaechter A, Ochsner PE, et al: Antimicrobial treatment of orthopedic implant-related infections with rifampin combinations. *Clin Infect Dis* 1992;14:1251–1253.

34. Drancourt M, Stein A, Argenson JN, et al: Oral rifampin plus ofloxacin for treatment of Staphylococcus-infected orthopedic implants. *Antimicrob Agents Chemother* 1993;37:1214–1218.

35. Murray WR: Use of antibiotic-containing bone cement. *Clin Orthop* 1984;190:89–95.

36. Bittar ES, Petty W: Girdlestone arthroplasty for infected total hip arthroplasty. *Clin Orthop* 1982;170:83–87.

37. Bourne RB, Hunter GA, Rorabeck CH, et al: A six-year follow-up of infected total hip replacements managed by Girdlestone's arthroplasty. *J Bone Joint Surg* 1984;66B:340–343.

38. Grauer JD, Amstutz HC, O'Carroll PF, et al: Resection arthroplasty of the hip. *J Bone Joint Surg* 1989;71A:669–678.

39. McElwaine JP, Colville J: Excision arthroplasty for infected total hip replacements. *J Bone Joint Surg* 1984;66B:168–171.

40. Waters RL, Perry J, Conaty P, et al: The energy cost of walking with arthritis of the hip and knee. *Clin Orthop* 1987;214:278–284.

41. Alexeeff M, Mahomed N, Morsi E, et al: Structural allograft in two-stage revisions for failed septic hip arthroplasty. *J Bone Joint Surg* 1996;78B:213–216.

42. Berry DJ, Chandler HP, Reilly DT: The use of bone allografts in two-stage reconstruction after failure of hip replacements due to infection. *J Bone Joint Surg* 1991;73A:1460–1468.

43. Buchholz HW, Engelbrecht H: Depot effects of various antibiotics mixed with Palacos resins. *Chirurg* 1970;41:511–515.

44. Nelson CL, Fitzgerald R Jr, Nelson JP, et al: Symposium: Antibiotic-impregnated acrylic composites. *Contemp Orthop* 1986;12:85–135.

45. Carlsson AS, Josefsson G, Lindberg L: Revision with gentamicin-impregnated cement for deep infections in total hip arthroplasties. *J Bone Joint Surg* 1978;60A:1059–1064.

46. Sanzén L, Carlsson AS, Josefsson G, et al: Revision operations on infected total hip arthroplasties: Two- to nine-year follow-up study. *Clin Orthop* 1988;229:165–172.

47. Garvin KL, Hanssen AD: Infection after total hip arthroplasty: Past, present, and future. *J Bone Joint Surg* 1995;77A:1576–1588.

48. Duncan CP, Beauchamp C: A temporary antibiotic-loaded joint replacement system for management of complex infections involving the hip. *Orthop Clin North Am* 1993;24:751–759.

49. Nestor BJ, Hanssen AD, Ferrer-Gonzalez R, et al: The use of porous prostheses in delayed reconstruction of total hip replacements that have failed because of infection. *J Bone Joint Surg* 1994;76A:349–359.

50. Lai KA, Shen WJ, Yang CY, et al: Two-stage cementless revision THR after infection: 5 recurrences in 40 cases followed 2.5-7 years. *Acta Orthop Scand* 1996;67:325–328.

51. Harris WH: Traumatic arthritis of the hip after dislocation and acetabular fractures: Treatment by mold arthroplasty. An end-result study using a new method of result evaluation. *J Bone Joint Surg* 1969;51A:737–755.

52. Kostuik J, Alexander D: Arthrodesis for failed arthroplasty of the hip. *Clin Orthop* 1984;188:173–182.

53. Fenelon GC, Von Foerster G, Engelbrecht E: Disarticulation of the hip as a result of failed arthroplasty: A series of 11 cases. *J Bone Joint Surg* 1980;62B:441–446.

54. Adams K, Couch L, Cierny G, et al: In vitro and in vivo evaluation of antibiotic diffusion from antibiotic-impregnated polymethylmethacrylate beads. *Clin Orthop* 1992;278:244–252.

55. Baker AS, Greenham LW: Release of gentamicin from acrylic bone cement: Elution and diffusion studies. *J Bone Joint Surg* 1988;70A:1551–1557.

56. Bayston R, Milner RD: The sustained release of antimicrobial drugs from bone cement: An appraisal of laboratory investigations and their significance. *J Bone Joint Surg* 1982;64B:460–464.

57. Brien WW, Salvati EA, Klein R, et al: Antibiotic impregnated bone cement in total hip arthroplasty: An in vivo comparison of the elution properties of tobramycin and vancomycin. *Clin Orthop* 1993;296:242–248.

58. DiMaio FR, O'Halloran JJ, Quale JM: In vitro elution of ciprofloxacin from polymethylmethacrylate cement beads. *J Orthop Res* 1994;12:79–82.

59. Elson RA, Jephcott AE, McGechie DB, et al: Antibiotic-loaded acrylic cement. *J Bone Joint Surg* 1977;59B:200–205.

60. Hill J, Klenerman L, Trustey S, et al: Diffusion of antibiotics from acrylic bone-cement in vitro. *J Bone Joint Surg* 1977;59B:197–199.

61. Kirkpatrick DK, Trachtenberg LS, Mangino PD, et al: In vitro characteristics of tobramycin-PMMA beads: Compressive strength and leaching. *Orthopedics* 1985;8:1130–1133.

62. Kuechle DK, Landon GC, Musher DM, et al: Elution of vancomycin, daptomycin, and amikacin from acrylic bone cement. *Clin Orthop* 1991;264:302–308.

63. Lautenschlager EP, Jacobs JJ, Marshall GW, et al: Mechanical properties of bone cements containing large doses of antibiotic powders. *J Biomed Mater Res* 1976;10:929–938.

64. Lautenschlager EP, Marshall GW, Marks KE, et al: Mechanical strength of acrylic bone cements impregnated with antibiotics. *J Biomed Mater Res* 1976;10:837–845.

65. Lawson KJ, Marks KE, Brems J, et al: Vancomycin vs tobramycin elution from polymethylmethacrylate: An in vitro study. *Orthopedics* 1990;13:521–524.

66. Masri BA, Duncan CP, Beauchamp CP, et al: Tobramycin and vancomycin elution from bone cement: An in vitro and in vivo study. *Orthop Trans* 1994;18:130.

67. Salvati EA, Callaghan JJ, Brause BD, et al: Reimplantation in infection: Elution of gentamicin from cement and beads. *Clin Orthop* 1986;207:83–93.

68. Seyral P, Zannier A, Argenson JN, et al: The release in vitro of vancomycin and tobramycin from acrylic bone cement. *J Antimicrob Chemother* 1994;33:337–339.

69. Wahlig H, Dingeldein E, Buchholz HW, et al: Pharmacokinetic study of gentamicin-loaded cement in total hip replacements: Comparative effects of varying dosage. *J Bone Joint Surg* 1984;66B:175–179.

70. Duncan CP, Masri BA: The role of antibiotic-loaded cement in the treatment of an infection after a hip replacement. *J Bone Joint Surg* 1994;76A:1742–1751.

71. Garvin KL, Evans BG, Salvati EA, et al: Palacos gentamicin for the treatment of deep periprosthetic hip infections. *Clin Orthop* 1994;298:97–105.

72. Abendschein W: Salvage of infected total hip replacement: Use of antibiotic/PMMA spacer. *Orthopedics* 1992;15:228–229.

73. Hovelius L, Josefsson G: An alternative method for exchange operation of infected arthroplasty. *Acta Orthop Scand* 1979;50:93–96.

74. Younger AS, Duncan CP, Masri BA, et al: The outcome of two-stage arthroplasty using a custom-made interval spacer to treat the infected hip. *J Arthroplasty* 1997;12:615–623.

75. Kreder HJ, Davey JR: Total hip arthroplasty complicated by tuberculous infection. *J Arthroplasty* 1996;11:111–114.

76. Spinner RJ, Sexton DJ, Goldner RD, et al: Periprosthetic infections due to Mycobacterium tuberculosis in patients with no prior history of tuberculosis. *J Arthroplasty* 1995;11:217–222.

Osteolysis: Cause and Effect

Raj K. Sinha, MD, PhD
Arun S. Shanbhag, PhD
William J. Maloney, MD
Carl T. Hasselman, MD
Harry E. Rubash, MD

Introduction

Osteolysis is the product of a particle-induced biologic process at the metal-bone or cement-bone interface, resulting in bone loss. Manifestations of this type of bone loss in patients range from new radiolucencies around previously well-fixed implants, which progress slowly and eventually result in mechanical instability, to rapidly expanding focal lesions that may or may not result in loosening. In the orthopaedic vernacular, the former process is generally termed "aseptic loosening" and the latter is widely known as "osteolysis." Because of the popular usage of these two terms, many orthopaedists mistakenly believe that each phenomenon represents a distinct clinical entity with dissimilar implications. However, research indicates that access to the metal-bone or cement-bone interface allows the same biologic phenomenon to result in both aseptic loosening and osteolysis.

Pathophysiology

The loosening of prosthetic components in the absence of infection has been a known clinical entity since the inception of joint replacement in the early 1960s. During revision of loose cemented cups, the implant invariably is surrounded by macrophage-laden fibrous tissue at the cement-bone interface.[1-5] Initially, this interfacial membrane was believed to form in response to the curing of acrylic cement. However, after evaluating tissues around failed prostheses, Willert and Semlitsch[6,7] proposed that loosening results from the macrophage response to wear debris. Wear particles generated within the joint space are phagocytosed and stored within cells in the joint capsule. Smaller particles (< 7 μm) generally are retained within macrophages, whereas larger nonphagocytosable particles are surrounded by foreign-body giant cells. Depending on the biocompatibility and toxicity of the debris material, there is a variable amount of cellular necrosis and associated infiltration by inflammatory cells. Particulate debris, cleared from the local area by the lymphatic drainage, has been recovered from regional lymph nodes.[8-10]

The generation of wear debris often exceeds the capacity of the capsule to clear or store the particles. In this case, all periprosthetic interfaces may be susceptible to infiltration by wear debris and granulation tissue.[7,11] The associated inflammation and interfacial bone loss can compromise bony fixation of the implant, resulting in loosening.[7,11] One manifestation of interfacial bone loss is a linear radiolucency about the implant, which may progress to circumferential canal enlargement and endosteal bone lysis. Alternately, the bone loss may appear to be focal, manifesting as a lytic, expansile lesion.[12-14] These focal lesions are associated with both stable and loose components, and they may progress in size.[12,15] If this process compromises the stability of the component, revision may be required. Revision may also be required for progressive bone loss in the absence of component instability.

Although Willert and Semlitsch's original observations involved cemented components, others have described a similar process adjacent to uncemented implants.[11,16-18] Schmalzried and associates[11] suggested that particulate wear debris generated at the articulation can be carried to all periprosthetic regions that are accessible to joint fluid. It has been further suggested that the flow pattern of the wear debris is determined by the degree of access to the interfaces.[19-21] Dispersion of particles along the interface results in linear osteolysis, whereas accumulation in discrete areas is thought to lead to focal osteolysis.

The pathology of the interfacial membrane has been studied extensively. Periprosthetic membranes with sheets of macrophages in a fibrous stroma intermingled with multinucleated giant cells, polymethylmethacrylate (PMMA) particles, and metallic wear debris are a common finding.[3,4,22,23] When interfacial tissues were placed in organ culture, they produced collagenase and prostaglandin E_2 (PGE_2),[24,25] both stimulators of osteoclastic bone resorption and matrix degradation in vivo. These data support the hypothesis of Willert and Semlitsch[7] that the interface tissue actively participates in bone resorption, possibly leading to loosening of the components.[24] Since this hypothesis was first proposed, numerous investigators have shown that the cellular activity within the membrane produces a variety of enzymes such as gelatinase, stromelysin and other metalloproteinases, prostaglandins, and cytokines such as interleukin-1α (IL-1α), IL-1β, IL-6 and tumor necrosis factor-α (TNF-α).[26–34]

Goodman and associates[26] reported that tissues around loose total hip replacement components were associated with significantly higher levels of PGE_2 than tissues around stable components. This finding supports those of other investigators, suggesting that PGE_2 and IL-1 are associated with osteolysis around loose prostheses.[26,28] Membranes from around loosened bipolar components have been shown to produce larger amounts of PGE_2 than those around loose total hip arthroplasties.[29] There appears to be no difference in the levels of various mediators between failed cemented and uncemented hip prostheses[31,34] or between failed titanium (Ti) and cobalt-chromium-molybdenum (Co-Cr-Mo) alloy components.[35] These findings reaffirm the hypothesis that the biologic response leading to interfacial bone loss results from exposure to particulate debris.

In the above studies, the pathologic process of linear versus focal osteolysis was not differentiated. However, Chiba and associates[32] specifically studied tissues retrieved from components with each particular radiographic appearance of osteolysis. Levels of IL-1, TNF-α, and IL-6 were significantly higher in granulomas from focal lesions than in those from regions of linear osteolysis. Focal osteolytic defects also contained more macrophages and ultra-high molecular weight polyethylene (UHMWPE) debris, possibly accounting for the increased levels of osteolysis-associated mediators. Thus, the particle burden and

the intensity of the biologic response seem to be associated with the radiographic appearance of the osteolysis. Nevertheless, the pathophysiologic process appears to be similar in both types of defects.

In the studies cited above, actual levels of biochemical mediators were quantified. In addition, in situ hybridization showed IL-1β protein to be bound to both macrophages and fibroblasts, whereas the messenger ribonucleic acid (mRNA) was detected only in macrophages.[30] This research also supports the primary role of the macrophage response to wear debris in the development of osteolysis.

In tissues around failed components, macrophages are the predominant cell type containing intracellular wear debris. Consequently, macrophages cultured with particles in vitro have been used to model specific events at the bone-implant interface. Such in vitro macrophage-particle experiments permit the systematic study of several variables.

Transformed or immortalized macrophage cell lines such as $P388D_1$, J774, IC-21, and RAW 267 have been used to study macrophage-particle interactions in vitro.[36–42] However, the transformed nature of these cell lines may limit the correlation of these studies to actual clinical events.[43] Macrophages in interfacial membranes are believed to be derived from the circulating peripheral blood monocytes. Subsequently, primary monocytes may be more appropriate for studying cellular events occurring in aseptic loosening.[44,45]

Early studies on macrophage-particle interactions focused primarily on the toxicities of particles having different compositions. Several investigators have found that most particles in vitro are cytotoxic to some extent. According to Haynes and associates,[46] the most cytotoxic particles are composed of Co-Cr-Mo, followed by Ti-alloy. Horowitz and associates[37,39,47] demonstrated that

PMMA particles (< 0.5 μm) inhibit DNA synthesis, and Shanbhag and associates[44] reported that UHMWPE particles retrieved from interfacial tissues or fabricated in the laboratory were less toxic to cells than PMMA particles. Investigators also have reported that particle-mediated cytotoxicity was dose-dependent.[41,44] Using similarly sized Co-Cr-Mo and Ti particles, Haynes and associates[46] found that Co-Cr-Mo particles had a limited ability to stimulate the release of inflammatory mediators or even inhibited their release, possibly because of cytotoxic effects. However, the less toxic Ti-alloy particles induced the synthesis and release of significant levels of PGE_2 and IL-1, IL-6, and TNF.[46]

Despite their inherent cytotoxicity, Co-Cr-Mo alloy particles can stimulate macrophages to release lysosomal enzymes such as β-glucuronidase and N-acetyl-β-D-glucose aminidase.[48] Glant and associates[40,49] and others[18] reported that $P388D_1$ macrophages challenged with PMMA and Ti particles released PGE_2 and IL-1 in culture medium. The secretion of PGE_2, IL-1, or TNF was reproducible with several different transformed and primary mouse peritoneal macrophages. Consistent with these findings was the release of the arachidonic acid metabolites PGE_1 and PGE_2 by $P388D_1$ cells cultured with PMMA particles.[39]

In addition to their composition and concentration, the size of the challenging particles can strongly influence the macrophage release of osteolytic mediators.[18,33,41] Horowitz and associates[18] noted that PMMA particles small enough to be phagocytosed (< 7 μm) will stimulate macrophages to release TNF, whereas larger particles will not. Within the phagocytosable range, the release of inflammatory mediators is also a function of particle size distribution. Fine particles appear to be more stimulatory than coarse particles in the osteolytic process.[6,22,27,33,39,50-52] Ti alloy, commercially pure (cp) Ti and UHMWPE particles retrieved from interface membranes, and fabricated UHMWPE particles in clinically relevant sizes were used to challenge human peripheral blood monocytes.[44,45,53] The metallic particles were more stimulatory for PGE_2, IL-1α, IL-1β, TNF-α, and IL-6 than both the retrieved and fabricated UHMWPE particles. The Ti alloy and cpTi particles also increased bone resorption from mouse calvaria in vitro, and they enhanced the proliferation of human dermal fibroblasts.

Whether it is termed aseptic loosening or osteolysis, interfacial bone loss occurs by the same pathologic process. The implication is that the various radiographic appearances represent different points on the continuum of a single pathologic process. This then raises the question: Why is bone loss manifested so differently in different patients? The answer may lie in the relationship between interfacial bone loss and several mechanical, genetic, and microenvironmental factors.

Mechanical Factors

Mechanical factors concern the stability of the interface. Fracture of the bone or cement mantle leads to loosening that can open conduits for particle migration around the interface. The "effective joint space" concept[11] underlines the importance of particle access in loosening of previously well-fixed components. The access of particles to the interfaces depends on such design features as stem shape, stem size, and extent of porous coating.

Microenvironmental Factors

Microenvironmental factors are patient-specific features, such as bone quality and nutrition, that affect healing. At the interface, the nature of the particulate debris also affects the degree of the inflammatory response. Particle characteristics such as size, shape, composition, and roughness all influence the degree and profile of the macrophage-induced cytokine

elaboration.[33,41,46,47] Further study will likely determine the most important trigger(s) for the development of osteolysis in individual patients.

Genetic Factors

Genetic factors, such as the major histocompatibility complex loci, could explain the variable nature of the immunologic response. That is, some patients may be more genetically susceptible than others to interfacial bone resorption. In addition, the regulation of the expression of osteogenic genes depends on material characteristics of the implant.[54,55] Thus, without circumferential bone ingrowth, the interface of cementless components is accessible to wear debris. Although many investigations are currently underway, no firm data yet exist to link specific genetic factors to osteolytic processes.

In summary, research has identified certain key features of the pathologic response leading to periprosthetic osteolysis. Wear debris generated by the articulating components stimulates macrophages to elaborate various cytokines. These cytokines subsequently result in osteoclast-mediated interfacial bone resorption. The size, shape, concentration, and composition of the particles, as well as their access to the interface, determine the intensity of the pathologic response and influence the radiographic appearance of the osteolysis.

Diagnosis

In patients who have undergone total joint replacement, the implication of radiographic osteolysis depends on the surgeon's point of view. Based on radiographic appearance, "aseptic loosening" was first identified around cemented components, and subsequently was defined as the development of a radiolucent line around a previously well-fixed prosthesis (Fig. 1).[56] The natural history of this radiolucency with cemented components is slow progression.[57] When the zone of radiolucency is wider than 2 mm,

or becomes circumferential, the prosthesis is considered to be at risk for loosening, and may already be clinically loose.[58] The radiolucency appears to progress from the intra-articular margin of the interface until it extends circumferentially. Alternatively, aseptic loosening may manifest as a circumferential periprosthetic endosteal scalloping of bone at the implant-bone or cement-bone interface. In addition to the thin zone of circumferential radiolucency, certain regions of the interface exhibit greater bone loss. It is possible that such focal areas of bone loss are more accessible to, or have a higher concentration of particles.[32] Regardless, aseptic loosening may appear as either a linear or expansile radiolucency. Once the component is loose, interfacial bone loss is progressive.[58]

"Osteolysis" is generally defined as a focal, often rapidly expanding radiolucency at the implant-bone or cement-bone interface[59] (Fig. 1). Such radiolucencies can represent small, clinically insignificant lesions that may not lead to loosening of the implant, such as with well-fixed, uncemented, fully porous-coated stems.[60] Alternately, the lytic lesion may progress to compromise fixation of cemented[61] and uncemented implants. Although the latter phenomenon rarely has been reported, the failure of the component is catastrophic. In addition, a common appearance of pelvic osteolysis in uncemented cups is that of a ballooning lesion that extends away from the component.[62] Despite interfacial bone loss, "osteolysis" results in loosening only when large amounts of structural bone loss occurs.

In patients with so-called aseptic loosening (ie, most commonly, a linear pattern of radiolucency typically associated with cemented components), a previously well-fixed implant has become loose. In patients with osteolysis (ie, the radiographic appearance of an expansile lytic lesion), there is focal loss of bone but the implant is stable. However, in

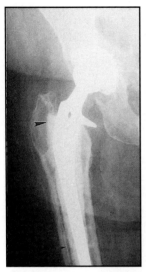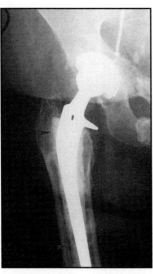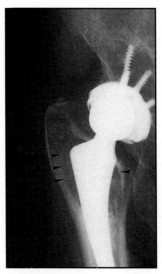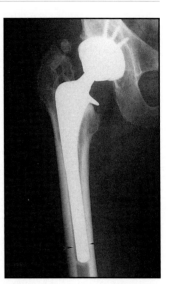

Fig. 1 Left, Radiograph demonstrating linear osteolysis (aseptic loosening) in the femur of a patient with a cemented stem (arrows). **Left center**, Radiograph of the same patient 6 months later, demonstrating progression of linear osteolysis (arrows). **Right center**, Radiograph demonstrating focal osteolysis in the proximal femur of a patient with a painless, stable femoral component (arrows). **Right**, Radiograph showing progressive osteolysis around an uncemented stem that has compromised stability of the component (arrows).

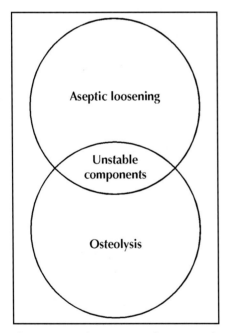

Fig. 2 Diagram depicting sets of patients with radiographic "aseptic loosening" and "osteolysis" that shows an overlapping subset of patients with both disease processes. Research shows that both processes are the same pathophysiologically, regardless of radiographic appearance, and that both may eventually lead to loosening of the component.

some patients, osteolysis may result in loosening (Fig. 2). Nevertheless, despite the different radiographic appearances, the same pathologic phenomena occur in both sets of patients. This implies that both "osteolysis" and "aseptic loosening" are terms that merely describe different manifestations of the same disease process. Therefore, it is important to realize that each manifestation represents osteolysis and interfacial bone loss. For the purposes of this discussion, linear osteolysis will refer to what was previously termed aseptic loosening, whereas focal or expansile osteolysis will refer to large, scalloped or balloon-like periprosthetic lesions.

Clinical Symptomatology

The majority of patients with osteolysis are asymptomatic when the resorptive process begins. In fact, extensive bone loss can occur with focal osteolysis in the absence of symptoms. Cemented components can cause increasing pain, which is suggestive of loosening but which is not apparent until the osteolysis has caused

severe bone loss.[62] Uncemented components may present initially with pain secondary to wear-debris induced synovitis or after periprosthetic fracture through the site of the lesion.[63,64] Osteolysis has been reported to occur as early as 12 months after implantation.[65] Once osteolysis has developed, it is likely to progress. If the component becomes loose, bone loss progresses more rapidly, resulting in defects larger than those seen with well-fixed components.[15] Therefore, most authors recommend routine serial, radiographic follow-up once osteolysis is identified.

Radiographic Appearance

Osteolysis is commonly described in characteristic patterns. On the acetabular side, the osteolytic regions may appear linear, focal, or expansile with both cemented and uncemented components.[11,60,62,65-73] Osteolysis also has been associated with both stable and unstable components.[62,66] Quite commonly, both the location and volume of bone loss will progress, resulting in extensive expansile

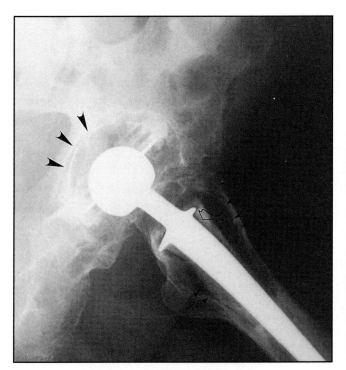 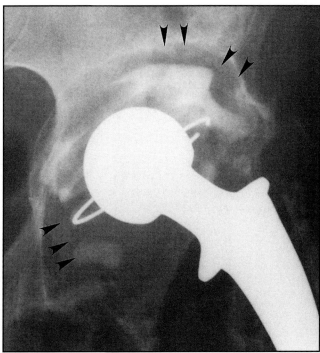

Fig. 3 Left, Linear osteolysis about a cemented socket, which has collapsed into the circumferential osteolytic cavity, giving the appearance of a thin linear region of radiolucency (large arrows). Also note the expansile osteolysis in femoral zones 8 and 14 (small arrows). The radiographic also demonstrates definite loosening of the femoral component as evidenced by stem-cement debonding (open arrow). **Right,** Focal osteolysis around a cemented cup, resulting in expansile lesion and subsequent catastrophic failure of the implant (arrows).

lesions involving the pelvis and femur.[15,74-76] An important caveat is that radiographs consistently underestimate the size of osteolytic lesions. In addition, the radiographic appearance differs depending on the mode of fixation.

Cemented Sockets
With cemented acetabular components, the path of least resistance for joint fluid and wear particles is at the cement-bone interface. As demonstrated in autopsy studies by Schmalzried and associates,[77] after the implantation of a cemented socket, the subchondral bone reconstitutes and acts as a partial barrier that prevents joint fluid and particles from gaining access to the trabecular bone of the ilium. The soft-tissue membrane created by the biologic reaction to wear particles dissects along the cement-bone interface, leading to disruption of this interface. As the interfacial disruption progresses to

the acetabular dome, fixation is lost. Radiographically, the osteolytic pattern is linear, and the radiolucency occurs at the cement-bone junction (Fig. 3). The component tends to migrate into the radiolucent areas in the superior and medial aspects of the acetabulum. Although cystic lesions are uncommon, bone loss can still be extensive, especially if the disease has been longstanding and untreated.

Zicat and associates[73] described patterns of osteolysis around all-polyethylene cemented components. In 12 of 63 patients, loosening necessitated revision of the cups within 7 years of implantation. Eight of these 12 cases (75%) had a circumferential linear pattern. Although 51 patients did not require revision of the acetabular component, 19 had unstable cups. Of these 19, four (22%) had a progressive linear pattern present in all three zones, and three (18%) had focal expansile lesions. These expansile lesions

occurred predominantly in zone III.[78] Failure of the cemented cups requiring revision was more often associated with a higher patient weight (66 versus 55 kg) and younger age at the time of implantation (44 versus 60 years).

Radiographically, the hallmarks of cemented socket loosening are circumferential radiolucency, a cracked cement mantle, or component migration.[58]

Cemented Stems
In arthroplasties with a cemented femoral component, the path of least resistance for particle migration on the femoral side is along the cement-metal or the cement-bone interface. Linear, expansile, and focal lesions all have been seen with both stable and unstable stems.[12,59,73,79,80] Several authors have demonstrated the potential for a passage to form at the stem-cement interface.[12,80] Anthony and associates[80] postulated that the formation

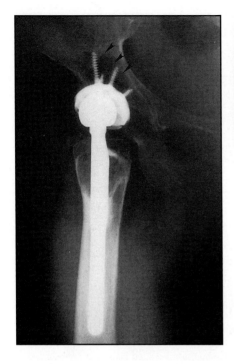
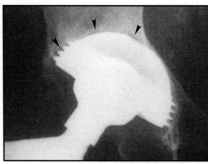

Fig. 4 Left, Rapidly expansile region of focal osteolysis adjacent to an uncemented socket (arrows). **Right,** Slowly progressive linear osteolysis around a threaded uncemented cup (arrows).

of a membrane within the passage may be a causative factor for the focal lytic lesions that develop around the distal aspect of an otherwise well-fixed cemented femoral component. They suggested that fluid and particles are driven along the interface by the high intra-articular pressures generated during normal gait and reach the cement-bone interface via defects in the cement mantle. The resulting biologic reaction can lead to focal osteolysis in the presence of a well-fixed cemented stem.

As with cemented acetabular components, particles can migrate along the cement-bone interface of femoral components. However, the consequences are quite different. In the absence of cement fracture or debonding at the cement-metal interface, the femoral component usually does not loosen, probably because the articular surface area for femoral components is much smaller and the surface area for fixation is much larger than that of the acetabular component.[19] Thus, 2 cm to 3 cm of disruption of the proximal cement-bone interface due to linear

osteolysis (ie, membrane formation) will not significantly compromise femoral component stability. In contrast, 2 cm to 3 cm of disruption at the cement-bone interface in a cemented socket is likely to have a significant effect on implant stability. Osteolysis around the proximal femur thus can result in progressive bone loss. With modern cementing technique, though, it is rarely the primary cause of loosening.[81,82] However, with stem debonding or cement fracture, cement debris is produced due to the instability of the implant. With adequate access to the cement-bone interface, the debris leads to the development of osteolysis as a secondary phenomenon.

Clinical studies of stems inserted using first-generation cementing techniques found osteolysis in all Gruen zones.[16,66] With second- and third-generation cementing techniques, radiolucencies at the cement-bone interface are primarily linear and are located in Gruen zones 1, 7, 8, and 14.[82] In addition, although the incidence of osteolysis in cemented stems is quite low, an increase

from 3% to 9% has been reported for the same patients between the 11-year and 15-year follow-up.[81-83]

Cemented stems are definitely loose when the component has migrated, a new radiolucency at the cement-metal interface has developed, the stem is deformed or fractured, or when the cement mantle is fractured.[56,59] A complete radiolucency at the cement-bone interface suggests probable loosening, whereas 50% to 99% radiolucency suggests possible loosening. Significantly, interpretation of the radiolucent line is critical in determining whether the radiographic manifestations are suggestive of linear osteolysis or remodeling.[84]

Cementless Sockets
The pattern of osteolysis around cementless sockets is a function of whether bone ingrowth has occurred. If the socket is stable and bone-ingrown, the path of least resistance is via noningrown areas (eg, gaps and/or fibrous tissue) and screw holes, which allow particles to migrate into the trabecular bone of the ilium, ischium, and pubis. This results in two patterns of osteolysis in bone-ingrown cups that may be related to the local particle concentration (Fig. 4). High particle loads may be more likely to result in the first pattern, which is rapidly growing expansile lesions with indistinct margins. The consequences of osteolysis in these cases is progressive bone loss. Loosening does not result until bone loss is extensive, and failure is usually acute and catastrophic. The patient usually remains clinically asymptomatic until the component loosens.

The second pattern of osteolysis is a more slowly growing lesion that has sclerotic margins. Sclerotic bone often forms at the implant-bone interface, probably as a result of micromotion. The pattern of osteolysis in this case is quite similar to that seen with cemented sockets. Linear osteolysis occurs with the implant migrating into the radiolucent area. In

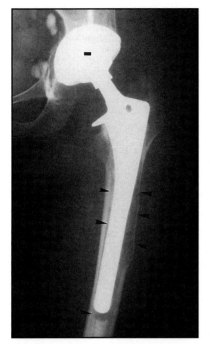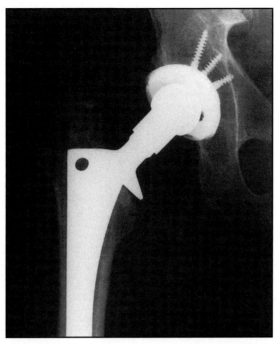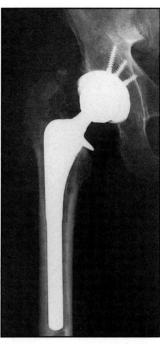

Fig. 5 Left, Typical radiographic appearance of progressive focal osteolysis about a noncircumferentially porous-coated Harris-Galante (Zimmer, Warsaw, IN) femoral component (arrows). **Center,** Typical radiographic appearance of proximal focal osteolysis in zones I and VII (arrows) adjacent to a stable Anatomic Medullary Locking (Depuy, Warsaw, IN) femoral component. **Right,** Radiographic demonstrating "windshield wiper" pattern of distal osteolysis in an uncemented femoral component. This pattern is believed to result from the concentration of particles in the diaphysis with subsequent loosening of the stem and toggling of the femur.

addition, if late migration of the component is noted in the absence of previous radiolucency, then fibrous fixation with progressive osteolysis should be assumed to have developed. The consequences of osteolysis in this case are progressive bone loss and clinical loosening.

The radiographic determination of whether a socket has bone ingrowth is quite difficult. Radiographic criteria of the type described for bone ingrown porous-coated cementless stems have not been delineated for cementless cups. A cementless socket that is radiographically stable is often presumed to be bone ingrown, although that may not be the case. Cementless sockets in which bone-ingrowth does not occur are predisposed to late migration.

In a study by Zicat and associates,[73] 71 of 74 one-piece metal-backed Anatomic Medullary Locking (AML, DePuy, Warsaw, IN) sintered-bead porous-coated cups, inserted with cementless techniques with three spikes and no screw holes, were well-functioning after 7 years. Fourteen (20%) had radiolucent lines in at least one zone, most commonly zone III. No component had circumferential linear osteolysis. One or more periarticular focal lesions occurred in 18% of the cups. Two cups (3%) also had osteolytic areas remote from the joint. Similarly, Porous Coated Anatomic (PCA, Howmedica, East Rutherford, NJ) cups have been associated with an equal incidence of focal osteolysis in all three zones.[68,71] Reports have noted the occurrence of nonprogressive radiolucent lines around Harris-Galante (HG-I, Zimmer, Warsaw, IN) cups, but no focal osteolysis has been noted at 7 to 11 years of follow-up.[13,85] Studies have shown that with screw-in cups, osteolysis occurs rapidly in a linear circumferential pattern with catastrophic migration of the compo-

nents.[86,87] In addition, regardless of cup type, both linear and expansile osteolysis has been noted about the fixation screws.[67,86,87] With the HG cups after 5 years, the use of screws for initial fixation showed one lesion in 83 cups (1.2%);[88] no osteolysis was identified in the same cup fixed without screws in 122 hips.[89] Thus, the patterns of osteolysis around uncemented cups depend on the cup design.

When uncemented cups are used, migration greater than 5 mm is consistent with definite loosening.[90] Migration may be difficult to detect because of the variation in imaging planes of radiographs. Roentgenographic stereophotogrammetric analysis is more accurate[91] but is not widely used. Migration may occur with associated fracture of transacetabular screws, shedding of the porous coating, or implant fracture. Progressive radiolucent lines suggest imminent loosening, whereas static lines are of less concern.[90]

Cementless Stems

As with cementless sockets, the pattern of osteolysis with cementless stems depends on whether bone ingrowth has occurred. In addition, the implant design is a major factor in the location of osteolytic lesions (Fig. 5). With patch-porous coated implants, the path of least resistance is often along the smooth portion of the stem into the diaphysis of the femur. Thus, these types of stems are prone to diaphyseal osteolysis, as demonstrated in studies in which partially porous-coated cylinders were implanted into the distal femur of rabbits.[21] Polyethylene particles then were injected into the joint, and the femora were harvested several weeks after surgery. Histologic analysis demonstrated that the bone-ingrown areas were relative barriers to the ingress of joint fluid and polyethylene debris. In contrast, a periprosthetic cavity with a membrane formed around the smooth portion of the stem. Polarized light microscopy demonstrated that this soft-tissue membrane contained abundant polyethylene particles. Similar findings have been noted in studies examining patch-porous coated stems that were implanted in humans.[12,15,66,85,92]

With circumferential porous-coated stems such as the AML or the PCA, focal osteolytic lesions occur most commonly in the proximal aspect of the femur. Occasionally, these lesions have presented as spontaneous fractures of the greater and lesser trochanter.[64] With AML femoral components, Zicat and associates,[73] and Engh and associates,[60] described primarily periarticular lesions occurring in zones 1 and 7 (greater and lesser trochanters, respectively). In these two studies, the clinical significance of the osteolysis was minimal. Osteolysis around the PCA stem also occurred in zones 1, 7, or both in some studies,[68,93] and in zones 1, 2, 3, and 7 in another study.[64]

In contrast, diaphyseal expansile osteolysis is much more common in patch-porous coated implants such as the original Harris-Galante porous-coated stem (HGP, Zimmer, Warsaw, IN),[92] the Anatomic Porous Replacement (APR-I, Intermedics Orthopedics, Austin, TX) stem,[94] and the initial S-ROM (Joint Medical Products, Stamford, CT) implant, which had a seam that allowed joint fluid to reach the diaphysis. For example, in a 5-year follow-up study of the HGP stem, Maloney and Woolson[76] reported a 52% incidence of femoral osteolysis. Sixty-seven percent of these lesions were in the diaphysis in Gruen zones 3, 4, and 5. Many other reports indicate a high incidence of osteolysis in all periprosthetic femoral zones of patients who received the HGP stem.[15,85,92] The consequences of osteolysis in these cases is progressive diaphyseal bone loss. Loosening can occur when significant support for the implant is lost along the smooth portion of the stem. Because load is then transferred across a small area of bone ingrowth, stress fracture of the ingrown area leading to implant loosening can occur and has been reported.[61,95] Thus, it is possible for the surgeon to predict the location, appearance, and prevalence of osteolysis as a function of the implant design.

If bone-ingrowth does not occur in a porous-coated cementless stem, a fibrous interface develops. Radiographically, sclerotic lines adjacent to the fibrous tissue suggest the presence of a partial barrier obstructing the access of fluid and particle to the endosteal surface of the femur. In these cases, linear osteolysis described as a "windshield wiper" pattern is often noted. Progressive loss of diaphyseal bone may occur, leading to expansion of the endosteal canal. These patients often have pain from the time of surgery that progressively worsens. Implant migration also suggests unstable fibrous ingrowth.

Uncemented stems are definitely loose if migration and subsidence are evident. Radiographic criteria for uncemented stems are in a state of evolution, but particular findings for individual implants have been described to help determine whether specific implants may be loose. Unstable PCA components demonstrate subsidence of greater than 2 mm, cortical hypertrophy, or cancellous hypertrophy at the stem tip (ie, pedestal formation).[96] Similarly, possible loosening of AML femoral components is indicated radiographically by widening circumferential radiolucencies adjacent to the porous surface, divergent lines of demarcation, shedding of the porous coating, absence of proximal stress shielding, or cortical hypertrophy with pedestal formation.[97] In addition, dynamic rotational computed tomography has been used to determine whether uncemented femoral components are loose.[98] In this technique, femoral component version is measured in maximal internal and external rotation. The component is considered loose if there is a difference of 2° or more between these angles.

Epidemiology
Acetabulum

The incidence of osteolysis in hip replacement is most easily described in terms of the components and their mode of fixation (Table 1). For cemented cups, the incidence of focal osteolysis has been reported to be from 0% to 19%, with loss of fixation occurring at rates between 0% and 44%.[13,57,82,99-106] Salvati and associates[99] reported on polyethylene cups implanted using first-generation cementing techniques. At 10 years, two of 54 patients (3.7%) demonstrated linear osteolysis at the cement-bone interface that led to component loosening; no patients had expansile osteolysis. Others have reported loosening rates due to linear osteolysis of 11% to 23% for first-generation cemented polyethylene cups after a minimum of 10 years.[57,105] MacKenzie and associates[106] used all-polyethylene cups implanted with second-generation cementing technique in patients with developmental dysplasia or chronic dislo-

Table 1 Incidence of osteolysis in acetabular components after total hip arthroplasty

Reference	Prosthesis*	No. of Hips	Average Follow-up (months)	Onset of Lysis (months)	Incidence (%)
Salvati et al[99]	1st-generation Charnley	54	120	N/A	0
Woolson and Maloney[107]	HGP	69	44	N/A	0
Martell et al[85]	HGP	121	67	50	2
Kim and Kim[68]	PCA	116	76	N/A	9
Hozack et al[102]	Metal-backed cemented cups	70	49	N/A	0
Schmalzried and Harris[115]	ARC or HGP	97	78	N/A	2
Goetz et al[92]	HGP	41	74	42	0
Schmalzried et al[89]	HGP	122	56	N/A	0
Owen et al[71]	PCA	95	< 60	< 60	8
		99	> 60	> 60	36
Engh et al[60]	AML	227	> 84	N/A	20
	Cemented AML	63	> 84	N/A	30
Fox et al[86]	T-Tap	68	72	> 36	87
Smith and Harris[108]	HGP	94	53	16	1
Xenos et al[110]	PCA	100	84	N/A	2
Learmonth et al[72]	PCA	104	50	36	1
Zicat et al[73]	AML	74	102	N/A	19
	Cemented cups	63	107	N/A	46
Mohler et al[104]	HGP	142	62	24-60	1
Nashed et al[111]	Ti head	15	79	N/A	35
	CoCr head	74	66	N/A	35
	Cemented polyethylene	24	113	N/A	0
	Cemented metal-backed	62	94	N/A	7
MacKenzie et al[106]	2nd-generation Charnley	37	192	N/A	19

*HGP = Harris-Galante porous-coated (Zimmer, Warsaw, IN); PCA = porous-coated anatomic (Howmedica, Rutherford, NJ); ARC = acetabular reconstruction component (Howmedica, Rutherford, NJ); AML = anatomic medullary locking (DePuy, Warsaw, IN); T-Tap = threaded titanium acetabular cup (Biomet, Warsaw, IN)

cation of the hip. They found focal osteolysis in seven of 37 patients (19%), and, in 16 of 59 patients (27%), linear osteolysis resulted in loosening after an average of 192 months. Second-generation cementing techniques fared no better in a study by Mulroy and associates,[82] with linear osteolysis leading to loosening in 44% of patients a minimum of 14 years after implantation. Some authors believe the rates of osteolysis will increase after longer follow-up, thus warranting a repeat evaluation of results.[81]

Acetabular components inserted without cement have shown better results at 5 to 7 years than those implanted with cement. The HGP cup consis-

tently has achieved very low intermediate and long-term rates of osteolysis and loosening (0% to 2%).[15,85,92,104,107-111] However, other uncemented cups have not performed as well. For the PCA cup, rates of focal osteolysis have ranged from 1% at 4 years to 36% after more than 5 years.[68,71,72,111] The same reports noted that loosening had an incidence of between 0% and 11%, but it was not attributed to osteolysis. However, certain variables in these studies have been implicated in the high rates of osteolysis. The patients tended to be younger with higher levels of activity, and 32-mm heads were commonly used. In addition, shedding of the porous coating can accel-

erate third-body wear. Engh and associates[60] and Zicat and associates[73] reported that focal osteolysis occurred in 20% of patients 84 to 102 months after receiving nonmodular AML cups with 32-mm heads, and the loosening rate was 4%.

Threaded cups such as the T-TAP (Biomet, Warsaw, IN) have also produced high rates of osteolysis (59 of 68 patients, 87%) and osteolysis-associated loosening (26 of 68, 38%) after only 6 years.[86] Similarly, 95 of 378 (25%) threaded Mecring (Mecron, Berlin, Germany) cups were found to be radiographically loose only 4 1/2 years after implantation.[87] Although initially quite stable, screw-in cups apparently cause a high

Hip

Table 2 Incidence of osteolysis in femoral components after total hip arthroplasty

Reference	Prosthesis*	No. of Hips	Average Follow-up (months)	Onset of Lysis (months)	Incidence (%)
Salvati et al[99]	1st-generation Charnley	54	120	N/A	11
Sutherland et al[100]	Muller	78	120	N/A	19
Woolson and Maloney[107]	HGP	69	44	N/A	22
Tanzer et al[15]	HGP	154	53	32	13
Martell et al[85]	HGP	121	67	50	18
Kim and Kim[68]	PCA	116	76	N/A	24
Hozack et al[102]	Trilock	70	49	N/A	0
	Dualock	71	52	N/A	0
Schmalzried and Harris[115]	HD-2 or Precoat	97	78	N/A	16
Owen et al[71]	PCA	95	< 60	< 60	7
		99	> 60	> 60	13
Goetz et al[92]	HGP	41	74	42	29
	Precoat	41	72	N/A	0
Engh et al[60]	AML, cementless cup	227	> 84	N/A	34
	AML, cemented cup	63	> 84	N/A	12
Smith and Harris[108]	HGP	94	53	16	31
Xenos et al[110]	PCA	100	84	N/A	25
Learmonth et al[72]	PCA	104	50	36	24
Zicat et al[73]	AML	74	102	N/A	32
Mohler et al[104]	Iowa	1941	N/A	24-120	1.5
Nashed et al[111]	BIAS, Ti head	15	79	N/A	87
	BIAS, CoCr head	74	66	N/A	22
	BIAS, cemented PE cup	24	113	N/A	0
	BIAS, cemented metal-backed	62	94	N/A	24
Mulroy et al[82]	Precoat	102	> 168	N/A	10
MacKenzie et al[106]	2nd-generation Charnley	37	192	N/A	8
Maloney and Woolson[76]	HGP	69	71	N/A	52

*HGP = Harris-Galante porous-coated (Zimmer, Warsaw, IN); PCA = porous-coated anatomic (Howmedica, Rutherford, NJ); HD-2 = Harris-Davey cobalt-chromium implant (Howmedica, Rutherford, NJ); AML = anatomic medullary locking (DePuy, Warsaw, IN); BIAS = biologic ingrowth anatomic system (Zimmer, Warsaw, IN)

concentration of local stress and possibly pressure necrosis. Bruijn and associates[87] also suggested that such stress causes bone resorption, decreased stability, increased micromotion, and greater access of wear particles to the metal-bone interface, resulting in rapidly progressive osteolysis. Regardless of the mechanism of failure, most studies have found that threaded acetabular cups fail at sufficiently high rates to preclude their continued use.

Femur
Whereas femoral components inserted with first-generation cementing techniques loosened at rates between 11% and 30%,[57,99,105] those inserted using second- or third-generation cementing techniques have enjoyed excellent results in terms of osteolysis, loosening, and revision rates. Several authors have reported the long-term incidence of focal osteolysis to be less than 8%, even in difficult reconstructions.[13,82,104,106]

Intermediate to long-term rates of loosening associated with osteolysis have increased from 1.5% or 3% to 7% at latest follow-up (Table 2).[13,81,82,104]

On the other hand, the incidence of osteolysis in femurs that received uncemented stems is quite high. The HGP prosthesis was associated with focal osteolysis rates of 13% to 52% over short to intermediate follow-up periods.[15,76,85,88,92,107,108] The incidence of loosening of these components has been between 8% and 32%. With the PCA stem,[68,71,72,110] the incidence of osteolysis was also quite high (13% to 25%) at 50 to 84 month follow-up. As noted earlier, osteolytic lesions occurred in periarticular Gruen zones 1, 2, and 7, and were not the cause of loosening. Rather, implant micromotion and shedding of the porous coating appeared to be responsible.[68,93] Although studies suggested high rates (32% to 34%) of osteolysis with the AML stem,[60,73] these lesions also were confined to zones 1 and 7, were quite small, and did not result in loosening. Nashed and associates[111] reported that osteolysis occurred in 13 of 15 (87%) arthroplasties using a BIAS (Zimmer, Warsaw, IN) stem with a titanium head and in 16 of 74 (22%) arthroplasties using a cobalt-chrome head. Loosening associated with osteolysis occurred in 40% and 14% of these patients, respectively. The incidence of osteolysis was 9% for the Identifit (Thackray, Leeds, England) stem without porous coating, although loosening was more frequent (28%) and was not entirely the product of osteolysis.[79]

Risk Factors

The likelihood that osteolysis will develop after total hip replacement currently is difficult to predict. However, based on several retrospective studies, it is possible to identify certain features that may place a patient at increased risk. These factors include young age at the time of replacement,[105] developmental dysplasia of the hip (DDH) or osteonecrosis (ON) as the primary cause of coxarthrosis,[85,106] relatively high patient activity, and high wear rates.[68,112] The diagnosis of ON or DDH may be less of a predisposing factor than the young age of these patients at the time of arthroplasty. Many studies have shown that young patients have higher rates of acetabular loosening and osteolysis,[112,113] although femoral loosening does not depend on age. MacKenzie and associates[106] reported that cemented

stems had an 85% survivorship at 15 years in patients with Crowe type II, III, or IV DDH. However, the cemented acetabulae had a survivorship of only 68% after the same interval. Osteolysis occurred adjacent to cups or stems in 55% of patients with ON, but only in 29% of those without ON.[85] Greater patient activity generates more wear debris, and particle load has been implicated in types of osteolysis.[32] Surgical risk factors include the types of implants used (see above) and poor cement technique.[114] The incidence of osteolysis has not consistently been associated with gender, weight, or postoperative range of motion.

References

1. Charnley J: The bonding of prostheses to bone by cement. *J Bone Joint Surg* 1964;46B: 518-529.

2. Charnley J, Follacci FM, Hammond BT: The long-term reaction of bone to self-curing acrylic cement. *J Bone Joint Surg* 1968;50B:822-829.

3. Mirra JM, Amstutz HC, Matos M, et al: The pathology of the joint tissues and its clinical relevance in prosthesis failure. *Clin Orthop* 1976;117:221-240.

4. Mirra JM, Marder RA, Amstutz HC: The pathology of failed total joint arthroplasty. *Clin Orthop* 1982;170:175-183.

5. Bullough PG, DiCarlo EF, Hansraj KK, et al: Pathologic studies of total joint replacement. *Orthop Clin North Am* 1988;19:611-625.

6. Willert HG, Semlitsch M: Tissue reactions to plastic and metallic wear products of joint endoprostheses, in Gschwend N, Debrunner HU (eds): *Total Hip Prosthesis.* Baltimore, MD, Williams & Wilkins, 1976, pp 205-239.

7. Willert HG, Semlitsch M: Reactions of the articular capsule to wear products of artificial joint prostheses. *J Biomed Mater Res* 1977;11:157-164.

8. Gray MH, Talbert ML, Talbert WM, et al: Changes seen in lymph nodes draining the sites of large joint prostheses. *Am J Surg Pathol* 1989;13:1050-1056.

9. Urban RM, Jacobs JJ, Gilbert JL, et al: Migration of corrosion products from modular hip prostheses: Particle microanalysis and histopathological findings. *J Bone Joint Surg* 1994;76A:1345-1359.

10. Sauer PA, Urban RM, Jacobs JJ, et al: Particles of metal alloys in the liver, spleen, and para-aortic lymph nodes of patients with total hip or knee replace-

ment prostheses. Proceedings of the American Academy of Orthopaedic Surgeons 63rd Annual Meeting, Atlanta, GA. Rosemont, IL, American Academy of Orthopaedic Surgeons, 1996, p 226.

11. Schmalzried TP, Jasty M, Harris WH: Periprosthetic bone loss in total hip arthroplasty: Polyethylene wear debris and the concept of the effective joint space. *J Bone Joint Surg* 1992;74A:849-863.

12. Maloney WJ, Jasty M, Harris WH, et al: Endosteal erosion in association with stable uncemented femoral components. *J Bone Joint Surg* 1990;72A:1025-1034.

13. Mohler CG, Callaghan JJ, Collis DK, et al: Early loosening of the femoral component at the cement-prosthesis interface after total hip replacement. *J Bone Joint Surg* 1995;77A:1315-1322.

14. Jacobs JJ, Kull LR, Frey GA, et al: Early failure of acetabular components inserted without cement after previous pelvic irradiation. *J Bone Joint Surg* 1995;77A:1829-1835.

15. Tanzer M, Maloney WJ, Jasty M, et al: The progression of femoral cortical osteolysis in association with total hip arthroplasty without cement. *J Bone Joint Surg* 1992;74A:404-410.

16. Willert HG, Bertram H, Buchhorn GH: Osteolysis in alloarthroplasty of the hip: The role of bone cement fragmentation. *Clin Orthop* 1990;258:108-121.

17. Willert HG, Bertram H, Buchhorn GH: Osteolysis in alloarthroplasty of the hip: The role of ultra-high molecular weight polyethylene wear particles. *Clin Orthop* 1990;258:95-107.

18. Horowitz SM, Doty SB, Lane JM, et al: Studies of the mechanism by which the mechanical failure of polymethylmethacrylate leads to bone resorption. *J Bone Joint Surg* 1993;75A:802-813.

19. Horikoshi M, Rubash HE, Macauley W: An analysis of the bone-cement and the bone-implant interface in failed cemented and cementless acetabular components after failed total hip arthroplasty, in Galante JO, Rosenberg AG, Callaghan JJ (eds): *Total Hip Revision Surgery.* New York, NY, Raven Press, 1995, pp 119-125.

20. Urban RM, Jacobs JJ, Sumner DR, et al: The bone-implant interface of femoral stems with non-circumferential porous coating. *J Bone Joint Surg* 1996;78A:1068-1081.

21. Bobyn JD, Jacobs JJ, Tanzer M, et al: The susceptibility of smooth implant surfaces to peri-implant fibrosis and migration of polyethylene wear debris. *Clin Orthop* 1995;311:21-39.

22. Vernon-Roberts B, Freeman MAR: Morphological and analytical studies of the tissues adjacent to joint prostheses: Investigations into the causes of loosening of prostheses, in Schaldach M, Hohmann D (eds): *Advances in Artificial Hip and Knee*

Joint Technology. Berlin, Germany, Springer-Verlag, 1976, pp 148-186.

23. Vernon-Roberts B, Freeman MAR: The tissue response to total joint replacement prostheses, in Swanson SAV, Freeman MAR (eds): *The Scientific Basis of Joint Replacement*. New York, NY, John Wiley & Sons, 1977, pp 86-129.

24. Goldring SR, Schiller AL, Roelke M, et al: The synovial-like membrane at the bone-cement interface in loose total hip replacements and its proposed role in bone lysis. *J Bone Joint Surg* 1983;65A:575-584.

25. Goldring SR, Jasty M, Roelke MS, et al: Formation of a synovial-like membrane at the bone-cement interface: Its role in bone resorption and implant loosening after total hip replacement. *Arthritis Rheum* 1986;29:836-842.

26. Goodman SB, Chin RC, Chiou SS, et al: A clinical-pathologic-biochemical study of the membrane surrounding loosened and nonloosened total hip arthroplasties. *Clin Orthop* 1989;244:182-187.

27. Howie DW: Tissue response in relation to type of wear particles around failed hip arthroplasties. *J Arthroplasty* 1990;5:337-348.

28. Thornhill TS, Ozuna RM, Shortkroff S, et al: Biochemical and histological evaluation of the synovial-like tissue around failed (loose) total joint replacement prostheses in human subjects and a canine model. *Biomaterials* 1990;11:69-72.

29. Kim KJ, Rubash HE: Large amounts of polyethylene debris in the interface tissue surrounding bipolar endoprostheses: Comparison to total hip prostheses. *J Arthroplasty* 1997;12:32-39.

30. Jiranek WA, Machado M, Jasty M, et al: Production of cytokines around loosened cemented acetabular components: Analysis with immunohistochemical techniques and in situ hybridization. *J Bone Joint Surg* 1993;75A:863-879.

31. Kim KJ, Rubash HE, Wilson SC, et al: A histologic and biochemical comparison of the interface tissues in cementless and cemented hip prostheses. *Clin Orthop* 1993;287:142-152.

32. Chiba J, Rubash HE, Kim KJ, et al: The characterization of cytokines in the interface tissue obtained from failed cementless total hip arthroplasty with and without femoral osteolysis. *Clin Orthop* 1994;300:304-312.

33. Gelb H, Schumacher HR, Cuckler J, et al: In vivo inflammatory response to polymethylmethacrylate particulate debris: Effect of size, morphology, and surface area. *J Orthop Res* 1994;12:83-92.

34. Shanbhag AS, Jacobs JJ, Black J, et al: Cellular mediators secreted by interfacial membranes obtained at revision total hip arthroplasty. *J Arthroplasty* 1995;10:498-506.

35. Dorr LD, Bloebaum R, Emmanual J, et al: Histologic, biochemical, and ion analysis of tissue and fluids retrieved during total hip arthroplasty. *Clin Orthop* 1990;261:82-95.

36. Rae T: A study on the effects of particulate metals of orthopaedic interest on murine macrophages in vitro. *J Bone Joint Surg* 1975;57B:444-450.

37. Horowitz SM, Frondoza CG, Lennox DW: Effects of polymethylmethacrylate exposure upon macrophages. *J Orthop Res* 1988;6:827-832.

38. Schindler R, Mancilla J, Endres S, et al: Correlations and interactions in the production of interleukin-6 (IL-6), IL-1, and tumor necrosis factor (TNF) in human blood mononuclear cells: IL-6 suppresses IL-1 and TNF. *Blood* 1990;75:40-47.

39. Horowitz SM, Gautsch TL, Frondoza CG, et al: Macrophage exposure to polymethyl methacrylate leads to mediator release and injury. *J Orthop Res* 1991;9:406-413.

40. Glant TT, Jacobs JJ, Molnar G, et al: Bone resorption activity of particulate-stimulated macrophages. *J Bone Miner Res* 1993;8:1071-1079.

41. Shanbhag AS, Jacobs JJ, Black J, et al: Macrophage/particle interactions: Effect of size, composition and surface area. *J Biomed Mater Res* 1994;28:81-90.

42. Macaulay W, Shanbhag AS, Marinelli R, et al: Nitric oxide release from murine macrophages when stimulated with particulate debris. *Trans Soc Biomat* 1995;18:307.

43. Sinha RK, Tuan RS: In vitro analysis of the bone-implant interface. *Semin Arthroplasty* 1993;4:194-204.

44. Shanbhag AS, Jacobs JJ, Black J, et al: Human monocyte response to particulate biomaterials generated in vivo and in vitro. *J Orthop Res* 1995;13:792-801.

45. Blaine TA, Rosier RN, Puzas JE, et al: Increased levels of tumor necrosis factor-alpha and interleukin-6 protein and messenger RNA in human peripheral blood monocytes due to titanium particles. *J Bone Joint Surg* 1996;78A:1181-1192.

46. Haynes DR, Rogers SD, Hay S, et al: The differences in toxicity and release of bone-resorbing mediators induced by titanium and cobalt-chromium-alloy wear particles. *J Bone Joint Surg* 1993;75A:825-834.

47. Horowitz SM, Doty SB, Lane JM, et al: Mechanism by which cement failure leads to bone resorption in aseptic loosening. *Orthop Trans* 1991;15:540-541.

48. Rae T: The biological response to titanium and titanium-aluminium-vanadium alloy particles: I. Tissue culture studies. *Biomaterials* 1986;7:30-36.

49. Glant TT, Jacobs JJ: Response of three murine macrophage populations to particulate debris: Bone resorption in organ cultures. *J Orthop Res* 1994;12:720-731.

50. Charnley J: Tissue reactions to implanted plastics, in Charnley J (ed): *Acrylic Cement in Orthoaedic Surgery*. Edinburgh, Scotland, E & S Livingstone, 1970, pp 1-9.

51. Forest M, Carlioz A, Vacher Lavenu MC, et al: Histological patterns of bone and articular tissues after orthopaedic reconstructive surgery (artificial joint implants). *Pathol Res Pract* 1991;187:963-977.

52. DiCarlo EF, Bullough PG: The biologic responses to orthopedic implants and their wear debris. *Clin Mater* 1992;9:235-260.

53. Maloney WJ, James RE, Smith RL: Human macrophage response to retrieved titanium alloy particles in vitro. *Clin Orthop* 1996;322:268-278.

54. Groessner-Schreiber B, Tuan RS: Enhanced extracellular matrix production and mineralization by osteoblasts cultured on titanium surfaces in vitro. *J Cell Sci* 1991;101:209-217.

55. Sinha RK: *Adhesion of Bone Cells to Orthopaedic Implant Materials*. Thomas Jefferson University, Philadelphia, PA, 1993. Thesis.

56. Gruen TA, McNeice GM, Amstutz HC: "Modes of Failure" of cemented stem-type femoral components: A radiographic analysis of loosening. *Clin Orthop* 1979;141:17-27.

57. Stauffer RN: Ten-year follow-up study of total hip replacement. *J Bone Joint Surg* 1992;64A:983-990.

58. Hodgkinson JP, Shelley P, Wroblewski BM: The correlation between the roentgenographic appearance and operative findings at the bone-cement junction of the socket in Charnley low friction arthroplasties. *Clin Orthop* 1988;228:105-109.

59. Harris WH, Schiller AL, Scholler JM, et al: Extensive localized bone resorption in the femur following total hip replacement. *J Bone Joint Surg* 1976;58A:612-618.

60. Engh CA, Hooten JP Jr, Zettl-Schaffer KF, et al: Porous-coated total hip replacement. *Clin Orthop* 1994;298:89-96.

61. Jasty M, Maloney WJ, Bragdon CR, et al: Histomorphological studies of the long-term skeletal responses to well-fixed cemented femoral components. *J Bone Joint Surg* 1990:72A:1220-1229.

62. Maloney WJ, Peters P, Engh CA, et al: Severe osteolysis of the pelvis in association with acetabular replacement without cement. *J Bone Joint Surg* 1993;75A:1627-1635.

63. Pazzaglia U, Byers PD: Fractured femoral shaft through an osteolytic lesion resulting from the reaction to a prosthesis: A case report. *J Bone Joint Surg* 1984;66B:337-339.

64. Heekin RD, Engh CA, Herzwurm PJ: Fractures through cystic lesions of the greater trochanter: A cause of late pain after cemenetless total hip arthroplasty. *J Arthroplasty* 1996;11:757-760.

65. Buechel FF, Drucker D, Jasty M, et al: Osteolysis around uncemented acetabular components of cobalt-chrome surface replacement hip arthroplasty. *Clin Orthop* 1994;298:202-211.

66. Jasty MJ, Floyd WE III, Schiller AL, et al: Localized osteolysis in stable, non-septic total hip replacement. *J Bone Joint Surg* 1986;68A:912-919.

67. Santavirta S, Konttinen YT, Bergroth V, et al: Aggressive granulomatous lesions associated with hip arthroplasty: Immunopathological studies. *J Bone Joint Surg* 1990;72A:252-258.

68. Kim YH, Kim VE: Uncemented porous-coated anatomic total hip replacement: Results at six years in a consecutive series. *J Bone Joint Surg* 1993;75B:6-13.

69. Kim YH, Kim VE: Cementless porous-coated anatomic medullary locking total hip prostheses. *J Arthroplasty* 1994;9:243-252.

70. Schmalzried TP, Guttmann D, Grecula M, et al: The relationship between the design, position, and articular wear of acetabular components inserted without cement and the development of pelvic osteolysis. *J Bone Joint Surg* 1994;76A:677-688.

71. Owen TD, Moran CG, Smith SR, et al: Results of uncemented porous-coated anatomic total hip replacement. *J Bone Joint Surg* 1994;76B:258-262.

72. Learmonth ID, Grobler GP, Dall DM, et al: Loss of bone stock with cementless hip arthroplasty. *J Arthroplasty* 1995;10:257-263.

73. Zicat B, Engh CA, Gokcen E: Patterns of osteolysis around total hip components inserted with and without cement. *J Bone Joint Surg* 1995;77A:432-439.

74. D'Antonio JA, Capello WN, Borden LS, et al: Classification and management of acetabular abnormalities in total hip arthroplasty. *Clin Orthop* 1989;243:126-137.

75. Paprosky WG, Perona PG, Lawrence JM: Acetabular defect classification and surgical reconstruction in revision arthroplasty: A 6-year follow-up evaluation. *J Arthroplasty* 1994;9:33-44.

76. Maloney WJ, Woolson ST: Increasing incidence of femoral osteolysis in association with uncemented Harris-Galante total hip arthroplasty: A follow-up report. *J Arthroplasty* 1996;11:130-134.

77. Schmalzreid TP, Kwong LM, Jasty M, et al: The mechanism of loosening of cemented acetabular components in total hip arthroplasty: Analysis of specimens retrieved at autopsy. *Clin Orthop* 1992;274:60-78.

78. DeLee JG, Charnley J: Radiological demarcation of cemented sockets in total hip replacement. *Clin Orthop* 1976;121:20-32.

79. Lombardi AV Jr, Mallory TH, Eberle RWW, et al: Failure of intraoperatively customized non-porous femoral components inserted without cement in total hip arthroplasty. *J Bone Joint Surg* 1995;77A:1836-1844.

80. Anthony PP, Gie GA, Howie CR, et al: Abstract: Localised endosteal bone lysis in relation to soundly fixed femoral components of cemented total hip replacements: A possible mechanism. *J Bone Joint Surg* 1990;72B:532.

81. Mulroy RD Jr, Harris WH: The effect of improved cementing techniques on component loosening in total hip replacement: An 11-year radiographic review. *J Bone Joint Surg* 1990;72B:757-760.

82. Mulroy WF, Estok DM, Harris WH: Total hip arthroplasty with use of so-called second-generation cementing techniques: A fifteen-year-average follow-up study. *J Bone Joint Surg* 1995;77A:1845-1852.

83. Harris WH, McCarthy JC, O'Neill DA: Femoral component loosening using contemporary techniques of femoral cement fixation. *J Bone Joint Surg* 1982;64A:1063-1067.

84. Kwong LM, Jasty M, Mulroy RD, et al: The histology of the radiolucent line. *J Bone Joint Surg* 1992;74B:67-73.

85. Martell JM, Pierson RH III, Jacobs JJ, et al: Primary total hip reconstruction with a titanium fiber-coated prosthesis inserted without cement. *J Bone Joint Surg* 1993;75A:554-571.

86. Fox GM, McBeath AA, Heiner JP: Hip replacement with a threaded acetabular cup: A follow-up study. *J Bone Joint Surg* 1994;76A:195-201.

87. Bruijn JD, Seelen JL, Feenstra RM, et al: Failure of the Mecring screw-ring acetabular component in total hip arthroplasty: A three to seven-year follow-up study. *J Bone Joint Surg* 1995;77A:760-766.

88. Schmalzried TP, Harris WH: The Harris-Galante porous-coated acetabular component with screw fixation: Radiographic analysis of eighty-three primary hip replacements at a minimum of five years. *J Bone Joint Surg* 1992;74A:1130-1139.

89. Schmalzried TP, Wessinger SJ, Hill GE, et al: The Harris-Galante porous acetabular component press-fit without screw fixation: Five-year radiographic analysis of primary cases. *J Arthroplasty* 1994;9:235-241.

90. Whirlow J, Rubash HE: Aseptic loosening in total hip arthroplasty, in Callaghan JJ, Dennis DA, Paprosky WG, et al (eds): *Orthopaedic Knowledge Update: Hip and Knee Reconstruction*. Rosemont, IL, American Academy of Orthopaedic Surgeons, 1995, pp 147-156.

91. Onsten I, Carlsson AS, Ohlin A, et al: Migration of acetabular components, inserted with and without cement, in one-stage bilateral hip arthroplasty: A controlled, randomized study using roentgenstereophotogrammetric analysis. *J Bone Joint Surg* 1994;76A:185-194.

92. Goetz DD, Smith EJ, Harris WH: The prevalence of femoral osteolysis associated with components inserted with or without cement in total hip replacements: A retrospective matched-pair series. *J Bone Joint Surg* 1994;76A:1121-1129.

93. Heekin RD, Callaghan JJ, Hopkinson WJ, et al: The porous-coated anatomic total hip prosthesis, inserted without cement: Results after five to seven years in a prospective study. *J Bone Joint Surg* 1993;75A:77-91.

94. Dorr LD, Gruen TA: Cement versus cementless fixation for total hip replacement in patients 65 and older. Proceedings of the American Academy of Orthopaedic Surgeons 61st Annual Meeting, New Orleans, LA. Rosemont, IL, American Academy of Orthopaedic Surgeons, 1994, p 250.

95. Jasty M, Bragdon C, Jiranek W, et al: Etiology of osteolysis around porous-coated cementless total hip arthroplasties. *Clin Orthop* 1994;308:111-126.

96. Callaghan JJ, Salvati EA, Pellicci PM, et al: Results of revision for mechanical failure after cemented total hip replacement, 1979 to 1982: A two to five-year follow-up. *J Bone Joint Surg* 1985;67A:1074-1085.

97. Engh CA, Bobyn JD: The influence of stem size and extent of porous-coating on femoral bone resorption after primary cementless hip arthroplasty. *Clin Orthop* 1988;231:7-28.

98. Berger R, Fletcher F, Donaldson T, et al: Dynamic test to diagnose loose uncemented femoral total hip components. *Clin Orthop* 1996;330:115-123.

99. Salvati EA, Wilson PD Jr, Jolley MN, et al: A ten-year follow-up study of our first one hundred consecutive Charnley total hip replacements. *J Bone Joint Surg* 1981;63A:753-767.

100. Sutherland CJ, Wilde AH, Borden LS, et al: A ten-year follow-up of one hundred consecutive Müller curved-stem total hip-replacement arthroplasties. *J Bone Joint Surg* 1982;64A:970-982.

101. Bosco JA, Lachiewicz PF, DeMasi R: Survivorship analysis of cemented high modulus total hip arthroplasty. *Clin Orthop* 1993;294:131-139.

102. Hozack WJ, Rothman RH, Booth RE Jr, et al: Cemented versus cementless total hip arthroplasty: A comparative study of equivalent patient populations. *Clin Orthop* 1993;289:161-165.

103. Havelin LI, Espehaug B, Vollset SE, et al: The effect of the type of cement on early revision of Charnley total hip prostheses: A review of eight thousand five hundred

and seventy-nine primary arthroplasties from the Norwegian Arthroplasty Register. *J Bone Joint Surg* 1995;77A:1543-1550.

104. Mohler CG, Kull LR, Martell JM, et al: Total hip replacement with insertion of an acetabular component without cement and a femoral component with cement: Four to seven-year results. *J Bone Joint Surg* 1995;77A:86-96.

105. Neumann L, Freund KG, Sorensen KH: Total hip arthroplasty with the Charnley prosthesis in patients fifty-five years old and less: Fifteen to twenty-one-year results. *J Bone Joint Surg* 1996;78A:73-79.

106. MacKenzie JR, Kelley SS, Johnston RC: Total hip replacement for coxarthrosis secondary to congenital dysplasia and dislocation of the hip: Long-term results. *J Bone Joint Surg* 1996;78A:55-61.

107. Woolson ST, Maloney WJ: Cementless total hip arthroplasty using a porous-coated prosthesis for bone ingrowth fixation:

3 1/2-year follow-up. *J Arthroplasty* 1992;7(suppl):381–388.

108. Smith E, Harris WH: Increasing prevalence of femoral lysis in cementless total hip arthroplasty. *J Arthroplasty* 1995;10:407-412.

109. Maloney WJ, Anderson MJ, Jacobs JJ, et al: Polyethylene wear and pelvic osteolysis in association with the Harris-Galante socket in primary total hip replacement. Proceedings of the American Academy of Orthopaedic Surgeons 63rd Annual Meeting, Atlanta, GA. Rosemont, IL, American Academy of Orthopaedic Surgeons, 1996, p 81.

110. Xenos JS, Hopkinson WJ, Callaghan JJ, et al: Osteolysis around an uncemented cobalt chrome total hip arthroplasty. *Clin Orthop* 1995;317:29-36.

111. Nashed RS, Becker DA, Gustilo RB: Are cementless acetabular components the

cause of excess wear and osteolysis in total hip arthroplasty? *Clin Orthop* 1995;317:19-28.

112. Amstutz HC, Campbell P, Kossovsky N, et al: Mechanism and clinical significance of wear debris-induced osteolysis. *Clin Orthop* 1992;276:7-18.

113. Sarmiento A, Ebramzadeh E, Gogan WJ, et al: Total hip arthroplasty with cement: A long-term radiographic analysis in patients who are older than fifty and younger than fifty years. *J Bone Joint Surg* 1990;72A:1470-1476.

114. Barrack RL, Mulroy RD, Harris WH Jr: Improved cementing techniques and femoral component loosening in young patients with hip arthroplasty: A 12-year radiographic review. *J Bone Joint Surg* 1992;74B:385-389.

115. Schmalzried TP, Harris WH: Hybrid total hip replacement: A 6.5-year follow-up study. *J Bone Joint Surg* 1993;75B:608-615.

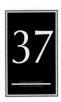

Osteolysis: Surgical Treatment

Harry E. Rubash, MD
Raj K. Sinha, MD, PhD
William J. Maloney, MD
Wayne G. Paprosky, MD, FACS

Introduction

Despite the increased understanding of the pathophysiology of osteolysis, its treatment and prevention remain challenging. Preventive measures already have been widely instituted, but their efficacy is to be determined. Time and detailed follow-up will render the eventual judgment on the current level of understanding. As with any relatively new field of inquiry, evolution is a key theme. Such is the case with the management of periprosthetic osteolysis, for which treatment schema are still developing. The current section provides a rational approach for the management of osteolysis in total hip arthroplasty.

When treating patients with osteolysis around a well-functioning total hip replacement, the surgeon must adhere to some basic tenets (Fig. 1).[1] The implication of the finding must be impressed on patients, and the importance of close follow-up cannot be overstated. Further, the reasons for the development of the lesions must be explored. The underlying cause of osteolysis is the generation of particulate debris in and around the joint space. Particle generation is influenced by patient factors (age, activity level, bone quality), implant considerations (threaded acetabular cups, noncircumferentially porous-coated femoral components, poor-quality polyethylene), and technical issues. Once the underlying mechanisms have been assessed, a decision for management must be made. Important

considerations in determining treatment include clinical symptoms, the location and likelihood of progression of the lesions, the degree of bone loss, and the status of fixation of the components. After all available data are reviewed, surgical intervention may be the best and most conservative form of treatment for a favorable clinical outcome. The surgeon must remove the osteolytic lesion and the sources of increased wear (so-called particle-generators, which include worn or loose polyethylene liners, scored or burnished femoral heads, Ti femoral heads, 32-mm heads, and others). Therefore, surgery should focus on the removal of granulomatous material, filling the defects with the appropriate graft material, and the possible exchange of components, depending on the extent of damage (Fig. 2). Wide exposure and attention to normal anatomy help the surgeon restore the appropriate biomechanical relationships.

Femoral Osteolysis
Classification

The American Academy of Orthopaedic Surgeons Committee on the Hip (COTH),[2] now referred to as the Committee on Hip and Knee Arthritis, has developed a classification of the defects produced by femoral osteolysis. Defects are classified as segmental, cavitary, or combined lytic. Segmental defects are those in which there is erosion of the supporting cortical shell of the femur.

These are subdivided into complete or partial deficiencies. Another type of segmental loss is the intercalary defect (ie, cortical window) in which cortical bone is intact above and below the defect. Cavitary defects represent contained lesions with excavation of the endosteal bone and an intact cortical shell. These can be classified as cancellous, in which only the cancellous medullary bone is eroded, or cortical, in which both cancellous and cortical bone have been eroded from within. Ectasia, another form of cavitary defect, results in marked dilatation of the femur with complete loss of cancellous bone and severe thinning of the cortex. In combined defects, cavitary and segmental defects coexist. Proximal combined defects are the most common femoral lesions caused by osteolysis.

For classification purposes, the level of the defect can be localized according to the COTH scheme. Level I is defined as proximal to the inferior aspect of the lesser trochanter. Level II is from the lesser trochanter to a point 10 cm distal, and level III is even further distal. Most defects are encountered in levels I and II, and those in level III are especially challenging.

The defects can be graded further by the severity of the bone loss. Grade I defects are those in which there would be complete contact between the host bone and the revision prosthesis. Grade II lesions have areas with incomplete contact, which do not compromise stability,

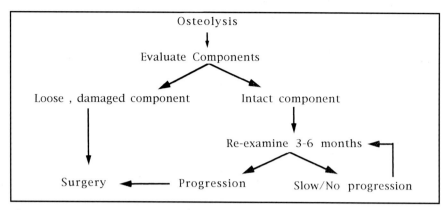

Fig. 1 Treatment algorithm for patients presenting with osteolysis.

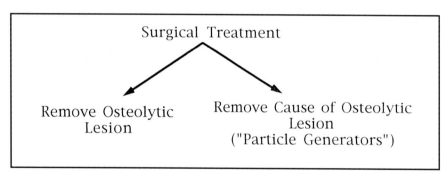

Fig. 2 Goals of surgical treatment for osteolysis.

although bulk allografts are often used to augment initial stability. In grade III defects, structural bone grafting is necessary to stabilize the prosthesis.

Management Approach

The initial considerations for managing osteolysis about femoral components are the location of the lesion, the likelihood of progression, and whether this will compromise fixation of the component. Current information suggests that linear osteolysis around cemented stems is often circumferential, involving all Gruen femoral zones, and that it will progress to the point of loosening. Observation at intervals of every 3 to 6 months is a reasonable approach until the patient becomes symptomatic or progressive lysis is observed radiographically. Although data are not available to help determine when observation should be abandoned in favor of surgery, sound sur-

gical judgment supports surgery when structural stability is threatened. Conditions threatening stability include loss of the proximal femoral cortex, including the calcar, and the presence of large osteolytic lesions that may predispose to periprosthetic fracture, such as those at the tip of the stem.

When osteolysis already has resulted in symptomatic loosening, the decision to operate is more straightforward, determined principally by the patient's degree of pain. If the component is loose, it clearly needs to be replaced. However, if the component is well-fixed (as with cementless implants), then further bone loss can result from injudicious removal. Thus, curettage and grafting of the lytic lesion, with retention of the stem, and exchange of the polyethylene liner are appropriate. Preliminary results indicate that this is a reasonable approach, although long-term data are not yet available.[1]

Engh and associates[1] have recently proposed guidelines for the management of femoral osteolysis (Fig. 3). They advocate revision of all loose stems. Definite loosening of cemented stems is indicated by migration or subsidence of the component, stem debonding, stem fracture or bending, or cement fracture.[3] Probable loosening is suggested by a circumferential radiolucency at the bone-cement interface.[3] For cementless components, migration and subsidence most reliably indicate a loose stem. Additional signs of instability include cortical or cancellous hypertrophy at the tip, distal pedestal formation, shedding of the porous coating, and radiolucency adjacent to the porous coating.

For well-fixed stems, surgery may be indicated if there is documented progression of osteolysis on serial radiographic examinations, which preferably are performed at 3 to 6 month intervals. Other factors that should be considered include the size and location of the lesion and patient age, activity, and medical status. For stems with focal and cavitary osteolysis only in zones 1 and 7, the lytic lesions may be grafted, although this has not uniformly been done in the past. In addition, the sources of the particles should be removed. This step may include changing the polyethylene liners in well-fixed acetabular cups, downsizing modular femoral heads to 26 or 28 mm, and replacing titanium heads with cobalt-chromium-molybdenum (Co-Cr-Mo) heads. For progressive lysis distal to zones 1 and 7, the stem and particle generator often require revision. For small focal lesions or linear osteolysis, we recommend observation if the patient is elderly and less active, and we reserve revision for physiologically young patients.

The location, extent, and type of porous coating also influences decision-making concerning uncemented stems.[4] For proximal focal lysis, if the component is proximally or fully porous-coated circumferentially, the lesion may be grafted with particulate graft and the particle generators should be removed. A noncircumferentially coated component may be retained in elderly, sedentary patients, with grafting of the lesions and removal of the particle generators. This approach may be used in young, active patients if the stem is well-fixed. However, if the stem is also a source of particles (eg, monoblock titanium, extensive fretting of the modular taper), then it should be revised as well. For lysis distal to zones 1 and 7, the stem and polyethylene usually should be revised. Because the distal lysis usually progresses with a noncircumferentially coated well-fixed stem, the stem should be revised. Cavitary lesions distal to the stem tip require revision of the stem because of the high risk of periprosthetic fracture. In addition, well-fixed stems that are small or designs prone to fracture should be revised before metal fatigue leads to breakage of the stem.[5] Distal lysis in extensively coated stems has not been reported; however, its appearance implies that the stem may be loose.

Surgical Treatment

Several surgical principles must be observed during revision of femoral components as a result of osteolysis. Wide exposure is necessary for full and accurate assessment of defects from within and from without the femoral canal. Extensive subperiosteal elevation of the overlying musculature may be required to gain access to the lytic lesions, or an extended osteotomy of the femur may be necessary, especially in cases of distally ingrown stems. Second, during revision, the osteolytic membrane should be removed in its entirety, followed by curettage of the canal to remove neocortex, thereby creating an appropriate bed of bone for either a cemented or uncemented component. All structural defects should be reinforced with structural strut grafts. Cortical femoral struts or intact distal femoral allografts may be used. In

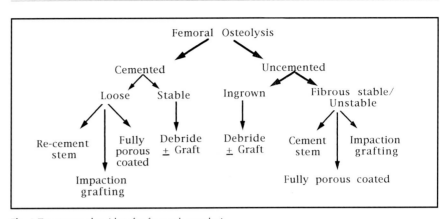

Fig. 3 Treatment algorithm for femoral osteolysis.

either case, the graft should be contoured meticulously with a high-speed burr to allow intimate contact with native bone. Once the cortex has been reestablished, the endosteal cavities can be filled with particulate allograft. Then, the neutral axis of the femur must be reestablished so that the revision stem can be placed in proper alignment. This can be accomplished by passing a beaded guide wire down the canal to the cancellous bone just proximal to the knee, a measure that also confirms the absence of breaches in the cortex. Finally, the sources of the particles inducing the osteolytic response must be addressed. Because they are associated with higher rates of polyethylene wear, titanium heads usually should be replaced with cobalt-chrome heads and 32-mm heads should be replaced with 28-mm heads and corresponding polyethylene liners. Also, monoblock stems with extensive scoring of the head generally should be replaced. Patient factors, such as age, activity, and medical status, also should be considered when making the decision whether to revise well-fixed components.

Results of Treatment

Reports of treatment specifically for osteolysis are few. Most common are those describing the results for revision of loose components after interfacial bone loss resulting from either linear or focal oste-

olysis. Nevertheless, a review of papers discussing revision of specific components provides some useful information regarding osteolysis management.

One revision option is to cement the revision component in place after adequate debridement. Although early reports on this approach were discouraging, recent improvement in cementing technique has resulted in acceptable results. For example, Pierson and Harris[6] used a variety of cemented components to treat 29 patients with osteolysis around fixed cemented stems. After 8.5 years, 25 components (86%) remained well-fixed, one was radiographically loose, and two were revised for loosening. Only two showed evidence of recurrent osteolysis (7%), with revision required for one of these. Using cemented femoral stems to treat linear osteolysis of cemented femoral components, Rubash and Harris[7] initially reported that after an average 6-year follow-up, one of 43 femoral components required revision, and 11% were judged to be radiographically loose. Estok and Harris[8] found in the same patients that after 11.5 years, 10.5% of the stems required revision for loosening, and an additional 10.5% were radiographically loose. Ten of 38 (26%) hips demonstrated recurrent osteolysis, although only one stem was loose. At the 15-year follow-up in the same group of patients, Mulroy and Harris[9] reported that seven of 33

(21%) required revision due to loosening associated with linear osteolysis. Two additional stems were radiographically loose, resulting in a failure rate of 27% after 15 years. Similarly, Raut and associates[10] revised 106 cemented femoral components with cemented stems. After an average of more than 6 years, three of 106 (3%) required revision for loosening, and another five (5%) were loose radiographically. Osteolysis to some degree recurred in 16% of the cases and was significant in 1.9%. Thus, revision with cemented femoral stems seems to be a satisfactory treatment when osteolysis leads to component loosening.

Alternatively, femoral components can be reinserted without cement to treat osteolysis. This approach was initiated because early reports of revision with recemented femoral stems were discouraging. Extensively porous-coated AML (De Puy, Warsaw, IN) femoral stems were used for revision in 174 patients with osteolysis.[11] After a minimum of 5 years, six required another revision for symptomatic loosening, and two were loose radiographically, resulting in a 7% failure rate. Greater degrees of bone stock deficiency correlated inversely with implant survivorship. Only 77% of the stems were functioning well in patients with severe bone loss, compared to a survivorship rate of 100% in mildly deficient femurs. Similarly, Engh and associates[12] found that cylindrical, extensively porous-coated AML stems performed better than the rectangular, proximally porous-coated New England Baptist (NEB) stems. At 24 to 72 months (mean, 26 months), 86% of the AML stems were bone ingrown and 13% were fibrous-stable, with only 1% loose. Of the NEB stems, 77% were bone ingrown, 8% were fibrous-stable, and 15% were loose. Again, regardless of component choice, bone stock at revision correlated inversely with the success rate. Hozack and associates[13] used a plasma-sprayed porous-coated Mallory-Head (Biomet, Warsaw,

IN) calcar femoral component to treat 72 patients with 154 osteolytic defects. After 2 to 5 years, 18% of the lesions had stabilized, 42% had regressed, 40% had healed, and none had progressed. The location of the lesion adjacent to the porous-coated region did not affect its healing potential. Additionally, the use of allograft paste to fill the lesions did not correlate with healing potential. In fact, several lesions healed without grafting, whereas others failed to heal even after grafting. Therefore, it is unclear whether routine grafting is required at the time of revision. Thus, fully porous-coated femoral components seem to be a satisfactory option for the treatment of loosening due to bone loss.

Because the degree of femoral bone loss affects implant stability, other treatment options are necessary when bone loss is severe. The use of massive structural allografts as a salvage procedure is one approach. McGann and associates[14] reported early success in five cases, yet speculated that further revision surgery would likely be required. Impaction grafting for massive osteolysis and loss of structural support has been described.[15-17] In this technique, cortical defects are strut grafted with cortical allografts secured by cerclage wires. Strut grafting is especially important for defects that will not be bypassed by the short polished stem. Crushed cancellous bone from femoral head or distal femoral condyles are packed tightly within the thinned femoral canal, creating a tube of bone. A series of wedge-shaped tamps then are used to further pack the bone and create a space for a collarless, polished, and tapered femoral component to be cemented in place. Revisions with this technique have shown encouraging early results. In addition, there is histologic evidence that remodeling occurs, with partial incorporation of the allograft and restoration of bone stock.[18] However, revision in the face of massive bone loss remains a difficult clinical problem.

Ideally, close follow-up and early surgical intervention will prevent these defects.

In summary, there are two keys to the effective treatment of femoral osteolysis. First, identify and remove the sources of the particles. Potential sources include worn polyethylene liners, modular junctions of metallic components, scored femoral heads, and fragmented cement. Third-body wear is the primary mechanism of wear in vivo, and the presence of any particulate matter predisposes to this modality. Second, treat the interfacial bone loss. Removal of loose components and the appropriate grafting of bony defects is often required. The issue of removing a well-fixed cementless stem with focal osteolysis should be addressed on an individual case basis using the guidelines described above.

Acetabular Osteolysis
Classification of Lytic Defects
Defect classification enables a systematic approach to acetabular lesions. Paprosky and associates[19] have developed a useful system that is based on the integrity of the acetabular rim and its ability to support an implanted component. Three types have been identified.

Type 1 defects involve minimal deformity and are completely supportive of a new cup. The superior dome and medial wall are usually intact. Ischial lysis is absent, suggesting that the posterior wall is structurally sound. Particulate allogeneic graft can be used to fill the holes because structural support is already present. An uncemented cup, often larger than previously used, is required.

Type 2 defects represent a distortion of the acetabular hemisphere. The anterior and posterior columns are intact, although the medial wall and/or superior dome may be destroyed, such that the component has migrated less than 2 cm. Cancellous bone may be replaced with sclerotic bone. A structural graft is not needed for type 2 defects. For reconstruc-

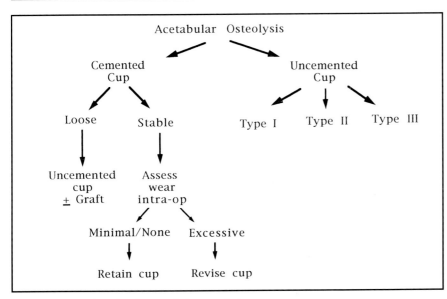

Fig. 4 Treatment algorithm for acetabular osteolysis.

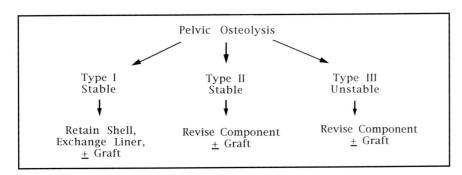

Fig. 5 Treatment algorithm for pelvic osteolysis in uncemented cups.

tion, the component can be placed in a "high hip-center" position. The defect can be filled with particulate graft, or a femoral head allograft may be fixed to the superior dome with screws. The new socket then is reamed, and a porous-ingrowth cup is press-fit in place. In addition, a variety of specialized cups are available to reconstruct nonstructural defects.

In type 3 defects, severe bone loss results in the absence of the supporting structures of the acetabulum, and greater than 2 cm of migration of the component occurs. Consequently, structural allografts must be used to provide structural support. Bulk distal or proximal femoral allografts must be fashioned

such that they can be secured to the ilium with screws or reconstruction plates. The component then is placed within the new allograft-host bone composite acetabulum. Approximately 60% of the host bone must be present for ingrowth to occur.[17] Otherwise, the cup should be secured with polymethylmethacrylate.

The COTH also developed a classification of acetabular deficiencies[2] with two basic categories: segmental and cavitary. Segmental defects result in complete loss of bone in some part of the acetabular hemisphere. These are subclassified into peripheral and central defects. Segmental defects generally require block allograft to provide struc-

tural support for the revision component. Cavitary deficiencies represent volumetric loss in the acetabular cavity, while the rim remains intact. These also can be subdivided on the basis of location. Particulate graft packed into the lesion often is sufficient for reconstruction of cavitary defects.

Management Approach

The algorithm in Figure 4 provides a systematic approach to the assessment and treatment of acetabular lysis. For cemented cups, the first step is to evaluate stability. Linear or focal osteolysis in two or three zones is associated with 71% and 94% incidences of loosening of the component, respectively.[20] A loose cemented cup must be revised, preferably with an uncemented cup. Bone stock deficiencies must be treated with appropriate grafting techniques. If the cup is stable, then the degree of wear should be evaluated. Worn liners with evidence of eccentric femoral head positioning within the cup should be replaced. In addition, 32-mm heads, which have been shown to have the highest degree of volumetric wear, and 22-mm heads, which have the highest degree of linear wear, should be replaced with 28-mm heads and corresponding liners.

Uncemented cups can be classified into three separate groups (Fig. 5). A type I cup is stable with focal osteolysis in discrete regions, including zones 1 and 3, and occasionally adjacent to screws (Fig. 6). The component usually can be retained, with particulate graft packed into the defect. In addition, the polyethylene liner should be replaced for all modular cups as long as the locking mechanism is functional. For nonmodular metal-backed cups, periodic observation of the osteolysis is appropriate, although a low threshold for revision is recommended when progression of the osteolysis is evident. Type II components are also stable by virtue specifically of

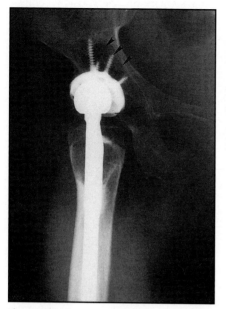 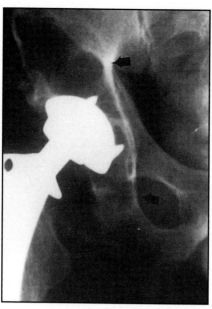

Fig. 6 Left, Example of a type I cup. The focal osteolysis has not compromised stability of the component. At surgery, the locking mechanism was intact, thus allowing simple exchange of the worn polyethylene liner. **Right,** Example of a type III cup. The focal osteolysis has become expansile, leading to superior and medial migration of the component. At surgery, the cup was grossly unstable.

bone ingrowth; however, the function of the cup is compromised. For example, the locking mechanism of the modular cup may be broken, there may be excessive backside wear of the shell, or the shell may be malpositioned. In such cases, the entire component should be removed, defects filled with the appropriate graft, and a new cup reimplanted without cement. Rarely, an all-polyethylene component can be cemented into the well-fixed acetabular shell, provided the thickness of polyethylene implanted is sufficient. Type III cups are unstable and usually have migrated into the osteolytic lesion (Fig. 6). Therefore, they must be exchanged. Any acetabular defects should be grafted appropriately. Additionally, threaded screw-in design cups are to be avoided for revision surgery because of their high rate of loosening.

Surgical Treatment
Wide exposure allows complete visualization of the cup and its periphery to facilitate removal of modular polyethylene liners. Type I cups can be retained, replacing the worn polyethylene liner. The appropriate extraction device to remove the polyethylene liner without damaging the locking mechanism should be available for each manufacturer's cup. If it is not, a useful technique is to drill a hole in the polyethylene liner and then place a screw in the hole. As the screw contacts the metal shell, it lifts the liner away from the shell, eventually disengaging it. The locking mechanism must be inspected to determine whether it is functional.

If the shell must be removed because of structural concerns or if it is a type II cup, then the entire acetabular rim must be accessible. The first step in removing the cup is to separate it from the underlying cement mantle or bone-ingrowth bed, using specially shaped osteotomes or gouges. Occasionally, the component must be removed piecemeal because the underlying bond with

cement or bone cannot be broken. This is more often the case with well-fixed uncemented cups than with cemented all-polyethylene cups. Care must be taken not to breach the medial wall during component removal, because doing so compromises structural support and threatens underlying pelvic structures. Generally, the cup cannot be removed until it is released past its widest diameter from underlying bone or cement.

The next step is to break the cement mantle to facilitate its removal. In cases in which there is a large amount of intrapelvic cement, forceful extraction from within the acetabulum could threaten to rupture underlying vessels. When of concern, this possibility may be evaluated preoperatively with computed tomography scan and/or contrast venography. If the cement is adherent to underlying vasculature, an intrapelvic surgical approach can be used to dissect the vessels free of cement or components.[21] After the cement is removed, all osteolytic membrane must be removed, especially within cement anchor holes or around screw holes. The appropriate grafting technique is used to correct the defects. If a structural graft is required, its trabeculae should be oriented to withstand axial compressive forces across the hip joint.[14]

Next, the acetabulum is prepared to accept a porous-ingrowth cup. The acetabular bed is reamed hemispherically in a manner that preserves as much host bone as possible and maximizes the area of bone-component contact. The subchondral or sclerotic bone should not be breached because this is the strongest bone and provides the initial stability. The cup should be placed as near the anatomic position as possible. Screw fixation may be required to enhance the initial stability of the cup. Provided that adequate stability of the component can be achieved, a 28-mm polyethylene liner is recommended. In certain situations, a polyethylene cup may need to be implanted with cemented fixation. These cases include when greater than 60% of the contact area between component and structural bone is allograft,[14] and when the pelvic bed has been previously irradiated,[22] among others.

Results of Treatment

The initial revisions of failed cemented acetabular components relied on the reimplantation of new cups using cement fixation. In general, the results with this approach have been poor. Among a group of young patients (average age, 50 years), Amstutz and associates[23] found that 71% of the revised cups had circumferential radiolucencies after 2 years, with 9% requiring repeat revision. Similarly, Pellici and associates[24] found progressive radiolucencies around eight of 99 recemented cups 3 years postimplantation. Of these 99 patients, 16 had progressive lucencies around the cups after an average of 8.1 years, and five were re-revised for loosening.[25] Kavanaugh and associates[26] reported on the 4.5-year average follow-up of 166 acetabular revisions with recemented Charnley cups. A complete radiolucent line was seen around 117 (71%) cups, and 15 (9%) had migrated. Of these, 20% were considered to be loose and an additional 18% were possibly loose radiographically. Callaghan and associates[5] also reported that radiolucencies occurred after 2 to 5 years adjacent to 75% of revised cups inserted with cement, and 34% progressed to become circumferential. In contrast, at 5 to 14 years, Marti and associates[27] found that only three of 80 (4%) revised cemented acetabular components had migrated and seven of 80 (9%) had circumferential lucencies, although an additional 48 of 80 (60%) had radiolucencies in at least one acetabular zone. Most reports suggest that the results of acetabulum revision with cemented cups for osteolysis and loosening are unsatisfactory.

The short- and intermediate-term results for acetabular revision using cementless components have been encouraging, and long-term data are expected to show satisfactory outcomes. Hedley and associates[28] used PCA (Howmedica, East Rutherford, NJ) components to revise 82 failed hip replacements. At 20 months, clinical results were good or excellent in 56 of 62 entirely uncemented arthroplasties and in 34 of 35 hybrid revisions. Four cups had migrated, and only two had circumferential radiolucencies, both of which were less than 1-mm wide. In the series of Emerson and associates,[29] 46 acetabula were revised with plasma-sprayed porous-coated hemispherical cups. After 22 months, seven (15%) had migrated minimally but stabilized radiographically. None required revision. Engh and associates[12] reported that one of 34 porous coated cups with three fixation spikes was loose after 4.4 years. In addition, the extent of bone damage correlated inversely with rate of success. Using the HGP (Zimmer, Warsaw, IN) fiber-metal porous-coated hemispherical cup for 23 cementless acetabular revisions, Harris and associates[30] reported that after more than 2 years, no cups had migrated and only one had a complete radiolucency. With the same component, Tanzer and associates[31] noted that two of 140 cups were loose at 3.4 years, both in patients with pelvic discontinuity. An additional five components had circumferential radiolucency, although none of these had migrated. Padgett and associates[32] further corroborated the success of cementless cups in a series using HGP cups in 124 revised acetabula. At 3.7 years, only one cup had migrated. Although radiolucent lines were seen in 81% of the cups and 10% of these were circumferential, none were wider than 2 mm.

Bone grafting plays an important role in acetabular revision. Allogeneic particulate graft from femoral heads or from distal femoral condyles can be used to fill cavitary lesions where bony support does not need to be augmented for reimplantation. When structural support is required, then bulk allograft bone must be used. The graft must be fashioned such that it provides support and can be secured to the native pelvic bone without the fixation devices interfering with placement of the revision cup.

Reports concerning grafting specifically for osteolytic lesions are sparse and preliminary. McGann and associates[14] reported the 14-month results for 75 consecutive socket revisions with the HGP cup. Sixty-four required grafting, with cancellous freeze-dried particulate allograft used in 45 cases, particulate autograft in 18 cases, and a nonstructural autograft in one case. Approximately 65% of the acetabular bed was host bone, and 94% of the sockets had 80% or greater coverage. Fixation screws were used in all 75 cases. Large, uncontained grafts resorbed one third of their volume routinely. Radiographically, contained defects incorporated and there was no difference in appearance between allograft and autograft. However, a high incidence of nonprogressive radiolucencies adjacent to the graft suggested that bone ingrowth does not occur at graft sites.

Preliminary data from Maloney and associates[33] suggest that liner exchange with debridement of the osteolytic lesion may be a satisfactory treatment option (Fig. 7). They debrided 46 lesions in 35 patients who had progressive lysis with stable cementless cups (type I). In addition, 34 of 46 defects were filled with particulate allograft. The particle generators were also removed. At a minimum of 2 years, all grafts had consolidated radiographically and no defects had progressed. Moreover, ungrafted lesions had healed. Data reported by Thomas Schmalzried corroborate those of Maloney (personal communication, 1996). Twenty-three hips with 30 pelvic lesions were reoperated. They left 15

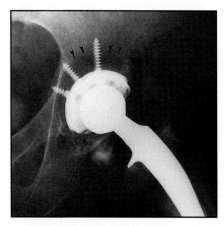 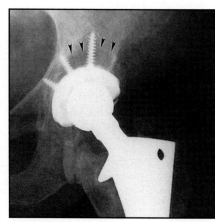

Fig. 7 Left, A patient with a type I cup. Although asymptomatic, this patient demonstrated progression of the lesion. The femoral stem was found to be loose at the time of surgery and was revised. However, the cup was well-fixed despite the osteolysis. Subsequently, the polyethylene liner was exchanged and the lesion was filled with particulate allografting through the screw holes (if the lesion is not accessible, there appears to be no need to graft it). **Right,** Radiograph 1 year later. The lesion has healed without evidence of progression.

considerable insight into osteolysis and its treatment. The development of improved models of osteolysis will enable the detailed study of particular treatment methods. These may include improved grafting materials and techniques, pharmalogic intervention, or immunologic modulation. In addition, the return to nonmodular femoral stems and the development of alternative bearing surfaces, such as improved polyethylene, ceramics, or highly polished metal-on-metal articulations, may reduce the generation of particulate debris. Although much has been learned about osteolysis in the previous decade, the prospects for a higher level of understanding remain.

uncemented cups in situ, and curretted the lesions. Eight cups were revised. Particulate allograft was used in 18 acetabula. No lesions progressed, 26 of 30 lesions had increased radiographic density, and all components remained well-fixed.

Finally, Paprosky described the use of bulk allografts to treat acetabular osteolysis with structural deficiencies (type III cups)(personal communication, 1996). Femoral head allografts were fashioned into a modified 7 shape and were secured to the ilium with 6.5-mm cancellous screws. Cementless hemispheric cups then were placed within the reconstructed acetabulum after reaming, and 50% to 70% host bone-cup contact was achieved. At 6 years, 45 of 48 reconstructions were stable and all grafts had incorporated.

Conclusions and Future Directions

In the preceding discussion, we have attempted to use the current level of understanding of the biologic basis for periprosthetic osteolysis to delineate its clinical features and outline the appropriate surgical management. Particulate debris from multiple sources induces macrophage-stimulated osteoclast-mediated interfacial bone loss. The degree of bone ingrowth or adequacy of the cement mantle determine the extent of access the particles have to the interface. As a result, the extent of access results in characteristic radiographic appearances for cemented and cementless components on both the acetabular and femoral sides. Cemented components tend to manifest linear osteolysis, whereas cementless components are more commonly associated with focal osteolysis. Once lytic defects have occurred, management depends on the stability of the components. Unstable components must be removed, while stable ones may be retained. The source of the wear debris must be identified and removed. Any interfacial bone loss must be treated with appropriate grafting techniques. Both cementless, cemented, and impaction grafting have been found to be successful on the femoral side, while uncemented cups are best used on acetabular side.

Future research should provide

References

1. Engh CA, Jacobs JJ, Peters P, et al: Osteolysis: Clinical manifestations and management. Proceedings of the American Academy of Orthopaedic Surgeons 63rd Annual Meeting, Atlanta, GA. Rosemont, IL, 1996, p 185.

2. D'Antonio J, McCarthy JC, Bargar WL, et al: Classification of femoral abnormalities in total hip arthroplasty. Clin Orthop 1993;296:133–139.

3. Harris WH, Schiller AL, Scholler JM, et al: Extensive localized bone resorption in the femur following total hip replacement. J Bone Joint Surg 1976;58A:612–618.

4. Engh CA, Bobyn JD: The influence of stem size and extent of porous coating on femoral bone resorption after primary cementless hip arthroplasty. Clin Orthop 1988;231:7–28.

5. Callaghan JJ, Salvati EA, Pellici PM, et al: Results of revision for mechanical failure after cemented total hip replacement, 1979 to 1982: A two to five-year follow-up. J Bone Joint Surg 1985;67A:1074–1085.

6. Pierson JL, Harris WH: Cemented revision for femoral osteolysis in cemented arthroplasties: Results in 29 hips after a mean 8.5-year follow-up. J Bone Joint Surg 1994;76B:40–44.

7. Rubash HE, Harris WH: Revision of nonseptic, loose, cemented femoral components using modern cementing techniques. J Arthroplasty 1988;3:241–248.

8. Estok DM II, Harris WH: Long-term results of cemented femoral revision surgery using second-generation techniques: An average 11.7-year follow-up evaluation. Clin Orthop 1994;299:190–202.

9. Mulroy WF, Harris WH: Revision total hip arthroplasty with use of so-called second-generation cementing techniques for aseptic loosening of the femoral component: A fifteen-year-average follow-up study. J Bone Joint Surg 1996;78A:325–330.

10. Raut VV, Siney PD, Wroblewski BM: Cemented Charnley revision arthroplasty for severe femoral osteolysis. *J Bone Joint Surg* 1995;77B:362–365.

11. Lawrence JM, Engh CA, Macalino GE: Revision total hip arthroplasty: Long-term results without cement. *Orthop Clin North Am* 1993;24:635–644.

12. Engh CA, Glassman AH, Griffin WL, et al: Results of cementless revision for failed cemented total hip arthroplasty. *Clin Orthop* 1988;235:91–110.

13. Hozack WJ, Bicalho PS, Eng K: Treatment of femoral osteolysis with cementless total hip revision. *J Arthroplasty* 1996;11:668–672.

14. McGann WA, Welch RB, Picetti GD III: Acetabular preparation in cementless revision total hip arthroplasty. *Clin Orthop* 1988;235:35–46.

15. Ling RS, Timperley AJ, Linder L: Histology of cancellous impaction grafting in the femur: A case report. *J Bone Joint Surg* 1993;75B:693–696.

16. Fowler JL, Gie GA, Lee AJ, et al: Experience with the Exeter total hip replacement since 1970. *Orthop Clin North Am* 1988;19:477–489.

17. Gie GA, Linder L, Ling RS, et al: Impacted cancellous allografts and cement for revision total hip arthroplasty. *J Bone Joint Surg* 1993;75B:14–21.

18. Nelissen RG, Bauer TW, Weidenhielm LR, et al: Revision hip arthroplasty with the use of cement and impaction grafting: Histological analysis of four cases. *J Bone Joint Surg* 1995;77A:412–422.

19. Paprosky WG, Perona PG, Lawrence JM: Acetabular defect classification and surgical reconstruction in revision arthroplasty: A 6-year follow-up evaluation. *J Arthroplasty* 1994;9:33–44.

20. Hodgkinson JP, Shelley P, Wroblewski BM: The correlation between the roentgenographic appearance and operative findings at the bone-cement junction of the socket in Charnley low friction arthroplasties. *Clin Orthop* 1988;228:105–109.

21. Petrera P, Trakru S, Mehta S, et al: Revision total hip arthroplasty with a retroperitoneal approach to the iliac vessels. *J Arthroplasty* 1996;11:704–708.

22. Jacobs JJ, Kull LR, Frey GA, et al: Early failure of acetabular components inserted without cement after previous pelvic irradiation. *J Bone Joint Surg* 1995;77A:1829–1835.

23. Amstutz HC, Ma SM, Jinnah RH, et al: Revision of aseptic loose total hip arthroplasties. *Clin Orthop* 1982;170:21–33.

24. Pellicci PM, Wilson PD Jr, Sledge CB, et al: Revision total hip arthroplasty. *Clin Orthop* 1982;170:34–41.

25. Pellicci PM, Wilson PD Jr, Sledge CB, et al: Long-term results of revision total hip replacement: A follow-up report. *J Bone Joint Surg* 1985;67A:513–516.

26. Kavanagh BF, Ilstrup DM, Fitzgerald RH Jr: Revision total hip arthroplasty. *J Bone Joint Surg* 1985;67A:517–526.

27. Marti RK, Schüller HM, Besselaar PP, et al: Results of revision of hip arthroplasty with cement: A five to fourteen-year follow-up study. *J Bone Joint Surg* 1990;72A:346–354.

28. Hedley AK, Gruen TA, Ruoff DP: Revision of failed total hip arthroplasties with uncemented porous-coated anatomic components. *Clin Orthop* 1988;235:75–90.

29. Emerson RH Jr, Head WC, Berklacich FM, et al: Noncemented acetabular revision arthroplasty using allograft bone. *Clin Orthop* 1989;249:30–43.

30. Harris WH, Krushell RJ, Galante JO: Results of cementless revisions of total hip arthroplasties using the Harris-Galante prosthesis. *Clin Orthop* 1988;235:120–126.

31. Tanzer M, Drucker D, Jasty M, et al: Revision of the acetabular component with an uncemented Harris-Galante porous-coated prosthesis. *J Bone Joint Surg* 1992;74A:987–994.

32. Padgett DE, Kull L, Rosenberg A, et al: Revision of the acetabular component without cement after total hip arthroplasty: Three to six-year follow-up. *J Bone Joint Surg* 1993;75A:663–673.

33. Maloney WJ, Rubash HE, Engh CA: Salvage procedure for severe pelvic osteolysis in association with uncemented acetabular replacement. *J Bone Joint Surg*, in press.

Prevention and Treatment of Venous Thromboembolic Disease Complications in Primary Hip Arthroplasty Patients

Guy D. Paiement MD

Incidence

Venous thromboembolism, a major cause of death among hospitalized patients, is estimated to be the direct cause of 100,000 deaths each year and to contribute to another 100,000. Venous thromboembolism is an unusual condition in the community. The incidence of symptomatic acute deep vein thrombosis (DVT) in the general population under the age of 50 is very low. It increases to 5.11 episodes per year per 1,000 males over the age of 50 living in the city.

Venous thromboembolism occurs primarily in hospitalized patients, complicating another clinical condition or its treatment. A study of pulmonary embolism (PE) in 16 acute care hospitals in central Massachusetts has reported an incidence of verified PE of 23 per 100,000 per year, with a case fatality rate of 12%.[1] Extrapolation of these data gives approximately 260,000 cases of clinically recognized PE each year in the United States, only for acute care hospitals. It is responsible for the death of 1% of all patients admitted to acute care hospitals.

The historic rate of venous thromboembolic complications in unprotected hip arthroplasty has been well documented in the 70s and the 80s, with large clinical series in which venography, pulmonary angiography, and autopsy were used as diagnostic endpoints. In these series, the DVT rate is 50%, with approximately half being proximal; the symptomatic non-fatal PE rate is between 5% and 20%; and the fatal PE rate is around 2%.

Some authors have recently reported a lower rate of fatal PE in hip arthroplasty patients, but it is difficult to determine if the incidence of the disease has truly diminished, if the patient population has changed (age, health status, etc.), or if prophylaxis measures are responsible for this reported decrease.[2] Venous thromboembolic disease remains a major cause of death and morbidity in these patients, and it is probably the most common preventable cause of death in elective hip arthroplasty patients.

Pathogenesis

Blood coagulation is a very complex process that has not been completely elucidated. Clot formation and fibrinolysis are in dynamic equilibrium, and this delicate balance prevents the subject from either bleeding or coagulating to death when the structural integrity of the vascular system is compromised.

The numerous factors that affect this delicate balance can be grouped under three general headings, known as the Virchow triad. They are vascular injury (endothelial damage), activation of blood coagulation (hypercoagulability), and venous stasis.

Many risk factors have been associated with venous thromboembolism. Some of these factors, such as age and inherited coagulation disorders, are intrinsic to the patient. Other factors, such as immobilization and estrogen supplementation, are more amenable to some control by the surgeon. Lower extremity orthopaedic procedures carry a risk of venous thromboembolism in and of themselves. Because of anatomic and physiologic reasons, this risk is greater than the risk associated with the surgical procedure itself. Conditions specific to these procedures are as follows. Twisting and folding of the common femoral vein during dislocation of the hip can distend and break the endothelial intercellular bridges, exposing collagen and other procoagulant substances to the blood flow. Retractors and surgical manipulations can cause extensive venous endothelial damage. A large increase in thromboplastin antigens has been observed with reaming and preparation of bone and the impacting of various implants. The heat generated during the polymerization of methacrylate may also cause some venous endothelial damage. Immobilization and bed rest, inevitable after hip arthroplasty, cause significant venous stasis.

Patient-related factors are also very important, and the effects of some of these factors on venous thromboembolic rates have been documented. Age is a very significant risk factor for venous thromboembolism, increasing progressively after the age of 20. Previous history of DVT or PE, metastatic malignancy, venous disease, tobacco use, and hormonal therapy (estrogen) have also been associated with an increased risk of venous thromboembolism in surgical patients. Research is being conducted regarding genetic risk factors, such as resistance to activated protein C, a condition present in 2% to 5% of the healthy Caucasian population. It is believed that this condition is associated with a sevenfold increase in the risk of DVT.

Nonpharmacologic Prophylaxis
General Preventive Measures
Among the few simple measures that can be implemented as a general protocol for these patients are adequate pain control to help motion, elevation of the foot of the bed, aggressive early mobilization, and active/passive ankle motion exercises.

Early Mobilization and Rehabilitation
Rehabilitation after hip arthroplasty is started earlier and is more aggressive today than it was 25 years ago. There is no published controlled study documenting its effect on thromboembolic disease. Early mobilization has such positive effects on patient rehabilitation that it has become the standard of care notwithstanding its possible beneficial effect on thromboembolic disease prevention.

Elastic Stockings
Elastic stockings increase the peak femoral vein flow by about 1.5 times the baseline, and they prevent blood stasis in venous aneurysm enlargements and saccular dilatations, which are often present in the deep venous system of older peo-

ple. Effective elastic stockings should provide a gradient of pressure greatest at the foot (15 to 18 mm Hg) and decreasing up the leg to about 5 mm Hg at the proximal thigh, should be devoid of garters, and should be available in a sufficient selection of sizes to fit most patients. Elastic bandages should be totally abandoned because they create garters, which have a venous tourniquet effect. No significant difference between above-the-knee and below-the-knee stockings has been found in the general surgery population. There is no published study using venography as a diagnostic end point in which the efficacy of elastic stockings alone is compared to a placebo in hip arthroplasty patients.

The routine use of graded-compression elastic stockings can only be considered as an adjuvant to an efficacious prophylaxis. Its cost effectiveness has not been studied, and it has no effect on de novo proximal thrombus formation, which is observed in hip arthroplasty patients.

Mechanical Prophylaxis
Sequential pneumatic compression accelerates venous emptying in the lower limb by increasing peak venous flow and stimulates the fibrinolytic system. It has the theoretical advantage of leaving the coagulation system undisturbed, therefore minimizing the bleeding risks. Sequential pneumatic compression is especially attractive for patients who are at very high risk of severe bleeding complications or for those with coagulation disorders that preclude the use of pharmacologic agents. This prophylaxis is efficacious in reducing overall DVT incidence in hip arthroplasty patients when venography is used as a diagnostic end point. It is not, however, as efficacious as low-dose warfarin in preventing proximal DVT in the same patients.

The arteriovenous impulse pump is a pneumatic device consisting of a chamber that is rapidly inflated in 0.4 seconds

against the sole of the foot, maintained inflated for 3.6 seconds, and deflated for 16 seconds. The device empties the venous plantar plexus (capacity of about 30 cc), and stimulates myovenous contraction. Tested in small series of hip arthroplasty patients, it has been reported to be effective.[3]

Both of these devices can cause discomfort, and there is a definite compliance problem in hip arthroplasty patients who are aggressively mobilized.

Pharmacologic Prophylaxis
Dextran
The antithrombotic properties of dextran have been known for more than 30 years. Suggested mechanisms of action include reduction of platelet function, coating of endothelial surfaces, stabilization of red blood cell suspension, and plasma volume expansion with subsequent blood viscosity decrease and weakening of the thrombus structure. Despite its efficacy, however, it has not gained wide acceptance as a prophylactic agent for routine administration because of its costs, its side effects (especially bleeding complications and congestive heart failure), and the need for intravenous administration.

Warfarin
Warfarin interferes with vitamin K metabolism in the liver and prevents the formation of functional clotting factors II, VII, IX, and X. It takes at least 36 hours to have a measurable effect, and 4 to 5 days to reach its full anticoagulation. Dose response to warfarin, especially in surgical patients, is hard to predict, and prothrombin time (PT) monitoring is necessary. The anticoagulant effect is expressed in INR (international normalized ratio) value, which corrects for the variability in sensitivity of the different reagents used in various institutions to measure PT.

Warfarin is one of the most commonly used forms of prophylaxis against thromboembolic disease in hip arthroplasty patients. The reported venographic rates for overall DVT are between 10% and 20%, and between 5% and 10% for proximal DVT. Major bleeds occur in 1% to 3% of the cases, and minor bleeds occur in 2% to 5%. In a series of 3,700 hip arthroplasty patients at UCLA, there were no fatal PE, 0.57% symptomatic nonfatal PE, and 1.6% major bleeds when warfarin was used for 10 to 14 days. Warfarin can be started safely either the night before surgery or after surgery. The clinical benefit of one approach versus the other has not been determined.

Heparin

Commercial heparin is a heterogeneous mixture of sulfated polysaccharide chains of molecular weights ranging from 3,000 to 30,000 daltons (mean 15,000). One third of the heparin, mostly low molecular weight fractions, binds to antithrombin III and is responsible for most of the anticoagulant activity at therapeutic levels. At the molecular level, heparin acts on antithrombin III by inducing a conformational change that unmasks an arginine center that, in turn, inhibits the active serine center of thrombin and other coagulation enzymes. After doing so, heparin dissociates from antithrombin III and can be reused.

High molecular weight heparin fractions, however, have a high affinity for platelets where they inhibit the aggregation. They also inhibit platelet function and the proliferation of vascular smooth-muscle cells. These fractions delay hypersensitivity reactions and increase the permeability of vessel walls. Finally, they have been implicated in the regulation of angiogenesis.

Low-Dose Unfractionated Heparin

Unfractionated heparin has been used as a prophylaxis in fixed low doses of 5,000 IU every 8 or 12 hours in hip arthroplasty patient populations. Some randomized trials have shown low-dose heparin prophylaxis to be ineffective (compared to a placebo) or not as effective (compared to warfarin or low molecular weight heparin) in reducing radiographic DVT rate.

Adjusted-Dose Unfractionated Heparin

The concept of adjusted dose heparin was developed when it became clear that low-dose unfractionated heparin was not as effective in hip arthroplasty patients as in general surgery patients. It increases the partial thromboplastin time (PTT) to the upper limit of the normal range or just a few seconds above it by frequently adjusting the multiple daily subcutaneous heparin doses. Adjusted-dose heparin is effective in reducing DVT incidence after hip arthroplasty, but it is complicated, labor intensive, and expensive (requiring admission 48 hours before surgery), and it carries a sizable bleeding risk.

Low Molecular Weight Heparin

Two observations have prompted the development of low molecular weight heparin (LMWH). First, it has been shown in animal models that LMWH produces less bleeding than standard heparin for the same antithrombotic effect. Second, LMWH does not prolong the PTT while retaining its anti-factor X activity.

The potential advantages of LMWH compared to unfractionated regular heparin are a more predictable dose response, a longer half life, and a hemorrhagic effect less than that of unfractionated heparin for a given antithrombotic effect.

LMWH is not an homogenous drug, but it contains only polysaccharide chains of less than 8,000 daltons. The many commercially available forms of LMWH are prepared by different processes. Because these preparations differ pharmacologically, they may not be clinically identical.

Clinical studies have reported a 60% to 80% overall radiographic DVT risk reduction in hip arthroplasty patients for

Table 1
Characteristics of low molecular weight heparin and warfarin

Warfarin	LMWH
Well established drug	Relatively new medication
Monitoring necessary	No monitoring necessary
Individualized variable dosage	Universal fixed dosage
Oral administration	Parenteral administration
Effective in hip surgery	Effective in hip surgery
Relatively safe	Relatively safe

LMWH when compared with a placebo. No significant increase in major bleeding complications was found, but a significant increase in minor bleeds (mostly subcutaneous hematomas) has been noted.[4]

Large studies have not demonstrated a significant difference between LMWH and warfarin in hip arthroplasty patients in terms of overall or proximal DVT rates, major bleeding events, or clinical thromboembolic events at 3 months after surgery. No pharmacoeconomic or cost effectiveness study has demonstrated a clear advantage in favor of one or the other prophylaxis. The characteristics of LMWH and warfarin are summarized in Table 1.

Surveillance and Diagnosis of Venous Thromboembolic Disease

Such typical clinical findings as leg pain, swelling, shortness of breath, and chest pain are present in less than half of the patients who have venous thromboembolism. Venous thromboembolism is often silent or misdiagnosed with PE being unsuspected in between 70% and 80% of patients diagnosed at autopsy.

The clinical diagnosis of DVT is therefore very difficult because typical symptoms and clinical signs are rarely

Table 2
Summary of three large clinical studies*

	Consortium USA	PASS Group Canada	CC Group Canada
Number of patients	3,012 (all hips)	1,024 (508 hips, 518 knees)	1,984 (1,142 hips, 842 knees)
Institutions	156	1	28
Prophylaxis	enoxaparin 1,516 patients warfarin 1,496 patients	warfarin 1,024 patients	enoxaparin 1,984 patients
Duration of prophylaxis	enoxaparin 7.5 days warfarin 7.0 days	9.7 days	9.0 days
Length of follow-up	90 days	90 days	90 days
Patients followed	100%	100%	100%
Symptomatic DVT	enoxaparin/warfarin		
Inpatient	0.3% / 1.1%	unknown	2.1%
Outpatient	2.5% / 1.9%	1.0%	2.0%
Total	2.8% / 3.0%		4.1%
Fatal pulmonary embolism	0.1% / 0.1%	none	0.2% (all knees)

*At the time of submission of this instructional course these three studies had not been published. Minor data discrepancies may be noted with the published articles.

present. Clinical examination of asymptomatic high risk patients for venous thrombus by the most experienced physicians has a sensitivity of 33% and a specificity of 50%. Assessment for DVT must be done by objective methods.

The gold standard remains venography, by which it is possible to detect both distal and proximal thrombi. Venography, however, is expensive and invasive, and it carries significant side effects, including superficial contrast dye thrombosis (3% of patients).

Duplex scanning provides an accurate alternative in symptomatic patients (sensitivity of 93% and specificity of 98% for proximal thrombi). This accuracy has not been consistently reproduced in asymptomatic high-risk patients, such as hip arthroplasty patients, in whom the reported sensitivities vary from 60% to 98%. A recent study has randomized 1,090 joint replacement patients (508 hips and 518 knees) on warfarin prophylaxis (average, 9 days) to duplex ultrasound compression or a sham procedure.

The examination was positive in 3.7% of the patients (19 out of 518) but was not confirmed by venography in six patients. The postdischarge rate of clinical events at 90 days was 0.8% in the negative ultrasound group and 1.0% in the sham group.

The relatively small size and the nonocclusive nature of many of these thrombi at the time of screening, as well as technical factors related to the operator experience, may explain these discrepancies. Routine duplex scanning for DVT surveillance in asymptomatic hip arthroplasty patients cannot be recommended at this moment, and it needs further study.

Clinical suspicion of PE needs objective confirmation. A chest radiograph, electrocardiograph, and arterial blood gas analysis may help to confirm an alternative diagnosis, such as pericarditis, rib fracture, or pneumothorax. A ventilation/perfusion quotient (V/Q) lung scan should be obtained to confirm the diagnosis. A normal V/Q scan rules out a PE,

and a high probability one is at least 90% accurate. An intermediate or low probability V/Q scan requires further investigation, such as a duplex ultrasound of the lower extremities, a venography, or a pulmonary angiography.[5]

Risk Period for Venous Thromboembolism

The postoperative risk period for venous thromboembolism has not been clearly defined, and the indication for postdischarge prophylaxis is controversial. Detectable thrombus formation after hip arthroplasty is noted at about 48 hours and peaks at 5 days (distal and proximal thrombi). There is a secondary peak for distal thrombi formation at 10 days. It is still generally accepted that efficacious venous thromboembolism prophylaxis during this period will prevent the majority of clinically important events, but it is not known how long the period of risk extends after joint replacement.

In today's health care environment, delivery systems are under enormous pressures to become more cost effective. This concern has has led to shorter hospital stays and early transfer to facilities with a lower level of care. In 1985, the average length of stay for hip replacement in the U.S. was 13.8 days; in 1995, it was 6.6 days, with half of patients going directly home alone after this short hospital stay.

Currently, even the most efficacious prophylaxis in hip arthroplasty patients carries an overall rate of DVT of 10% to 15% (proximal DVT 3% to 7%) as determined by routine venography at the time of discharge. There is an urgent need for information regarding the indication for the post acute care prophylaxis against venous thromboembolism.

Recent European studies have looked at the rate of venographic DVT following discharge. One study randomized 179 hip arthroplasty patients with a negative venogram at 14 days postoperatively to receive either a placebo or enoxaparin for another 21 days, after which a second venography was performed. DVT was detected in 7.1% of the enoxaparin patients and in 19.3% of the placebo patients. There were no deaths or symptomatic PE during the study period.

Another study randomized 233 patients to a placebo (116 patients) or enoxaparin (117 patients) after the whole group had received enoxaparin for 9 days while in the hospital. Patients underwent a venography 21 days after randomization, and the DVT rate was 39% in the placebo group versus 18% in the treatment group. There were no deaths, but the rates of symptomatic DVT were 9% in the placebo group and 2% in the treatment group. Two other smaller studies have confirmed the high rate of venographic DVT in hip arthroplasty patients after discharge from the hospital. The question to be answered is how these figures translate in terms of clinical outcomes.

Three large clinical series have recently reported the incidence of postdischarge clinical events after joint replacement. Pertinent data are summarized in Table 2.

These three similar clinical studies include 6,020 patients (4,662 hips and 1,358 knees) who received in-hospital prophylaxis (warfarin or enoxaparin) for an average of 7 to 10 days. All patients were followed up for at least 90 days. The overall fatal PE rate was 0.1% , and the symptomatic DVT rate after discharge was 2.0%

Treatment of Venous Thromboembolic Disease

The main goal of DVT treatment is essentially to prevent fatal PE, recurrent venous thrombosis, and postphlebitic syndrome. The latter condition seems to be rare in hip arthroplasty patients with asymptomatic DVT.

The standard protocols and guidelines for treatment of DVT and PE have been developed for symptomatic patients. Asymptomatic proximal thrombi are usually treated like symptomatic ones (5 days of iv heparin and 3 months of warfarin). This is the prudent way to manage these asymptomatic thrombi. Recent large clinical series have demonstrated the efficacy and the safety of the use of outpatient low molecular weight heparin followed by warfarin in the treatment of symptomatic proximal DVT compared to inpatient intravenous unfractionated heparin followed by warfarin.

The treatment of distal thrombi (symptomatic or not) remains controversial because there is no consensus as to how many of these thrombi will propagate proximally and eventually cause a symptomatic, potentially fatal PE. The rate of proximal extension, without treatment, has been reported to range from 0 to 40%. Most experts recommend full treatment of symptomatic distal DVT. There is no consensus on the management of asymptomatic distal DVT. The spectrum of recommended treatment goes from benign neglect to monitoring of proximal extension by serial duplex ultrasound to full treatment.

Summary

This chapter is a brief and incomplete overview of a rapidly changing field. The following points are helpful for the management of hip arthroplasty patients. There is no clinically significant difference between warfarin and enoxaparin prophylaxis in terms of efficacy (venographic or clinical events) and safety. Hip arthroplasty patients should receive warfarin or enoxaparin for at least 7 to 10 days postoperatively. There is a high rate of postdischarge venographic DVT even if prophylaxis is used for 7 to 10 days after surgery. There is a 2% rate of postdischarge symptomatic DVT if prophylaxis is used for 7 to 10 days after surgery. There is a 0.1% rate of postdischarge fatal PE at 90 days postoperatively if prophylaxis is used for 7 to 10 days after surgery. The value of routine predischarge surveillance for DVT is not clear at this moment.

References

1. Anderson FA Jr, Wheeler HB, Goldberg RJ, et al: A population-based perspective of the hospital incidence and case-fatality rates of deep vein thrombosis and pulmonary embolism: The Worcester DVT study. *Arch Intern Med* 1991; 151:933–938.

2. Williams HR, Macdonald DA: Audit of thromboembolic prophylaxis in hip and knee surgery. *Ann R Coll Surg Engl* 1997;79:55–57.

3. Santori FS, Vitullo A, Stopponi M,et al: Prophylaxis against deep-vein thrombosis in total hip replacement. Comparison of heparin and foot impulse pump. *J Bone Joint Surg* 1994;76B:579–583.

4. Turpie AG, Levine MN, Hirsh J, et al: A randomized controlled trial of a low-molecular-weight heparin (enoxaparin) to prevent deep-vein thrombosis in patients undergoing elective hip surgery. *New Engl J Med* 1986;315:925–929.

5. Dalen JE, Hirsh J (eds):Fourth ACCP consensus conference on antithrombotic therapy, *Chest* 1995;108(suppl):225s–522s.

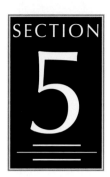

SECTION 5

Knee, Ankle, and Foot

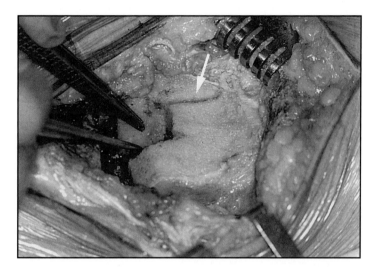

Algorithm for Anterior Knee Pain

Michael A. Kelly, MD

Algorithms have gained recent interest in the management of common clinical problems. An algorithm involves the systematic approach to defining a problem, creating a differential diagnosis, and then establishing a treatment protocol for the specific diagnosis. Anterior knee pain is a common clinical complaint with a broad differential diagnosis. There is little consensus, either in the orthopaedic literature or among orthopaedic surgeons specializing in patellofemoral disorders, regarding the diagnosis and treatment issues involved in anterior knee pain. This project is the work of a group of orthopaedic surgeons, including Drs. Michael Kelly, John Fulkerson, Michael Rock, and Michael Stuart, who attempted to create a clinical algorithm (Fig. 1) for the diagnosis and treatment of anterior knee pain. As suggested by this controversial topic, the development of this algorithm required compromises within the group to reach a consensus in the form of the final algorithm. We believe it represents a logical approach to diagnosing anterior knee pain and rendering treatment specific to this diagnosis. However, variations in nonsurgical treatment and specific surgical procedures are represented. An attempt was made to present specific surgical indications and procedures in accordance with existing orthopaedic literature.

The differential diagnosis of anterior knee pain is broad and varied. The initial evaluation is based on the standard orthopaedic approach and includes a careful history and physical examination with appropriate radiographic evaluation. In patients with anterior knee pain the history may provide information that will suggest a likely diagnosis. Patients with patellar instability tend to have specific complaints that may be related to a more discrete event. Peripatellar syndromes may cause pain at specifically associated anatomic locations, such as the tibial tubercle in Osgood-Schlatter's syndrome. More commonly, anterior knee pain complaints may be vague, insidious in onset, bilateral, and aggravated with prolonged sitting, stair climbing, or running/walking on inclines. Additionally, symptoms may be related to direct trauma or overuse.

In addition to a standard knee examination, the algorithm recommends specific clinical tests that may prove helpful in establishing a diagnosis in patients with anterior knee pain. It should be emphasized that these tests complement a routine complete knee examination. Lateral tilting of the patella characterized by a tight lateral retinaculum may be evaluated by the passive patellar tilt test.[1-3] Normally, when the lateral border of the patella is lifted while the knee is kept passively extended, the lateral patellar edge should rise to the horizontal plane or slightly past. Failure of the patella to reach the horizontal is indicative of a tight lateral retinaculum. Careful assessment of patellofemoral tracking is critical. The alignment of the quadriceps muscle, patella, and patellar tendon in extension is determined by the quadriceps angle (Q angle).[1] Normal values of the Q angle are approximately 10° in men and 15° in women. This Q angle can also be measured at 90° of flexion, and this measurement is known as the tubercle sulcus angle or TSA. The tibial tubercle rotates internally beneath the femur as the knee flexes and the patella is engaged in the femoral sulcus. The normal TSA is 0°, with measurements greater than 10° considered abnormal.[3] The TSA is my preferred method of assessing the quadriceps angle. Kolowich and associates[3] have discussed evaluation of patellar glide. The patella is divided into longitudinal quadrants. Medial/lateral patellar mobility is then assessed with the knee at 20° to 30° of flexion. Normal patellar mobility in this plane should not exceed two quadrants. Decreased medial glide is suggestive of a tight lateral retinaculum; increased lateral glide indicates laxity of the medial retinacular structures, possibly seen with lateral subluxation or dislocation of the patella. Apprehension may be demonstrated with extreme lateral patellar displacement.

A careful and thorough palpation of the anatomic structures involved in the differential diagnosis of anterior knee pain may be crucial in establishing the diagnosis. This is particularly true in the diagnosis of peripatellar disorders such as prepatellar bursitis, plica, retinacular pain, Osgood-Schlatter or Sinding-Johansson-Larsen syndrome, patellar or quadriceps tendinitis, and iliotibial band syndrome. Neuromata in the lateral reti-

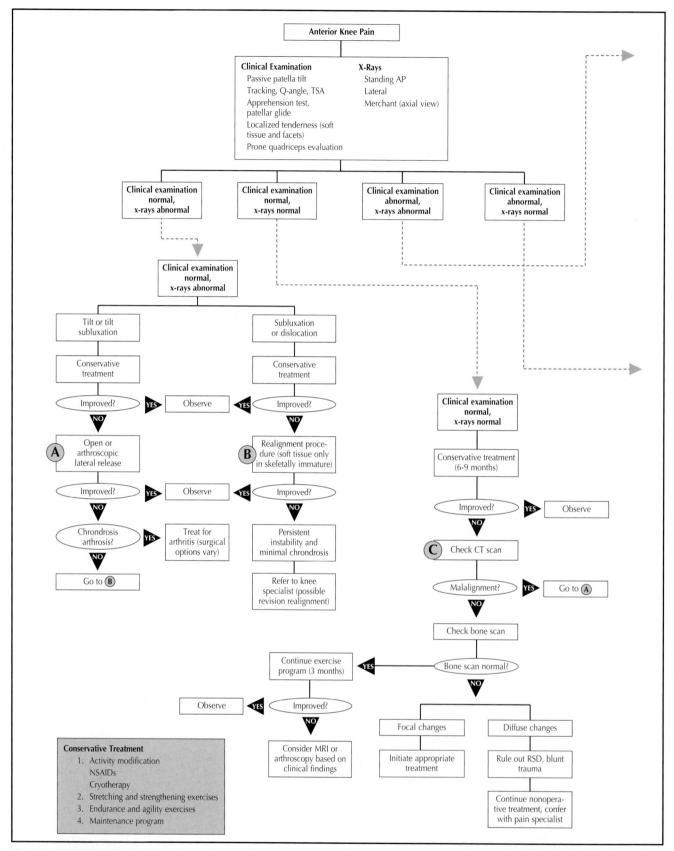

Fig. 1 Anterior knee pain algorithm. (Reproduced with permission from Kelly MA, Scuderi JR: Management of patellofemoral pain. *Orthop Spec Ed* 1997;3:37-40.)

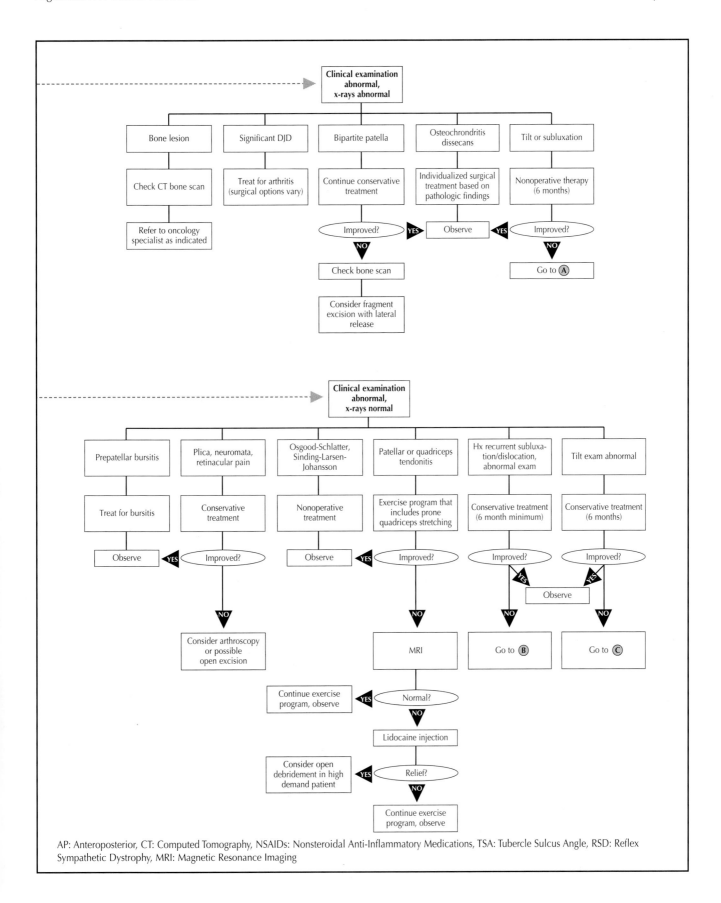

AP: Anteroposterior, CT: Computed Tomography, NSAIDs: Nonsteroidal Anti-Inflammatory Medications, TSA: Tubercle Sulcus Angle, RSD: Reflex Sympathetic Dystrophy, MRI: Magnetic Resonance Imaging

naculum have been described as a source of anterior knee pain.[2] Additionally, neuromata associated with previous surgical scars may be a source of focal pain symptoms or associated with a reflex sympathetic dystrophy (RSD) condition.[4] Although uncommon, RSD of the knee typically involves the patellofemoral compartment.[5,6]

Excessive tightness of the quadriceps extensor mechanism is determined by placing the patient prone with the knees flexed as far as is tolerable while the pelvis is stabilized.[2] Normally, symmetric flexion is possible and each heel can be brought to or near the buttocks on full flexion. The inability to flex freely is an important consideration in designing an appropriate rehabilitation plan. Again, it must be stressed that these tests were emphasized in the algorithm to allow accurate diagnosis of anterior knee pain, but the knee examination should also include the typical patellofemoral examination and all tests necessary to establish the presence or absence of other pathologic entities in the knee, such as meniscal lesions and ligamentous instability.

Radiographic evaluation is important in evaluating anterior knee pain.[7] The recommended views in this algorithm include standing anteroposterior (AP), lateral, and axial views of the patellofemoral compartment. Although the standing AP view of the knee may provide little information regarding the patellofemoral compartment, it is useful in assessing tibiofemoral degenerative joint disease and knee alignment. Patellar height is best assessed on the lateral view. The Insall-Salvati ratio of the patellar tendon length and the height of the patella is useful for determining patella alta.[8] An axial view of the patellofemoral compartment is mandatory in the assessment of anterior knee pain. A variety of axial views have been described. In this algorithm we have suggested the use of a Merchant axial view. This view, which is well standardized,[9] is taken with the knee flexed 45° and the X-ray beam projected caudal at an angle of 30° from the plane of the femur. This same technique may be applied with the knee at 30° flexion. This latter view allows evaluation of patellar alignment, both subluxation and lateral tilt, as well as the anatomy of the femoral sulcus. It may be helpful both in determining the diagnosis and in planning the treatment of patellar malalignment conditions. Because of the lack of sensitivity of axial views, we have suggested the use of computed tomography (CT) for further assessment of possible patellofemoral malalignment in patients whose symptoms persist despite normal axial radiographs.[10] Schutzer and associates[11] have described the use of CT of the patellofemoral joint at 15°, 30°, and 45° of flexion to demonstrate malalignment. As can be seen, this test is used for patients who fail to respond to nonsurgical treatment programs after 6 to 9 months. Based on our present clinical practice, we anticipate that the need for CT scans will be uncommon in this algorithm. However, it is important to demonstrate malalignment of the patella before recommending any surgical realignment procedures, and CT may be helpful in this setting.

In more complex situations, the algorithm suggests the use of magnetic resonance imaging (MRI) and bone scans. While MRI has been proposed to evaluate both articular cartilage lesions and patellofemoral alignment, we believe that the recommended use of MRI in this algorithm is both efficient and cost effective. Bone scans may be useful in specific situations as proposed by Dye and Boll.[12] Others have suggested their usefulness for suspected reflex sympathetic dystrophy involving the knee.[5] Finally, undiagnosed anterior knee pain that has failed to respond to prolonged nonsurgical treatment (after 9 to 12 months) may indicate the need for surgical arthroscopy.[13]

The treatment protocols in this algorithm are designed to provide a specific clinical diagnosis and to emphasize nonsurgical treatment. This emphasis reflects our understanding that greater than 90% of patients with anterior knee pain will respond successfully to nonsurgical measures. A complete review of nonsurgical treatment is beyond the spectrum of this algorithm. Use of a broad range of nonsurgical treatment is suggested, including activity modification, nonsteroidal anti-inflammatory agents, stretching and strengthening exercises, and endurance and agility exercises with a maintenance exercise program.[14] The importance of a carefully outlined nonsurgical approach is stressed. However, the algorithm does allow for individual variations in accomplishing such goals as prescribed by individual physicians or physical therapists. No single program of nonsurgical treatment is universally accepted, and this algorithm was designed to encourage the careful and thoughtful planning of each program.

The algorithm is initially divided into four categories based on the individual history, clinical examination, and radiographic evaluation. Each of these four parameters is determined to be considered either normal or abnormal. The patient's suspected clinical diagnosis, or in some cases lack of specific diagnosis, will allow categorization within one of these four groups. A treatment plan is prescribed. In this algorithm, treatment is typically nonsurgical for 3 to 6 months. Clinical assessment of the patient will then determine whether the patient has improved or has not improved. This determination will dictate the next step in the algorithm. The algorithm is self-explanatory from this point. In diagnostic categories in which surgery may be considered, the surgical recommendation may be specific or may only suggest a specific surgical procedure. A large number of patellar realignment procedures have been described in the literature.[2,15–20] No single patellar realignment procedure has gained a consensus as the preferred procedure, either in the orthopaedic literature or among involved orthopaedic surgeons. Acknowledging this fact, the algorithm recommends patellar realignment for recurrent subluxation or dislocation of the patella after failure of nonsurgical treatment. However, the specific procedure to be used is to be determined by the treating orthopaedic surgeon. Similarly, there is no consensus in the surgical treatment of patellofemoral arthritis. No specific recommendation is established in this algorithm. While the diversity of opinion and special considerations that typify this patient population did not allow for appropriate recommendations from the consulting group, the surgical options are listed for consideration.[1,3,16,21,22]

In summary, nonsurgical treatment of anterior knee pain is stressed in this algorithm regardless of diagnosis. Surgical indications for specific disorders within this algorithm are specified after failure of nonsurgical treatment. The surgical procedures indicated allow for individual surgeon preference as supported by the orthopaedic literature or present investigations. The proposed algorithm (Fig. 1) for the treatment of anterior knee pain allows a thoughtful approach to this problem, and it should assist in establishing a specific diagnosis and treatment plan for the management of these patients.

References

1. Aglietti P, Buzzi R, Insall JN: Disorders of the patellofemoral joint, in Insall JN, Windsor RE, Scott WN, et al (eds): Surgery of the Knee, ed 2. New York, NY, Churchill Livingstone, 1993, pp 241–385.

2. Fulkerson JP, Hungerford DS, Ficat RP (eds): Disorders of the Patellofemoral Joint, ed 2. Baltimore, MD, Williams & Wilkins, 1990.

3. Kolowich PA, Paulos LE, Rosenberg TD, et al: Lateral release of the patella: Indications and contraindications. Am J Sports Med 1990;18: 359–365.

4. Poehling GG, Pollock FE Jr, Koman LA: Reflex sympathetic dystrophy of the knee after sensory nerve injury. Arthroscopy 1988;4:31–35.

5. Cooper DE, DeLee JC: Reflex sympathetic dystrophy of the knee. J Am Acad Orthop Surg 1994;2:79–86.

6. Cooper DE, DeLee JC, Ramamurthy S: Reflex sympathetic dystrophy of the knee: Treatment using continuous epidural anesthesia. J Bone Joint Surg 1989;71A:365–369.

7. Math KR, Ghelman B, Potter HG: Imaging of the patellofemoral joint, in Scuderi GR (ed): The Patella. New York, NY, Springer-Verlag, 1995, pp 83–125.

8. Insall J, Salvati E: Patella position in the normal knee joint. Radiology 1971;101:101–104.

9. Merchant AC, Mercer RL, Jacobsen RH, et al: Roentgenographic analysis of patellofemoral congruence. J Bone Joint Surg 1974;56A: 1391–1396.

10. Fulkerson JP, Schutzer SF, Ramsby GR, et al: Computerized tomography of the patello-femoral joint before and after lateral release or realignment. Arthroscopy 1987;3:19–24.

11. Schutzer SF, Ramsby GR, Fulkerson JP: Computed tomographic classification of patellofemoral pain patients. Orthop Clin North Am 1986;17:235–248.

12. Dye SF, Boll DA: Radionuclide imaging of the patellofemoral joint in young adults with anterior knee pain. Orthop Clin North Am 1986; 17:249–262.

13. Greenfield MA, Scott WN: Arthroscopic evaluation and treatment of the patellofemoral joint. Orthop Clin North Am 1992;23:587–600.

14. McConnell J: The management of chondromalacia patellae: A long term solution. Aust J Physiotherapy 1986;32:215–223.

15. Cox JS: Evaluation of the Roux-Elmslie-Trillat procedure for knee extensor realignment. Am J Sports Med 1982;10:303–310.

16. Fulkerson JP: Anteromedialization of the tibial tuberosity for patellofemoral malalignment. Clin Orthop 1983;177:176–181.

17. Insall JN, Aglietti P, Tria AJ Jr: Patellar pain and incongruence: II. Clinical application. Clin Orthop 1983;176:225–232.

18. Kelly MA: Operative treatment: Proximal realignment. Sports Med Arthroscopy Rev 1994;2: 243–249.

19. Scuderi GR: Surgical treatment for patellar instability. Orthop Clin North Am 1992;23: 619–630.

20. Scuderi G, Cuomo F, Scott WN: Lateral release and proximal realignment for patellar subluxation and dislocation: A long-term follow-up. J Bone Joint Surg 1988;70A:856–861.

21. Fulkerson JP, Becker GJ, Meaney JA, et al: Anteromedial tibial tubercle transfer without bone graft. Am J Sports Med 1990;18:490–496.

22. Kelly MA, Insall JN: Patellectomy. Orthop Clin North Am 1986;17:289–295.

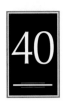

Patellar Instability in the School Age Athlete

Carl L. Stanitski, MD

Patellar instability manifests itself in a spectrum of presentations that range from occasional subluxation to chronic, complete dislocation. The true incidence and prevalence of various types of patellar instability among school-age athletes (6 to 18 years of age) is unknown. Lesser degrees of instability, especially subluxation, are commonly misdiagnosed. Instability data in immature athletes are often interspersed in reports of adult patients who have a mixture of acute or recurrent dislocations. This paper focuses on children and adolescents whose patellar instability is not associated with such congenital or syndromic conditions as Down syndrome, Ehlers-Danlos syndrome, and multiple epiphyseal dysplasia. The vast majority of patellar dislocations are lateral. Medial dislocation is quite rare and is usually the result of a direct blow or as an iatrogenic consequence of an over-vigorous lateral release.[1,2] Intra-articular dislocations are quite rare.

In the spectrum of athletic knee injuries, an acute dislocation often receives more attention, because most patellar instability sports injuries are acute ones. It has been suggested that Casey's (of the immortal strike-out fame) inept performance was due to an acute patellar dislocation.[3] Recurrent patellar instability, on the other hand, may prevent a student athlete from being able to participate in a chosen sport.

Terminology describing the setting for patellar instability is confusing, and the terms malalignment, maltracking, and instability are used interchangeably. This imprecise nosology makes it difficult to compare works between authors and to discuss diagnostic and treatment venues.[4] Malalignment is an abnormal static relationship between the patella, its associated soft tissues, and the femoral and tibial axes. The malalignment may be asymptomatic. Maltracking is an expression of the dynamic relationships of the above noted tissues during active and passive motions. Such maltracking may also be asymptomatic. Both malalignment and maltracking present with a spectrum of magnitudes.

Patellar instability is classified according to mechanism of instability, frequency of recurrence, and interval between recurrences. The mechanism of injury may be from direct percussion from a sports object (bat, ball, helmet, goal-post) or an opponent's or teammate's body. It also may occur indirectly from a rapid, noncontact deceleration or change of direction maneuver. The precipitating force should be categorized as major or minor. I classify recurrences as initial, second, and, after that, chronic. Frequency of recurrences are graded as daily, weekly, monthly, or infrequent. In addi-

tion to classifying the direction of dislocation, the magnitude of instability (subluxated, dislocated) and the ease of reduction (spontaneous, sedation required) are important points for consideration (Table 1). Using these classification parameters allows more directed analysis of treatment options.

Many of the reported series of acute patellar dislocations are limited by such design flaws as small number of patients, broad patient age range, differing mechanisms of injury, initial versus recurrent status, and varying methods of treatment. Although a benign course has historically been expected following an acute patellar dislocation in adolescence, a critical review of the reported cases in this age group suggests that this optimism is not justified.[5-12] Recurrent dislocation rates vary between 17% and 44%, and failure to return to previous levels of sports activity is reported to be as high as 55%.[6-8,11-13] Causes of such a dismal outcome include persistent instability and unrecognized intra-articular injury.

Anatomy

By the end of the embryonic period (8 weeks), an adult form knee is present, including a well-developed quadriceps

Table 1 Patellar instability classification				
Onset	Mechanism	Interval	Frequency	Reduction
Acute	Direct (contact)	Initial	Daily	Spontaneous
Recurrent	Indirect	First recurrence	Weekly	Sedation
	Major force	Second recurrence	Monthly	Anesthesia
	Minor force	Chronic	Infrequent	

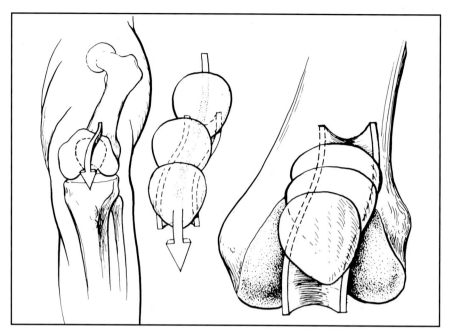

Fig. 1 Toroidal path of the patella from extension to flexion. (Reproduced with permission from Stanitski CL: Patellofemoral mechanism, in Stanitski CL, DeLee JC, Drez D (eds): *Pediatric and Adolescent Sports Medicine*. Philadelphia, PA, WB Saunders, vol 3, 1994, p 307.)

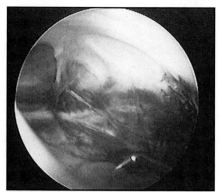

Fig. 2 Arthroscopic view of a medial retinacular tear seen after an acute patellar dislocation.

and patellar mechanism with intimate relations between the femur and tibia. Joint motion has begun. The patella traverses a toroidal path, one that requires motion along all three axes simultaneously (Fig. 1). This motion occurs from early engagement of the patella in the femoral trochlea at 5° of flexion to full seating at 90° of flexion.

Normal joint stability occurs through a complex interaction of static and dynamic joint stabilizers, which provide four-quadrant balance. Static stability is provided by joint congruence and lower extremity alignment. Dynamic stability is a function of muscle forces, primarily from the quadriceps and hamstrings, but ankle/foot and hip/spine mechanisms also play major roles in the integrated, articulated lower extremity. Defects of the lateral trochlear margin or trochlear depth cause loss of the normal bone restraints to patellar travel. If lateral soft tissues are tight and/or if medial soft-tissue structures are incompetent, soft-tissue balance is lost and instability occurs.

Pathophysiology
The underlying expression of both acute and chronic instability is the loss of the normal four-quadrant vector balance, and this loss produces primary and secondary deficits. Soft-tissue changes occur extra- and intra-articularly. Extra-articular sites of compromise include the medial quadriceps mechanism at either the patellar-medialis junction or at the medialis-adductor convergence, more specifically the medial patellofemoral ligament (Fig. 2). In medial dislocations, the lateral quadriceps retinaculum is damaged. Intra-articular soft tissues that may be damaged include menisci or, more commonly, the anterior cruciate ligament, especially in a noncontact, change of direction, deceleration type injury. Intra-articular hard-tissue injury is a common associated finding, caused by the concussive and shear effects of the dislocation and relocation, either from a direct blow or from quadriceps contraction. Articular injuries range from in situ cartilage damage or stable osteochondral lesions to

completely displaced osteochondral loose bodies. Once a major acute dislocation occurs, the stage is set for retinacular attenuation, loss of the medial vector, repeat articular damage, quadriceps insufficiency from pain, and progressive loss of the normal quadriceps/hamstring balance, with recurrent dislocation and articular compromise.

Clinical History
By the time the child begins scholastic age sports, most underlying congenital, syndromic, and developmental causes of patellar instability have been recognized. Classification of the nature of the instability is done using the parameters stated above. Previous treatments and their effects are recorded. The degree of functional instability (interference with daily nonsports tasks) is ascertained. Symptoms of the opposite knee and both hips are investigated. The nature of the pain is closely questioned to rule out stigmata of reflex sympathetic dystrophy. Constant pain, especially burning-type, out of proportion to the injury, coupled with hypersensitivity to touch, is prima facie evidence of this not uncommon but frequently missed condition in children and adolescents. Risk factors, such as ligamentous laxity, previous untreated dislocations, and significant lower extremity malalignment, should be discussed.

Chapter 40

Physical Examination

Patient cooperation with the examination will vary with the patient's acuity and the severity of the instability. Ideally, the patient should be gowned or dressed in shorts, to allow evaluation of the entire lower extremity during stance and gait. In stance, lower extremity angular or rotatory malalignments are assessed. The use of 'Q'angle measurements as a predictor of risk for dislocation has been inconsistent. In patients with lateral malalignment, the 'Q' angle will actually be less, not greater, than the broad range of normal values. Both knees are examined and signs of generalized ligamentous laxity are tested. A hip examination is done to rule out concomitant knee and hip disease or symptoms referred from the hip. Knee stability, active and passive motion, and sites of focal retinacular tenderness are identified. In patients with nonacute recurrent instability, the patient commonly precisely indicates loci of pain as opposed to the 'grab sign' ie, grasping the entire anterior knee when asked to pinpoint the site of pain, a sign commonly seen in patients with idiopathic anterior knee pain. This is in contrast to the apprehension test, which is precipitated by the examiner's attempt to translate the patella. With instability, apprehension sign is usually positive. With the patient and the physician seated facing one another, the patient's knee is taken through a passive and active range of motion as comfort permits. I find that palpation of the patella as it passes through the femoral sulcus is the most helpful evaluation of patellar tracking. Displacement of the patella to determine tilt and/or translation usually cannot be done in the acute setting. No normative values of tilt or translation (glide) have been determined for children or adolescents. A gap may be palpable at the site of the retinacular tear. The opposite knee, if asymptomatic, is a useful control. In cases of recurrent instability, diminished quadriceps bulk and definition is a reflec-

tion of lower extremity muscle atrophy and weakness. This condition usually is not limited to the quadriceps or more specifically, as is often suggested, the vastus medialis obliquus. An effusion is usually present following an acute dislocation. If a significant tear has occurred in the quadriceps mechanism, the hemarthrosis will be dispersed into the thigh's soft tissues, which can lead the inexperienced observer to assume that, in the absence of an effusion, no intra-articular injury occurred.

Imaging

Initial standard radiographs should include anteroposterior, lateral, tunnel, and skyline views, the latter in less than 30° of flexion, because all but the most grossly unstable patellae will assume a midline position with more than 30° of flexion. Static views, like those described by Lauren and Merchant, provide information about patellar and femoral sulcus size and configuration but, by their static nature, provide little information about dynamic instability. Patellar orientation (tilt, translation) may be distorted by effusion or positioning.[14] Patella alta is difficult to document in skeletally immature patients because of the amount of nonossified patella and tibial tubercle, which render standard landmarks invalid. In recurrent cases, previous evidence of injury, such as medial, nonarticular patellar avulsion fracture, is often seen. Chondral and osteochondral in situ injuries as well as loose bodies are rarely visible radiologically.[10,15] Dainer and associates[16] reported 29 cases of acute patellar dislocations in adolescents and young adults assessed arthroscopically, and they found osteochondral defects more than 5 mm in diameter that had not been seen on radiographs. In a personal series of 48 adolescent patients with primary, noncontact, acute patellar dislocation, comparison was made between articular injury findings on radiographs and those documented at arthroscopy. Arthroscopy

identified articular injury that ranged from articular contusion to osteochondral loose bodies 4 mm to 20 mm in size in 71% of the patients. Only 23% of the articular lesions were identified on radiographs. Osteochondral loose bodies were identified radiographically in only 29% of the cases, and recognition was independent of fragment size. In this group of patients, routine radiographs were of limited value in assessing articular injury, and arthroscopy documented significant, unexpected articular damage.

Use of specialized imaging techniques should be reserved for assessment of recurrent cases. Magnetic resonance imaging (MRI) should not be used as a screening tool because, with the current technology, specificity of articular imaging is often lacking. This specificity limitation was demonstrated by Virolainen and associates,[17] who studied 25 young adult military conscripts with acute patellar dislocation who had evidence of articular injury on arthroscopic examination in 19 of 25 patients. Eleven of the 25 patients' standard radiographs showed articular damage, but only one of the 11 injuries seen on standard radiographs was documented by MRI studies. Sallay and associates[13] reported that MRI is more sensitive in detecting lateral femoral condylar damage than patellar surface injury. Kirsch and associates[18] reported good results using MRI to detect articular injury in patients following acute patellar dislocation, but the MRI correlated with findings at surgery in only 26%. Further refinements of MRI techniques may clarify the role of this imaging modality in diagnosis and management of patellar instability. Use of computed tomography (CT) scans to differentiate three patterns of instability (tilt, translation, and tilt plus translation) reported by Fulkerson and associates is helpful in recurrent cases.[19-21] Guzzanti and associates[22] demonstrated that these patterns may change with dynamic CT views, ie, views made with and without quadriceps contraction.

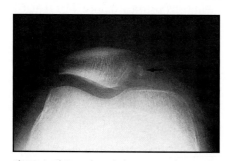

Fig. 3 Avulsion of medial, nonarticular patellar segment (arrow) in a patient with recurrent patellar dislocation.

Despite the multiple attempts to image the patellofemoral articulation to document instability factors, it has not been possible, to date, to show these relationships in a functional, ie, weightbearing, dynamic, reproducible manner.

Subluxation

Patellar subluxation represents a point on the instability spectrum and reflects the mechanism of injury and/or the patient's anatomic predisposition. The diagnosis is often difficult, with the patient relating a vague history of knee 'feeling like it's going out' or a feeling of 'weakness'. Findings at clinical examination vary depending on the magnitude of the instability, which can range from mild to moderate. Imaging studies are often of little help, especially in the pre-adolescent. CT scan with the knee between 10° and 15° of flexion can be of value. Patients with subluxation commonly respond to a nonsurgical management program designed to restore quadriceps strength and lateral retinacular flexibility. Passive mobilization of the lateral retinaculum to increase medial patellar translation coupled with progressive resistance quadriceps exercises in a comfortable arc of motion (often provided by a closed kinetic chain protocol) are the mainstays of the rehabilitation program. Curative claims with use of a variety of knee braces or taping techniques have not been borne out by objective scrutiny. If,

after 8 weeks, a nonsurgical program fails with a compliant patient, surgical intervention is required to prevent persistent recurrent instability with secondary articular injury. Surgical treatment requires balance of the four quadrant vector forces, usually by lateral release and medial capsular imbrication with vastus medialis obliquus transfer.

Dislocation

An acute patellar dislocation is a dramatic, memorable event. Epidemiologic data on the exact number of patients who go on to frequent, functionally disabling instability is sparse in both skeletally immature and mature populations.[6-8,12] Recurrence rates appear to be related to the underlying etiology (significant trochlear dysplasia and/or malalignment, laxity) and chronic quadriceps mechanism attenuation and imbalance. In a recently reported study[10] of adolescent patients with initial lateral, acute patellar dislocation, those patients with nonpathologic generalized laxity had two and one half times fewer articular injuries documented arthroscopically than did a similar cohort with nongeneralized laxity. Patients with bilateral instability usually have unequal involvement, which may be from separate etiologies. Nonetheless, bilaterality must be considered a risk factor that diminishes the prognosis for a successful outcome independent of treatment. Activity demands play a major role in potential recurrences, with many patients choosing to avoid activities that could cause symptomatic instability. Although not enough patients have been studied to provide adequate statistical power, it seems probable that patients who sustain a medial patellar, nonarticular avulsion fracture (Fig. 3) have a lower rate of recurrence because of bone union as opposed to those with soft-tissue diastasis within the quadriceps mechanism envelope. Vähäsarja and associates[11] evaluated 48 patients who underwent 57 patellar realignment procedures for

recurrent instability. At a mean follow-up of 4 years, 23% had required reoperation. Results were not dependent on preoperative radiologic parameters. In most series of young adults, results following surgical reconstruction diminished with time. The significant demands on those patients who were active military recruits may account for some of the injuries.[23]

Initial treatment following an acute patellar dislocation should include as atraumatic a patellar reduction as is possible to avoid a second insult to the articular surfaces of the patella and femur. Sedation, to allow patient relaxation and cooperation, is often needed in children. If an intra-articular loose body is seen on the pre- or postreduction radiographs, arthroscopic assessment of the articular surfaces should be done, with management of the fragment as indicated by its size, source location, and condition, ie, comminution, salvageability of the articular surface, and the amount of subchondral bone amenable to fixation. At the same time, direct repair of the medial retinacular defect is done under arthroscopic control as suggested by Small and associates.[24] This repair involves a small incision over the medial retinaculum for suture retrieval and closure. Lateral release is done only if lateral tilt remains after medial reconstruction. If persistent medial subluxation exists, it may be due to over-vigorous lateral release. If lateral subluxation persists, the medial reconstruction was inadequate and a formal open medial reconstruction may be required.

If no loose fragment is seen on the radiographs, knee aspiration may be done to provide patient comfort. The hemarthrotic fluid is assessed for evidence of fat, which would indicate marrow space invasion from an osteochondral injury, either in situ or from an unstable loose fragment not visible radiologically. If evidence of osteochondral injury is lacking, a period of immobilization with crutch-protected partial weightbearing gait for 3 to 5 days is recommended, with reexamination after that time. Lack of improvement, as evidenced by persistent pain, effusion, and loss of motion, may be caused by an unrecognized intra-articular injury and calls for more aggressive management, including arthroscopy.

Over 115 surgical techniques have been reported for management of recurrent patellar instability, almost all dealing with skeletally mature patients. The sheer number of these procedures bears testimony to the lack of definition of the problem and to a misunderstanding of the individualized needs of the patient, especially if the added factor of growth is included. Reconstructive techniques are designed to normalize the static and dynamic four-quadrant balance that is lost with repeat episodes of instability, and which is necessary for normal function. The procedures provide release of the lateral tether, augmentation of the medial vector, and correction of the malalignment, alone or, as is usually the case, in combination (Table 2). Peripatellar reconstructions include lateral retinacular release, medial capsular imbrication, vastus medialis obliquus advancement, and semitendinosis transfer.[25] Infrapatellar techniques include patellar ligament transfer, either in part, via the Roux-Goldthwaite method, which is preferred in skeletally immature patients, or completely, using the Roux-Elmslie-Trillat tibial tubercle rotationplasty.[23,26] More significant tibial tubercle osteotomy and transfer, eg, Fulkerson technique, is uncommonly needed as an initial reconstruction. The Hauser procedure is not recommended because of the significant potential for compartment syndrome and patella infera associated with it.[27] In unique cases, femoral and/or tibial osteotomies combined with soft-tissue balancing procedures may be required to correct major malalignment.

Postoperative rehabilitation focuses on gaining a controlled arc of motion with progressive restoration of lower extremity strength and endurance, partic-

ularly the quadriceps/hamstring ratio. Agility exercises and gradual completion of sport-specific tasks are done prior to return to sport. The patient and family must be aware of the prolonged 3- to 4-month major rehabilitative effort required after patellar mechanism reconstruction. Loss of large segments of weightbearing femoral articular surfaces requires special consideration, which may include fresh osteochondral allograft, 'mosaicplasty,' or autologous chondrocyte implantation reconstructions. All of these techniques must be considered experimental at this time and lack documentation of long-term efficacy.

Summary

In 1945, Haxton[28] observed that, "it seems likely that more has been written about the patella relative to its size than about any other bone in the human body." Patellar instability represents a broad spectrum of conditions and etiologies. Diagnosis of the lesser degrees of instability may be difficult. Acute patellar dislocation causes large compressive and shear loads on the articular surface, with resultant damage often underestimated by standard radiographs. Inaccurate diagnosis and laissez faire treatment result in a vicious cycle of continued imbalance, recurrent instability, and repeat articular injury. Management of recurrent patellar instability must be individualized, taking into account the patient's anatomic assets and liabilities. One must keep in mind Malgaigne's notation of over a century and a half ago, "...when I searched along past and present authors for the origins of the doctrines generally accepted today concerning dislocations of the patella, I was surprised to find among them such a dearth of facts with such an abundance of opinions."[19]

References

1. Busch MT, DeHaven KE: Pitfalls of the lateral retinacular release. *Clin Sports Med* 1989;8:279.

Table 2 Surgical intervention	
Condition	**Intervention**
Suprapatellar	Lateral release
	Medial capsuloplasty
	Vastus medialis obliquus
	transfer
	Hamstring transfer
Infrapatellar	Patellar tendon transfer
	Partial; Goldthwaite
	Rotational; Trillat
Combination	Supra + infrapatellar
	Femoral, tibial
	osteotomies
No malalignment	Medial capsuloplasty
	Vastus medialis obliquus
	transfer
	± Lateral release
	± Hamstring transfer
Malalignment	Patellar tendon transfer
	Goldthwaite
	Trillat
	Hamstring transfer
	Femoral osteotomy
	Tibial osteotomy

2. Hughston JC, Flandry F, Brinker M, Terry GC, Mills JC: Surgical correction of medial subluxation of the patella. Am J Sports Med 1996; 24:486–491.

3. Gross RM: Acute dislocation of the patella: The Midville mystery. *J Bone Joint Surg* 1986;68A:780.

4. Stanitski CL: Management of patellar instability [editorial]. *J Pediatr Orthop* 1995;15:279–280.

5. Cash JD, Hughston JC: Treatment of acute patellar dislocation. *Am J Sports Med* 1988;16:244–249.

6. Cofield RH, Bryan RS: Acute dislocation of the patella: Results of conservative treatment. *J Trauma* 1977;17:526–531.

7. Hawkins RJ, Bell RH, Anisette G: Acute patellar dislocations: The natural history. *Am J Sports Med* 1986; 14:117–120.

8. McManus F, Rang M, Heslin DJ: Acute dislocation of the patella in children: The natural history. *Clin Orthop* 1979;139:88–91.

9. Nietosvaara Y, Aalto K, Kallio PE: Acute patellar dislocation in children: Incidence and associated osteochondral fractures. *J Pediatr Orthop* 1994;14:513–515.

10. Stanitski CL: Articular hypermobility and chondral injury in patients with acute patella dislocation. *Am J Sports Med* 1995; 23:146–150.

11. Vähäsarja V, Kinnueen P, Lanning P, Serlo W: Operative realignment of patellar malalignment in children. *J Pediatr Orthop* 1995;15:281–285.

12. Rorabeck C, Bobechko WP: Acute dislocation of the patella with osteochondral fracture: A review of eighteen cases. *J Bone Joint Surg* 1976;58B:237–240.

13. Sallay PI, Poggi J, Speer KP, Garrett WE: Acute dislocation of the patella. *Am J Sports Med* 1996;24:52–60.

14. Kujala UM, Österman K, Kormano M, Komu M, Nelimarkka O, Hurme M, Taimela S: Patellofemoral relationships in recurrent patellar dislocation. *J Bone Joint Surg* 1989;71B:788–792.

15. Vainionpaa S, Laasonen E, Patilala H, et al: Acute dislocation of the patella: Clinical, radiographic and operative findings in 64 consecutive cases. *Acta Orthop Scand* 1986;57:331–333.

16. Dainer RD, Barrack RL, Buckley SL et al: Arthroscopic treatment of acute patellar dislocation. *Arthroscopy* 1988;4:267–271.

17. Virolainen H, Visure T, Kuusela T: Acute dislocation of the patella: MR findings. *Radiology* 1993;189:243–246.

18. Kirsch MD, Fitzgerald SW, Friedman H, Rogers LF: Transient lateral patellar dislocation: Diagnosis with MR imaging. *Am J Roentgenol* 1993;161:109–113.

19. Fulkerson JP, Hungerford D: *Disorders of the Patellofemoral Joint*. Baltimore, MD, Williams & Williams, 1990.

20. Fulkerson JP: Patellofemoral alignment. *J Bone Joint Surg* 1990;72A:1424.

21. Schutzer SF, Ramsby GR, Fulkerson JP: The evaluation of patellofemoral pain using computerized tomography. *Clin Orthop* 1986;204:287–93.

22. Guzzanti V, Gigant A, DiLazzaro A et al: Patellofemoral malalignment in adolescents. *Am J Sports Med* 1994;22:55–60.

23. Cox JS: An evaluation of the Roux-Elmslie-Trillat procedure for knee extensor realignment. *Am J Sports Med* 1982;9:425.

24. Small, NC, Glogau, AI, Berezin, MA: Arthroscopically assisted proximal extensor mechanism realignment of the knee. *Arthroscopy* 1993; 9(1):63

25. Hall JE, Micheli LJ, McNamara GB, Jr: Semitendinosus tenodesis for recurrent subluxation or dislocation of the patella. *Clin Orthop* 1979;144:31.

26. Pappas AM, Anas P, Toczylowski HM Jr: Asymmetrical arrest of the proximal tibial physis and genu recurvatum deformity. *J Bone Joint Surg* 1984;66A:575–81.

27. Chrisman OD, et al: A long-term prospective study of the Hauser and Roux-Goldthwaite procedures for recurrent patellar dislocation. *Clin Orthop* 1979;144:27.

28. Haxton R: The function of the patella and the effects of excision. *Surg Gynocol Obstet* 1945;80:389–95.

Anterior Cruciate Ligament Injuries in the Skeletally Immature Patient

Ian K. Y. Lo, MD

David M. Bell, MD

Peter J. Fowler, MD, FRCSC

Introduction

Complete disruption of the anterior cruciate ligament (ACL) in the skeletally immature patient is being diagnosed with increasing frequency.[1-10] This increase has been attributed to a better understanding and greater clinical suspicion of ACL tears, and to the preadolescent athlete's higher level of skill and participation.[11,12] Unfortunately, information regarding the natural history of ACL injury in this subset of patients is limited. The severity of the disability associated with ACL disruption in the young patient compared to that resulting from the same injury in the adult is unclear. The long-term prognosis and the issue of whether cartilage injury, meniscal tears, and early arthrosis commonly noted in the ACL-injured adult are similar also remain poorly understood.[13] The onset of maturation relative to age is extremely variable,[14,15] but few studies have investigated the relationship between prognosis and the true level of skeletal immaturity.

The literature reporting long-term outcomes after nonsurgical treatment regimens for ACL injuries in the skeletally immature indicates a poor prognosis with respect to return to sports and long-term sequelae.[5,9,12,16-21] Most reports describe episodes of giving way, inability to return to previous level of athletic participation, and meniscal tears. As has been documented in adults, repeated episodes of giving way with secondary meniscal and articular cartilage damage may predispose patients to early arthrosis.[13,22,23] It is likely that patients without any treatment would do worse than those treated nonsurgically with rehabilitation and bracing. Thus, it is presumed that the natural history of the untreated ACL injury in the skeletally immature patient consists of severe functional disability and permanent long-term sequelae.

In addition, the efficacy and potential risks of surgical treatment to the growing knee are not well documented. It is unknown whether the reconstruction techniques used in adults are as effective in the young patient, or whether they carry special risks such as growth arrest, early graft failure, or early arthrosis. The success of surgical treatment of the injured skeletally immature knee needs to persist far into maturity, despite the variables of growth and bone development. Therefore, a solid understanding of ACL injury in the young patient is needed to prevent loss of function and early arthrosis, and to delineate appropriate treatment options.

Diagnosis

Much recent literature has described many of the subtle complexities of the ACL injury in adults. This has led to a higher index of suspicion of ACL injury, resulting in prompter and more appropriate treatment. It is not known if the symptoms or physical findings of ACL injury in the skeletally immature differ from those in the adult, but it can be assumed that they are similar. Just as in the adult, arthrometer measurements should substantiate the diagnosis. The differential diagnosis of anterior knee instability in the young patient includes tibial eminence fractures, periarticular fractures, constitutional laxity, and congenital absence of the ACL. It is important to examine the contralateral knee to assist in ruling out these other entities. The timing of the injury, either acute or chronic, should also be noted.

Arthroscopy has assisted in the determination of ACL tears, especially in the acute period.[6] Examination under anesthesia for laxity and pivot shift, and arthroscopic visualization of the ligament to assess partial or complete tears can assist in determining an appropriate treatment plan. An acute hemarthrosis in the young knee alerts the clinician to a major joint injury, and arthroscopic examination of the knee for an acute hemarthrosis has shown ACL ligament injury in 47% of cases.[24]

Advances in imaging have enhanced the ability to identify ACL tears. Magnetic resonance imaging has assisted the clinician in detecting ACL tears with a high level of specificity and sensitivity. With a knowledge of the symptom complex and physical examination, an ACL tear can be diagnosed.

Assessment of Skeletal Maturity

It is important to define the patient's true level of skeletal immaturity, because this and physiologic physeal closure are variable with respect to age.[9,15,25] The young patient may have significant growth

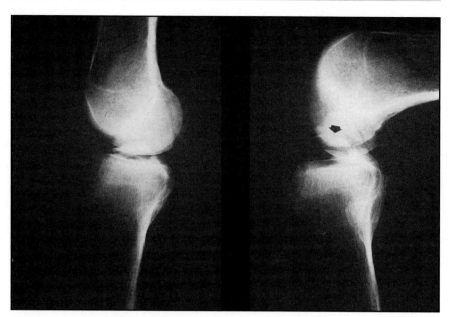

Fig. 1 Lateral radiographs demonstrating tibial spine avulsion.

remaining, and surgical procedures near the physis, such as ACL repair or reconstruction may increase the risk for deformity and leg-length discrepancy. The patient can be assessed chronologically for age, and physiologically for signs of development, including secondary sexual characteristics such as menarche and pigmented pubic and axillary hair as noted by Tanner and Davies,[25] and cessation of change in shoe size. Family height can be used as an appropriate estimate of growth potential. In addition, the patient can be assessed radiographically for determination of bone age using Risser's sign in the pelvis or examination of hand and wrist on an AP view of the wrist, comparing the findings to known standards in an atlas.[14]

Roche and associates[15] studied radiographic patterns of maturation of the knee to develop a formula for knee-specific estimates of skeletal age. Skeletal age estimates based on the knee should be superior to those based on the wrist, especially when predicting longitudinal growth potential or planning surgical procedures about the knee. Roche noted radiographic knee maturation patterns

such as "capping" of the metaphysis by the epiphysis, which precedes physiologic physeal fusion. Information about a patient's skeletal maturity is crucial in delineating a treatment plan for ACL injuries and in determining risks to the physis with surgical treatment.

Tibial Eminence Fractures

Tibial eminence fractures represent a unique variant of ACL disruption (Fig. 1), where the bony insertion of the ligament on the intercondylar tibial eminence is avulsed. Rinaldi and Mazzarella[26] noted that, in the skeletally immature patient, the tibial spine offers less resistance than the ACL substance to traction forces. Thus, an injury that could cause a mid-substance tear in the adult can result in an avulsion of the tibial spine in the skeletally immature.

Meyers and McKeever[27] noted that the most common mechanism of injury is a fall from a bicycle or motorcycle and stated that a child with a swollen knee following a fall from a bicycle should be considered to have a fracture of the intercondylar eminence until proven otherwise. Other mechanisms include sports

injuries and pedestrian-motor vehicle trauma.[28] Many authors have reported collateral ligament and meniscal injuries with tibial spine avulsions.[27,29–32]

Meyers and McKeever[30] classified tibial spine fractures (Fig. 2), with type 1 fractures having minimal or no displacement and type 2 fractures having anterior hinging of one third to one half of the tibial eminence. Type 3 fractures are completely displaced from the fracture bed and type 3+ fractures have rotational malalignment. Zaricznyj[32] further noted a type 4 fracture, in which the displaced fragment is comminuted.

Treatment of Tibial Eminence Fractures

Type 2 and type 3 fractures can usually be treated with closed reduction and immobilization. Aspiration of a tense hemarthrosis is necessary to allow the knee to be brought closer to full extension. Many authors recommend immobilization in approximately 20° of flexion in a long leg cast for 4 to 6 weeks.[27,31,33–35] Micheli[11] and Micheli and Foster[31] stated that the fracture fragment is subject to the least tension at 15° to 30° of flexion and that further extension to 0° results in displacement of the fragment. This empiric observation has been supported by biomechanical studies, which demonstrate the lowest in-vitro strain at 35° of flexion.[36–40] Others have recommended immobilization in full extension to allow the femoral condyles to compress the fragment into its fracture bed.[28,34,35,41] Roberts[42] stated that the terminal 5° of extension mechanically reduces the tibial eminence fracture by direct contact with the lateral femoral condyle. The reduction must be confirmed fluoroscopically or under direct vision, by either arthroscopic or open methods, in order to determine the knee position that optimizes the reduction.

If reduction following closed manipulation is unsatisfactory, then open or arthroscopic reduction may be neces-

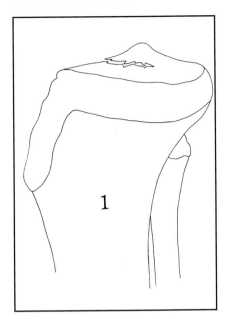
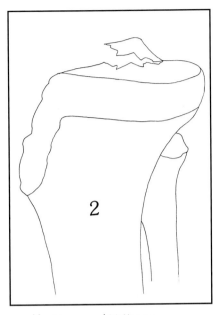
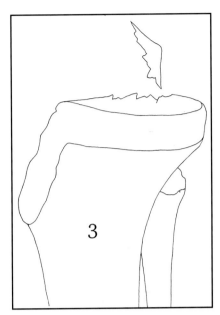

Fig. 2 Classification of tibial spine fractures as proposed by Meyers and McKeever.

sary.[27,28,30,33,41,43] The fracture fragment and bed are debrided of interposed soft tissue, including meniscus or cartilage, which may be preventing proper seating of the fracture fragment. Arthroscopic fixation (Fig. 3) of the fracture fragment may be accomplished using a heavy absorbable suture woven through the anteromedial and anterolateral portions of the ACL fracture fragment.[34,35,44,45] These sutures are then tied anteriorly through drill holes in the proximal tibial epiphysis. Immobilization in extension for approximately 2 weeks is followed by range-of-motion exercises.

Frequently, the fracture fragment is larger than it appears radiographically. If the fracture fragment is of sufficient size, fixation may be achieved with 3.5-mm cannulated screws or smooth pin fixation placed in retrograde fashion from the anterior epiphysis.[32,45] Trans-epiphyseal fixation is not recommended because of the risk of anterior growth arrest and hyperextension deformity of the knee.[46] Some authors have recommended suturing the anterior horn of the lateral meniscus or the medial meniscus to the fragment.[28,45]

It is important to emphasize that whether reduction is achieved by closed technique or by internal fixation, the avulsed anterior cartilaginous component can still become displaced. Therefore, regardless of the method of reduction, a period of immobilization in extension is essential.

The overall results following adequate reduction of the tibial spine are good to excellent.[27,30,33,43] Sequelae following tibial spine fractures may include residual ACL laxity and loss of terminal knee extension.[28,41] Residual ACL laxity may be secondary to a number of factors, including secondary hypertrophy and lengthening of the tibial spine, functional ACL lengthening, or associated ACL injury. In a primate study, Noyes and associates[47] demonstrated disruption of normal collagen architecture of ACL fibers in which failure of the ACL had occurred at the tibial spine. At long-term follow up of 45 patients with open reduction of tibial eminence fractures, Wiley and Baxter[28] found minimal side to side differences in anterior laxity in type I injuries with a mean difference of 1 mm, but more significant side to side differ-

ences in type II (3 mm) and type III (4 mm) injuries. Greater laxity (5 mm) was noted in patients who suffered pedestrian-motor vehicle trauma. Willis and associates[41] found mean side to side differences of 1 mm, 3.5 mm, and 4.5 mm, in 56 patients with types I, II, and III tibial spine avulsions, respectively, at 2- to 8-year evaluations. Two of these patients were treated by cast in 20° of flexion, 36 with aspiration or arthroscopy and closed reduction in extension, and 18 with open reduction and internal fixation. Functional results were good, however, with 84% returning to the same level of sports and 98% without complaints of giving way.

Also, loss of terminal knee extension may result following tibial spine fractures.[27,43] Lengthening and hypertrophy of the tibial spine can occur secondary to hyperemia or residual displacement and can provide a bony block to extension. In Wiley and Baxter's[28] series of 45 patients, all patients had some decrease in extension (range, 4° to 15°), and 64% of the patients were symptomatic. Willis and associates[41] reported no significant (> 10°) loss of extension.

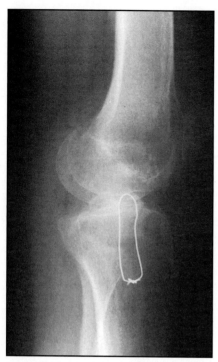

Fig. 3 Technique of arthroscopic suture fixation of tibial eminence fractures.

Treatment of ACL Injury

Treatment of ACL injury in the immature knee must take into account the developmental aspects of the growing knee, namely the fragility of the physis and the grave consequences of physeal damage. The long-term function and wide range of potential demands on the knee in the patient's future must be carefully considered as treatment is planned.

Nonsurgical Treatment

Due to the risk of physeal damage with surgical treatment, nonsurgical treatment has been used in the skeletally immature patient.[11,31] One treatment plan is to use rehabilitation and bracing to defer surgical treatment until skeletal maturity. Most reports indicate that patients treated nonsurgically have a poor prognosis with respect to return to sports and long-term sequelae.[16–18,20] Angel and Hall[1] reviewed 22 ACL-deficient skeletally immature patients at an average follow-up of 51

months, and no patient with a complete ACL tear was able to return to sports at a preinjury level. McCarroll and associates[6] treated 16 patients with quadriceps and hamstring rehabilitation and bracing. Nine were unable to return to sports, and all 16 patients had giving way episodes.

Also, many long-term consequences have been reported in ACL-deficient skeletally immature patients, including repeated giving way episodes, meniscal damage, and early arthrosis. Graf and associates[19] treated eight patients with rehabilitation and bracing. At a follow-up of only 2 years, all eight patients had symptoms of giving way, and seven of eight patients had developed new meniscal tears. Mizuta and associates[7] treated 18 patients with rehabilitation and bracing. At a minimum follow-up of 36 months, all patients were symptomatic: 17 had giving way episodes, nine had evidence of secondary meniscal tears, and 11 had evidence of early degenerative arthritis.

It is difficult to quantify the success of nonsurgical treatment in the literature, because demands on the ACL-deficient knee vary according to activity. It is also unclear whether associated lesions, such as cartilage damage, patellofemoral pain, or meniscal lesions, are responsible for treatment failures in the goal of returning to sports. Nonetheless, most reports indicate that the success of nonsurgical treatment of ACL insufficiency in the skeletally immature is poor. Despite adequate rehabilitation and bracing, the majority of active patients will develop symptomatic instability, be unable to return to sports, sustain meniscal tears, and suffer long-term sequelae of articular damage.

Surgical Treatment

There have been reports of many surgical treatment options including primary repair, extra-articular procedures, intra-articular procedures without transphyseal graft tunnels, and intra-articular procedures using transphyseal tunnels.

Primary ACL Repair

DeLee and Curtis[48] reported on three patients who underwent primary ACL repair through sutures tied across the physis. At 21-month follow-up, all had clinical laxity and two of the three had subsequent episodes of giving way. Engebretsen and associates[49] reviewed eight patients 3 to 8 years following primary repair and found that all experienced a decreased level of activity and five of the eight demonstrated gross instability at clinical examination. Grontvedt and associates[14] noted that results of primary ACL repair in the skeletally immature are no better than those in adults. In summary, the results of primary repair in children are poor. Permanent plastic deformation and early degeneration of the ligament as may contribute to failure.

Extra-Articular Reconstruction

Extra-articular procedures have been used for ACL-deficient knees in adults in the past. The advantage of these techniques in skeletally immature patients is that drilling across the physis is not required. In 1988, McCarroll and associates[6] reported on a group of 24 skeletally immature patients with midsubstance ACL disruptions treated surgically. Ten underwent extra-articular procedures, with tenodesis of the iliotibial band in three and a modified Andrews iliotibial band tenodesis in seven. At a mean follow-up of 26 months, five of 10 patients experienced mild instability during sports activity. Subsequent reports by McCarroll and associates[21] confirmed deteriorating results with extra-articular techniques, and these are no longer recommended by the authors as stabilizing procedures in children.

In a follow-up of two skeletally immature patients who underwent extra-articular reconstruction, Graf and associates[19] reported that both had developed recurrent instability and secondary meniscal damage. It appears that extra-articular reconstruction in the skeletally immature as either temporizing or definitive treatment does not prevent subsequent instability and reinjury.

Intra-Articular Reconstructions

To determine the risk of drilling a graft tunnel across the physis, Guzzanti and associates[50] performed 21 semitendinosus reconstructions in a rabbit model through tibial and femoral tunnels 2 mm in diameter. This procedure caused damage to 11% of the femoral physis in the frontal plane and 3% of its cross-sectional area, yet no alteration in growth or axial deviation was noted in the femur at the 6-month evaluation. Tibial physis cross section analysis revealed 12% damage in the frontal plane and 4% involvement of its cross-sectional diameter. Two tibiae subsequently developed valgus deformities, and one tibia became shortened. Stadlemaier and associates[51] found no evidence of alteration of growth plate anatomy with fascia lata autografts placed in tunnels drilled across the femoral and tibial physes in dogs. The safe threshold for tibial and femoral physeal tunnels in humans has yet to be determined.

In adults, the most effective treatment of the symptomatic ACL-deficient knee is intra-articular reconstruction of the ACL with anatomic graft placement. To consider intra-articular ACL reconstruction with its risk of physeal injury, young patients must be divided into those approaching skeletal maturity, who have little growth remaining, and those prepubescent children who have "wide open" physes with significant growth remaining. The more skeletally mature group can be offered intra-articular reconstructions with minimal risk of growth arrest or deformity, because physiologic physeal closure is imminent.

The treatment of the less skeletally mature group with significant growth remaining, however, is controversial. The risks of early physeal closure, limb-length discrepancy, and angular deformity are higher, and intra-articular ACL reconstruction through transphyseal drill holes has historically been discouraged. Many clinicians have advocated nonsurgical treatment until skeletal maturity draws closer. Unfortunately, compliance with a nonsurgical treatment plan of limited activity and bracing is often low in active children. In addition, it appears that this group of patients is at a particularly high risk for recurrent instability, with associated meniscal tears. Also, the potential for the occurrence of secondary arthritic changes while surgical stabilization is delayed is a concern.

Nontransphyseal Intra-Articular Reconstructions

In an attempt to provide knee stability while reducing the risk of physeal damage, Brief[52] developed a technique of ACL reconstruction without the use of transphyseal drill holes. The semitendinosus and gracilis tendon grafts were left with their distal attachments intact and passed into the knee joint under the anterior horn of the medial meniscus. The graft was fixed to the lateral femoral condyle epiphysis by staples in the over-the-top position. All patients also had extra-articular iliotibial band tenodesis. In this report of nine patients with a mean age at reconstruction of 17.2 years at 3- to 6.5-year follow up, no patient had a pivot shift and eight of the nine were without symptoms of instability. At follow-up, all patients had a 1+ Lachman's test and 1+ anterior drawer test, which may indicate graft stretching. Six of nine patients were able to return to sports at their preinjury level, but with bracing and precautions.

Parker and associates[8] reported their results in five patients who had ACL reconstruction using hamstring tendons placed in a groove over the front of the tibia and over the top of the femur. At a mean follow-up of 33 months, four of five patients had returned to their previous level of competitive sports. No patient had a positive pivot shift test; two patients had a 1+ Lachman's test. Instrumented laxity measurements revealed a mean side-to-side difference of 3.6 mm ± 1.9 mm. Radiographic follow-up revealed symmetric closure of three growth plates and two that remained symmetrically open. Leg-length discrepancies of 1.0 cm were noted in all five patients.

Despite its low risk to the physis, this technique is acknowledged to be nonisometric and nonanatomic. The long-term success of the graft remains unknown.

Intra-Articular Reconstruction With Transphyseal Graft Tunnels

Similar to the reconstruction techniques used in adults, intra-articular reconstruction with transphyseal drill holes has been used in skeletally immature patients.[21,53-55] Most series have used soft-tissue grafts, such as hamstring tendon autograft and Achilles tendon or fascia lata allograft. The use of bone-patellar tendon-bone grafts has also been reported.[21]

Lipscomb and Anderson[54] reviewed 24 patients who underwent open semitendinosus and gracilis reconstruction using a transphyseal tibial drill hole and a femoral epiphyseal drill hole. There were 11 patients with completely open physes and 13 patients with partially open physes. At mean follow-up of 35 months, 15 of 24 had returned to their preinjury level of activity. The mean instrumented side-to-side laxity difference was 1.6 mm. Orthoroentgenograms revealed a limb-length discrepancy of 5 to 10 mm in five patients, one patient with a 13 mm difference, and one patient with a 20 mm difference, which was attributed to inadvertent stapling across the tibial and femoral physes during graft fixation. When considering the smaller discrepancies, it is important to remember that 77% of the normal population have a mean leg-length discrepancy of 7 mm, and in 7% to 8% of normal patients a 12.5 mm or greater leg-length

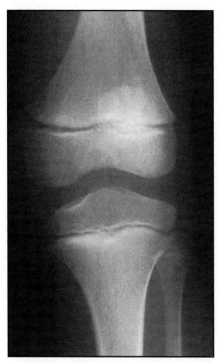

Fig. 4 AP radiograph of a typical patient with "wide open" physes. (Reproduced with permission from Lo IKY, Fowler PJ, Miniaci A, et al: The outcome of operatively treated anterior cruciate ligament disruptions in the skeletally immature child. Presented at the Canadian Orthopaedic Association Annual Scientific Meeting, Quebec City, Quebec, May, 1996. *Arthroscopy* 1997;13:627–634.)

discrepancy is noted.[15,56]

In 1988, McCarroll treated selected young patients surgically with intra-articular reconstruction using bone-patellar tendon-bone autograft and a concomitant extra-articular procedure for "reinforcement" with excellent clinical results and no growth disturbances.[6] In 1994, McCarroll and associates[21] reported their experience of 60 patients and proposed a protocol for the management of ACL disruptions in the skeletally immature. In general, patients who were Tanner stage 1 or 2, with evidence of skeletal immaturity represented by "wide open" physes, no occurrence of the adolescent growth spurt, and a significant height discrepancy (10 to 15 cm shorter when compared to grown siblings or parents), were treated

nonsurgically. Thirty-eight patients fit this criteria and were initially treated with a program of rehabilitation, bracing, and activity modification for a mean time of 29 months (range, 3 to 120). Symptomatic meniscal tears developed in 27 of the 38 patients.

Patients were treated surgically if there was radiographic evidence of skeletal maturity, the adolescent growth spurt had occurred, height was similar to parents and siblings (within 2.5-5.0 cm), and Tanner stage was at least 4. Central bone-patellar tendon-bone grafts 10 mm in width were used, with transphyseal tibial and femoral tunnels. Results of reconstruction were good, with 55 of 60 patients returning to sports and no reports of giving way. In addition, no growth disturbances or angular deformities were noted. The mean postoperative gain in height was only 2.3 cm, which is consistent with this group's skeletal maturity.

In 1994, Andrews and associates[53] reported on the use of 7-mm fascia lata or Achilles tendon allograft through transphyseal tibial drill holes and over-the-top positioning on the femur. At a mean follow-up of 58 months, all eight patients demonstrated symmetric closure of the growth plates, with no clinically significant limb-length discrepancy on orthoroentgenograms. The mean height increase postoperatively was 4.55 cm.

Lo and associates[55] reviewed ACL reconstruction in cases of extreme skeletal immaturity. From a larger series of 19 skeletally immature children who had undergone ACL reconstruction, five patients with evidence of "wide open" physes on plain radiographs were identified (Fig. 4). The mean age was 12.9 years, with the youngest patient 8 years of age at the time of reconstruction (Fig. 5). All patients had tibial tunnels of 6 mm or less in diameter drilled across an open tibial physis, with graft placement in an over-the-top position on the femur. All grafts were of soft tissue. Three of the reconstructions used hamstring tendons and

two used quadriceps prepateller fascia-patellar tendon. The Kennedy Ligament Augmentation Device (LAD™) was used in four cases. At a mean follow-up of 7.4 years, no patient had a positive anterior drawer, Lachman, or pivot shift test. All patients had instrumented laxity side-to-side differences of ≤ 3 mm, and the mean was 1.0 mm ± 1.6 mm. MRI demonstrated that four tibial physes had closed in a symmetric fashion and one remained open (Fig. 5). Orthoroentgenograms revealed no significant leg-length discrepancy (-0.8 mm ± 3.4 mm) or angular deformity. International Knee Documentation Committee evaluation scores were grade A (normal) in four and grade C (abnormal) in one. Four of five patients had returned to their preinjury activity level and one could participate only in light activities. The one patient with a poorer result had a 12-mm loose body identified by MRI from a patellar osteochondral fracture suffered post-reconstruction. The mean height gained postoperatively was 14.3 cm (range 7.5 cm to 28.5 cm), which is consistent with the true skeletal immaturity of the group.

It is evident that intra-articular reconstructions with soft tissue grafts can be performed with low risk of physeal injury in young patients either approaching or a significant time from skeletal maturity. While the use of bony grafts across the physis in the younger skeletally immature patient has not been reported, these are contraindicated when there is significant growth remaining.

Summary

Anterior cruciate ligament injury in the skeletally immature is becoming increasingly recognized and reported. History taking and physical examination based on the principles of ACL injuries in adults, with adjuncts such as arthroscopy and MRI, are effective in diagnosing ACL injury in the young patient. Evaluation of the young patient's true level of skeletal immaturity by comparison with family

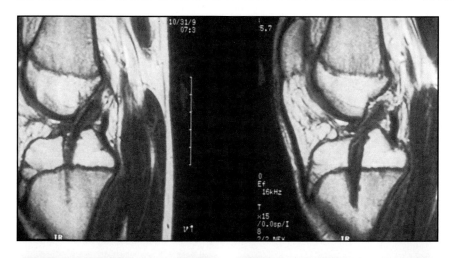

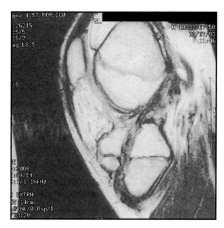

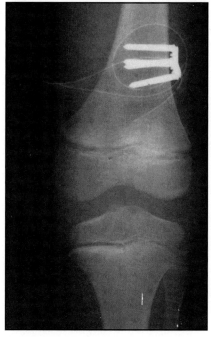

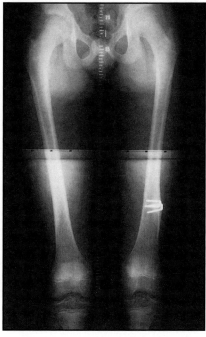

Fig. 5 Our youngest patient reconstructed at age 8. T-2 weighted coronal MRI revealing symmetric open tibial physis at, **top left**, 4.5 years postoperative, and **top right**, 6 years postoperative. Serial long leg films reveal no angular deformity or leg-length discrepancy and migration of staple fixation. (Reproduced with permission from Lo IKY, Fowler PJ, Miniaci A, Kirkley A: The outcome of operatively treated anterior cruciate ligament disruptions in the skeletally immature child. Presented at the Canadian Orthopaedic Association Annual Scientific Meeting, Quebec City, Quebec, May, 1996. *Arthroscopy* 1997;13:627–634.) **Bottom left**, 1 year postoperative, and **bottom right**, 4.5 years postoperative.

growth history, examination for signs of sexual maturity, and radiographic evaluation is critical. The risk of physeal damage with surgical treatment is related to the immaturity of the distal femoral and proximal tibial physes.

The functional results of nonsurgical treatment of ACL injury, either as an attempt at definitive treatment or as a temporizing plan until skeletal maturity occurs, are poor and the risks of reinjury and further meniscal and cartilage damage are significant. Surgical treatment for primary repair or extra-articular recon-

struction alone has not proven to be efficacious. In the adolescent patient who is approaching skeletal maturity, risk of physeal injury is low and intra-articular reconstruction can be performed as in the adult patient. Results with respect to decreased laxity and return to athletic activities mirror those described in adults.

In patients with significant growth remaining, however, surgical treatment carries much higher risks of physeal damage and subsequent deformity. Yet, as noted above, intra-articular reconstruc-

tion in truly skeletally immature patients using a soft-tissue graft through a transphyseal tibial tunnel of moderate or small diameter and the over-the-top position on the femur has not been shown to cause early physeal closure, limb-length discrepancy, or angular deformity. In humans, the maximum diameter of graft tunnel that will not cause physeal closure has not been determined. Animal studies have shown that the tibial physis can be very sensitive to drilling. Therefore it is wise to use moderate tunnel diameters. Bone-patellar tendon-bone grafts have been used with success in patients closer to skeletal maturity. Their use has not been reported in the very skeletally immature knee and cannot be recommended because of the presumed high risk of physeal closure with a bone plug traversing the physis.

It is hoped that improved understanding of the ACL injury in the skeletally immature patient will provide treatment options that will restore enduring knee function and prevent early arthrosis.

References

1. Angel KR, Hall DJ: Anterior cruciate ligament injury in children and adolescents. *Arthroscopy* 1989;5:197–200.

2. DeLee JC: ACL insufficiency in children, in Feagin JA Jr (ed): *The Crucial Ligaments: Diagnosis and Treatment of Ligamentous Injuries About the Knee.* New York, NY, Churchill Livingstone, 1988, pp 439–447.

3. Gallagher SS, Finison K, Guyer B: The incidence of injuries among 87,000 Massachusetts children and adolescents: Results of the 1980-81 Statewide Childhood Injury Prevention Program Surveillance System. *Am J Public Health* 1984;74:1340–1347.

4. Goldberg B: Pediatric sports medicine, in Scott WN, Nisonson B, Nicholas JA (eds): *Principles of Sports Medicine.* Baltimore, MD, Williams & Wilkins, 1984, pp 403–426.

5. Matz SO, Jackson DW: Anterior cruciate ligament injury in children. *Am J Knee Surg* 1988;1:59–65.

6. McCarroll JR, Rettig AC, Shelbourne KD: Anterior cruciate ligament injuries in the young athlete with open physes. *Am J Sports Med* 1988;16:44–47.

7. Mizuta H, Kubota K, Shiraishi M, et al: The conservative treatment of complete tears of the anterior cruciate ligament in skeletally immature patients. *J Bone Joint Surg* 1995;77B: 890–894.

8. Parker AW, Drez D Jr, Cooper JL: Anterior cruciate ligament injuries in patients with open physes. *Am J Sports Med* 1994;22:44–47.

9. Stanitski CL: Anterior cruciate ligament injury in the skeletally immature patient: Diagnosis and treatment. *J Am Acad Orthop Surg* 1995;3:146–158.

10. Sullivan JA: Ligamentous injuries of the knee in children. *Clin Orthop* 1990;255:44–50.

11. Micheli LJ: Pediatric and adolescent sports injuries: Recent trends. *Exerc Sport Sci Rev* 1986;14:359–374.

12. Nottage WM, Matsuura PA: Management of complete traumatic anterior cruciate ligament tears in the skeletally immature patient: Current concepts and review of the literature. *Arthroscopy* 1994;10:569–573.

13. Hawkins RJ, Misamore GW, Merritt TR: Followup of the acute non-operated isolated anterior cruciate ligament tear. *Am J Sports Med* 1986;14:205–210.

14. Grontvedt T, Engebretsen L, Benum P, et al: A prospective, randomized study of three operations for acute rupture of the anterior cruciate ligament: Five-year follow-up of one hundred and thirty-one patients. *J Bone Joint Surg* 1996;78A:159–168.

15. Roche AF, Wainer H, Thissen D (eds): *Skeletal Maturity: The Knee Joint as a Biological Indicator.* New York, NY, Plenum Medical, 1975.

16. Bradley GW, Shives TC, Samuelson KM: Ligament injuries in the knees of children. *J Bone Joint Surg* 1979;61A:588–591.

17. Chick RR, Jackson DW: Tears of the anterior cruciate ligament in young athletes. *J Bone Joint Surg* 1978;60A:970–973.

18. Clanton TO, DeLee JC, Sanders B, et al: Knee ligament injuries in children. *J Bone Joint Surg* 1979;61A:1195–1201.

19. Graf BK, Lange RH, Fujisaki CK, et al: Anterior cruciate ligament tears in skeletally immature patients: Meniscal pathology at presentation and after attempted conservative treatment. *Arthroscopy* 1992;8:229–233.

20. Kannus P, Järvinen M: Knee ligament injuries in adolescents: Eight-year follow-up of conservative management. *J Bone Joint Surg* 1988;70B; 772–776.

21. McCarroll JR, Shelbourne KD, Porter DA, et al: Patellar tendon graft reconstruction for midsubstance anterior cruciate ligament rupture in junior high school athletes: An algorithm for management. *Am J Sports Med* 1994;22: 478–484.

22. Hart JAL: Abstract: Meniscal injury associated with acute and chronic ligamentous instability of the knee joint. *J Bone Joint Surg* 1982;64B: 119.

23. Jones RE, Henley MB, Francis P: Nonoperative management of isolated grade III collateral ligament injury in high school football players. *Clin Orthop* 1986;213:137–140.

24. Stanitski CL, Harvell JC, Fu F: Observations on acute knee hemarthrosis in children and adolescents. *J Pediatr Orthop* 1993;13:506–510.

25. Tanner JM, Davies PS: Clinical longitudinal standards for height and height velocity for North American children. *J Pediatr* 1985;107: 317–329.

26. Rinaldi E, Mazzarella F: Isolated fracture-avulsions of the tibial insertions of the cruciate ligaments of the knee. *Ital J Orthop Traumatol* 1980;6:77–83.

27. Meyers MH, McKeever FM: Fracture of the intercondylar eminence of the tibia. *J Bone Joint Surg* 1970;52A:1677–1684.

28. Wiley JJ, Baxter MP: Tibial spine fractures in children. *Clin Orthop* 1990;255:54–60.

29. DeLee JC: Ligamentous injury of the knee, in Stanitski CL, DeLee JC, Drez D Jr (eds): *Pediatric and Adolescent Sports Medicine.*

Philadelphia, PA, WB Saunders, 1994, vol 3, pp 406–432.

30. Meyers MH, McKeever FM: Fracture of the intercondylar eminence of the tibia. *J Bone Joint Surg* 1959;41A:209–222.

31. Micheli LJ, Foster TE: Acute knee injuries in the immature athlete, in Heckman JD (ed): *Instructional Course Lectures 42.* Rosemont, IL, American Academy of Orthopaedic Surgeons, 1993, pp 473–481.

32. Zaricznyj B: Avulsion fracture of the tibial eminence: Treatment by open reduction and pinning. *J Bone Joint Surg* 1977;59A:1111–1114.

33. Molander ML, Wallin G, Wikstad I: Fracture of the intercondylar eminence of the tibia: A review of 35 patients. *J Bone Joint Surg* 1981;63B:89–91.

34. Rask BP, Micheli LJ: Knee ligament injuries and associated derangements in children and adolescents, in Fu FH, Harner CD, Vince KG, et al (eds): *Knee Surgery.* Baltimore, MD, Williams & Wilkins, 1995, pp 365–381.

35. Warner JJP, Micheli LJ: Pediatric and adolescent musculoskeletal injuries, in Grana WA, Kalenak A (eds): *Clinical Sports Medicine.* Philadelphia, PA, WB Saunders, 1991, pp 490–498.

36. Kennedy JC, Hawkins RJ, Willis RB: Strain gauge analysis of knee ligaments. *Clin Orthop* 1977;129:225–229.

37. Meglan D, Zuelzer W, Buck W, et al: The effects of quadriceps force upon strain in the anterior cruciate ligament. *Trans Orthop Res Soc* 1986;11:55.

38. Noyes FR, Grood ES, Butler DL, et al: Clinical laxity tests and functional stability of the knee: Biomechanical concepts. *Clin Orthop* 1980;146: 84–89.

39. Smith BA, Livesay GA, Woo SL: Biology and biomechanics of the anterior cruciate ligament. *Clin Sports Med* 1993;12:637–670.

40. Takeda Y, Xerogeanes JW, Livesay GA, et al: Biomechanical function of the human anterior cruciate ligament. *Arthroscopy* 1994;10:140–147.

41. Willis RB, Blokker C, Stoll TM, et al: Long-term follow-up of anterior tibial eminence fractures. *J Pediatr Orthop* 1993;13:361–364.

42. Roberts JM: Avulsion fractures of the proximal tibial epiphysis, in Fowler PJ, Kennedy JC (ed): *The Injured Adolescent Knee.* Baltimore, MD, Williams & Wilkins, 1979.

43. Baxter MP, Wiley JJ: Fractures of the tibial spine in children: An evaluation of knee stability. *J Bone Joint Surg* 1988;70B:228–230.

44. Kogan M, Amendola A: Arthroscopic suture fixation of displaced tibial intercondylar eminence fractures. *Arthroscopy* 1997;13:301–306.

45. Roberts JM: Operative treatment of fractures about the knee. *Orthop Clin North Am* 1990;21: 365–379.

46. Mylle J, Reynders P, Broos P: Transepiphysial fixation of anterior cruciate avulsion in a child: Report of a complication and review of the literature. *Arch Orthop Trauma Surg* 1993;112: 101–103.

47. Noyes FR, DeLucas JL, Torvik PJ: Biomechanics of anterior cruciate ligament failure: An
analysis of strain-rate sensitivity and mechanisms of failure in primates. *J Bone Joint Surg*
1974;56A:236–253.

48. DeLee JC, Curtis R: Anterior cruciate ligament
insufficiency in children. *Clin Orthop*
1983;172:112–118.

49. Engebretsen L, Svenningsen S, Benum P: Poor
results of anterior cruciate ligament repair in
adolescence. *Acta Orthop Scand* 1988;59:
684–686.

50. Guzzanti V, Falciglia F, Gigante A, et al: The
effect of intra-articular ACL reconstruction on
the growth plates of rabbits. *J Bone Joint Surg*
1994;76B:960–963.

51. Stadlemaier DN, Arnoczky SP, Dodds H, et al:
The effect of drilling and soft tissue grafting
across open growth plates: A histologic study.
Am J Sports Med 1995;23:431–435.

52. Brief LP: Anterior cruciate ligament reconstruction without drill holes. *Arthroscopy*
1991;7:350–357.

53. Andrews M, Noyes FR, Barber-Westin SD:
Anterior cruciate ligament allograft reconstruc-
tion in the skeletally immature athlete. *Am J
Sports Med* 1994;22:48–54.

54. Lipscomb AB, Anderson AF: Tears of the anterior cruciate ligament in adolescents. *J Bone
Joint Surg* Am 1986;68:19–28.

55. Lo IKY, Fowler PJ, Miniaci A, et al: The outcome of operatively treated anterior cruciate
ligament disruptions in the skeletally immature. Presented at the Canadian Orthopaedic
Association Annual Scientific Meeting,
Quebec City, Quebec, May, 1996. *Arthroscopy*
1997;13:627–634.

56. Nichols PJR: Short-leg syndrome. *Br Med J*
1960;1:1863–1865.

Revision Anterior Cruciate Ligament Reconstruction

Eric W. Carson, MD
Peter T. Simonian, MD
Thomas L. Wickiewicz, MD
Russell F. Warren, MD

Introduction

Anterior cruciate ligament (ACL) injury and subsequent reconstruction are increasingly common.[1] After primary ACL reconstruction, long-term good to excellent results range from 75% to more than 90%.[2–5] However, because a substantial group of patients will have an unsatisfactory outcome, with pain and arthritis,[2,3,6] loss of motion,[7–10] and graft failure,[2–4,6] the need for revision ACL reconstruction continues to increase. Successful revision surgery begins with a methodical and organized approach. A complete understanding of the etiology for these failures is essential. A thorough preoperative evaluation, consisting of a detailed history, physical examination, and radiographic examination, is required. Despite adequate planning, the degree of unpredictability is significantly increased with revision surgery; therefore, an understanding of described ACL revision techniques is invaluable.[11–17]

Etiology of Failed ACL Reconstruction

Before the etiology of ACL reconstruction failure can be discussed, it must first be defined. Several factors must be considered, including limited motion,[7–10,18] recurrent instability,[2–4,6] and/or arthrosis.[2,3,6]

Loss of Motion/Arthrofibrosis

Motion loss is the most common complication following intra-articular ACL reconstruction.[7–10,18–23] The reported incidence of motion loss is variable, probably because of the different criteria used to define it and variations between studies in timing and in the techniques used for reconstruction. Sachs and associates[23] reported a 24% incidence of loss of extension greater than 5° following ACL reconstruction. Loss of extension is typically more detrimental than loss of flexion, particularly in the high-performance athlete. Loss of extension may be more disabling than the preoperative instability. Typically, patients with extension loss tend to have limited success with physical therapy, to ambulate with an abnormal bent leg gait, and to have patellofemoral pain secondary to increased force at the joint.[23]

Etiologic factors for loss of motion include intercondylar notch scarring (approximately 50% of all cases), non-anatomic graft placement, capsulitis with ligament scarring or calcification, concomitant ligament surgery, anterior nodule or Cyclops lesion, immobilization, infection, and/or reflex sympathetic dystrophy. Before considering revision surgery, correct identification of the etiologic factor is crucial.[11,12,14–16,17,24–28]

Once the etiology for the loss of motion has been determined, a logical treatment plan can be formulated. The inflammatory phase of the knee is critical. Surgical intervention must be avoided when the knee is highly inflamed in order to avoid further compromise to the range of motion. The surgeon's primary goal should be to obtain a maximal, painless range of motion of the knee before attempting any type of surgery. A staged procedure may be required. The goal of the first stage is to obtain functional motion, and the second stage addresses any recurrent instability, if present.

Particular attention must be paid to capsulitis or arthrofibrosis, conditions associated with periarticular inflammation and swelling related to an exaggerated healing response. Patients often complain of pain and stiffness, resulting in quadriceps inhibition. On physical examination, there can be loss of motion, reduced patellar mobility, increased warmth, and diffused swelling of the knee. If these problems are not recognized, the patient may progress to patella baja, eventually leading to infrapatellar contracture syndrome.[8,29] Treatment goals are directed at early diagnosis and reduction of the inflammatory reaction. Aggressive and forceful manipulation should be avoided. In the acute phase of these conditions, treatment involves the use of nonsteroidal anti-inflammatory drugs and gentle range of motion. In the fibrotic phase, if there has been no improvement after 3 months, arthroscopic debridement should be considered. Extension should be obtained first, followed by flexion. At times a second arthroscopic debridement may be needed to regain flexion. The final and most advanced phase, infrapatellar contracture syndrome, often requires open debridement and releases.[8]

Recurrent Instability

The incidence of recurrent instability after a primary ACL reconstruction has been reported to range from 0.7% to 8%.[2-5] Identifying the cause of recurrent instability can be difficult. Johnson and associates[13] have attempted to classify the causes into three categories: (1) technical errors, (2) failure of graft incorporation, and (3) recurrent trauma.

Traumatic Arthritis

One goal of ACL reconstruction is to prevent or postpone the development of traumatic arthritis. Whether this goal is attainable with ACL reconstruction is controversial and is likely related to patient selection.[30] Questions regarding the effectiveness of ACL reconstruction are related to the many factors that can contribute to the development of arthritis. These include the age and activity level of the patient, the effect of the initial trauma (including meniscal and occult osteochondral injuries), and the progressive damage to cartilage secondary to instability. Bone bruises are of particular interest, because they are evident in 80% of acute ACL injuries.[31,32] These injuries typically occur on the anterolateral femoral condyle and the posterolateral tibial plateau. A bone bruise is a blunt injury that involves the bone marrow, the subchondral bone, and the overlying cartilage surface. Even if there are no visible changes to the articular surface, changes

may have occurred at the histologic and ultrastructural level.

In patients with instability and arthritis, differentiation between instability and pain can be difficult. However, it is important to differentiate these symptoms to provide appropriate treatment.

Technical Considerations

Surgical errors that can cause ACL failure include nonanatomic tunnel placement, graft impingement, inappropriate graft tension, and failure of fixation.

Tunnel Placement

With the advent of the endoscopic ACL reconstructive technique, an increasing number of failed procedures have been recognized that are secondary to nonanatomic tunnel placement. Nonanatomic tunnels affect normal knee kinematics. An improperly placed femoral or tibial tunnel will cause poor graft isometry, and the resultant excessive length changes in the graft can lead to recurrent laxity or loss of motion as the knee is captured. Either laxity or loss of motion will increase stress on the graft, resulting in its eventual failure.[25,33-39]

Because the femoral attachment of the ACL is close to the axis of rotation of the knee, small changes in the position of the femoral tunnel have a significant effect. The ideal position of the femoral tunnel should be as posterior as possible without violating the cortical posterior wall. The most common technical error is incorrect positioning of the femoral tunnel. Particularly with use of the endoscopic one-incision technique, the femoral tunnel can be placed in too anterior a position. This typically occurs because it is difficult to visualize the most posterior aspect of the femoral notch (the "over-the-top" position). Anterior placement of the femoral tunnel, which leads to excessive lengthening and tension on the ACL graft when the knee is flexed, often results in failure through the graft fixation site, through the substance of the

graft, through restriction of motion, and/or by excessive stress on the articular surfaces of the knee joint. Conversely, a more posterior position on the femur, "over the top," once commonly used, has a less detrimental effect, although there is a length increase in extension and slight looseness in flexion.

Placement of the tibial tunnel, which originally was not thought to be critical to the success of ACL surgery, has subsequently been shown to have a profound effect. The original anterior eccentric position was found to cause impingement on the intercondylar roof, loss of extension, and increased graft failure.[20,25,36,39-41] Currently, the preferred position is posteromedial on the ACL footprint.[36,40] Particular attention must be given to knees that have a vertical intercondylar roof or significant recurvaturm; these require a more posterior tunnel placement and roofplasty to avoid impingement. However, an extreme posterior placement of the tibial tunnel can result in excessive laxity in flexion, possible impingement with the posterior cruciate ligament (PCL), or injury to the PCL with drilling. Also, a nonisometric vertical orientation, which usually controls anterior translation, may not control internal rotation and can result in persistent instability.

Medial or lateral misorientation of the tibial tunnel can lead to graft failure. Medial displacement can cause articular damage to the medial tibial plateau. Lateral displacement can result in impingement against the medial aspect of the lateral femoral condyle, causing tunnel divergence, with graft abrasion and wear resulting in graft failure.

Notchplasty

An inadequate notchplasty may result in impingement.[40-42] Through a similar mechanism of abrasion on the lateral femoral condyle or the roof, repetitive trauma may result in gradual ligament attrition and eventual failure. Plain radiographs, computed tomography (CT), or magnetic resonance imaging (MRI) can aid in the preoperative assessment of notch architecture and intercondylar osteophytes.[42,43] A notchplasty that is too large can distort the anatomic position of the femoral tunnel placement. To avoid this risk, some surgeons advocate no notchplasty.

Graft Tensioning

Graft tensioning is another potential cause of failure. The optimal intraoperative tension is unknown.[44,45] Many factors are responsible for graft tension.[46,47] These include the type of graft material, the length of the graft, tunnel placement, physiologic joint laxity, the type of graft fixation, and the knee angle at time of fixation. Inadequate graft tension can lead to an incompetent and nonfunctioning graft; overtensioning can result in overconstraint, resulting in decreased motion and/or delayed revascularization, myxoid degneration, and ultimate failure.[46-48]

Graft Fixation

Initial graft fixation must be secure enough to hold the graft in position during biologic graft incorporation.[28,49-52] Fixation strength depends on the type of fixation device used. When used correctly, the interference screw has been shown to provide stronger graft pullout strength than other types of fixations, such as staples, suture fixation around a post, or a soft-tissue washer and screw.[28,49,50,52,53] However, the use of interference screws does involve potential pitfalls, including poor fixation secondary to improper sizing of bone plugs or to osteopenic bone stock, divergent or convergent screw placement relative to the bone plug, and/or failure of the graft to heal within the tunnel.[28,49,50,52-54]

Improper Diagnosis/ Multiple Ligament Injuries

The success of any surgical procedure is dependent on proper diagnosis. Diag-

nosis is of particular importance in cases involving combined ligament injuries.[55,56] ACL graft failure can occur if there are other ligament and/or soft-tissue injuries that are not recognized and treated. Gersoff and Clancy[57] have estimated that associated posterolateral laxity is present in 10% to 15% of chronic ACL-deficient knees. Failure to diagnose such associated secondary or tertiary restraint injuries will cause increased loads on the newly reconstructed ACL. Conditions such as previous subtotal or complete meniscectomy or a triple varus knee also can subtly alter the knee joint kinematics and lead to ligament failure, if additional procedures, such as high tibial osteotomy or, possibly, a meniscal allograft are not also done.[58,59]

Graft Material

The type of graft used also has a role in the possible failure of the reconstructed ACL. Currently the autogenous bone-patella tendon-bone is the graft of choice for many surgeons. Recently, other sources of autogenous tissue, such as multiple loops of the semitendinosus and gracilis tendons, have gained increased popularity. In years past, many surgeons were reluctant to use these graft sources because of concerns regarding their strength when used as a single tendon.[60] Some surgeons used augmenting devices in conjunction with these grafts. However, more recent data have shown that the quadruple semitendinosus and gracilis construct may be stronger and stiffer than bone-patellar tendon-bone.[61,62]

The role of allograft material continues to develop as we gain a better understanding of its basic science.[14,15,63-67] Irradiating allografts can decrease disease transmission, but the effect is dose dependent.[68,69] The high doses of radiation required to neutralize the human immunodeficiency virus have been shown to decrease the mechanical properties of the graft and possibly reduce the rate of graft incorporation.[68,70,71]

Complete replacement synthetic ligaments (Dacron, Gore-Tex) were used routinely through the 1980s, with promising early results. However, this use of these synthetics has been abandoned because of a significant number of complications, including massive synovitis, infection, mechanical failure or loosening, tunnel osteolysis, and ligament rupture through attrition.[11,16,72-74] Once recommended for revision ligament surgery, these synthetic grafts are now rarely used. Augmentation devices (LAD and Leeds-Keio) have fared better by providing early stability while the graft is incorporating.[64,66,75] However, concerns have been raised regarding stress-shielding related to the stiffer mechanical properties of these devices and their possible detrimental effect on revascularization of the graft.[66,76]

Failure of Graft Incorporation

Another cause of reconstruction failure occurs when the graft fails to incorporate. The graft source can affect the rate of incorporation. It is widely believed that soft-tissue graft to tunnel incorporation takes longer than bone autologous bone plug to tunnel incorporation, but this belief is controversial.[77]

Allograft material may also take longer to incorporate,[65] and differing methods of graft fixation may also impact the rate of graft incorporation. The immune response may also affect the incorporation of allograft material and it may result in bone tunnel osteolysis; however, this has not been proven.[27,78,79] Both histologic studies and biomechanical studies have demonstrated that allograft material is incorporated more slowly than autograft material.

Aside from the differences in graft material and fixation, explanations for delayed graft incorporation include avascularity related to impingement, improper tensioning of the graft, and poor tunnel placement. At the time of revision, the graft may appear intact. However, closer examination often reveals that these grafts are nonfunctional and are unable to take up tension when stressed. When ligament augmentation devices are used, they may stress-shield the graft and delay its incorporation.[66,76]

Traumatic Causes of Graft Failure

Graft failure related to recurrent trauma occurs infrequently. Sources of trauma that can cause recurrent laxity include overaggressive rehabilitation or premature return to competitive sports. The process of graft incorporation and ligamentization involves three stages—inflammation, remodeling, and maturation. During the first year after reconstruction, the graft strength and stiffness have been reported to be 30% to 50% of that of original ACL.[80,81] Excessive loads during this time can lead to plastic deformation and elongation. A clear and simple physician-directed rehabilitation program and protection of the graft during this period help to avoid such complications.[10,82,83]

Significant trauma, another source of graft failure, occurs in patients who have exhibited a complete restoration of functional stability and have returned to preinjury competitive level. The traumatic event is similar to the initial event, often with a "pop," immediate hemarthrosis, and increased anterior laxity. The other causes of graft failure, described previously, can make the knee more susceptible to recurrent trauma.

Experience at the Hospital for Special Surgery

Recently, the experience at the Hospital for Special Surgery (HSS) was reviewed. The study included 87 patients who had failed ACL surgeries during a 7-year period from 1989 to 1996. Grafts used for revision included 62 autografts (56 bone-patella tendon-bone, five hamstring tendons, and one iliotibial band) and 25 fresh frozen bone-patella tendon-bone allografts.

The etiology of the failed ACL included 41 technical errors, 22 traumatic reinjuries, seven grafts that failed to incorporate, eight related to missed associated injuries (alignment or combined ligamentous pattern), and four related to loss of motion. The mean time between primary ACL and revision was 2.7 years (range, 6 months to 13 years). Overall mean follow-up from time of revision ACL procedure was 2.1 years (range, 3 months to 6 years), including 52 patients with a minimum follow-up of 2 years, of whom 43 were available to respond to a questionnaire and undergo physical examination. The HSS Knee Ligament Evaluation revealed 62.8% good/excellent results, compared to 95.5% in the primary ACL group, a statistically significant difference. Objective laxity tests revealed a 3.1 mm mean side-to-side difference at 30°. No difference was noted between the use of allograft or autograft in the revised ACL group.

Preoperative Evaluation

The preoperative plan includes a detailed history, physical examination, and radiographic assessment to determine the type of failure, the etiology of failure, and whether the patient is a candidate for revision. If revision surgery is considered, the patient must be told what this entails and given a realistic understanding of what to expect. Revision surgery is technically more demanding than primary ACL reconstructions, the results are not equivalent, and the patient needs to know this.

The history should include a detailed sequence of events from the initial injury to the present time and should state the current status of the knee. Information should include the mechanism of the primary injury, timing from injury to surgery, and specifics about the postoperative period, including the rehabilitation program, the return to preinjury level, reinjury, and any complications. Crucial information from medical records should

include the type of graft and fixation (including the specific manufacturer and model) used, as well as the status of articular cartilage and menisci. Patients with significant osteochondral or previous subtotal or complete meniscectomy may present with the primary complaint of pain and have concurrent laxity. The treatment and prognosis for this group of patients are very different from that given to those who only have increased laxity and a primary complaint of instability.

Next, a comprehensive knee examination should be performed. The examination should include an analysis of gait and overall alignment, including attention to the double or triple varus knee. The basic knee examination should evaluate the range of motion and all translational and rotatory instability patterns; these findings should be compared to the contralateral extremity.

Radiographic evaluation should include an anteroposterior view, a lateral view, a notch view, a Merchant view, and a weightbearing posteroanterior view at 45° of flexion.[84] The femoral and tibial tunnels, as seen on the anteroposterior and lateral radiographs, can be evaluated for position, osteolysis or enlargement, possible graft impingement, and the type of hardware used for graft fixation. Patella height (alta/baja) can also be evaluated with these radiographs. The weightbearing radiograph at 45° of flexion can give information with regard to joint space narrowing and early degenerative changes, as well as information on the notch architecture. Information gained regarding the graft position and the degree of notch stenosis will be useful when performing the revision notchplasty. Full length radiographs can be used to assess the overall alignment if there is a significant component of varus. Other imaging modalities that can be used include scintigraphy, for evaluation of early degenerative changes; CT, which is helpful in detailing and defining bone loss; and MRI.[31,32] MRI can be very accurate in evaluating the ACL graft integrity and location and in assessing any associated meniscal, ligamentous, and chondral pathology.[85–87]

Revision Surgery

Once the decision has been made to proceed with the revision ACL surgery, several preparation steps must be taken. The need for specific equipment for removal of the graft and graft fixation as well as the need for allograft materials must be anticipated. Certain circumstances are best treated in a staged fashion, for example, the need to bone graft large osteolytic bone tunnel defects or the need to manipulate and/or debride the knee to regain motion prior to the definitive revision reconstructive procedure. Incisions must be carefully planned around the previous scars. Technical considerations specific to revision ACL surgery include removal of hardware and prosthetic ligaments, revision notchplasty, placement of tunnels, and graft fixation.[11–17]

Removal of Graft Fixation/ Prosthetic Graft

For revision surgery, equipment used for both primary and revision ACL must be made available. Hardware removal is not always necessary, especially if the original tunnels were positioned incorrectly. When necessary, hardware in the tibia can usually be removed through old incisions. Complete removal of all soft tissue and bone around hardware, particularly around the aperture of interference screws, is needed to properly seat the appropriate size and type of screw. Without such a maneuver, the screw head or aperture may be damaged and stripped, requiring extensive bone removal in order to retrieve the interference screw. On the femoral side this complication could significantly compromise placement of the new tunnel, necessitating bone grafting and a staged procedure. When converting a two-incision technique to an endoscopic technique,

the screw can often be left in place. The new femoral tunnel, being divergent, tends to miss the old screw. Femoral screws, when placed endoscopically, usually must be removed because of their proximity to the new tunnel. However, screws that were placed too anterior on the femur are best left alone if they do not hinder the drilling of the new tunnel. Removing these screws can weaken the bone and cause a large bone defect on the femur. Multiple sized screw drivers should also be available.

Removal of a prosthetic ligament can be very challenging. The surgeon must have a thorough understanding of the techniques used to implant the various types of prosthetic ligament substitute. Preoperative CT or MRI is helpful in evaluating bone loss and osteolysis. If there is significant bone osteolysis of the tunnels, a staged procedure with an autogenous iliac bone graft of the tunnels is recommended, followed by revision ACL procedure in 12 to 16 weeks, once the graft has matured.

The removal of Gore-Tex or Dacron ligament presents a special set of problems. Gore-Tex grafts have been associated with significant inflammatory reaction secondarily to the creation of fibers or particles of synthetic material, which have been shown to destroy both bone and cartilage. The ligament must be removed en bloc. Any technique that creates particles must be avoided to prevent osteolysis or cartilage damage after reconstructing the ACL. Bone gauges that match the diameter of the tunnel can be passed to disrupt the bone attachments. Similar techniques can be used for Dacron grafts that have significant bone ingrowth.

Removal of ligament augmentation devices, which are usually fixed at one end, can also be technically demanding. Previous operative reports may indicate which end of the device is fixed. An attempt should be made to remove the entire prosthesis.

Revision Notchplasty

Revision notchplasty is necessary in almost all revision ACL reconstructions, particularly when dealing with failures that resulted from impingement. The over-the-top position must be visualized before drilling the new femoral tunnel. Careful review of the plain radiographs will give detailed information of the notch architecture and help determine the amount of bone to be removed. The notch can sometimes regrow after the initial notchplasty. Additionally, there is a loss of the normal landmarks of the notch, which can lead to excessive bone removal. Such a complication can lead to articular incongruencies between the patellofemoral or tibiofemoral articulation or lateralization of the anatomic attachment site of the ACL. To ensure that an adequate notchplasty has been performed prior to graft placement, tunnel expanders (Instrument makers, Okemos, MI) can be used to perform an impingement test.[88] With the appropriate sized tunnel expander within the tibial tunnel the knee can be ranged to assess clearance and to note if there are any areas of impingement.

Bone Tunnels

Often the most demanding aspect of revision ACL surgery involves the placement of the new tunnels. The location of new tibial and femoral tunnels must be approached in a systematic fashion. At revision, once the notchplasty has been performed and the "over-the-top" position well visualized, the position of the old tunnel can be assessed with regard to the ideal anatomic placement. If the original tunnel was in an optimal location, it can be redrilled. The most common surgical error resulting in ACL failure is anterior placement on the femur via an endoscopic technique. In this situation, the new tunnel can often be placed completely posterior to the original tunnel without interference. Cases in which the original tunnel is only slightly anterior or posterior to the optimal position must be individualized depending on the extent to which the original and the new tunnels overlap.

Another problem with revision ACL surgery is tunnel enlargement, a problem that has been observed with autografts, with allografts (particularly those treated with ethylene oxide), and with synthetic grafts (Gore-Tex). Treatment options for tunnel bone loss include use of an allograft with larger bone plugs or staged bone grafting with tricortical iliac bone.

Graft Fixation

Fixation must hold the graft in position until the it has been incorporated in the tibial and femoral tunnels. During the early postoperative period, graft fixation is the weakest link in the system. There are various techniques for graft fixation to accommodate specific conditions at revision ACL surgery. Bone-to-bone fixation with an interference screw has been shown to be the strongest technique. However, if there is bone loss or osteopenia related to compromised tunnel placement or if a semitendinosus/gracilis tendons or Achilles tendon graft is used, alternative or supplemental modes of fixation may be required. These include such fixation techniques as two interference screws, an over-sized interference screw, suturing over a post, a Hughston button, or staple fixation in a bone trough. The Endobutton (Acufex, Mansfield, OH) can be used as a salvage technique to circumvent poor fixation in the femoral tunnel or a violated posterior cortex. The fixation relies on the anterolateral femoral cortex and does not depend on fixation within the tunnel.

Conclusion

An increasing number of ACL revision procedures are being performed each year. Performing these revisions is a challenging experience and cannot be approached in the same manner as a primary ACL reconstruction. A well-orga-

nized preoperative plan is of great importance. Through a detailed history, comprehensive physical examination and review of medical records, the etiology of failure is determined and a plan for revision formulated. The surgeon must be familiar with the many revision ACL reconstructive techniques, including removal of hardware or synthetic graft material, notchplasty, manipulation of the tibial and femoral tunnels for optimal placement, and graft fixation. In addition to complete planning, intraoperative flexibility is required to allow the surgeon to adjust to unanticipated findings, which may require an innovative solution.

References

1. Miyasaka KC, Daniel DM, Stone ML, et al: The incidence of knee ligament injuries in the general population. Am J Knee Surg 1991;4:3–8.
2. Harter RA, Osternig LR, Singer KM, et al: Long-term evaluation of knee stability and function following surgical reconstruction for anterior cruciate ligament insufficiency. Am J Sports Med 1988;16:434–443.
3. Howe JG, Johnson RJ, Kaplan MJ, et al: Anterior cruciate ligament reconstruction using quadriceps patellar tendon graft: Part I. Long-term followup. Am J Sports Med 1991;19:447–457.
4. Kornblatt I, Warren RF, Wickiewicz TL: Long-term followup of anterior cruciate ligament reconstruction using the quadriceps tendon substitution for chronic anterior cruciate ligament insufficiency. Am J Sports Med 1988;16:444–448.
5. Kaplan MJ, Howe JG, Fleming B, et al: Anterior cruciate ligament reconstruction using quadriceps patellar tendon graft: Part II. A specific sport review. Am J Sports Med 1991;19:458–462.
6. Holmes PF, James SL, Larson RL, et al: Retrospective direct comparison of three intraarticular anterior cruciate ligament reconstructions. Am J Sports Med 1991;19:596–600.
7. Harner CD, Irrgang JJ, Paul J, et al: Loss of motion after anterior cruciate ligament reconstruction. Am J Sports Med 1992;20:499–506.
8. Paulos LE, Rosenberg D, Drawbert J, et al: Infrapatellar contracture syndrome: An unrecognized cause of knee stiffness with patella entrapment and patella infera. Am J Sports Med 1987;15:331–341.
9. Graf B, Uhr F: Complications of intra-articular anterior cruciate reconstruction. Clin Sports Med 1988;7:835–848.
10. Shelbourne KD, Wilckens JH, Mollasbashy A, et al: Arthrofibrosis in acute anterior cruciate ligament reconstruction: The effect of timing

of reconstruction and rehabilitation. Am J Sports Med 1991;19:332–336.
11. Greis PE, Johnson DL, Fu FH: Revision anterior cruciate ligament surgery: Causes of graft failure and technical considerations of revision surgery. Clin Sports Med 1993;12:839–852.
12. Johnson DL, Fu FH: Anterior cruciate ligament reconstruction: Why do failures occur? in Jackson DW (ed): Instructional Course Lectures 44. Rosemont, IL, American Academy of Orthopaedic Surgeons, 1995, pp 391–406.
13. Johnson DL, Harner CD, Maday MG, et al: Revision anterior cruciate ligament surgery, in Fu FH, Harner CD, Vince KG, et al (eds): Knee Surgery. Baltimore, MD, Williams & Wilkins, 1994, pp 877–895.
14. Noyes FR, Barber-Westin SD, Roberts CS: Use of allografts after failed treatment of rupture of the anterior cruciate ligament. J Bone Joint Surg 1994;76A:1019–1031.
15. Safran MR, Harner CD: Revision ACL surgery: Technique and results utilizing allografts, in Jackson DW (ed): Instructional Course Lectures 44. Rosemont, IL, American Academy of Orthopaedic Surgeons, 1995, pp 407–415.
16. Steadman JR, Seemann MD, Hutton KS: Revision ligament reconstruction of failed prosthetic anterior cruciate ligament, in Jackson DW (ed): Instructional Course Lectures 44. Rosemont, IL, American Academy of Orthopaedic Surgeons, 1995, pp 417–429.
17. Wirth CJ, Kohn D: Revision surgery after failed anterior cruciate ligament repair. Orthopade 1993;22:399–404.
18. Strum GM, Friedman MJ, Fox JM, et al: Acute anterior cruciate ligament reconstruction: Analysis of complications. Clin Orthop 1990;253:184–189.
19. Jackson DW, Schaefer RK: Cyclops syndrome: Loss of extension following intra-articular anterior cruciate ligament reconstruction. Arthroscopy 1990;6:171–178.
20. Fullerton LR Jr, Andrews JR: Mechanical block to extension following augmentation of the anterior cruciate ligament: A case report. Am J Sports Med 1984;12:166–168.
21. Irrgang JJ, Harner CD: Loss of motion following knee ligament reconstruction. Sports Med 1995;19:150–159.
22. Recht MP, Piraino DW, Cohen MA, et al: Localized anterior arthrofibrosis (cyclops lesion) after reconstruction of the anterior cruciate ligament: MR imaging findings. Am J Roentgenol 1995;165:383–385.
23. Sachs RA, Daniel DM, Stone ML, et al: Patellofemoral problems after anterior cruciate ligament reconstruction. Am J Sports Med 1989;17:760–765.
24. Weber SC: Case report: Revision anterior cruciate ligament reconstruction. Arthroscopy 1994;10:700–701.
25. Howell SM, Taylor MA: Failure of reconstruction of the anterior cruciate ligament due to impingement by the intercondylar roof. J Bone Joint Surg 1993;75A:1044–1055.

26. Vergis A, Gillquist J: Graft failure in intra-articular anterior cruciate ligament reconstructions: A review of the literature. *Arthroscopy* 1995;11:312–321.

27. Berg EE: Tibial bone plug nonunion: A cause of anterior cruciate ligament reconstructive failure. *Arthroscopy* 1992;8:380–384.

28. Doerr AL Jr, Cohn BT, Ruoff MJ, et al: A complication of interference screw fixation in anterior cruciate ligament reconstruction. *Orthop Rev* 1990;19:997–1000.

29. Noyes FR, Wojtys EM, Marshall MT: The early diagnosis and treatment of developmental patella infera syndrome. *Clin Orthop* 1991;265:241–252.

30. Daniel DM, Stone ML, Dobson BE, et al: Fate of the ACL-injured patient: A prospective outcome study. *Am J Sports Med* 1994;22:632–644.

31. Spindler KP, Schils JP, Bergfeld JA, et al: Prospective study of osseous, articular, and meniscal lesions in recent anterior cruciate ligament tears by magnetic resonance imaging and arthroscopy. *Am J Sports Med* 1993;21:551–557.

32. Speer KP, Spritzer CE, Bassett FH III, et al: Osseous injury associated with acute tears of the anterior cruciate ligament. *Am J Sports Med* 1992;20:382–389.

33. Howell SM, Clark JA: Tibial tunnel placement in anterior cruciate ligament reconstructions and graft impingement. *Clin Orthop* 1992;283:187–195.

34. Howell SM, Berns GS, Farley TE: Unimpinged and impinged anterior cruciate ligament grafts: MR signal intensity measurements. *Radiology* 1991;179:639–643.

35. Howell SM, Barad SJ: Knee extension and its relationship to the slope of the intercondylar roof: Implications for positioning the tibial tunnel in anterior cruciate ligament reconstructions. *Am J Sports Med* 1995;23:288–294.

36. Jackson DW, Gasser SI: Tibial tunnel placement in ACL reconstruction. *Arthroscopy* 1994;10:124–131.

37. Yaru NC, Daniel DM, Penner D: The effect of tibial attachment site on graft impingement in an anterior cruciate ligament reconstruction. *Am J Sports Med* 1992;20:217–220.

38. Hoogland T, Hillen B: Intra-articular reconstruction of the anterior cruciate ligament: An experimental study of length changes in different ligament reconstructions. *Clin Orthop* 1984;185:197–202.

39. Romano VM, Graf BK, Keene JS, et al: Anterior cruciate ligament reconstruction: The effect of tibial tunnel placement on range of motion. *Am J Sports Med* 1993;21:415–418.

40. Howell SM, Clark JA, Farley TE: Serial magnetic resonance study assessing the effects of impingement on the MR image of the patellar tendon graft. *Arthroscopy* 1992;8:350–358.

41. Tanzer M, Lenczner E: The relationship of intercondylar notch size and content to notchplasty requirement in anterior cruciate ligament surgery. *Arthroscopy* 1990;6:89–93.

42. Howell SM, Clark JA, Farley TE: A rationale for predicting anterior cruciate graft impingement by the intercondylar roof: A magnetic resonance imaging study. *Am J Sports Med* 1991;19:276–282.

43. LaPrade RF, Burnett QM II: Femoral intercondylar notch stenosis and correlation to anterior cruciate ligament injuries: A prospective study. *Am J Sports Med* 1994;22:198–203.

44. Burks RT, Leland R: Determination of graft tension before fixation in anterior cruciate ligament reconstruction. *Arthroscopy* 1988;4:260–266.

45. Bylski-Austrow DI, Grood ES, Hefzy MS, et al: Anterior cruciate ligament replacements: A mechanical study of femoral attachment location, flexion angle at tensioning, and initial tension. *J Orthop Res* 1990;8:522–531.

46. Gertel TH, Lew WD, Lewis JL, et al: Effect of anterior cruciate ligament graft tensioning direction, magnitude, and flexion angle on knee biomechanics. *Am J Sports Med* 1993;21:572–581.

47. Yoshiya S, Andrish JT, Manley MT, et al: Graft tension in anterior cruciate ligament reconstruction: An in vivo study in dogs. *Am J Sports Med* 1987;15:464–470.

48. Muneta T, Lewis JL, Stewart NJ: Load affects remodeling of transplanted, autogenous bone-patellar tendon-bone segments in a rabbit model. *J Orthop Res* 1994;12:138–143.

49. Kurosaka M, Yoshiya S, Andrish JT: A biomechanical comparison of different surgical techniques of graft fixation in anterior cruciate ligament reconstruction. *Am J Sports Med* 1987;15:225–229.

50. Matthews LS, Soffer SR: Pitfalls in the use of interference screws for anterior cruciate ligament reconstruction: Brief report. *Arthroscopy* 1989;5:225–226.

51. Manaster BJ, Remley K, Newman AP, et al: Knee ligament reconstruction: Plain film analysis. *Am J Roentgenol* 1988;150:337–342.

52. Brown CH Jr, Hecker AT, Hipp JA, et al: The biomechanics of interference screw fixation of patellar tendon anterior cruciate ligament grafts. *Am J Sports Med* 1993;21:880–886.

53. Steiner ME, Hecker AT, Brown CH Jr, et al: Anterior cruciate ligament graft fixation: Comparison of hamstring and patellar tendon grafts. *Am J Sports Med* 1994;22:240–247.

54. Jomha NM, Raso VJ, Leung P: Effect of varying angles on the pullout strength of interference screw fixation. *Arthroscopy* 1993;9:580–583.

55. Marks PH, Harner CD: The anterior cruciate ligament in the multiple ligament-injured knee. *Clin Sports Med* 1993;12:825–838.

56. O'Brien SJ, Warren RF, Pavlov H, et al: Reconstruction of the chronically insufficient anterior cruciate ligament with the central third of the patellar ligament. *J Bone Joint Surg* 1991;73A:278–286.

57. Gersoff WK, Clancy WG Jr: Diagnosis of acute and chronic anterior cruciate ligament tears. *Clin Sports Med* 1988;7:727–738.

58. O'Neill DF, James SL: Valgus osteotomy with anterior cruciate ligament laxity. *Clin Orthop* 1992;278:153–159.

59. Noyes FR, Barber SD, Simon R: High tibial osteotomy and ligament reconstruction in varus angulated, anterior cruciate ligament-deficient knees: A two- to seven-year follow-up study. *Am J Sports Med* 1993;21:2–12.

60. Noyes FR, Butler DL, Grood ES, et al: Biomechanical analysis of human ligament grafts used in knee-ligament repairs and reconstructions. *J Bone Joint Surg* 1984;66A:344–352.

61. Aglietti P, Buzzi R, Zaccherotti G, et al: Patellar tendon versus doubled semitendinosus and gracilis tendons for anterior cruciate ligament reconstruction. *Am J Sports Med* 1994;22:211–218.

62. Brown CH Jr, Steiner ME, Carson EW: The use of hamstring tendons for anterior cruciate ligament reconstruction: Technique and results. *Clin Sports Med* 1993;12:723–756.

63. Daniel DM: Use of allografts after failed treatment of rupture of the anterior cruciate ligament. *J Bone Joint Surg* 1995;77A:1290.

64. Amendola A, Fowler P: Allograft anterior cruciate ligament reconstruction in a sheep model: The effect of synthetic augmentation. *Am J Sports Med* 1992;20:336–346.

65. Jackson DW, Grood ES, Goldstein JD, et al: A comparison of patellar tendon autograft and allograft used for anterior cruciate ligament reconstruction in the goat model. *Am J Sports Med* 1993;21:176–185.

66. Noyes FR, Barber SD: The effect of a ligament-augmentation device on allograft reconstructions for chronic ruptures of the anterior cruciate ligament. *J Bone Joint Surg* 1992;74A:960–973.

67. Olson EJ, Harner CD, Fu FH, et al: Clinical use of fresh, frozen soft tissue allografts. *Orthopedics* 1992;15:1225–1232.

68. Rasmussen TJ, Feder SM, Butler DL, et al: The effect of 4 Mrad of gamma irradiation on the initial mechanical properties of bone-patellar tendon-bone grafts. *Arthroscopy* 1994;10:188–197.

69. Gibbons MJ, Butler DL, Grood ES, et al: Effects of gamma irradiation on the initial mechanical and material properties of goat bone-patellar tendon-bone allografts. *J Orthop Res* 1991;9:209–218.

70. Buck BE, Malinin TI: Human bone and tissue allografts: Preparation and safety. *Clin Orthop* 1994;303:8–17.

71. Buck BE, Resnick L, Shah SM, et al: Human immunodeficiency virus cultured from bone: Implications for transplantation. *Clin Orthop* 1990;251:249–253.

72. Paulos LE, Rosenberg TD, Grewe SR, et al: The GORE-TEX anterior cruciate ligament prosthesis: A long-term followup. *Am J Sports Med* 1992;20:246–252.

73. Woods GA, Indelicato PA, Prevot TJ: The Gore-Tex anterior cruciate ligament prosthesis: Two versus three year results. *Am J Sports Med* 1991;19:48–55.

74. Shelbourne KD, Whitaker JH, McCarroll JR, et al: Anaterior cruciate ligament injury: Evaluation of intraarticular reconstruction of acute tears without repair. Two to seven year followup of 155 athletes. *Am J Sports Med* 1990;18:484–489.

75. Jackson DW, Grood ES, Arnoczky SP, et al: Cruciate reconstruction using freeze dried anterior cruciate ligament allograft and a ligament augmentation device (LAD): An experimental study in a goat model. *Am J Sports Med* 1987;15:528–538.

76. Yoshiya S, Andrish JT, Manley MT, et al: Augmentation of anterior cruciate ligament reconstruction in dogs with prostheses of different stiffnesses. *J Orthop Res* 1986;4:475–485.

77. Rodeo SA, Arnoczky SP, Torzilli PA, et al: Tendon-healing in a bone tunnel: A biomechanical and histological study in the dog. *J Bone Joint Surg* 1993;75A:1795–1803.

78. Fahey M, Indelicato PA: Bone tunnel enlargment after anterior cruciate ligament replacement. *Am J Sports Med* 1994;22:410–414.

79. Linn RM, Fischer DA, Smith JP, et al: Achilles tendon allograft reconstruction of the anterior cruciate ligament-deficient knee. *Am J Sports Med* 1993;21:825–831.

80. Clancy WG Jr, Narechania RG, Rosenberg TD, et al: Anterior and posterior cruciate ligament reconstruction in rhesus monkeys. *J Bone Joint Surg* 1981;63A:1270–1284.

81. Drez DJ Jr, DeLee J, Holden JP, et al: Anterior cruciate ligament reconstruction using bone-patellar tendon-bone allografts: A biological and biomechanical evaluation in goats. *Am J Sports Med* 1991;19:256–263.

82. Noyes FR, Mangine RE, Barber SD: The early treatment of motion complications after reconstruction of the anterior cruciate ligament. *Clin Orthop* 1992;277:217–228.

83. Cosgarea AJ, Sebastianelli WJ, DeHaven KE: Prevention of arthrofibrosis after anterior cruciate ligament reconstruction using the central third patellar tendon autograft. *Am J Sports Med* 1995;23:87–92.

84. Rosenberg TD, Paulos LE, Parker RD, etal: The forty-five-degree posteroanterior flexion weight-bearing radiograph of the knee. *J Bone Joint Surg* 1988;70A:1479–1483.

85. DeHaven KE: Diagnosis of acute knee injuries with hemarthrosis. *Am J Sports Med* 1980;8:9–14.

86. Noyes FR, Bassett RW, Grood ES, et al: Arthroscopy in acute traumatic hemarthrosis of the knee: Incidence of anterior cruciate tears and other injuries. *J Bone Joint Surg* 1980;62A:687–685.

87. Warren RF: Meniscectomy and repair in the anterior cruciate ligament-deficient patient. *Clin Orthop* 1990;252:55–63.

88. Johnson DL, Miller MD, Fu FH: The arthroscopic "impingement test" during anterior cruciate ligament reconstruction. *Arthroscopy* 1993;9:714–717.

43

Management of Chronic Posterolateral Rotatory Instability of the Knee: Surgical Technique for the Posterolateral Corner Sling Procedure

John P. Albright, MD
Andrew W. Brown, MD

Introduction

The term posterolateral rotatory instability (PLRI) of the knee describes a spectrum of pathologic states of ligamentous laxity, in which the lateral tibial plateau subluxates posterior to the lateral femoral condyle when an external rotational force is applied to the knee (Fig. 1). When the point of subluxation is reached, the patient will recognize the associated weakness and posterolateral pain. In its mildest form, it is merely a finding during physical examination of a gliding motion, which is determined to be excessive only when it is compared to the patient's opposite side. When a clinically significant degree of laxity exists, the examiner can hold the foot in external rotation, apply valgus pressure, and move the knee from a fully extended position into 20° or 30° of flexion to demonstrate the subluxation. This subluxation often presents as the sudden translational acceleration of the tibia on the femur that the patient associates with episodes of giving way and that we know as a reverse pivot-shift phenomenon. Further flexion with the leg in valgus and external rotation will increase the patient's complaint of pain and weakness in the posterolateral corner of the knee. Complicating the picture is the wide variety of ligament injuries that are often present; PLRI is rarely an isolat-

ed finding. The diagnosis of PLRI is uncommon not only because of its inherent rarity but also because the physical examination can be confusing or subtle in the face of multidirectional patholaxity in the knee. Indeed, the diagnosis of PLRI is usually considered as a secondary pattern of instability to the diagnosis of cruciate ligament pathology. The diagnosis of PLRI requires a sound physical examination of the knee as well as a high index of suspicion, because, if left untreated, it can lead to failure of cruciate reconstructions. Hughston and associates[1] were instrumental in drawing attention to this area as a source of instability as well as to the difficulty in making the diagnosis of injury to this area.

Clinically, functional instability is known to result either acutely (from hyperextension-varus injuries) or gradually, in association with other ligament injury patterns. Patients with mild PLRI present with a subtle entity, commonly overlooked on physical examination. Often this represents an insidiously developing entity that may take a few months or even a few years to become severe enough to be symptomatic. Patients with the most severe degree of laxity present a dramatic clinical picture and experience violent and painful pivot-shift subluxations with every step. This

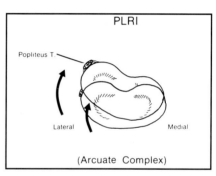

Fig. 1 Top view of pathologic posterior displacement of the lateral tibial plateau on the lateral femoral condyle with laxity of the arcuate complex.

severe chronic state is the most difficult to correct surgically. Thus early diagnosis is the key to successful treatment of PLRI as well as to prevention of the known consequence of untreated PLRI on what would otherwise be successful cruciate reconstructions.[2]

In the mid 1970s, a novel soft-tissue procedure, the posterolateral corner sling procedure (PLCS), was developed by the senior author (JPA) that has, in our experience, proven to be a very reliable method for eliminating PLRI and the reverse pivot-shift phenomenon. The procedure involves creation of an extra-articular sling that extends from a point on the posterior tibia, immediately medial to the proximal tibiofibular articulation, then anteriorly and superiorly to an isometric point on the femur. In addition, other procedures that have been described for both acute and chronic PLRI will also be described.

Anatomy

An understanding of the anatomy of the posterolateral corner of the knee is important for conceptualizing pathology as well as for planning and executing surgical exploration and repair. The first modern discussion of the posterolateral corner was presented by Seebacher and associates,[3] who described the posterolateral corner as having three layers. The first layer consists of the iliotibial band and the biceps femoris tendon. The second layer consists of the quadriceps retinaculum and the lateral patellofemoral ligaments. The third and most important layer consists of the lateral collateral ligament (LCL), the fabellofibular ligament, the popliteus, and the arcuate ligament. They described variations in cadaveric dissections with regard to the reinforcement of the lateral corner of the joint capsule, with 13% having an arcuate ligament alone, 20% the fabellofibular ligament alone, and 67% having both. Watanabe and associates[4] also performed cadaveric dissections of the posterolateral aspect of the knee in 115 specimens and found that 38.3% showed a fabellofibular ligament with a fibular origin of the popliteus, 35.7% had an arcuate ligament and a fibular origin of the popliteus, 12.2% had a fibular origin of the popliteus only, 7.8% showed all three components, 3.5% had a fabellofibular ligament with an arcuate ligament, 1.7% had a fabellofibular ligament alone, and 0.9% had an arcuate ligament alone. Finally, Sudasna and Harnsiriwattanagit[5] described their findings in the dissection of 50 cadavers. They found the fabellofibular ligament in 34 specimens, the popliteofibular ligament in 49, and a thin membranous arcuate in 12 knees. Thus, the

complex anatomy of this region is variable.

In spite of this region's complexity, until recently there had been no comprehensive surgical approach to this area. Terry and LaPrade[6] described in great detail their findings of 30 cadaveric and 71 patient dissections of this region. They describe a surgical approach to the region using as needed a series of three fascial incisions and a lateral capsular incision for visualization of the various components of the posterolateral knee complex. The first fascial incision bisects the iliotibial band. The second lies along the posterior aspect of the iliotibial band and the edge of the short head of the biceps femoris. The third fascial incision lies along the posterior border of the long head of the biceps femoris with dissection of the peroneal nerve. Finally, a capsular incision can be made into the knee at the anterior edge of the LCL. We have found this incision to be particularly helpful in assessing the lateral meniscus and the popliteal tendon. Using this approach, the authors described in detail the iliotibial tract, the biceps femoris muscle, the fibular collateral ligament, the midthird lateral capsular ligament, the fabellofibular ligament, the posterior arcuate ligament, the popliteus muscle complex, the lateral coronary ligament, and the posterior capsule.

The biceps femoris complex may also be injured in the setting of PLRI. Its importance was reviewed by Marshall and associates[7] who speculated on the dynamic effect the muscle may have on the LCL. Terry and LaPrade[8] described this complex based on the findings in 30 cadavers and 82 patients explored for injuries to this region. They described the long head of the biceps femoris with a reflected arm, a direct arm, an anterior arm, and a lateral and anterior aponeurosis. The short head was found to have a proximal attachment to the long head, a capsular arm, a confluence of the biceps and the capsulo-osseus layer of the ilio-

tibial tract, a direct arm, an anterior arm, and a lateral aponeurosis. They correlated injuries to the region to increased anterior translation. We feel that this area should be assessed during reconstruction and that injury to this area may preclude the successful use of a Clancy procedure to correct PLRI.

Biomechanics

Our understanding of the various portions of the posterolateral complex as they relate to stability have been elucidated from a number of serial sectioning studies from multiple authors.[9-15] Gollehon and associates[16] showed that sectioning of the posterior cruciate ligament (PCL) alone did not affect varus or external rotation, whereas the additional sectioning of the LCL and the deep ligaments of the posterolateral corner caused a large increase in posterior translation and varus rotation. External rotation increased at angles of flexion greater than 30°. Grood and associates[17] showed that isolated sectioning of the posterolateral complex resulted in increased external rotation of the knee at 30° and 90° of flexion, with greater changes noted at 30°, 13° versus 5.3°, respectively. When the PCL was also sectioned, further increases were noted, with greater changes noted with the knee at 90°, with external rotation increased by 18.0° at 30° and 20.9° at 90° of flexion.

Markolf and associates[9] showed that sectioning of the LCL and posterolateral structures increased lateral opening of the knee and created increased forces on the anterior cruciate ligament (ACL) with internal rotation and increased forces on the PCL with external rotation.

Noyes and associates[13] confirmed increased external rotation of the tibia with respect to the femur when the posterolateral ligaments were sectioned. They also confirmed the increase noted with the addition of PCL sectioning. However, they also noted subluxation of both the lateral and medial tibiofemoral compartments, further evidence of the complexity of instability resulting from injuries to this region. Veltri and associates[14] compared posterolateral sectioning with either PCL or ACL sectioning and showed that external rotation at 30° of flexion might not be reliable in diagnosing ACL and PLRI injuries, because primary varus, primary posterior translation, and coupled external rotation were increased in both patterns of sectioning. Thus, the diagnosis in the setting of multiple ligament injuries can be confusing to the uninitiated.

Recently, interest has focused on the popliteal complex and the popliteofibular ligament in particular. The importance of the popliteus has long been known. In selective cutting experiments, Veltri and associates[15] showed greater instability when the popliteus, the popliteofibular ligament, and posterolateral structures were sectioned together as assessed by primary posterior translation, varus rotation, external rotation, and coupled external rotation. Maynard and associates[10] showed that a force of 424 N was required to cause failure of the popliteofibular ligament, providing further evidence of its importance. It is also interesting to note that the anatomic studies previously mentioned, in spite of their variability in other structures, showed this ligament to be present in over 90% of the specimens studied.

Preoperative Evaluation and Surgical Planning

In isolated cases of severe arcuate complex pathology, the following clinical findings are usually present; varus laxity, a positive dial test at 30° and 90° of flexion, a posterior lateral drawer test, and a reverse pivot-shift. The degree of direct lateral laxity due to LCL deficiency must be carefully evaluated, because a separate surgical correction may also be required. The presence of intra-articular pathology is highly likely. It should be documented and treated arthroscopically prior to the extracapsular dissection. The coexistence of other planes of instability is also quite frequent. In our experience, the most frequent ligamentous deficiency to accompany PLRI is ACL deficiency with anterolateral rotatory instability (ALRI). Less frequently, PCL deficiency with direct posterior laxity is present. The combination of PCL and the arcuate ligament complex insufficiency makes for the most dramatic findings on dial and reverse pivot shift testing. The dial test is then likely to be greater at 90° than at 30°. Acutely injured knees may show anteromedial contusions or abrasions with posterolateral tenderness.[18]

Findings During Physical Examinations

Patients with demonstrable reverse pivot shifts demonstrate impressively abnormal gaits. High adduction moments can create a dramatic varus thrust.[19] Abnormal gait can manifest with pivot shifting with every step. Patients will internally rotate at the knee to avoid subluxation. External rotation makes knee more unstable.

PLRI

The external rotation dial tests (at 30° and 90° of flexion) are known from the previously cited biomechanical studies to be abnormal in the face of posterolateral complex pathology. External rotation is greater on the involved side as can be seen by dialing the foot and tibia through the knee at both 30° and 90° of flexion. The test is most easily performed with the patient prone. A difference of greater than 5° to 10°, noted by both the examiner and the patient, should be considered clinically significant. Care must be taken to ensure that the apparent difference is not a result of malpositioning on the examination table. The differential diagnosis of a positive dial test is anteromedial rotatory instability (AMRI) versus PLRI. With isolated posterolateral complex injury, the dial test shows the greatest increase in external rotation over the opposite side at 30° of knee flexion. When a PCL tear is also present, the magnitude of an increased dial test will be greater overall and is most pronounced at 90° of knee flexion.

Posterolateral Drawer Test (90°)

Straight posterior laxity does not exist without PCL insufficiency. However, rotational laxity can be detected during the posterior drawer test if the leg is not controlled for rotation or if the posterior force is applied from the lateral hand. Described as coupled external rotation, this rotational laxity is known to be increased with posterolateral injury.[14,20]

Modified Lachman Test (30°)

We perform this using a standard Lachman test: a 30° anterior drawer with tibial hand placed medially. We then repeat the test with the hands switched so that tibial hand is placed laterally. A gross apparent difference in displacement may appear when PLRI is present.

Reverse Pivot Shift Test

We perform this test starting with the leg in maximum extension. The foot is then externally rotated, a valgus stress is applied and the knee is slowly flexed to 90°. A pivot shift of the tibial plateau posteriorly, felt as a sudden transitional acceleration, denotes a positive reverse pivot shift test. We prefer to start in full extension and move to flexion and subluxation rather than starting in flexion with the tibia subluxed, because this is more comfortable for the patient at the initiation of the examination and limits reflexive spasm. The pivot should occur in the first 30° of flexion. This test can be mistaken for anterior pivot shift subluxation. When performing the anterior pivot shift maneuver, ask the patient at what point the knee feels out of place. When a patient has PLRI instead of ALRI you will find that when you think the knee is "in," the patient feels it is "out." Conversely,

Table 1 Posterolateral Rotatory Instability (PLRI) Grading System			
Grade PLRI	Dial Test	90° Subluxation	30° Reverse Pivot Shift
Grade I	Positive		
Grade II	Positive	Positive	
Grade III	Positive	Positive	Positive

when you think that the knee is "out," the patient thinks that it is "in." The patient's perceptions are critical in the examination of a multiligamentous injury. Cooper[21] found that this test was positive in 35% of asymptomatic knees examined under anesthesia. Jakob and associates[22] felt that a positive test was significant if found in one knee only.

Posterolateral Subluxation
Even though clinically significant PLRI exists, often the sudden acceleration of the reverse pivot shift is not demonstrable. In this instance, the feeling of the patient that the tibia is posteriorly subluxed on the lateral femoral condyle will increase as the externally rotated leg is flexed toward 90°. Confirmation of subluxation is obtained when the primary source of discomfort is the posterolateral aspect of the knee and relief is obtained by release of external rotation only with the knee held at 90° of flexion with maintained valgus stress.

PLRI Grading system
Recognizing that PLRI can present as a spectrum of laxity with no specific physical finding pathognomonic we grade the patient based on the presence or absence of concurrent physical findings[20,23] (Table 1).

Varus Laxity
When reverse pivot shift is present, there will also be some laxity with varus stress at 20° flexion. Severity of direct varus laxity and its functional significance will vary.

This factor and assessment of the opposite leg are important considerations in determining the need for valgus osteotomy.

External Rotation Recurvatum Test
As described by Hughston and Norwood,[20] this is present only when the PCL is damaged in addition to the arcuate complex, and gross laxity of the LCL exists.

Opposite Leg Assessment
Examination of the opposite leg will help in determining the best surgical plan. If it appears that excessive varus stress was placed on the lateral and posterolateral structures prior to injury, then proximal tibial valgus osteotomy may be indicated. This osteotomy can be done as a closing wedge laterally, as a dome, or as a medial opening wedge. The advantage of the latter two procedures is that adequate space is left for the tibial tunnel for the PLCS.

Hyperextension
Although its presence may not predict anything about patients who develop this problem, we have seen individuals who had hyperlaxity at the knee with the ability to hyperextend who developed secondary varus laxity and PLRI on a chronic plastic deformation basis after they first ruptured the ACL and an atempt was made to treat the ACL injuries nonsurgically. Thus, this may be a relative contraindication to conservative management of an ACL rupture in the face of subtle findings of posterolateral corner injury.

Varus Alignment
We routinely obtain full-length weight-bearing films of both legs to assess anatomic alignment and to look for lateral joint line opening. Preoperative calculations can be useful if the decision is made intraoperatively to perform a valgus osteotomy.

The LCL reconstruction must not be anticipated to end up tighter than the uninvolved knee. Will the repetitive lateral stresses of weightbearing prove too much for the reconstructed tissue? Often, this question cannot be answered. Evaluation of the dynamics of the patient's gait can prove helpful.

Varus Thrust
When varus alignment is present on the uninvolved side, look closely for varus thrust during stance phase of gait. Experience has shown that the presence of varus thrust on the uninvolved side precludes a good result of any soft-tissue procedure unless a valgus proximal tibial osteotomy is done first. An involved knee with varus laxity but without varus thrust or gross varus alignment will probably do well without an osteotomy.

Surgical Planning
Recently, magnetic resonance imaging has been shown to be effective in visualizing the posterolateral corner of the knee. This may prove useful in evaluating this area for acute tears of the posterolateral complex.[24]

In any case of multidirectional instability of the knee, it is recommended that surgical correction of each component of instability be planned preoperatively. This is particularly important for estimating the duration of the entire operation and in planning for judicious use of the tourniquet. Diagnostic arthroscopy and the PLCS procedure can be accomplished together in under 2 hours. However, each additional finding that requires surgical correction will add to the total length of the case. For instance,

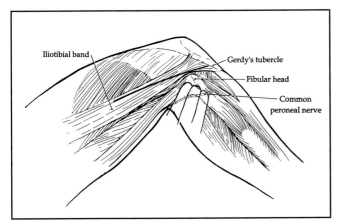

Fig. 2 Lateral view of knee flexed 70° to 80°. The incision is shown as it begins at Gerdy's tubercle and extends proximally up the mid thigh region. The location of the peroneal nerve can be identified as it becomes superficial to the fibular shaft approximately 3 finger breadths from the fibular head.

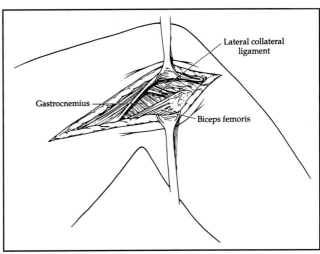

Fig. 3 Beneath the iliotibial band, the lateral collateral ligament and the tendinous portion of the lateral head of the gastrocnemius lie adjacent to each other.

when an ACL reconstruction with patellar tendon autograft, a single meniscus excision/repair, and an LCL reconstruction are added to the above two-step procedure, a target time of 5 hours should be anticipated. In this instance, a split surgical team approach could be used to cut down surgical time.

Baker and associates[25,26] were the first to report on the surgical treatment of posterolateral instability of the knee. They recommended repair of acutely injured structures. When this repair could not be achieved because of tissue incompetence or chronicity, they recommended anterior and superior advancement of the arcuate ligament. Hughston and Jacobson[23] also recommended repair and proximal advancement of the arcuate complex.

Clancy and associates[27] have described biceps tenodesis for PLRI. This procedure, in theory, advances and tensions the posterolateral structures while addressing varus laxity. Biomechanical studies have confirmed this, but other authors have questioned sacrificing the dynamic stabilizing effect of the tendon as well as the quality of posterolateral tissue that is advanced secondarily.[28,29] Salvage in the

face of a failed biceps tenodesis may be quite difficult. We feel that this procedure has utility and have used it successfully. Additionally, when performed with a PCL reconstruction, the procedure could in theory reduce dynamic stress on the graft.

Noyes and Barber-Westin[28] have described repair of the posterolateral complex with allograft augmentation as well as allograft reconstruction as dictated by the quality and volume of tissue encountered at surgery. They reported a successful outcome in 16 of 21 patients as measured by stress radiographs and physical examination.

Veltri and Warren[30] have recently described a procedure similar to the PLCS. They augment the popliteus tendon either with reinforcement by grafting or by total replacement with a sling similar to ours. They also note the importance of the popliteofibular ligament and recommend its concurrent reconstruction as well, and they also describe use of a sling to reconstruct this ligament.

Here we present our results of the PLCS with a review of technical considerations and our postoperative protocol.

Description of the Surgical Procedure
The Approach
With the knee flexed 45°, the skin incision courses from just distal to Gerdy's tubercle (Fig. 2), along the iliotibial band (ITB) onto the midlateral aspect of the distal thigh. Before the posterolateral corner is dissected, it is important to identify and protect the peroneal nerve. It is most readily identified three finger breadths below the fibular head where it becomes superficial as it wraps around the fibula (Fig. 2). Maintenance of the knee in a flexed position keeps the nerve out of the operative field during the procedure described below.

The most important anatomic structures that need to be exposed for this approach are best located by first identifying the LCL from its femoral to its fibular attachment (Fig. 3). Lying immediately posterior to the LCL is the tendinous portion of the lateral head of the gastrocnemius. The plane between the tendon of the lateral head of the gastrocnemius (Fig. 4) and the LCL is developed from the femoral insertions to 2 to 3 cm below the lateral joint line. The gastrocnemius is retracted posteriorly to expose

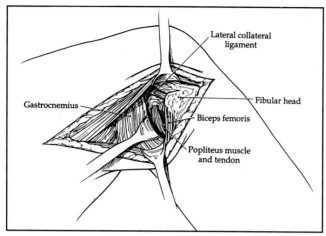

Fig. 4 When the gastrocnemius is retracted, the popliteus can be found coursing obliquely. The muscle originates on the posterior aspect of the proximal tibia and inserts on the femur just inferior and anterior to the lateral collateral ligament. The popliteofibular ligament is not depicted.

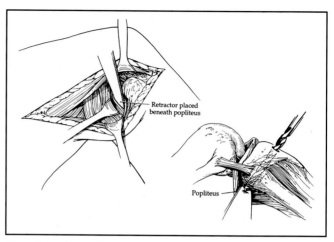

Fig. 5 Once the popliteus is mobilized posteriorly, a retractor is inserted to expose the site where the tunnel will exit.

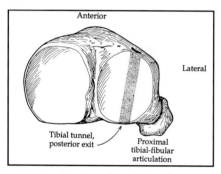

Fig. 6 Superior view of the tibia to illustrate relationship of tunnel to proximal tibiofibular joint. When an iliotibial band autograft is used, the anterior aspect of the tunnel should be in line with Gerdy's tubercle as shown here. When the posterolateral corner sling procedure is to be combined with a Losee type anterior sling, the entry portal should be medial to Gerdy's tubercle in the interval between the tubercle and the patellar tendon.

the structures deep to it. Careful dissection is then carried out in order to identify the capsule and the popliteus tendon.

The popliteus tendon should be clearly delineated as it courses obliquely across this interval. In the deep distal portion of the wound it fans out as a wide muscle belly to its origin on the posterior aspect at the tibia distal to the capsule. The popliteofibular ligament normally would be seen as a fibrous band coursing from the posterior aspect of the fibular head to the tendinous portion of the popliteus. The popliteus tendon disappears near the joint line as it dives deep to a thickening in the capsule, into the popliteal foramen. This foramen can be observed from above during the arthroscopic inspection of the lateral gutter and the posterior corner of the lateral meniscus. If help is needed to locate the popliteus tendon, it is most readily visualized from the top of the foramen through a vertical incision into the joint capsule at the anterior edge of the LCL. The narrowest of the Cave retractors (or a hemostat) can then be passed retrograde through the foramen to help identify the course of the tendon in the area of interest. Once the portion of the tendon inferior to the joint line has been identified, an incision is made along its anterior border and the entire tendon is bluntly freed from the adjacent tissues. This maneuver is continued until the popliteus can be swept posteriorly enough to expose the posterolateral corner of the tibia. The

popliteofibular ligament is most often torn in these cases, but otherwise must be either retracted or incised.

The Tunnel

A retractor is then placed beneath the popliteus to identify the target area on the posterior aspect of the tibia and to protect the soft tissue from the exiting drill while the tunnel is being created (Fig. 5). With the posterior tibia exposed, a 3/32 guide pin is passed from near Gerdy's tubercle to the desired point on the exposed tibia. The pin should exit at least 1 to 1.5 cm beneath the articular surface of the lateral tibial plateau and at least 1 cm medial to the proximal tibiofibular articulation (Fig. 6). This placement may be accomplished free hand or with the help of one of the latest large arc versions of the tibial guides available for endoscopic ACL reconstruction. Having achieved proper guide pin placement, a tunnel 6 to 8 mm in diameter is established with a cannulated drill. The size of the tunnel depends on the size of the patient as well as of the graft but usually is 6, 7, or 8 mm in diameter. The location of the anterior starting point of the tunnel must be sufficiently inferior to the tibial articular surface and medial to the tibiofibular joint to avoid compromising their integrity. If it is necessary to incorporate an anterior Losee type extracapsular sling allograft to help control ALRI (due to a concomitant ACL deficiency), the starting point should be at, or slightly medial to, Gerdy's tubercle.

The Graft

Allografts and autografts have proven successful for this procedure. Freeze dried and fresh frozen (and irradiated) ITB and Achilles tendon allografts have been used. At least at the time of implantation, fresh frozen tissue is notably stronger than the freeze dried grafts. Among the allografts, Achilles tendons are the easiest to work with and probably the stronger of the two alternatives. For autografts, the central slip of the ITB is the most convenient to use, both because of its length and because of its attachment to Gerdy's tubercle. If ITB autograft is being used, care must be taken to make sure that sufficient length of graft is harvested. While usually around 18 cm, an accurate estimate of the length needed can be made by running a suture through the tunnel and up to the proposed femoral attachment site. If an ITB or Achilles tendon allograft is used, anterior tibial fixation must be achieved prior to searching for and securing the isometric femoral attachment.

Creating the Sling

The extracapsular posterolateral corner sling is created by passing a graft through the tibial tunnel from front to back with lead end anchor sutures and suture passers. The graft then exits its bony tunnel to emerge anterior to the lateral head of the gastrocnemius and popliteal tendon (Fig. 7). From this point, the graft runs to a point on the femur that will prevent pathologic posterior subluxation of the lateral tibial plateau in an isometric fashion. This isometric point is initially estimated by placing a Steinmann pin

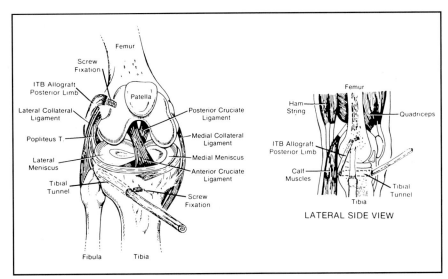

Fig. 7 The posterior sling is accomplished by passing the graft from anterior to posterior in the tunnel. (Shown here is an allograft that must first be fixed to the tibia.) The posterior limb that exits the tunnel is brought up to an isometric point on the femur.

slightly superior and anterior to the femoral attachment of the lateral collateral ligament. The proposed graft placement site is then tested for isometry by first placing the knee at 90° of flexion, rotating the foot 10° to 15° internally, and then tensioning the soft-tissue unit over the Steinmann pin locator.

Placement Testing

Two tests are performed. The first test is performed by maintaining the internal rotation of the foot while the knee is run through a complete range of flexion and extension. Successful placement will result in equal tension of the graft throughout a complete range of motion from at least 0 to 120° of flexion. A migration of more than a few millimeters throughout the entire range should be considered unacceptable. In the second test, the thigh is supported and the knee is flexed to the degree (usually at least 45° of flexion) that produced the most dramatic reverse pivot-shift preoperatively. By grasping the foot (without varus stress) the reverse pivot shift phenomenon is recreated when there is no tension placed on the PLCS graft. Tightening the

graft should eliminate the posterior subluxation. This test can be repeated throughout the entire range of flexion. Care must be taken to make sure that any varus laxity from lateral joint line opening is taken up in the tensioning process. Once satisfactory placement has been identified, the graft is secured with a screw and soft tissue washer on the lateral femur. When LCL reconstruction is also needed, a tunnel through the femur for the PLCS will avoid abutment of the two screws laterally.

Considerations in the Presence of Complex Multidirectional Laxity: ACL Deficiency With ALRI

Most frequently, PLRI is seen in conjunction with ACL deficiency and ALRI. In this situation, concomitant intra-articular reconstruction of the ACL is imperative. This reconstruction can be carried out in any manner the surgeon wishes. Even an over-the-top graft should not preclude anchoring the extracapsular sling on the lateral femoral condyle. If the ACL tunnel is to exit on the lateral femoral cortex, care should be taken to insure that it is located as high as possible

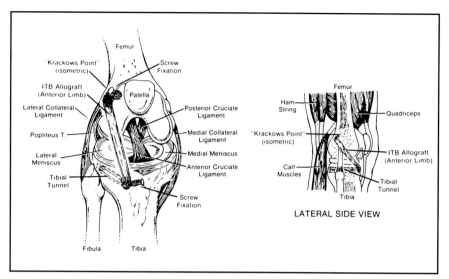

Fig. 8 If an anterior extracapsular sling is needed to help control anterolateral rotatory instability, the anterior limb of the allograft is taken back to Krackow's point.

above the flair of the distal femoral metaphysis. This placement is particularly important to avoid a conflict between the ACL graft tunnel location and the screw fixation of the PLCS. Until the arthroscopically assisted intra-articular ACL reconstruction is completed, it is particularly important to maintain a water-tight joint by avoiding any incisions into the lateral capsule.

Because it is difficult to establish a neutral point for the lateral compartment in the presence of both anterior and posterior lateral rotary instability, the manner in which the grafts are tightened is critical. It is our experience that the best way to find this neutral tibial-femoral relationship is to achieve ACL graft fixation first with the knee held in full extension equal to the opposite leg. This should be accomplished without varus deformity and in the very slight external rotation of the screw-home position seen in terminal extension. Once the proper positioning and graft tension are identified in this position, the knee is maintained in the same rotation as the knee joint is flexed to about 20° and the graft is tightened and secured with interference screws. Having achieved this fixation, the PLCS proce-

dure can be tensioned against the ACL. Particular care must be given to avoid creating unphysiologic internal rotation from the PLCS graft.

If an allograft is being used for the PLCS and a Losee type extracapsular reinforcement of the ACL reconstruction is desired, an anterior extracapsular sling is run from the anterior tibial tunnel exit to a point near Krackow's isometric point on the femoral condyle (Fig. 8). This sling is secured after the PLCS has been secured. The isometric point is also located with and tested over a Steinmann pin. However, in this situation, neutral and even slight external rotation is maintained throughout the range of motion. Krackow's point was described as isometric in relationship to the ITB attachment at Gerdy's tubercle. It is located posterior to the femoral attachment of the LCL and near the gastrocnemius tendon. More specifically, it is usually found to be 1 cm distal and posterior to the septum for the lateral thigh.

Varus Laxity

If varus laxity presents a significant problem, attention should also be directed to the fibular collateral ligament. Unless

there is extreme varus alignment or a dynamic thrust during gait, soft-tissue reconstruction should be successful, obviating the need for a tibial osteotomy. If the ligament is intact but just lax, it is tightened by the proximal advancement of its femoral attachment on a cortical bone block. If there is insufficient LCL tissue or if there is a need for augmentation of an acutely ruptured ligament, this can be accomplished in one of two ways. First, as described by Clancy and associates,[27] all or part of the biceps tendon can be left attached to the fibula and dissected proximally after the peroneal nerve has been identified at its posterior border. The tendon is then screwed to the femoral origin of the LCL. Another alternative to this reconstruction is to use an Achilles tendon allograft. This method first involves the shaping of a tapered 6 to 7 mm bone plug cylinder from the calcaneus. This is such a small bone plug that shaping with a Midas Rex (or other high-powered) bur is recommended over the use of rongeurs in order to avoid shattering the bone. A taper is designed with the narrow end at the tendon attachment and the wider diameter located at the calcaneal end. This graft is then run from front to back through a tapered tunnel in the fibular head (7 to 8 mm tapering to 6 mm) that runs parallel to the lateral knee joint line. The proximal portion is then fixed over a soft tissue screw and washer at the LCL femoral attachment.

Posterior Cruciate Ligament Deficiency with Posterior Laxity

Similar to the situation of ACL deficiency, the PCL should be reconstructed prior to the PLCS procedure. A particularly difficult situation to deal with involves both ACL and PCL deficiency as well as medial collateral ligament (MCL) and LCL laxity. Simultaneous tightening of both cruciate constructs with repeated testing of anteroposterior laxity is a critical first step. The PLRI and varus components can be addressed only after intra-articular ligament stability has been achieved.

Postoperative Management

Postoperative management should be individualized, but the plan should generally include a moderate early range of motion (eg, 0 to 90°), protection from external rotation, and avoidance of varus stress for at least 6 to 8 weeks. The patient is kept nonweightbearing if there is varus alignment. Often, a cast brace is indicated to maximize rotational and medial-lateral control during this critical period. A functional knee brace with straps placed in a manner similar to those used for the posterior cruciate reconstructions and a lateral heel and sole wedge are prescribed for use at 6 to 8 weeks postoperatively. Progress should be cautious. Patients must be warned that any loosening may require them to resume wearing a cast. A 9- to 12-month rehabilitation time period is anticipated. The rehabilitation period should not be considered over until there are firm endpoints on examination and the patient has resumed full activity.

Study Population[31]

Between 1984 and 1990, 33 patients underwent this procedure, 30 of whom were available for follow-up evaluation. Twenty nine of this 30 study-group members have been assessed for an average of 4 (2 to 7) years postsurgery. One patient is included in the study with less than a 2-year follow-up, because she became an early postoperative failure when she went "zip skiing" 3 months after surgery.

Evaluation Methods

Instability was assessed using varus and external rotation stresses, anterior and reverse pivot shift tests, and the "Hughston external rotation recurvatum test." Varus alignment was determined with weightbearing radiographs. Clinical outcomes were determined for each patient by noting postoperative changes

in the International Knee Documentation Committee's (IKDC) Knee Rating System.

Results

Preoperative Status

Ninety-seven percent (29/30) of the patients in this study had at least a combination ALRI and PLRI as well as slight varus laxity prior to surgical reconstruction. An insidious onset of impairment was common, with growing problems of control over the patients' increasingly complex pathologic laxity becoming clinically detectable an average of 3.5 years after injury. The appearance of PLRI was associated with a distinct worsening of functional status to the point of subluxation episodes, which occurred many times each day, and persistent pain and/or swelling.

In all patients, a positive external rotation dial test, as well as a reverse pivot shift subluxation was demonstrated. Varus laxity was also almost always present (29/30), and 50% of the patients (15/30) had varus alignment demonstrated in the normal leg on weightbearing radiographs. Eight LCL ruptures were also found, as well as five PCL ruptures.

Postoperative Status

The IKDC knee rating scores improved an average of 20 points (from 50 to 70) postoperatively. The preoperative function level and the intra-articular pathology greatly influenced the postoperative results. The low average group scores fail to reflect the success of the procedure partly because of the use of the very unforgiving IKDC format, which evaluates all patients in comparison with the function level of the normal, competitive athlete. The only patients whose results were in the excellent range were those eight who were totally without intra-articular pathology (eg, normal menisci and pristine articular surfaces in all three compartments.)

One third of the postoperative scores

for the group remained in the poor category. In addition to accumulating joint pathology, this was partly due to the accumulation of intra-articular pathology and partly due to residual laxity, with only 16/30 (53%) gaining a knee that was completely stable in all directions initially. This figure elevated to 22/30 (73%) after six of the patients with initial failures underwent additional stabilizing type procedures. Five patients in this "poor" postoperative score category also had some sort of residual laxity.

However, a closer look reveals that it was not the PLCS that was at fault. As a matter of fact, looking more specifically at the PLCS, it proved most reliable of all procedures. In 87% (26/30) of all patients, the PLRI was reduced to the point of elimination of the reverse pivot shift, and in all patients in whom the reverse pivot had been eliminated, there was a dramatic improvement in the quality of their lives, as they now could walk without fear of painful, dramatic subluxations with every step. In all 26 cases, it also corrected hyperextension. In 87% (13/15) of cases it reduced varus laxity, and good functional results were even noted in the remaining two, despite persistence of varus laxity. Eight of these 15 were considered to have ruptured the LCL and seven of these were considered to be severe enough to require grafting.

Our results imply that this procedure is indicated for patients with mild to moderate varus alignment, because when used in patients without a varus thrust it did not produce less than satisfactory end results. It is true that many of the ten patients with a varus alignment on weightbearing experienced a more prolonged and demanding rehabilitation program, involving casting and/or nonweightbearing. However, in the end, the results were rewarding. All three of the elite athletes in this study group successfully returned to full competition in football or basketball.

Only two individuals went on to subsequent valgus tibial osteotomies. One osteotomy was done because of failure of the ACL and because of medial compartment degeneration following meniscectomy. At the time of follow-up, three patients demonstrated excessive varus related to narrowing of the medial joint space.

Complications

Complications were frequent in this group. Several patients required manipulation and/or open debridement of the infrapatellar fat pad because of infrapatellar fibrosis and patella baja. Three of these had meniscal repairs. Another patient became acutely infected after a fall onto the incision site and incurred a secondary or retrograde contamination. Because of the alternative option for a knee fusion, the patient requested a regrafting after waiting 3 years free of signs of infection.

Conclusion

The complex instability of multidirectional instability is quite disabling. While not the only procedure usually required, the PLCS procedure effectively eliminates PLRI and reverse pivot shift subluxations and reduces hyperextension and varus laxity. The complexity of the preoperative status of these patients kept the overall postoperative scores low. Intervention prior to development of joint surface pathology is recommended.

References

1. Hughston JC, Andrews JR, Cross MJ, et al: Classification of knee ligament instabilities: Part II. The lateral compartment. *J Bone Joint Surg* 1976;58A:173–179.
2. O'Brien SJ, Warren RF, Pavlov H, et al: Reconstruction of the chronically insufficient anterior cruciate ligament with the central third of the patellar ligament. *J Bone Joint Surg* 1991;73A:278–286.
3. Seebacher JR, Inglis AE, Marshall JL, et al: The structure of the posterolateral aspect of the knee. *J Bone Joint Surg* 1982;64A:536–541.
4. Watanabe Y, Moriya H, Takahashi K, et al: Functional anatomy of the posterolateral structures of the knee. *Arthroscopy* 1993;9:57–62.
5. Sudasna S, Harnsiriwattanagit K: The ligamentous structures of the posterolateral aspect of the knee. *Bull Hosp Jt Dis Orthop Inst* 1990;50:35–40.
6. Terry GC, LaPrade RF: The posterolateral aspect of the knee: Anatomy and surgical approach. *Am J Sports Med* 1996;24:732–739.
7. Marshall JL, Girgis FG, Zelko RR: The biceps femoris tendon and its functional significance. *J Bone Joint Surg* 1972;54A:1444–1450.
8. Terry GC, LaPrade RF: The biceps femoris muscle complex at the knee: Its anatomy and injury patterns associated with acute anterolateral-anteromedial rotatory instability. *Am J Sports Med* 1996;24:2–8.
9. Markolf KL, Wascher DC, Finerman GA: Direct in vitro measurement of forces in the cruciate ligaments: Part II. The effect of section of the posterolateral structures. *J Bone Joint Surg* 1993;75A:387–394.
10. Maynard MJ, Deng X, Wickiewicz TL, et al: The popliteofibular ligament: Rediscovery of a key element in posterolateral stability. *Am J Sports Med* 1996;24:311–316.
11. Nielsen S, Helmig P: The static stabilizing function of the popliteal tendon in the knee: An experimental study. *Arch Orthop Trauma Surg* 1986;104:357–362.
12. Nielsen S, Rasmussen O, Ovesen J, et al: Rotatory instability of cadaver knees after transection of collateral ligaments and capsule. *Arch Orthop Trauma Surg* 1984;103:165–169.
13. Noyes FR, Stowers SF, Grood ES, et al: Posterior subluxations of the medial and lateral tibiofemoral compartments: An in vitro ligament sectioning study in cadaveric knees. *Am J Sports Med* 1993;21:407–414.
14. Veltri DM, Deng XH, Torzilli PA, et al: The role of the cruciate and posterolateral ligaments in stability of the knee: A biomechanical study. *Am J Sports Med* 1995;23:436–443.
15. Veltri DM, Deng XH, Torzilli PA, et al: The role of the popliteofibular ligament in stability of the human knee: A biomechanical study. *Am J Sports Med* 1996;24:19–27.
16. Gollehon DL, Torzilli PA, Warren RF: The role of the posterolateral and cruciate ligaments in the stability of the human knee: A biomechanical study. *J Bone Joint Surg* 1987;69A:233–242.
17. Grood ES, Stowers SF, Noyes FR: Limits of movement in the human knee: Effect of sectioning the posterior cruciate ligament and posterolateral structures. *J Bone Joint Surg* 1988;70A:88–97.
18. DeLee JC, Riley MB, Rockwood CA Jr: Acute posterolateral rotatory instability of the knee. *Am J Sports Med* 1983;11:199–207.
19. Noyes FR, Schipplein OD, Andriacchi TP, et al: The anterior cruciate ligament-deficient knee with varus alignment: An analysis of gait adaptations and dynamic joint loadings. *Am J Sports Med* 1992;20:707–716.
20. Hughston JC, Norwood LA Jr: The posterolateral drawer test and external rotational recurvatum test for posterolateral rotatory instability of the knee. *Clin Orthop* 1980;147:82–87.
21. Cooper DE: Tests for posterolateral instability of the knee in normal subjects: Results of examination under anesthesia. *J Bone Joint Surg* 1991;73A:30–36.
22. Jakob RP, Hassler H, Staeubli HU: Observations on rotatory instability of the lateral compartment of the knee: Experimental studies on the functional anatomy and pathomechanism of the true and the reversed pivot shift sign. *Acta Orthop Scand* 1981;191(suppl):1–32.
23. Hughston JC, Jacobson KE: Chronic posterolateral rotatory instability of the knee. *J Bone Joint Surg* 1985;67A:351–359.
24. Yu JS, Salonen DC, Hodler J, et al: Posterolateral aspect of the knee: Improved MR imaging with a coronal oblique technique. *Radiology* 1996;198:199–204.
25. Baker CL Jr, Norwood LA, Hughston JC: Acute combined posterior cruciate and posterolateral instability of the knee. *Am J Sports Med* 1984;12:204–208.
26. Baker CL Jr, Norwood LA, Hughston JC: Acute posterolateral rotatory instability of the knee. *J Bone Joint Surg* 1983;65A:614–618.
27. Clancy WG Jr, Meister K, Craythorne CB: Posterolateral corner collateral ligament reconstruction, in Jackson DW (ed): *Reconstructive Knee Surgery.* New York, NY, Raven Press, 1995, pp 143–159.
28. Noyes FR, Barber-Westin SD: Surgical reconstruction of severe chronic posterolateral complex injuries of the knee using allograft tissues. *Am J Sports Med* 1995;23:2–12.
29. Wascher DC, Grauer JD, Markoff KL: Biceps tendon tenodesis for posterolateral instability of the knee: An in vitro study. *Am J Sports Med* 1993;21:400–406.
30. Veltri DM, Warren RF: Operative treatment of posterolateral instability of the knee. *Clin Sports Med* 1994;13:615–627.
31. Albright JP, Tearse DS, Dodds JA: Chronic posterolateral instability of the knee: Evaluation of the posterolateral corner sling procedure. *Orthop Trans* 1994;18:746.

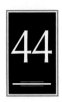

The Role of Allografts in Repair and Reconstruction of Knee Joint Ligaments and Menisci

Frank R. Noyes, MD
Sue D. Barber-Westin, BS
David L. Butler, PhD
Ross M. Wilkins, MD, MS

Introduction

Allograft tissue is a popular substitute tissue used in reconstructing torn or deficient knee ligament structures. In a survey of 36 United States tissue banks, conducted from 1990 through 1992, over 16,000 bone-patellar ligament-bone, Achilles tendon, and fascia lata allografts had been implanted.[1] Since 1986, encouraging clinical results have been reported by many authors following replacement of the anterior cruciate ligament (ACL) both in short-term studies averaging 1 to 4 years after surgery,[2–16] and in longer studies averaging 5 to 11 years after surgery.[17–20] Clinical outcome following allogeneic ACL reconstruction has been compared with that following autogenous reconstruction, with conflicting results. Some studies have found no statistically significant differences between graft types in outcome 1 to 5 years after surgery.[21–24] Others have reported significant differences between graft types for anterior stability[14] and other factors[25] after surgery.

Only a few authors have described the use of allografts for reconstruction of a ruptured posterior cruciate ligament (PCL), either as a single procedure[26,27] or in combination with ACL repair following knee dislocation.[28–30] Allografts have also been used to replace deficient medial, lateral, and posterolateral knee ligamentous structures.[31–33]

Implantation of human meniscus allografts has received significant attention in the past several years; however, disagreement is apparent among authors concerning the outcome of this procedure.[34–45] Currently, no clear consensus exists concerning tissue processing, long-term function, indications, or the efficacy of this procedure.

The objectives of this chapter are to review pertinent literature and present current knowledge concerning the biomechanical and clinical principles surrounding the use of allografts for knee ligament reconstruction. Issues pertaining to disease transmission, graft sterilization, clinical outcome, and indications for the use of allografts will be discussed, as well as our preferred surgical techniques for the implantation of allografts for ACL, PCL, and lateral collateral ligament (LCL) ruptures. Finally, a brief review of current meniscal allograft investigations will be presented.

Allograft Considerations

After knee ligament rupture and the subsequent need for reconstruction, several factors must be considered when selecting an autograft or allograft for replacement. The ideal ligament graft should have sufficient strength and other biomechanical properties, should attempt to approximate normal anatomic structure, should have the potential for biologic healing and eventual incorporation by the host, and should have the ability to respond to normal stresses to provide knee stability. Autograft tissues fulfill many of these requirements, which explains why these are the most frequently used ligament substitute. At present, artificial ligament replacements have not proven satisfactory. In certain select circumstances, allograft tissues may be chosen for ligament reconstruction. Allografts can be sized to meet a specification, and no autogenous structures are used. In theory, there is an ample supply of allograft tissue, with lessened morbidity to the patient regarding the surgical procedure.

Conversely, allografts have certain inherent disadvantages. It was originally believed that few immunologic processes were involved with the implantation of devitalized frozen tissues. Even though it is extremely rare for immunologic processes to become clinically relevant, sophisticated studies have shown that, in some instances, there is a slow chronic response to foreign frozen tissue.[46,47] The allograft also undergoes a remodeling process that requires months, which is presumed to be much slower than that undergone by autograft replacements.[3,4,48] During this incorporation period, the graft is vulnerable to failure if extremes of stress are encountered. In addition, as with any transplantable tissue, there is a risk of bacterial and viral disease transmission.[49-51]

Allograft Processing and Sterilization

Three different methods are used to process and preserve bone and soft-tissue allografts. These are deep freezing (-70° C), freeze drying (lyophilization), and cryopreservation (cryoprotectant plus controlled-rate freezing). Generally, cryopreservation is reserved for cartilaginous structures and is used in an attempt to preserve living cells in the thawed tissue at the time of surgery. Even in the best of situations, only about 50% of the cells survive, and they no longer function in a metabolically normal fashion.[44] Deep freezing without cryopreservation is an excellent preservation technique that decreases the antigenicity of the graft and maintains its structural integrity. Once frozen, however, the graft must remain frozen until use. In freeze drying, or lyophilization, water within the biologic substance is replaced with alcohol. The alcohol is then sublimed from the tissue by a vacuum process, leaving it essentially dehydrated, stiff, and inert. Freeze-dried products can be stored at room temperature for many years, and they must be rehydrated upon use. In general, a minimum of 24 hours is required to totally rehydrate a structure as large as a tendon or ligament graft. It is often impractical to start rehydration of the graft prior to the actual start of the surgical procedure. In some instances, an impatient surgeon manipulates rehydrating tissue prematurely, which can fracture the collagen bundles and decrease the ultimate strength of the graft. Overall, we prefer and recommend the use of deep frozen tendon graft material.

In discussing the sterilization of grafts, several types of microbes need to be considered, including bacteria, fungi, and viruses. The majority of tissue currently used for ligament allograft replacement is procured under strictly aseptic conditions. These grafts undergo repeated bacterial and fungal culturing episodes to assure sterility in regard to those agents. Of greater concern is the possibility of viral contamination through clinically undetectable infection in the donor. Because viruses are extremely difficult to culture, especially in low numbers, culturing methods have not been effective in detecting viral particles in tissue.

Two widely used processes have been employed to sterilize allograft tissue. The first involves the use of ethylene oxide, which has been shown to be effective in sterilizing bacterial, fungal, and viral particles on nonporous surfaces such as surgical instruments. However, ethylene oxide has been shown to be ineffective in eradicating the feline leukemia virus from feline bone, an often-used human immunodeficiency virus (HIV) analog system.[51] In fact, the investigators were able to actually grow active virus after attempted sterilization with ethylene oxide in the feline model. Additionally, ethylene oxide-sterilized ACL allografts have been shown to produce reactive synovial and bony changes after implantation.[52,53] Therefore, this method of sterilization is not recommended for virus sterilization of biologic tissues.

Gamma radiation has been used for many years to sterilize substances that have bacterial contamination, and it is quite effective in eradicating fungi and bacterial species.[54] It has also been shown to decrease the infectivity of viral particles found on surfaces, in solutions, and in artificial infection models of allograft tissue.[55-57] However, it has been difficult to establish an irradiation level that will sterilize the graft against HIV and hepatitis viral infections,[58] without altering its mechanical properties.[59] While even 1 Mrad of gamma irradiation inactivates large classes of micoorganisms[54,56,60-64] including some viruses, Conway and associates[65] estimated that more than 3.6 Mrads of gamma irradiation may be needed to inactivate all but one in a million HIV-infected bone cells. This level is nearly twice the level of irradiation that the typical tissue bank applies to allograft tissues.[58,66] Moreover, Fideler and associates[57] showed that HIV-infected patellar ligament allografts subsequently irradiated to 2.5 Mrads were not uniformly sterilized, based on polymerase chain reaction testing.

Methods to Evaluate the Effects of Allograft Sterilization and Remodeling After Surgery

For an allograft to function successfully as a ligament replacement in the knee, the tissue must be able to withstand the lower functional loads of normal daily activity, the higher functional loads of vigorous activity, and traumatic failure forces, such as those that produced the original ligament injury.[59,67-69] Changes in the allograft caused by initial sterilization and remodeling after surgery can influence how well the allograft responds to these forces over time.

The in vivo response of sterilized and healing allografts to multiple force ranges are simulated in the laboratory, and the resultant changes in tissue and joint biomechanics are evaluated. Changes in tissue biomechanics caused by lower functional loads are simulated by performing viscoelastic static or cyclic creep tests (Fig. 1). Static creep tests involve applying a small constant load to the tissue and recording how much the graft stretches over time. Cyclic creep testing involves applying varied loads between zero (or some small amount) and a larger peak load. The cyclic test is performed at a frequency like that of normal gait and peak loads are similar to force levels—either those applied by the surgeon during implantation or those incurred later by the patient. The effects of higher functional loads, delivered to the allograft to simulate more vigorous activities of daily living, are usually assessed by recording the linear stiffness or slope of the allograft's force-deformation curve (Fig. 2). The effects of

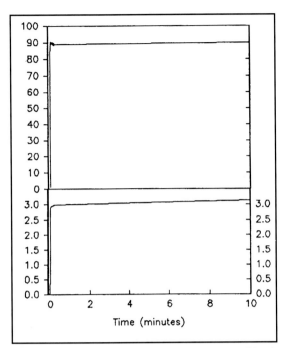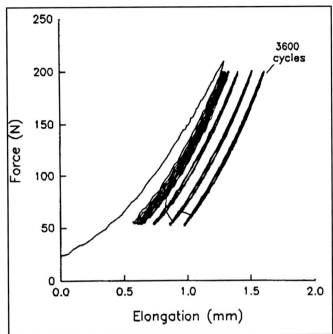

Fig. 1 Changes in tissue biomechanics at lower functional loads. **Left,** Typical static creep response for a 2 Mrad-irradiated human patellar tendon-bone (PTB) unit. The top plot shows the application of a 90-N force in less than 1 second. The bottom plot shows the initial PTB unit elongation, followed by slow elongation up to 10 min. **Right,** Typical cyclic creep response curve for an irradiated human PTB unit. Note the increase in elongation as the PTB unit is cycled for up to 1 h (3,600 cycles). (Reproduced with permission from Rasmussen TJ, Feder SM, Butler DL, et al: The effects of 4 Mrad of gamma irradiation on the initial mechanical properties of bone-patellar tendon-bone grafts. *Arthroscopy* 1994;10:188–197.)

traumatic failure loads are determined by monitoring the maximum force and deformation developed by the graft as well as the energy from the area under the loading curve to graft rupture (Fig. 2).

A second means of evaluating the performance of a treated or remodeling allograft is to determine how the treatment affects knee joint biomechanics. Three measures that represent altered joint mechanics are the knee's anterior-posterior displacement, its stiffness, and the contribution of the structure as a percentage of total joint load.[4,70,71] Tibiofemoral displacement and stiffness are measured at a specific applied load, typically a value like that imposed during an anterior drawer or Lachman test (Fig. 3). The percentage force contribution is computed at increments of controlled joint displacement.

By evaluating how treatment changes the tissue initially and over time, and by determining how the graft alters the function of the joint, biomechanical investigators can help the surgeon and therapist provide rational assessments of various treatment modalities. Inferior or marginally acceptable methods can be discarded, and more promising treatments pursued.

Effects of Preservation and Sterilization on Initial Tissue and Joint Properties

Tissue banks are challenged with providing surgeons and hospitals with allograft tissues that have been unaffected during transport and storage. Tissue preservation methods, such as freezing and freeze-drying, assure the tissue bank that allograft tendons will not degrade during

shipment, and also allow the hospital to store the specimens until the surgeon is ready to use them. Although frozen tissue must be maintained in dry ice during transport and kept properly frozen during storage, freeze-dried grafts can be transported and stored at room temperature. The mechanical and structural changes produced by these treatments are of obvious concern to all who deal with such grafts. Prior studies by several authors[72-74] have demonstrated that freezing alone has minimal effects on tendon, ligament, and bone mechanical properties, as long as the specimens are not repeatedly frozen and thawed. Bright and Burchardt,[75] Haut and Powlison,[76] Pelker and associates,[73] and Triantafyllou and associates[77] have also shown that freeze-drying alone produces only modest changes in tendon and bone biomechan-

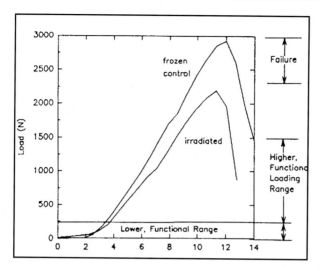

Fig. 2 Effects of higher functional loads and traumatic failure loads on allograft tissue response. Typical load-elongation curves for an irradiated and a contralateral frozen control human patellar tendon-bone unit generated during an axial failure test. Note the lower and higher functional loading regions and failure region. The effects of irradiation become more pronounced with increasing load level. (Reproduced with permission from Rasmussen TJ, Feder SM, Butler DL, et al: The effects of 4 Mrad of gamma irradiation on the initial mechanical properties of bone-patellar tendon-bone grafts. *Arthroscopy* 1994;10:188–197.)

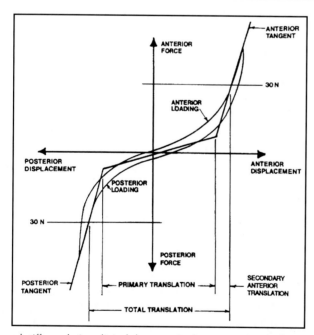

Fig. 3 Laxity and stiffness during clinical drawer or Lachman test. A typical anterior-posterior (AP) force-displacement curve for a goat knee, from which total AP translation, primary AP translation, and secondary anterior translation are determined. Anterior stiffness, in this case, is calculated from a line tangent to the loading curve at 30 N of anterior force. (Reproduced with permission from Holden JP, Grood ES, Butler DL, et al: Biomechanics of fascia lata ligament replacements: Early postoperative changes in the goat. *J Orthop Res* 1988;6:639–647.)

ics, with more pronounced effects after implantation.[48,78,79] A problem with freeze-drying is the necessity to rehydrate the specimen at surgery prior to implantation and to determine when the rehydration is complete. Preservation effects do require an understanding of the potential interactions with the process selected for tissue sterilization.

Surgeons, engineers, and tissue banks have been concerned with the mechanical alterations that might occur with high levels of irradiation.[59,80] It is known that high levels of gamma irradiation severely weaken large bone allografts before surgery. For example, cortical bone loses significant strength in bending and torsion if it is sterilized to more than 3 Mrads.[55,77,81] Therefore, it is not surprising that soft tissues might be similarly affected. Early soft-tissue irradiation studies[82,83] suggested that treatment-related changes do occur in patellar ligament allografts. Using paired goat patellar ligament-bone units, we showed that, compared to freezing alone, 3 Mrads of irradiation decreased the mechanical properties of maximum failure force by 27% and the energy to maximum force by 40%. Smaller reductions were noted in the material properties of maximum stress (15%) and energy per unit volume to maximum force (19%).[84] Haut and Powlison[76] and De Deyne and Haut[85] found that a combination of 2 Mrads of irradiation and freeze-drying reduced human patellar ligament mechanical properties, especially when the grafts were freeze-dried before irradiation. Thus, tissue banks and surgeons were forced to deal with the conflicting facts that high levels of gamma irradiation were required for viral sterilization, but that these high levels were detrimental to mechanical integrity.

We further addressed these issues by studying how higher levels of gamma irradiation alter the initial mechanical and material properties of goat and human patellar ligament-bone allografts before surgery. First, we determined the effects of up to 8 Mrads of gamma irradiation on goat patellar ligament allograft dimensions, mechanical and material properties, and collagen mature hydroxypyridinium cross-link density.[80] After bisecting left and right patellar ligament-bone units from ten animals to permit intra-animal comparisons, each left ligament half was frozen and then exposed to 4, 6, or 8 Mrads of gamma irradiation. The right ligament halves served as frozen controls (0 Mrads). Each patellar ligament-bone specimen was then failed in tension, after which its soft-tissue midsubstance was processed to measure collagen content and hydroxypyridinium cross-link density. We found dose-dependent reductions in allograft mechanical properties (Fig. 4). At 4 Mrads, decreases were found in maximum failure load (46%; $p < 0.01$) and stiffness (18%; $p < 0.05$). Reductions in material properties are shown in Figure 5. At 4 Mrads, reductions were found in maximum stress (37%; $p < 0.005$) and modulus (8%; $p > 0.05$). These results were consistent with those of the lower-dosage study by Gibbons and associates,[84] which are included as dashed lines in Figures 4 and 5. There were no decreases found in hydroxypyridinium cross-link density until 6 or more Mrads of irradiation ($p < 0.05$) were used.

In the second in vitro study, we exposed pairs of frozen, bisected human patellar ligament-bone allografts to either zero or 4 Mrads of gamma irradiation sterilization.[59] Each specimen was subjected to lower functional loads, higher functional loads, and then to failure. The effects of lower functional loads were assessed from static and cyclic creep tests, and the effects of higher functional loads and failure were obtained from a high rate, tensile failure test. Irradiation to 4 Mrads had no effect on static or cyclic creep ($p > 0.05$), with increases of 0.1 mm after 10 minutes of constant load and less than 0.5 mm after 3,600 cycles of

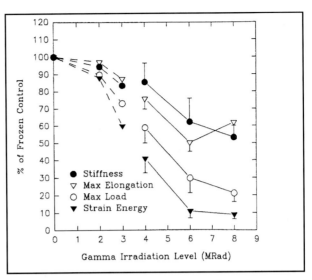

Fig. 4 Average dose-dependent response curves for four mechanical properties (solid lines), expressed as percentages of values for contralateral frozen controls. Normalized data for 2 and 3 Mrads of irradiation (broken lines) from our earlier study[84] are also plotted; that study used different testing conditions. Note the nearly linear decline in all curves between 2 and 6 Mrads. (Reproduced with permission from Salehpour A, Butler DL, Proch FS, et al: Dose-dependent response of gamma irradiation on mechanical properties and related biochemical composition of goat bone-patellar tendon-bone allografts. *J Orthop Res* 1995;13:848–906.)

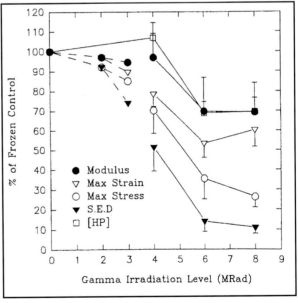

Fig. 5 Average dose-dependent response curves for all four material properties (solid lines), expressed as percentages of values for contralateral frozen controls. Normalized data for 2 and 3 Mrads (broken lines) from our earlier study[84] are also plotted; that study used different testing conditions. Note the nearly linear decline in all curves between 2 and 6 Mrads. S.E.D. = strain energy density and HP = hydroxypyridinium cross-link density. (Reproduced with permission from Salehpour A, Butler DL, Proch FS, et al: Dose-dependent response of gamma irradiation on mechanical properties and related biochemical composition of goat bone-patellar tendon-bone allografts. *J Orthop Res* 1995;13:848–906.)

oscillating load (Fig. 1). The treatment did, however, reduce linear stiffness (12%; $p < 0.025$) and maximum force (26%; $p < 0.001$) (Fig. 2). These results indicated that high levels of irradiation produced negligible changes in tissue performance at small loads, but graft behavior was altered under higher forces. While high levels of irradiation appeared to be deleterious, this study did not predict graft performance during the early healing and later collagen remodeling phases after cruciate ligament reconstruction.

We then asked whether the irradiation-induced reductions in patellar ligament stiffness might also reduce the knee's anterior restraining forces and intra-articular graft forces during anterior displacement of the tibia.[86] We treated paired goat patellar ligament allografts with three levels of gamma irradiation (0 versus 4 Mrads or 0 versus 6 Mrads) prior to ACL reconstruction. Intra-articular graft pre-tension (22 N) and flexion angle (50° from full extension) were controlled at implantation. We then performed 1,000 cyclic anterior drawer tests with the knee at 25° from full extension and measured cyclic anterior restraining force as well as intra-articular graft force using an implantable force transducer.[87–89] We found that knees reconstructed with grafts irradiated to 4 Mrads relaxed to 89% of the initial anterior force after 1,000 cycles compared to knees reconstructed with previously frozen grafts, which had relaxed to 73% of the initial anterior restraining force. Intra-articular graft forces followed a similar trend, with more pronounced relaxation in the control ligaments (62% of the initial graft force) than in the treated tissues (78% of the initial graft force). Differences in relaxation between the treated and control groups for anterior force and graft force were significant ($p < 0.05$) after 500 and 50 anterior displacement cycles, respectively. Thus, the data showed that irradiated grafts maintained their load

during cycling and demonstrated less viscoelasticity during loading.

Effect of Patellar Ligament Sterilization on Graft Remodeling After Implantation

We have also examined how two levels of ^{60}Co gamma irradiation (2 and 4 Mrads) influence allograft biomechanics and dimensions as well as grafted knee mechanics in the goat model 6 months after surgery.[90–92] We first evaluated the effects of 2 Mrads on these measures. Frozen, gamma-irradiated grafts were implanted in one knee of recipient goats and paired, frozen control grafts were implanted in the opposite knee. Surgeries were phased 8 weeks apart, but the experimental design permitted us to evaluate the grafts and knees an average 6 months after surgery. We found no significant effects of 2 Mrads of gamma irradiation on anterior-posterior knee translation or anterior knee stiffness. We also observed no significant differences in any graft dimension, mechanical property, or material property assessed.

Previous studies of ACL reconstruction have never, to our knowledge, reported the graft's contribution to resisting anterior-posterior translations compared to other joint structures. We developed a technique, modified from an earlier study,[70] to quantify these contributions for paired goat knees containing either frozen or frozen, 2 Mrad-irradiated allografts. After measuring anterior knee laxity and joint stiffness in the 6-month grafted, but otherwise intact, knee during anterior-posterior drawer, structures were sequentially sectioned without removing the knee from the tester. The anterior displacement test was repeated after each cut. The ACL allograft remained intact throughout testing, permitting its subsequent mechanical testing in axial tension. The percentage contribution at a predetermined anterior displacement was computed from the precut to postcut drop in

anterior force. Changes in anterior knee stiffness and anterior-posterior translations were also recorded after each cut. Frozen control and irradiated grafts were not significantly different ($p > 0.05$) in their percentage contributions to anterior restraining force, both contributing 50% to 62% of the total restraining force. We interpreted these results to indicate that after implantation irradiated allografts and frozen allografts function in a similar manner.

Our final study sought to investigate the effects of 4 Mrads of gamma irradiation on graft and knee biomechanics 6 months after surgery.[92,93] Paired patellar ligament allografts were procured, with left grafts irradiated to 4 Mrads and right grafts serving as frozen controls. Using a balanced design, we phased bilateral ACL reconstructions 8 weeks apart to allow return of near-normal gait. At 6 months, limbs were procured and frozen to -30° C for later evaluation. Anterior-posterior selective cutting tests were performed to determine the percentage contributions of the graft to anterior displacement. Graft area and length were measured, and each specimen failed in tension at a high strain rate. We again found no significant differences between treated and control grafts, with both grafts providing approximately 50% to 60% of total restraining force at 30 N anterior force and 50% to 65% of total restraining force at 50 N anterior force. A significant ($p < 0.05$) decrease in anterior knee stiffness was found in the knees containing irradiated grafts at both 30 and 50 N of anterior force. During subsequent failure testing of the graft-bone specimens, graft stiffness significantly ($p = 0.025$) decreased by 30% due to the treatment. No other mechanical or material properties were significantly affected by irradiation. In summary, 2 Mrads of irradiation showed no significant effect on anterior knee stiffness 6 months postoperatively. At 4 Mrads, both grafts provided equal contributions to resisting anterior translation, however, irradiation reduced knee stiffness by 33% to 40%.

Disease Transmission and Allograft Sterilization

Surgeons and patients remain justifiably concerned about the possibility of disease transmission after implanting soft-tissue allografts. To date, only one account of transmission of HIV has been documented following knee ligament allograft reconstruction.[94] The donor tissue was processed in 1985 at a tissue bank certified by the American Association of Tissue Banks after screening negative for the virus through family interview, medical history review, and enzyme-linked immunosorbent assay HIV antibody testing. The bone-patellar ligament-bone graft was frozen and was not processed or sterilized. Interestingly, three patients who received a total of four other soft-tissue allografts from this same donor (fascia lata, Achilles tendon, patellar ligament), which were processed and freeze-dried all tested negative for HIV.

Two cases of transmission of hepatitis C following patellar ligament allograft reconstruction have also been reported.[95] These grafts were frozen and were not processed or sterilized. Neither of the recipients had been tested for the antibody to hepatitis C preoperatively, and both tested positive for the antibody after surgery. In the same study, one other soft-tissue allograft and 11 bone allografts, which had been processed and irradiated, did not transmit the hepatitis C virus.

These cases[95,96] of viral disease transmission are similar in that the grafts were not processed, were transplanted without removal of blood and bone marrow, and did not receive any type of secondary sterilization. Similar soft-tissue allografts that had been processed and that received either ethylene oxide or irradiation sterilization did not transmit either hepatitis C or HIV in these reports.

Reducing the risk of transmission of HIV and other viral infections through transplantation of musculoskeletal allografts depends on several factors. Since the one reported case of HIV transmission, which occurred in 1985, there have been no known reports of this virus in at least 500,000 musculoskeletal allograft cases.[97] The only other known transmission of a viral infection, which occurred in 1991, involved the above-mentioned hepatitis C incidents. We recommend that surgeons take the following steps to reduce the risk of disease transmission. First, an understanding of the standards of tissue banks is essential. We recommend purchasing allografts only from banks that are accredited by the American Association of Tissue Banks and that have complied with the Food and Drug Administration regulations issued in 1993.[1] Second, the most advanced test for detection of viral diseases is the polymerase chain reaction assay,[97] an in vitro method of DNA amplification powerful enough to detect one infected cell in a population of 10^6 uninfected cells.[98] This is a more sensitive screening test than the antibody test, and may detect the HIV antibody within 20 to 25 days after exposure.[99,100] The decision for use of allograft sterilization with gamma irradiation rests with the surgeon. However, the Centers for Disease Control report that "although some physical and chemical agents have been shown to reduce the likelihood of isolating virus from treated solid tissues, conclusive evidence that those processes render solid tissue completely safe yet structurally intact is lacking."[101]

The current American Association of Tissue Banks recommended irradiation dosage is between 1.5 and 2.5 Mrads, although the Association acknowledges that some resistant spore-forming organisms and viruses may survive more than 2.5 Mrads.[102] Fideler and associates[57] reported in 1994 that doses of 2.0 to 2.5 Mrads did not inactivate HIV, as the viral DNA was detectable in bone marrow attached to bone-patellar ligament-bone grafts. These authors reported that DNA of HIV was not detectable in allografts treated with 3.0 to 4.0 Mrads of irradiation, and they concluded that at least 3.0 Mrads is required for sterilization. Conway and associates[103] calculated that approximately 3.6 Mrads is required to inactivate HIV in bone allografts. Although there is no absolute assurance regarding viral sterility, the senior author (FRN) has previously recommended 4.0 Mrads of irradiation for Achilles tendon and bone-patellar ligament-bone allografts,[19] recognizing the dose-dependent reductions in allograft biomechanics that occur above 2.0 Mrads.

Anterior Cruciate Ligament Allograft Reconstruction

Since Shino and associates[13] first report appeared on allografts for ACL reconstruction in 1986, an abundance of information and outcome data have been published describing results of this operation.[2–12,14–20,50,104] It is difficult to compare these studies because of discrepancies in length of follow-up, allograft tissues, secondary sterilization procedures, and rating systems employed to ascertain outcome. Bone-patellar ligament-bone grafts are the most popular allogeneic tissue described in the literature for ACL reconstruction. Fewer authors have used fascia lata or Achilles tendon tissues. Many different secondary sterilization techniques have been employed, including none (fresh-frozen), freeze-drying, ethylene oxide, a combination of freeze-drying and ethylene oxide, or irradiation. Of these sterilization procedures, deleterious effects on allograft healing have been attributed to ethylene oxide.[52,53,105]

Results

In our review of the current literature, we found 16 studies that provided joint arthrometer anterior-posterior displacement data following ACL allograft reconstruction. Table 1 shows the vari-

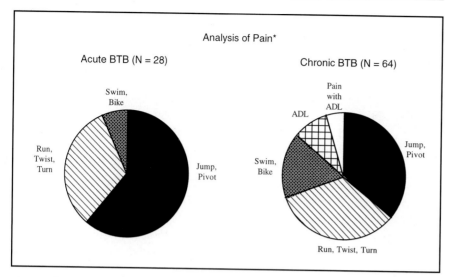

Fig. 6 Differences found between patients with acute and chronic anterior cruciate ligament ruptures after reconstruction for pain. The scale provides a rating for the highest activity level patients can achieve without incurring pain. BTB = bone-patellar tendon-bone; LAD = ligament augmentation device; EA = extra-articular; ADL = activities of daily living.

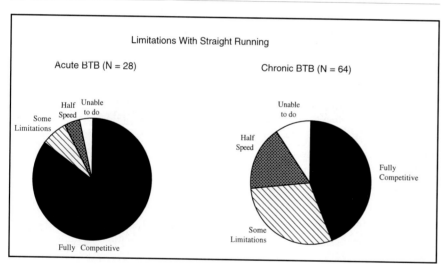

Fig. 7 Differences found between patients with acute and chronic anterior cruciate ligament ruptures after reconstruction for straight running.

ability in population characteristics, allograft tissues, methods of sterilization, force levels, and methods of data reduction that exists in these reports. We did not include studies that provided only mean displacement data in this assessment. The variability present in the reports listed in Table 1 accounts for the large range of percent of patients (19% to 86%) in the normal stability category (less than 3 mm of difference between the involved and noninvolved knee).[106] In knees with chronic ACL deficiency, an iliotibial band extra-articular procedure added to an allograft reconstruction resulted in lower amounts of displacement than did an allograft alone.[6] However, the addition of a ligament augmentation to allograft reconstructions did not reduce displacements.[107] The

effect of irradiation on anterior-posterior displacement, in comparison to fresh-frozen or other secondary sterilization procedures, has not been formally addressed in the literature. Four studies[14,21,23,24] have compared displacement data following allograft and autograft reconstruction; three[21,23,24] found no statistically significant difference between graft types, and one[14] found lower displacements in the allograft group.

Discrepancies also exist in the literature concerning the effect of allograft ACL reconstruction in patients with acute ruptures compared to those with chronic deficiency. Some authors reported no difference in results,[14,53] others found significant differences,[17,108] and still others combined these subgroups without assessing the effect of this variable on results.[4,16,23,24] We recommend assessing these subgroups separately, as we found that significant differences existed at follow-up in subjective symptom and function scores (Figs. 6 and 7). Patients with chronic ACL-deficiency often had a multitude of preexisting symptoms, and many had prior meniscectomy and presented with articular cartilage damage, which complicated treatment and, in some instances, contributed to poorer results.[76] The goals of ACL reconstruction in these individuals often differ from those for patients with acute ruptures who choose surgical intervention early after injury. Our displacement data also showed that significant differences existed at follow-up between these subgroups (Table 1), because patients with acute ruptures had lower anterior-posterior displacements than did those with chronic deficiency (except for patients who had an iliotibial band extra-articular procedure with the allograft).

In reviewing studies that assessed acute and chronic ACL ruptures separately and provided objective arthrometer data, the following conclusions may be reached. First, in a study we published with a mean follow-up of 7 years, allo-

Table 1
Joint arthrometer testing following anterior cruciate ligament allograft reconstruction

Author/Reference	No. Patients Tested, LF	Allograft Tissue, Sterilization	Arthrometer Results (Involved-Noninvolved) Force level	Distribution of Patients	Authors' Comments Regarding Displacement Data
Noyes et al[7]	42 A, 25-67 mos	BTB: FF	89N	83% < 3mm, 13% 3-5 mm, 4% > 5mm	BTB Significantly lower AP
		FL: FD + ETO	89N	53% < 3 mm, 42% 3-5 mm, 5% > 5mm	displacements than FL
Indelicato et al[4]	41 A & C, 24-36 mos	BTB:FD	89N	85% < 3 mm, 15% 3-5 mm	No significant difference FD and FF
		BTB: FF	89 N	84% < 3 mm, 15% 3-5 mm	BTB allografts
Noyes and Barber[6]	96 C, 23-54 mos	BTB: 2.5 Mrad Irr	89N	54% < 3 mm, 34% 3-5 mm, 12% > 5 mm	BTB + EA significantly lower AP
		Same, + ITB EA	89 N	74% < 3 mm, 22% 3-5 mm, 4% > 5 mm	displacements than BTB alone
Roberts et al[53]	31 A & C, 24 mos	BTB: FD + ETO	134 N	19% ≤ 3 mm, 55% 3-7 mm, 26% > 7 mm	Cannot recommend ETO
Olson et al[10]	23, 30-58 mos	BTB: FF	89 N	65% < 3 mm, 17% 3-5 mm, 17% ≥6 mm	
Noyes and Barber[107]	101 C, 23-53 mos	BTB: 2.5 Mrad Irr	89N	53% < 3 mm, 34% 3-5.5 mm, 13% ≥6 mm	LAD not effective in reducing AP
		Same, + LAD	89 N	53% < 3 mm; 30% 3-5.5 mm, 17% ≥6 mm	displacements
Indelicato et al[5]	40 C, 24-40 mos	BTB: FF	89 N	93% ≤ 5 mm, 7% ≥6 mm	
Meyers et al[104]	28, 24 mos	FL: FD	89 N	93% ≤ 4 mm, 7% > 4 mm	
Saddemi et al[23]	18 A & C, 24 mos	BTB: 2.0 Mrad Irr	178 N	86% < 3 mm, 9% 3-5 mm, 5% > 5 mm	No difference allografts and BTB autografts
Linn et al[112]	29 A & C, 18-44 mos	AT: FF	Manual maximum	69% < 2 mm, 28% 2-4 mm, 3% 5-7 mm	
Levitt et al[17]	181 A & C, 57 mos	AT or BTB FF or FD	Not given	87% ≤ 5 mm, 13% > 5 mm	No difference AT and BTB
Noyes et al[8]	57 C, 42 mos	BTB: 2.5 Mrads Irr	134 N	53% < 3 mm, 30% 3-5 mm, 17% ≥6 mm	ACL revision procedures
Pritchard et al[20]	39 A & C, 11 yrs	FL: FD + EA	134 N	82% ≤ 3 mm, 18% 3-5 mm	
Harner et al[21]	64 A & C, 30-75 mos	BTB: FF	134 N	94% ≤ 5 mm, 6% > 5 mm	No difference allografts and BTB autografts
Noyes and Barber-Westin[19]	68 A, 7 yrs	BTB: FF FL: FD+ ETO	89 N 89N	82% < 3 mm, 14% 3-5.5 mm, 4% >5.5 mm 78%<3 mm, 23% 3-5.5 mm	No deterioration in later results both BTB and FL
Stringham et al[24]	31 A & C, 13-57 mos	BTB: FF	Manual maximum	70% ≤ 3 mm, 22% ≤ 5 mm, 7% ≤ 6 mm	No statistical difference BTB allografts and autografts

LF = length of follow-up, A = acute, C = chronic, BTB = bone-patellar tendon-bone, FL = fascia lata, AT = achilles tendon, FF = fresh frozen, FD = freeze-dried, Irr = irradiated, ETO = ethylene oxide, ITB = illotibial band, EA = extra-articular, LAD = ligament augmentation device, AP = anteroposterior

grafts demonstrated the ability to restore stability in 78% and 82% (fascia lata and bone-patellar ligament-bone grafts, respectively) of knees with acute ruptures.[19] Sixty-eight patients were evaluated twice, and the early (2- to 4-year) results were compared with the later (5- to 9-year) results. No change or deterioration was found in the second evaluation for anterior-posterior displacements, patellofemoral crepitus, subjective pain and jump function scores, or the overall rating. The graft failure rate was 14%. We concluded that these favorable results justified the use of allografts for reconstruction of acute ACL rupture when the surgeon and patient choose this approach. We do note that our current study on bone-patellar ligament-bone autografts[109] in a consecutive series of 94

patients operated on by the senior author (FRN) showed a failure rate of 8% in knees with acute ruptures, which was lower than that found for allografts.

Second, allografts implanted in knees with chronic ACL ruptures restored stability in a lower percentage than in those with acute ruptures. Three[6,8,107] of four[5] studies that focused solely on chronic ruptures reported that 53% to 54% had less than 3 mm of increased displacement at a minimum of 2 years after surgery. Still, patients reported significant improvements in symptoms and functional limitations and returned to typically light sports activities. Failure rates ranged from 12% to 17% when allografts were used alone or with a ligament augmentation device, and were reduced to 4% when used with an iliotibial band

extra-articular procedure.

Third, allografts may be used in ACL revision operations when other graft alternatives are not available or chosen.[8,110,111] We prospectively followed 66 consecutive knees that had a bone-patellar ligament-bone allograft revision operation for a mean of 42 months postoperatively.[8] Arthrometer testing showed 53% had less than 3 mm of increased anterior-posterior displacement, 30% had 3 to 5 mm of increase, and 17% had 6 mm or more. Statistically significant improvements were found between the preoperative and follow-up subjective symptom and function scores. Patients that had articular cartilage damage had lower subjective scores than those that had normal appearing cartilage. Good short-term results were also reported by Safran and

Harner,[111] who followed up 35 patients an average of 2 years postoperatively. All patients in their series showed improvement in subjective symptoms and functional limitations and in arthrometer testing.

Complications involving immunologic reactions after ACL allograft reconstruction have been reported only in grafts sterilized with ethylene oxide. Pinkowski and associates[105] reported that freeze-dried ethylene oxide-sterilized grafts produced a measurable immune response in four of eight patients studied. Jackson and associates[52] found that seven of 109 patients (6.4%) developed symptoms that strongly suggested a nonspecific or immune-mediated response after implantation. Roberts and associates[53] noted that eight of 36 patients developed large tibial or femoral cysts, evident on radiographs, and had complete dissolution of the ethylene oxide-sterilized allograft. All of these investigators concluded that use of freeze-dried ethylene oxide-sterilized allografts is not recommended for ACL reconstruction.

A noticeable increase in the size of femoral and tibial tunnels following ACL allograft reconstruction was noted in one study, which used Achilles tendon allografts. Linn and associates[112] reported that nearly all of the 35 patients in their series who received a fresh-frozen Achilles tendon allograft had an increase in the size of the femoral and tibial tunnels 2 to 4 years postoperatively. The increase was unexplainable and did not correlate with any subjective or objective findings, including anterior-posterior displacement. Still, the authors recommended Achilles tendon allograft reconstruction only as a salvage procedure. In our series of 68 patients who had either fascia lata or bone-patellar ligament-bone allograft reconstruction, three knees had an increase in the size of the tibial tunnel and no knee had more than a 2 mm increase in the size of the femoral tunnel an average of 7 years postoperatively.[19] Shino and associates[13] found no abnormalities in the size or appearance of the femoral and tibial tunnels 2 years postoperatively in 31 patients who received a variety of allogeneic tendons.

In summary, in our experience, allografts are used less frequently than autograft tissues because of cost considerations, disease transmission issues, and improvements in surgical technique for the implantation of autografts, which have lessened the morbidity of the procedure. The current indications for allografts in ACL reconstruction are revision procedures and special situations, such as when suitable autogenous tissues are not available or during multiple ligament reconstructive procedures in which the autogenous tissues are used for other ligaments, such as the posterior cruciate or collaterals.

Preferred Technique
We prefer to use irradiated bone-patellar ligament-bone tissues for ACL allograft reconstruction. An endoscopic procedure uses one limited 2-cm incision on the tibia just adjacent to the patellar ligament to allow placement of the allograft. The allograft is preconditioned in the operating room in a sterile ligament-stretching device, which holds the graft under a constant force of 89 N for 20 minutes prior to implantation.

The bone portion is usually 22 to 25 mm long, 10 mm wide, and 6 to 8 mm deep; the ligament portion is 10 mm wide. Fixation is accomplished with an interference screw at both the tibial and femoral sites.

In select cases of allograft reconstruction in patients who have had failed multiple ligament reconstructive procedures, who have continued ACL deficiency, and who are competitive athletes or weigh over 200 lbs, we often use an iliotibial band extra-articular procedure in addition to the allograft reconstruction to improve stability results.[6] A Losee-type tenodesis of the iliotibial band is performed, modified by inserting the proximal part of the strip of the iliotibial band through an osseous tunnel in the lateral femoral condyle. The strip averages 12 mm in width. The defect in the iliotibial band is closed, and a lateral release is performed to relieve tension on the patellofemoral joint. Fixation is accomplished with sutures and a four-prong staple securing one arm of the graft to Gerdy's tubercle after passage through the femoral site. However, in these select cases we still prefer, if possible, to use an autograft. Note that the quadriceps tendon-patellar bone graft is frequently available, which avoids the necessity for an extra-articular procedure.

Posterior Cruciate Ligament Reconstruction
The use of allografts for posterior cruciate ligament (PCL) reconstruction has been discussed by only a few authors.[26,27,89] Miller and Harner[89] presented their preferred surgical technique and noted that Achilles tendon allografts were their first choice for PCL replacement. Clinical follow-up data were not available for assessment. Bullis and Paulos[26] briefly described 12-month follow-up results for 20 patients who received PCL Achilles tendon allograft reconstruction. At follow-up, 75% had resumed at least light sports, and 60% had 5 mm or less of posterior drawer on manual testing. The authors recommended that allografts could be used for PCL reconstruction when autogenous tissues are not available.

Results
We previously reviewed in detail our experience with PCL allograft reconstructions.[27] Twenty-five patients were treated either with an allograft reconstruction alone (ten patients) or with an allograft-ligament augmentation device composite (15 patients). All fresh frozen allografts received 2.5 Mrads of gamma irradiation prior to implantation. Ten patients had an acute PCL rupture;

15 had chronic ruptures. Postoperatively, no statistically significant differences were found between the allograft alone group and the composite group for anterior-posterior displacements, symptoms, functional limitations, sports activity levels, or the overall rating score. The ligament augmentation device provided no benefit to the reconstruction. The arthrometer data showed that, at 20° of flexion, all of the knees with acute ruptures had less than 3 mm of increased displacement. In knees with chronic deficiency, 60% had less than 3 mm and 40% had 3 to 5.5 mm of increase. At 70° of knee flexion, none of the knees with acute ruptures had less than 3 mm of increased displacement, 60% had 3 to 5.5 mm, and 40% had 6 mm or more. In the knees with chronic deficiency, 25% had an increase of less than 3 mm, 12% had 3 to 5.5 mm, and 63% had 6 mm or more. Patients with acute ruptures showed significantly better symptom and functional outcome than those with chronic deficiency. We concluded that the PCL allograft reconstruction restored posterior stability in the majority of patients at low functional knee flexion angles but not at higher flexion angles. Our current recommendation for PCL reconstruction is to use autogenous tissues (quadriceps-tendon bifid graft), reserving allografts for those cases for which suitable autogenous tissues are not available.

Preferred Technique
The PCL allograft reconstruction is performed as an arthroscopically assisted procedure with an Achilles tendon-bone allograft. A 2-cm skin incision is made over the medial femoral condyle, and a second 2-cm incision is made over the medial tibia adjacent to the tibial tubercle. The osseous portion of the allograft may be secured to the femoral condyle site with an interference screw or fixed to the posterior tibia by a limited posteromedial approach, with the gastrocnemius muscle and neurovascular structures reflected

laterally. The collagenous portion of the graft is split into a bifid graft with half of the graft (occupying the distal femoral PCL footprint) tensioned at 90° of flexion and the other half of the graft (occupying the proximal portion of the PCL footprint) tensioned at 10° of flexion. The purpose is to fill the PCL anatomic footprint with collagenous tissue and to tension a major portion of the PCL graft in flexion to decrease postoperative graft forces and to allow better control of posterior tibial subluxation with knee flexion.[113]

Lateral Ligament Reconstructions
The use of allografts to reconstruct ruptured lateral ligament structures has been reported by only a few authors,[31,114] and we are aware of only one report that provided clinical follow-up data of this procedure.[31] The indications are based on the quality and integrity of the lateral collateral ligament (LCL) and posterolateral tissues determined at the time of surgery. In cases in which a definitive, but slack, LCL of normal width and integrity is identified (at least 5 to 7 mm in width), the popliteus attachments to the fibula (popliteal-fibular ligament) and tibia are intact, and the posterolateral structures judged to be of adequate thickness (3 to 4 mm), a proximal advancement may be performed.[33] In cases in which the LCL is deficient as a result of prior gross disruption and poor healing and is not of normal width, or if considerable scar tissue to the lateral and posterolateral structures is identified, an allograft or autograft augmentation of the LCL and posterolateral tissues may be performed.

Results
We reported results of the LCL allograft procedure previously.[31] Twenty-one consecutive patients who had this procedure were followed a mean of 42 months postoperatively. All had chronic LCL deficiency, 13 also had ACL deficiency; three had PCL deficiency; and three had medial col-

lateral ligament deficiency. All of the concomitant deficient ligaments were reconstructed during the LCL allograft procedure. Additionally, a plication or advancement of the remaining posterolateral tissues was performed in all patients. Fifteen of the allografts used for the LCL reconstruction received 2.5 Mrads of gamma irradiation prior to implantation. The results showed that 16 knees (76%) had a functional LCL reconstruction, three (14%) had partial function, and two (10%) failed. All but one of the 13 patients who had a concomitant ACL reconstruction had function or partial function of that ligament restored. Of the three PCL reconstructions, one was functional, one was partially functional, and one failed. Subjectively, significant improvements were found for symptoms and functional limitations at follow-up. We concluded that the procedure was effective in restoring lateral and posterolateral complex function in the majority of knees.

Preferred Technique
A straight lateral incision approximately 15 cm in length centered over the lateral joint line is used. The incision extends distally to allow exposure to the fibular head and peroneal nerve, and proximally to allow exposure of the attachment of the LCL to the femur. The skin flaps are mobilized to protect the vascular and neural supply to the skin. After identifying the attachment of the iliotibial band, an incision is made along the anterior border of the iliotibial band and continued proximally, overlying the vastus lateralis. The attachment of the iliotibial band to the lateral intramuscular septum is preserved. An inferior incision is made along the posterior aspect of the iliotibial band and the attachments overlying the biceps muscle.

The peroneal nerve is identified proximally and is carefully dissected, proceeding distally around the fibular neck to a point 2 cm distal to the neck, where the nerve enters the anterior tibial muscle

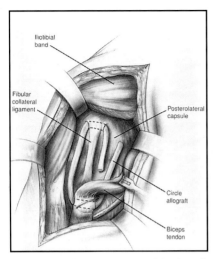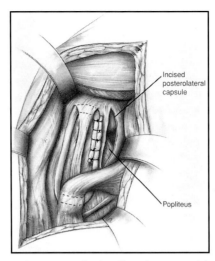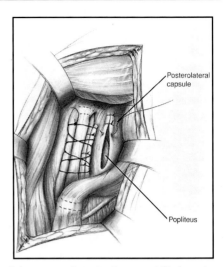

Fig. 8 Allograft reconstruction of the lateral cruciate ligament. **Left,** The allograft is inserted through bony tunnels in the femur and fibula and lies next to the stretched and slack LCL. **Center,** Suture of allograft arms and remaining ligament tissues. **Right,** A vest-over-pants plication of the posterolateral complex to the LCL reconstruction. (Reproduced with permission from Noyes FR, Roberts CS: High tibial osteotomy in knees with associated chronic ligament deficiencies, in Jackson DW (ed): *Reconstructive Knee Surgery.* New York, NY, Raven Press, 1995, pp 185–210.)

compartment. The peroneal nerve is protected throughout the surgical procedure. The fibular head and neck region is exposed anteriorly and posteriorly by subperiosteal dissection. Approximately 12 to 15 mm of the proximal fibula is exposed. A 6-mm drill hole is made anteriorly and posteriorly at the head-neck junction in the center of the fibula. A drill guide is used to ensure that the soft tissues are protected. A straight curette is used to dilate the 6-mm cortical hole from anterior to posterior, compressing the cancellous bone. The tibiofibular joint capsule is not disturbed.

At the femoral attachment of the LCL, a 6-mm drill hole is made just anterior and posterior to the ligament's insertion. The drill hole is deepened 10 mm, leaving approximately 8 mm of the LCL attachment. The lateral femoral cortex is preserved at the ligament attachment site. A curved curette is used to make a bony tunnel underneath the ligament insertion without removing excess bone.

An Achilles tendon allograft, 6 to 7 mm in diameter, is prepared. The graft is measured to allow sufficient length (19 to

20 mm) for the proximal and distal posterior arms of the circle graft to overlap, which adds additional collagenous tissue to the posterolateral aspect of the joint. Two interlocking closed loop sutures of No. 2 Ticron (Davis and Feck, Danbury, CT) are sutured into both ends of the allograft. The graft is initially stretched for 15 minutes under an 89 N load in a ligament stretching device.

An incision is made vertically just behind the LCL into the posterolateral capsule, just anterior to the arcuate complex. The tissues of the posterolateral capsule, arcuate ligament complex, and LCL are carefully inspected. Either a simple vest-over-pants capsular plication or a proximal advancement of the posterolateral complex on the femur is performed based on the quality and integrity of these tissues.

The allograft is inserted through the bony tunnel in the femur and fibula and lies next to the stretched and slack LCL (Fig. 8, *left*). The allograft is placed under slight tension with the knee at 30° of flexion, neutral tibial rotation, and with the lateral side of the joint closed. Multiple

interrupted sutures are used through the posterior overlapped arms of the allograft (Fig. 8, *center*). The slack LCL is interposed between the anterior and posterior arms of the circled allograft, and horizontal sutures are placed between both structures (Fig. 8, *right*). The knee is taken through a range of motion of 0° to 90°. Normal internal-external rotation is determined at 30° of flexion to avoid overconstraining the joint. The posterolateral plication or advancement is then performed under sufficient tension to allow 0° of extension without hyperextension. The vertical incision between the LCL allograft and the posterolateral structures is closed throughout.

The purpose of this procedure is to provide the first arm of the lateral reconstruction and replace important tensile bearing tissues laterally and posterolaterally. It is then possible to perform either plication or advancement of the posterolateral complex, which is also sutured to the allograft reconstruction, producing a dense collagenous plate of tissues extending from the LCL around the posterolateral corner of the knee joint.

In cases of severe disruption to the lateral and posterolateral tissues, graft substitutions of the LCL and posterolateral structures are required. Our preferred graft choice is a bone-patellar ligament-bone substitution for the LCL and a semitendinosus-gracilis double graft substitution of the popliteus-arcuate complex.[32] Alternative graft choices include allografts, or an iliotibial band autogenous graft.

Allografts in the Dislocated Knee

Use of allografts may be indicated in the reconstruction of the dislocated knee in which multiple ligament ruptures are present. In these knees, the surgeon may prefer to reduce the morbidity of the procedure and not harvest autogenous tissues, or autogenous tissues may be used to reconstruct one cruciate and allogeneic tissues to reconstruct the other cruciate. In the worst cases, a severely ruptured medial collateral ligament or LCL may also require graft augmentation, thereby complicating the procedure. Allografts offer an attractive graft source in these knees because of their availability and because they reduce operating time and morbidity in already traumatized knees.

To our knowledge, results of allografts used to reconstruct one or both cruciates in the dislocated knee have been provided in only three series in the literature.[28–30] Shapiro and Freedman[30] used fresh-frozen Achilles tendon or bone-patellar ligament-bone allografts to reconstruct both cruciates in seven patients. Five patients sustained 17 concomitant orthopaedic injuries; two of these had arterial injuries and three developed peroneal nerve palsy. Patients used a continuous passive motion machine postoperatively. An average of 51 months postoperatively, only one patient had significant pain, three patients had giving-way, and all had returned to work or school. Arthrometer testing at 20° of flexion showed that three patients

had less than 3 mm of increased anterior-posterior displacement and four patients had 5 mm or more of increase. Two patients required manipulation, and two others had arthroscopic lysis of adhesions for arthrofibrosis. At follow-up, three of these patients lacked 3° to 5° of extension and three had 105° to 115° of flexion. The authors concluded that reconstruction of both cruciate ligaments can minimize pain and improve functional outcome, but that arthrofibrosis is a common complication and manipulation is frequently necessary.

Fanelli and associates[28] used a combination of allografts and autografts to reconstruct both cruciates in a series of 20 knees. Irradiated allografts were used to reconstruct 14 of the PCLs, and four of the ACLs. Both acute (ten knees) and chronic (ten knees) injuries were included in the series. Nineteen patients had concomitant medial or lateral ligament ruptures. An arthroscopic technique was employed, followed by 3 weeks of immobilization. At a minimum of 2 years after surgery, no differences were found in rating scales or arthrometer measurements between the acute and chronic injuries, or between PCL autograft and allograft subgroups. On manual testing, improvements were noted in 11 knees that had a grade I posterior drawer (increase 5 mm) test and in nine knees that had a normal drawer test. However, on objective arthrometer testing, no statistically significant improvement was found in posterior displacement measurements from the preoperative values. Significant improvements were found in the mean anterior displacements between the preoperative and follow-up evaluations. The authors concluded that the results of the ACL reconstructions were more predictable than those of PCL reconstructions.

We recently reviewed our series of 11 consecutive patients who had concomitant reconstruction of both cruciate ligaments following total knee dislocation.[29] Irradiated or fresh-frozen allografts were

used to reconstruct ten ACLs, nine PCLs, and one LCL. Six patients also required repair or reconstruction of the medial ligamentous structures, and five had reconstruction or advancement of posterolateral complex tissues. Seven patients had acute injuries and were operated on a range of 7 to 28 days after the injury (Group 1), and four patients had chronic ruptures and received the operation a range of 13 to 31 months following injury (Group 2). All 11 patients returned for follow-up a mean of 4.8 years postoperatively (range, 2.5 to 9 years).

All ligament ruptures were surgically addressed. All patients were placed into a program of immediate knee motion and rehabilitation. The program included protection against early weightbearing or vigorous activity, because these knees had multiple gross instabilities. A full lower extremity, hinged double-upright brace was used for at least 12 weeks postoperatively. Knee motion in the range of 10° to 90° was allowed for the first 4 postoperative weeks and was then gradually increased to 135° by the twelfth postoperative week. No or only toe-touch weightbearing was allowed for the first 4 postoperative weeks. Then, a gradual increase was permitted, with full weightbearing allowed by the twelfth to sixteenth postoperative week. Knee hyperextension was avoided for 6 months postoperatively, and as they resumed weightbearing patients were assigned to a specific gait retraining program designed to avoid knee hyperextension. Hamstring exercises were avoided for the first 12 postoperative weeks to avoid excessive posterior shear forces and protect the PCL grafts. Running was discouraged for the first 10 to 12 postoperative months, and patients in whom articular cartilage deterioration was found during the reconstruction were counseled to return to only light recreational activities.

At follow-up in Group 1, the results of joint arthrometer and subluxation testing showed that only one of 22 (5%) ligament reconstructions failed. All but one of the patients in this group had less than 3 mm of increased total anterior-posterior displacement at 20° and 70° of knee flexion. The one knee in which the ACL graft failed had 11 mm of increased anterior-posterior displacement at 20° of flexion. One knee had 3.5 mm of increase at 70° of flexion.

In Group 2, three of 12 (25%) reconstructive procedures failed. These included two PCL reconstructions and one posterolateral split biceps tendon transposition. All patients in this group had less than 3 mm of increased displacement at 20° of flexion. At 70°, two patients had less than 3 mm and two patients had more than 6 mm of increased displacement.

Five patients, all from Group 1, required treatment intervention for early postoperative knee motion limitations. Nine of the 11 patients had a full range of motion at follow-up. One patient lacked 5° of both flexion and extension and one had only 100° of total knee flexion.

At follow-up, the subjective questionnaire findings determined that five of the seven patients in Group 1 had no limitations with daily or sports activities. None of these patients had experienced a giving-way reinjury since the operation. Three patients had returned to strenuous sports activities; three, to swimming or bicycling only; and one had not returned to athletics. The patient rating of the knee condition showed that three patients rated their knee as normal; two, good; and two, poor.

In Group 2, the subjective questionnaire analysis showed that three patients had no symptoms with daily activities but had symptoms with any sports activity, and one patient had no symptoms with swimming or bicycling but could not perform any other athletic activity. Importantly, these patients all demonstrated articular cartilage damage during the reconstruction procedure and between the symptoms arising from the

knee arthrosis and our counseling, most decided to avoid any sports activity. The patient rating of the knee condition showed that one patient rated the knee as very good; one, good; and two, fair.

We concluded that simultaneous ACL and PCL reconstruction, performed with associated medial or lateral repair or reconstruction, is warranted to restore function to all ligament structures. Even though an immediate knee motion program was used, many patients experienced difficulty regaining motion and required manipulation or arthroscopic debridement, which was performed early postoperatively and which was effective in restoring full motion and preventing permanent arthrofibrosis. An arthroscopic approach for the ACL and PCL substitution procedure can be used in select knees, if one side (medial or lateral ligaments) is not disrupted and if there is sufficient soft-tissue healing to allow the procedure. In select cases in which soft-tissue damage is extreme and early reconstruction inadvisable, we allow for early soft-tissue healing and knee motion during this delay of 2 to 3 weeks by using appropriate brace protection. We proceed with ligament reconstruction after the initial trauma to the tissue is stabilized and knee motion regained. The goal is to lessen the postoperative knee motion complications frequently encountered after major ligament reconstruction in dislocated knees.

Meniscal Allografts

At the time of writing, there were no long-term clinical studies in the English literature pertaining to outcome of meniscal allografts. Table 2 shows the wide variability among investigations concerning tissue processing, length of follow-up, secondary sterilization, and methods of evaluation of these allografts. While many studies have found good healing at the allograft-host interface,[115-119] others report correlations between allograft degeneration or failure

and joint arthrosis.[41,42] Importantly, because there are no long-term studies at present, no conclusions can be reached concerning the procedure's ability to prevent articular cartilage deterioration.

We recently presented the largest consecutive series of meniscal allografts followed prospectively for at least 2 years postoperatively.[41] Ninety-six fresh-frozen, irradiated meniscus allografts were implanted arthroscopically into 82 patients who had a prior meniscectomy. The mean patient age was 29 years (range, 13 to 45 years). Twenty-nine menisci in 28 patients were removed prior to the 2-year follow-up evaluation, and these were excluded except for the calculation of the overall rate of failure and the histologic analysis. Therefore, 67 menisci (57 medial and ten lateral) in 62 patients were studied. Fifty-four patients also had ACL deficiency, and 50 of these were reconstructed. All 62 patients returned for evaluation a mean of 30 months postimplantation (range, 22 to 58 months). The meniscal allografts were evaluated by magnetic resonance imaging (MRI) in 60 patients a mean of 28 months postoperatively and by follow-up arthroscopy in 35 patients a mean of 16 months postoperatively. A classification of meniscal healing was devised using MRI and arthroscopy criteria. All patients were also rated on the Cincinnati Knee Rating System.

The overall meniscal healing rates for all 96 menisci were nine (9%), healed; 30 (31%), partially healed; 56 (58%), failed; and one (2%), unknown. The overall healing rates for the 67 menisci that survived for at least 2 years postoperatively were nine (13%), healed; 30 (45%), partially healed; 27 (40%), failed; and one (2%), unknown. A significant relationship was found between the overall healing rates and the arthrosis rating on MRI ($p < 0.001$). Patients with femoral condylar spurring and tibial plateau concavity had higher rates of failure than those with normal appearing tibiofemoral joints.

Table 2
Clinical outcome studies following meniscal allograft implementation

Author/Reference	No. Menisci Followed	Tissue Processing, Sterilization	Length of Follow-up	Evaluation Methods	Results, Authors' Conclusions
Locht et al[37]	5	Fresh	24 months	Clinical only	No clinical evidence allograft tearing
Keene et al[116]	1	Fresh	6 months	Arthroscopy	Healed periphery only
Milachowski et al[40]	20	FF, FD	6-30 months	Arthroscopy (14) Arthrography (6)	One failure, no operative complications
Zukor et al[44]	14	Fresh	12 months	Arthroscopy (10)	Minor tears frequent but no failures
Meyers et al[38]	2	Fresh	24 months	Clinical only	Cannot recommend, no data on survival
Milachowski et al[39]	22	FF, FD, & Irrad	4-30 months	Arthroscopy (16) Arthrography (6)	Both types menisci decreased in size, fresh-frozen better results
Zukor et al[45]	28	Fresh	1-8.5 years	Arthroscopy (10) Arthrotomy (5)	No reoperations/failures due to meniscus
De Boer and Koudstaal[24]	1	Cryo	12 months	Arthroscopy	Meniscus survived, patient asymptomatic
Garrett[35]	28	Fresh or Cryo	2-24 months	Arthroscopy	Eight cases failed due to arthrosis
Shelton[43]	10	Cryo	< 12 months	Arthroscopy (2)	Two failures, no data on long-term survival
Rubins et al[117]	42	Cryo	6-18 months	Arthroscopy (8)	Graft/host interface healed, symptom relief
Wojtys and Carpenter[119]	9	Unknown	14-40 months	Arthroscopy	Excellent meniscal-capsular healing, pain relief
Veltri et al[118]	11	Cryo	8 months	Arthroscopy (7)	Allografts can be expected to heal at periphery
De Boer and Koudstaal[115]	3	Cryo	12, 20, 24 months	Arthroscopy	Allograft failure due to factors responsible for vascularization, joint instability or malalignment
Noyes and Barber-Westin[41]	96	Irrad	22-58 months	MRI (60) Arthroscopy (64)	9% healed, 31% partially healed. Failures correlated with joint arthrosis
Potter et al[42]	24	Fresh	3-41 months	MRI (24) Arthroscopy (19)	63% degeneration posterior horn. Correlation displacement/degeneration with joint arthrosis

FF = fresh frozen, FD = freeze-dried, Irrad = irradiated, Cryo = cryopreserved, MRI = magnetic resonance imaging

At follow-up arthroscopy, ten of the 35 grafts observed had small tears, and six of these required partial meniscectomy. Histologic evaluations of the failed specimens typically showed minimal cellular repopulation of the central core and on both the tibial and femoral surfaces. In the majority, the predominant cell type was a fibrocyte. Abnormal, disorganized collagen orientation was also found in several specimens.

Thirty-eight of the 50 knees that had ACL reconstruction were stable at follow-up. Statistically significant improvements were found for symptoms and functional limitations with activities of daily living and sports ($p < 0.05$). These improvements were attributed to restoration of knee stability and not the meniscal allograft procedure.

We believe multiple factors may have led to the high failure rate of the meniscal allografts in this study. These include the minimal cellular repopulation of the allograft central core, the disorganized collagen orientation and predominant fibrocyte cellular structure found in several of the failed specimens, and a possible increase in water content as reported by Jackson and Simon.[120] All of these factors are indicators of a disorder in the remodeling process required for subsequent meniscal function after implantation.

Based on these findings, we reserve meniscal allograft transplantation to symptomatic knees in young individuals in whom advanced joint arthrosis has not occurred. The high failure rate precludes our recommendation of this procedure in asymptomatic postmeniscectomized patients at this time. We acknowledge that these conclusions apply only to the type of meniscus allografts and procedures described in this study. Hopefully, as more research is performed and success rates for meniscus allografts demonstrate higher healing rates, the procedure will become an important development to decrease postmeniscectomized knee arthrosis in the future.

Conclusion/Recommendations

In our practice, we prefer the use of autogenous tissues (bone-patellar ligament-bone, quadriceps tendon-bone, semitendinosus-gracilis) for knee ligament reconstruction. However, allografts play a role in major ligament reconstructive procedures in which multiple substitutions or revisions are required. In the dislocated knee, allografts may offer an advantage in reconstructing the PCL. As well, allografts offer an appropriate substitute for LCL and posterolateral reconstructions in chronically deficient multiply operated knees. In this evolving field, the surgeon should be aware of issues pertaining to graft processing and risks of disease transmission to select the appropriate ligament reconstructive procedure with the least risk and morbidity to the patient.

References

1. Vangsness CT Jr, Triffon MJ, Joyce MJ, et al: Soft tissue for allograft reconstruction of the human knee: A survey of the American Association of Tissue Banks. *Am J Sports Med* 1996;24:230–234.

2. Barber-Westin SD, Noyes FR: The effect of rehabilitation and return to activity on anterior-posterior knee displacements after anterior cruciate ligament reconstruction. *Am J Sports Med* 1993;21:264–270.

3. Defrere J, Franckart A: Freeze-dried fascia lata allografts in the reconstruction of anterior cruciate ligament defects: A two- to seven-year follow-up study. *Clin Orthop* 1994;303:56–66.

4. Indelicato PA, Bittar ES, Prevot TJ, et al: Clinical comparison of freeze-dried and fresh frozen patellar tendon allografts for anterior cruciate ligament reconstruction of the knee. *Am J Sports Med* 1990;18:335–342.

5. Indelicato PA, Linton RC, Huegel M: The results of fresh-frozen patellar tendon allografts for chronic anterior cruciate ligament deficiency of the knee. *Am J Sports Med* 1992;20:118–121.

6. Noyes FR, Barber SD: The effect of an extra-articular procedure on allograft reconstructions for chronic ruptures of the anterior cruciate ligament. *J Bone Joint Surg* 1991;73A:882–892.

7. Noyes FR, Barber SD, Mangine RE: Bone-patellar ligament-bone and fascia lata allografts for reconstruction of the anterior cruciate ligament. *J Bone Joint Surg* 1990;72A;1125–1136.

8. Noyes FR, Barber-Westin SD, Roberts CS: Use of allografts after failed treatment of rupture of the anterior cruciate ligament. *J Bone Joint Surg* 1994;76A:1019–1031.

9. Noyes FR, Mangine RE, Barber S: Early knee motion after open and arthroscopic anterior cruciate ligament reconstruction. *Am J Sports Med* 1987;15:149–160.

10. Olson EJ, Harner CD, Fu FH, et al: Clinical use of fresh, frozen soft tissue allografts. *Orthopedics* 1992;15:1225–1232.

11. Shino K, Inoue M, Horibe S, et al: Maturation of allograft tendons transplanted into the knee: An arthroscopic and histological study. *J Bone Joint Surg* 1988;70B:556–560.

12. Shino K, Inoue M, Nakamura H, et al: Arthroscopic follow-up of anterior cruciate ligament reconstruction using allogeneic tendon. *Arthroscopy* 1989;5:165–171.

13. Shino K, Kimura T, Hirose H, et al: Reconstruction of the anterior cruciate ligament by allogeneic tendon graft: An operation for chronic ligamentous insufficiency. *J Bone Joint Surg* 1986;68B:739–746.

14. Shino K, Nakata K, Horibe S, et al: Quantitative evaluation after arthroscopic anterior cruciate ligament reconstruction: Allograft versus autograft. *Am J Sports Med* 1993;21:609–616.

15. Valenti JR, Sala D, Schweitzer D: Anterior cruciate ligament reconstruction with fresh-frozen patellar tendon allografts. *Int Orthop* 1994;18:210–214.

16. Wainer RA, Clarke TJ, Poehling GG: Arthroscopic reconstruction of the anterior cruciate ligament using allograft tendon. *Arthroscopy* 1988;4:199–205.

17. Levitt RL, Malinin T, Posada A, et al: Reconstruction of anterior cruciate ligaments with bone-patellar tendon-bone and achilles tendon allografts. *Clin Orthop* 1994;303:67–78.

18. Noyes FR, Barber-Westin SD: The treatment of acute combined ruptures of the anterior cruciate and medial ligaments of the knee. *Am J Sports Med* 1995;23:380–389.

19. Noyes FR, Barber-Westin SD: Reconstruction of the anterior cruciate ligament with human allograft: Comparison of early and later results. *J Bone Joint Surg* 1996;78A:524–537.

20. Pritchard JC, Drez D Jr, Moss M, et al: Long-term followup of anterior cruciate ligament reconstruction using freeze-dried fascia lata allografts. *Am J Sports Med* 1995;23:593–596.

21. Harner CD, Olson E, Irrgang J, et al: Allograft versus autograft anterior cruciate ligament reconstruction: 3- to 5-year outcome. *Clin Orthop* 1996;324:134–144.

22. Lephart SM, Kocher MS, Harner CD, et al: Quadriceps strength and functional capacity after anterior cruciate ligament reconstruction: Patellar tendon autograft versus allograft. *Am J Sports Med* 1993;21:738–743.

23. Saddemi SR, Frogameni AD, Fenton PJ, et al: Comparison of perioperative morbidity of anterior cruciate ligament autografts versus allografts. *Arthroscopy* 1993;9:519–524.

24. Stringham DR, Pelmas CJ, Burks RT, et al: Comparison of anterior cruciate ligament reconstructions using patellar tendon autograft or allograft. *Arthroscopy* 1996;12:414–421.

25. Snyder-Mackler L, Delitto A, Bailey SL, et al: Strength of the quadriceps femoris muscle and functional recovery after reconstruction of the anterior cruciate ligament: A prospective, randomized clinical trial of electrical stimulation. *J Bone Joint Surg* 1995;77A:1166–1173.

26. Bullis DW, Paulos LE: Reconstruction of the posterior cruciate ligament with allograft. *Clin Sports Med* 1994;13:581–597.

27. Noyes FR, Barber-Westin SD: Posterior cruciate ligament allograft reconstruction with and without a ligament augmentation device. *Arthroscopy* 1994;10:371–382.

28. Fanelli GC, Giannotti BF, Edson CJ: Arthroscopically assisted combined anterior and posterior cruciate ligament reconstruction. *Arthroscopy* 1996;12:5–14.

29. Noyes FR, Barber-Westin SD: Reconstruction of the anterior and posterior cruciate ligaments after knee dislocation: Use of early protected postoperative motion to decrease arthrofibrosis. *Am J Sports Med* 1997;25:769–778.

30. Shapiro MS, Freedman EL: Allograft reconstruction of the anterior and posterior cruciate ligaments after traumatic knee dislocation. *Am J Sports Med* 1995;23:580–587.

31. Noyes FR, Barber-Westin SD: Surgical reconstruction of severe chronic posterolateral complex injuries of the knee using allograft tissues. *Am J Sports Med* 1995;23:2–12.

32. Noyes FR, Barber-Westin SD: Treatment of complex injuries involving the posterior cruciate and posterolateral ligaments of the knee. *Am J Knee Surg* 1996;9:200–214.

33. Noyes FR, Roberts CS: High tibial osteotomy in knees with associated chronic ligament deficiencies, in Jackson DW (ed): *Reconstructive Knee Surgery*. New York, NY, Raven Press, 1995, pp 185–210.

34. De Boer HH, Koudstaal J: The fate of meniscus cartilage after transplantation of cryopreserved nontissue-antigen-matched allograft: A case report. *Clin Orthop* 1991;266:145–151.

35. Garrett JC: Abstract: Free meniscal transplantation: A prospective study of 44 cases. *Arthroscopy* 1993;9:368–369.

36. Garrett JC: Meniscal transplantation: A review of 43 cases with 2- to 7-year follow-up. *Sports Med Arthroscopy Rev* 1993;1:164–167.

37. Locht RC, Gross AE, Langer F: Late osteochondral allograft resurfacing for tibial plateau fractures. *J Bone Joint Surg* 1984;66A:328–335.

38. Meyers MH, Akeson W, Convery FR: Resurfacing of the knee with fresh osteochondral allograft. *J Bone Joint Surg* 1989;71A:704–713.

39. Milachowski KA, Weismeier K, Wirth CJ: Homologous meniscus transplantation: Experimental and clinical results. *Int Orthop* 1989;13:1–11.

40. Milachowski KA, Weismeier K, Wirth CJ, et al: Meniscus transplantation: Experimental study and first clinical report. *Am J Sports Med* 1987;15:626.

41. Noyes FR, Barber-Westin SD: Irradiated meniscus allografts in the human knee: A two to five year follow-up study. *Orthop Trans* 1995;19:417.

42. Potter HG, Rodeo SA, Wickiewicz TL, et al: MR imaging of meniscal allografts: Correlation with clinical and arthroscopic outcomes. *Radiology* 1996;198:509–514.

43. Shelton WR: Meniscal allotransplantation: An arthroscopically assisted technique. *Arthroscopy* 1993;9:361.

44. Zukor D, Brooks P, Gross A, et al: Abstract: Meniscal allografts. Experimental and clinical study. *Orthop Rev* 1988;17:522.

45. Zukor DJ, Cameron JC, Brooks PJ, et al: The fate of human meniscal allografts, in Ewing JW (ed): *Articular Cartilage and Knee Joint Function: Basic Science and Arthroscopy*. New York, NY, Raven Press, 1990, pp 147–152.

46. Stevenson S, Horowitz M: The response to bone allografts. *J Bone Joint Surg* 1992;74A:939–950.

47. Stevenson S, Li XQ, Martin B: The fate of cancellous and cortical bone after transplantation of fresh and frozen tissue-antigen-matched and mismatched osteochondral allografts in dogs. *J Bone Joint Surg* 1991;73A:1143–1156.

48. Jackson DW, Grood ES, Arnoczky SP, et al: Freeze dried anterior cruciate ligament allografts: Preliminary studies in a goat model. *Am J Sports Med* 1987;15:295–303.

49. Nemzek JA, Arnoczky SP, Swenson CL: Retroviral transmission in bone allotransplantation: The effects of tissue processing. *Clin Orthop* 1996;324:275–282.

50. Simonds RJ, Holmberg SD, Hurwitz RL, et al: Transmission of human immunodeficiency virus type 1 from a seronegative organ and tissue donor. *N Engl J Med* 1992;326:726–732.

51. Withrow SJ, Oulton SA, Suto TL, et al: Evaluation of the antiretroviral effect of various methods of sterilizing/preserving corticocancellous bone. *Orthop Trans* 1990;15:226.

52. Jackson DW, Windler GE, Simon TM: Intraarticular reaction associated with the use of freeze-dried ethylene oxide-sterilized bone-patella tendon-bone allografts in the reconstruction of the anterior cruciate ligament. *Am J Sports Med* 1990;18:1–10.

53. Roberts TS, Drez D Jr, McCarthy W, et al: Anterior cruciate ligament reconstruction using freeze-dried, ethylene oxide-sterilized, bone-patellar tendon-bone allografts: Two year results in thirty-six patients. *Am J Sports Med* 1991;19:35–41.

54. Sommer RE: The effects of ionizing radiation on fungi, in *Manual on Radiation Sterilization of Medical and Biological Materials*. Vienna, Austria, International Atomic Energy Agency, 1973, pp 73–79.

55. Bright RW, Smarsh JD, Gambill VM: Sterilization of human bone by irradiation, in Friedlaender GE, Mankin HJ, Sell KW (eds): *Osteochondral Allografts: Biology, Banking, and Clinical Applications*. Boston, MA, Little Brown, 1983, pp 223–232.

56. Christensen EA, Kristensen H, Sehested K: Radiation sterilisation, in Russell AD, Hugo WB, Ayliffe GAJ (eds): *Principles and Practice of Disinfection, Preservation and Sterilisation*. Oxford, England, Blackwell Scientific, 1982, pp 513–533.

57. Fideler BM, Vangsness CT Jr, Moore T, et al: Effects of gamma irradiation on the human immunodeficiency virus: A study in frozen human bone-patellar ligament-bone grafts obtained from infected cadavera. *J Bone Joint Surg* 1994;76A:1032–1035.

58. Strong DM, Sayers MH, Conrad EU III: Screening tissue donors for infectious markers, in Friedlaender GE, Goldberg VM (eds): *Bone and Cartilage Allografts: Biology and Clinical Applications*. Park Ridge, IL, American Academy of Orthopaedic Surgeons, 1991, pp 193–209.

59. Rasmussen TJ, Feder SM, Butler DL, et al: The effects of 4 Mrad of gamma irradiation on the initial mechanical properties of bone-patellar tendon-bone grafts. *Arthroscopy* 1994;10:188–197.

60. Bridges AE, Olivo JP, Chandler VL: Relative resistances of microorganisms to cathode rays: II. Yeasts and molds. *Appl Microbiol* 1956;4:147–149.

61. Darmady EM, Hughes KE, Burt MM, et al: Radiation sterilization. *J Clin Pathol* 1961;14:55–58.

62. Gibbs CJ Jr, Gajdusek DC, Latarjet R: Unusual resistance to ionizing radiation of the viruses of kuru, Creutzfeldt-Jakob disease, and scrapie. *Proc Natl Acad Sci USA* 1978;75:6268–6270.

63. Koh WY, Morehouse CT, Chandler VL: Relative resistances of microorganisms to cathode rays: I. Non sporeforming bacteria. *Appl Microbiol* 1956;4:143–146.

64. Wright KA, Trump JG: Co-operative studies in the use of ionizing radiation for sterilization and preservation of biological tissue, twenty years experience, in *Sterilization and Preservation of Biological Tissues by Ionizing Radiation*. Vienna, Austria, International Atomic Energy Agency, 1970, pp 107–118.

65. Conway B, Tomford W, Mankin HJ, et al: Radiosensitivity of HIV-1: Potential application to sterilization of bone allografts. *AIDS* 1991;5:608–609.

66. Lord CF, Gebhardt MC, Tomford WW, et al: Infection in bone allografts: Incidence, nature and treatment. *J Bone Joint Surg* 1988;70A:369–376.

67. Butler DL: Evaluation of fixation methods in cruciate ligament replacement, in Griffin PP (ed): *Instructional Course Lectures XXXVI*. Park Ridge, IL, American Academy of Orthopaedic Surgeons, 1987, pp 173–178.

68. Lewis JL, Lew WD, Shybut GT, et al: Biomechanical function of knee ligaments, in Finerman G (ed): American Academy of Orthopaedic Surgeons *Symposium on Sports Medicine: The Knee*. St. Louis, MO, CV Mosby, 1985, pp 152–168.

69. Noyes FR, Butler DL, Grood ES, et al: Biomechanical analysis of human ligament grafts used in knee-ligament repairs and reconstructions. *J Bone Joint Surg* 1984;66A:344–352.

70. Butler DL, Noyes FR, Grood ES: Ligamentous restraints to anterior-posterior drawer in the human knee: A biomechanical study. *J Bone Joint Surg* 1980;62A:259–270.

71. Feder SM, Butler DL, Holden JP: A technique for the evaluation of the contributions of knee structures to knee mechanics in the knee that has a reconstructed anterior cruciate ligament. *J Orthop Res* 1993;11:448–451.

72. Noyes FR, Grood ES: The strength of the anterior cruciate ligament in humans and Rhesus monkeys: Age-related and species-related changes. *J Bone Joint Surg* 1976;58A:1074–1082.

73. Pelker RR, Friedlaender GE, Markham TC, et al: Effects of freezing and freeze-drying on the biomechanical properties of rat bone. *J Orthop Res* 1984;1:405–411.

74. Woo SL, Orlando CA, Camp JF, et al: Effects of postmortem storage by freezing on ligament tensile behavior. *J Biomech* 1986;19:399–404.

75. Bright RW, Burchardt H: The biomechanical properties of preserved bone grafts, in Friedlaender GE, Mankin HJ, Sell KW (eds): *Osteochondral Allograft: Biology, Banking, and Clinical Application*. Boston, MA, Little Brown and Company, 1983, pp 241–247.

76. Haut RC, Powlison AC: Order of irradiation and lyophilization on the strength of patellar tendon allografts. *Trans Orthop Res Soc* 1989;14:514.

77. Triantafyllou N, Sotiropoulos E, Triantafyllou JN: The mechanical properties of the lyophylized and irradiated bone grafts. *Acta Orthop Belg* 1975;41(suppl 1):35–44.

78. Jackson DW, Grood ES, Arnoczky SP, et al: Cruciate reconstruction using freeze dried anterior cruciate ligament allograft and a ligament augmentation device (LAD): An experimental study in a goat model. *Am J Sports Med* 1987;15:528–538.

79. Webster DA, Werner FW: Freeze-dried flexor tendons in anterior cruciate ligament reconstruction. *Clin Orthop* 1983;181:238–243.

80. Salehpour A, Butler DL, Proch FS, et al: Dose-dependent response of gamma irradiation on mechanical properties and related biochemical composition of goat bone-patellar tendon-bone allografts. *J Orthop Res* 1995;13:898–906.

81. Pelker RR, Friedlaender GE, Markham TC: Biomechanical properties of bone allografts. *Clin Orthop* 1983;174:54–57.

82. Butler DL, Noyes FR, Walz KA, et al: Biomechanics of human knee ligament allograft treatment. *Trans Orthop Res Soc* 1987;12:128.

83. Paulos LE, France EP, Rosenberg TD, et al: Comparative material properties of allograft tissues for ligament replacement: Effects of type, age, sterilization and preservation. *Trans Orthop Res Soc* 1987;12:129.

84. Gibbons MJ, Butler DL, Groos ES, et al: Effects of gamma irradiation on the initial mechanical and material properties of goat bone-patellar tendon-bone allografts. *J Orthop Res* 1991;9:209–218.

85. De Deyne P, Haut RC: Some effects of gamma irradiation on patellar tendon allografts. *Connect Tissue Res* 1991;27:51–62.

86. Haridas B, Butler DL, Doxey CM, et al: Effects of allograft gamma irradiation on the cyclic anterior/posterior response of the reconstructed goat knee. *Trans Orthop Res Soc* 1994;19:627.

87. Glos DL, Butler DL, Groos ES, et al: In vitro evaluation of an implantable force transducer (IFT) in a patellar tendon model. *J Biomech Eng* 1993;115:335–343.

88. Xu WS, Butler DL, Stouffer DC, et al: Theoretical analysis of an implantable force transducer for tendon and ligament structures. *J Biomech Eng* 1992;114:170–177.

89. Miller MD, Harner CD: The anatomic and surgical considerations for posterior cruciate ligament reconstruction, in Jackson DW (ed): *Instructional Course Lectures 44.* Rosemont, IL, American Academy of Orthopaedic Surgeons, 1994, pp 431–440.

90. Butler DL, Oster DM, Feder SM, et al: Effects of gamma irradiation on the biomechanics of patellar tendon allografts of the ACL in the goat. *Trans Orthop Res Soc* 1991;16:205.

91. Oster DM, Groos ES, Feder SM, et al: Anterior translation and ACL graft tension in the goat knee: Effects of flexion angle and initial tension at the time of graft installation. *Trans Orthop Res Soc* 1991;16:600.

92. Schwartz HE, Butler DL, Matava MJ, et al: Gamma irradiation affects the biomechanics and biochemistry of the goat ACL allograft at 6 months post surgery. *Trans Orthop Res Soc* 1996;21:772.

93. Schwartz HE, Butler DL Matava MJ, et al: Effects of 4Mrad of gamma irradiation on goat ACL allograft and knee biomechanical properties at 6 months post surgery. *Trans Orthop Res Soc* 1995;20:632.

94. American Association of Tissue Banks: HIV Transmission incident described by LifeNet's Bottenfield. *Am Assoc Tissue Banks NL* 1991;14:1–2.

95. Conrad EU, Gretch DR, Obermeyer KR, et al: Transmission of the hepatitis-C virus by tissue transplantation. *J Bone Joint Surg* 1995;77A:214–224.

96. Asselmeier MA, Caspari RB, Bottenfield S: A review of allograft processing and sterilization techniques and their role in transmission of the human immunodeficiency virus. *Am J Sports Med* 1993;21:170–175.

97. Tomford WW: Transmission of disease through transplantation of musculoskeletal allografts. *J Bone Joint Surg* 1995;77A:1742–1754.

98. Persing DH, Landry ML: In vitro amplification techniques for the detection of nucleic acids: New tools for the diagnostic laboratory. *Yale J Biol Med* 1989;62:159–171.

99. Busch MP: HIV and blood transfusions: Focus on seroconversion. *Vox Sang* 1994;67(suppl 3):13–18.

100. Busch MP, Eble BE, Khayam-Bashi H, et al: Evaluation of screened blood donations for human immunodeficiency virus type 1 infection by culture and DNA amplification of pooled cells. *N Engl J Med* 1991;325:1–5.

101. Centers for Disease Control: Guidelines for preventing transmission of human immunodeficiency virus through transplantation of human tissue and organs. *Morbid Mortal Weekly Rep* 1994;43:1–17.

102. American Association of Tissue Banks: *Technical Manual for Surgical Bone Banking.* McLean, VA, American Association of Tissue Banks, 1989.

103. Conway B, Tomford WW, Hirsch MS, et al: Effects of gamma irradiation on HIV-1 in a bone allograft model. *Trans Orthop Res Soc* 1990;15:225.

104. Meyers JF, Caspari RB, Cash JD, et al: Arthroscopic evaluation of allograft anterior cruciate ligament reconstruction. *Arthroscopy* 1992;8:157–161.

105. Pinkowski JL, Reiman PR, Chen SL: Human lymphocyte reaction to freeze-dried allograft and xenograft ligamentous tissue. *Am J Sports Med* 1989;17:595–600.

106. Daniel DM, Malcom LL, Losse G, et al: Instrumented measurement of anterior laxity of the knee. *J Bone Joint Surg* 1985;67A:720–726.

107. Noyes FR, Barber SD: The effect of a ligament-augmentation device on allograft reconstructions for chronic ruptures of the anterior cruciate ligament. *J Bone Joint Surg* 1992;74A:960–973.

108. Noyes FR, Barber SD: Allograft reconstruction of the anterior and posterior cruciate ligaments: Report of ten-year experience and results, in Heckman JD (ed): *Instructional Course Lectures 42.* Rosemont, IL, American Academy of Orthopaedic Surgeons, 1993, pp 381–396.

109. Noyes FR, Barber-Westin SD: A comparision of results in acute and chronic anterior cruciate ligament ruptures of arthroscopically-assisted autogenous patellar tendon reconstruction. *Am J Sports Med* 1997;25:460–471.

110. Mayday MG, Harner CD, Fu FH: Revision ACL surgery: evaluation and treatment, in Applewhite LB (ed): *The Crucial Ligament: Diagnosis and Treatment of Ligamentous Injuries about the Knee,* ed 2. New York, NY, Churchill Livingstone, 1994, pp 711–723.

111. Safran MR, Harner CD: Revision ACL surgery: technique and results utilizing allografts, in Jackson DW (ed): *Instructional Course Lectures 44.* Rosemont, IL, American Academy of Orthopaedic Surgeons, 1995, pp 407–415.

112. Linn RM, Fischer DA, Smith JP, et al: Achilles tendon allograft reconstruction of the anterior cruciate ligament-deficient knee. *Am J Sports Med* 1993;21:825–831.

113. Galloway MT, Grood ES, Mehalik JN, et al: Posterior cruciate ligament reconstruction: An in vitro study of femoral and tibial graft placement. *Am J Sports Med* 1996;24:437–445.

114. Clancy WG Jr, Sutherland TB: Combined posterior cruciate ligament injuries. *Clin Sports Med* 1994;13:629–647.

115. De Boer HH, Koudstaal J: Failed meniscus transplantation: A report of three cases. *Clin Orthop* 1994;306:155–162.

116. Keene GC, Paterson RS, Teague DC: Advances in arthroscopic surgery. *Clin Orthop* 1987;224:64–70.

117. Rubins D, Barrett JP Jr, Hayter R: Abstract: Arthroscopic meniscal allograft transplantation. *Arthroscopy* 1993;9:356–357.

118. Veltri DM, Warren RF, Wickiewicz TL, et al: Current status of allograft meniscal transplantation. *Clin Orthop* 1994;303:44–55.

119. Wojtys EM, Carpenter JE: Abstract: Meniscal replacement: Early experience. *Arthroscopy* 1994;10:337.

120. Jackson DW, Simon M: Biology of meniscal allograft, in Mow BC, Arnoczky SP, Jackson DW (eds): *Knee Meniscus: Basic and Clinical Foundations.* New York, NY, Raven Press, 1992, pp 141–152.

Running Injuries: A Biomechanical Approach

Tom F. Novacheck, MD

Approximately 30 million Americans run for recreation or competition. A marathon runner takes an average of 25,000 steps during a race. At each step his or her body is subjected to a ground reaction force that is several times body weight. A 50 mile-per-week runner may take as many as 3 million strides each year. Each year between a quarter and half of runners will sustain an injury that is severe enough to cause a change in practice or performance.[1] This injury may lead the runner to seek consultation, alter training, or use medication. Often, it is the number of repetitions that is problematic. A variety of intrinsic and extrinsic factors have been blamed for the development of these types of injuries.[2-4]

In addition, particular patterns of injury have been noted. James and Jones[3] noted the six injury sites shown in Figure 1 that accounted for almost 75% of complaints. Interestingly, although one might assume intuitively that particular anatomic abnormalities lead to specific injury patterns (eg, hyperpronation predisposing to posterior tibial syndrome or genu varum leading to iliotibial band syndrome), few such relationships have been found.

The quandary for the last 10 to 15 years has been how to make more sense out of why and how injuries occur. Greater understanding, which will improve diagnosis and counseling, will come from new biomechanical information collected at gait analysis laboratories.[5,6] In the last two decades, this type of

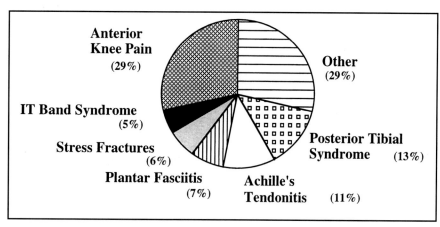

Fig. 1 Most common sites of distance running injuries.

analysis has been used primarily either for research or for clinical evaluation of walking abnormalities in pediatric orthopaedics and in amputees. Gait analysis laboratories can now measure three-dimensional motion, using computerized motion measurement systems, and can calculate net joint moments by combining motion analysis with force plate data. Newer systems that can capture data at greater than 200 Hz now make it possible to evaluate sports biomechanics.

This type of new dynamic biomechanical information, when combined with an appreciation of the physiology and pathophysiology of the musculoskeletal system, will shed light on the genesis of overuse musculoskeletal injuries associated with running. This chapter includes information on (1) the biomechanics of human locomotion; (2)

the biomechanics, physiology, and pathophysiology of tendon; and (3) soft-tissue stresses for some musculotendinous structures frequently injured in long distance runners, which are the tendons that make up the knee extensor mechanism, the iliotibial band, the Achilles tendon, and the plantar fascia.

Biomechanics of Forward Human Locomotion

How do we go from a standstill to maximum forward velocity during sprinting? How does the movement strategy change between walking and running locomotion? The demarcation between walking and running (Fig. 2, point A) occurs when periods of double support during the stance phase of the gait cycle (both feet are simultaneously in contact with the ground) give way to two periods of double float (neither foot is touching the

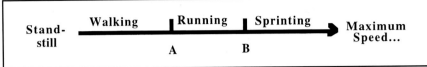

Fig. 2 Forward human locomotion. Point A is the demarcation between walking and running. Point B is where the initial contact changes from the hindfoot to the forefoot.

ground). Generally as speed increases further, the point of initial contact changes from the hindfoot to the forefoot (Fig. 2, point B). This change typically marks the distinction between running and sprinting. In practicality, the difference between running and sprinting is in the goal to be achieved. Running is performed over longer distances, for endurance, and with conservation of energy (aerobic). Jogging, road racing, and marathons are examples. Not all distance runners, however, maintain a hindfoot initial contact. Sprinting activities are done over shorter distances and at faster speeds, with the goal of covering a relatively short distance in the shortest period of time possible without regard for maintaining aerobic metabolism. Elite sprinters perform with a forefoot initial contact, and in fact, the hindfoot may never contact the ground.

The Gait Cycle

The gait cycle is the basic unit of measurement in gait analysis.[7] The gait cycle begins when one foot comes in contact with the ground and ends when the same foot contacts the ground again. These points in time are referred to as initial contact. For the purposes of this chapter, stance phase will be plotted before the swing phase (not all authors follow this convention). Stance ends when the foot is no longer in contact with the ground. Toe off marks the beginning of the swing phase of the gait cycle. Each of these phases is subdivided further as seen in Figure 3. In walking, the stance phase accounts for more than 50% of the gait cycle, which means that there are two

periods of double support (Fig. 4), one at the beginning and one at the end of stance phase. In running, because toe off occurs before 50% of the gait cycle is completed, there are no periods when both feet are in contact with the ground. Instead, both feet are airborne at the same time twice during the gait cycle, at the beginning and at the end of swing,[8] and this is referred to as double float. The timing of toe off depends on speed. Less time is spent in stance as the athlete moves faster. In our study, toe off occurred at 39% and 36% of the gait cycle for running and sprinting, respectively. Faster runners and elite sprinters spend much less time in stance than that. World class sprinters have been shown to toe off at as early as 22% of the gait cycle.[9]

Potential and Kinetic Energy

In addition to these distinctions, the relationship between potential and kinetic energy differs critically in walking and running activities (Fig. 5). In walking, the two are out of phase. When potential energy is high, kinetic energy is low, and vice versa. In running, the two are in phase. An appreciation of this difference makes it possible to understand why walking has been referred to as controlled falling (from the zenith of the center of mass in midstance to its nadir during double support), while running has been likened to an individual on a pogo stick,[10] propelling oneself from a low point during the middle portion of stance (stance phase reversal) to a peak during double float.

As a result of this difference between walking and running, the body complete-

ly alters the methods it uses to maintain energy efficiency. Large fluctuations in total energy going into and out of the system would be disadvantageous regardless of the pace of movement. In walking, efficiency is maintained by the effective interchange between potential and kinetic energy, which are out of phase. In running, in which the two are in phase, this is not possible. Instead, efficiency is primarily maintained in two ways,[5,11,12] first, by the storage and later return of elastic potential energy by the stretch of elastic structures (especially tendons), and second, by the transfer of energy from one body segment to another by two joint muscles such as the rectus femoris and the hamstrings.

I will elaborate on the significance of the first of these two points in later sections on the physiology of tendons and the pathophysiology of chronic running injuries.

Kinematics

Kinematics is the description of movement without consideration for the forces that cause that movement. This type of analysis can be done in different ways. In our laboratory at Gillette Children's Specialty Healthcare, the computer system uses retroreflective markers that are placed on particular landmarks of the trunk and lower extremities (Fig. 6). These markers, by reflecting infrared light (from emitters in the corners of the room), allow the video camera system to track their position. Their specific locations in space are determined by a computer software system. From these marker locations, specific body segment positions and joint movements can be determined. This information can be shown in a graph (Fig. 7). As clinicians, we have a qualitative understanding of what normal knee motion is. This type of analysis provides an objective way to quantify the position of various joints at different points in the gait cycle as well as the degree of move-

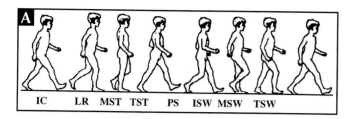

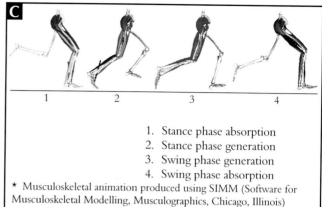

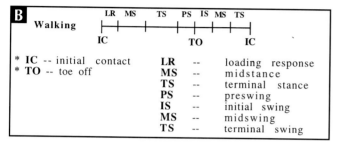

1. Stance phase absorption
2. Stance phase generation
3. Swing phase generation
4. Swing phase absorption

★ Musculoskeletal animation produced using SIMM (Software for Musculoskeletal Modelling, Musculographics, Chicago, Illinois)

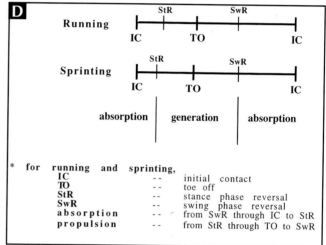

Fig. 3 The gait cycle. **A,** Walking figure. **B,** Walking gait cycle. **C,** Running figure. **D,** Running gait cycle. (IC = initial contact, TO = toe off, LR = loading response, MST = midstance, TST = terminal stance, PS = preswing, IS = initial swing, MSW = midswing, TSW = terminal swing, StR = stance phase reversal, SWR = swing phase reversal, absorption = from SWR through IC to StR, generation = from StR through TO to SwR) (Figure 3A is reproduced with permission from Gage JR: Normal gait, in *Gait Analysis in Cerebral Palsy*. London, England, MacKeith Press, 1991, pp 61–100.) (Figures 3B and 3D are reproduced with permission from Novacheck F: Walking, running, and sprinting: Three-dimensional analysis of kinematics and kinetics, in Jackson DW (ed): *Instructional Course Lectures 44*. Rosemont, IL, American Academy of Orthopaedic Surgeons, 1995, pp 497–506.)

Kinetics

Kinetics is the study of the forces that are responsible for movement. This information is gathered by using forceplates in the running surface to measure the ground reaction force (GRF). The GRF is the equal and opposite force exerted on one another by the foot and the ground. In running, the GRF is characterized by a short duration initial spike followed by a broader wave that peaks in midstance (Fig. 8).[5,6,10]

Inverse dynamics is a series of mathematical equations that incorporates joint positions (motion analysis), the size and direction of the GRF (forceplate), and the mass and location of the center of mass of each of the body segments (anthropometric data) to calculate net joint moments about the hip, knee, and ankle.

A moment, also known as a force couple, is expressed in Newton-meters. It is a force that acts at a distance about an axis of rotation to cause an angular acceleration about that axis (Fig. 9). Once again, this information can be shown in a graph (Fig. 10). External moments include the GRFs and inertial forces mentioned previously. Internal moments are those produced within the body, and they may be generated by muscle, ligament, or joint capsule. These moments are calculated using inverse dynamics. At this time, current modeling techniques do not allow

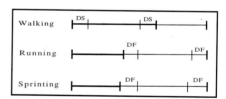

Fig. 4 Double support (DS)/Double float (DF). (Reproduced with permission from Novacheck F: Walking, running, and sprinting: Three-dimensional analysis of kinematics and kinetics, in Jackson DW (ed): *Instructional Course Lectures 44*. Rosemont, IL, American Academy of Orthopaedic Surgeons, 1995, pp 497–506.)

the calculation of individual tissue forces. Insight into the magnitude and timing of the net joint moments, however, does provide insight into which tissues are subjected to the highest stresses.

Joint power is the product of the net

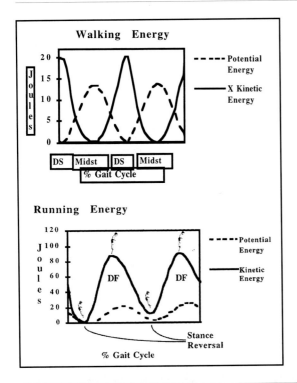

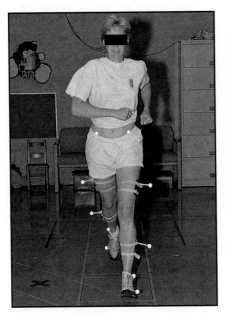
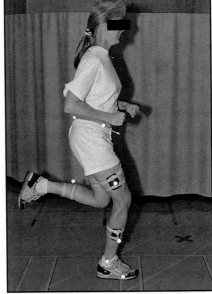

Fig. 5 Potential and kinetic energy interactions during walking and running.

Fig. 6 Runner being tested with markers on force plates. Note the retroreflective markers in specific locations over key bony landmarks and the forceplates in the running surface.

joint moment and the joint angular velocity (Power = Force × distance × omega) and is expressed in Watts/kg (Fig. 11). This type of analysis provides insight into which musculotendinous structures are responsible for deceleration and also makes it possible to identify the timing and location of sources of power for forward movement. This information has been presented in detail in previous *Instructional Course Lectures* volumes.[8,12] To summarize, the main sources of power

input are the gastrocnemius-soleus complex, at push-off; the quadriceps, in the first half of the generation phase (just after stance phase reversal); the hip extensors, in late swing/early stance; the hip flexors, at push off and early swing; and the hip abductors, in the first half of the generation phase (just after stance phase reversal). Interestingly, each of these musculotendinous units absorbs power by stretching (eccentric) just before they shorten (concentric) to generate power.

Recent animal studies have indicated that the changes in the length of the muscle belly itself are relatively minimal.[13] Instead, the muscles function as tensioners of the musculotendinous springs, their tendons. Most of the change in length comes from the stretch and recoil of their respective tendons. Therefore, most of the work is done by the tendons. Tendons are, in fact, excellent biologic springs (Fig. 12). In this way, we should begin to think of tendons as springs, and of muscles as the tensioners of the springs.[14] This concept makes the analogy of a runner to a person on a pogo stick make even more sense. If we consider the Achilles tendon, for example, we can begin to understand the way that it stretches during the first portion of the stance phase of the gait cycle, and then recoils, to return that energy back to the individual at the time of push-off. Its function is similar to that of the spring of the pogo stick (except that the tendon stretches under tension while the pogo stick spring compresses under pressure). The energy that it absorbs is returned back to the system. I will elaborate on these concepts in the next section on the physiology of tendon.

We can begin to draw some conclusions based on biomechanics. R. McNeil Alexander[10] found that the forceplate measures approximately 100 joules ground reaction force when a person is running at 4.5 meters per second. He calculated that 35 joules are stored as strain

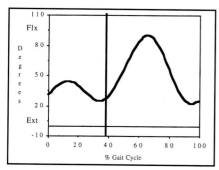

Fig. 7 Kinematic graph. The gait cycle is plotted along the X axis from one initial contact to the next. We choose to depict this in percent, but it could also be shown as a function of time. The vertical line in the midportion of the graph (in this case at 39%) represents the time of toe off. To the left of that line is stance phase. Swing phase is to the right. The measure of the degrees of movement is depicted along the Y axis of the particular joint being considered (in this case the knee). This type of graph provides answers to questions such as "What is the position of the knee at the time of contact with the ground?", "What is the total range of motion of the knee during running?", or "What is the maximum degree of knee extension that occurs during running?".

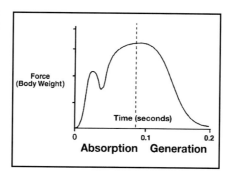

Fig. 8 Ground reaction forces during running. Note that the ground reaction forces can only be measured during the stance phase portion of the gait cycle when the foot is in contact with the ground. Therefore, this graph depicts only the stance phase of gait.

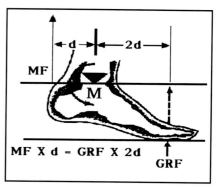

Fig. 9 Sagittal plane ankle moment diagram (MF = muscle force, GRF = ground reaction force). (Reproduced with permission from Gage JR: Normal gait, in *Gait Analysis in Cerebral Palsy*. London, England, MacKeith Press, 1991, pp 61–100.)

energy in the heelcord and 17 joules in the arch of the foot. More is stored in the stretch of the quadriceps and patellar tendons. As a result, less than half of this energy has to be removed by the muscles acting as brakes and returned by them doing work. The muscles must still exert tension, but they shorten/lengthen less.

Until this type of biomechanical analysis of the forces created in running was available, the forces that create the tissue trauma responsible for chronic injuries were not known. This lack of knowledge led to inaccurate assumptions. The greatest of these was that most injuries were caused by the high impact forces that occurred at the time of heelstrike. As a result, a tremendous amount of research has focused on footwear and the running surface and how those two factors alter the impact of heelstrike.[15-21] By reviewing Figure 8, it is easy to see

that the passive forces associated with heelstrike are smaller and shorter in duration than the larger, active force phase that occurs during the latter three fourths of the stance phase.[6] While attenuating the shock of ground contact is still important, one must understand that absorption doesn't occur instantaneously, like a bowling ball landing on a cement sidewalk. Instead, several different tissues dissipate this force over time during the first half of stance phase, thereby minimizing the shock to the body.[22] These tissues include the Achilles tendon, the plantar fascia, the quadriceps mechanism, and the hip abductors.

It is notable that this list includes many of the sites most commonly injured in distance runners, showing the extent to which inverse dynamics has advanced the art of biomechanical evaluation. It now seems more likely that most chronic injuries from jogging are related to the high forces that occur in mid and late stance.[15] Based on these calculations, training with eccentric knee exercise and concentric plantarflexion can be recommended to help avoid injury. We now have an appreciation for the biomechanical stresses that can provide insight into the etiology of some of the most common injury patterns. These biomechani-

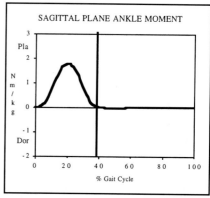

Fig. 10 Moment graph. Just as in the kinematic plot (Fig. 7), the gait cycle is depicted along the X-axis in percent. The moment is depicted along the Y-axis. Internal moments are plotted. The moment is measured in Newton-meters, and for standardization, they are commonly divided by body weight (Newton-meters/kg). Deflections above the zero line represent (in this example) net plantarflexor moments. The ankle plantarflexors are dominant at that time. Deflections below the line represent predominance of the ankle dorsiflexors which, as you can see, is not measurable at any point during the running gait cycle. This type of graph provides answers to questions such as "Which group of muscles is predominant at stance phase reversal?", or "What is the maximum moment that this individual's ankle plantarflexors are able to produce?".

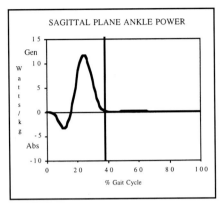

Fig. 11 Sagittal plane ankle power. Once again, the gait cycle is plotted along the X-axis. Power, in Watts/kg body weight, is plotted on the Y-axis. Positive power indicates that power is being generated by the muscle group that is predominant at that time at that joint (concentric contraction). Deflection below the zero line, negative power, indicates power absorption or eccentric muscle activity. This type of graph provides answers to questions such as "Do the ankle plantarflexors function eccentrically and if so, when?", "When do they function concentrically?", or "How much power do the ankle plantarflexors generate just prior to push-off?".

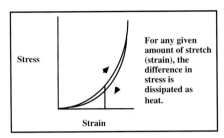

Fig. 12 Hysteresis curve for tendon. If subjected to stretch (stress), the tendon elongates (strain)—arrow directed up and to the right. The energy is stored as elastic potential energy. If the amount of deformation is within the physiologic range, the tendon will recoil returning the majority of the energy absorbed during stretching (arrow directed down and to the left). Of the energy used to stretch them, tendons generally return 90% to 95% as kinetic energy. The remainder is dissipated as heat.

cal data will be presented in the final section of this chapter. Before that discussion, further insight can be gained by reviewing the anatomy, physiology, and biomechanical behavior of tendons.

Biomechanics, Physiology, and Pathophysiology of Tendons: Insights into Injury Mechanisms

Tendons are relatively avascular. They are made up of 30% collagen, 2% elastin, and 68% water. The cells incorporated in the tendon are tenocytes. The tendon has a breaking point similar to that of steel. When first formed, the tropocollagen molecules have no cross-links between them. Cross-links develop between the 6th and 14th days. Fibrils, laid down randomly at first, later come to lie parallel to the tensile forces of the tissue. When tendons are first formed, they are not as strong, and, if they are immobilized too

long after an injury, they can lose 20% to 40% of their ground substance. Early motion helps to align collagen fibers, improving tensile strength and gliding. Training also increases the tensile and maximum static strength of tendons. Exercise increases collagen synthesis, the number and size of the fibrils, and the concentration of metabolic enzymes.[23]

With aging, the enzymes essential for collagen formation decrease. Repair of soft tissue is delayed in older individuals. Collagen becomes tougher, tensile strength is reduced, fibers shrink, the tendon stiffens, and the tendon is more likely to tear.[23,24]

Tendons are subjected to large tensile forces. As discussed before, if the forces are in the physiologic range, tendons deform and then return to their original state (Fig. 13). Tendons are stronger than muscles and withstand larger forces. Longer fibers elongate more. The greater the cross-sectional area, the larger the load that can be withstood without deformation.[25] Tendons that go around corners are subject to greater strain and are more likely to have interference with their blood supply. Tendons, being viscoelastic,

are rate and size dependent.[26] Maximum load capacity and tear resistance peak in the third decade, after which both decrease with age.[23]

A sports injury occurs with the loss of cells or extracellular matrix resulting from sports-induced trauma. There is a failure of cell matrix adaptation to load exposure, which can be caused either by sudden overload or by accumulative overload secondary to cyclic overuse. Injuries caused by cyclic overuse have been variously referred to as cumulative trauma disorders or cumulative cell matrix adaptive responses.[24] With acute injuries, a sudden crisis causes failure either through aberrant tissue or as a result of high strain rates.[27] The slow insidious onset that characterizes chronic injuries implies an antecedent subthreshold spectrum of structural damage. This damage eventually leads to a crisis episode, often heralded by pain and/or signs of inflammation. These injuries are characterized by a persistence of symptoms without resolution. It is worthwhile to note that pain has assumed a disproportionate emphasis in the definition of inflammation, to the extent that any painful structure is immediately presumed to be inflamed.

With a regenerative response, repair produces new tissue that is structurally and functionally identical to normal tissue. In degenerative response, the new tissue produced is of a lower or less functional form. This tissue, which is more vulnerable to either cyclic or sudden overloading leading to mechanical fatigue and failure, represents a profound imbalance in cell matrix homeostasis. Heat generated within the tendon may cause tenocyte necrosis promoting degeneration.[28]

The four pathologic conditions that make up the spectrum of tendinopathy are (1) paratenonitis, an inflammation of only the paratenon (friction); (2) tendinosis, intratendinous degeneration due to atrophy; (3) paratenonitis with tendinosis, paratenon inflammation associated with intratendinous degeneration; and (4) tendinitis, symptomatic degeneration of the tendon with vascular disruption and inflammatory repair response.[24] With tendon overload/overuse, an initial adaptive cell matrix response occurs. With continued abusive sports activity, two detrimental microscopic consequences occur. Matrix degradation increases, and inadequate matrix is synthesized (Fig. 14). Factors that influence this process are hypoxia, poor nutrition, hypovascularity, hormonal factors, chronic inflammation, and aging. With increased matrix degradation and inadequate matrix synthesis, a feedback loop, the tendinosis cycle, is entered whereby tendon degeneration and microtears occur alternately, as shown in Figure 14. Ultimately, there is structural deterioration, partial tissue failure, and a potential for complete tissue rupture.

Periodization in athletic training is currently recommended and is based on the principle of transition.[24,27] A sports injury is most likely to occur when the athlete experiences any change in mode or use of the involved part. This is a rate-dependent process. If training is within the physiologic range, there is cellular homeostasis with an overall anabolic response. With insufficient training, there is disuse/deconditioning, leading to a catabolic response that can ultimately cause injury. Overtraining can also cause a catabolic response leading to injury. Transitional risks include increased performance level; improper training; changes in equipment; environmental changes (new surfaces, different training altitudes); alterations in frequency, intensity, or duration of training; attempts to master new techniques; return to sport too soon after injury; and body growth.

Soft-Tissue Stresses for Specific Musculotendinous Units

As discussed previously, the state of the art has indeed advanced beyond the eval-

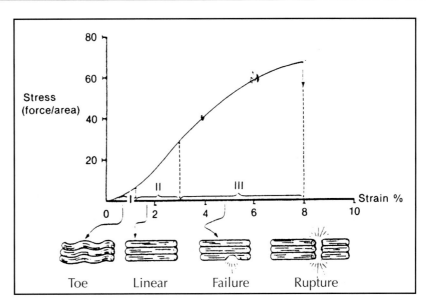

Fig. 13 Stress/strain curve for tendon. (1) Toe region constitutes the 0 to 2% strain (stretch). The wavy configuration disappears in this region. Collagen fibers are crimped, and they straighten. (2) The second region is a physiologic zone where collagen fibers deform and respond linearly to load. If stress is less than 4%, it returns to its original length. The size and number of fibers determine the force the tendon can withstand. (3) In the third region, between 4% and 8% strain, collagen fibers can begin to slide past one another as cross-links start to fail. This is also referred to as the microscopic failure region. (4) The fourth region, macroscopic failure, occurs above 8% strain. There is tensile failure of the fibers and sheer failure between the fibers. There is a three to fourfold difference between loads that are well tolerated in the physiologic range (2nd) and those that cause failure. (Reproduced with permission from Curwin S, Staniski WD (eds): *Tendinitis: Its Etiology and Treatment.* Lexington, MA, DC Health, 1984.)

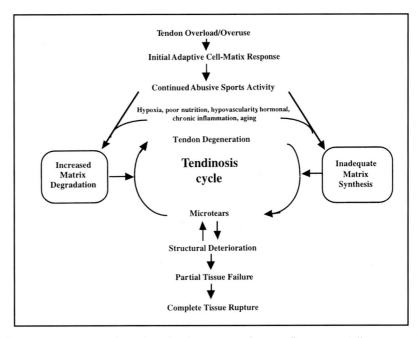

Fig. 14 The tendinosis cycle. (Adapted with permission from Leadbetter WB: Cell-matrix response in tendon injury. *Clin Sports Med* 1992;11:533–578.)

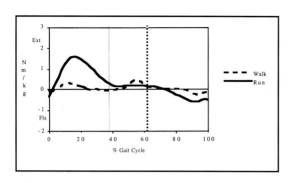

Fig. 15 Sagittal plane knee moment (walking versus running).

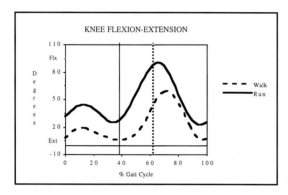

Fig. 16 Sagittal plane knee kinematic (walking versus running).

uation of kinematic variables and the ground reaction force under the support foot. We can gain a better appreciation for the etiology of some of the common injuries by evaluating the forces to which the soft tissues are subjected. Inverse dynamics allows the evaluation of net joint moments about the hip, knee, and ankle, and provides insight into the location and timing of these soft-tissue stresses.[6,11,12] One should remember, however, that actual stress levels within specific musculotendinous structures cannot currently be calculated. The development of improved models will allow accurate calculation of individual tissue stresses. Four of the most common overuse injuries are anterior knee pain, iliotibial band syndrome, Achilles' tendinopathy, and plantar fasciitis. Biomechanical data relative to these injuries are as follows.

Anterior Knee Pain

The extensor mechanism of the knee is the most common site of chronic running injury. Different anatomic sites

within this structure can be involved.[29] Pain may be caused by periarticular soft-tissue degeneration/inflammation or by excessive stress on the patellofemoral articular cartilage. A thorough examination of the extensor mechanism assesses quadriceps development, contracture, and vastus medialis oblique position, as well as patellar position, tracking, stability, and mobility. The examiner also looks for a painful arc and areas of point tenderness. This area is a common site of chronic injury because the extensor mechanism of the knee functions eccentrically to absorb 42% of the actively absorbed energy associated with ground contact.[12]

The knee moment during this part of the gait cycle shows that there is a net knee extensor moment that is five times greater in running than it is in walking (Fig. 15). Figure 16 shows that at the time the knee extensor moment is the greatest, the knee is also flexed more in the runner (about 45°). This is about twice the amount of flexion that occurs in walking

(22°). This increased flexion creates a significantly higher amount of stress on the quadriceps muscles, quadriceps tendon, and the patellar tendon.[30] In addition, the compression force on the patellofemoral articular cartilage is increased. In the skeletally immature or growing athlete, the growth centers about the patella and at the tibial tubercle are subjected to these stresses. Therefore, Osgood-Schlatter's disease and jumper's knee are common.[31] Typically, these forces do not exceed the single event injury threshold, but the cumulative effects of subthreshold stresses over time may be sufficient to damage the soft-tissue structures about the knee.

Iliotibial Band Syndrome

Friction of the iliotibial (IT) band over the lateral femoral condyle is thought to cause this syndrome. The runner presents with tenderness along the lower end of the IT band along the outside of the knee.[6] The ground reaction force normally falls medial to the knee joint during single limb support in any activity. An external varus moment is produced. The IT band stabilizes the knee against this external force by generating an internal valgus moment to help maintain an upright position. The knee valgus moment (calculated in the coronal plane) is two and one half times greater in running than it is in walking (Fig. 17).

At the time that this peak occurs, the knee is at its maximum degree of stance phase flexion—about 45° (Fig. 16). Therefore, there is a high knee valgus moment at the time that the knee is flexed. This degree of flexion places the iliotibial band directly over the lateral femoral condyle, where it is most susceptible to a friction injury. It is well known that IT band syndrome is more common in runners who have a neutral or varus knee alignment. The ground reaction force is in a more medial position because of this anatomic variation. The external varus moment is therefore larger, and the IT band must generate a larger valgus moment to balance it, which increases the amount of friction. This is an excellent example of how one can begin to understand how a common chronic injury pattern occurs. The combination of the kinematic and kinetic data provides the insight into both the joint position and the joint forces that create the tissue stress responsible for injury.

Achilles Tendinopathy

The Achilles tendon and its insertion are frequent sites of chronic injury in athletes. Pain along the course of the tendon is the most frequent presenting complaint. Tenderness, with or without swelling, along its course is common. Acute ruptures are almost always preceded by a prodromal period of low grade pain.[6,32,33]

The Achilles tendon is another anatomic structure that stretches during the first half of stance phase and recoils later in a spring-like fashion. It stores energy as it is stretched and efficiently returns 90% of this energy at the time of push off.[10] If initial contact is on the forefoot, the eccentric function of the gastrocnemius/soleus/Achilles tendon complex is exaggerated as the heel is slowly lowered to the ground. The gastrocnemius/soleus generates greater ankle plantarflexor moments during running than it does during walking (Fig. 18).

Because few other structures are involved, peak Achilles tendon forces can be estimated. They are in the range of six to eight times body weight.[10] Peak moments occur not at initial contact, but in midstance. They are generated by the powerful contraction of the gastrocnemius/soleus complex–not by the shock of initial contact with the ground. These injuries are caused by the active muscle forces of midstance, not by the passive impact forces at the time of initial contact. Shoe wear and the type of running surface are much less important factors in the genesis of this type of injury than is commonly believed. Shoewear may play

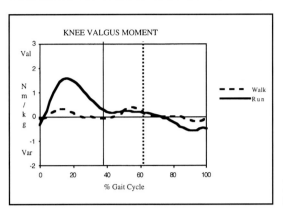

Fig. 17 Coronal plane knee moment (walking versus running).

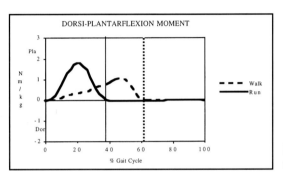

Fig. 18 Sagittal plane ankle moment (walking versus running).

a role in decreasing locally increased stress for an individual running on an uneven surface or for a hyperpronator. If the shoe can control the position of the hindfoot, it may decrease the localized stresses both along the medial aspect of the Achilles' tendon and further up the kinetic chain.[3,32,34]

Plantar Fasciitis

The plantar fascia functions in much the same way as the Achilles tendon. It stores elastic potential energy when it stretches and efficiently returns the majority of it later in the cycle. Pain, especially on rising in the morning, is the most common presenting symptom. Tenderness, either along its course or at its origin on the medial aspect of the calcaneal tuberosity, is a typical finding on examination.[6] Stress in the plantar fascia can be as high as three times body weight.[10] Peak stress occurs around midstance, when most of the weightbearing forces have been transferred from the hindfoot to the ball of the

foot. Excessive pronation increases the traction along the medial part of the plantar fascia, predisposing it to excessive stress and injury.

Conclusion

An appreciation for the biomechanics of running activities and the physiology of the musculoskeletal system sheds light on the pathophysiology of overuse musculoskeletal injuries associated with running. The list of possible contributing factors to chronic running injuries can be overwhelming. The goal of this chapter has been to help the reader better understand these concepts by coupling new information regarding the biomechanics of normal running with previously available knowledge of the musculoskeletal tissue response to mechanical stress. Because a recent change in the training program is frequently an inciting factor, the concept of the safe, healthful transitional training window is a key component of management and prevention.

The three-dimensional kinematic and kinetic data cited briefly here to explain various potential areas of injury are dealt with in much greater detail elsewhere.[11,12] This information is essential for an understanding of the intricacies of running gait. A knowledge of normal is prerequisite to understanding what can go wrong. Only in this way can an insightful management plan addressing shoewear, orthotics, exercise, or training modifications be recommended.

Acknowledgements

The author wishes to acknowledge Joyce Phelps Trost and Mary Trost for their assistance in the development and preparation of this manuscript and the staff of the Motion Analysis Laboratory at Gillette Children's Specialty Healthcare (200 East University Ave, St. Paul, MN 55101), where the information on which this chapter is based was gathered.

References

1. Hoeberigs JH: Factors related to the incidence of running injuries: A review. *Sports Med* 1992;13:408–422.

2. Renstrom AFH: Mechanism, diagnosis, and treatment of running injuries, in Heckman JD (ed): *Instructional Course Lectures 42*. Rosemont, IL, American Academy of Orthopaedic Surgeons, 1993, pp 225–234.

3. James SL, Jones DC: Biomechanical aspects of distance running injuries, in Cavanagh PR (ed): *Biomechanics of Distance Running*. Champaign, IL, Human Kinetics, 1990, pp 249–269.

4. Grana WA, Kalenak A: Running injuries. *Clin Sports Med* 1991:458–465.

5. Vaughan CL: Biomechanics of running gait. *Crit Rev Biomed Eng* 1984;12:1–48.

6. Winter DA, Bishop PJ: Lower extremity injury: Biomechanical factors associated with chronic injury to the lower extremity. *Sports Med* 1992;14:149–156.

7. Gage JR: An overview of normal walking, in Greene WB (ed): *Instructional Course Lectures XXXIX*. Park Ridge, IL, American Academy of Orthopaedic Surgeons, 1990, pp 291–303.

8. Ounpuu S: The biomechanics of running: A kinematic and kinetic analysis, in Greene WB (ed): *Instructional Course Lectures XXXIX*. Park Ridge, IL, American Academy of Orthopaedic Surgeons, 1990, pp 305–318.

9. Mann RA, Hagy J: Biomechanics of walking, running, and sprinting. *Am J Sports Med* 1980;8:345–350.

10. Alexander RM (ed): *The Human Machine*. New York, NY, Columbia University Press, 1992, pp 74–87.

11. Novacheck TF: The biomechanics of running and sprinting, in Guten GN (ed): *Running Injuries*. Philadelphia, PA, WB Saunders, 1997, pp 4–19.

12. Novacheck TF: Walking, running, and sprinting: A three-dimensional analysis of kinematics and kinetics, in Jackson DW (ed): *Instructional Course Lectures 44*. Rosemont, IL, American Academy of Orthopaedic Surgeons, 1995, pp 497-506.

13. Roberts TJ, Marsh RL, Weyand PG, et al: Muscular force in running turkeys: The economy of minimizing work. *Science* 1997;275:1113–1115.

14. McMahon TA: Spring-like properties of muscles and reflexes in running, in Winters JM, Woo SLY (eds): *Multiple Muscle Systems: Biomechanics and Movement Organization*. New York, NY, Springer-Verlag, 1990, pp 578–590.

15. Winter DA: Moments of force and mechanical power in jogging. *J Biomech* 1983;16:91–97.

16. Cavanagh PR (ed): *The Running Shoe Book*. Mountain View, CA, Anderson World, 1980.

17. Nigg BM, Denoth J, Luethi S, et al: Methodological aspects of sport shoe and sport floor analysis, in Matsui H, Kobayashi K (eds): *Biomechanics VIII: Proceedings of the Eighth International Congress of Biomechanics*, Nagoya, Japan. Champaign, IL, Human Kinetics, 1983.

18. Nigg BM: External force measurements with sport shoes and playing surfaces, in Nigg BM, Kerr BA (eds): *Biomechanical Aspects of Sport Shoes and Playing Surfaces*. Calgary, Canada, University of Calgary, 1983, p 11.

19. Bates TF, Osternig LR, Sawhill JA, et al: Design of running shoes, in Shoup TE, Thacker JG (eds): *International Conference on Medical Devices and Sports Equipment*. New York, NY, ASME, 1980.

20. Bates BT, Osternig LR, Sawhill JA, et al: An assessment of subject variability, subject-shoe interaction, and the evaluation of running shoes using ground reaction force data. *J Biomech* 1983;16:181–191.

21. Clarke TE, Frederick EC, Cooper LB: Biomechanical measurement of running shoe cushioning properties, in Nigg BM, Kerr BA (eds): *Biomechanical Aspects of Sport Shoes and Playing Surfaces*. Calgary, Canada, University of Calgary, 1983, p 25.

22. Novacheck TF, Trost JP: Videotape: *Running: Injury Mechanisms and Training Strategies*. St. Paul, MN, Gillette Children's Specialty Healthcare Foundation, 1997.

23. O'Brien M: Functional anatomy and physiology of tendons. *Clin Sports Med* 1992;11:505–520.

24. Leadbetter WB: Cell-matrix response in tendon injury. *Clin Sports Med* 1992;11:533–578.

25. Booth FW, Gould EW: Effects of training and disuse on connective tissue. *Exerc Sport Sci Rev* 1975;3:83–112.

26. Brewer BJ: Mechanism of injury to the musculotendinous unit, in Reynolds FC (ed): American Academy of Orthopaedic Surgeons *Instructional Course Lectures XVII*. St. Louis, MO, CV Mosby, 1960, p 354.

27. Kibler WB: Clinical implications of exercise: Injury and performance, in Schafer M (ed): *Instructional Course Lectures 43*. Rosemont, IL, American Academy of Orthopaedic Surgeons, 1994, pp 17–24.

28. Wilson AM, Goodship AE: Abstract: The role of exercise-induced hyperthermia in the pathogenesis of tendon degenerative change. *J Bone Joint Surg* 1992;74B(suppl 2):228.

29. James SL: Running injuries to the knee. *J Am Acad Orthop Surg* 1995;3:309–318.

30. Andriacchi TP, Kramer GM, Landon GC: The biomechanics of running and knee injuries, in Finerman G (ed): *Symposium on Sports Medicine: The Knee*. St. Louis, MO, CV Mosby, 1985, pp 23–32.

31. Järvinen M: Epidemiology of tendon injuries in sports. *Clin Sports Med* 1992;11:493–504.

32. Clement DB, Taunton JE, Smart GW: Achilles tendinitis and peritendinitis: Etiology and treatment. *Am J Sports Med* 1984;12:179–184.

33. Galloway MT, Jokl P, Dayton OW: Achilles tendon overuse injuries. *Clin Sports Med* 1992;11:771–782.

34. Snyder-Mackler L: Scientific rationale and physiological basis for the use of closed kinetic chain exercise in the lower extremity. *J Sport Rehab* 1996;5:2–12.

Running Injuries of the Knee

Stan L. James, MD

Since the running boom began in the 1970s, and particularly after the 1972 Olympics, when Frank Shorter won the marathon, a plethora of running injuries has ensued.[1,2] The prime site for these injuries is the knee, which accounts for approximately 30% of running injuries. In 1978, James and associates,[3] published a follow-up report on 180 runners. They found that the knee was the most common site of injury, and this has remained true through the years, with percentages varying little from that initial figure. In 1985, McKenzie and associates[4] reported that the incidence of knee injuries in runners had increased from 18%, in studies performed a few years earlier, to 50%. It was their impression that the improved construction of running shoes, which probably played some role in reducing the number of leg and foot injuries, was less effective in protecting the knee.

Two thirds of running-related injuries are caused by training errors.[3] A weekly mileage of 20 to 25 miles seems to separate the occasional runner from the serious runner, and there is an increased incidence of injuries in more serious runners.[5] Because two thirds of running injuries are the result of training error, the single most important aspect of the history is an analysis of the runner's training program. The examiner must be able to communicate with runners in their own terms. Without a knowledge of training techniques or what is appropriate or inappropriate, the physician is at a definite handicap in addressing running injuries. This, along with a knowledge of the biomechanics of running is the cornerstone for successful treatment of running injuries. Noake's *Lore of Running*,[6] Galloway's *Book on Running*,[7] Higdon's *Run Fast*,[8] and Guten's *Running Injuries*[9] are four resources that I recommend highly. Noake's *Lore of Running*, perhaps the most comprehensive resource available, covers all aspects of running and includes information on training as well as physiologic and medical considerations.

It is interesting that injuries are not restricted to beginning runners but occur just as frequently, or perhaps even more so, in elite runners. Over the past 25 years I have found that elite runners make basically the same mistakes that beginning runners make, and they have essentially the same type of injuries. The most common training errors are high mileage, high intensity, and sudden changes in the program. There is also a tendency toward reinjury once an area has been injured.

The body is a tremendously adaptable mechanism, but it does require time to accommodate to a change in stress patterns. This accommodation time differs for each individual. To a lesser extent, shoes, surfaces, terrain, and anatomic factors also play a role in injury. In a 1978 report by James and associates[3] we had hoped to establish an injury pattern based on anatomic factors. Unfortunately, we did not find that any specific anatomic or biomechanical variance, such as compensatory pronation, genu varum, or muscle contracture, necessarily correlated with a specific injury. This remains true. Through the years, we have found that any specific anatomic variation can create any of a number of injuries.

It is frustrating to find the same basic cause for an injury recur repeatedly and frequently in the same individual, making that person seem incapable of seeing an obvious training mistake. My theory is that most runners are afraid to deviate from the high mileage, high intensity program that has become so popular and that this keeps them from seeking out an optimal individualized training program. By optimal, I mean the least amount of training that will still maximize the runner's abilities. This approach is a hard philosophy to sell. The questions to be addressed are these. Why go beyond this optimal point and risk illness or injury? If a 10,000-meter runner can train to the best of his or her ability on perhaps 70 miles per week, why run 100 miles per week and risk injury? Maximum training benefit has been found to lie between 80 to 90 km training per week (48 to 57 miles),[10] so why run more?

Many runners have a "mind-body" communication gap. Regardless of how logical a program may seem intellectually, the body, by creating injury or illness, will reject it if it is too stressful. There are few accidents or acts of God relating to injuries or illness; instead, most are self-inflicted when the runner exceeds the body's capacity to withstand physical stress.

Runners can maximally train their body for a given event at a mileage and intensity far below "the line," beyond which injury and/or illness becomes a serious risk factor. Nature has a buffer zone for everyone, and as long as individuals do not try to train on or very near "the line," training will continue, with very few interruptions, which should be the goal of any program. How is an optimal training level found? Unfortunately, for the most part it is achieved empirically. An astute coach can be extremely helpful, but usually the individual must seek the ideal personal training program by educated guess or trial and error. Errors can be useful as long as they become learning experiences for the runner and not habitual recurrences, which unfortunately is frequently the case. A runner, by reviewing his or her training log, will often find a clue to the type of workout schedule that produced an optimal performance.

Not everyone requires a structured training program. A general game plan, with the specifics of each day's training determined just before the workout, may be a better option for the average runner. Granted, a competitive runner, peaking for a specific event, will benefit from a personalized, more structured schedule, but many of those who run for general fitness and recreation fare better with less structure. My advice to these people is to ignore a predetermined time, distance, and intensity for workouts. Simply playing off the body's feeling for a given day's workout may actually be the ultimate in long-term training sophistication. Unfortunately, however, many individuals prefer a very structured program.

Some general guidelines for an appropriate training schedule, particularly for the runner who wants to maintain a high degree of fitness year after year but perhaps doesn't respond well to structured programs is as follows. The philosophy of alternating hard and easy days has been proven time and again to be an effective method of training. This doesn't necessarily mean that every other day should be a maximum effort to ultimate fatigue, but that relatively hard workouts should be interspersed with easier workouts. Many people tend to have a somewhat harder day and a somewhat easier day, but never maximize the effects with a really hard workout. Most runners do extremely well with two or three quality workouts a week, for example, one workout that has some element of quickness, another at moderate pace and distance, and a third with a distance run appropriate to the individual. Workouts for speed and strength may vary from fartlek runs to formal interval workouts, depending on the runner's stage of training and conditioning.

Transition times, when the training program will be changed from shorter distance to longer distance or from slower workouts, to faster workouts, can put the runner at risk for injury. Many runners who try to increase their training do so too fast (10% per week is maximum). They pay too much attention to the response of the aerobic system and neglect the needs of the musculoskeletal system for adaptation. I describe this as the theory of the "engine and chassis" with the engine representing the cardiorespiratory adaptations to training and the chassis as the musculoskeletal adaptations to training. The weak link, the adaptation of the chassis (musculoskeletal system), can cause a breakdown as the runner focuses on training the engine (aerobic systems). It is not unusual for aerobic capacity to exceed musculoskeletal capacity. This situation is typified by competitive cross country skiers, who finish the competitive season in the early spring with superb aerobic fitness and then try to make a rapid transition to running. Although their aerobic conditioning is excellent, the musculoskeletal system is not ready for the loads imposed by running. These individuals must supplement their program with alternative forms of aerobic exercise as they gradually and safely increase their running mileage to an appropriate level.

Several alternative forms of exercise can benefit a runner not only by adding variety to a program but also by providing a safe mechanism for that need to get in extra work and also to help maintain conditioning during periods of injury. *Cross-Training for Sports*,[11] by Moran and McGlynn, is an excellent resource. Perhaps the best form of alternative training that transfers quite readily to running and is also an excellent mode of maintaining conditioning is aqua jogging, or running in the water. There are also several machines now on the market, such as cross-country ski simulators and stair-step machines, that can provide beneficial alternative methods of training.

Total body fitness should not be ignored. Too many runners have excellent lower extremities but a poorly developed upper body. Resistance training should be a part of every runner's routine regimen. I don't advocate a heavy power lifting program; a well-designed circuit course that covers all the muscle groups of the body will suffice. The body's strength stems from the larger, powerful muscles of the trunk and hips and flows sequentially to smaller, less powerful, but faster muscle groups in the extremities. This conformation creates a summation of forces that propels the body over the running surface more efficiently and represents a total body effort, not just an isolated effort of the lower extremities.

The History

Because 60% of injuries are due to training errors, the training program must be thoroughly analyzed. Look for sudden changes in duration, frequency, or intensity of training. The history must include current complaints, past running injuries, running experience, training patterns, and running terrain. Has cross training been used? What type and how often? Has there been a sudden increase in mileage? Has there been previous injury and is there a tendency for recurrence? An increase of 10% in the number of miles run per week is about the maximum that can be tolerated safely. Many complaints are caused by attempts to compensate for a previous injury, an injury that may not, at the time of evaluation, be the most prominent problem. It is important to know where and when the pain occurs in the run. For example, is it worse running uphill or downhill, and does it vary with the intensity of the run? Does the pain occur during the swing phase or the support phase of the running stride?

The history of previous injuries and their treatment must be investigated, because injuries tend to recur. It is also important to identify the make and style of running shoe and to find if a shoe change or the particular type of shoe being worn might be related to the injury. Also note if orthotic devices are being used or have ever been used, and if so, whether they were of any benefit, and how they were fabricated.

Physical Examination

The most important point in the physical examination is to include the entire lower extremity from pelvis to toes. Often when the runner complains of knee pain, examiners concentrate on the knee itself, although the problem itself may lie either distal or proximal to the knee (Outline 1). Keep in mind that growth abnormalities in alignment or anatomy of the lower extremity, including the knee, may not always be readily apparent at examination. Running imposes repetitive forces on the lower extremity, and even minor variations from normal can be exaggerated by this activity.

Begin the examination by evaluating alignment in the frontal and transverse

planes during stance, walking, and, if possible, running. An even better method is to make a video of the individual while running in order to analyze the patient's gait in slow motion or stop action. With this technique, abnormalities in gait are frequently noted that cannot be seen by direct observation.

The level of the iliac wings gives some indication of whether or not there is a leg-length discrepancy, but the presence of a leg-length discrepancy does not necessarily mean that is what is causing a problem. I have seen runners with up to 2 cm of shortening who had no problems whatsoever. Extremity length should be measured from the anterior-superior iliac spine to the medial malleolus and, if needed, I would recommend the use of radiographs.

Patellar dynamics are particularly important and should be assessed with the patient walking. The examiner should look for evidence of patellar malalignment or transverse-plane rotational abnormalities. The presence of squinting patellae (patellae that incline somewhat to the midline when the feet are placed parallel) suggests rotational malalignment, particularly proximally, with a femoral neck anteversion and associated femoral torsion. Ankle dorsiflexion should be assessed both with the knee extended and with the knee flexed. Chronic gastrocnemius-soleus complex tightness is frequently found in runners and, with the foot in neutral position, dorsiflexion is frequently limited to no more than a neutral position. There should be at least 10° of dorsiflexion during support phase, or compensatory foot pronation will be required to provide adequate dorsiflexion through the subtalar/midtarsal joint. The overall alignment and configuration of both feet should be noted with the patient standing and walking.

Heel-leg alignment and heel-forefoot alignment are extremely important to evaluate.[12] With the subtalar joint in neu-

---

Outline 1
Causes of knee pain in runners

Anterior Knee Pain

Patellar tilt/maltracking
Patellar instability
Quadriceps and patellar tendinopathy
Pathologic plica

Other Conditions

Meniscal lesion
Bursitis
Stress fracture
Osteoarthritis
Iliotibial band friction syndrome
Popliteal tenosynovitis
Ligament instability

---

tral position, forefoot supination or pronation is sought in relation to the hindfoot. Subtalar joint motion normally should allow approximately 8° of eversion and 25° of inversion (ie, a ratio of about 1:3). Any disruption of this ratio is associated with compensatory pronation of the foot and can be secondary to a tibia vara, tightness of the gastrocnemius-soleus complex muscles with limited ankle dorsiflexion, an inherent heel varus, or forefoot supination in relation to the hindfoot. All of these conditions require compensatory pronation to place the forefoot plantigrade on the surface. When compensatory pronation is present, the tibia is held internally rotated in an obligatory fashion for longer than normal, which, it has been speculated, creates a rotational mistiming at the knee between the tibia, patella, and femur.[3] In such cases, the patient complains of knee pain, but the source of the problem is distal, at the foot.

Inspecting the runner's shoes for wear patterns and distortions is also extremely important. It is not unusual to find heels that are worn, particularly on the lateral side, or heel counters that are badly distorted. Shoes must be replaced before excessive wear occurs.

Runners with knee pain frequently have several anatomic variations present.

A classic example of such variations occurs in the miserable malalignment[3] group, who usually present with a complaint of knee pain associated with running. Examination reveals femoral neck anteversion with a greater range of internal hip rotation than external hip rotation, genu varum, squinting patellae, excessive Q angle, tibia vara, functional equinus with tight gastrocnemius-soleus muscle groups, and often a compensatory pronation of the feet.

Finally, the examiner should carry out a very thorough knee examination. Because many problems are associated with the extensor mechanism, it must be examined in detail. Patellar position, tracking, stability, crepitus, and areas of tenderness should be noted.

Radiographic Examination

If indicated, routine radiographic examination includes at least four views: a weightbearing anteroposterior view, a lateral view in 45° of flexion, a tangential view of the patella, and a notch view in either the weightbearing or nonweightbearing position. Such studies are not required for obvious tendinopathy or soft-tissue conditions, but if any degenerative condition, patellofemoral malalignment, or other bony abnormalities or injury is suspected, a complete examination is certainly warranted. Other imaging studies such as magnetic resonance imaging (MRI) or triple phase bone scan may be indicated in certain instances. Computed tomographic arthrography, as described by Fulkerson,[13] is frequently helpful in analyzing patellofemoral abnormalities.

Anterior Knee Pain

The problem referred to in the lay literature as runner's knee, which is called chondromalacia in the professional literature, is a nonspecific diagnosis for anterior knee pain. Anterior knee pain, the most common knee complaint in runners, requires a very thorough extensor

mechanism examination. Quadriceps development; muscle contractures; vastus medialis obliquus position and development; and patellar position, tracking, stability, and mobility must all be noted, as well as any painful arc of motion, the Q angle, noting fat pad tenderness or crepitus, and quadriceps and patellar tendon tenderness.

Keep in mind that anterior knee pain is generally resolved conservatively. Only after failure of a reasonable period of conversative treatment should appropriate surgery be considered.

Maltracking/Patellar Tilt

Even mild maltracking or tilt of a minimal degree can cause pain as a result of the accumulative effect of the high patellofemoral joint forces in running. Excessive lateral pressure syndrome or patellar tilt is characterized by diffuse anterior knee pain, but often runners indicate that the patella is the major site of discomfort. Clinical examination of the patellar tracking may not reveal anything particularly remarkable, but palpation of the lateral retinaculum often reveals tenderness. There may also be tightness of the lateral retinaculum and iliotibial band. When this occurs, the lateral border of the patella cannot be brought to the horizontal plane on examination with the knee fully extended and the quadriceps relaxed. The examiner stabilizes the medial patella with the fingers of both hands, uses the thumbs to pull up on the lateral patella, and observes the degree of mobility present. If the condition has been persistent, there may be crepitus and tenderness along the lateral patellar border, which indicates the possibility of degenerative changes in the lateral facet articular cartilage.

An axial view of the patella, such as the Merchant view or Laurin view,[14] normally shows the patella concentrically positioned in the sulcus without tilt or subluxation. Fulkerson[13] has described a technique for using computed tomogra-

phy to determine patellar alignment but, in some cases, the actual maltracking of the patella may require arthroscopic diagnosis.

Once the diagnosis of patellar tilt or maltracking has been made, a conservative treatment program should be initiated initially. If after 6 months of conservative treatment there is no reduction in the symptoms and the diagnosis is clinically and radiographically confirmed, surgery may be considered. An arthroscopic or open lateral retinacular release is effective for treatment of patellar tilt, particularly when there is minimal or no articular cartilage involvement of the patella. This procedure is not particularly efficacious in the absence of patellar tilt or lateral placement of the patella. Although an arthroscopic lateral release may seem relatively benign, it is important to stress to the runner that 8 to 12 weeks of rehabilitation may be required before a return to running can be allowed.

Patellar Instability

Patellar instability, a condition associated with anterior knee pain in runners, may be characterized by episodes of instability, but rarely involves dislocation. Even minor patellar subluxation or lateral maltracking can alter the normal distribution of patellofemoral joint compression forces, creating pain with or without actual articular cartilage damage.[15] Some factors associated with instability are a lax medial retinaculum, weak vastus medialis obliquus, high Q angle, shallow sulcus, patella alta, genu valgum, femoral neck anteversion, and compensatory pronation. Symptoms of giving way may be present, but anterior knee pain is the most common complaint.

The diagnosis of patellar instability can usually be made on the basis of the history and clinical examination alone. The physical examination determines patellar position, tracking, and stability. It is important to observe patellar tracking during active knee extension and flexion with the patient sitting. Lateral placement of the patella or lateral displacement at the termination of extension, the J sign, suggests maltracking. With the knee positioned in 30° of flexion, lateral pressure applied to the patella will detect the presence of lateral instability. The patella should remain secure in the sulcus at 30° of flexion. A Q angle of more than 20° indicates a tendency for abnormal lateral displacement of the patella by the quadriceps. Determination of the congruence angle on a Merchant view of the patella may reveal patellar subluxation. A lateral radiograph of the knee in 30° of flexion will determine the presence of patella alta, which is often associated with instability. The normal ratio of patellar length to patellar tendon length should be no more than 1:1.2.

The more subtle forms of maltracking and subluxation can be managed with quadriceps rehabilitation and by emphasizing closed chain exercises rather than open chain exercises, which can aggravate patellar problems by overloading the patellofemoral joint. A program prescribed by a knowledgeable physical therapist or physician should be faithfully pursued for at least 3 months before any surgical treatment is considered. Most runners become symptom free and can return to training after such a rehabilitation program, but continuation of rehabilitation exercises may be necessary for an indefinite period even after the patient has returned to training and is asymptomatic.

For the small group of patients for whom surgical intervention is considered, arthroscopic lateral retinacular release, with a patellar chondroplasty, if indicated, is the option selected most often. Ideally the patellar articular surface will not be seriously involved, because damage here can have a deleterious effect on the runner's future. A lateral release is compatible with a return to running and is preferable to more extensive procedures. Although many runners anticipate

a much shorter course because the procedure does not seem to be terribly complicated, 8 to 12 weeks of rehabilitation is required before a return to running. Because this rehabilitation period seems rather prolonged, it must be thoroughly explained to runners.

Distally, a medial tibial tubercle transfer or anteromedialization of the tibial tubercle, as described by Fulkerson,[13] may be indicated. Proximally, medial retinacular reefing can be carried out in addition to the lateral retinacular release, but this must be done with care to avoid creating a tight medial retinaculum and patellar tilt or rotation. It has been my experience that the result following extensive proximal and distal realignment of the extensor mechanism is unpredictable in terms of the ability to return to serious distance running. A simple procedure, such as a lateral release, gives a better prospect for a return to training. In large part, the result will be determined by the extent of patellofemoral joint degenerative changes or chondral damage from repeated episodes of subluxation or chronic maltracking.

Quadriceps and Patellar Tendinopathy

Quadriceps tendon tendinosis and patellar tendon (ligament) tendinosis are often referred to as jumper's knee,[16] and the latter condition is frequently encountered in runners. The area involved is the tendon insertion at the distal pole of the patella. Excessive forces at the ligament insertion result in microruptures and, in some cases, local areas of deep tendon degeneration or tendinosis. The microtears can lead to structural deterioration with partial tissue failure.[17] In some instances there is a complete rupture of the tendon, but this is not common. Tendinosis at the tendon insertion distally on the tibial tubercle is far less common in runners. Quadriceps tendon tendinosis is associated with pain at the

insertion site of the quadriceps tendon proximally on the patella and its location is usually more lateral than medial. Runners with patellar tendon tendinosis often indicate an area of tenderness and pain at the distal pole of the patella. Localized swelling may also be noted, particularly when the symptoms are acute. Typically, pain comes on gradually during the course of a run. The initial symptoms may be mild enough not to interrupt the training program, but with time they can become more persistent and may eventually lead to cessation of running.

Physical examination of quadriceps tendinosis reveals tenderness directly over the insertion site of the quadriceps tendon, generally over the lateral aspect of the tendon. There may also be associated crepitus, particularly if there is a prominent lateral epicondylar ridge on the femur or perhaps even an osteophyte from some degenerative patellofemoral joint changes. Squatting places increased tension on the tendon and often is as painful as running.

With patellar tendon tendinosis, the pain is located directly over the distal pole of the patella and is best palpated with the patient's knee in full extension and the quadriceps relaxed. Pressure is applied to the proximal pole of the patella to tilt up the distal pole so the patellar tendon insertion may be easily palpated and the tenderness localized. With the knee flexed, this area frequently is not tender. Occasionally swelling or induration of the soft tissues is also noted and there may an increased Q angle. The Q angle may be observed to change dramatically during the support phase of gait, with compensatory pronation when there is increased obligatory tibial rotation present during the support phase of running. With compensatory pronation, internal tibial rotation is both excessive and prolonged and may place eccentric traction on the patellar tendon leading to tendinosis.

Routine radiographic findings are often normal, although in some instances the distal pole may be elongated or have a fragmented tip. Occasionally ectopic bone or calcific deposits are noted in the tendon but these are rare. Ultrasonography and magnetic resonance imaging (MRI) are the best ways to delineate an intratendinous lesion, but these studies are usually reserved for cases in which at least 3 months of conservative treatment has failed and surgery is being contemplated. Ultrasonography is quite specific and less expensive than MRI, but MRI delineates the lesion, which is usually located posteriorly at the insertion site, more clearly.

Unless the process is advanced, both patellar and quadriceps tendinosis often can be resolved conservatively by using the treatment protocol discussed later in this chapter. Curwin and Stanish[18] described a rehabilitation program for tendinosis that had a success rate of about 90%. Unfortunately, their results were less successful with patellar tendon tendinosis, with only 30% of patients experiencing relief, but I often ask runners to at least try this program to see if they might achieve relief. In my experience, once a lesion has developed that is visible on MRI or ultrasonography, the chances of resolving it are quite slim if distance running is continued.

Failure of a conservative program after 3 to 6 months offers the runners two choices. One is to discontinue the activity; the other is surgical exploration of the involved area and excision of any abnormal tissue. If the lesion is quite large, it may be necessary to reattach the tendon to freshened bone. Fortunately, in most patients the area of involvement is relatively small and the defect can be closed with imbrication. The surgical technique for quadriceps tendon tendinosis is similar to that used for patellar tendon tendinosis. If an osteophyte or prominent epicondylar ridge is present, it is removed to decompress the area.

Pathologic Plica

A pathologic plica is another cause of anterior knee pain in runners. Most commonly it involves the medial peripatellar plica, which becomes fibrotic and rubs or snaps over the medial femoral condyle and may be impinged between the condyle and the overlying patella. Occasionally, a suprapatellar plica, located deep to the quadriceps tendon, may become symptomatic as well. Pain usually comes on gradually with distance running. However, it can be acute and associated with sudden changes in training routine such as more intense, short-interval workouts. Even snapping and buckling may be noted. The patient may also report that sitting is painful. The pain is rather diffuse but often a runner can localize it to the medial retinacular area or suprapatellar area.

A common physical finding is localized tenderness over the medial femoral condyle adjacent to the medial border of the patella. There is frequently a palpable snap and sometimes crepitus noted over a tender, palpable, medial fibrotic cord. Full knee flexion may elicit suprapatellar pain. An effusion is not usual with a plica syndrome and, if present, other interarticular causes should be considered. There may be a tendency to overdiagnosis this condition, but it is also important to remember that a truly pathologic plica can mimic a number of other conditions in the joint.

The treatment protocol will be discussed under treatment. Active knee resistive exercises, which will irritate the plica, should be avoided. It may be necessary to confirm the diagnosis by arthroscopic inspection of the joint, with excision of the fibrotic band if present. This procedure usually entails very little loss of training for the runner. If at the time of arthroscopic examination the suspected plica is not thickened, avascular, and widened (over 12 mm), Ewing[19] has suggested it probably is not the cause of the problem, and other sources of the pain should be sought diligently.

Other Conditions
Meniscal Lesions

Meniscal lesions, although quite unusual in younger runners, become more of a problem for runners who are middle-aged and older. The diagnosis of meniscal tears in runners is like that for any athlete with this condition. Runners who are middle-aged and older often complain of an insidious onset of pain, although, in some instances, there may be an inciting incident such as a misstep or a twist. There may be a history of joint effusion and/or catching. Locking episodes are less common in older runners, unless they have developed a flap tear or bucket hand tear, which happens infrequently.

The physical signs, which sometimes include a small effusion, usually involve joint line tenderness over the involved area, most commonly in the posterior medial portion of the medial meniscus. In my experience, McMurray's test has been positive in about half of the patients. Arthrography has fallen into disuse with the current tendency to use MRI, but if a radiologist is available who is very competent at arthrography, arthrography is more cost effective and, in my mind, virtually as reliable as MRI for medial meniscal lesions.

Meniscal lesions lend themselves to arthroscopic surgery,[20] generally with a relatively short interruption (4 to 6 weeks) in the training program, which is acceptable to most runners. In some instances, a meniscal repair is indicated, particularly in younger runners. An appropriate rehabilitation program must be supervised, as discussed later in this section.

Bursitis

Bursitis most commonly involves the pes anserine bursa, and Vochel's bursa, which is deep to the superficial portion of the medial collateral ligament. Tenderness with Vochel's bursitis is immediately below the joint line deep to the superficial portion of the medial collateral ligament. Pes anserine bursitis is a bit more distal and its symptoms are tenderness and, in some instances, crepitus and perhaps also a sense of fullness. Active knee flexion with resistance may cause pain. These two conditions must be differentiated from a medial meniscal lesion, in which the tenderness is more directly over the joint line as opposed to being localized more distally. Both types of bursitis usually respond promptly to conservative measures and, in some instances, a steroid injection may be of help. I have never had the experience of doing surgery on either of these conditions. These are not common running injuries.

Stress Fractures

A proximal medial tibial stress fracture must also be considered in differentiation of knee pain in runners. Most tibial stress fractures occur in the middle and distal thirds, however. Tibial stress fractures are usually associated with localized tenderness on palpation and swelling. A triple phase bone scan is the best early diagnostic tool. Once the diagnosis has been made, the treatment is rest until symptoms abate, which usually involves a period of some 6 to 10 weeks.

Osteoarthritis

With the advent of the running boom in the mid 1970s there has been a significant increase in the number of older runners. It is not unusual to find very dedicated runners in the 6th and 7th decade and older. The frequency of osteoarthritic conditions increases with increasing age. They also can occur in younger runners, particularly if there has been chondral damage to one of the articular surfaces of the knee. Most current studies involving the etiology of arthritis in the lower extremities or particularly the knee do not clearly implicate running itself as an etiologic factor in a normal knee.[21,22]

The relationship between running and osteoarthrosis aside, once degenera-

tive changes are established, the running program must be carefully customized and monitored. A frequent question that I have from runners is whether or not running will accelerate a known osteoarthritic condition. The answer is, yes, it can. To a great extent the risk depends on the running program. For the most part runners are unwilling to accept the advice to give up running, but they frequently will accept the advice to modify the program and to try and find one they can tolerate with minimal insult to the joint. Sometimes it's best to first allow them to try to find a program that their knees will tolerate. Then, if they are unable to do so, it may be easier for them to decide to discontinue running rather than just being arbitrarily told they must stop.

With significant degenerative changes, low-impact aerobic activities are possible alternatives to running. These activities include ski machines, swimming, aerobic water exercises, biking, and race walking, either in lieu of running or to supplement running. Often I have patients run only once or twice a week and derive the rest of their conditioning from nonimpact or very low-impact activities. By reducing mileage, intensity, and duration, they frequently can find a level of running that is tolerated. I caution runners that persistent pain and recurrent swelling, are signs that their knee is not tolerating running well, and they may have to discontinue it.

Minimal arthroscopic joint debridement to remove bothersome osteophytes, degenerative menisci, and loose bodies may help symptomatically but probably offers no long-term improvement. The condition still persists. In my experience, extensive chondroplasty procedures and abrasion chondroplasty procedures have not been effective in allowing a return to serious running (over 20 to 25 miles).

Iliotibial Band Friction Syndrome

Iliotibial band friction syndrome, the most common problem involving the lateral

aspect of the knee in runners,[23] is usually initiated by an extra long run and is particularly aggravated by running downhill. This syndrome is characterized by pain over the lateral aspect of the knee, which often starts after a mile or two into a run and then becomes worse for the duration of the run. The pain may cease completely after the run has ended. Sometimes it occurs only with downhill running. Often participation in other sports activities is absolutely pain free. The cause is an area of irritation beneath the iliotibial band (ITB) as it glides back and forth over the lateral femoral condyle, which in some instances may be prominent enough to create an underlying synovitis.

On physical examination, there is tenderness directly over the distal ITB at the level of the lateral femoral condyle. Swelling and crepitus can occur in the area but are rare. The usual symptom is simply an area of tenderness. Genu varum and/or tibia varum, heel varus, forefoot supination, and compensatory pronation can play a role in the initiation of ITB syndrome. Tibia varum creates increased tension on the ITB as it crosses the lateral femoral condyle. The ITB attaches at Gerdy's tubercle, which is rotated forward and inward with compensatory pronation, and this, too, probably places more tension on the ITB. Hip abductor weakness with early muscle fatigue may cause exaggerated pelvic sag during the support phase. As the pelvis sags away from the support extremity, increased tension is placed on the ITB. These conditions increase friction between the ITB and the lateral femoral condyle and lead to an underlying synovitis. Tenderness is typically present about 2 to 3 cm proximal to the joint line and directly over the lateral femoral condyle along the distal portion of the ITB. In a meniscal lesion, the tenderness is more directly over the joint line, and in popliteal tenosynovitis, the tenderness is directly posterior to the fibular collateral ligament laterally.

Ober's test may be positive for ITB tightness, but a better test is performed with the patient lying on his or her side with the affected knee up. Pressure is applied to the lateral femoral condyle and the knee is moved through a range of motion of about 30° to 45°, which positions the tensed ITB directly over the lateral femoral condyle and accentuates the pain.

In addition to the modalities usually used in the treatment of runners' injuries in general, a corticosteroid injection or phonophoresis (ultrasound with topical hydrocortisone) in the area of involvement may help resolve the condition, particularly in the acute phase. Other techniques include stretching the ITB and strengthening the abductor musculature. Consideration may also be given to orthotics and shoe change.

Surgery may be indicated in patients with intractable symptoms. Even if the surgeon is certain that the condition is ITB friction syndrome, I think it is worth arthroscoping the joint so that the lateral compartment may be carefully inspected to rule out a meniscal lesion. Other disorders, such as a pathologic lateral plica, can also occur, but are very rare. If no other cause is identified, an open procedure similar to that described by Noble[24] is performed to release the posterior 2 cm of the iliotibial band at the level of the lateral condyle, where it has the most tension over the femoral condyle. In my experience, this procedure has been effective and usually allows a return to running within about 4 weeks. However, as is the case for many surgical procedures used to treat runners' injuries, there are no well-controlled prospective clinical studies that unequivocally show this to be efficacious. Fortunately, most cases can be resolved conservatively.

Popliteal Tenosynovitis

Popliteal tenosynovitis is another cause of lateral knee pain but is seen less frequently than ITB friction syndrome. It is, however, important to consider as a differential diagnosis for lateral knee pain. Popliteal tenosynovitis involves the popliteal tendon posterolaterally and may be either transient or chronic. The onset is often associated with downhill running, in which the popliteus restrains the femur, preventing it from translating anteriorly on the tibia.

Examination reveals tenderness directly over the popliteal tendon just posterior to the fibular collateral ligament. Placing the lower extremity in a figure 4 position places the fibular collateral ligament under tension, and the popliteal tendon can be easily palpated immediately behind the fibular collateral ligament.

Treatment is conservative and is similar to that used for ITB friction syndrome. I have never found surgery necessary for a patient with this condition.

Ligamentous Instability

Ligamentous instability of the knee is not a common problem caused by running, even among competitive runners. However, some runners may have ligamentous instability, particularly an anterior cruciate ligament deficit, which was incurred in other sports, such as downhill skiing. If the menisci remain intact, there are no recurrent episodes of instability with swelling and pain, and the activity of running is confined to good surfaces, the knee may function well without difficulty in spite of the instability, but close monitoring is required on the part of both the physician and the runner. Personally I have had several runners who incurred an anterior cruciate ligament injury from other activities but were still able to run comfortably and without problems. They had only minor instability on clinical examination, there were no clinical signs or MRI evidence of meniscal injury, and these people have done well.

I cannot emphasize enough that most knee injuries in runners can be resolved with the use of conservative methods. Surgery should be undertaken when its need is clearly indicated, but only after a trial of conservative treatment has failed. Nigg[25] suggests that most effective biomechanical strategies to reduce load and stress on a locomotor system involve the following factors: (1) the movement, such as a change in running style; (2) the surface (soft versus hard); (3) the shoe, current shoes designs provide considerable variability in cushion and motion control of the foot; and (4) the frequency of repetitive movement (mileage, pace, or duration of running).

Treatment Protocol

I recommend a treatment protocol (Outline 2) that is adaptable to virtually all runners' injuries, including those involving the knee. The physician is to choose a treatment from this protocol and apply it to the condition in an appropriate fashion. Based on my years of personal experience in treating running injuries, this approach has proven quite effective.

Training Program

Earlier in this section, considerable emphasis was devoted to training and training principles and to the fact that about two thirds of runners' injuries are the result of an error in the training program. Thus it seems logical that training must be an area of emphasis in treating any runner's injury. Evaluating and modifying the training program as necessary will often resolve many of the runner's injuries. Being told to rest is the last piece of advice runners generally want to hear, but at times it is necessary. Instead of stopping, runners generally prefer to modify their program by reducing the frequency, intensity, and duration of their running. A reduced running program or one that has to be stopped can be supplemented or replaced by running in water with a flotation device. This exercise is an excellent form of nonweightbearing cross training for running during rehabilitation; it allows the runner to maintain a reasonably high level of aerobic conditioning, and, at the same time, maintains lower extremity muscle strength and endurance along with joint mobility. Many local coaches prescribe workouts in the water that are often similar to workouts that would be taken on the track. Other modes of low-impact training include cross-country ski devices, steppers, biking, and rowing, all of which can help supplement a runner's modified program.

Anatomic and Biomechanical Variations

A thorough assessment of the entire lower extremity is mandatory. Although the complaint is at the knee, concentrating on the site of complaint about the knee can cause the examiner to overlook the actual etiologic factor that is causing the pain.[26] Thus, it is important to look both distally and proximally from the knee to note any anatomic or biomechanical variations that may be of significance. It is also important to learn how to evaluate foot function.[3] Many knee problems or complaints of pain are related to abnormal foot function. Disruption of the normal ratio between supination and pronation of the foot during stance phase alters the normal obligatory tibial rotation and the tibial-femoral rotational relationship at the knee.

Shoe Modification

Shoes generally come in three classifications: those that control motion, those that provide support, and those that cushion the foot. Most running shoe manufacturers have shoes that fit into these three classifications. A motion control shoe helps the wearer control subtalar joint motion for compensatory pronation. Support shoes are for individuals who do not require much control, and cushioned shoes are for runners with rigid feet that require more flexibility and protection from contact. Usually an orthotist or shoe repair shop can modify running shoes to relieve such special problems as leg-length discrepancies. Changing the hardness of the midsole and heel wedge and using a variable hardness heel wedge can change foot mechanics by altering the rate of pronation. This change influences knee function by altering the amount and duration of obligatory tibial rotation during pronation. However, heel wedge and midsole cushioning do very little to alter the ground reaction forces generated during the propulsive phase of the support phase. These cushions are primarily effective during the short impact phase. Much emphasis has been placed by shoe manufacturers on the cushioning or shock-absorbing effect on impact during running. Actually, this is less significant than the vertical ground reaction forces experienced later, during the propulsive phase. At this point, the midsole hardness probably has minimal effect on the forces being generated.

The temperature effect on midsole materials has not been seriously considered by the industry. Because characteristics vary widely from cold to warm, a shoe that provides cushioning in normal conditions may not do so when it is cold. Likewise, in extremely warm conditions a motion control shoe may function more as a cushion type shoe. After approximately 300 miles, shoes begin to lose their effectiveness even though the wear may not be visible.

Muscle Reconditioning and Flexibility

Restoration of muscle strength, endurance, and balance of the entire lower extremity is essential after injury or surgery. After a runner's return to competition, I have seen many situations in which a muscle group deficit has persisted because of a lack of specific reconditioning during rehabilitation. Runners must use specific exercises to restore muscle strength and endurance to affected muscle groups, or deficits will persist.

Flexibility is also important and sustained stretching is another aspect of conditioning that must not be ignored. Although there are no data in the literature that support the beneficial aspects of stretching for injury prevention, most physicians, coaches, and athletes do feel it is important. Tightness or contracture of the hamstrings and gastrocnemius-soleus muscle groups is very common among distance runners. Taunton and associates[27] stress the importance of appropriate rehabilitation to restore muscle strength and endurance. When speaking of restoration of muscle strength, it is important to emphasize the entire lower extremity, starting at the hip and proceeding distally. Muscular deficiency is often the cause when a runner complains of a lower extremity that does not feel right or is not tracking right. A runner's inability to define the complaint specifically may mean that it is caused by muscle imbalance.

Orthotic Devices

Since the running boom in the 1970s, orthotic devices have become popular modalities for treating running injuries. Few data are available regarding their efficacy,[12] but I have found them to be effective, particularly for medial tibial stress syndrome, tibial stress fractures, and plantar fasciitis, as well as such knee problems as patellofemoral pain. The theory behind the insertion of an orthotic device into the shoe is that it controls

Table 1
Return to running protocol

Week	Activity
1	Walk 1 to 2 miles, alternating 1 minute fast and 1 minute normal
2	Walk 2 to 3 miles, alternating 1.5 minutes fast and 1.5 minutes normal. You may also replace the fast walking with jogging
3	Continue week 2 and if doing well, substitute (not add) a 10-minute jog every other day in lieu of walk/jog
4	Same as 3, but jog 15 minutes every other day in lieu of walk/jog
5	Jog 15 minutes one day and 25 minutes the next
6	Jog 20 minutes one day and 30 minutes the next
7	Jog 20 minutes one day and 35 minutes the next
8	Jog 20 minutes one day and 40 minutes the next
9	Resume training at appropriate duration, intensity, and frequency

subtalar joint motion, maintaining it at or near the neutral position with a more normal inversion/eversion ratio, which should be 3:1 or 4:1.[3] Orthotics can also reduce compensatory pronation and its effect on obligatory tibial rotation. They may also function as shock absorbers by using appropriate materials to reduce some of the impact at foot strike. Their primary function, however, appears to be related to subtalar joint motion.

Orthotic devices basically are classified as noncontrolling, partially controlling, or fully controlling. Noncontrolling, or accommodative, devices provide shock absorption and minimal control, such as is required by the cavus foot. Partially controlling devices correct mild compensatory pronation and are generally fabricated from more resilient or flexible materials. Fully controlling devices are to correct severe compensatory pronation, and they are probably more effective when fabricated from more rigid materials.

The market has been flooded with orthotic devices over the past few years, many of which are not well designed or particularly useful. If you are prescribing orthotic devices, be certain that the manufacturer's instructions for taking appropriate molds of the foot are followed implicitly, because a bad mold of the foot will result in a bad orthotic device.

Medications and Physical Therapy

Medications such as nonsteroidal anti-inflammatory agents can help by reducing pain and inflammation, but analgesics should never be used just to allow an individual to run. Occasionally, diminishing doses of corticosteroids will relieve acute soft-tissue conditions. The area about the knee where I have found an injection in an acute situation to be most helpful is with ITB syndrome. However, they do not help chronic ITB syndrome. Steroids must not be injected directly into tendinous tissues.

Physical therapy must be directed specifically to the condition involved. Here again, the entire lower extremity musculature must be taken into consideration. Most anterior knee pain problems can be resolved with appropriate exercises. Closed chain exercises should be emphasized in anterior knee pain. For the most part, active knee extension exercises are to be avoided.

Light, flexible knee sleeves are tolerated reasonably well in runners, but more restrictive bracing and taping are not well tolerated. A counterforce band may be used for patellar tendon tendonopathy; I have not found these devices to be particularly effective.

Surgery

The vast majority of runners' injuries can be managed conservatively, but this program must be adequately supervised. Then, if it fails, the runner, the coach, and the physician will feel comfortable considering surgical treatment. Surgical indications in runners do not differ from those in the general population. Surgery is generally used as a last resort, particularly in elite runners, except for certain conditions, such as a meniscal lesion or loose body, that can be managed effectively with early arthroscopic surgery. Conservative treatment does not require unusual or unwarranted delay, but it does involve taking a methodical approach to problems. It is important to inform the runner when a condition is present that could terminate running in spite of well-indicated surgery.

In the knee, the most common surgical conditions relate to the extensor mechanism, menisci, plica, and degenerative changes. Explain the procedure in detail so that the runner can make an informed decision and will not have unrealistic expectations of the result.

Rehabilitation

Once surgery has been carried out, the surgeon must direct the postoperative rehabilitation program with the athlete, the trainer or physical therapist, and the coach. All too often, the results of surgery are negated by too rapid a return to running without adequate and careful rehabilitation. Similar problems can occur after recovery from an injury without surgery. My personal rules of thumb for returning to running after a period of missed training from whatever cause is as follows: (1) missed training of 1 week or less, resume an appropriate training program, but monitor it very closely and correct any training errors; (2) if 1 to 2 weeks, reduce the training 25% for the first week of return and then resume an appropriate training program, (3) if 2 to 3 weeks, reduce the training 50% for the first week of return, 25% the second week and then resume training; (4) if the period of missed training is 4 weeks or more, use the protocol shown in Table 1. When it is modified depending upon the individual situation, I have found this program quite satisfactory. It emphasizes a graduated return to running after a significant lay off following injury or surgery. It is important to point out to the runner that the purpose of this protocol is to condition the injured area, not to substitute for aerobic conditioning, which can be maintained with the cross training activities already mentioned. The runner should use an easy, comfortable pace, perhaps 7 to 10 minutes per mile and should also plan a rest day every 7 to 10 days. Instruct the runner not to be concerned about the amount of mileage, because the program is based primarily on time rather than distance. During the course of the graduated buildup, the runner can hold at a given level or even drop back a level if necessary. The program can be varied to meet individual needs. In some instances runners can move ahead 1 week or 2 if they are progressing very well. Levels can be shortened or lengthened depending on progress. If there are problems, tell the runner to stop and reevaluate the situation. Remember that general strengthening and flexibility exercises for the rest of the body should not be neglected.

Summary

Running injuries of the knee are very common. Significant risk factors for injuries are high mileage, previous injury, and rapid change in the program. Because two thirds of running injuries are training related, training is an important aspect of the history. In the case of knee injuries, the examination must include the entire lower extremity and not concentrate only on the knee. Most running injuries, whether in the knee or elsewhere, are managed conservatively, but, as with any condition, surgery is sometimes indicated. During rehabilitation from injury or surgery, the physician must supervise the rehabilitation and the return to running to avoid reinjury.

References

1. VanMechelen W: Running injuries: A review of the epidemiological literature. *Sports Med* 1992;14:320–335.

2. Lysholm J, Wiklander J: Injuries in runners. *Am J Sports Med* 1987;15:168–171.

3. James SL, Bates BT, Osternig LR: Injuries to runners. *Am J Sports Med* 1978;6:40–50.

4. McKenzie DC, Clement DB, Taunton, JE: Running shoes, orthotics and injuries. *Sports Med* 1985;2:334–347.

5. Hoeberigs JH: Factors related to the incidence of running injuries: A review. *Sports Med* 1992; 13:408–422.

6. Noakes T (ed): *Lore of Running*, ed 3. Champaign, IL, Leisure Press, 1991.

7. Galloway J (ed): *Galloway's Book on Running*. Bolinas, CA, Shelter Publications, 1984.

8. Higdon H (ed): *Run Fast: How to Train for a 5-K or 10-K Race*. Emmaus, PA, Rodale Press, 1992.

9. Guten GN (ed): *Running Injuries*. Philadelphia, PA, WB Saunders, 1997.

10. Wilmore JH, Costill DL (eds): *Physiology of Sport and Exercise*. Champaign, IL, Human Kinetics, 1994, p 152.

11. Moran GT, McGlynn G (eds): *Cross-Training for Sports*. Champaign, IL, Human Kinetics, 1997.

12. Jones DC, James SL: Foot orthoses, in Baxter DE (ed): *The Foot and Ankle in Sport*. St. Louis, MO, Mosby-Year Book, 1995, pp 369–378.

13. Fulkerson JP: Patellofemoral pain disorders: Evaluation and management. *J Am Acad Orthop Surg* 1994;2:124–132.

14. Laurin CA, Dussault R, Levesque HP: The tangential x-ray investigation of the patellofemoral joint: X-ray technique, diagnostic criteria and their interpretation. *Clin Orthop* 1979;144:16–26.

15. Boden BP, Pearsall AW, Garrett WE Jr, et al: Patellofemoral instability: Evaluation and management. *J Am Acad Orthop Surg* 1997;5:47–57.

16. Blazina ME, Kerlan RK, Jobe FW, et al: Jumper's knee. *Orthop Clin North Am* 1973;4:665–678.

17. Leadbetter WB: Aging effects upon the repair and healing of athletic injury, in Gordon SL, Gonzalez-Mestre X, Garrett WE Jr (eds): *Sports and Exercise in Midlife*. Rosemont, IL, American Academy of Orthopaedic Surgeons, 1993, pp 177–233.

18. Curwin S, Stanish WD: Clinical results, in *Tendinitis: Its Etiology and Treatment*. Lexington, MA, Collamore Press, 1984, pp 157–181.

19. Ewing JW: Plica: Pathologic or not? *J Am Acad Orthop Surg* 1993;1:117–121.

20. Foos GR, Fox JM: Arthroscopy of the knee in runners, in Guten GN (ed): *Running Injuries*. Philadelphia, PA, WB Saunders, 1997, pp 93–111.

21. Lane NE, Michel B, Bjorkengren A, et al: The risk of osteoarthritis with running and aging: A 5-year longitudinal study. *J Rheumatol* 1993;20: 461–468.

22. Paty JG Jr: Arthritis and running, in Guten GN (ed): *Running Injuries*. Philadelphia, PA, WB Saunders, 1997, pp 189–200.

23. Messier SP, Edwards DG, Martin DF, et al: Etiology of iliotibial band friction syndrome in distance runners. *Med Sci Sports Exerc* 1995;27: 951–960.

24. Noble CA: The treatment of iliotibial band friction syndrome. *Br J Sports Med* 1979; 13:51–54.

25. Nigg BM: Biomechanics, load analysis and sports injuries in the lower extremities. *Sports Med* 1985;2:367–379.

26. James SL, Jones DC: Biomechanical aspects of distance running injuries, in Cavanagh PR (ed): *Biomechanics of Distance Running*. Champaign, IL, Human Kinetics Books, 1990, pp 249–269.

27. Taunton JE, Clement DB, Smart GW, et al: Non-surgical management of overuse knee injuries in runners. *Can J Sport Sci* 1987; 12:11–8.

Achilles Tendon Problems In Runners

Donald C. Jones, MD

Incidence

Disorders of the Achilles tendon are very common in the running athlete, with a reported incidence ranging from 6.5% to 18.7%.[1-3] Welsh and Clodman[4] found that, of competitive track athletes with chronic Achilles tendinitis, 16% were forced to abandon their sports prematurely, while 54% continued to compete despite significant discomfort.

Achilles tendon injuries also occur in other sports, such as basketball, racquetball, soccer, football, and badminton. The mean age of patients with these injuries is between 24 and 30 years of age.[1,5,6]

Terms used to describe inflammation about the Achilles tendon and paratenon vary, which has led to considerable confusion when reviewing the literature. The classification used by Puddu and associates[7] provides a simple, but functional, arrangement. Peritendinitis refers to inflammation of the paratenon without an associated inflammatory response within the tendon. Peritendinitis with tendinosis describes a second stage of inflammation, in which both the Achilles tendon and paratenon are involved. The third stage, tendinosis, refers to asymptomatic degenerative lesions within the Achilles tendon, but without alteration of the paratenon. These changes may consist of mucoid or fatty change and/or fibroid degeneration, cartilage metaplasia, calcification, or bone metaplasia. Arner

and associates[8] described these changes in biopsies taken at the time of repair of acute ruptures in asymptomatic patients.

Anatomy

The gastrocnemius and soleus muscles form the common Achilles. The gastrocnemius muscle originates from both the lateral and medial femoral condyles, and the soleus muscle originates from the posterior surface of the tibia and the fibula.

The soleus and gastrocnemius muscles contribute separately to the formation of the Achilles tendon. The gastrocnemius muscle segment ranges from 11 to 26 cm in length, and the soleus muscle portion measures 3 to 11 cm. The narrowest part of the tendon is 4 cm proximal to its insertion.

The tendinous portion of the triceps surae complex has a relatively poor blood supply, consisting primarily of longitudinal arteries that course the length of the tendon complex. These arteries are supplemented by vessels from the mesotenon. Studies have shown the least vascular area to be 2 to 6 cm above the insertion of the Achilles tendon into the calcaneus. As a result, this area of poor vascularity is susceptible to chronic inflammation and rupture.[1,9-11]

The Achilles tendon fibers rotate laterally as they descend. Cummins and associates[12] describe three patterns of rotation. In the most common pattern,

the gastrocnemius muscle contributes two thirds of the fibers posteriorly and the soleus muscle contributes the remaining one third. In the second most common pattern, the gastrocnemius and the soleus muscle each contribute half of the fibers. In the least frequent pattern, the soleus muscle makes up the posterior two thirds and the gastrocnemius muscle the remaining one third. This rotation of the Achilles tendon plays an important part in the development of pathologic conditions.

Contributing Factors

The etiology of Achilles tendon disorders can be singular or multifactorial. According to Clement and associates,[1] the primary etiologic factors include training errors, such as an increase in training mileage, a single severe competitive session (10 km or a marathon), a sudden increase in training intensity, repetitive hill running, recommencement of training after an extended period of inactivity, and running on uneven or slippery terrain.

However, biomechanical variations, such as miserable malalignment, genu varum, and cavus foot, can also contribute to increased stress on the Achilles tendon and resultant bursitis. Excessive pronation of the forefoot has been implicated as the major biomechanical factor in running-induced injuries.[1,13,14]

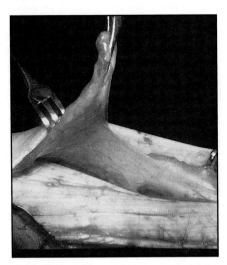

Fig. 1 Thickened hyperemic paratenon (peritendinitis).

An understanding of the biomechanics of the foot and ankle can help clarify the causal relationship between hyperpronation of the foot and Achilles tendon problems. In the initial phase of gait, the foot contacts the ground in supination. This supinated position results in a locked subtalar and midfoot joint, producing a very rigid structure. The rigidity of the foot provides the sturdy platform needed to absorb the tremendous amount of force transferred across the hindfoot at impact. Immediately after heel strike, the runner's body weight progresses over the center of the foot, and passive pronation is initiated. The calcaneus moves laterally, the talus drops off medially, and the forefoot begins to abduct. At this point, the foot becomes more flexible. As the body weight reaches the midline, maximum pronation is achieved and the hindfoot and forefoot are very flexible. Described as a "bag of bones," the foot is now capable of adapting to most unlevel running surfaces. As the weight transfer continues toward the toe-off position, the foot supinates and once again becomes a rigid lever for the function of push-off.

During this cycle, total range of motion of the subtalar joint, according to

James and associates,[15] is 31°, with 23° of inversion and 8° of eversion. This subtalar motion creates a "whipping" action of the tendon and the resultant shear forces across the Achilles tendon can result in chronic inflammation about the Achilles tendon complex.

Realizing that excessive hindfoot motion is not desirable in patients with Achilles problems, a decrease in subtalar motion is desirable in symptomatic patients. A number of studies have demonstrated that use of an orthosis can decrease this extreme motion.[16-18] The reduction of maximum eversion with an orthosis ranges from 6% to 12%. It is therefore assumed that the reduction of this extreme subtalar joint motion and the resultant "Achilles whip" can benefit patients with Achilles discomfort.

Achilles Tendon Disorders
Musculotendinous Junction Injury
Injuries to the musculotendinous junction are quite infrequent. These injuries usually occur in younger individuals with tight heel cords. Because of the excellent blood supply to this area, these injuries usually heal quite quickly.[15] Frequently, a decrease in vigorous activities for a short period of time is adequate treatment. However, on rare occasion, short-term immobilization is necessary. Total time from injury to recovery varies from 2 to 4 weeks.

Peritendinitis
The Achilles tendon is surrounded by the paratenon, not a synovial sheath. This paratenon is a loose, fatty, areolar tissue, which plays an important role in vascularization of the Achilles tendon.

Peritendinitis may result from abnormal biomechanics as previously described, or it may be caused by friction between the Achilles tendon and the adjacent tendon sheath. This friction may result from either intrinsic or extrinsic pressure. Examples of extrinsic causes of friction are ill-fitting shoes or poorly

applied tape about the ankle, which crimps the Achilles tendon. Intrinsic irritation may result from direct compression by a distal posterior tibial exostosis.

Symptoms of Achilles peritendinitis consist primarily of pain in the Achilles tendon area that is aggravated by activity and relieved by rest. The involved area may be only several centimeters in length or it can involve the entire tendon from its insertion to the musculotendinous junction.

Initial treatment of Achilles peritendinitis should consist of ice massage, contrast baths, and anti-inflammatory medication. If there is an alignment problem, orthoses that place the hindfoot in subtalar neutral are appropriate. With adequate conservative treatment, the athlete is usually asymptomatic in a relatively short period of time.

In more advanced or chronic cases, the paratenon becomes fibrotic and stenosed. An attempt may be made to dissect the adhered surrounding paratenon from the Achilles tendon. This is accomplished by placing a needle between the paratenon and Achilles tendon and rapidly injecting 15 ml of local anesthetic into the subparatenon space, creating a mechanical lysis of the adhesions. However, if this treatment fails, surgical decompression may be required.

The involved tendon is exposed through a medial peripatellar incision. Usually the involved paratenon is hyperemic, thickened, and somewhat adherent to the underlying tendon (Fig. 1). However, the paratenon may not be thickened and may only demonstrate a slight brownish blush over the tender area. Completely excise the involved paratenon medially, laterally, and posteriorly. Leave the anterior paratenon and fatty tissue intact, as this is a major area of blood supply to the tendon. Histology of the excised paratenon will frequently show only a relatively minimal acute inflammatory reaction, but a significant amount of hypervascularity.

Rehabilitation following open lysis of adhesions consists of immediate active and passive range of motion of the ankle along with protected weightbearing for 10 to 14 days. Two weeks postoperatively, full weightbearing is allowed and a vigorous rehabilitation program, consisting of range of motion, strengthening, and proprioception education, is initiated. The patient is allowed to return to a gradual running program at 6 to 8 weeks after surgery.

Peritendinitis and Tendinosis

As mentioned earlier, in some cases both the paratenon and Achilles tendon exhibit inflammation. Involvement of the Achilles tendon can be secondary to interstitial microscopic failure or obvious central necrosis with mucoid degeneration. As opposed to isolated peritendinitis, which frequently involves tenderness along the entire Achilles tendon, the combination of peritendinitis and tendinosis usually presents with a localized area of tenderness 2 to 6 cm above the insertion.[5,13,19] Swelling and nodular deformity may also be present (Fig. 2).

In the acute stage, pain is present with prolonged running and high impact-type activities, while lesser activities are asymptomatic. However, in chronic cases, pain may be present during both training and daily activities.

In the absence of nodular deformity, it may be difficult to differentiate between pure peritendinitis and peritendinitis with tendinosis. It is extremely important that this distinction be made. In peritendinitis alone, there is no need to violate the tendon at the time of surgical intervention. On the other hand, if peritendinitis and tendinosis exist together, the tendon must be opened and debrided. Evaluation by magnetic resonance imaging (MRI) is extremely helpful preoperatively in determining whether or not tendinosis is a component of the Achilles disorder (Fig. 3).

The conservative measures men-

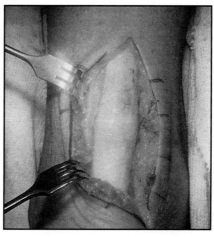

Fig. 2 Nodular deformity of the Achilles tendon (tendinosis).

tioned above are usually effective in resolving the problem. If not, a 1- to 2-week period of immobilization in a walking cast may be of benefit. If conservative treatment is unsuccessful after 6 months, surgery is an option for those athletes unable to train at the desired or needed level.

Expose the Achilles tendon through a posteromedial incision. Excise the paratenon and palpate the Achilles tendon for nodular deformities. In a tendon that is quite normal looking, but symptomatic, a preoperative MRI is helpful in locating the area of tendinosis.

A longitudinal incision is made through the tendon for a twofold purpose: (1) to see if there is an area of central necrosis or inflamed tissue that should be excised, and (2) to stimulate the healing reaction. After excising the involved area, the tendon is closed with absorbable sutures. If the defect is large, the tendon may require augmentation. Options include a plantaris weave,[20] a turn-down flap, or a flexor hallucis longus transfer.

Postoperatively, the period of immobilization depends on the amount of tissue excised. If a small defect is present, the patient is rigidly immobilized for 2 weeks, followed by mobilization in a

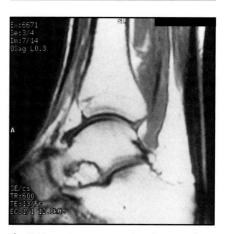

Fig. 3 Magnetic resonance imaging reveals change in the Achilles tendon consistent with tendinosis.

removable boot for an additional 2 to 4 weeks. With a larger defect, 4 to 6 weeks of rigid immobilization may be necessary.

Athletes who undergo this type of surgery must exercise great patience. It is not uncommon for the recovery process to require 4 to 6 months for total rehabilitation and the ability to return to vigorous training.

Posterior Heel Pain

Pain along the posterior wall of the calcaneus is not uncommon in runners. Although not seen as frequently as pain in the Achilles tendon, posterior heel pain can be extremely limiting to the athlete. Conditions that cause posterior heel pain include retrocalcaneal bursitis and tendinosis, pre-insertional Achilles tendinitis, and pre-tendinous Achilles bursitis.

Anatomic Considerations

Familiarity with the anatomy of the hindfoot is important in understanding the etiology and treatment of hindfoot discomfort. The posterior calcaneus has three surfaces—posterior, middle posterior, and superior. The posterior surface is a continuation of the tuberosity of the calcaneus with the plantar aponeurosis, the flexor retinaculum, and the flexor digitorum brevis muscle. The middle posterior surface is where the Achilles tendon has its most proximal insertion, with the tendon fanning out into both medial and lateral expansions. It is important to understand that the insertion of the Achilles tendon extends much further inferiorly than is frequently appreciated. The fact that this insertion extends onto the plantar aspect of the calcaneus is a very important consideration when performing a partial retrocalcaneal ostectomy. The superior surface of the calcaneus extends from the talar articulation to the posterior border. Just above this border is the pre-Achilles fat pad, which occupies a portion of Kaeger's triangle.

The nerve supply of the posterior calcaneal area originates from the medial surocutaneous nerve, a combined branch from the tibial nerve, and the communicating branch of the common peroneal nerve. Vascularity of the posterior aspect of the calcaneus consists of both the medial calcaneal branches of the posterior tibial artery and the peroneal artery.

Numerous variations of posterior calcaneal morphology have been described. It is important to recognize the three most common variations in the shape of the superior tuberosity of the calcaneus: (1) hyperconcave, (2) normal, and (3) hypoconcave.

Two separate bursa reside along the posterior calcaneal wall. The adventitious superficial pre-Achilles tendinous bursa separates the Achilles tendon from the overlying skin and is present in about 50% of individuals. It becomes inflamed secondary to chronic irritation from external compression of shoe wear. The second bursa, the retrocalcaneal bursa, is present at birth and lies between the posterosuperior aspect of the calcaneus and the overlying Achilles tendon. This bursa is horseshoe shaped, with medial and lateral arms that extend distally along the medial and lateral edge of the Achilles tendon. With average measurements of 2 mm in length by 4 mm in width by 8 mm

in depth, it is a significant structure. The synovial lining in the proximal portion abuts against the Achilles fat pad. The anterior bursa wall is composed of fibrocartilage, while the posterior wall is indistinguishable from the epitenon of the Achilles tendon. Interestingly, the retrocalcaneal bursa has a consistently characteristic bursal fluid. Canoso and associates[21] demonstrated that the normal retrocalcaneal bursal fluid has a low cellular content, with predominantly mononuclear cells and a good mucin clot. The hyaluronic acid content of the fluid is noted to be higher than that of the fluid found in the olecranon and prepatellar subcutaneous bursa. The average volume of fluid in a normal retrocalcaneal bursa is 1.22 ml.

Retrocalcaneal Bursitis

Retrocalcaneal bursitis is inflammation of the retrocalcaneal bursa. I have biopsied multiple Achilles tendons distal to the inflamed retrocalcaneal bursa and have consistently found chronic inflammation. Therefore, the entity referred to as "retrocalcaneal bursitis" is actually retrocalcaneal bursitis and distal Achilles tendinitis. This condition can develop as the result of a systemic inflammatory disease process, direct pressure from shoe wear, or altered mechanics of the foot and ankle.

When treating a running athlete with recalcitrant retrocalcaneal bursitis, always exclude the possibility of a systemic inflammatory disease as the cause of the symptoms before considering surgical intervention. This is especially important if the process is bilateral. The overall instance of retrocalcaneal bursitis with rheumatoid arthritis is estimated to be between 2% and 10%.[22]

As previously stated, biomechanical abnormalities can also potentiate the development of retrocalcaneal bursitis. The most common associated abnormalities are rigid plantarflexed first ray, rearfoot varus, and hyperrotation. The

abnormal motion created by these deformities can lead to increased shear stress at the osseous soft tissue interface along the posterosuperior aspect of the calcaneus, resulting in traumatic inflammation of the retrocalcaneal bursa and the adjacent Achilles tendon.

Although a heel prominence may be contributory, it is not uncommon to see retrocalcaneal bursitis develop in runners without an associated calcaneal deformity. The bursa may become inflamed as the result of heel counter compression or secondary to a "nutcracker" effect of the Achilles and the calcaneus on the bursa during repeated episodes of forced ankle dorsiflexion. It is for this reason that many long distance runners who use uphill running (as a training method) develop retrocalcaneal bursitis-type symptoms. A deadly combination for a long distance runner is abnormal biomechanics of the hindfoot in tandem with maltraining.

Diagnosis

Signs of retrocalcaneal bursitis include swelling and erythema over the posterosuperior calcaneal tuberosity. Palpation of this area reveals tenderness both medial and lateral to the Achilles tendon along the extended arms of the retrocalcaneal bursa. Fluid within the bursa is occasionally ballotable. Infrequently, there is tenderness along the Achilles tendon above the bursa; however, most frequently there is tenderness distal to the retrocalcaneal bursa. The pain is aggravated by dorsiflexion of the ankle beyond the neutral position and is relieved by plantarflexion.

Clinical examination usually confirms the diagnosis of retrocalcaneal bursitis; however, when difficulty in diagnosis arises, an MRI and bone scan may be helpful. An MRI will show an enlarged, inflamed bursa (Fig. 4), while a bone scan (Fig. 5) will demonstrate marked increased uptake along the superior wall of the posterior calcaneus.

Treatment

The heel counter must first be inspected. If there is any evidence of extrinsic compression, the foot wear must be modified. Once the extrinsic pressure has been relieved, ice, nonsteroidal anti-inflammatory medication, and a 3/8- to 1-in temporary heel lift may help to relieve the symptoms. Because lower extremity malalignment may be a factor, mechanical problems, such as tibial vara, functional equinus, tight hamstrings or calf muscles, and cavus foot, must be excluded as an aggravating factor. Training mileage should be decreased and the use of a soft, stable running surface encouraged. If the symptoms are not relieved at this point, the ankle and the retrocalcaneal bursa may require immobilization in a short leg cast for 3 to 4 weeks. However, once the cast is removed, the treating physician must be very careful not to incorporate dorsiflexion exercises too rapidly into the physical therapy.

An injection of steroid solution into the retrocalcaneal bursa has been advocated. However, Kennedy and Willis,[23] who reported on the effects of local steroid injection into tendons, found the most significant effect of such an injection to be collagen necrosis, with the return of normal tensile strength not occurring in the tendon for 14 days after the injection. This effect puts the tendon at risk for rupture for a period of 2 weeks postinjection. Even though the injection is into the bursa, not the Achilles tendon, there is always the concern that some of the steroid solution may come in contact with the Achilles tendon. I, personally, avoid this form of treatment.

Historically, three procedures have been advocated for this condition. Ippolito and Ricciardi-Pollini[24] described three patients with this condition. They removed the retrocalcaneal bursa and reported complete clinical relief of symptoms. Keck and Kelley[25] also reported on a series of patients who gained complete relief from simple bursal excision.

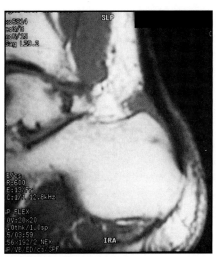

Fig. 4 Inflamed, enlarged retrocalcaneal bursa.

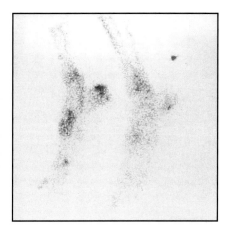

Fig. 5 Increased uptake along superior aspect of calcaneus consistent with retrocalcaneal bursitis.

Zadek[26] advocated a wedge osteotomy of the calcaneus. A dorsally based wedge of calcaneus is removed from the proximal half posteriorly, and the dorsal osteotomy site is closed, thereby foreshortening the calcaneus and theoretically decreasing the pressure across the calcaneal Achilles interface.

Stanley James and I have found that a partial retrocalcaneal ostectomy is a reliable procedure when dealing with this problem.[27] The objective of this procedure is to relieve pain by removing the underlying intrinsic source of irritation and pressure. Because of the associated Achilles tendinitis, bony decompression of the bursal area and distal Achilles tendon is mandatory. For this reason, we do not feel that simple excision of the bursa is adequate.

When surgically treating retrocalcaneal bursitis and Achilles tendinitis, controversy remains relating to the ideal incision. Numerous surgical approaches have been advocated. The most common incision used for this approach is a longitudinal incision parallel to the Achilles tendon. However, a lazy-L, reverse J-shape, and transverse incision also have been suggested. I recommend using two incisions, a parallel medial incision and a

lateral longitudinal incision (Fig. 6). Of a large number of failed retrocalcaneal ostectomies seen in my office, most occurred following the use of a single incision, which in many instances does not allow adequate visualization of the calcaneus and the Achilles tendon.

The technique for partial ostectomy using two incisions is as follows. The patient is placed in a prone position with a bolster placed under the distal leg. Longitudinal incisions are made from the insertion of the Achilles tendon to 7 to 10 cm proximal on either side of the Achilles tendon. Carry the incision distal to the superior portion of the plantar heel skin. Great care is taken to avoid damage to the sural nerve, which lies approximately 1 to 2 cm anterior to the lateral border of the Achilles tendon. The retrocalcaneal area and the superior aspects of the calcaneus are then exposed by a combination of blunt and sharp dissection. Once the tendon has been adequately exposed to the insertion site, which is much more distal than is generally appreciated, an oblique partial ostectomy of the superior angle of the calcaneus is carried out. The ostectomy begins approximately 1 cm anterior to the superior angle and then angles well downward past the point of tenderness.

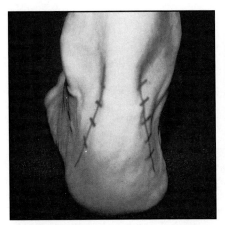

Fig. 6 Double incision technique used for partial retrocalcaneal ostectomy.

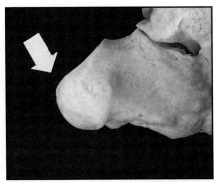

Fig. 7 Ostectomy must be perpendicular to the longitudinal axis of the calcaneus.

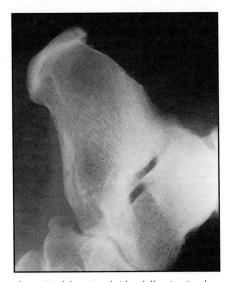

Fig. 8 Painful retained ridge following inadequate partial retrocalcaneal ostectomy.

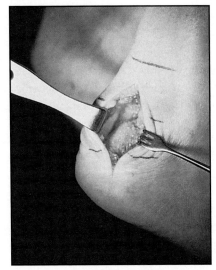

Fig. 9 Area of decompression between the posterior calcaneus and Achilles tendon.

Occasionally, a fairly large piece of posterior calcaneus must be resected in order to decompress the individual area of tendon. Kodziej and Nunley presented a study in which they showed that up to 75% of the length of insertion site may be resected without fear of tendon failure (Kolodziej P, Nunley JA, personal communication).

The reciprocating saw blade must be observed through both incisions so that the cut does not angle to one side or the other, but remains perpendicular to the longitudinal axis of the calcaneus (Fig. 7).

The inflamed bursa is removed in tandem with the bony fragment.

Often a ridge of bone is left at the distal insertion site (Fig. 8). This must be carefully removed with a small curette or rongeur so that no irritating prominence remains below the distal Achilles tendon. Next, the medial and lateral margins of the calcaneus are chamfered with small osteotomes and rasped smooth. The posterior calcaneus is repeatedly palpated through the overlying skin to make certain that all bony ridges and bony prominences are removed. With dorsiflexion of

the ankle, a visible space between the calcaneus and the adjacent Achilles insures adequate decompression (Fig. 9). Prior to closure, the Achilles tendon is inspected for inflamed or necrotic areas that require resection. The wound is closed in a routine fashion over a hemovac. A postoperative film should be taken (Fig. 10).

Insertional Achilles Tendinitis

It is not uncommon in the Masters age group runner to encounter insertional Achilles tendinitis associated with a calcific projection.[22] This projection, frequently referred to as a "fish hook" osteophyte (Fig. 11), is related to an inward angulation of the lower half of the posterior calcaneal tuberosity, which causes the Achilles tendon to begin its insertion at an anatomically low point. The resultant abnormal traction in the lower half of the posterior tuberosity produces a reactive osteosclerosis and formation of a prominent spur. This calcification may become very painful as a result of local pressure and associated Achilles inflammation. At the time of surgery, it is not uncommon to note erosion of the central portion of the Achilles tendon at the site of the fish hook osteophyte. Therefore, the pain in this condition is caused not only by extrinsic pressure on a prominent calcaneal spur, but also by the associated Achilles tendinitis and erosion.

A long period of conservative care is essential before considering surgery. We have found the previously mentioned conservative forms of care to be beneficial. In addition, in recalcitrant cases, I find that immobilizing the foot and ankle in a short leg walking cast is frequently beneficial.

If surgery is necessary, great care must be taken with skin retraction, because this condition usually occurs in older individuals and skin necrosis and wound breakdown are serious threats. If adequate circulation is present, two incisions may be used for the purpose of debridement, as in the cases of retrocalcaneal bursa treat-

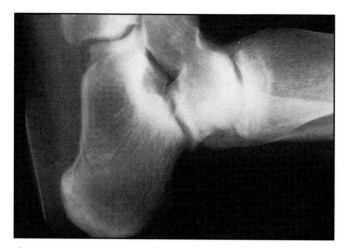

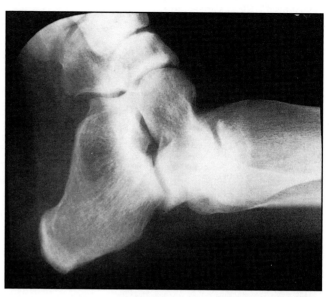

Fig. 10 Pre- and postoperative film.

ment. Baxter and Thigpen,[28] who use a single longitudinal central incision for debridement, have found the results satisfactory.

Superficial Peritendinous Achilles Bursitis (pump bumps)

Superficial peritendinous Achilles bursitis develops secondary to chronic inflammation caused by direct compression from shoes or blunt trauma. As mentioned in the discussion on anatomy, this bursa is present only 50% of the time. The location of the bursa corresponds to the upper edge of the offending shoe heel counter. It is not uncommon to see associated thickened and inflamed skin overlying the irritated superficial bursa. Clinically, it is important to realize that this pump bump may exist with or without underlying intrinsic pressure from a hyperconvex retrocalcaneal tuberosity. A bony prominence of this sort is best evaluated radiographically.

Conservative measures are almost always effective. A 3/16-in heel lift and modification of the shoe heel counter will usually suffice. The heel counter may be raised, lowered, or softened in an attempt to decrease the direct pressure and irritation.

If surgery is warranted, the offending prominent superior portion of the calcaneus can usually be removed through a single incision.

Heel Pain

The most common causes of heel pain in the runner are plantar fasciitis, nerve entrapment about the heel, and fat pad trauma/atrophy. These disabling entities are most frequently seen in distance runners, because most distance runners are midfoot strikers, while most sprinters are forefoot strikers.

Plantar Fasciitis

Plantar fasciitis is a term used to describe a painful condition located about the posterior medial surface of the foot just distal to the attachment of the plantar fascia to the calcaneus. It is caused by microtears and chronic inflammation where the plantar fascia attaches to the medial tubercle of the calcaneus.

During the early phase of plantar fasciitis, the symptoms occur gradually and are of relatively low intensity. However, as the patient continues to train, the pain becomes more noticeable and can cause serious disability for the athlete. The patient gives a history of

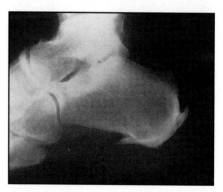

Fig. 11 Calcific insertional tendinosis, the "fish hook" osteophyte.

severe pain in the morning upon rising. The pain decreases with initial walking activities; however, it quickly returns with activities such as walking on hard surfaces, prolonged running, or climbing. If the athlete continues to run despite the pain, the gait pattern is usually altered. In order to decrease the stress on the plantar fascia, the foot assumes a fixed supinated and inverted posture from foot strike to toe-off. Because of overloading of the lateral column of the foot in this supinated position, the runner may also develop lateral foot pain.

Physical examination usually reveals maximum tenderness over the medial edge of the plantar fascia just distal to its insertion into the calcaneus. Interestingly, considerable pressure may be required to locate the exact area of tenderness.

Tightness of the Achilles tendon is frequently noted in this condition. Leg-length inequality may also be a precipitating factor. If one leg is longer than the other, heel pain is more frequently seen in the shorter leg.

Conservative Treatment As with most running injuries, the cornerstone of nonsurgical treatment is alteration of training. Cycling and deep water running activities are effective in maintaining the cardiovascular fitness of the athlete and produce very little stress across the inflamed plantar fascia. In addition to these low impact cardiovascular work-outs, abbreviated running workouts may also be continued. A stretching program, ice massage, and nonsteroidal anti-inflammatory medication are also recommended. The use of a night splint that holds the foot in 5° of dorsiflexion has also been helpful. Because the night splint prevents the foot from lying in the equinus position during sleep, the plantar fascia is not allowed to contract. Therefore, the hindfoot is much less painful in the morning. In recalcitrant cases, short-term full immobilization in a short leg walking cast is recommended. If a biomechanical abnormality such as hyperpronation, miserable malalignment, or a rigid cavus deformity is identified, orthoses are recommended.

In patients with continuing refractory symptoms, a steroid injection may be beneficial. However, great care must be taken when injecting this area with steroid solution. Multiple steroid injections may predispose the runner to plantar fascia rupture, which is not a benign complication. Disruption of the plantar fascia attachment from the calcaneus may have a detrimental effect on function. Daly and associates[29] demonstrated a change in both arch height and the ratio of arch height to arch length following complete plantar fascia release. With

complete fascial rupture, increased compressive forces are transmitted to the dorsal aspect of the midfoot, while decreased flexion forces occur across the metatarsal phalangeal joint complex. Midfoot pain and metatarsalgia can result.

Surgical Treatment If the patient has 10 to 12 months of pain recalcitrant to conservative treatment, surgery is an option. An oblique incision 3 to 4 cm in length is made just distal and medial to the heel pad, near the junction of the thicker plantar heel pad skin. This incision must be anterior to the medial calcaneal branch of the posterior tibial nerve. Inadvertent injury to this branch of the posterior tibial nerve will result in a postoperative neuroma. Dissection proceeds through subcutaneous tissue. The medial and lateral borders of the proximal plantar fascia are identified. The medial 50% of the plantar fascia is incised 1 to 2 cm distal to its origin from the calcaneus. If a large heel spur is present, it may be removed. If a smaller heel spur is present, the more extensive dissection required for its excision is not indicated. Surgical removal of this heel spur is controversial, because numerous studies have indicated that such spurs play very little role in pain associated with plantar fasciitis.[29,30]

The tourniquet is released and hemostasis established. The wound is closed with interrupted sutures. Postoperatively, the patient is kept nonweightbearing for 1 week. Progressive weightbearing in a postoperative shoe is allowed as tolerated 1 week postoperatively. The sutures are removed in 10 to 14 days. No repetitive impact loading activities are allowed for a total of 6 weeks. It is not unusual for the rehabilitation process to take up to 3 months before the patient is able to carry out high-impact loading activities.

Nerve Entrapments About the Heel
Heel pain can also result from nerve entrapment syndromes. Perhaps the best known nerve entrapment syndrome in

this area is tarsal tunnel syndrome. Tarsal tunnel syndrome is characterized by neurogenic pain described as burning in nature. In differentiating tarsal tunnel syndrome from plantar fasciitis, there is no tenderness over the medial tubercle in tarsal tunnel syndrome, but there is a positive Tinel sign over the posterior tibial nerve as it passes under the laciniate ligament. Nerve conduction studies are also quite helpful in making the diagnosis.

The most frequent nerve entrapment syndrome causing heel pain in the runner is entrapment of the first branch of the lateral plantar nerve.[31,32] Entrapment of this nerve occurs as the nerve changes from a vertical to a horizontal direction and passes under the heavy deep fascia of the abductor hallucis muscle. The abductor hallucis muscle is frequently hypertrophied in runners, which contributes to the entrapment process. The pathognomonic sign of entrapment of the first branch of the lateral plantar nerve is tenderness along its course, in association with burning, shooting pain from the ankle to the heel. No numbness is present with this entrapment process. Unlike plantar fasciitis, there is no early morning pain and no increase in symptoms when the patient arises after a prolonged period of sitting. Although no cutaneous sensory deficit occurs, motor weakness of the abductor digiti quinti may occasionally be detected. However, electrodiagnostic studies, electromyography, and nerve conduction studies are not helpful in making a diagnosis of entrapment of the first branch of the lateral nerve.[28,33-35]

Conservative Treatment Conservative treatment for athletes with this problem consists of modification of running activities, contrast baths, nonsteroidal anti-inflammatory medication, and ice massage. As with plantar fasciitis, if excessive pronation is present, a semi-rigid orthosis may decrease the stresses across the compressed nerve.

Baxter and Thigpen[28] have shown an 82% success rate in patients with this condition treated surgically. Baxter and Pfeffer[34] published a series that included 59 heels in 53 patients, with 89% excellent or good results following surgery.

Surgical Treatment A 4- to 5-cm oblique incision is made over the proximal abductor hallucis muscle, with the incision centered along the course of the first branch of the lateral plantar nerve. As with all incisions in this area, care must be taken to avoid damage to the medial calcaneal sensory nerve branches, which course posterior to this incision. The superficial fascia of the abductor hallucis muscle is exposed. This fascia is then divided. The abductor muscle belly is retracted superiorly with a right-angle retractor. The deep fascia of the abductor hallucis is exposed. The inferior edge of the deep fascia is incised, exposing the area where the nerve is compressed between this tight fascia and the medial border of the quadratus plantae muscle. Care should be taken to completely divide the fascia from inferior to superior. If the heel spur is felt to add additional compression to the nerve, it is removed as well. Leave the abductor hallucis muscle belly intact. At this point, the nerve should be thoroughly decompressed and a small hemostat should fit easily along the course of the nerve without impingement dorsally or plantarward. The plantar fascia is not incised unless there are associated symptoms of plantar fasciitis or the medial edge of the plantar fascia is compressing the nerve. Return to activities varies between 4 to 12 weeks.

Heel Pad Pain

Fat pad atrophy in the athlete can result from multiple steroid injections or repeated trauma. The pain is usually quite diffuse. There is no morning pain as seen in plantar fasciitis, and there is no neurogenic pain as seen in nerve entrapment syndromes.

On clinical examination, the heel paid is usually quite flat and relatively thin. Unfortunately, there is no surgical treatment for this entity. Treatment consists of cushioned heel cups and shock-absorbent sneakers or inserts. In some cases, a plastic heel cup may be helpful.

References

1. Clement DB, Taunton JE, Smart GW: Achilles tendinitis and peritendinitis: Etiology and treatment. Am J Sports Med 1984;12:179–184.
2. Krissoff WB, Ferris WD: Runners' injuries. Phys Sports Med 1979;7:55–64.
3. Jones DC, James SL: Overuse injuries of the lower extremity: Shin splints, iliotibial band friction syndrome, and exertional compartment syndromes. Clin Sports Med 1987;6:273–290.
4. Welsh RP, Clodman J: Clinical survey of Achilles tendinitis in athletes. Can Med Assoc J 1980;122:193–195.
5. Denstad TF, Roaas A: Surgical treatment of partial Achilles tendon rupture. Am J Sports Med 1979;7:15–17.
6. Nelen G, Martens M, Burssens A: Surgical treatment of chronic Achilles tendinitis. Am J Sports Med 1989;17:754–759.
7. Puddu G, Ippolito E, Postacchini F: A classification of Achilles tendon disease. Am J Sports Med 1976;4:145–150.
8. Arner O, Lindholm A, Lindvall N: Roentgen changes in subcutaneous rupture of the Achilles tendon. Acta Chir Scand 1959;116:496–500.
9. Gillies H, Chalmers J: The management of fresh ruptures of the tendo Achillis. J Bone Joint Surg 1970;52A:337–343.
10. Inglis AE, Sculco TP: Surgical repair of ruptures of the tendo Achillis. Clin Orthop 1981;156:160–169.
11. Lotke PA: Ossification of the Achilles tendon: Report of seven cases. J Bone Joint Surg 1970;52A:157–160.
12. Cummins EJ, Anson BJ, Carr BW, et al: The structure of the calcaneal tendon (of Achilles) in relation to orthopedic surgery: With additional observations on the plantaris muscle. Surg Gynecol Obstet 1946;83:107–116.
13. Clancy WG Jr, Neidhart D, Brand RL: Achilles tendonitis in runners: A report of five cases. Am J Sports Med 1976;4:46–57.
14. Buchbinder MR, Napora NJ, Biggs EW: The relationship of abnormal pronation to chondromalacia of the patella in distance runners. J Am Podiatry Assoc 1979;69:159–162.
15. James SL, Bates BT, Osternig LR: Injuries to runners. Am J Sports Med 1978;6:40–50.
16. Bates BT, Osternig LR, Mason MS, et al: Foot orthotic devices to modify selected aspects of lower extremity mechanics. Am J Sports Med 1979;7:338.
17. Cavanagh PR (ed): The Running Shoe Book. Mountain View, CA, Anderson World, 1980.
18. Clarke TE, Frederick EC, Cooper LB: Biomechanical measurement of running shoe cushioning properties, in Nigg BM, Kerr BA (eds): Biomechanical Aspects of Sports Shoes and Playing Surfaces. Calgary, Canada, University of Calgary, 1983, pp 25–34.
19. Fox JM, Blazina ME, Jobe FW, et al: Degeneration and rupture of the Achilles tendon. Clin Orthop 1975;107:221–224.
20. Lynn TA: Repair of the torn Achilles tendon, using the plantaris tendon as a reinforcing membrane. J Bone Joint Surg 1966;48A:268–272.
21. Canoso JJ, Wohlgethan JR, Newberg AH, et al: Aspiration of the retrocalcaneal bursa. Ann Rheum Dis 1984;43:308–312.
22. Turlik MA: Seronegative arthritis as a cause of heel pain. Clin Podiatr Med Surg 1990;7:369–375.
23. Kennedy JC, Willis RB: The effects of local steroid injections on tendons: A biomechanical and microscopic correlative study. Am J Sports Med 1976;4:11–21.
24. Ippolito E, Ricciardi-Pollini PT: Invasive retrocalcaneal bursitis: A report of three cases. Foot Ankle 1984;4:204–208.
25. Keck SW, Kelly PJ: Bursitis of the posterior part of the heel: Evaluation of surgical treatment of eighteen patients. J Bone Joint Surg 1965;47A:267–273.
26. Zadek I: An operation for the cure of achillobursitis. Am J Surg 1939;43:542–546.
27. Jones DC, James SL: Partial calcaneal ostectomy for retrocalcaneal bursitis. Am J Sports Med 1984;12:72–73.
28. Baxter DE, Thigpen CM: Heel pain: Operative results. Foot Ankle 1984;5:16–25.
29. Daly PJ, Kitaoka HB, Chao EY: Plantar fasciotomy for intractable plantar fasciitis: Clinical results and biomechanical evaluation. Foot Ankle 1992;13:188–195.
30. Sarrafian SK: Functional characteristics of the foot and plantar aponeurosis under tibiotalar loading. Foot Ankle 1987;8:4–18.
31. Rubin G, Witten M: Plantar calcaneal spurs. Am J Orthop 1963;5:38–41;53–55.
32. Lapidus PW, Guidotti FP: Painful heel: Report of 323 patients with 364 painful heels. Clin Orthop 1965;39:178–186.
33. Kenzora JE: The painful heel syndrome: An entrapment neuropathy. Bull Hosp Jt Dis Orthop Inst 1987;47:178–189.
34. Baxter DE, Pfeffer GB: Treatment of chronic heel pain by surgical release of the first branch of the lateral plantar nerve. Clin Orthop 1992;279:229–236.
35. Schon LC, Glennon TP, Baxter DE: Heel pain syndrome: Electrodiagnostic support for nerve entrapment. Foot Ankle 1993;14:129–135.

48

High Tibial Osteotomy and Distal Femoral Osteotomy for Valgus or Varus Deformity Around the Knee

Matthew J. Phillips, MD
Kenneth A. Krackow, MD

Introduction

Osteoarthritis of the knee is a common medical condition that affects a large number of individuals who are middle aged and older. One percent of males and 0.9% of females aged 55 to 64, 2% of males between 65 and 74, and 6.6% of females between 65 and 74 are afflicted with this debilitating disease.[1] Varus or valgus malalignment of an extremity may predispose a person to degenerative joint disease, or malalignment may be the sequela of asymmetric joint wear. Treatment options for individuals with osteoarthritis of the knee include medical management, debridement (either arthroscopic or open), osteotomy, unicompartmental knee arthroplasty, and total knee arthroplasty.

Medical management consists of oral medication, injection therapy, assistive devices, weight loss, physical therapy, and activity modification. Although the benefits of these interventions have been well documented,[2] the current state of nonsurgical therapy for osteoarthritis involves symptomatic treatment only. No modality yet exists for the medical prevention or reversal of osteoarthritis, and the treatments that are currently available typically have a finite usefulness and are associated with significant costs.[3]

While open debridement is rarely performed today, there has been a growing interest in arthroscopic debridement for the treatment of osteoarthritis of the knee, largely because of the relative ease of the procedure and the short surgical recovery required. The variable results of arthroscopic debridement may relate to technique and also to the preoperative condition of the degenerative knee.[4] Merchan and Galindo[5] found that 75% of their patients improved with arthroscopic treatment, compared to only 16% who had not undergone arthroscopy. The average age of their patients was 56 years. Rand,[6] however, reported only 39% improvement at 3.8 years, and 57% of his patients had undergone total joint arthroplasty by 3 years.

The success of knee replacement surgery in the treatment of osteoarthritis of the knee has been well documented in the literature.[7-11] Outcomes following unicompartmental knee replacement surgery vary widely, and its role remains controversial.[12] Many surgeons prefer unicompartmental arthroplasty for elderly patients with unicompartmental disease because of reported excellent initial results and ease of recovery, and because it has fewer complications than high tibial osteotomy.[13]

Total knee arthroplasty has become the major surgical treatment for osteoarthritis of the knee in the United States. Two hundred and fifty thousand knee replacements are performed annually,[14] with cost estimates as high as $10 billion.[15] With 10- to 15-year survival rates of 95% quoted in the literature, it is difficult to argue against the success of the procedure itself.[9] Complications do exist, however.[16] Perhaps the single greatest concern, as the lower age limit for arthroplasty continues to drop, is that of longevity. Recent reports indicate that long-term results of total knee arthroplasty in younger individuals may differ from those obtained with an older, less active population.[17-19] The potential for mechanical failure, in conjunction with a changing economic climate, may contribute to a renewed interest in osteotomy as a treatment for osteoarthritis, especially in the younger, more active patient. Furthermore, autogenous cartilage transplant may lead to a new indication for osteotomy: biologic resurfacing in conjunction with osteotomy to address any underlying deformity.

Pathophysiology of Osteoarthritis

As opposed to the inflammatory arthropathies, osteoarthritis is felt to be primarily a mechanical problem.[20] Tibial or femoral deformity, intra-articular defects, trauma, osteonecrosis, ligamentous laxity, and absence of menisci can all produce unfavorable mechanical situations that lead to the development of osteoarthritis.[21-24] Significant laboratory data suggest that malalignment plays a definite role in osteoarthritis.[23,25-27] Current theory is that malalignment, by placing abnormal stresses on articular cartilage, leads to biochemical alterations in the cartilage. These changes include increased water content, decreased proteoglycan content, and variation in the collagen network, ultimately resulting in degradation of the material properties of the articular cartilage.[28] It is not unreasonable, therefore, to believe that correction of malalignment can stop or slow this pathologic process. Osteotomy may also alleviate symptoms

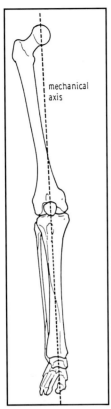

Fig. 1 The mechanical axis is a line that passes from the center of the hip to the center of the ankle.

by unloading the forces on the subchondral bone[29] and relieving intraosseous venous hypertension,[30] as well as by decreasing the stress on incipient microfractures in the subchondral bone.[31]

Normal Alignment

A knowledge of normal alignment is a prerequisite for understanding osteotomy surgery. The mechanical axis, a phrase frequently used when discussing alignment, is defined as a line passing from the center of the hip to the center of the ankle (Fig. 1).[32] Although it is generally believed that this line should pass through the center of the knee in the normal individual, several studies have shown this to be an approximation. Hsu and associates[33] showed the normal or average mechanical axis to be 1.2° of varus; Moreland and associates[34] found it

to be 1.3° of varus. This varus alignment results in about 60% of the load being transmitted through the medial compartment during weightbearing.[35] To us, these studies raise an issue of semantics. Is the slight varus normal, or does it simply represent averaging in a population disproportionately prone to varus rather than valgus gonarthrosis?

The distal femur is in approximately 3° of valgus relative to the mechanical axis, and the proximal tibia is in 3° of varus.[32] Because of this, the transverse axis of the knee lies at an angle of 3° from the perpendicular, which allows the knee joint to parallel the ground during gait.[32] The relationship of the femur to the tibia, the orientation of the joint line, and the location and type of deformity are all important considerations in osteotomy surgery.

History of Osteotomy of the Knee

According to Grelsamer,[23] reports of osteotomies can be found in the German literature of the nineteenth century. Most of the earliest reports in modern English literature are descriptions of proximal tibial valgus osteotomies for the treatment of osteoarthritis with varus deformity. In 1958, Jackson[36] wrote of proximal tibial osteotomy for the treatment of osteoarthritis. In 1961, Jackson and Waugh[37] described a domed tibial osteotomy performed distal to the tibial tuberosity for osteoarthritis. In 1962, Wardle[38] published his results of a tibial osteotomy done 10 cm distal to the tibial tuberosity for osteoarthritis with varus. Fourteen of 17 patients had good pain relief. Wardle stated that this surgery had been done in Liverpool since the time of Sir Robert Jones. Gariepy,[39] at the joint meeting of the Orthopaedic Associations in 1964, described a high tibial valgus osteotomy "done from the outer side after subperiosteal excision of the head of the fibula." He reported on 22 osteotomies in 13 patients with 1- to 7-

year follow-up. He described two delayed unions but otherwise good results. Coventry's[40] classic description of the modern closing wedge osteotomy appeared in the *Journal of Bone and Joint Surgery* in July 1965. Since then, several large series have reported good to excellent 5-year results with proximal tibial valgus osteotomy.[31,41,42] Coventry has reported a 60% success rate at 10 years and, more recently, Yasuda and associates[43] found 88% of 56 knees satisfactory at 6 years and 63% satisfactory at 10 to 15 years. Bouharras and associates[44] noted 74% good and excellent 5-year results and 64% good and excellent 10-year results. Of 193 tibial osteotomies reported by Lootvoet and associates,[45] 71% were good results at an average follow-up of 8 years.

The role of osteotomy has since expanded to include proximal tibial varus osteotomy[46–48] as well as distal femoral varus osteotomy for the treatment of lateral osteoarthritis with valgus deformity. Distal femoral valgus osteotomy is seldom used to treat medial compartment osteoarthritis.

Indications for Surgery

In the 1960s, with surgical treatment options for arthritis limited, osteotomy was indicated for all types of arthritic joint conditions.[49] As medium and long-term results of osteotomy began to appear in the literature along with the development of total knee arthroplasty, the indications and contraindications for osteotomy have gradually been defined. The following list has been compiled from the literature and is widely, although perhaps not universally, accepted.[23,31,49–52]

Age Although many authors quote 65 years of age as being the upper limit for osteotomy consideration, no single numeric value can be given. A better term might be "long life expectancy."[50] This indication may continue to change as the longevity of knee arthroplasty increases. The increasing life-expectancy of patients must also be considered.

Weight Although obesity may be associated with poor long-term survivorship following knee replacement[19,53] and thus may be perceived as an indication for osteotomy, patients of normal weight are more suitable candidates for osteotomy than obese patients.[23,31] In fact, Coventry[31] recommended treatment of obesity to be a prerequisite for osteotomy surgery. Similarly, at least two recent studies[54,55] show no correlation between results of total knee replacement and patient weight at 7 and 10 years, respectively.

Range of Motion Most authors consider range of motion to be an important factor, but, again, exact numbers are variable. Bochner[49] states 90° of flexion and less than 15° of flexion contracture are necessary preoperatively. Grelsamer[23] quotes a 100° arc of motion as ideal and Krackow[50] describes "severely diminished range of motion in conjunction with significant flexion contracture" as being a "negative with respect to the osteotomy option."

Activity Level In general, a patient's desire to return to an activity that would be prohibited following knee replacement would incline a surgeon toward osteotomy consideration if other necessary conditions were in order.[50]

Type of Disease Osteotomy is best reserved for osteoarthritis or posttraumatic arthritis or for the correction of deformity prior to the development of degenerative changes within the joint. Inflammatory arthritis is generally a contraindication.[31,41] Although early, unicompartmental arthritis may present an ideal situation for osteotomy,[49] complete loss of articular cartilage, patellar osteophytes, and tricompartmental disease with primarily unicompartmental involvement are not absolute contraindications to the surgery.[50] For patients with severe patellofemoral arthritis, Maquet[56] described a barrel-vault osteotomy, which allowed elevation of the tibial tubercle in conjunction with valgus correction. In 1981, Bourguignon[57] reported on two patients treated with combined high tibial valgus osteotomy and a true Maquet tibial tubercle elevation. One patient had an excellent result, the other only a fair result. Since then, both Insall[58] and Hofman and associates[59] have reported larger series with poor results and high complication rates. The combined procedure is probably best reserved for extremely unusual cases, and may be questionable even for these cases.

Instability Although instability must be appreciated preoperatively in the context of planning, it should not be considered an absolute contraindication to surgery. Coventry[31] stated that all knees with moderate loss of cartilage medially or laterally have some medial/lateral laxity. The ligament on the concave side becomes relatively lax and the convex ligament may be stretched. Medial instability can be corrected by opening wedge osteotomy,[60] combined medial opening/lateral closing wedge osteotomy,[50] or ligament advancement.[61]

Coventry[31] felt that instability secondary to anterior cruciate ligament (ACL) disruption was rare in osteoarthritis patients. Along with the increasing awareness of the arthritic knee with ACL deficiency has come experience with combined osteotomy and ligament reconstructions. The senior author (KAK) has historically used an extra-articular ACL reconstruction in combination with osteotomy for knees with significant pivot shift.[50,62]

Recently, Neuschwander and associates,[63] Noyes and associates,[64] and O'Neill and James[65] have reported good short- to medium-term results with combined intra-articular ACL reconstruction and high tibial osteotomy. Both Noyes and associates[64] and Miller and Fu[66] stress, however, that these are salvage procedures, that they are not designed to return an athlete to sports, and that the long-term results remain unknown. One rare cause of instability, an intra-articular osseous defect, may respond to intra-articular osteotomy.[35]

Patient Assessment

A thorough history and physical examination should be performed on every patient. The previously mentioned factors: age, weight, range of motion, activity level, type of arthritis, and presence of instability must all be considered. Any medical issues that impact on the patient's life expectancy should be noted, as decreased life expectancy will tend to favor arthroplasty. Weightbearing, 3-ft standing radiographs should be obtained on all patients to assess the degree of deformity in the anteroposterior (AP) plane. AP, lateral, and Merchant patellar views should be obtained in order to assess details of the articular surface, to detect the presence of patellofemoral disease, to visualize loose bodies, and to look for evidence of crystalline disease. An appreciation of any flexion, extension, or rotational deformities should also be made, because any of these can affect the apparent varus/valgus on the 3-ft radiograph.[23,67] Varus and valgus stress views are also recommended by some authors.[68]

Examination of the patient's gait is also important. While 3-ft standing radiographs can give an estimate of directions of forces through the knee, these forces can change significantly during gait. During gait, the ground reaction force is directed medial to the mechanical axis toward the umbilicus, resulting in a varus moment at the knee.[23] This increased varus moment is exhibited as a varus thrust on examination and may not be completely eliminated by a valgus osteotomy.[69,70]

Recent literature has offered some criticisms of the traditional static planning for osteotomy. Andriacchi[71] has published on the dynamics of knee realignment as have Tetsworth and

Paley.[26] Chao and Sim[72] used a computer program to aid in preoperative planning. Shaw and Moulton[73] were openly critical of tibial osteotomy, stating that "its biomechanical basis is fundamentally flawed." Although static planning may not be ideal, detractors have not provided any proven or practical alternatives nor have they come up with an overall better planning arrangement or a generally different set of planning targets.

Heel wedges and, more recently, unloader braces have been used to try preoperatively to predict the success of osteotomy. We have had success using the previously published technique of offset casting.[74] This technique has proven to be simpler and much more cost effective than custom bracing and also eliminates the variable of hindfoot motion, which is present when using heel wedges.

We offer specific warning with regard to two subgroups of patients when considering an osteotomy. These are patients receiving worker's compensation and patients with minimal varus who have already undergone a partial or complete medial meniscectomy. Both of these sets of patients have, in our hands, had less satisfactory results with osteotomy and with total knee replacement. That is not to say that the procedure cannot be done on these patients, but only that the surgeon and patient both must be aware of the reality of the situation when planning further treatment.

Specific Types of Osteotomy

Valgus proximal tibial osteotomy for primarily unicompartmental arthritis with varus deformity is the most common osteotomy performed for arthritis. The classic closing lateral wedge osteotomy described by Coventry[40] remains the most popular method used in this country.[75] The technique is relatively simple, and it has a high rate of healing due to the large surface area of cancellous bone.[76] The tibial tuberosity can be dis-

placed anteriorly if there is associated patellofemoral arthrosis.[59,76] Also, the osteotomy is performed close to the joint near the origin of the deformity in most instances. Potential disadvantages include shortening of the leg and lateral collateral laxity,[61] as well as infrapatellar scarring and patella baja,[77] increased q-angle,[75] limited correction,[76] and predisposition to fracture because of the size of the proximal fragment.[78]

A closing wedge can also lead to offset, which can affect future total knee replacement, especially if a tibial stem was needed. This problem can be avoided by shifting the fragments (shaft lateral), although this will certainly lessen the inherent stability of having an intact medial side. The location of the osteotomy relative to the joint can be a key factor. Closer osteotomies allow for larger correction, a broader surface for healing, and less offset, but they can lead to an avascular segment proximally, and also can make a fracture into the joint more likely. The farther away from the joint the osteotomy is made, the greater the offset. Healing may be slower, and the fragment may begin to involve the tibial tubercle. Less likely problems include injury to the anterior tibial artery and possibly anterior compartment syndrome. Cosmesis may also be of concern to some patients. The issue of cosmesis is a more common problem with valgus osteotomies than with varus osteotomies, and patients should be forewarned. In particular, infrapatellar scarring and patella baja may make exposure more difficult during future total knee replacement.[77] The size of the proximal fragment may also limit fixation options and make treatment of nonunions difficult.[76,78] Nonunions themselves are relatively rare. Myrnerts[79] had an incidence of 1.3%. Bauer and associates[80] stated 1.5%. Tjornstrand and associates[81] quoted 3.6%.

The medial opening wedge osteotomy with iliac crest bone grafting has been described.[60] This technique can be used

to tighten the medial collateral ligament (MCL).[60,61] Potential disadvantages include lengthening of the leg, displacement of the patella distally, and possible nonunion,[23] as well as typical bone graft donor site morbidity. A combined medial opening and lateral closing wedge osteotomy may provide the advantage of tightening the MCL and also eliminates the risk of bone graft donor site morbidity.[50] The thickness of the wedge needed for a given angle of correction is also one half of that needed with a standard closing wedge osteotomy.[23]

Various other forms of osteotomy have also been described. Jakob and Murphy[68] recommend an osteotomy behind the tibial tubercle, which they believe offers high rates of healing, allows for greater angular correction, and avoids the infrapatellar fat pad scarring associated with exposure problems during subsequent total knee replacement. Nakhostine and associates[82] described an oblique proximal tibial osteotomy, which preserves the medial cortex and iliotibial band insertion and allows for early weightbearing.

Dome-shaped osteotomies have been performed both proximal[83,84] and distal to the tibial tuberosity.[76] The reported advantages include accuracy, adjustability, and stability.[76,85] Also, no bone is resected, and these osteotomies permit anterior/posterior translation. The proximal type may lead to medial translation of the distal fragment, however, and neither type allows for torsional corrections.[76] Any osteotomy performed distal to the tubercle has disadvantages, including the possibility of creating a secondary angular deformity due to the location of the osteotomy away from the primary site of angular deformity,[76] as well as a slower rate of healing than occurs with an osteotomy through the more proximal, cancellous bone.[75] Because of the asymmetric shape of the tibia, accurate dome osteotomies usually require some type of jig or curved saws. Any dome osteotomy performed above the MCL insertion may have limited correction potential due to tightening of the ligament.

Methods of fixation of proximal tibial osteotomies include casts,[80] staples,[40] and plates and screws,[75] as well as external fixation.[86] Any type of fixation ultimately relies to a large degree on the quality of bone. In deformity, the concave-side bone sees more stress and is, therefore, more dense. The convex-side bone is less dense and often surprisingly soft intraoperatively. Casts allow for some fine tuning of correction, but require frequent follow-up, are cumbersome, and promote short-term stiffness, which may prolong rehabilitation. The cast alone must be viewed as less predictable. The potential for overcorrection in a cast exists if the patient starts with 3° to 5° of overcorrection and the already soft lateral bone implodes further. Casts are rarely used today as a sole source of fixation. Laterally placed staples provide adequate fixation if the medial stability remains intact, but this form of fixation may require supplementation with either bracing or casting. Plate fixation provides stability but generally requires more exposure of soft-tissues at the time of surgery. Blade plates are inherently more stable than T and L plates but are more difficult to place. T and L plates have both buttress and antidistraction properties, but they do not prevent far-side movement in the absence of bone and soft-tissue stability. There is growing interest in the use of external fixation for deformity correction.[86] Unilateral[87] and ring[88] fixators are most frequently employed within this group. External fixators allow gradual, precise adjustment of correction.[70] Major drawbacks of external fixators include inconvenience, pin care requirements, and the risk of pin tract infection near the site of a possible future total knee replacement.[70]

Our first choice for fixation is staples, although we occasionally choose a blade plate for larger individuals. Coventry[89] described use of a stepped staple for tibial osteotomy in 1969. In the German literature in 1978, Ebel[90] reported good results in 54 osteotomies using a single staple and stated that "internal fixation by plates or other devices is superfluous." He felt that the broad contact area of cancellous metaphyseal bone, along with one staple, provided enough stability for motion and weightbearing. Wildner and associates[91] reported a method-related complication rate of 1.1% and concluded that staples were reliable and safe. In a retrospective study of 223 high tibial osteotomies, Hsu and associates[33] concluded that buttress plating afforded no advantage over staple fixation. Knee scores were not statistically different. The staple group had shorter hospital stays but longer overall rehabilitation times.[92] The infection rate was higher in the group treated with buttress plates (9.3% compared to 0.8%). Buttress plates did not change the risk of nonunion or the recurrence of varus deformity.

We have found that two or three lateral Coventry staples provide adequate fixation. An additional anteromedial staple can be placed through a separate small incision if medial stability is in question. Compression can be obtained using staples according to the senior author's previously published technique.[93] Following surgery we keep patients in a Jones dressing and knee immobilizer, allowing toe-touch weightbearing, for 2 weeks. At that point, the immobilizer is removed three times daily by the patient and gentle active range of motion is begun. Patients are seen every 2 weeks and radiographs are taken. When radiographic evidence of healing can be seen, we advance the patients to weightbearing and wean them from crutches. Use of the immobilizer can also be discontinued when radiographic healing is apparent. Most patients require no formal physical therapy.

To allow for unrestricted correction of tibial deformity, the fibula must be untethered. Fibular management can be accomplished in several ways. Fibular osteotomy can be performed either through the fibular shaft[94] or, more proximally, in the region of the fibular head and neck.[23] Osteotomy of the shaft can be performed in the proximal, middle, or distal third of the fibula.[76] Each region has its own risks relative to injury to the peroneal nerve and its branches.[23,76,94,95] An especially high risk of injury to the branch of the peroneal nerve to the extensor hallucis longus between 7 and 15 cm distal to the head of the fibula has been noted by Kirgis and Albrecht.[94] The proximal osteotomy can provide an opportunity to tighten a lax lateral collateral ligament by advancing its insertion. Care must be taken to avoid the peroneal nerve in the region of the fibular neck.[76,96] Resecting the fibular head[40] and dividing the proximal tibia-fibular joint are two other techniques used to free the tibia for correction, but these procedures can be associated with lateral collateral laxity.[76]

The senior author's preference for fibular management is to extend the wedge-shaped osteotomy laterally through the fibula. This step removes a trapezoidal piece of fibular head and allows the LCL attachment to remain intact. With this technique, we have not found fixation to be necessary and have not noted lateral instability.

Reports vary regarding the degree of correction needed to obtain satisfactory results. Hernigou and associates[60] stated that 3° to 6° of valgus mechanical axis deviation correlated with successful outcome. Tjornstrand and associates[97] believed that deviation of 4° was necessary, and 5° has been proposed by Aglietti and associates.[98] Up to 8° has been reported to be acceptable by Torgerson and associates[99] and by Vainionpaa and associates.[96] Miniaci and associates[100] recommend an osteotomy that places the new mechanical axis through the middle third of the lateral compartment of the knee, and they have described a technique to determine the desired angle of correction based on the preoperative radiographs. Bauer and associates[80] estimated that 1 mm of resected bone equaled approximately 1° of correction, and many surgeons have followed this general guideline. We attempt to overcorrect to approximately 2° to 4° of valgus mechanical axis deviation. For example, a patient with 10° of mechanical axis varus would have a 12° to 14° closing wedge osteotomy. Both overcorrection and undercorrection have been associated with poorer results.[101]

Proximal Tibial Varus Osteotomy

Results of proximal tibial varus osteotomy have not equaled those of proximal tibial valgus osteotomy.[47,102] The natural valgus tibiofemoral orientation has led many authors to conclude that 12° to 15° of valgus deformity is the upper limit for consideration of a varus proximal tibial osteotomy.[46,103,104] Exceeding 12° to 15° of valgus correction or 10° of resultant joint line obliquity tends to result in lateral subluxation of the tibia and may contribute to poor results.[83,104,105] MCL laxity can also occur if a wedge is removed from the proximal tibia above the MCL insertion. MCL advancement on the tibial side can address this problem. However, proximal tibial varus osteotomy still has a role in the valgus, osteoarthritic knee.[103] Small degrees of deformity (ie, less than 12°) and specific situations, such as malunion of a proximal tibial fracture when the deformity is primarily below the level of the knee joint, can be indications for proximal tibial varus osteotomy.

Distal Femoral Varus Osteotomy

The limitations of proximal tibial varus osteotomy have led several authors to recommend distal femoral varus

osteotomy as the treatment of choice for the painful valgus knee. Healy and associates[47] reported 93% good or excellent results at an average follow-up of 4 years in 15 knees with osteoarthritis treated with distal femoral varus osteotomy. McDermott and associates[48] had 92% successful results at 4 years. Less successful results have been published by Johnson and Bodell[106] and Conrad and associates.[107]

Here, too, the desired degree of correction is variable, although it is more uniform than with proximal tibial valgus osteotomy. Several authors recommend correcting the valgus knee to a 0° tibiofemoral angle.[48,108] Morrey and Edgerton[108] also describe as a goal having the mechanical axis medial to the midportion of the medial plateau. The senior author (KAK) has typically aimed for approximately 4° of mechanical axis varus. This alignment seems to be well tolerated both clinically and cosmetically. In fact, the issue of cosmesis has only been a positive factor with distal femoral osteotomy in our experience. It has led us to the observation that small amounts of varus deformity are acceptable to patients, generally going unnoticed by them. Small amounts of valgus deformity, on the other hand, are usually readily apparent to even the untrained eye, and are cosmetically less acceptable to patients.

The distal femoral osteotomy is usually a medial closing wedge, although it can be performed through a lateral approach as well. We prefer a medial, subvastus-type exposure through our typical anterior total knee incision, which we move just slightly medial. This technique avoids the problem of skin bridges, should subsequent total knee replacement be necessary.

Distal femoral varus osteotomies have traditionally been fixed with angle blade plates.[105] We use a 90° blade plate placed medially. As with proximal tibial valgus osteotomy, some reports describe good

results using external fixation.[109] With the exception of peroneal nerve injury, which has not been a reported problem, complications at the femur are essentially the same as for proximal tibial osteotomy: delayed or nonunion, infection, and under- and overcorrection are the main concerns. Although the numbers are small, conversion to total knee replacement has been successful following satisfactory distal femoral osteotomy.[47,48,108]

Conclusion

Both high tibial and distal femoral osteotomy are useful procedures for varus and valgus deformity around the knee, most frequently in association with unicompartmental arthritis. Immediate to long-term results, concerns regarding durability of metal and plastic implants, and the promise of biologic resurfacing indicate that there is, and will continue to be, a role for osteotomy in the treatment of knee pathology.

References
1. Heck DA: Evaluation of the patient with an arthritic knee: History, examination, structured assessment, and radiologic evaluation, in Callaghan JJ, Dennis DA, Paprosky WG, et al (eds): *Orthopaedic Knowledge Update: Hip and Knee Reconstruction*. Rosemont, IL, American Academy of Orthopaedic Surgeons, 1995, pp 241–244.
2. Oddis CV: New perspectives on osteoarthritis. *Am J Med* 1996;100:10S–15S.
3. Gabriel SE, Crowson CS, O'Fallon WM: Costs of osteoarthritis: Estimates from a geographically defined population. *J Rheumatol* 1995;43(suppl):23–25.
4. Novak PJ, Bach BR Jr: Selection criteria for knee arthroscopy in the osteoarthritic patient. *Orthop Rev* 1993;22:798–804.
5. Merchan EC, Galindo E: Arthroscope-guided surgery versus nonoperative treatment for limited degenerative osteoarthritis of the femorotibial joint in patients over 50 years of age: A prospective comparative study. *Arthroscopy* 1993;9:663–667.
6. Rand JA: Role of arthroscopy in osteoarthritis of the knee. *Arthroscopy* 1991;7:358–363.
7. Ranawat CS, Flynn WF Jr, Deshmukh RG: Impact of modern technique on long-term results of total condylar knee arthroplasty. *Clin Orthop* 1994;309:131–135.
8. Rand JA: Comparison of metal-backed and all-polyethylene tibial components in cruciate

condylar total knee arthroplasty. *J Arthroplasty* 1993;8:307–313.

9. Scuderi GR, Insall JN, Windsor RE, et al: Survivorship of cemented knee replacement. *J Bone Joint Surg* 1989;71B:798–803.

10. Vince KG, Insall JN, Kelly MA: The total condylar prosthesis: 10- to 12-year results of a cemented knee replacement. *J Bone Joint Surg* 1989;71B:793–797.

11. Whiteside LA: Cementless total knee replacement: Nine- to 11-year results and 10-year survivorship anaysis. *Clin Orthop* 1994;309:185–192.

12. Scott RD, Chmell MJ: Unicompartmental total knee arthroplasty, in Callaghan JJ, Dennis DA, Paprosky WG, et al (eds): *Orthopaedic Knowledge Update: Hip and Knee Replacement.* Rosemont, IL, American Academy of Orthopaedic Surgeons, 1995, pp 251–254.

13. Broughton NS, Newman JH, Baily RA: Unicompartmental replacement and high tibial osteotomy for osteoarthritis of the knee: A comparative study after 5-10 years' follow-up. *J Bone Joint Surg* 1986;68B:447–452.

14. Silverton CD, Rosenberg AG: Long-term results in total knee arthroplasty, in Callaghan JJ, Dennis DA, Paprosky WG, et al (eds): *Orthopaedic Knowledge Update: Hip and Knee Reconstruction.* Rosemont, IL, American Academy of Orthopaedic Surgeons, 1995, pp 303–316.

15. Lavernia CJ. Drakeford MK, Tsao AK, et al: Revision and primary hip and knee arthroplasty: A cost analysis. *Clin Orthop* 1995;311:136–141.

16. Huo MH, Sculco TP: Complications in primary total knee arthroplasty. *Orthop Rev* 1990;19:781–788.

17. Cadambi A, Engh GA, Dwyer KA, et al: Osteolysis of the distal femur after total knee arthroplasty. *J Arthroplasty* 1994;9:579–594.

18. Robinson EJ, Mulliken BD, Bourne RB, et al: Catastrophic osteolysis in total knee replacement: A report of 17 cases. *Clin Orthop* 1995;321:98–105.

19. Tsao A, Mintz L, McRae CR, et al: Failure of the porous-coated anatomic prosthesis in total knee arthroplasty due to severe polyethylene wear. *J Bone Joint Surg* 1993;75A:19–26.

20. Radin EL, Burr DB, Caterson B, et al: Mechanical determnants of osteoarthrosis. *Semin Arthritis Rheum* 1991;21(suppl 2):12–21.

21. Allen PR, Denham RA, Swan AV: Late degenerative changes after meniscectomy: Factors affecting the knee after operation. *J Bone Joint Surg* 1984;66B:666–671.

22. Fairbank TJ: Knee joint changes after meniscectomy. *J Bone Joint Surg* 1948;30B:664–670.

23. Grelsamer RP: Unicompartmental osteoarthritis of the knee. *J Bone Joint Surg* 1995;77A:278–292.

24. King D: The function of semilunar cartilages. *J Bone Joint Surg* 1936;18:1069–1076.

25. Reimann I: Experimental osteoarthritis of the knee in rabbits induced by alteration of the load-bearing. *Acta Orthop Scand* 1973;44:496–504.

26. Tetsworth K, Paley D: Malalignment and degenerative arthropathy. *Orthop Clin North Am* 1994;25:367–377.

27. Wu DD, Burr DB, Boyd RD, et al: Bone and cartilage changes following experimental varus or valgus tibial angulation. *J Orthop Res* 1990;8:572–585.

28. Mankin HJ, Mow VC, Buckwalter JA, et al: Form and function of articular cartilage, in Simon SR (ed): *Orthopaedic Basic Science.* Rosemont, IL, American Academy of Orthopaedic Surgeons, 1994, pp 1–44.

29. Harris WR, Kostuik JP: High tibial osteotomy for osteo-arthritis of the knee. *J Bone Joint Surg* 1970;52A:330–336.

30. Arnoldi CC, Lemperg K, Linderholm H: Intraosseous hypertension and pain in the knee. *J Bone Joint Surg* 1975;57B:360–363.

31. Coventry MB: Osteotomy above the knee for degenerative and rheumatoid arthritis: Indications, operative technique, and results. *J Bone Joint Surg* 1973;55A:23–48.

32. Krackow KA: Approaches to planning lower extremity alignment for total knee arthroplasty and osteotomy about the knee. *Adv Orthop Surg* 1983;7:69–88.

33. Hsu RW, Himeno S, Coventry MB, et al: Normal axial alignment of the lower extremity and load-bearing distribution at the knee. *Clin Orthop* 1990;255:215–227.

34. Moreland JR, Bassett LW, Hanker GJ: Radiographic analysis of the axial alignment of the lower extremity. *J Bone Joint Surg* 1987;69A:745–749.

35. Kleining R, Hax PM: Intraligamentous elevating osteotomies for posttraumatic deformities about the knee, in Hierholzer G, Müller KH (eds): *Corrective Osteotomies of the Lower Extremity After Trauma.* Berlin, Germany, Springer-Verlag, 1985, pp 233–238.

36. Jackson JP: Abstract: Osteotomy for osteoarthritis of the knee. *J Bone Joint Surg* 1958;40B:826.

37. Jackson JP, Waugh W: Tibial osteotomy for osteoarthritis of the knee. *J Bone Joint Surg* 1961;43B:746–751.

38. Wardle EN: Osteotomy of the tibia and fibula. *Surg Gynecol Obstet* 1962;115:61–64.

39. Gariepy R: Abstract: Genu varum treated by high tibial osteotomy. *J Bone Joint Surg* 1964;46B:783–784.

40. Coventry MB: Osteotomy of the upper portion of the tibia for degenerative arthritis of the knee: A preliminary report. *J Bone Joint Surg* 1965;47A:984–990.

41. Insall JN, Joseph DM, Msika C: High tibial osteotomy for varus gonarthrosis: A long-term follow-up study. *J Bone Joint Surg* 1984;66A:1040–1048.

42. Healy WL, Riley LH Jr: High tibial valgus osteotomy: A clinical review. *Clin Orthop* 1986;209:227–233.

43. Yasuda K, Majima T, Tsuchida T, et al: A ten- to 15-year follow-up observation of high tibial osteotomy in medial compartment osteoarthrosis. *Clin Orthop* 1992;282:186–195.

44. Bouharras M, Hoet F, Watillon M, et al: Results of tibial valgus osteotomy for internal femoro-tibial arthritis with an average 8-year follow-up. *Acta Orthop Belg* 1994;60:163–169.

45. Lootvoet L, Massinon A, Rossillon R, et al: Upper tibial osteotomy for gonarthrosis in genu varum: Apropos of a series of 193 cases reviewed 6 to 10 years later. *Rev Chir Orthop Reparatrice Appar Mot* 1993;79:375–384.

46. Coventry MB: Upper tibial osteotomy for osteoarthritis. *J Bone Joint Surg* 1985;67A:1136–1140.

47. Healy WL, Anglen JO, Wasilewski SA, et al: Distal femoral varus osteotomy. *J Bone Joint Surg* 1988;70A:102–109.

48. McDermott AG, Finklestein JA, Farine I, et al: Distal femoral varus osteotomy for valgus deformity of the knee. *J Bone Joint Surg* 1988;70A:110–116.

49. Bochner R: Indications and alternatives to total knee replacement, in Laskin RS (ed): *Total Knee Replacement.* London, England, Springer-Verlag, 1991, pp 17–24.

50. Krackow KA (ed): *The Technique of Total Knee Arthroplasty.* St. Louis, MO, CV Mosby, 1990.

51. Brueckmann FR, Kettelkamp DB: Proximal tibial osteotomy. *Orthop Clin North Am* 1982;13:3–16.

52. Coventry MB, Ilstrup DM, Wallrichs SL: Proximal tibial osteotomy: A critical long-term study of eighty-seven cases. *J Bone Joint Surg* 1993;75A:196–201.

53. Ranawat CS, Flynn WF Jr, Saddler S, et al: Long-term results of the total condylar knee arthroplasty: A 15-year survivorship study. *Clin Orthop* 1993;286:94–102.

54. Mont MA, Mathur SK, Krackow KA, et al: Cementless total knee arthroplasty in obese patients: A comparison with a matched control group. *J Arthroplasty* 1996;11:153–156.

55. Partio E, Orava T, Lehto MU, et al: Survival of the Townley knee: 360 cases with 8 (0.1-15) years' follow-up. *Acta Orthop Scand* 1994;65:319–322.

56. Maquet P: Valgus osteotomy for osteoarthritis of the knee. *Clin Orthop* 1976;120:143–148.

57. Bourguignon RL: Combined Coventry-Maquet tibial osteotomy: Preliminary report of two cases. *Clin Orthop* 1981;160:144–148.

58. Insall JN: Patella pain syndromes and chondromalacia patellae, in Murray DG (ed): *American Academy of Orthopaedic Surgeons Instructional Course Lectures XXX.* St. Louis, MO, CV Mosby, 1981, pp 342–356.

59. Hofman AA, Wyatt RW, Jones RE: Combined Coventry-Maquet procedure for two-compartment degenerative arthritis. *Clin Orthop* 1984;190:186–191.

60. Hernigou P, Medevielle D, Debeyre J, et al: Proximal tibial osteotomy for osteoarthritis with varus deformity: A ten to thirteen-year follow-up study. *J Bone Joint Surg* 1987;69A:332–354.

61. Paley D, Bhatnagar J, Herzenberg JE, et al: New procedures for tightening knee collateral ligaments in conjunction with knee realignment osteotomy. *Orthop Clin North Am* 1994;25:533–555.

62. Krackow KA, Brooks RL: Optimization of knee ligament position for lateral extraarticular reconstruction. *Am J Sports Med* 1983;11:293–302.

63. Neuschwander DC, Drez D Jr, Paine RM: Simultaneous high tibial osteotomy and ACL reconstruction for combined genu varum and symptomatic ACL tear. *Orthopedics* 1993;16:679–684.

64. Noyes FR, Barber SD, Simon R: High tibial osteotomy and ligament reconstruction in varus angulated, anterior cruciate ligament-deficient knees: A two- to seven-year follow-up study. *Am J Sports Med* 1993;21:2–12.

65. O'Neill DF, James SL: Valgus osteotomy with anterior cruciate ligament laxity. *Clin Orthop* 1992;278:153–159.

66. Miller MD, Fu FH: The role of osteotomy in the anterior cruciate ligament-deficient knee. *Clin Sports Med* 1993;12:697–708.

67. Krackow KA, Pepe CL, Galloway EJ: A mathematical analysis of the effect of flexion and rotation on apparent varus/valgus alignment at the knee. *Orthopedics* 1990;13:861–868.

68. Jakob RP, Murphy SB: Tibial osteotomy for varus gonarthrosis: Indication, planning, and operative technique, in Eilert RE (ed): *Instructional Course Lectures XLI*. Park Ridge, IL, American Academy of Orthopaedic Surgeons, 1992, pp 87–93.

69. Harrington IJ: Static and dynamic loading patterns in knee joints with deformities. *J Bone Joint Surg* 1983;65A:247–259.

70. Johnson F, Leitl S, Waugh W: The distribution of load across the knee: A comparison of static and dynamic measurement. *J Bone Joint Surg* 1980;62B:346–349.

71. Andriacchi TP: Dynamics of knee malalignment. *Orthop Clin North Am* 1994;25:395–403.

72. Chao EY, Sim FH: Computer-aided preoperative planning in knee osteotomy. *Iowa Orthop J* 1995;15:4–18.

73. Shaw JA, Moulton MJ: High tibial osteotomy: An operation based on a spurious mechanical concept. A theoretic treatise. *Am J Orthop* 1996;25:429–436.

74. Krackow KA, Galloway EJ: A apreoperative technique for predicting success after varus or valgus osteotomy at the knee. *Am J Knee Surg* 1989;2:164–170.

75. Murphy SB: Tibial osteotomy for genu varum: Indications, preoperative planning, and technique. *Orthop Clin North Am* 1994;25:477–482.

76. Paley D, Maar DC, Herzenberg JE: New concepts in high tibial osteotomy for medial compartment osteoarthritis. *Orthop Clin North Am* 1994;25:483–498.

77. Katz MM, Hungerford DS, Krackow KA, et al: Results of total knee arthroplasty after failed proximal tibial osteotomy for osteoarthritis. *J Bone Joint Surg* 1987;69A:225–233.

78. Schatzker J, Burgess RC, Glynn MK: The management of nonunions following high tibial osteotomies. *Clin Orthop* 1985;193:230–233.

79. Myrnerts R: High tibial osteotomy with over-correction of varus malalignment in medial gonarthrosis. *Acta Orthop Scand* 1980;51:557–560.

80. Bauer GC, Insall J, Koshino T: Tibial osteotomy in gonarthrosis (osteo-arthritis of the knee). *J Bone Joint Surg* 1969;51:1545–1563.

81. Tjornstrand B, Hagstedt B, Persson BM: Results of surgical treatment for non-union after high tibial osteotomy in osteoarthritis of the knee. *J Bone Joint Surg* 1978;60A:973–977.

82. Nakhostine M, Friedrich NF, Muller W, et al: A special high tibial osteotomy technique for treatment of unicompartmental osteoarthritis of the knee. *Orthopedics* 1993;16:1255–1258.

83. Maquet PGJ (ed): *Biomechanics of the Knee: With Application to the Pathogenesis and the Surgical Treatment of Osteoarthritis*, ed 2. New York, NY, Springer-Verlag, 1984.

84. Sundaram NA, Hallett JP, Sullivan MF: Dome osteotomy of the tibia for osteoarthritis of the knee. *J Bone Joint Surg* 1986;68B:782–786.

85. Kettelkamp DB, Leach RE, Nasca R: Pitfalls of proximal tibial osteotomy. *Clin Orthop* 1975;106:232–241.

86. Grill F: Correction of complicated extremity deformities by external fixation. *Clin Orthop* 1989;241:166–176.

87. Price CT: Unilateral fixators and mechanical axis realignment. *Orthop Clin North Am* 1994;25:499–508.

88. Catagni MA, Guerreschi F, Ahmad TS, et al: Treatment of genu varum in medial compartment osteoarthritis of the knee using the Ilizarov method. *Orthop Clin North Am* 1994;25:509–514.

89. Coventry MB: Stepped staple for upper tibial osteotomy. *J Bone Joint Surg* 1969;51A:1011.

90. Ebel R: High tibial osteotomy for gonarthrosis. *Z Orthop* 1978;116:716–724.

91. Wildner M, Peters A, Hellich J, et al: Complications of high tibial osteotomy and internal fixation with staples. *Arch Orthop Trauma Surg* 1992;111:210–212.

92. Hee HT, Low CK, Seow KH, et al: Comparing staple fixation to buttress plate fixation in high tibial osteotomy. *Ann Acad Med Singapore* 1996;25:233–235.

93. Krackow KA, Mecherikunnel P: Influence of bone staple design on interfragmentary compression. *Orthopedics* 1991;14:751–755.

94. Kirgis A, Albrecht S: Palsy of the deep peroneal nerve after proximal tibial osteotomy: An anatomical study. *J Bone Joint Surg* 1992;74A:1180–1185.

95. Soejima O, Ogata K, Ishinishi T, et al: Anatomic considerations of the peroneal nerve for division of the fibula during high tibial osteotomy. *Orthop Rev* 1994;23:244–247.

96. Vainionpaa S, Laike E, Kirves P, et al: Tibial osteotomy for osteoarthritis of the knee: A five to ten-year follow-up study. *J Bone Joint Surg* 1981;63A:938–946.

97. Tjornstrand BA, Egund N, Hagstedt BV: High tibial osteotomy: A seven-year clinical and radiographic follow-up. *Clin Orthop* 1981;160:124–136.

98. Aglietti P, Rinonapoli E, Stringa G, et al: Tibial osteotomy for the varus osteoarthritic knee. *Clin Orthop* 1983;176:239–251.

99. Torgerson WR Jr, Kettelkamp DB, Igou RA Jr, et al: Tibial osteotomy for the treatment of degenerative arthritis of the knee. *Clin Orthop* 1974;101:46–52.

100. Miniaci A, Ballmer FT, Ballmer PM, et al: Proximal tibial osteotomy: A new fixation device. *Clin Orthop* 1989;246:250–259.

101. Matthews LS, Goldstein SA, Malvitz TA, et al: Proximal tibial osteotomy: Factors that influence the duration of satisfactory function. *Clin Orthop* 1988;229:193–200.

102. Harding ML: A fresh appraisal of tibial osteotomy for osteoarthritis of the knee. *Clin Orthop* 1976;114:223–234.

103. Coventry MB: Proximal tibial varus osteotomy for osteoarthritis of the lateral compartment of the knee. *J Bone Joint Surg* 1987;69A:32–38.

104. Maquet P: The treatment of choice in osteoarthritis of the knee. *Clin Orthop* 1985;192:108–112.

105. Healy WL, Wasilewski SA, Krackow KA: Distal femoral varus osteotomy for the painful valgus knee. *Tech Orthop* 1989;4:47–52.

106. Johnson EW Jr, Bodell LS: Corrective supracondylar osteotomy for painful genu valgum. *Mayo Clin Proc* 1981;56:87–92.

107. Conrad EU, Soudry M, Insall JN: Supracondylar femoral osteotomy for valgus knee deformities. *Orthop Trans* 1985;9:25–26.

108. Morrey BF, Edgerton BC: Distal femoral osteotomy for lateral gonarthrosis, in Eilert E (ed): *Instructional Course Lectures XLI*. Rosemont, IL, American Academy of Orthopaedic Surgeons, 1992, pp 77–85.

109. Knapp DR Jr, Price CT: Correction of distal femoral deformity. *Clin Orthop* 1990;255:75–80.

Periprosthetic Fractures Adjacent to Total Knee Implants: Treatment and Clinical Results

Gerard A. Engh, MD
Deborah J. Ammeen, BS

The unique characteristics that predispose patients to periprosthetic fractures make treatment difficult and unpredictable. Severe osteoporosis makes fracture fixation precarious. The typical elderly and debilitated patient must be mobilized rapidly to avoid medical complications brought on by prolonged bed rest and inactivity. However, walking with protected weightbearing often is impossible because of multiple-joint involvement, neurologic disorders, and systemic illness.

In most instances, early and definitive treatment is preferable to a prolonged period of bed rest and inactivity. Periprosthetic fractures may occur intraoperatively or postoperatively. The best treatment technique depends on whether the fracture is identified intraoperatively or postoperatively as well as on its location and severity. Common fracture-repair techniques, such as those involving use of a plate and screws, intramedullary rods, and external fixators, have been associated with variable rates of success. This paper examines the role of different techniques for management of the fracture and revision of the component in the treatment of periprosthetic fractures.

Intraoperative Periprosthetic Fractures of the Femur, Tibia, and Patella

Periprosthetic fractures that occur during a knee-replacement arthroplasty are rarely as challenging to treat as fractures that occur in the postoperative period. Most intraoperative fractures are neither displaced nor comminuted, the stability of the components is rarely altered, and the fractures are not associated with soft-tissue trauma. Treatment techniques that permit the patient to exercise safely during the early postoperative period should lead to an optimum clinical outcome. Usually, screws are adequate for stabilizing the fracture, and the patient may safely proceed with an unaltered rehabilitation protocol.

Femoral Fractures

When a fracture that splits the condyles occurs while the surgeon is making the box cut for a posterior stabilized component (Fig. 1, *left*), a transcondylar cancellous bone screw can be used to stabilize the fracture. One screw usually is sufficient, because the cement and the femoral component provide additional

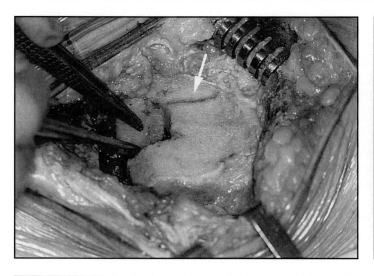

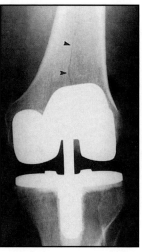

Fig. 1 Left, A condylar split fracture (arrow) that occurred while the box-shaped section was being prepared for insertion of a posterior stabilized implant. **Right,** Radiograph showing a condylar split fracture (arrowheads). The fracture typically is identified on a routine follow-up radiograph, and it heals uneventfully.

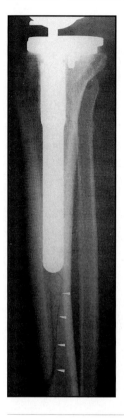

Fig. 2 Radiograph showing a fracture of the tibial shaft (arrowheads). The fracture was caused by impingement of the stem that was not recognized intraoperatively.

stability. If the metaphyseal bone is soft, a washer should be added. If the condyle is displaced or comminuted, the fracture is best treated with a long-stemmed femoral component that stabilizes the condyle to the diaphysis. A press-fit stem is optimum, but the stem can be inserted with cement as long as the cement is kept away from the fracture site.

A fracture of the anterior femoral cortex can occur when the cortex is perforated accidentally while the surgeon is inserting an intramedullary alignment rod. This fracture is a result of the rod perforating the anterior bow of the femur when the bone is severely osteoporotic. The perforation occurs in the transitional zone between cancellous metaphyseal and cortical diaphyseal bone in the suprapatellar region. If such a fracture occurs, a long-stemmed implant that bypasses the perforation should be used. If the fracture is identified initially on postoperative radiographs (Fig. 1, *right*) or if a long-stemmed component is not available at

the time of the operation, protected weightbearing is advisable for a minimum of 6 to 8 weeks.

Intraoperative fractures may occur during a revision of a previously inserted prosthesis when the surgeon is preparing bone that has been severely damaged by osteolysis or by migration of the component. It is important to anticipate such a complication and to select the appropriate component for the revision. The implant should provide stable fixation with a stem that bypasses the metaphyseal fracture, fills the diaphyseal bone segment, and relieves stress on the distal aspect of the femur. The stem should be fluted and cylindrical to provide rotational stability; it should not be cemented at the level of the fracture or proximal to it because the cement can interfere with union by reducing axial loads, which are needed to stimulate fracture healing. Cement may extrude into the fracture itself. Extruded cement should be removed with an osteotome, and cancellous bone graft should be applied to bridge the fracture site. Protected weightbearing in the early postoperative period is beneficial to stimulate fracture-healing.

Tibial Fractures

Tibial fractures caused by impingement of the stem respond well to nonsurgical treatment. These fractures usually are vertical and are not associated with the severe soft-tissue trauma that occurs with a high-velocity injury. Nondisplaced fractures heal with protected weightbearing. A hinged knee brace is optional, but knee motion should not be postponed.

Vertical fractures of the metaphyseal segment often are the result of the surgeon impacting an implant with peripheral pegs or fins. The fragments of this fracture of the tibial rim usually reapproximate anatomically. Although fixation of the tibial component with cement generally is satisfactory to protect the fracture, a cancellous bone screw can be placed for additional stabilization. Ac-

tivities should be modified in the early postoperative period.

A tibial shaft fracture can occur with impingement of the stem into the diaphysis. This fracture may angulate (Fig. 2) and displace if protected weightbearing is not instituted. However, the periosteum should be minimally disrupted and fracture healing should be uneventful after closed reduction and treatment with a cast. Fractures of the middle third of the tibia are best treated with a patellar ligament-bearing cast that permits knee flexion. A cast-brace or brace that permits knee motion but provides additional support proximal to the knee is indicated for fractures of the proximal third of the tibia. Use of a cast or brace, or both, is recommended for a period of 3 months. Weightbearing should be encouraged for anatomically aligned fractures.

Patellar Fractures

Intraoperative fractures of the patella most often are the result of removal of a stable patellar implant from osteoporotic bone at the time of a revision. Vertical fractures usually are stable and require no internal stabilization. However, transverse fractures are of far greater concern as they can interrupt the integrity of the extensor mechanism. A tension-band-wire technique can be used to stabilize fracture fragments and to permit early limited motion. A patellar component should not be reimplanted if the fractured patella requires surgical repair. If satisfactory stability cannot be obtained intraoperatively and confirmed by passive flexion of the knee to 90°, the unstable fracture fragments should be excised and the extensor mechanism should be augmented with a semitendinosus tendon graft[1] or replaced with an extensor mechanism allograft.[2]

Clinical Results

Because intraoperative fractures are rare, the outcomes of treatment have been largely unreported. However, Lombardi and associates[3] reported the results for 41 intercondylar distal femoral fractures. Thirty-five of these fractures were incidental findings on postoperative radiographs; they healed with no changes during a standard physical-therapy protocol for rehabilitation. The other six fractures were identified intraoperatively; they were treated with a long-stemmed femoral component or screw fixation, or both, and healed without complication. The postoperative regimen was not modified for these six patients.

Postoperative Periprosthetic Femoral Fractures

Systemic factors often predispose a patient to a supracondylar fracture of the femur and also jeopardize the results of conventional treatment. The typical patient is elderly, has osteoporosis, and occasionally has neurologic dysfunction with or without osteoarthrotic involvement of other joints. Therefore, when a treatment option is chosen, consideration must be given to multiple factors, including the status of the prosthetic fixation, the degree of comminution of the fracture, the proximity of the fracture to the prosthetic component, the longitudinal alignment of the limb, the degree of displacement of the fracture, and the extent of osteoporosis. The modification of Neer's fracture-classification system described by Lewis and Rorabeck[4] is useful for planning and analyzing the results of treatment of supracondylar periprosthetic fractures. However, fracture-classification systems do not take into account individual patient variables, which must be considered when the best method for stabilization of the fracture is being selected. In addition, the classification scheme of Lewis and Rorabeck does not include a category for supracondylar fractures for which attempts at stabilization have been unsuccessful. These fractures are categorized as type III, with the assumption that the prosthesis will fail if stabilization has been unsuccessful.

Type I: Undisplaced Supracondylar Fractures

If a type-I fracture is stable, the prosthesis is intact and functioning well, and the patient can walk safely while wearing a cast or cast-brace, then the knee is best treated closed and with range-of-motion exercises. The patient must have enough strength in the upper extremities to walk safely with protected weightbearing until the fracture has healed. Follow-up radiographs are necessary to ensure that overall alignment of the limb is not altered by angulation of the fracture. If displacement occurs and realignment becomes necessary, the fracture must be reduced and must be stabilized with a fixation device.

Surgical intervention is necessary to stabilize an undisplaced type-I fracture in patients who cannot tolerate a cast or cast-brace, cannot support part of their weight with walking aids, or cannot proceed with range-of-motion exercises. Many internal fixation devices are available for undisplaced or minimally displaced fractures. Intramedullary fixation devices that minimally disrupt the fracture hematoma are ideal. Rush rods and Zickel supracondylar rods are particularly applicable to nondisplaced fractures with minimum comminution. When a more stable fracture configuration with internal fixation is indicated, retrograde nailing, followed by locking, with an intramedullary supracondylar rod or a blade-plate may be used. A blade-plate is a third option for the treatment of type-I fractures, but it requires considerably more dissection and periosteal stripping in the region of the fracture.

Rush Rods For optimum stabilization of the fracture and firm purchase of the rods in the femoral condyles, Ritter and associates[5] recommended use of Rush condylar rods with a larger, flatter surface in the hooked area. The fracture is reduced with a counter bolster placed under the femur, and the reduction is checked with image intensification. The

lateral rod is placed first, with use of an awl angled at 30°, so that it enters near the femoral epicondyle. The awl is advanced in the longitudinal plane of the femur, and the rod, 4.7 mm in diameter, is introduced through the awl. A second rod is inserted into the distal fragment through the opposite epicondyle. The rods are advanced simultaneously across the fracture to the mid-diaphyseal level of the femur. Stress on the rods is relieved by bending them 3 to 5 cm from the exposed tip. The bent tip then is buried in the soft tissues. Use of a knee immobilizer and protected weightbearing with crutches or a walker are continued until the fracture has healed, usually for an interval of 3 months.

Zickel Supracondylar Rods The technique for insertion of a Zickel supracondylar rod is similar to that used for the Rush rod.[6,7] After the fracture has been reduced under image intensification, the surgeon introduces an awl distal to the epicondyle and as close as possible to the femoral component. A hole is placed more anteriorly in the lateral condyle, and a 90° rod of variable diameter (5, 7.5, or 11 mm) is inserted manually through the hole. Simultaneously, a 75° medial rod is passed across the fracture. These rods are driven alternately over short distances until both are flush with the cortex. Holes are predrilled for insertion of 6.4-mm compression screws. Postoperative management includes protected weightbearing and limited knee motion.

Clinical Results of Use of Rush and Zickel Supracondylar Rods In one study, Rush condylar rods were used successfully for the treatment of displaced periprosthetic supracondylar fractures in 22 patients; the fractures healed in 3 to 4 months.[5] Two fractures healed in 15° of valgus because of technical error. The patients recovered an average of 108° of knee flexion.

Zickel rods incorporate condylar screws for fracture stability. In soft condylar bone, this is an advantage over the marginal stability provided by a stress-relieved Rush rod. However, the results of use of Zickel rods for the treatment of periprosthetic supracondylar fractures have not been reported, to our knowledge.

Clinical Results of Nonsurgical Treatment In reviewing the English-language literature, Chen and associates[8] noted that 30 nondisplaced supracondylar fractures had been treated with traction or a cast, or both. Twenty-five patients were satisfied with the result. The results were not reported in terms of function or knee motion. Moran and associates[9] reported an average loss of 8° of motion in association with five type-I fractures; all five united with nonsurgical treatment. Merkel and Johnson[10] reported that six of six type-I fractures treated with a cast healed without surgical intervention. The results were not reported in terms of range of motion or knee function.

Early knee motion is necessary to optimize the functional results of nonsurgical treatment of type-I fractures. However, the results of bracing and early, limited motion have not been reported, to our knowledge. With early motion, malunion and nonunion can occur. Because these are the likely modes of failure of nonsurgical treatment, meticulous follow-up evaluation is essential.

Type II: Displaced Supracondylar Fractures

Surgical intervention is indicated for type-II supracondylar fractures that have resulted in unacceptable alignment of the extremity or the components. The fracture must be aligned correctly and stabilized to permit early motion of the knee and at least partial weightbearing. Variables to consider when selecting a fracture-fixation device include displacement and angulation, alignment of the extremity, bone quality, bone deformity, and the type of knee implant that is in place. Particular attention to the extent of bone damage in the distal condylar fragment is important when selecting the best method of fixation. Many internal fixation devices have been used successfully.

Plate-and-Screw Fixation Fracture plates, cobra plates, buttress plates, blade-plates, and condylar screws have been used successfully to stabilize periprosthetic supracondylar fractures. If a plate-and-screw option is selected, the condylar fragment must be large enough and of sufficient bone density to provide rigid distal fixation.

The proximity of the femoral component to the fracture must be considered when a fixation device is selected. Although a distal condylar screw is probably the easiest device to use, it is bulky and may be difficult to place in a more distal comminuted fracture. A condylar buttress plate offers the greatest flexibility but the least secure fixation. Often, a relatively thin blade-plate is the best option as it can be placed close to the lugs and the anterior flange of the component. The fracture can angulate with any of these devices, but it is less likely to do so with a blade-plate, which must migrate through bone to cause loss of alignment. Therefore, a blade-plate usually is the best of the plate-and-screw options available for the fixation of comminuted distal condylar fractures. If fracture stability is not clearly evident intraoperatively, the condylar fragment should be augmented with bone graft or bone cement to enhance internal fixation.

Plate-and-screw fixation is performed with use of a sterile tourniquet on the proximal aspect of the thigh. The fracture is exposed through a lateral or extended anterior approach. Periosteal stripping should be minimized to avoid devascularization of the bone. Interfragmentary lag-screws are placed anterior to posterior, with use of fluoroscopic imaging, to stabilize comminuted condylar fragments. Whenever the condylar segment has been fractured, stability of the components must be assessed. If stability has been lost, the fracture is classified as type III and a revision is the appropriate treatment option.

The first step is to secure the fixation device to the condylar fragment. If a condylar buttress plate is selected, then two or three 6.5-mm fully threaded cancellous-bone screws are placed through the appropriate right or left plate. If a 95° blade-plate is inserted, a guide-wire is positioned, with use of fluoroscopy, parallel to the joint surface in the coronal plane. The blade then is inserted as far distally in the condylar segment as permitted by the proximity of the femoral component. Attachment of the plate proximal to the fracture with use of bicortical screws reestablishes the anatomic valgus angulation of the distal aspect of the femur in relation to the mechanical axis of the knee. When a condylar screw is used, it should be angled posteriorly from lateral to medial over a guide-wire. Fluoroscopy is used to determine whether the position of the condylar screw is satisfactory.

The fracture is reduced and stabilized by applying bone-holding forceps to the plate and the proximal fragment. Fracture stability is assessed with the knee in flexion and extension and with application of varus and valgus stress. If the fracture is not stable, an augmentation procedure (the addition of bone graft or bone cement to the condylar fragment) should be used in conjunction with reinsertion of the fixation device into the condylar segment. This is done before the plate is attached to the proximal fragment with transcortical screws. A minimum of three bicortical screws must be placed proximal to the fracture.

An augmentation procedure can be used to enhance the stability of fracture fixation by securing the distal fragment more rigidly. Healy and associates[11] advocated making a window in the lateral surface of the lateral femoral condyle (Fig. 3). Autogenous graft, allograft, or bone

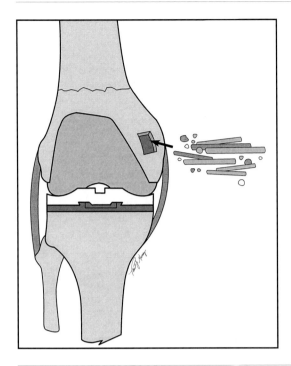

Fig. 3 A cortical window can be made in the femoral condyle and used for impacting bone graft or introducing bone cement to enhance fracture stabilization.

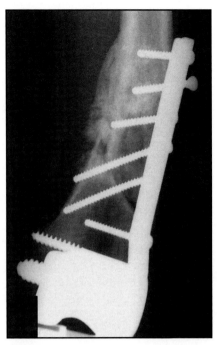

Fig. 4 Fracture stabilization has been lost with disruption at the plate-bone junction and varus angulation.

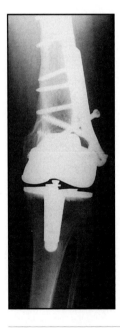

Fig. 5 A supracondylar fracture with varus angulation may affect the durability of the prosthesis.

cement then is impacted or injected into the metaphysis. Alternatively, low-viscosity bone cement can be injected through drill-holes in the condylar fragment with a standard 20-ml syringe.[12] The fixation device is inserted before the cement hardens. The fracture is reduced, and the plate is secured to the proximal fragment with bicortical screws.

Clinical Results of Use of Plates and Screws The clinical results of treatment with plates and screws have been satisfactory in approximately two thirds of reported cases. The best results of which we are aware were reported by Healy and associates,[11] who found that 18 of 20 fractures healed after treatment with a blade-plate, a condylar screw, or a buttress plate. Bone graft was used to enhance the fixation of 15 fractures. The postoperative Knee Society scores were as good as the scores before the fracture. Two patients needed a reoperation, but both ultimately had fracture-healing after reinsertion of a condylar screw-plate combined with autogenous bone-grafting. Zehntner and Ganz[12] reported success with use of condylar buttress plates

in six patients, two of whom had an augmentation procedure with injection of bone cement and bone graft. Four of the six patients had rheumatoid arthritis with multiple-joint involvement. All six patients regained their preoperative walking status, including the four who had depended on crutches. In another study, 17 of 20 fractures united after treatment with a compression plate, with or without bone graft.[13]

The clinical results in other studies involving treatment of these fractures with plates and screws have not been as successful. Figgie and associates[14] reported nonunion of five of ten fractures treated with a plate and screws, with failure of fixation occurring at the plate-bone junction (Fig. 4). Cordeiro and associates[15] reported varus angulation in three patients who were managed with a plate and screws (Fig. 5). Nielsen and associates[16] described failure of plate-and-screw fixation in three of three patients; the failures were due to infection, formation of a fistula, and a loose plate in one patient each.

Moran and associates[9] reported on 15

displaced fractures that had been treated with open reduction and internal fixation. The method of fixation was a 95° blade-plate in nine fractures, a lateral buttress plate in three, double-plating in two, and a dynamic condylar screw in one.

Table 1

Intercondylar distances of commonly used total condylar knee implants

Implant	Intercondylar Distance (mm)
Miller-Galante (Zimmer, Warsaw, IN)	12
Insall-Burstein (Zimmer)	14 to 19
Biomet (Warsaw, IN)	22
Intermedics (Austin, TX)	18
AMK (DePuy, Warsaw, IN)	14 to 17
Osteonics (Allendale, NJ)	19
PFC (Johnson & Johnson, New Brunswick, NJ)	20
Kirschner wires (Timonium, MD)	20
Genesis (Smith & Nephew Richards, Memphis, TN)	20
Duracon (Howmedica, Rutherford, NJ)	12 to 16

(Reproduced with modification from Jabczenski FF, Crawford M: Retrograde intramedullary nailing of supracondylar femur fractures above total knee arthroplasty: A preliminary report of four cases. *J Arthroplasty* 1995;10:95–101.)

Ten of the 15 patients regained satisfactory function after fracture healing. Three fractures healed with 2 cm of intentional femoral shortening. Iliac-crest grafts were used in six patients. Five of the 15 repairs failed, including three in patients who had a nonunion and required additional surgical treatment and two in patients who had a malunion and decreased knee function.

In summary, complications of treatment that have resulted in failure of the fixation or in a poor outcome are angulation of the fracture (malunion), migration of the condylar screw or the plate, nonunion, poor knee motion, and infection.

External Fixators External fixators have been used successfully but usually are contraindicated in the treatment of supracondylar femoral fractures. The goal of this treatment is satisfactory fixation that permits early motion and, at a minimum, walking with protected weightbearing. Because the external fixator cannot cross the knee joint, the pins frequently are placed close to the implant. The pins cannot avoid binding the quadriceps muscle and impeding motion of the knee. Infected pin sites that potentially expose the knee to infection also are common with use of this treatment.

Clinical Results of Use of External Fixators Three patients who were managed with a Hoffmann external fixator (Howmedica, Rutherford, NJ) had early motion and a good clinical result.[10] Walking with support and range-of-motion exercises were started within 1 week after application of the external fixator. The range of motion averaged 101° after the fractures healed, and all three knees were pain-free.

Supracondylar Intramedullary Rods When a supracondylar rod is used for fracture fixation, it is helpful to make anteroposterior and lateral radiographs of both the fractured and the contralateral femur. These radiographs are used to determine the correct diameter and length of the supracondylar intramedullary rod. If the intramedullary canal cannot be visualized on preoperative radiographs, fluoroscopy can be performed intraoperatively, with the rod (still in its sterile package) placed over the injured femur to ensure that at least two locking screws can be inserted proximal to the fracture. Supracondylar rods are available in lengths of 15, 20, and 25 cm. In most instances, the longest rod is used

because it centers itself in the isthmus and decreases the risk of fracture malalignment.

The Supracondylar Intramedullary Nail (Smith and Nephew Richards, Memphis, TN) is a stainless-steel fixation device that is available in diameters of 11, 12, or 13 mm. The type of knee prosthesis that is in place must be identified to determine if the intercondylar space is wide enough to accommodate insertion of a supracondylar rod. A minimum intercondylar distance of 12 mm is necessary. The distance between the condyles of most implants is 15 to 20 mm[17] (Table 1). The Miller-Galante I prosthesis (Zimmer, Warsaw, IN) in a small size is an exception. If the prosthesis cannot be identified, a notch or sunrise radiograph can be used to measure the intercondylar distance. If neither the intercondylar distance nor the type of implant can be determined, an alternative method of fixation must be used. It is very important to remember that posterior stabilized femoral components with closed housings and long-stemmed femoral components prohibit retrograde intramedullary nailing.

Insertion of a supracondylar intramedullary rod requires that the patient be placed supine on a radiolucent operating table, with the injured lower limb draped free of the table. A bolster is positioned under the thigh to flex the knee 50°. Traction is applied to reduce the fracture, and reduction is confirmed with C-arm fluoroscopic imaging. Comminuted fragments should be fixed with cannulated lag-screws with buttress washers before the intramedullary rod is inserted. These screws should be positioned carefully so that they do not interfere with insertion of the rod.

The intercondylar notch is exposed through either a medial parapatellar arthrotomy or a midline patellar ligament-splitting incision. A curved awl is used to locate the original intramedullary femoral guide-hole. An intramedullary guide-pin is passed into the femoral canal, and a cannulated reamer can be used for limited intramedullary reaming. A reamer is used to enlarge the entry hole so that it is 1 mm more in diameter than the diameter of the selected rod.

The rod and the external guide are coupled to confirm that the holes correspond. The assembled device then is passed over the guide-pin with the apex directed anteriorly. For most fractures, the distal end of the rod should be inserted 1 to 2 mm beyond the surface of the intercondylar notch. Alternatively, the rod may be left protruding by 1 cm for severely comminuted fractures located close to the femoral component, so that the condylar locking screws can be placed more distally in the femur. The protruding segment of the rod is removed at the end of the procedure with a high-speed carbide burr.

Fracture reduction should be confirmed fluoroscopically before the 5 mm condylar locking screws are inserted. The two most distal 5-mm screws are placed first, followed by a minimum of two proximal locking screws. A trocar pin (a standard instrument provided with the supracondylar rod) can help to decrease migration of the drill. When removing the drill, the surgeon must be careful not to advance or rotate the rod before inserting the proximal locking screws.

When a patient has large thighs there may be excessive soft-tissue pressure on the targeting guide, causing the guide-holes to drift. Drifting can be prevented by retaining the 8-mm drill sleeve over the last screw to stabilize the rod-guide assembly while the proximal screws are being placed. A 4-mm hole is drilled through both cortices, and bicortical screws of appropriate length are inserted.

Clinical Results of the Use of Supracondylar Intramedullary Rods
Rolston and associates[18] reported excellent clinical results after treatment of four type-II fractures with a supracondylar rod. Early motion was permitted for

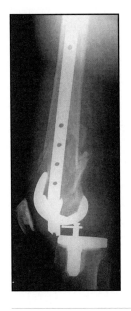
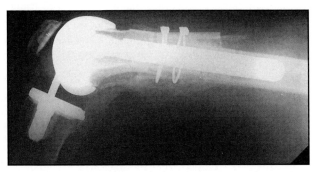

Fig. 6 Left, Radiograph, made 2 weeks postoperatively, showing loss of stabilization of a supracondylar fracture when the supracondylar rod migrated into the knee joint. **Right,** A composite consisting of an allograft and a long-stemmed femoral component was used to reconstruct the distal aspect of the femur after stabilization of the fracture with a supracondylar rod had failed. A canal-filling stem (Coordinate Knee System; DePuy, Warsaw, IN) with a diameter of 18 mm and a length of 195 mm was inserted.

three of the four patients. A hinged knee brace and partial weightbearing were prescribed for 6 to 8 weeks. These authors cited several advantages of the supracondylar rod as compared with plate-and-screw fixation. The advantages included decreased operative time, better access to the fracture without periosteal stripping, minimum disturbance of the fracture hematoma, more rigid fixation, and the ability to assess and revise the femoral component if it was loose or damaged.

McLaren and associates[19] reported good clinical results and fracture-healing with use of supracondylar rods in seven patients. Six of these patients used steroids on an ongoing basis because of rheumatoid arthritis and polyarticular involvement. The fractures occurred within 2 cm of the flange of the femoral component. In one patient, polymethylmethacrylate was used to improve fixation to the distal fragment. To achieve the desired screw location in the distal fragment, the surgeon left 1 cm of the rod exposed. The prominent portion of the rod then was removed with a high-speed carbide burr to avoid impingement against the patella or the tibia. Four patients recovered their preoperative

motion, while three lost 10° to 20° of knee flexion. A stress fracture at the site of the most proximal locking screw healed uneventfully in one patient.

Additional reports have documented good clinical results with use of supracondylar rods in small numbers of patients.[17,20,21] In the experience of the senior one of us (GAE), one of four patients managed with a supracondylar rod had migration of the rod through the intercondylar notch, causing loss of fixation (Fig. 6, *left*). Early motion and weightbearing were not factors as this patient was managed postoperatively with a knee immobilizer. In retrospect, the fixation should have been augmented with bone graft or bone cement.

Complications that can occur with use of supracondylar rods for the treatment of periprosthetic fractures include migration of the rod into the knee joint, femoral shortening, nonunion, loss of motion, and infection.

Type III: Displaced or Undisplaced Supracondylar Fractures
A supracondylar fracture adjacent to a loose or failing total knee implant can be treated in one of two ways: like a type-II fracture, with revision of the implant at a

later date, or with revision of the implant as part of the fracture stabilization. If the surgeon performs a revision, the implant should be replaced with a long-stemmed femoral component, a custom-made component or tumor prosthesis, or an allograft-implant composite that also replaces the damaged distal aspect of the femur. A stable tibial component can be retained if the femoral component used for the revision is of the same design and will articulate correctly with the tibial component in situ. Usually, dome-shaped patellar components should not be revised as they articulate satisfactorily with most femoral components used for revision.

It is prudent to have an implant or an allograft available that will replace the damaged bone of the distal aspect of the femoral condyles in revision procedures. Removal of the femoral component from the site of a comminuted supracondylar fracture in osteoporotic bone may result in considerable bone loss. This situation may not become evident until the femoral component has been removed. Excessive bone loss makes it difficult to adequately secure the implant to the damaged distal aspect of the femur. Use of a prosthesis that replaces the condyles or an allograft-implant composite is indicated if the condyles are too comminuted to provide satisfactory support for a revision component.

Early intervention and revision of the femoral component to one with a canal-filling stem are the best options for treatment of most type-III fractures. Because patients who have periprosthetic fractures usually are elderly and debilitated from systemic disease, it is very important to allow them to be out of bed as soon as possible. This is particularly true for patients in whom attempts at stabilizing the fracture have failed and for those who cannot be allowed out of bed without an additional procedure being performed. The exceptional patient who should not have early intervention is one

who will benefit from delayed revision. In this situation, the fracture can be reduced and internally fixed so that the patient can walk safely until the revision has been performed.

There are two advantages to delaying a revision procedure. First, revision of a knee that has an anatomically healed supracondylar fracture is far easier than revision of one that has unstable condylar fragments. Second, a standard revision implant can be used rather than a tumor replacement, a custom-made implant, or a large structural allograft. Implants without prosthetic constraints have a greater chance of long-term stability.

The surgical technique for this revision procedure involves opening the knee through a standard midline approach to provide access to the supracondylar fracture as well as to the knee. The goals are to preserve bone of the distal aspect of the femur for optimum fixation of the femoral component and to use the least constrained implant that provides adequate stability of the knee. Implants with higher levels of both varus-valgus and anterior-posterior stability should be available. Unstable fracture fragments should be excised and used as bone graft unless they are large enough to attach to stable fragments. The intramedullary canal of the femur is opened with progressively larger reamers until a tight fit has been obtained. The stem should be long enough to achieve a tight fit in the canal in the diaphyseal segment of the femur. A stem that is at least 150 mm long is optimum (Fig. 6, right).

Whenever a custom-made condylar tumor prosthesis or a rotating-hinge implant is selected, the rotation and length of the femoral component must be determined before fixation with cement. With the knee in flexion, the femoral component must be rotated to a position perpendicular to the long axis of the tibia for patellofemoral stability. The femoral canal then is plugged and lavaged, followed by cement pressuriza-

tion. The appropriate level of the joint line can be restored by intercalating an allograft between the distal aspect of the femur and the long-stemmed revision component. The allograft should be step-cut for rotational stability of the distal aspect of the femur. The step-cuts of the distal aspect of the femur and the allograft must preserve the correct rotation of the femur at a 90° angle to the tibia in order to maintain stability of the knee in flexion.

As an alternative treatment, the femoral component can be customized. A long-stemmed revision component can be modified by adding holes to the stem for medullary bicortical transfixion screws. A condylar replacement segment can be added to a rotating-hinge implant. In some situations, the intercondylar distance or the width of the intercondylar box of a posterior stabilized femoral component can be enlarged with a metal-cutting burr, permitting insertion of a supracondylar rod for fracture fixation. A customized component was used successfully in three of three patients,[22] four of four patients,[23] and one of one patient.[24]

Clinical Results Satisfactory outcomes have been reported consistently with use of a variety of implants and techniques to treat periprosthetic femoral fractures proximal to a total knee implant with revision of the component. In a comprehensive review of the literature, McLaren and associates[19] found that standard long-stemmed revision components were used most frequently. Of 25 knees so treated, 24 had a satisfactory outcome[19] (Table 2). Cordeiro and associates[15] reported on five fractures that were treated with a revision with a custom-made long-stemmed component; all five healed with a good result. Kraay and associates,[25] used a large segmental allograft and a long-stemmed, semiconstrained knee prosthesis in seven patients to reconstruct bone defects after a supracondylar fracture. All seven patients had a satisfactory outcome. Three patients died of unrelated causes before the 2-year follow-up examination, but at the latest evaluation all had had a satisfactory result. Cement fixation with canal-plugging and pressurization was used to stabilize the implant. The graft united with host bone in only one patient, although none of the others had notable resorption or mechanical failure. Two patients needed bracing for knee instability.[25]

Postoperative Periprosthetic Tibial Fractures

Periprosthetic tibial fractures have been reported in conjunction with early total knee-implant designs such as the Geometric and the Polycentric components (both manufactured by Howmedica).[26] The fractures were believed to have resulted from fatigue failure of the tibia secondary to axial malalignment and improper orientation of the component. The design of these early implants concentrated stresses on the adjacent cancellous bone. Rand and Coventry[26] reported on 15 knees that needed a revision arthroplasty because of loosening of the tibial component.

Tibial stress fractures are unlikely to occur if the implant is well aligned and metal-backed. However, fatigue fractures can occur in either the tibia or the femur when a patient who essentially could not walk before the total knee arthroplasty is mobilized immediately afterward. If the patient has an onset of pain in the leg during rehabilitation, radiographs should be examined to rule out a fracture. If the knee is unprotected, fatigue fractures will develop progressive angulation and even nonunion. The knee should be protected with a brace or cast, and activities should be modified until union is complete as confirmed by bridging endosteal new bone on follow-up radiographs. These fractures do not involve the fixation interface of the tibial component and, therefore, are not associated with loosening of the component.

Table 2
Summary of statistics from the meta-analysis of supracondylar fractures occurring proximal to sites of total knee arthroplasties

Treatment Method	Satisfactory Outcomes		
	Total	No.	Percent
Closed reduction	123	70	57
Open reduction	63	42	67
External fixation	6	4	
Intramedullary nailing	6	6	
Revision with long-stemmed femoral component	25	24	96

(Reproduced with permission from McLaren AC, Dupont JA, Schroeber DC: Open reduction internal fixation of supracondylar fractures above total knee arthroplasties using the intramedullary supracondylar rod. *Clin Orthop* 1994;302:194–198.)

Postoperative Periprosthetic Patellar Fractures

Patellar fractures result from fatigue failure caused by bone that has been weakened first by the patellar resection and second by the patellar prosthesis altering stresses on the bone.[27] Malalignment of the implant may impart additional stresses that contribute to patellar fracture.[28] The clinical presentation of a fractured patella can be a coincidental finding on a routine follow-up examination, a sudden disruption of knee function associated with fairly major trauma, or an insidious onset of progressive weakness and giving-way of the knee. The asymptomatic fracture is the most common type. The fracture can be either transverse or vertical. Often, it is not detected on clinical examination but, rather, on routine follow-up radiographs. There is no soft-tissue injury or disruption of the extensor mechanism.

A displaced fracture of the patella may or may not be associated with trauma such as a fall. The fracture usually is transverse and can occur through the body of the patella or as an avulsion fracture of the superior or inferior pole. When the quadriceps mechanism contracts suddenly, the patella may fracture or the extensor mechanism may rupture. In this situation, the fall may be the result rather than the cause of the fracture. The patient commonly describes the injury by

stating, "I caught my toe and my knee gave way," "my foot slipped," or "my knee just wouldn't hold me and I fell on it." In these instances, fracture or disruption of the patella may have led to the trauma. The patient is unable to support weight on the injured extremity.

With the insidious avulsion fracture, the patient describes difficulty with climbing stairs, progressive instability of the knee, and a fear of falling. Usually, no injury is associated with this type of fracture. A variable amount of the extensor mechanism has been avulsed with a small fragment of bone. This fragment and the abnormal position of the patella are visible on the lateral radiograph.

Treatment Options

The treatment of a periprosthetic patellar fracture depends on the stability of the patellar implant and the integrity of the extensor mechanism. Whether or not to revise a loose patellar component depends on the type of fracture (transverse or vertical), the displacement and comminution of the fracture fragments, and the quality of the remaining bone after the implant has been removed.

An asymptomatic nondisplaced patellar fracture identified on a routine follow-up radiograph requires no specific treatment. Earlier radiographs should be reviewed to determine if the fracture was present but not identified at a previous

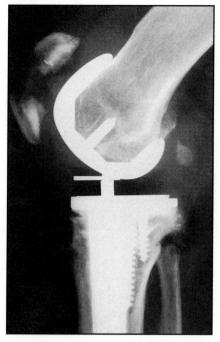
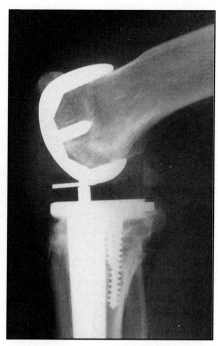

Fig. 7 Left, A transverse mid-substance fracture of the patella with an unstable patellar component. Repair required removal of the patellar component, excision of the unstable bone fragments, and an augmentation repair of the extensor mechanism. **Right,** Maximum flexion to 80° after repair of the fracture. Most of the patellar bone has been excised, and the extensor mechanism has been repaired with a semitendinosus graft.

office visit. The knee should be examined for any extensor lag or tenderness around the patella.

When a nondisplaced or minimally displaced patellar fracture, particularly a transverse fracture, is identified in a patient who has had a recent onset of symptoms or a known injury, treatment is required to permit fracture healing without displacement of the fragments. The integrity of the extensor mechanism is determined by palpating the knee for defects and tenderness as well as by evaluating the patient's ability to perform a straight-leg raise. A hemarthrosis may be present, but usually it does not need to be aspirated. A cylinder cast should be applied with the knee in 5° of flexion. The knee is comfortable in this position because the posterior aspect of the capsule is relaxed. The cast is worn for 6 weeks. The patient may begin isometric quadriceps exercises and may walk with

full weightbearing immediately. Range-of-motion and antigravity exercises begin after the cast has been removed. After the patient has regained 90° of flexion without an extensor lag, quadriceps-strengthening exercises with weights may be initiated.

Vertical fractures are inherently more stable than transverse fractures and rarely affect the function of the extensor mechanism. The patellar component usually remains fixed to the larger fragment. The fracture is minimally symptomatic and often is an unsuspected finding on a radiograph. If tenderness, swelling, or discoloration are present, a cylinder cast or a knee brace that limits flexion is recommended for 6 weeks. No treatment is necessary if a vertical fracture appears to be old and is asymptomatic. A negative technetium-99m bone scan may help to determine the age of the fracture, although the scan may remain positive

for as long as two years after the fracture.

Patients who have a displaced transverse periprosthetic fracture of the patella that is more than 2 cm long usually have an acute disabling injury (Fig. 7, *left*). A large hemarthrosis is present, and the knee is painful. The patient is unable to lift the lower limb. A defect is palpable in the patella. Lateral and Merchant radiographs of the patella confirm the fracture and the relative stability of the patellar component.

A displaced transverse fracture through the middle third of the patella should be surgically repaired. Routine methods of fixation, such as tension-band wiring, may not be possible because of the patellar component. Therefore, the patellar component should be removed if the fracture cannot be stabilized and the extensor mechanism cannot be optimally repaired (Fig. 7, *right*). Repairs of the fracture and the patellar retinaculum should be protected with a cylinder cast for 8 to 12 weeks.

A patient who has a fracture of the superior or inferior pole of the patella and disruption of the quadriceps or the patellar ligament also may have an acute injury. Radiographically, the patella is displaced in an alta position with a fracture of the inferior pole (Fig. 8) and in an infera position with a fracture of the superior pole. A stable repair of the extensor mechanism is essential. A Bunnell or Krackow[29] type of locking stitch is placed in the disrupted ligament with nonabsorbable sutures. The sutures are passed through vertical drill holes in the patella and are tied over the anterior surface of the patella. A tension-band wire extending from the inferior pole of the patella to the tibial tubercle protects the surgical repair of the inferior pole avulsion fracture. If the knee cannot be passively flexed 75° without disrupting the surgical repair, augmentation of the repair with a semitendinosus tendon graft should be considered.

Avulsion fractures of the inferior pole

of the patella can occur without a known injury. Patients report weakness, giving-way of the knee, difficulty with climbing stairs, and falling. Patients who had been doing well describe increasing difficulty with all activities. A cane or walker becomes necessary for support. The physical examination reveals an extensor lag and quadriceps weakness.

An avulsion fracture of the inferior pole of the patella should be treated as a rupture of the patellar ligament. A semitendinosus graft is prepared by detaching the tendon at its musculotendinous junction.[1] A transverse 48-cm drill hole is made in the inferior pole of the patella. The ligament is routed from its insertion through the drill hole in the patella and is attached either through a second 48-cm transverse drill hole in the tibial tubercle or to the periosteum and the patellar ligament at the tubercle. With the knee flexed at 45°, the sutures are secured. A cerclage wire extending from the patella to the tibial tubercle is used to protect the repair (Fig. 9). The limb is placed in a cylinder cast for 6 weeks, during which time weightbearing activities are permitted. When the cast is removed, a brace is used to limit flexion to 60° for an additional 6 weeks.

Rarely is the patellar component loose unless the fracture is transverse through the mid-substance of the patella. When a displaced fracture is repaired, a loose component should be removed. A stable patellar component should be removed if it interferes with repair of the fractured patella. We believe that a prosthesis should not be inserted in a patella in which a fracture has been repaired because the implant weakens the repair and imparts greater stress on the extensor mechanism, making the patient prone to a refracture after resuming full activities.

Clinical Results
Nondisplaced and minimally displaced fractures of the patella that are incidental findings on routine follow-up examina-

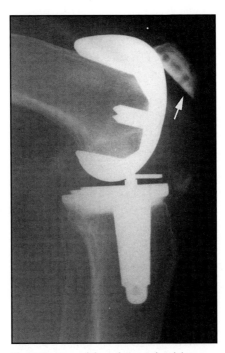

Fig. 8 Fracture of the inferior pole of the patella (arrow) with obvious patella alta and abnormal tilt. An augmentation repair of the patellar ligament is indicated.

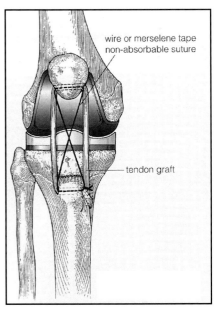

wire or merselene tape
non-absorbable suture

tendon graft

Fig. 9 Reconstruction of the patellar ligament with use of nonabsorbable sutures. (Reproduced, with permission from Cadambi A, Schmidt R: The extensor mechanism in revision total knee arthroplasty, in Engh GA, Rorabeck CH (eds): *Revision Total Knee Arthroplasty*. Baltimore, MD, Williams & Wilkins, 1997, p 217.)

tion and that require no specific treatment usually remain asymptomatic. Patients retain a good range of knee motion, with no quadriceps weakness or extensor lag.[30] Goldberg and associates[31] classified these fractures into four types. Fourteen knees that had a type-I fracture (through the middle of the patellar body or through the superior pole of the patella and not involving the implant or the extensor mechanism) and two that had a type-IIIB fracture (through the inferior pole without rupture of the patellar ligament) were rated as having a good or excellent result after nonsurgical treatment. Patients were managed with anti-inflammatory medications and a knee immobilizer along with partial weightbearing. Similarly, Brick and Scott[32] reported a good result in six patients in whom a periprosthetic patellar fracture was protected with a knee immobilizer for 6 weeks. The average flexion of these six knees after the fracture was 100°. Of

seven patients who had a nondisplaced fracture (three of whom were managed nonsurgically and four with a patellectomy), all had a good clinical result.[33] Although the patients obtained good flexion, the four who had had a patellectomy had a 75% decrease in the strength of the quadriceps muscle.

The results of surgical treatment of displaced patellar fractures with an extensor lag have been poor. Hozack and associates[33] reported poor results for four of six patients in whom a displaced fracture had been treated with a patellectomy. Likewise, the results were poor for two of four patients who had been managed with fragment excision and for two of two who had been managed with internal fixation. Only one of seven patients who had a displaced fracture and an extensor lag at the time of the operation had a satisfactory result. Brick and Scott[32] reported failure of fixation of three of four patellar fractures that had been treated with open reduction. Five patients who had been managed with a partial or total patellectomy had complications, including infection, a loose prosthesis, a functionally fused knee, and persistent weakness of the extensor mechanism. Grace and Sim[34] reported three complications after surgical treatment of eight patellar fractures; the complications included a ruptured quadriceps tendon, a second fatigue fracture in a repaired patella, and a *Staphylococcus aureus* infection. Goldberg and associates[31] reported a poor result for 13 of 19 knees that had been treated surgically, including five of seven that had had a fracture of the inferior pole of the patella, four of six that had had a midbody fracture involving the implant, and four of six that had had a fracture-dislocation of the patella.

References

1. Cadambi A, Engh GA: Use of a semitendinosus tendon autogenous graft for rupture of the patellar ligament after total knee arthroplasty: A report of seven cases. *J Bone Joint Surg* 1992;74A:974–979.

2. Emerson RH Jr, Head WC, Malinin TI: Reconstruction of patellar tendon rupture after total knee arthroplasty with an extensor mechanism allograft. *Clin Orthop* 1990;260:154–161.

3. Lombardi AV Jr, Mallory TH, Waterman RA, et al: Intercondylar distal femoral fracture: An unreported complication of posterior-stabilized total knee arthroplasty. *J Arthroplasty* 1995;10:643–650.

4. Lewis PL, Rorabeck CH: Periprosthetic fractures, in Engh GA, Rorabeck CH (eds): *Revision Total Knee Arthroplasty*. Baltimore, MD, Williams & Wilkins, 1997, pp 275–295.

5. Ritter MA, Keating EM, Faris PM, et al: Rush rod fixation of supracondylar fractures above total knee arthroplasties. *J Arthroplasty* 1995;10:213–216.

6. Barker LG, Ryan WG, Paul AS, et al: Zickel supracondylar nail to treat supracondylar fracture of the femur in patients with total knee replacements. *Int J Orthop Trauma* 1993;3:183–185.

7. Rosenfield AL, McQueen D: Zickel supracondylar fixation device and Dall-Miles cables for supracondylar fractures of the femur following total knee arthroplasty. *Tech Orthop* 1991;6:86–88.

8. Chen F, Mont MA, Bachner RS: Management of ipsilateral supracondylar femur fractures following total knee arthroplasty. *J Arthroplasty* 1994;9:521–526.

9. Moran MC, Brick GW, Sledge CB, et al: Supracondylar femoral fracture following total knee arthroplasty. *Clin Orthop* 1996;324:196–209.

10. Merkel KD, Johnson EW Jr: Supracondylar fracture of the femur after total knee arthroplasty. *J Bone Joint Surg* 1986;68A:29–43.

11. Healy WL, Siliski JM, Incavo SJ: Operative treatment of distal femoral fractures proximal to total knee replacements. *J Bone Joint Surg* 1993;75A:27–34.

12. Zehntner MK, Ganz R: Internal fixation of supracondylar fractures after condylar total knee arthroplasty. *Clin Orthop* 1993;293:219–224.

13. Culp RW, Schmidt RG, Hanks G, et al: Supracondylar fracture of the femur following prosthetic knee arthroplasty. *Clin Orthop* 1987;222:212–222.

14. Figgie MP, Goldberg VM, Figgie HE III, et al: The results of treatment of supracondylar fracture above total knee arthroplasty. *J Arthroplasty* 1990;5:267–276.

15. Cordeiro EN, Costa RC, Carazzato JG, et al: Periprosthetic fractures in patients with total knee arthroplasties. *Clin Orthop* 1990;252:182–189.

16. Nielsen BF, Petersen VS, Varmarken JE: Fracture of the femur after knee arthroplasty. *Acta Orthop Scand* 1988;59:155–157.

17. Jabczenski FF, Crawford M: Retrograde intramedullary nailing of supracondylar femur fractures above total knee arthroplasty: A preliminary report of four cases. *J Arthroplasty* 1995;10:95–101.

18. Rolston LR, Christ DJ, Halpern A, et al: Treatment of supracondylar fractures of the femur proximal to a total knee arthroplasty: A report of four cases. *J Bone Joint Surg* 1995;77A:924–931.

19. McLaren AC, Dupont JA, Schroeber DC: Open reduction internal fixation of supracondylar fractures above total knee arthroplasties using the intramedullary supracondylar rod. *Clin Orthop* 1994;302:194–198.

20. Henry SL: Management of supracondylar fractures proximal to total knee arthroplasty with the GSH supracondylar nail. *Contemp Orthop* 1995;31:231–238.

21. Murrell GA, Nunley JA: Interlocked supracondylar intramedullary nails for supracondylar fractures after total knee arthroplasty: A new treatment method. *J Arthroplasty* 1995;10:37–42.

22. Howes JP, Sakka SA, Riley TBH: A modified prosthesis with an interlocking nail stem for the treatment of supracondylar femoral fractures after total knee replacement: A report of three cases. *Orthop Intern Edition* 1995;3:303–308.

23. Madsen F, Kjaersgaard-Andersen P, Juhl M, et al: A custom-made prosthesis for the treatment of supracondylar femoral fractures after total knee arthroplasty: Report of four cases. *J Orthop Trauma* 1989;3:332–337.

24. Maniar RN, Umlas ME, Rodriguez JA, et al: Supracondylar femoral fracture above a PFC posterior cruciate-substituting total knee arthroplasty treated with supracondylar nailing: A unique technical problem. *J Arthroplasty* 1996;11:637–639.

25. Kraay MJ, Goldberg VM, Figgie MP, et al: Distal femoral replacement with allograft/prosthetic reconstruction for treatment of supracondylar fractures in patients with total knee arthroplasty. *J Arthroplasty* 1992;7:7–16.

26. Rand JA, Coventry MB: Stress fractures after total knee arthroplasty. *J Bone Joint Surg* 1980;62A:226–233.

27. Scott RD, Turoff N, Ewald FC: Stress fracture of the patella following duopatellar total knee arthroplasty with patellar resurfacing. *Clin Orthop* 1982;170:147–151.

28. Figgie HE III, Goldberg VM, Figgie MP, et al: The effect of alignment of the implant on fractures of the patella after condylar total knee arthroplasty. *J Bone Joint Surg* 1989;71A:1031–1039.

29. Krackow KA, Thomas SC, Jones LC: A new stitch for ligament-tendon fixation: Brief note. *J Bone Joint Surg* 1986;68A:764–766.

30. LeBlanc JM: Patellar complications in total knee arthroplasty: A literature review. *Orthop Rev* 1989;18:296–304.

31. Goldberg VM, Figgie HE III, Inglis AE, et al: Patellar fracture type and prognosis in condylar total knee arthroplasty. *Clin Orthop* 1988;236:115–122.

32. Brick GW, Scott RD: The patellofemoral component of total knee arthroplasty. *Clin Orthop* 1988;231:163–178.

33. Hozack WJ, Goll SR, Lotke PA, et al: The treatment of patellar fractures after total knee arthroplasty. *Clin Orthop* 1988;236:123–127.

34. Grace JN, Sim FH: Fracture of the patella after total knee arthroplasty. *Clin Orthop* 1988;230:168–175.

Fractures of the Femur, Tibia, and Patella
After Total Knee Arthroplasty:
Decision Making and Principles of Management

Cecil H. Rorabeck, MD, FRCSC
Richard D. Angliss, MB, BS, FRACS
Peter L. Lewis, FRACS

Introduction

Fracture complicating total knee arthroplasty (TKA), either intraoperatively or postoperatively, is uncommon. When fracture occurs, however, management and rehabilitation can be difficult and technically demanding. Loss of prefracture function is common despite anatomic reconstruction. With the increase in arthroplasty, specifically revision arthroplasty, these fractures are becoming more common. This chapter presents an overview of the problem, discusses management principles, and offers algorithms for the treatment of periprosthetic fractures based on anatomic location and prosthesis integrity.

Periprosthetic fractures are usually characterized by location according to the prosthetic component in direct proximity to the fracture. The fracture can occur intraoperatively or postoperatively and, in the latter group, may be traumatic or stress related. The primary factors in the decision as to the most appropriate form of management for a specific fracture are fixation of the prosthetic components, fracture location, and bone quality. The expectations and demands of the individual patient must also be considered.

Intraoperative Fractures

Fractures of the femur, tibia, and patella can occur during routine primary TKA; however, these injuries are more commonly related to revision arthroplasty. Intraoperative fracture is less common than postoperative fracture. Specific technical aspects and prosthetic design characteristics may make fracture more likely.

Femoral Fractures

Proximal Femur Fracture of the femoral neck has been reported in association with TKA[1] and is more likely in patients with rheumatoid arthritis or osteoporotic bone. The condition is almost certainly related to the force of femoral impaction: Femoral neck fracture is a rare complication that will be missed unless specifically sought. It should be suspected in patients who are slow to mobilize or who complain of hip and thigh pain after routine TKA.

Femoral Shaft Fractures of the femoral shaft may occur with the use of stemmed implants, usually during revision. The impaction of a slightly oversized or misdirected stem generates stresses that can lead to catastrophic frac-

ture, or a propagating fracture that may not be recognized clinically. Impaction is more likely in bone of poor quality. For this reason, the routine use of intraoperative radiographs with stemmed implants is to be encouraged. Intraoperative fracture fixation may be required to ensure implant stability and alignment. An example of a fracture at the tip of a revision stem is shown in Figure 1. Stresses from the introduction of the stemmed implant resulted in catastrophic failure of the bone, requiring internal stabilization to maintain fixation and alignment. In this case, strut allograft and cerclage wires provided good stability for both prosthesis and fracture.

Femoral shaft fracture and perforation are also possible with the use of intramedullary referenced femoral components. Once again, these problems are more likely in osteoporotic bone; and they may occur in patients with preexisting femoral shaft deformity or canal narrowing. The risk is lessened by careful preoperative assessment of femoral shape and canal dimensions on full femur radiographs in two planes. In such cases, proper placement of the distal femoral guide hole is crucial to safe passage of the

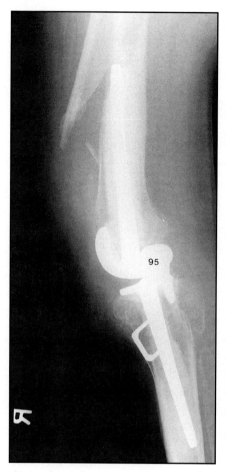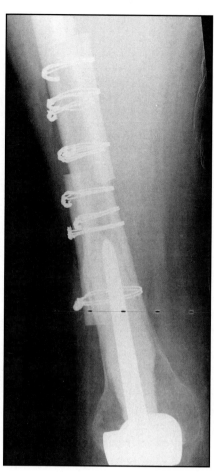

Fig. 1 Left, Supracondylar fracture at the tip of a revision femoral stem. **Right,** Fixation of the fracture with open reduction and allograft strut for structural support.

intramedullary guide.

Condylar and Supracondylar Fractures The risk of fracture around the supracondylar regions during TKA is greater in the revision setting or if there is significant bone loss or osteoporosis. Apart from these patient factors, technical factors (anterior femoral notching and medial placement of the femoral component) and prosthetic design factors (posterior cruciate substituting cut-out) play important roles. Fracture of the medial condyle is more frequent than true supracondylar fracture; however, both are possible, particularly if femoral impaction is excessive or misdirected.

In general, intraoperative fractures in this region should be managed with osteosynthesis, to restore the damaged anatomy, and careful completion of the arthroplasty. The use of a stemmed femoral component to protect the reconstruction is advised. Occasionally, more complicated reconstruction with bone graft or metal augmentation may be required; however, this is usually in revision situations.

Tibial Fractures
Tibial Metaphysis and Shaft Tibial fractures during total knee replacement are uncommon, particularly in the primary setting. Vertical split fractures can occur with impaction when oversized stemmed components are used or when components are malaligned. Revision surgery increases the risk of this type of fracture, as does the use of an extended

tibial tubercle osteotomy for exposure. In general, these fractures may not be recognized at the time of surgery, and will be seen on postoperative radiographs. Management is conservative, with protected weightbearing for 6 to 8 weeks, if the component is well fixed and stable. Normal rehabilitation of range of motion is usually possible. Peripheral rim fractures may also be seen in association with bone deficiency or osteoporosis. These fractures should be managed conservatively if the component and the fracture are stable.

As in the femur, the use of canal-filling stemmed implants during revision arthroplasty increases the risk of intraoperative fracture. These components are often necessary to ensure implant stability and support, but the use of intraoperative radiography is advised to ensure that occult fractures are detected and stabilized at the time of surgery.

Tibial Tubercle Fractures Tibial tubercle avulsion is more common intraoperatively if the knee range of motion is significantly restricted before surgery. In the patellar tendon, stripping along the subperiosteal plane is common, but in osteoporotic bone the failure can be through the tubercle itself. This piece of bone is often small, making secure reattachment difficult. Avulsion may be quite sudden, usually occurring with initial patellar eversion and flexion of the knee. In the tight knee, medial dissection to the midcoronal plane and consideration of proximal quadriceps release or extended tubercle osteotomy may avoid this problem. Established avulsion should be repaired with screws or tension wires and reinforced with soft-tissue repair and postoperative splinting. Active quadriceps activity should be avoided for 6 weeks.

Patellar Fractures
Fracture of the patella during surgery has become more common with the use of patellar clamps during resurfacing. The

incidence is higher in thin patellae or if excessive resection has been performed. A higher incidence of intraoperative fracture is also seen with the use of pegged and press-fit cementless components. Peripheral rim fracture (usually lateral) is more common with the use of inset patellar components.

Management of the fracture depends on the integrity of the extensor mechanism. Longitudinal fractures with an intact mechanism and stable component can be managed conservatively without special postoperative protection. Transverse fractures or those with extensor disruption should be repaired with wire or screw fixation to allow early postoperative mobilization.

Postoperative Fractures
Overview
Periprosthetic fractures around TKA present several management problems. The initial diagnosis is not usually difficult, but may present late, particularly in elderly patients with limited mobility and multiple joint disease. In most patients, a predisposing factor to fracture can be identified. It is important to explore the reasons for fracture to reduce the risk of recurrence and to guide the choice of management. The final decision as to which treatment option is the most appropriate will rest on assessment of the fracture location, the prosthesis fixation, and the quality of the bone around the fracture.

The assessment of prosthesis fixation is perhaps the prime determinant in this decision-making process. It is unusual to accept a loose or grossly malaligned prosthesis and treat the fracture alone. With a fracture around a well-fixed and well-aligned component, however, management is more likely to be open or closed without disturbing the prosthesis. The determination of component fixation is not always obvious, and great care should be taken to establish this before definitive treatment is commenced. Special imaging techniques such as tomography and ultrasound may be necessary to clarify the situation.

As with any fracture, the issue of bone quality is paramount if consideration is given to internal fixation. Poor quality of bone around a fracture site may be the result of a generalized process, such as rheumatoid arthritis or osteoporosis, or may be the result of the fracture itself. Poor bone quality will make rigid internal fixation less predictable, and in some cases will constitute a contraindication to open techniques. Poor bone stock can make revision arthroplasty necessary, even if the components are well fixed.

With the majority of fractures around a prosthesis, the choice of treatment will be between closed management and open fixation with or without prosthesis revision. The indications for closed reduction and open reduction may overlap somewhat, and examples can be found throughout the literature to support both techniques. Treatment algorithms can be presented as broad guidelines to help with this decision; however, fractures must be considered individually.

Femoral Fractures
Supracondylar femoral fracture following TKA has been well covered in recent literature reviews[2-7] including meta-analysis reviews from McLaren and associates[8] and Chen and associates.[9] The overall incidence ranges from 0.3% to 2.5% in these series. A summary of predisposing factors for supracondylar fracture after TKA is presented in Outline 1.

Patient factors present the most common predisposition to fracture. Osteoporosis is a common feature in the population undergoing TKA and is almost universal in those with inflammatory arthritis, which has been associated with a higher incidence of postoperative supracondylar fracture.[6,10] In their review, Culp and associates[2] point to the association between neurologic disorders and fracture. These disorders include obvious predispositions such as epilepsy, Parkinson's disease, and ataxia, and also the less obvious, such as cervical myelopathy and myasthenia gravis.

The other large group of predisposing factors are those associated with technical aspects of the TKA itself. Revision arthroplasty has a higher incidence of fracture than primary surgery.[4] Anterior femoral notching has been implicated by some authors as a predisposing factor;[2,10] however, others do not find an increased incidence.[11] It would seem reasonable that focal stress risers of any cause would predispose to fracture in this area. A report of fracture through a large polyethylene granuloma by Rand[12] highlights this focal etiology. Most of these fractures are associated with relatively low energy trauma such as tripping or twisting

---

Outline 1
Predisposing factors to supracondylar fractures

Systemic	Osteoporosis
	Senile
	Disuse
	Drug-induced
	Chronic disease
	Rheumatoid arthritis
	Neurologic disorders
	Seizures
	Parkinson's disease
	Cerebral palsy
	Polio
	Ataxia
Local	Revision surgery
	Anterior notching
	Malalignment
	Polyethylene wear granuloma
Prosthesis design	
Direct trauma	

Outline 2
Classification of periprosthetic supracondylar fractures

Type 1	Undisplaced fracture–Prosthesis stable
Type 2	Displaced fracture–Prosthesis stable
Type 3	Displaced or undisplaced fracture–Prosthesis loose or failing

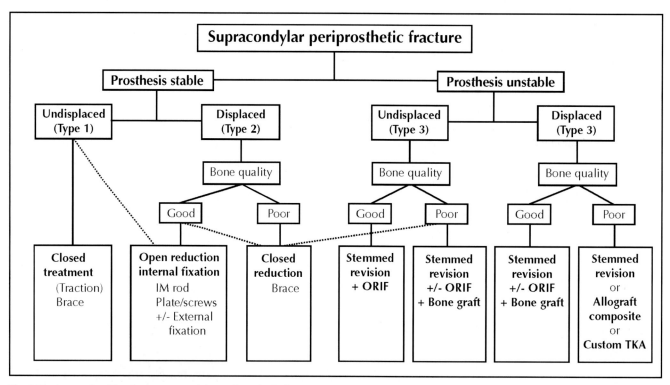

Fig. 2 Treatment algorithm for suprancondylar periprosthetic fractures.

injuries. Restricted range of flexion in the replaced knee also increases the risk of supracondylar fracture. Forced flexion of a prosthetic joint with a limited range of movement produces flexion stresses in the femur above the implant. High-energy trauma, of course, may lead to periprosthetic fracture, and is included here for completeness.

Management A classification of supracondylar periprosthetic fractures is presented in Outline 2. This classification is based on both fracture pattern and prosthesis integrity and is intended as a guide in management decision making. As previously stated, the fixation of the implant is the most important factor in deciding which technique to employ; however, location of the fracture and bone quality are also integral. Many reviews cover the experience with various methods of periprosthetic fracture management in the supracondylar region. Closed reduction,[6,7] open reduction and fixation,[3,13] intramedullary fixation,[14–16]

external fixation,[17] and revision[18–20] have all been advanced for specific indications.

The aim of treatment is to provide the patient with a well-healed fracture with correct alignment and adequate knee motion (at least 90°). Some shortening may be accepted (up to 2 cm). Alignment should be within 5° in the coronal plane and 10° in the sagittal plane.

The treatment algorithm in Figure 2 can serve as a guide to management. The risks of surgery must be balanced against the economic reality of prolonged conservative treatment, and the trend over the last 5 years has been toward open reduction and rigid internal fixation of these fractures.[4,5,13,16,21] This treatment provides early stability, allowing active mobilization of the patient and the joint and thus decreasing the cost and complications of bed rest and hospitalization as opposed to closed techniques.[22,23] Closed treatment, however, remains the appropriate method for minimally displaced fractures with stable configuration and

well-fixed components (type 1 and some type 2). Fractures with poor bone quality may also be better managed conservatively because the risk of failure of internal fixation is high. The most important principle is the maintenance of alignment of both the fracture and the prosthesis until union. Some would employ skeletal traction until callus appears and then cast bracing until union is achieved; however, as the cost of prolonged hospital stays continues to increase, early bracing with close outpatient review has become the standard. Restriction of weightbearing for a minimum of 6 weeks has been advised.[24]

Internal fixation allows accurate alignment and fracture reduction. The risks of deep infection and wound breakdown, however, must be considered. Chen and associates[9] estimate a 5% incidence of life- and limb-threatening complications from open reduction (compared to 1% for closed techniques). Fixation can be achieved with a plate and screws or variations (blade plate, condylar screws, etc). An example of fixation with a dynamic condylar screw and plate system is shown in Figure 3. This technique involves extensive soft-tissue stripping and significant morbidity. Intramedullary devices designed specifically for supracondylar fracture fixation have recently been reported in association with periprosthetic fractures.[14,15,25] These devices can be inserted through the knee; cross fixation allows early stability. Figure 4 shows preoperative and postoperative radiographs of a supracondylar femoral fracture fixed with an intramedullary nail and cross fixation. Early mobilization and discharge from the hospital were appropriate because of rigid fracture fixation. These devices cannot be used with posterior stabilized femoral components because access to the intramedullary canal is blocked by the implant. Osteoporosis is a relative contraindication in using this technique, although fixation may be stable enough to allow mobilization.

Open and semi-open techniques are advised for patients with type II fractures or those in whom prolonged bed rest is contraindicated. Figure 5 shows malunion of displaced fractures of both the tibia and femur around a stable prosthesis. Revision surgery in this situation is technically difficult and may require bulk replacement of the distal femur.

Loosening, malalignment, or instability of the prosthetic components in the presence of poor bone stock are contraindications to the use of closed or isolated open fixation in most patients. It is sometimes desirable to achieve fracture union and then address prosthetic problems, but usually it is best to combine fracture fixation with revision of the knee prosthesis. Use of stemmed revision components combined with direct fixation of the fracture provides reliable correction of both problems.[4,24] Diaphyseal fit is important and the stem should extend well above the fracture. Cement around the stem and fracture should be

avoided, because it may interfere with fracture union. Bone grafting may be needed at the time of revision to augment bone stock. In fractures associated with gross comminution, bone loss, soft bone, or tumor, custom prostheses may be useful to replace the distal end of the femur.[19,20] A similar indication exists for the use of a composite allograft/prosthesis construction.[18]

Complications Chen and associates[9] have stated that the complication rate for both surgical and closed intervention is about 30%. In the nonsurgical group, nonunion (16%) and malunion (10%) are relatively common, as are complications related to prolonged bed rest and casting. Figure 6 shows a fracture above a well-fixed femoral component that was well aligned initially. As union progressed, alignment was lost and the final result was a gross malunion that required osteotomy and revision of the prosthesis. These complications are not as common in the surgical group, with nonunion estimated at about 12%. Reoperation for infection, bone grafting, and even arthrodesis may range up to 13%. Knee stiffness is a problem initially in both groups. If rigid internal fixation is achieved, early motion with continuous passive motion equipment and supervised physiotherapy is beneficial.

Tibial Fractures
Periprosthetic fracture of the tibia is uncommon. The literature offers largely anecdotal studies, most of which use stemmed implants for revision surgery around the fracture.[26] Fractures after extended tubercle osteotomy have also been reported.[27] The incidence of rim and plateau fractures may be underestimated because these may present as florid tibial component loosening and subsidence. Rand and Coventry[28] have reported stress fracture of the medial tibial plateau with varus alignment of the prosthesis, leading to prosthesis failure.

Predisposing factors for tibial fracture

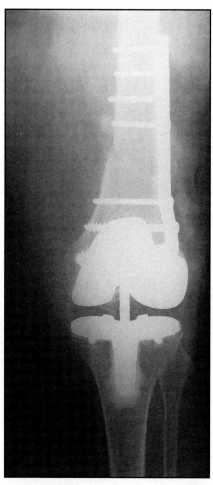

Fig. 3 Open reduction and internal fixation of a supracondylar fracture with condylar screw and plate. Refracture of the femur at the proximal end of this plate required replating with a longer device.

are similar to those for the femur. Tibial tubercle osteotomy and local stress risers caused by short stemmed implants are more specific to this region and may be added to the list presented in Outline 1. An example of fracture through a granulomatous cyst around a tibial implant is shown in Figure 7. A similar case involving the femur has been reported by Rand.[12]

Management As with femoral fractures, the integrity of the prosthetic fixation and the bone quality are the primary factors in deciding the most appropriate treatment option. If the prosthesis is well

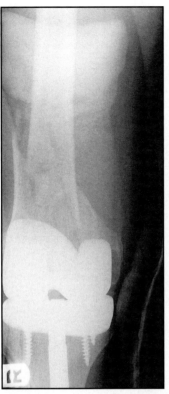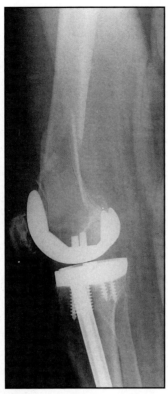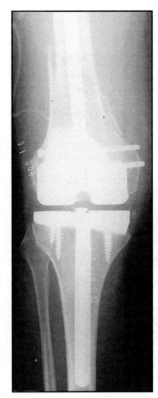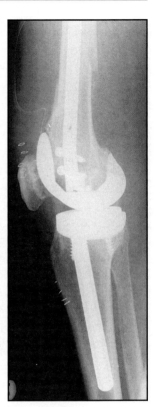

Fig. 4 Left, Anteroposterior and lateral radiographs of a supracondylar periprosthetic fracture. **Right,** Rigid fixation is achieved with an intramedullary nail inserted through the knee with percutaneous cross fixation.

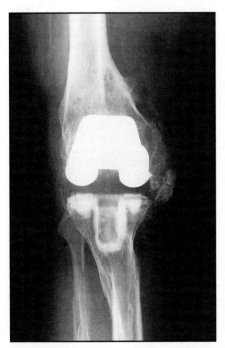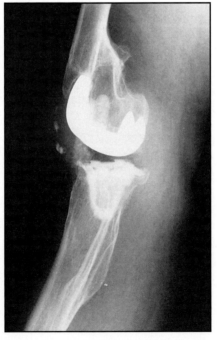

Fig. 5 Anteroposterior and lateral radiographs showing malunion of displaced fractures of femur and tibia with translation and loss of alignment. Revision requires major reconstruction and stemmed implants.

fixed and the fracture pattern stable and in good alignment, closed techniques are performed. A long leg cast, followed by a hinged cast brace when the fracture has adequate stability, should maintain the position. Protected weightbearing for at least 6 weeks is advised.

Fractures of the shaft of the tibia distal to a well-fixed prosthesis can occasionally be managed closed. If these fractures are unstable or position is lost, then intramedullary fixation from below is preferable to open fixation with plate and screws because it avoids soft-tissue stripping around the fracture site. When bone stock is poor, it may sometimes be necessary to revise the tibial component even though it remains well fixed. Fractures of the plateau and metaphysis may be associated with loss of component fixation. In some cases, stability and early mobilization can be achieved with minimal internal fixation.

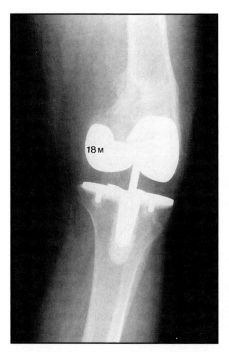

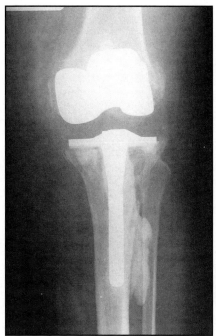

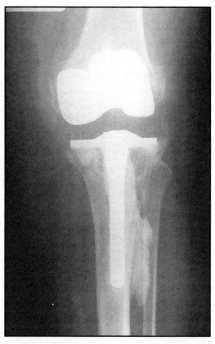

Fig. 6 Malunion of an initially undisplaced supracondylar fracture. Revision surgery and osteotomy were required.

Fig. 7 Anteroposterior and lateral radiographs showing fracture through a polyethylene granuloma around a tibial prosthesis. Revision arthroplasty was required.

Revision should be performed if the prosthesis is loose. Use of stemmed components with or without bone grafting would seem to be the treatment of choice of this group. The algorithm presented for femoral fractures in Figure 2 can also be applied to tibial fractures.

Patellar Fractures

Fractures of the patella are the most frequent periprosthetic fractures encountered with TKA, although even they are not common. Patellar fractures can occur without resurfacing of the patella (incidence 0.05%), but are obviously more common if resurfacing has been undertaken (incidence 0.33 %).[13] There are several extensive reviews of patella fractures occurring after TKA,[29-34] and this complication is discussed in broader reviews of patellar problems after TKA in several other reports.[35-38]

Patella fractures are usually traumatic or stress fractures, with the latter being more common. Stress fractures are usu-

ally transverse or longitudinal (usually laterally based). Examples of stress fractures of resurfaced patellae are shown in Figure 8. The predisposing factors for stress fracture of the patella are presented in Outline 3. Patient-related factors are similar to those for supracondylar femoral fracture (eg, osteoporosis, rheumatoid arthritis, etc); however, the incidence of patellar fracture is also increased in males and active patients. Insall implicates excessive range of motion in the early postoperative period as a predisposing factor.[24] Implant factors are related to the type of component used. Deep central pegs and press-fit cementless components are believed to increase fracture risk. The increased stresses associated with posterior stabilized prostheses may render the patella more liable to stress fracture.

Technical factors such as excessive bone resection or resurfacing of thin (< 13 mm) patellae are predisposing factors, along with revision surgery, heat necrosis

from cement, and patellar devascularization. Lateral release of the patellar retinaculum has been implicated as a predisposing factor to stress fracture of the patella.[39] Scuderi and associates[40] have used technetium bone scanning to record postoperative vascularity of the patella. They found an incidence of "cold" patellae in 56.4% of those who had undergone lateral release and in 15% of those in whom this procedure had not been performed. A similar study by Ritter and Campbell,[41] however, failed to reproduce this finding. They found patellar fracture to be less common after lateral release.

Treatment A classification of patellar fractures is presented in Outline 4. This classification relies on the integrity of the extensor mechanism and fixation of the patellar component as a guide to management decision making. The extensor mechanism is the key in this process.

An algorithm of a management pathway after a periprosthetic fracture of the patella is presented in Figure 9.

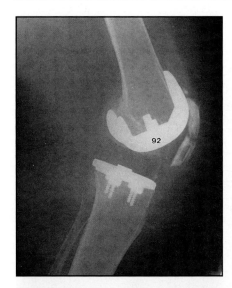
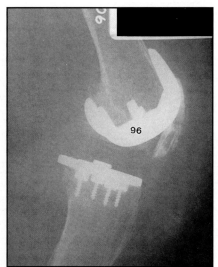
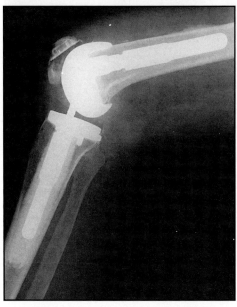
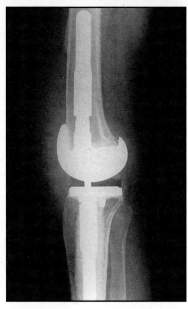

Outline 3
Predisposing factors to patellar fracture after TKA

Patient factors	Osteoporosis
	Rheumatoid arthritis
	Male
	Active
	Excessive range of motion
Implant factors	Patellar replacement/non-replacement
	Central peg
	Cementless
	Posterior cruciate ligament substituting prosthesis
	Inset design
	Osteolysis
Technical factors	Excessive resection
	Inadequate resection
	Anterior patellar perforation
	Revision
	Malalignment
	Patella subluxation
	Devascularization of patella

Outline 4
Classification of patellar fractures[12]

Type 1	Extensor mechanism intact Not extending to implant interface
Type 2	Extensor mechanism disrupted or extension to implant interface
Type 3	Inferior pole fracture Patellar ligament rupture Patellar ligament intact
Type 4	Associated patellar dislocation

Fig. 8 Top left, Patellar stress fracture with loose component. **Top right,** Long-term follow-up with preservation of the patellar implant. Extensor function was considered satisfactory. **Bottom left,** Patellar stress fracture with maltracking of the fragments and loose component. **Bottom right,** Patellectomy was required.

Transverse and vertical fractures represent the majority of presentations. As with other fracture sites, the prime discriminator is the fixation of the prosthetic component. Extensor mechanism integrity is also central to the selection of appropriate treatment.

The typical stress-induced patella fracture does not hamper function of the extensor mechanism and therefore can be treated conservatively (Fig. 8, *top*). These fractures are often insidious in onset and are seen only on routine radiographic follow-up. Even comminuted posttraumatic fractures do not usually disrupt the extensor mechanism and, as long as the component is stable, can be managed nonsurgically. Install recommends 6 weeks in a plaster cylinder with full weightbearing for these fractures.[34]

Fractures that produce significant extensor lag or are displaced by more than 2 cm should be repaired to restore the integrity of the extensor mechanism. Tension band wiring or use of lag screws are the techniques of choice and the repair should be protected postoperatively as for any patellar fracture. If the component is loose, then removal without replacement is advised because of the unreliable refixation of the component with healing fracture. In severely comminuted fractures or those producing maltracking of the fragments, patellectomy is sometimes required (Fig. 8, *bottom*).

The results of conservative treatment for patellar fractures are generally good.

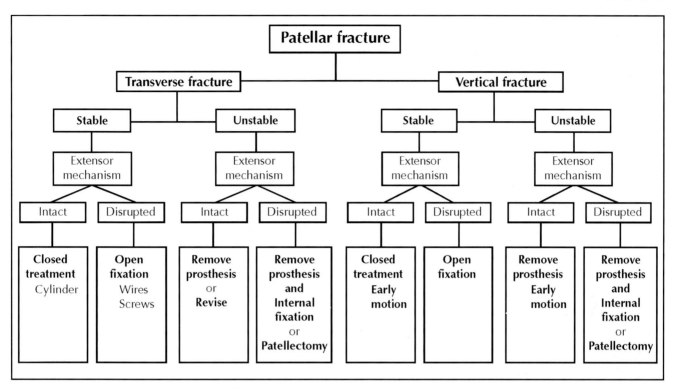

Patellar fracture

Transverse fracture — Vertical fracture

Stable | Unstable | Stable | Unstable

Extensor mechanism

Intact | Disrupted | Intact | Disrupted | Intact | Disrupted | Intact | Disrupted

| Closed treatment Cylinder | Open fixation Wires Screws | Remove prosthesis or **Revise** | Remove prosthesis and **Internal fixation** or **Patellectomy** | Closed treatment Early motion | Open fixation | Remove prosthesis Early motion | Remove prosthesis and **Internal fixation** or **Patellectomy** |

Fig. 9 Treatment alogrithm for periprosthetic patellar fractures.

Immobilization of a TKA for 6 weeks may lead to slight decrease in the overall knee score; however, final range of movement and the need for walking aids is not significantly changed from the prefracture situation.[30,32,33] Extensor disruption or patellar dislocation associated with fracture, on the other hand, lead to significant increase in the need for walking aids, loss of extensor power, and loss of movement range.

Conclusion

Periprosthetic fractures represent difficult management problems in most cases. Fractures around a TKA may present as catastrophic failure or more subtle stress fracture, and the surgeon is provided with a spectrum of management options. The decision whether or not to perform surgery will be based on the location of the fracture, the displacement of the fracture, the fixation and stability of the prosthesis, and the quality of the bone around the fracture and prosthesis. Loss of func-

tion and the expectations for treatment in the individual patient are also considerations. The management pathways described provide a general guide to treatment, but the needs of the individual patient will dictate the final choice and outcome.

References

1. Fipp G: Stress fractures of the femoral neck following total knee arthroplasty. *J Arthroplasty* 1988;3:347–350.

2. Culp RW, Schmidt RG, Hanks G, et al: Supracondylar fracture of the femur following prosthetic knee arthroplasty. *Clin Orthop* 1987;222:212–222.

3. DiGioia AM III, Rubash HE: Periprosthetic fractures of the femur after total knee arthroplasty: A literature review and treatment algorithm. *Clin Orthop* 1991;271:135–142.

4. Figgie MP, Goldberg VM, Figgie HE III, et al: The results of treatment of supracondylar fracture above total knee arthroplasty. *J Arthroplasty* 1990;5:267–276.

5. Healy WL, Siliski JM, Incavo SJ: Operative treatment of distal femoral fractures proximal to total knee replacements. *J Bone Joint Surg* 1993;75A:27–34.

6. Merkel KD, Johnson EW Jr: Supracondylar fracture of the femur after total knee arthroplasty. *J Bone Joint Surg* 1986;68A:29–43.

7. Sisto DJ, Lachiewicz PF, Insall JN: Treatment of supracondylar fractures following prosthetic arthroplasty of the knee. *Clin Orthop* 1985;196:265–272.

8. McLaren AC, Dupont JA, Schroeber DC: Open reduction internal fixation of supracondylar fractures above total knee arthroplasties using the intramedullary supracondylar rod. *Clin Orthop* 1994;302:194–198.

9. Chen F, Mont MA, Bachner RS: Management of ipsilateral supracondylar femur fractures following total knee arthroplasty. *J Arthroplasty* 1994;9:521–526.

10. Aaron RK, Scott R: Supracondylar fracture of the femur after total knee arthroplasty. *Clin Orthop* 1987;219:136–139.

11. Ritter MA, Faris PM, Keating EM: Anterior femoral notching and ipsilateral supracondylar femur fracture in total knee arthroplasty. *J Arthroplasty* 1988;3:185–187.

12. Rand JA: Supracondylar fracture of the femur associated with polyethylene wear after total knee arthroplasty: A case report. *J Bone Joint Surg* 1994;76A:1389–1393.

13. Zehntner MK, Ganz R: Internal fixation of supracondylar fractures after condylar total knee arthroplasty. *Clin Orthop* 1993;293:219–224.

14. Jabczenski FF, Crawford M: Retrograde intramedullary nailing of supracondylar femur fractures above total knee arthroplasty: A preliminary report of four cases. *J Arthroplasty* 1995;10:95–101.

15. Murrell GA, Nunley JA: Interlocked supracondylar intramedullary nails for supracondylar fractures after total knee arthroplasty: A new treatment method. *J Arthroplasty* 1995;10:37–42.

16. Ritter MA, Keating EM, Faris PM, et al: Rush rod fixation of supracondylar fractures above total knee arthroplasties. *J Arthroplasty* 1995;10:213–216.

17. Biswas SP, Kurer MH, Mackenney RP: External fixation for femoral shaft fracture after Stanmore total knee replacement. *J Bone Joint Surg* 1992;74B:313–314.

18. Kraay MJ, Goldberg VM, Figgie MP, et al: Distal femoral replacement with allograft/prosthetic reconstruction for treatment of supracondylar fractures in patients with total knee arthroplasty. *J Arthroplasty* 1992;7:7–16.

19. MacEachern AG, Ling RS: Ununited supracondylar fracture of the femur following Attenborough stabilized gliding knee arthroplasty treated by distal femoral replacement. *Injury* 1983;15:214–216.

20. Madsen F, Kjaersgaard-Andersen P, Juhl M, et al: A custom-made prosthesis for the treatment of supracondylar femoral fractures after total knee arthroplasty: Report of four cases. *J Orthop Trauma* 1989;3:332–337.

21. Short WH, Hootnick DR, Murray DG: Ipsilateral supracondylar femur fractures following knee arthroplasty. *Clin Orthop* 1981;158:111–116.

22. Delport PH, Van Audekercke R, Martens M, et al: Conservative treatment of ipsilateral supracondylar femoral fracture after total knee arthroplasty. *J Trauma* 1984;24:846–849.

23. Nielsen BF, Petersen VS, Varmarken JE: Fracture of the femur after knee arthroplasty. *Acta Orthop Scand* 1988;59:155–157.

24. Insall JN, Haas SB: Complications of total knee arthroplasty, in Insall JN, Windsor RE, Scott WN, et al (eds): *Surgery of the Knee*, ed 2. New York, NY, Churchill Livingstone, 1993, vol 2, pp 891–934.

25. Rolston LR, Christ DJ, Halpern A, et al: Treatment of supracondylar fractures of the femur proximal to a total knee arthroplasty: A report of four cases. *J Bone Joint Surg* 1995;77A:924.–931.

26. Cordeiro EN, Costa RC, Carazzato JG, et al: Periprosthetic fractures in patients with total knee arthroplasties. *Clin Orthop* 1990;252:182–189.

27. Leblanc JM: Patellar complications in total knee arthroplasty: A literature review. *Orthop Rev* 1989;18:296–304.

28. Rand JA, Coventry MB: Stress fractures after total knee arthroplasty. *J Bone Joint Surg* 1980;62A:226–233.

29. Figgie HE III, Goldberg VM, Figgie MP, et al: The effect of alignment of the implant on fractures of the patella after condylar total knee arthroplasty. *J Bone Joint Surg* 1989;71A:1031–1039.

30. Goldberg VM, Figgie HE III, Inglis AE, et al: Patellar fracture type and prognosis in condylar total knee arthroplasty. *Clin Orthop* 1988;236:115–122.

31. Grace JN, Sim FH: Fracture of the patella after total knee arthroplasty. *Clin Orthop* 1988;230:168–175.

32. Hozack WJ, Goll SR, Lotke PA, et al: The treatment of patellar fractures after total knee arthroplasty. *Clin Orthop* 1988;236:123–127.

33. Tria AJ Jr, Harwood DA, Alicea JA, et al: Patella fractures in posterior stabilized knee arthroplasties. *Clin Orthop* 1994;299:131–138.

34. Windsor RE, Scuderi GR, Insall JN: Patella fractures in total knee arthroplasty. *J Arthroplasty* 1989;4(suppl):S63–S67.

35. Brick GW, Scott RD: The patellofemoral component of total knee arthroplasty. *Clin Orthop* 1988;231:163–178.

36. Healy WL, Wasilewski SA, Takei R, et al: Patellofemoral complications following total knee arthroplasty: Correlation with implant design and patient risk factors. *J Arthroplasty* 1995;10:197–201.

37. Martin JW, Whiteside LA: Tibial tubercle osteotomy for exposure in difficult total knee replacement. Proceedings of the American Academy of Orthopaedic Surgeons 62nd Annual Meeting, Orlando, FL. Rosemont, IL, American Academy of Orthopaedic Surgeons, 1995, pp 397.

38. Lynch AF, Rorabeck CH, Bourne RB: Extensor mechanism complications following total knee arthroplasty. *J Arthroplasty* 1987;2:135–140.

39. Scott RD, Turoff N, Ewald FC: Stress fracture of the patella following duopatellar total knee arthroplasty with patellar resurfacing. *Clin Orthop* 1982;170:147–151.

40. Scuderi G, Scharf SC, Meltzer LP, et al: The relationship of lateral releases to patella viability in total knee arthroplasty. *J Arthroplasty* 1987;2:209–214.

41. Ritter MA, Campbell ED: Postoperative patellar complications with or without lateral release during total knee arthroplasty. *Clin Orthop* 1987;219:163–168.

SECTION

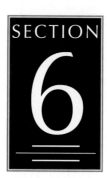

6

Articular Cartilage

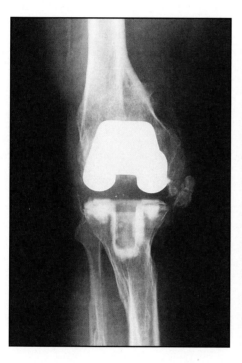
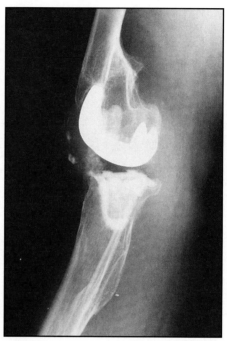

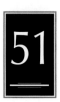

Cartilage and Bone Development

David J. Zaleske, MD

Introduction

There have been several reviews of growth plate development and physiology.[1-4] One intriguing feature of the growth plate is its interface between the basic and clinical sciences of endochondral bone formation.[5] As molecular genetics and molecular development studies elucidate the mechanisms underlying morphogenesis and cytodifferentiation, a fundamental understanding of cartilage and bone is also evolving: how these tissues are formed; how their formation is regulated; and molecular explanations for abnormalities in their formation and regulation.[6] Such knowledge holds the promise of precise intervention in pathologic conditions. Ultimately, some new therapies, such as the revision of an abnormal enzyme to ameliorate abnormalities of the musculoskeletal system that would otherwise result, may not be strictly surgical.[7] Also, some surgical reconstructions that are currently limited by lack of tissue availability may become possible with the advent of engineered tissue, tissue designed and produced combining biology and engineering as a functional substitute for the deficient tissue.[8] An understanding of how tissue is created during normal development is fundamental to this effort.[9,10] A synergistic combination of the use of animal models and an understanding of molecular development will be necessary prior to clinical application.[11-14] The purpose of this chapter is to review the development of bone and cartilage from the vantage point of limb morphogenesis, to indicate how various factors, such as genes and growth factors, are orchestrated in the production of shape, and to review how several abnormalities of cartilage, including physeal cartilage, are understood at the molecular level.

Vertebrate Development

Vertebrate development has been studied descriptively for centuries.[9] The vertebrate skeleton has three main lineages. The craniofacial skeleton is derived from the neural crest. The axial skeleton is derived from the sclerotome of the somites. The appendicular skeleton is derived from the lateral plate mesoderm that will participate in the formation of limb buds. The focus of this chapter will be on limb development as a model system for endochondral bone formation.

Aristotle noted it is advantageous to use the chick in studying development, because part of the shell can be removed from a fertile egg and the events observed directly. Darwin was impressed by the similarities among vertebrate limbs put to various uses throughout phylogeny. In the early part of this century, Morgan began his work with *Drosophila*, which would put genetics on a quantitative basis. Simultaneously, Spemann initiated his studies into experimental embryology and described alterations in shape that can be engendered in amphibian embryos by the transplantation of tissues with specific activity.[15] Morgan was awarded the Nobel prize in 1933;

Spemann in 1935. Molecular genetics exploded with the description of the structure of DNA by Watson and Crick. Continuation of tissue transplantation and ablation experiments in developmental biology led to models of development that were experimentation at the level of tissue interactions. One notable example is the chick limb. However, developmental biology was not to be recognized with another Nobel prize until 1995.[16] In completing a loop, Lewis, Nusslein-Volhard, and Wieschaus were recognized for describing homeobox genes—genes that altered body segmentation in *Drosophila*. Such molecular development might be viewed as a curiosity were it not for the fact that developmentally active genes are highly conserved phylogenetically.

Homeobox genes and other developmentally important genes, which were discovered in *Drosophila*, with its well-described genetics and observable development, were then sought and found functioning in analogous roles in other organisms, including vertebrates. The tissue interaction experiments, such as those that explored chick limb development, can now be repeated and reinterpreted at the molecular level. The situation is synergistic: molecular biology provides the mechanistic explanation for previously described animal models, but the molecular biology alone would be uninterpretable were it not for previously described experiments at the level of the organism. The mouse, a mammal

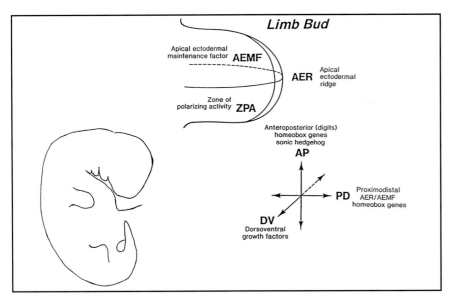

Fig. 1 Diagram of a 4-week-old human embryo at lower left corner, side view, and enlargement of limb bud with axes (PD, proximodistal; AP, anteroposterior; DV, dorsoventral). (Reproduced with permission from Zaleske DJ: Development of components of the skeletal system, in *Principles of Orthopaedic Practice.* New York, NY, McGraw Hill, 1997.)

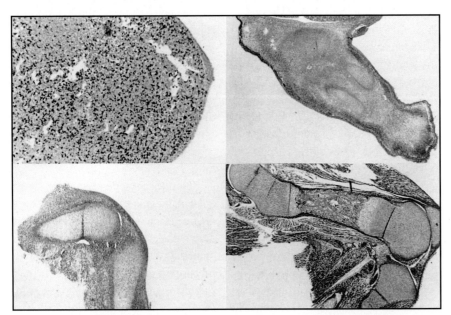

Fig. 2 Composite of four key stages in the development of the veretebrate limb. **Top left,** Autoradiograph of a hindlimb bud from a 3 day chick embryo, ×100. No mesenchymal condensations are present. **Top right,** Hindlimb from a 13 day mouse embryo, ×40. Mesenchymal condensations are forming. **Bottom left,** Hindlimb from a 15 day mouse embryo, ×40. The condensations are beginning to chondrify, and early joint cavitation is occurring in the knee region. **Bottom right,** Hindlimb from an 18 day mouse fetus, ×40. The chondroepiphyses of the proximal and distal femur and the proximal tibia are visible. The primary ossification center of the femur is visible at the midshaft. (Reproduced with permission from Zaleske DJ: Development of components of the skeletal system, in *Principles of Orthopaedic Practice.* New York, NY, McGraw Hill, 1997.)

whose development has clear analogies to *Homo sapiens,* has become an extremely important model system in this regard. The mouse has a well-described genetics with known chromosomal homologies, and the capability to create transgenic and knockout mice has proven very powerful in unraveling developmental mechanisms.[17,18]

Descriptive Embryology

Descriptive embryology is essential to understanding molecular development as a program. While timing may vary, events in limb development at the tissue and cellular levels have marked similarities among vertebrates.[19] In *Homo sapiens,* limb development begins as an outpouching at the lateral body wall at 4 weeks of gestation, and limb morphogenesis is completed at 8 weeks (Fig. 1). At 4 weeks, the limb bud, as seen at the light microscopic level, is undifferentiated mesoderm covered by a jacket of surface ectoderm (Fig. 2, *top left*). A genetic and epigenetic network is established along the three axes of the limb bud. These factors, of course, can only be varied experimentally in animal work (chick and mice being particularly valuable for the reasons noted above), but many lines of evidence indicate that the basic mechanisms are shared by *Homo sapiens.* Outgrowth along the proximodistal (PD) axis is governed by the interaction between a thickening of the ectoderm at the distal end of the limb bud, the apical ectodermal ridge (AER), and the underlying mesoderm, which in turn secretes an apical ectodermal maintenance factor (AEMF). By ablation experiments in the developing chick limb, it was demonstrated that all outgrowth ceases when the AER is removed.[19] The underlying mesoderm adjacent to the AER, a region termed the progress zone, is maintained in an undifferentiated, rapidly proliferating state.[20] Condensations of mesenchyme, the recognizable precursors of the skeletal anlagen, are formed on the proximal side of the progress zone as outgrowth of the limb proceeds. The condensations are formed in a proximal to distal sequence (Fig. 2, *top right*). This phenomenon has been reexamined at the molecular level. Fibroblast growth factors (FGF-1, FGF-2, FGF-4) can induce ectopic limb buds on the flanks of chick embryos.[21] In a limb bud culture system using mouse limb buds, FGF-4 was demonstrated to mediate the outgrowth function of the AER.[22] It is interesting that, in this same system, bone morphogenetic protein-2 (BMP-2) served an inhibitory function.[22] There is also a requirement for BMP signaling in interdigital cell death.[23]

Homeobox Genes

As stated previously, homeobox (*Hox*) genes have been identified as controlling body segmentation in *Drosophila*. These genes produce transcription factors that contain a highly conserved 60 amino acid sequence or homeobox that binds to DNA and regulates its transcription. Homeobox genes occur in clusters, have been highly phylogenetically conserved, and share intriguing geographic properties on the genome and during expression in embryogenesis. Homeobox genes located at the 3´ end of a cluster in the genome are expressed earlier in development and more anteriorly in the embryo. The expression of the homeobox genes precedes the appearance of the mesenchymal condensations. Nomenclature for the homeobox genes has evolved to recognize similarities throughout phylogeny.[24] Two homeobox genes seem to be important in the evolution of the PD axis. *Msx1 (Hox 7)* is expressed in the progress zone and *Msx2 (Hox 8)* is expressed in the AER.[25]

The digits are specified along the anteroposterior (AP) axis of the limb bud. Again, in earlier experiments in tissue ablation and transplantation in the chick, a zone of tissue at the posterior border of the limb bud was noted to possess polarizing activity, crucial to ordering the digits. This zone of polarizing activity (ZPA) was noted to be capable of producing digit duplications when transplanted to the anterior border of the limb bud.[26] Once more this tissue activity has been elucidated to the molecular level. A vertebrate gene, *Sonic hedgehog* (*Shh*), which is related to a *Drosophila* gene, mediates this polarizing activity.[27] Retinoic acid, when applied to the anterior limb bud, has also been shown to be capable of producing digit duplications; retinoic acid also induces *Shh*.[25,27]

Expression of the homeobox genes *HoxD* (*HOXD* in humans) correlates with the specification of digits along the AP axis.[25] While the mechanism of regulation is complex, it would appear that a developmental cascade involving *Shh* and retinoic acid in turn leads to a sequential expression of *HoxD* genes that specify the digits. In humans, it has been demonstrated that mutations in *HOXD13* lead to the transformation of metacarpals and metatarsals into small carpal and tarsal-like structures.[28] This would be consistent with the hypothesis that homeobox genes work to control the mass of mesenchyme that is programmed to condense and the subsequent local growth of that mesenchyme.

The dorsoventral (DV) axis is established by a secreted protein, *WNT7a*, which in turn activates another homeobox gene.[29] The limb pattern is therefore established by an interactive program of genes, the products of which are transcription factors for other genes, signaling molecules, receptors, and local growth regulatory factors. Mesenchymal condensations are the tissue-level result of this information network, patterned from a proximal to distal sequence as the anlagen or recognizable precursors of the skeletal elements to follow. It should be recognized that the morphogenetic program is not a static grid or blueprint that instructs cells to condense at a particular location but rather is a very dynamic three-dimensional spreadsheet.[30] Cells are receivers, processors, and distributors of information, with time being the fourth dimension. Disruptions of this complicated system would in theory result from an abnormality of any single factor. This principle will be illustrated in practice with clinical correlations at the conclusion of this paper.

Limb Development

As limb development continues, the mesenchymal condensations begin to chondrify (Fig. 2, *bottom left*). The interzone regions between the anlagen begin to break down in the process of joint cavitation, which is also beginning to be examined at the molecular level.[31] The articular cartilage is derived from the interzone, whereas the physeal and epiphyseal cartilages are derived from the cartilaginous anlagen. At the end of the embryonic period and beginning of the fetal period (8 weeks in *Homo sapiens*), the chondrocytes at the mid-shafts of the cartilaginous anlagen of the long bones become hypertrophic and elicit vascular invasion, and formation of the primary centers of ossification begins (Fig. 2, *bottom right*). The transformation from small round chondrocytes to hypertrophic chondrocytes is a theme put to use at various locations, including within the growth plate itself.[32-34] The molecular regulation of this transformation will be discussed below. At this stage, the articular cartilage, epiphyseal cartilage, and physeal cartilage are contiguous in a single cartilaginous mass. It can be appreciated that this cartilaginous mass at either end of a long bone is already quite heterogeneous, with separate chondrocytic populations for articulation, growth of the articular surface, growth of the chondroepiphysis, and growth of the long bone.

The appearance and growth of the secondary center of ossification within the chondroepiphysis demarcates these populations more clearly, but their functional heterogeneity was established

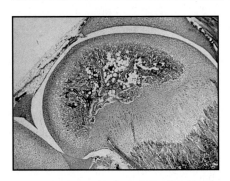

Fig. 3 Distal femoral chondroepiphysis from a 10 day postnatal mouse, ×40. The secondary center of ossification has now formed. The growth plate is clearly defined between the secondary center of ossification and the metaphysis. (Reproduced with permission from Zaleske DJ: Development of components of the skeletal system, in *Principles of Orthopaedic Practice*. New York, NY, McGraw Hill, 1997.)

much earlier by the developmental events described above (Fig. 3). In humans, the secondary centers of ossification generally appear postnatally, the single exception being that of the distal femur, which appears at 36 weeks of gestation. The round or small bones of the carpus and tarsus ossify at various times pre- and postnatally to form the equivalent of the primary centers of ossification of the long bones. Because these bones have generally spherical growth plates and never form secondary centers of ossification, their growth plates, unlike the growth plates of long bones, are never revealed as radiolucent lines between (radiopaque) osseous tissue on conventional radiography. In cases of intoxication with heavy metal, such as lead, all growth plates, including these spherical growth plates of small bones, avidly accumulate the ingested marker at the zone of provisional ossification.

Growth Plate Development

With the formation of the secondary center of ossification and its growth to occupy a large part of the chondroepiphysis, the physeal cartilage becomes a growth plate (Fig. 3). It should be recognized that the cytodifferentiation of the growth plate was clearly present even at the light microscopic level, prior to the formation of the secondary center of ossification (Figs. 2, *top right*, and 3). The functional heterogeneity of all articular and proliferating cartilage resulted from the earlier events in development. Endochondral

bone follows the pattern that is the net result of all these embryologic events precisely orchestrated in space and time.

The zones of the growth plate have been divided into reserve, proliferative, upper hypertrophic, lower hypertrophic, and zone of provisional calcification. The biochemical functions of these zones have been studied in detail, with much of the original work having been performed by orthopaedic scientists.[1]

The resting, or reserve, zone at one time was thought to provide the new cells entering into the columnar progression to hypertrophic cells at the metaphyseal side of the growth plate, but the work of Kember demonstrated that the kinetic activity was confined to the proliferative zone.[35-37] The reserve zone appears to function in lipid and glycogen storage and may serve as a structure to limit the advance of the secondary center of ossification on the epiphyseal side.

The proliferative zone is dedicated to rapid, ordered cell division and matrix production. Cell division is clearly central to the continual movement of the growth plate away from the advancing ossification of the metaphysis. Matrix functions are also critical.[38] Proteoglycan size—large at the proliferative zone to small at the hypertrophic zone—is important in hydration and in regulating the calcification of the matrix.[39] Collagen is important in maintaining the columnar arrangement of the chondrocytes, thus bringing order and direction to the kinetic activity. The predominant collagen type is type II; type

X collagen seems to be important in endochondral ossification, because its expression is limited to the terminal hypertrophic chondrocytes.[40,41]

In the upper hypertrophic zone, cell swelling begins, another key parameter in determining rate of growth.[33,34] Calcium begins to be accumulated in the mitochondria of the chondrocytes of the upper hypertrophic zone.

In the lower hypertrophic zone, cell swelling continues. Proteoglycan size decreases, rendering the matrix calcifiable as calcium is discharged by the mitochondria. There is an abrupt appearance of type X collagen. Angiogenesis proceeds at the zone of provisional calcification. Bone is first formed as the primary spongiosa. Type I collagen, the bone collagen, is synthesized by the osteoblasts. Remodeling proceeds with resorption of the primary spongiosa by osteoclasts and formation of the secondary spongiosa. The remodeling process is particularly active at the metaphysis but continues throughout life being the net result of genetic, inductive, and mechanical factors.

Cartilage

The regulation of cartilage proliferation determines the shape that the skeleton attains at maturity. It has long been recognized that cartilage proliferation is under hormonal or endocrine control. Notable anabolic or up-regulators include growth hormone, which acts through the somatomedins or insulin-like growth factor I (IGF-I), thyroxine, parathyroid hormone, and sex steroids.[2,4] Vitamins that have important regulatory functions are A, C, and D. Vitamin A is required for normal chondrocyte maturation. Vitamin C is necessary for normal collagen synthesis. Vitamin D and its metabolites are necessary for the normal mineralization at the hypertrophic side of the growth plate. These factors interact in complex ways to control growth at the systemic level.

An increasingly important topic is

the control of growth at the local level. One of the important aspects underlying this local control is the mass of cells recruited for growth in the original anlagen. As discussed previously, this recruitment or programming is the net result of a cascade of developmentally active genes, including the homeobox genes, inductive factors, and growth factors. Relative to the mammalian growth plate, which may be viewed as the terminal extension at either end of the primary center of ossification, the concept that the mass of cells recruited for proliferation is a factor in regulating growth, has recently been verified experimentally.[42] The differential rate of growth at different growth plates could be attributed to the size and cellular density of the proliferative zone and cell cycle time. It follows that the regulation of conversion from the small cell chondrocyte phenotype to the hypertrophic phenotype and the associated extracellular matrix changes constitute another important regulator of growth. A negative feedback loop has been demonstrated that governs this conversion.[43,44]

The gene *Sonic hedgehog (Shh)* and its importance in development has been discussed above. A related gene *Indian hedgehog (Ihh)* was noted to be expressed in the prehypertrophic chondrocytes of the cartilage anlagen. *Ihh* indirectly controls the rate at which chondrocytes differentiate into the hypertrophic phenotype. *Ihh* signals the perichondrium and induces another signaling molecule, parathyroid hormone-related protein (PTHrP). The receptor for PTHrP also responds to parathyroid hormone (PTH). The PTH/PTHrP receptor is expressed in several areas including bone, kidney, and proliferating chondrocytes. The PTHrP directly slows the conversion of proliferating to hypertrophic chondrocytes, thus completing an *Ihh*-PTHrP negative feedback loop. This function represents a very significant example of the autocrine/paracrine control of growth, in which sig-

naling molecules are produced and act on the same cells or on cells near their site of production. It is interesting to note that the PTH/PTHrP receptor thus will respond to either an endocrine pathway (PTH) or a paracrine pathway (PTHrP). Exactly how all the endocrine and autocrine/paracrine signals are integrated remains unclear. Also, the role that physical force plays in the control of the growth plate has been recognized as important since the enunciation of the Hueter-Volkmann principle.[45] Its interaction with both pathways will also require elucidation.[46,47]

Growth Hormones

Another example of interaction between endocrine and autocrine/paracrine pathways is regulation of the growth plate by growth hormone. Although growth hormone is a fundamental regulator of skeletal growth, its action on the growth plate is not direct.[4] Growth hormone is synthesized by the pituitary. Released into the circulation, it stimulates the liver, which in turn synthesizes and releases IGF-I (somatomedin). IGF-I then causes the growth plate to produce further IGF-I, which has a positive autocrine or paracrine proliferative effect on growth plate chondrocytes.

To return to the very factors that were crucial in the histogenesis of the growth plate, fibroblast growth factors and transforming growth factor-beta (TGF-β) have important autocrine and paracrine regulatory functions in the growth plate.[48] Basic fibroblast growth factor (bFGF) and IGF-I have a synergistic effect on cell division of growth plate chondrocytes.[49] The site of action of bFGF seems to be on less mature, proliferative chondrocytes. It will be recalled that FGF was important in the induction and outgrowth of the limb bud. TGF-β appears to be another important autocrine/paracrine regulator of chondrocyte maturation. The TGF-β superfamily includes the bone morphogenetic

proteins. The transition from cartilage to bone is at least partly under the control of this class of molecules; once more correlation can be made to *Drosophila* molecular genetics and development.[50]

Abnormal Growth

Although far from complete, this outline of molecular cartilage and bone development may now be used to correlate abnormalities in the pathways with clinical conditions.[51,52] The chondrodysplasias in particular will be the focus of this correlation. It might be anticipated that as specific pathogenetic mechanisms are elucidated they will be located in various groups in the developmental pathways.[53] Such has indeed been the case, and examples now exist in several categories: (1) structural molecules; (2) metabolism; (3) local regulators; (4) systemic regulators; (5) gene identified but pathogenetic mechanism not established; and (6) gene linkage established but specific gene not yet identified.

Structural Molecules

Because type II collagen is the major collagen in cartilage, it is logical to assume that many chondrodysplasias result from defects in either the quality or quantity of this molecule, and this is indeed the case. Abnormalities in type II collagen underlie achondrogenesis II/hypochondrogenesis, some types of spondyloepiphyseal dysplasia, Kniest dysplasia, and some forms of Stickler syndrome.[54,55] Abnormalities in type IX collagen are found in some of the kindreds of Fairbanks multiple epiphyseal dysplasia.[56] Mutations in type X collagen cause the Schmid-type chondrometaphyseal dysplasia.[57] In a subset of Stickler syndrome distinct from that associated with the type II collagenopathy, a mutation has been described in type XI collagen.[58] Finally, a quite heterogeneous group of type I collagenopathies have been described throughout the spectrum of osteogenesis imperfecta.[52]

Metabolism

The prototypical example of a defect in cartilage metabolism is diastrophic dwarfism. The mutation that underlies this condition is in a gene encoding a sulfate transporter molecule, the diastrophic dysplasia sulfate transporter.[59] This mutation leads to an undersulfation of proteoglycans. Although this undersulfation exists throughout the body, its most apparent dramatic impact is on cartilage. It will be remembered that proteoglycan size and hydration were important factors in the function of the growth plate. The disturbance in growth that results from this defect in cartilage metabolism produces the short stature and particularly severe equinovarus deformities seen in this condition.

Local Regulators

Achondroplasia is the prime example of a disturbance in local control of cartilage growth. It has been apparent for some time that achondroplasia is a defect in endochondral bone growth. The molecular basis has now been established as an abnormality in fibroblast growth factor receptor.[3,60,61] Unlike the molecular heterogeneity that underlies osteogenesis imperfecta, most cases of achondroplasia occur because of a mutation in a single base pair resulting in a single amino acid substitution in the receptor.

Parathyroid hormone-related protein (PTHrP) has been noted for its importance in the regulation of cartilage transition from small cell to hypertrophic phenotype. A mutation in the PTHrP receptor resulting in a constitutively active state has been described as the defect behind Jansen-type chondrometaphyseal dysplasia.[62,63] This type has a radiographic similarity to rickets. The constitutively active receptor allows a too rapid conversion of chondrocytes to the hypertrophic phenotype and, because it is the shared receptor for PTH, leads to hypercalcemia and hypophosphatemia with normal levels of PTH.

Systemic Regulators

The mucopolysaccharidoses result from systemic enzymatic defects that have variable effects on proliferating cartilage.[64] To variable degrees they share a spondyloepiphyseal dysplasia phenotype.

Gene and Mechanism Disorders

Campomelic dysplasia is a disorder with an identified gene but an unknown mechanism.[65,66] There is an association with sex reversal. Stature is markedly shortened, with delayed ossification and kyphosis of the thoracic spine. The gene, *SOX9*, is expressed in condensing mesenchyme but not in cartilage.

Developmental abnormalities that are caused by failure to recruit and program mesenchyme appropriately might be included either in the fifth category, identified gene with unknown mechanism, or in the final one, linkage established but gene unidentified. The abnormal branching and growth pattern attributed to *HOXD13* is an example of the former.[28] A complex polysyndactyly mapping to 7q36 is an example of the latter.[67]

Conclusion

The considerable information that has been garnered regarding cartilage and bone development may now be taken further to the level of molecular genetics, molecular development, and molecular signal transduction in several areas. Much work remains to be done before there is a complete molecular explanation for musculoskeletal development. Given the current rate of advance, this explanation may be available in the not too distant future. Even given such knowledge, treatments and their timing may vary markedly. Provision of a circulating hormone, such as growth hormone, postnatally is already possible. Correcting a structural molecule or receptor with somatic distribution postnatally will prove more challenging. The possibility of regenerating autogeneic cartilage coupled with orthopaedic surgical techniques should allow us to provide our patients with treatments that currently do not exist. Ultimately, clinical care will be improved by a fundamental understanding of the development of cartilage and bone.

References

1. Brighton CT: Longitudinal bone growth: The growth plate and its dysfunctions, in Griffin PP (ed): *Instructional Course Lectures XXXVI*. Park Ridge, IL, American Academy of Orthopaedic Surgeons, 1987, pp 3–25.

2. Iannotti JP, Goldstein S, Kuhn J, et al: Growth plate and bone development, in Simon SR (ed): *Orthopaedic Basic Science*. Rosemont, IL, American Academy of Orthopaedic Surgeons, 1994, pp 185–217.

3. Robertson WW Jr: Newest knowledge of the growth plate. *Clin Orthop* 1990;253:270–278.

4. Trippel SB: Basic science of the growth plate. *Curr Opin Orthop* 1990;1:279–288.

5. Rosenberg LC: Editorial: The physis as an interface between basic research and clinical knowledge. *J Bone Joint Surg* 1984;66A:815–816.

6. Erlebacher A, Filvaroff EH, Gitelman SE, et al: Toward a molecular understanding of skeletal development. *Cell* 1995;80:371–378.

7. Evans CH, Robbins PD: Possible orthopaedic applications of gene therapy. *J Bone Joint Surg* 1995;77A:1103–1114.

8. Langer R, Vacanti JP: Tissue engineering. *Science* 1993;260:920–926.

9. Sledge CB, Zaleske DJ: Developmental anatomy of joints, in Resnick D, Niwayama G, (eds): *Diagnosis of Bone and Joint Disorders*, ed 2. Philadelphia, PA, WB Saunders, 1988, vol 2, pp 604–624.

10. Crelin ES: Development of the musculoskeletal system. *Clin Symp* 1981;33:1–36.

11. Wolohan MJ, Zaleske DJ: Hemiepiphyseal reconstruction using tissue donated from fetal limbs in a murine model. *J Orthop Res* 1991;9:180–185.

12. Barr SJ, Zaleske DJ, Mankin HJ: Physeal replacement with cultured chondrocytes of varying developmental time: Failure to reconstruct a functional or structural physis. *J Orthop Res* 1993;11:10–19.

13. Barr SJ, Zaleske DJ: Physeal reconstruction with blocks of cartilage of varying developmental time. *J Pediatr Orthop* 1992;12:766–773.

14. Savarese JJ III, Brinken BW, Zaleske DJ: Epiphyseal replacement in a murine model. *J Pediatr Orthop* 1995;15:682–690.

15. Hamburger V (ed): *The Heritage of Experimental Embryology: Hans Spemann and the Organizer Viktor Hamburger.* New York, NY, Oxford University Press, 1988.

16. Roush W: Nobel prizes: Fly development work bears prize-winning fruit. *Science* 1995;270:380–381.

17. Hanahan D: Transgenic mice as probes into complex systems. *Science* 1989;246: 1265–1275.

18. Majzoub JA, Muglia LJ: Knockout mice. *N Engl J Med* 1996;334:904–907.

19. Hinchliffe JR, Johnson DR (eds): *The Development of the Vertebrate Limb: An Approach Through Experiment, Genetics and Evolution.* Oxford, England, Clarendon Press, 1980.

20. Summerbell D, Lewis JH, Wolpert L: Positional information in chick limb morphogenesis. *Nature* 1973;244:492–496.

21. Cohn MJ, Izpisua-Belmonte JC, Abud H, et al: Fibroblast growth factors induce additional limb development from the flank of chick embryos. *Cell* 1995;80: 739–746.

22. Niswander L, Martin GR: FGF-4 and BMP-2 have opposite effects on limb growth. *Nature* 1993;361:68–71.

23. Zou H, Niswander L: Requirement for BMP signaling in interdigital apoptosis and scale formation. *Science* 1996;272: 738–741.

24. Scott MP: Vertebrate homeobox gene nomenclature. *Cell* 1992;71:551–553.

25. Tabin CJ: Retinoids, homeoboxes, and growth factors: Toward molecular models for limb development. *Cell* 1991;66: 199–217.

26. Saunders JW, Gasseling M: Ectodermal-mesenchymal interaction in the origin of limb symmetry, in Fleischmajer R, Billingham RE (eds): *Epithelial-Mesenchymal Interactions.* Baltimore, MD, Williams & Wilkins, 1968, pp 78–97.

27. Riddle RD, Johnson RL, Laufer E, et al: Sonic hedgehog mediates the polarizing activity of the ZPA. *Cell* 1993;75: 1401–1416.

28. Muragaki Y, Mundlos S, Upton J, et al: Altered growth and branching patterns in synpolydactyly caused by mutations in HOXD13. *Science* 1996;272:548–551.

29. Riddle RD, Ensini M, Nelson C, et al: Induction of the LIM homeobox gene Lmx1 by WNT7a establishes dorsoventral pattern in the vertebrate limb. *Cell* 1995; 83:631–640.

30. Duboule D: How to make a limb? *Science* 1994;266:575–576.

31. Storm EE, Huynh TV, Copeland NG, et al: Limb alterations in brachypodism mice due to mutations in a new member of the TGF beta-superfamily. *Nature* 1994;368:639–643.

32. Floyd WE III, Zaleske DJ, Schiller AL, et al: Vascular events associated with the appearance of the secondary center of ossification in the murine distal femoral epiphysis. *J Bone Joint Surg* 1987;69A:185–190.

33. Buckwalter JA, Mower D, Ungar R, et al: Morphometric analysis of chondrocyte hypertrophy. *J Bone Joint Surg* 1986;68A: 243–255.

34. Hunziker EB, Schenk RK, Cruz-Orive LM: Quantitation of chondrocyte performance in growth-plate cartilage during longitudinal bone growth. *J Bone Joint Surg* 1987;69A:162–173.

35. Kember NF: Cell kinetics and the control of growth in long bones. *Cell Tissue Kinet* 1978;11:477–485.

36. Kember NF: Cell division in endochondral ossification: A study of cell proliferation in rat bones by the method of tritiated thymidine autoradiography. *J Bone Joint Surg* 1960;42B:824–839.

37. Kember NF: Cell population kinetics of bone growth: The first ten years of autoradiographic studies with tritiated thymidine. *Clin Orthop* 1971;76:213–230.

38. Buckwalter JA: Proteoglycan structure in calcifying cartilage. *Clin Orthop* 1983;172: 207–232.

39. Ehrlich MG, Armstrong AL, Neuman RG, et al: Patterns of proteoglycan degradation by a neutral protease from human growth-plate epiphyseal cartilage. *J Bone Joint Surg* 1982;64A:1350–1354.

40. Burgeson RE, Nimni ME: Collagen types: Molecular structure and tissue distribution. *Clin Orthop* 1992;282:250–272.

41. Sandell LJ, Sugai JV, Trippel SB: Expression of collagens I, II, X, and XI and aggrecan mRNAs by bovine growth plate chondrocytes in situ. *J Orthop Res* 1994;12: 1–14.

42. Wilsman NJ, Farnum CE, Leiferman EM, et al: Differential growth by growth plates as a function of multiple parameters of chondrocytic kinetics. *Trans Orthop Res Soc* 1996;21:90.

43. Vortkamp A, Lee K, Lanske B, et al: Regulation of rate of cartilage differentiation by Indian Hedgehog and PTH-related protein. *Science* 1996;273:613–622.

44. Lanske B, Karaplis AC, Lee K, et al: PTH/PTHrP receptor in early development and Indian Hedgehog-regulated bone growth. *Science* 1996;273:663–666.

45. Hueter C: Anatomische Studien an den Extremitatengelenken Neugeborener und Erwachsener. *Virchows Archiv* 1862;25: 572–599.

46. Carter DR, Wong M: Mechanical stresses and endochondral ossification in the chondroepiphysis. *J Orthop Res* 1988;6: 148–154.

47. Greco F, de Palma L, Specchia N, et al: Growth-plate cartilage metabolic response to mechanical stress. *J Pediatr Orthop* 1989;9:520–524.

48. Jingushi S, Scully SP, Joyce ME, et al: Transforming growth factor-beta and fibroblast growth factors in rat growth plate. *J Orthop Res* 1995;13:761–768.

49. Trippel SB, Wroblewski J, Makower AM, et al: Regulation of growth-plate chondrocytes by insulin-like growth-factor I and basic fibroblast growth factor. *J Bone Joint Surg* 1993;75A:177–189.

50. Kaplan FS, Hahn GV, Zasloff MA: Heterotopic ossification: Two rare forms and what they can teach us. *J Am Acad Orthop Surg* 1994;2:288–296.

51. Rimoin DL: Molecular defects in the chondrodysplasias. *Am J Med Genet* 1996; 63:106–110.

52. Cole WG: Etiology and pathogenesis of heritable connective tissue diseases. *J Pediatr Orthop* 1993;13:392–403.

53. Spranger J: Pattern recognition in bone dysplasias, in Papadatos CJ, Bartsocas CS (eds): *Endocrine Genetics and Genetics of Growth.* New York, NY, Alan R Liss, 1985, pp 315–342.

54. Spranger J, Winterpacht A, Zabel B: The type II collagenopathies: A spectrum of chondrodysplasias. *Eur J Pediatr* 1994;153: 56–65.

55. Rimoin DL, Cohn DH, Eyre D: Clinical-molecular correlations in the skeletal dysplasias. *Pediatr Radiol* 1994;24:425–426.

56. Briggs MD, Choi H, Warman ML, et al: Genetic mapping of a locus for multiple epiphyseal dysplasia (EDM2) to a region of chromosome I containing a type IX collagen gene. *Am J Hum Genet* 1994;55: 678–684.

57. Warman ML, Abbott M, Apte SS, et al: A type X collagen mutation causes Schmid metaphyseal chondrodysplasia. *Nat Genet* 1993;5:79–82.

58. Vikkula M, Mariman EC, Lui VC, et al: Autosomal dominant and recessive osteochondrodysplasias associated with the COL11A2 locus. *Cell* 1995;80:431–437.

59. Hastbacka J, de la Chapelle A, Mahtani MM, et al: The diastrophic dysplasia gene encodes a novel sulfate transporter: Positional cloning by fine-structure linkage disequilibrium mapping. *Cell* 1994;78: 1073–1087.

60. Shiang R, Thompson LM, Zhu Y-Z, et al: Mutations in the transmembrane domain of FGFR3 cause the most common genetic form of dwarfism, achondroplasia. *Cell* 1994;78:335–342.

61. Le Merrer M, Rousseau F, Legeai-Mallet L, et al: A gene for achondroplasia-hypochondroplasia maps to chromosome 4p. *Nat Genet* 1994;6:318–321.

62. Schipani E, Kruse K, Juppner H: A constitutively active mutant PTH-PTHrP receptor in Jansen-type metaphyseal chondrodysplasia. *Science* 1995;268:98–100.

63. Schipani E, Langman CB, Parfitt AM, et al: Constitutively activated receptors for parathyroid hormone and parathyroid hormone-related peptide in Jansen's metaphyseal chondrodysplasia. *N Engl J Med* 1996;335:708–714.

64. Neufeld EF, Muenzer J: The mucopolysaccharidoses, in Scriver CR, Beaudet AL, Sly WS, et al (eds): *The Metabolic and Molecular Basis of Inherited Disease*, ed 7. New York, NY, McGraw-Hill-Health Professions Division, 1995, vol 2, pp 2465–2494.

65. Tommerup N, Schempp W, Meinecke P, et al: Assignment of an autosomal sex reversal locus (SRA1) and campomelic dysplasia (CMPD1) to 17q24.3-q25.1. *Nat Genet* 1993;4:170–174.

66. Foster JW, Dominguez-Steglich MA, Guioli S, et al: Campomelic dysplasia and autosomal sex reversal caused by mutations in an SRY-related gene. *Nature* 1994;372:525–530.

67. Tsukurov O, Boehmer A, Flynn J, et al: A complex bilateral polysyndactyly disease locus maps to chromosome 7q36. *Nat Genet* 1994;6:282–286.

52

Autocrine Regulation of Articular Cartilage

Randy N. Rosier, MD, PhD
Regis J. O'Keefe, MD

Introduction

The articular cartilage of diarthrodial joints is a remarkable tissue in many regards. The matrix of this tissue is designed to allow joint movement with extremely low friction, and it can withstand high levels of repetitive loading while efficiently transfering these mechanical loads to the underlying subchondral bone. The cartilage of most joints can be expected to function for a lifetime of use, although age-related changes in the cells and matrix occur. One unique feature of articular cartilage is the isolation of the cells composing it from each other and from other cell types, afforded by the collagen and proteoglycan-containing matrix that constitutes the majority of the tissue volume. One of the few tissues in the body that has no vascular supply, it derives its nutrition instead from the synovial fluid. Although metabolically active in matrix maintenance and remodeling, adult articular chondrocytes do not demonstrate significant proliferation under normal conditions. This extremely low rate of proliferation may be one of the reasons why articular cartilage is one of the only tissues from which malignant neoplasms are not known to arise.

Articular chondrocytes derive embryologically from uncommitted mesenchymal cells, which differentiate to form the cartilaginous anlagen of the bones. During fetal development, the process of endochondral ossification transforms the

majority of this cartilaginous model into bone, with the physis and cartilaginous epiphyses persisting into postnatal life. At skeletal maturity, following secondary epiphyseal ossification center development and later fusion of the physes, the only remaining cartilaginous portion of the bone is the articular surface, which remains throughout life. Thus, the articular chondrocytes and the chondrocytes that produce the primary and secondary ossification centers and physes develop from common chondrogenic precursors, although they differ markedly in their terminal state of differentiation. Articular chondrocytes and those capable of endochondral bone formation, such as growth plate chondrocytes, represent different pathways of terminal cartilage differentiation. Once the cells are committed to one of these pathways, the phenotype is not readily reversible, although under some circumstances this can occur. For example, in degenerative arthritis, chondrocytes recapitulate developmental events of endochondral bone formation, with chondrocyte proliferation (cloning) and hypertrophy with expression of type X collagen and alkaline phosphatase.[1]

Reactivation of endochondral ossification in the deep layer of the articular cartilage may contribute in part to the subchondral sclerosis often observed radiographically in degenerative arthritis. This reversion to the endochondral ossification pathway demonstrates some degree of plasticity in the phenotype.

Similarly, when chondrocytes or explants of growth plate are placed in an articular defect, the surface layers take on the appearance and phenotype of articular cartilage.[2] The matrix and synovial fluid environment undoubtedly play extremely important roles in the maintenance of the articular chondrocyte phenotype.

Articular cartilage contains a number of important matrix macromolecules, which confer its unique biological and mechanical properties. The major organic component is type II collagen, a fibrillar collagen, which provides the tensile strength of the tissue. Type II collagen is accompanied by a number of other minor collagens, including types IX, XI, and VI.[3] Type IX collagen is a nonfibrillar collagen with a glycosaminoglycan-containing moiety. The type IX collagen molecules coat the surface of the type II molecules, with the glycosaminoglycan moiety extending from the surface of the molecule, where it is thought to interact with other matrix components and may also regulate type II fibril formation.[3] Type XI collagen has been proposed to regulate type II fibril diameter in cartilage, and is associated with smaller diameter fibrils.[4] Type VI collagen is located in the pericellular region of the articular chondrocytes, and may be involved in cell-matrix interactions.[5] The other major macromolecules of articular cartilage are proteoglycans, most in the form of aggregates of proteoglycan monomers (aggrecan) bound to a hyaluronic acid backbone by a noncovalent association with a link glycoprotein.[3] The highly charged, polysulfated glycosaminoglycan components of the aggrecan molecules attract cations and water, resulting in osmotic pressure in the tissue due to the constraint of the molecular configuration caused by containment within the collagen meshwork. These properties of the proteoglycans provide the compressive strength of the tissue to withstand mechanical loading. The articular cartilage has a highly ordered tissue structure, with a flattened layer of chondrocytes at the surface and tangential arrangement of the surface layers of collagen. Within the transitional zone, the collagen fibrils assume a more random orientation, and the cells a more rounded morphology. In the deep or radial zone, the fibrils are oriented perpendicular to the joint surface and interface with the subchondral bone.[3]

Growth Factors

The isolation of articular chondrocytes from direct contact with other cell types (including vascular elements, which are found in nearly every other tissue type) suggests that the cellular regulation of phenotype may be largely determined at a local level. A large number of studies have investigated the phenotypic effects of growth factors and cytokines on articular chondrocytes, as well as the autocrine expression and regulation of these molecules, and the list of local regulatory molecules continues to expand. The major growth factors that have been studied include insulin-like growth factors (IGFs), transforming growth factor-betas (TGF-ßs), fibroblast growth factors (FGFs), parathyroid hormone related protein (PTHrP), platelet-derived growth factor (PDGF), epidermal growth factor (EGF), and the bone morphogenetic proteins (BMPs).[6-25] Cytokines have also been studied, and in many ways the distinctions between these protein-signaling molecules and growth factors

are subtle, although most cytokines were originally discovered in cells of the immune or hematopoietic systems. Cytokines that have been investigated in articular cartilage as both phenotypic effectors and chondrocyte autocrine products include tumor necrosis factor alpha (TNFα), interleukins (including IL1, IL4, IL6, IL8, IL10, and IL11), and colony-stimulating factors such as macrophage colony-stimulating factor (MCSF). Although some basal expression of these cytokines has been described in normal articular cartilage, in general these factors appear to be involved in matrix degradation in response to injury or disease, and are induced or upregulated under these circumstances.[14,26-30] The most important autocrine growth factors that appear to regulate normal articular chondrocyte phenotype are IGF-I, TGF-ßs, FGFs, and, possibly, the BMPs.

Insulin-Like Growth Factors

One of the first growth factors to be identified as an important autocrine regulator of articular cartilage was IGF-I. This factor is produced in cartilage in response to systemic stimulation by growth hormone, and it mediates the anabolic effects of growth hormone on the tissue.[7,8,31] IGF-I regulation is complex, with a number of IGF-binding proteins also being produced in cartilage. These proteins compete with receptors for binding in the extracellular matrix and help control the steady state levels of IGF-I acting on the cells.[32-34] IGF-II has also been identified in cartilage, and it has similar anabolic effects.[35] The major reported effects of IGF-I on articular cartilage are a stimulation of proteoglycan synthesis and cellular proliferation.[7,8,16,21,36] These effects are undoubtedly of great importance during growth and development, and they may help stimulate controlled enlargement of the articular surface. An additional anabolic effect of IGF-I is the stimulation of type II colla-

gen synthesis. IGF-I also inhibits expression of matrix metalloproteinases (MMPs), which degrade proteoglycans.[37] IGF-I is also an important mediator of DNA and proteoglycan synthesis by chondrocytes committed to the endochondral ossification pathway, such as in the growth plate.[7] Thus, the anabolic effects of IGF-I on chondrocytes are similar, whether the cells are committed to maturation or terminally differentiated articular function. The systemic overproduction of growth hormone seen in acromegaly causes enlargement and thickening of the articular cartilage in adults, consistent with the anabolic effects of IGF-I on this tissue. PDGF and EGF both have mitogenic effects on articular chondrocytes and have been demonstrated to be present in this tissue, but, overall, these molecules appear to play a less important role in chondrocyte regulation.[21,38,39]

Transforming Growth Factor-Beta

TGF-ß is a ubiquitous and pleiotropic regulatory protein that is expressed in articular cartilage and has potent effects on chondrocyte phenotype. The TGF-ß superfamily includes five isoforms of TGF-ß, characterized by secretion in a latent propeptide form that requires extracellular cleavage for activation. The BMPs, activins, and some of the growth and differentiation factors (GDF) are also members of this family. The active TGF-ß proteins are disulfide-bonded dimeric molecules in the 20 to 30 kd molecular weight range, which bind to a number of types of cell surface receptors. Greater than 90% of secreted TGF-ß is in a latent form. There is also a latent TGF-ß binding protein in the extracellular matrix of cartilage, which associates with the latent molecule and inhibits activation.[40,41] TGF-ß can be activated by heat, by acid exposure, and, in vivo in cartilage, by matrix metalloproteinase (MMP) activity. A significant proportion of TGF-ß is retained in the cartilaginous matrix around chondrocytes. The dominant effects of TGF-ß on chondrocytes are anabolic, with stimulation of proteoglycan synthesis and, under most conditions, stimulation of DNA synthesis.[10,13,14,17,21] The latter effect depends on factors such as culture conditions and the presence of serum components.[16] In addition, TGF-ß has an anti-catabolic effect on cartilage matrix degradation, and it has been shown to upregulate tissue inhibitors of matrix metalloproteinases (TIMPs) and to inhibit MMP expression.[14,17,42,43] When exogenous TGF-ß is injected into joints in vivo, the effect on the cartilage is a stimulation of proteoglycan synthesis, but it also results in an inflammatory synovitis that over the longer term leads to secondary cartilage degeneration.[38] Applications of TGF-ß as a potential stimulatory molecule in articular cartilage repair may be limited by its adverse effects on the synovium, although recently successful repair of articular defects with TGF-ß applied in a specific matrix with liposomes has been reported.[3] In contrast, intra-articular injections of PDGF have little effect on articular cartilage or synovium.[38]

Three major TGF-ß receptors have been identified, and all are present in articular cartilage.[44] The type I and type II receptors form signaling heterodimers; the type III receptor is a cell surface proteoglycan that may be involved in storage or presentation of the protein to the signaling receptors. The heterodimeric receptor autophosphorylates following ligand binding, and functions as a serine/threonine kinase.[41] The downstream signaling pathways are incompletely understood. Regulation of protein kinase C by TGF-ß in cartilage has been reported, and mitogen-activated protein (MAP) kinase has also been implicated.[45,46] Recently, a family of signaling proteins called SMADs has been identified. Following activation by TGF-ß receptor binding, these proteins are translocated to the nucleus where they function as transcriptional regulators.[47]

All four of the major TGF-ß isoforms have been identified in cartilage, and differential regulation of the individual isoforms by other growth factors has been described.[40] For instance, in one study PDGF stimulated TGF-ß2 and TGF-ß3 but not TGF-ß1.[23] Similarly, IL6 stimulated TGF-ß1 mRNA but had a minimal effect on TGF-ß3 and no effect on TGF-ß2, and IL1 inhibited TGF-ß1 but strongly upregulated TGF-ß3 in articular chondrocytes.[48] Thus, the regulation of TGF-ß in cartilage, as well as in other skeletal tissues, is extremely complicated. Furthermore, TGF-ß activation is under regulation, as is expression of latent TGF-ß binding protein, which adds further layers of complexity.[49] Vitamin D metabolites may serve as one modulator of these latter functions.[50,51] TGF-ß1 and TGF-ß3 knock-out mice have been engineered, but they have not demonstrated any major skeletal or cartilaginous phenotypic abnormalities, except for defective palatogenesis in the TGF-ß3 null mice. This probably reflects functional redundancy among the TGF-ß family members, and makes assessment of the role of the specific isoforms in articular cartilage more difficult. The TGF-ß1 null mice develop progressive inflammatory lesions in multiple organ systems, and the TGF-ß3 null mice exhibit defective pulmonary development.[52,53]

Fibroblast Growth Factor

FGF is another important autocrine growth factor in articular cartilage. Basic FGF (FGF2), probably the dominant isoform, is highly bound by heparin-like molecules in the cartilaginous matrix. FGF functions as a mitogen for articular chondrocytes, and has been shown to have synergistic interactions with IGF-I.[9,10,16,22,24] However, unlike IGF-I and TGF-ß, FGF suppresses, rather than stimulates, proteoglycan synthesis. In a study of the effects of IGF-I and FGF2

on cartilage explants, IGF-I maintained normal mechanical properties in culture, while FGF2 treatment led to a decline in the mechanical properties of the explants.[54] FGF has also been shown to stimulate articular enlargement in young rats when injected intra-articularly.[15] FGF stimulates TGF-ß release in articular chondrocytes, but does not affect mRNA levels.[23] The FGF receptor family has been implicated in a number of skeletal dysplasias that affect growth plate function and endochondral ossification, but articular defects have not been associated with these. FGF receptors function as tyrosine kinases, but downstream signaling events are incompletely characterized. Mutations of FGFR3 leading to constitutively active receptors have been identified as the defect that causes achondroplasia and thanatophoric dysplasia.[55] FGF overexpression in transgenic models also causes bone abnormalities, but disruption of articular cartilage structure has not been reported. Thus, the role of FGF in articular cartilage is currently not clear, because it appears to have more profound effects on chondrocytes in the endochondral ossification pathway in overexpression models. However, the large amount of FGF bound in the cartilaginous matrix may have some function in pathologic conditions, as in cartilage injury and repair. Intra-articular delivery of FGF2 in animal models has been shown to stimulate cartilage repair and migration of mesenchymal stem cells into articular defects.[56,57]

Bone Morphogenetic Proteins

BMPs are a subset of the TGF-ß superfamily that have recently been identified as important autocrine factors. The BMPs are dimeric secreted signaling molecules, like TGF-ß, but are not secreted in a latent form.[58] Recently, however, extracellular binding proteins, noggin and chordin, have been identified, which inhibit BMP function and may, therefore, regulate its activity.[59] Type I and type II BMP receptors form heterodimeric signaling serine/threonine kinases, although the downstream signals are not fully elucidated.[60] Recent evidence suggests that the SMAD family of molecules may be involved in signal transduction.[61] The effect of BMPs on undifferentiated mesenchymal cells is to induce chondrogenesis, and when BMPs are implanted ectopically, the entire cascade of endochondral ossification is induced.[62] BMP-1 differs from the other family members in that it does not induce endochondral ossification, and it possesses a metalloproteinase activity. Recently, BMP-1 has been demonstrated to function as the C-propeptidase of type I and probably types II and III collagen.[63] BMP-1 is constitutively expressed in articular cartilage, where its proteolytic activity likely plays a role in extracellular collagen processing.[64]

In addition to the chondrogenic differentiating effects that BMPs have on undifferentiated mesenchymal cells, these growth factors also exhibit regulatory effects on the phenotype of differentiated chondrocytes. In one study, BMP-2 and BMP-3 maintained proteoglycan synthesis in articular cartilage explants to a level similar to that of explants treated with TGF-ß and IGF-I,[19] and other studies have also demonstrated stimulation of proteoglycans and maintenance of articular phenotype by BMP-3 and BMP-4.[18,65] Not surprisingly, BMP receptor expression has also been demonstrated in articular chondrocytes.[18] Vgr-1, a murine homolog of BMP-6, is expressed in hypertrophic chondrocytes, and a similar family member, BMP-7, has been shown to enhance the differentiation of chondrocytes committed to the maturation pathway, with stimulation of type X collagen.[66,67] However, BMP-7 does not stimulate hypertrophic phenotype in articular chondrocytes,[68] and, overall, the expression and effects of BMPs in articular cartilage have not been extensively investigated.

Parathyroid Hormone Related Protein

Parathyroid hormone related protein (PTHrP) has recently been identified as an important autocrine/paracrine growth factor in cartilage, primarily associated with endochondral bone development. In embryonic bone development, PTHrP functions as a paracrine factor, being produced at high levels in the articular and epiphyseal chondrocytes as well as the cells of the perichondrium.[69] The PTHrP produced in these locations acts on PTHrP receptors within the developing growth plate to stimulate cellular proliferation and inhibit hypertrophy. The expression of PTHrP in the epiphysis is stimulated by production of a signaling molecule, Indian hedgehog (*IHH*) within the proliferating zone of the growth plate. PTHrP in turn suppresses production of *IHH*, creating a paracrine feedback loop.[70,71] In genetically engineered mice in which the PTHrP gene is deleted, the animals suffer from deranged endochondral ossification, with impaired long bone growth, histologic evidence of diminished chondrocyte proliferation in the growth plate, and premature chondrocyte hypertrophy.[72] The defect is lethal in the immediate postnatal period, putatively due to inadequate rib cage development to allow respiration. There are not, however, obvious defects in the articular cartilage, which suggests that this tissue may not be a target for PTHrP action. Expression of PTHrP in the epiphysis and articular cartilage diminishes with age postnatally, and adult articular cartilage does not express PTHrP.[73] Regulation of endochondral ossification in the adolescent growth plate may depend to a greater extent on autocrine production of PTHrP within the lower proliferating and upper hypertrophic zones, where low levels of the protein are expressed. The role of PTHrP in articular cartilage is unclear, with conflicting data on articular chondrocyte responsiveness to PTHrP. Adolescent chick articular

chondrocytes have been reported to lack phenotypic changes or cyclic adenosine 5'-monophosphate (c-AMP) elevation in response to PTH or PTHrP,[12] while articular chondrocytes from young rats exhibited responsiveness.[74] While age or species dependence may account for these reported discrepancies, the lack of articular abnormalities in the knock-out mouse model supports a paracrine rather than an autocrine role of the PTHrP produced in the articular cartilage. PTHrP is re-expressed in degenerative articular cartilage in arthritis, and, therefore, it may play some role in mediating cellular changes associated with injury and repair processes in this tissue.[75]

Growth Factors and Articular Cartilage Degeneration

During injury and repair processes in articular cartilage, a number of changes occur in the patterns of expression of growth factors and cytokines. Although there is an increase in production of IGF-I and expression of IGF-I receptor by articular arthritic cartilage,[32,76] responsiveness of the cells to exogenous IGF-I decreases.[39] This is probably due to the markedly enhanced expression of IGF binding proteins, particularly IGFBP3 and IGFBP5, which diminish the amount of IGF-I available for receptor interaction.[32] IL6 is expressed in arthritic, but not in normal cartilage, and its expression is enhanced by IL1 and TNF, which are mediators of cartilage matrix degradation.[27,29,76,77] IL1 and TNF produced by synovium may be major mediators of cartilage catabolism in inflammatory arthritis. In addition, there is endogenous expression of IL1 and TNF by chondrocytes of degenerating cartilage, which may contribute to MMP stimulation and matrix breakdown through an autocrine mechanism. IL6 antagonizes IL1-mediated cartilage breakdown, and its expression in arthritic cartilage may represent a repair response.[78] Mechanical loading of articular cartilage also stimulates IL6 expression, and this cytokine may function in the regulation of the response of matrix metabolism to stress.[79] Other cytokines expressed by articular chondrocytes under conditions of injury or arthritis include IL4, IL8, IL10, IL11, leukemia inhibitory factor (LIF), MCSF, and granulocyte MCSF (GMCSF), but the function of these numerous factors is currently unclear.[26,27,80,81,82]

Conclusion

Articular cartilage depends on a large number of autocrine factors to maintain chondrocyte phenotype and normal matrix metabolism. Normal cartilage expresses IGF-I, FGF2, and all 4 major isoforms of TGF-ß, which are probably among the most important local regulators of articular chondrocyte function. The major effects of TGF-ß and IGF-I are anabolic, with stimulation of proteoglycan synthesis, type II collagen synthesis, and cellular proliferation. FGF is mitogenic, but suppresses proteoglycan synthesis, and may be involved in cartilage repair or injury response given its sequestration in the cartilaginous matrix. The regulation of these growth factors in normal cartilage is complex, and interactive effects occur, including synergistic stimulations and co-regulations of growth factor expression by one another. PTHrP is produced in embryonic and young articular cartilage, but it may not directly affect the articular chondrocyte, acting instead in a paracrine fashion on the adjacent growth plate to stimulate proliferation and prevent premature chondrocyte hypertrophy. In adult articular cartilage, PTHrP expression disappears, although it may be re-expressed during cartilage degeneration or response to injury. BMPs have recently been identified in cartilage, and generally exhibit anabolic effects, although their role in regulation of normal cartilage metabolism or injury and repair remains unclear. Cytokines such as IL1 and TNF promote cartilage matrix degradation. IL1 and TNF are not expressed at significant levels in normal cartilage, but are produced in arthritic or injured cartilage. These factors induce expression of other cytokines such as IL6, which may function in moderating their catabolic effects on the cartilage matrix. A wide spectrum of other cytokines and growth factors has been demonstrated in articular chondrocytes, but the physiologic and pathophysiologic functions of these factors remain to be determined.

References

1. Walker GD, Fischer M, Gannon J, et al: Expression of type-X collagen in osteoarthritis. *J Orthop Res* 1995;13:4–12.

2. Umehara T: Immunohistochemical localization of transforming growth factor-beta 1 in growth plate freshly transplanted into a full-thickness defect in articular cartilage. *Nippon Seikeigeka Gakkai-Zasshi* 1994;68:790–797.

3. Buckwalter JA, Mankin HJ: Articular cartilage: Part I. Tissue design and chondrocyte-matrix interactions: Part II. Degeneration and osteoarthrosis, repair, regeneration, and transplantation. *J Bone Joint Surg* 1997;79A:600–632.

4. Keene DR, Oxford JT, Morris NP: Ultrastructural localization of collagen types II, IX, and XI in the growth plate of human rib and fetal bovine epiphyseal cartilage: Type XI collagen is restricted to thin fibrils *J Histochem Cytochem* 1995;43:967–979.

5. Hagiwara H, Schroter-Kermani C, Merker HJ: Localization of collagen type VI in articular cartilage of young and adult mice. *Cell Tissue Res* 1993;272:155–160.

6. Trippel SB, Chernausek SD, Van Wyk JJ, et al: Demonstration of type I and type II somatomedin receptors on bovine growth plate chondrocytes. *J Orthop Res* 1988;6:817–826.

7. Trippel SB, Corvol MT, Dumontier MF, et al: Effect of somatomedin-C/insulin-like growth factor I and growth hormone on cultured growth plate and articular chondrocytes. *Pediatr Res* 1989;25:76–82.

8. Luyten FP, Hascall VC, Nissley SP, et al: Insulin-like growth factors maintain steady-state metabolism of proteoglycans in bovine articular cartilage explants. *Arch Biochem Biophys* 1988;267:416–425.

9. Froger-Gaillard B, Charrier AM, Thenet S, et al: Growth-promoting effects of acidic and basic fibroblast growth factor on rabbit articular chondrocytes aging in culture. *Exp Cell Res* 1989;183:388–398.

10. Inoue H, Kato Y, Iwamoto M, et al: Stimulation of cartilage-matrix proteoglycan synthesis by morphologically transformed chondrocytes grown in the presence of fibro-

blast growth factor and transforming growth factor-beta. *J Cell Physiol* 1989;138:329–337.

11. Sailor LZ, Hewick RM, Morris EA: Recombinant human bone morphogenetic protein-2 maintains the articular chondrocyte phenotype in long-term culture. *J Orthop Res* 1996;14:937–945.

12. Crabb ID, O'Keefe RJ, Puzas JE, et al: Differential effects of parathyroid hormone on chick growth plate and articular chondrocytes. *Calcif Tissue Int* 1992;50:61–66.

13. Morales TI, Roberts AB: Transforming growth factor beta regulates the metabolism of proteoglycans in bovine cartilage organ cultures. *J Biol Chem* 1988;263:12828–12831.

14. Lum ZP, Hakala BE, Mort JS, et al: Modulation of the catabolic effects of interleukin-1 beta on human articular chondrocytes by transforming growth factor-beta. *J Cell Physiol* 1996;166:351–359.

15. Shida J, Jingushi S, Izumi T, et al: Basic fibroblast growth factor stimulates articular cartilage enlargement in young rats in vivo. *J Orthop Res* 1996;14:265–272.

16. Trippel SB: Growth factor actions on articular cartilage. *J Rheumatol* 1995;43(suppl):129–132.

17. Morales TI: Transforming growth factor-beta and insulin-like growth factor-1 restore proteoglycan metabolism of bovine articular cartilage after depletion by retinoic acid. *Arch Biochem Biophys* 1994;315:190–198.

18. Luyten FP, Chen P, Paralkar V, et al: Recombinant bone morphogenetic protein-4, transforming growth factor-beta 1, and activin A enhance the cartilage phenotype of articular chondrocytes in vitro. *Exp Cell Res* 1994;210:224–229.

19. Luyten FP, Yu YM, Yanagishita M, et al: Natural bovine osteogenin and recombinant human bone morphogenetic protein-2B are equipotent in the maintenance of proteoglycans in bovine articular cartilage explant cultures. *J Biol Chem* 1992;267:3691–3695.

20. Loveys LS, Gelb D, Hurwitz SR, et al: Effects of parathyroid hormone-related peptide on chick growth plate chondrocytes. *J Orthop Res* 1993;11:884–891.

21. Mankin HJ, Jennings LC, Treadwell BV, et al: Growth factors and articular cartilage. *J Rheumatol* 1991;27(suppl):66–67.

22. Osborn KD, Trippel SB, Mankin HJ: Growth factor stimulation of adult articular cartilage. *J Orthop Res* 1989;7:35–42.

23. Villiger PM, Lotz M: Differential expression of TGF beta isoforms by human articular chondrocytes in response to growth factors. *J Cell Physiol* 1992;151:318–325.

24. Posever J, Phillips FM, Pottenger LA: Effects of basic fibroblast growth factor, transforming growth factor-beta 1, insulin-like growth factor-1, and insulin on human osteoarthritic articular cartilage explants. *J Orthop Res* 1995;13:832–837.

25. Peracchia F, Ferrari G, Poggi A, et al: IL-1 beta-induced expression of PDGF-AA isoform in rabbit articular chondrocytes is modulated by TGF-beta 1. *Exp Cell Res* 1991;193:208–212.

26. Tanabe BK, Abe LM, Kimura LH, et al: Cytokine mRNA repertoire of articular chondrocytes from arthritic patients, infants, and neonatal mice. *Rheumatol Int* 1996;16:67–76.

27. Henrotin YE, De Groote DD, Labasse AH, et al: Effects of exogenous IL-1 beta, TNF alpha, IL-6, IL-8 and LIF on cytokine production by human articular chondrocytes. *Osteoarthritis Cartilage* 1996;4:163–173.

28. van de Loo FA, Joosten LA, van Lent PL, et al: Role of interleukin-1, tumor necrosis factor alpha, and interleukin-6 in cartilage proteoglycan metabolism and destruction: Effect of in situ blocking in murine antigen- and zymosan-induced arthritis. *Arthritis Rheum* 1995;38:164–172.

29. Malfait AM, Verbruggen G, Almqvist KF, et al: Coculture of human articular chondrocytes with peripheral blood mononuclear cells as a model to study cytokine-mediated interactions between inflammatory cells and target cells in the rheumatoid joint. *Vitro Cell Dev Biol Anim* 1994;30A:747–752.

30. Campbell IK, Ianches G, Hamilton JA: Production of macrophage colony-stimulating factor (M-CSF) by human articular cartilage and chondrocytes: Modulation by interleukin-1 and tumor necrosis factor alpha. *Biochim Biophys Acta* 1993;1182:57–63.

31. Jansen J, van Buul-Offers SC, Hoogerbrugge CM, et al: Characterization of specific insulin-like growth factor (IGF)-I and IGF-II receptors on cultured rabbit articular chondrocyte membranes. *J Endocrinol* 1989;120:245–249.

32. Olney RC, Tsuchiya K, Wilson DM, et al: Chondrocytes from osteoarthritic cartilage have increased expression of insulin-like growth factor I (IGF-I) and IGF-binding protein-3 (IGFBP-3) and -5, but not IGF-II or IGFBP-4. *J Clin Endocrinol Metab* 1996;81:1096–1103.

33. Olney RC, Wilson DM, Mohtai M, et al: Interleukin-1 and tumor necrosis factor-alpha increase insulin-like growth factor-binding protein-3 (IGFBP-3) production and IGFBP-3 protease activity in human articular chondrocytes. *J Endocrinol* 1995;146:279–286.

34. Olney RC, Smith RL, Kee Y, et al: Production and hormonal regulation of insulin-like growth factor binding proteins in bovine chondrocytes. *Endocrinology* 1993;133:563–570.

35. Wang E, Wang J, Chin E, et al: Cellular patterns of insulin-like growth factor system gene expression in murine chondrogenesis and osteogenesis. *Endocrinology* 1995;136:2741–2751.

36. Tyler JA: Insulin-like growth factor 1 can decrease degradation and promote synthesis of proteoglycan in cartilage exposed to cytokines. *Biochem J* 1989;260:543–548.

37. Rogachefsky RA, Dean DD, Howell DS, et al: Treatment of canine osteoarthritis with insulin-like growth factor-1 (IGF-1) and sodium pentosan polysulfate. *Osteoarthritis Cartilage* 1993;1:105–114.

38. Hulth A, Johnell O, Miyazono K, et al: Effect of transforming growth factor-beta and platelet-derived growth factor-BB on articular cartilage in rats. *J Orthop Res* 1996;14:547–553.

39. Verschure PJ, Joosten LA, van der Kraan PM, et al: Responsiveness of articular cartilage from normal and inflamed mouse knee joints to various growth factors. *Ann Rheum Dis* 1994;53:455–460.

40. Jakowlew SB, Dillard PJ, Winokur TS, et al: Expression of transforming growth factor-betas 1-4 in chicken embryo chondrocytes and myocytes. *Dev Biol* 1991;143:135–148.

41. Kingsley DM: The TGF-beta superfamily: New members, new receptors, and new genetic tests of function in different organisms. *Genes Dev* 1994;8:133–146.

42. Su S, Dehnade F, Zafarullah M: Regulation of tissue inhibitor of metalloproteinases-3 gene expression by transforming growth factor-beta and dexamethasone in bovine and human articular chondrocytes. *DNA Cell Biol* 1996;15:1039–1048.

43. Gunther M, Haubeck HD, van de Leur E, et al: Transforming growth factor beta 1 regulates tissue inhibitor of metalloproteinases-1 expression in differentiated human articular chondrocytes. *Arthritis Rheum* 1994;37:395–405.

44. Glansbeek HL, van der Kraan PM, Vitters EL, et al: Correlation of the size of type II transforming growth factor beta (TGF-beta) receptor with TGF-beta responses of isolated bovine articular chondrocytes. *Ann Rheum Dis* 1993;52:812–816.

45. Sylvia VL, Mackey S, Schwartz Z, et al: Regulation of protein kinase C by transforming growth factor beta 1 in rat costochondral chondrocyte cultures. *J Bone Miner Res* 1994;9:1477–1487.

46. Yamaguchi K, Shirakabe K, Shibuya H, et al: Identification of a member of the MAPKKK family as a potential mediator of TGF-beta signal transduction. *Science* 1995;270:2008–2011.

47. Lagna G, Hata A, Hemmati-Brivanlou A, et al: Partnership between DPC4 and SMAD proteins in TGF-beta signalling pathways. *Nature* 1996;383:832–836.

48. Villiger PM, Kusari AB, ten Dijke P, et al: IL-1 beta and IL-6 selectively induce transforming growth factor-beta isoforms in human articular chondrocytes. *J Immunol* 1993;151:3337–3344.

49. Miyazono K, Ichijo H, Heldin CH: Transforming growth factor-beta: Latent forms, binding proteins and receptors. *Growth Factors* 1993;8:11–22.

50. Boyan BD, Schwartz Z, Parker-Snyder S, et al: Latent transforming growth factor-beta is produced by chondrocytes and activated by extracellular matrix vesicles upon exposure to 1,25-(OH)2D3. *J Biol Chem* 1994;269:28374–28381.

51. Schwartz Z, Bonewald LF, Caulfield K, et al: Direct effects of transforming growth factor-beta on chondrocytes are modulated by vitamin D metabolites in a cell maturation-specific manner. *Endocrinology* 1993;132:1544–1552.

52. Boivin GP, O'Toole BA, Ormsby IE, et al: Onset and progression of pathological lesions in transforming growth factor-beta 1-deficient mice. *Am J Pathol* 1995;146:276–288.

53. Kaartinen V, Voncken JW, Shuler C, et al: Abnormal lung development and cleft palate in mice lacking TGF-beta 3 indicates defects of epithelial-mesenchymal interaction. *Nat Genet* 1995;11:415–421.

54. Sah RL, Trippel SB, Grodzinsky AJ: Differential effects of serum, insulin-like growth factor-I, and fibroblast growth factor-2 on the maintenance of cartilage physical properties during long-term culture. *J Orthop Res* 1996;14:44–52.

55. Stoilov I, Kilpatrick MW, Tsipouras P: A common FGFR3 mutation is present in achondroplasia but not in hypochondroplasia. *Am J Med Genet* 1995;55:127–133.

56. Cuevas P, Burgos J, Baird A: Basic fibroblast growth factor (FGF) promotes cartilage repair in vivo. *Biochem Biophys Res Commun* 1988;156:611–618.

57. Hunziker EB, Rosenberg LC: Repair of partial-thickness defects in articular cartilage: Cell recruitment from the synovial membrane. *J Bone Joint Surg* 1996;78A:721–733.

58. Hogan BL: Bone morphogenetic proteins: multifunctional regulators of vertebrate development. *Genes Dev* 1996;10:1580–1594.

59. Hemmati-Brivanlou A, Melton D: Vertebrate embryonic cells will become nerve cells unless told otherwise. *Cell* 1997;88:13–17.

60. Liu F, Ventura F, Doody J, et al: Human type II receptor for bone morphogenic proteins (BMPs): Extension of the two-kinase receptor model to the BMPs. *Mol Cell Biol* 1995;15:3479–3486.

61. Liu F, Hata A, Baker JC, et al: A human Mad protein acting as a BMP-regulated transcriptional activator. *Nature* 1996;381:620–623.

62. Wozney JM, Rosen V, Celeste AJ, et al: Novel regulators of bone formation: Molecular clones and activities. *Science* 1988;242:1528–1534.

63. Kessler E, Takahara K, Biniaminov L, et al: Bone morphogenetic protein-1: The type I procollagen C-proteinase *Science* 1996;271:360–362.

64. Reynolds SD, Rosier RN, Puzas JE, et al: Differential expression and localization of BMP1 and tolloid in the chick. *J Bone Miner Res* 1995;10(suppl 1):163.

65. Harrison ET Jr, Luyten FP, Reddi AH: Osteogenin promotes reexpression of cartilage phenotype by dedifferentiated articular chondrocytes in serum-free medium. *Exp Cell Res* 1991;192:340–345.

66. Lyons KM, Pelton RW, Hogan BL: Patterns of expression of murine Vgr-1 and BMP-2a RNA suggest that transforming growth factor-beta-like genes coordinately regulate aspects of embryonic development. *Genes Dev* 1989;3:1657–1668.

67. Chen P, Vukicevic S, Sampath TK, et al: Osteogenic protein-1 promotes growth and maturation of chick sternal chondrocytes in serum-free cultures. *J Cell Sci* 1995;108:105–114.

68. Chen P, Vukicevic S, Sampath TK, et al: Bovine articular chondrocytes do not undergo hypertrophy when cultured in the presence of serum and osteogenic protein-1. *Biochem Biophys Res Commun* 1993;197:1253–1259.

69. Lee K, Deeds JD, Segre GV: Expression of parathyroid hormone-related peptide and its receptor messenger ribonucleic acids during fetal development of rats. *Endocrinology* 1995;136:453–463.

70. Lanske B, Karaplis AC, Lee K, et al: PTH/PTHrP receptor in early development and Indian hedgehog-regulated bone growth. *Science* 1996;273:663–666.

71. Vortkamp A, Lee K, Lanske B, et al: Regulation of rate of cartilage differentiation by Indian hedgehog and PTH-related protein. *Science* 1996;273:613–622.

72. Amizuka N, Warshawsky JE, Henderson D, et al: Parathyroid hormone related peptide-depleted mice show abnormal epiphyseal cartilage development and altered endochondral bone formation. *J Cell Biol* 1994;126: 1611–1623.

73. Tsukazaki T, Ohtsuru A, Enomoto H, et al: Expression of parathyroid hormone-related protein in rat articular cartilage. *Calcif Tissue Int* 1995;57:196–200.

74. Tsukazaki T, Ohtsuru A, Namba H, et al: Parathyroid hormone-related protein (PTHrP) action in rat articular chondrocytes: Comparison of PTH(1-34), PTHrP(1-34), PTHrP(1-141), PTHrP(100-114) and antisense oligonucleotides against PTHrP. *J Endocrinol* 1996;150:359–368.

75. de Mesy-Jensen KL, Hicks DG, Reynolds PR, et al: Immunolocalization of PTHrP in chicken and human growth plate and articular cartilage. *Trans Orthop Res Soc* 1994;19:417.

76. Middleton J, Manthey A, Tyler J: Insulin-like growth factor (IGF) receptor, IGF-I, interleukin-1 beta (IL-1 beta), and IL-6 mRNA expression in osteoarthritic and normal human cartilage. *J Histochem Cytochem* 1996;44: 133–141.

77. Guerne PA, Carson DA, Lotz M: IL-6 production by human articular chondrocytes: Modulation of its synthesis by cytokines, growth factors, and hormones in vitro. *J Immunol* 1990;144:499–505.

78. Shingu M, Miyauchi S, Nagai Y, et al: The role of IL-4 and IL-6 in IL-1-dependent cartilage matrix degradation. *Br J Rheumatol* 1995;34: 101–106.

79. Mohtai M, Gupta MK, Donlon B, et al: Expression of interleukin-6 in osteoarthritic chondrocytes and effects of fluid-induced shear on this expression in normal human chondrocytes in vitro. *J Orthop Res* 1996;14:67–73.

80. Alsalameh S, Firestein GS, Oez S, et al: Regulation of granulocyte macrophage colony stimulating factor production by human articular chondrocytes: Induction by both tumor necrosis factor-alpha and interleukin 1, downregulation by transforming growth factor beta and upregulation by fibroblast growth factor *J Rheumatol* 1994;21:993–1002.

81. Campbell IK, Ianches G, Hamilton JA: Production of macrophage colony-stimulating factor (M-CSF) by human articular cartilage and chondrocytes: Modulation by interleukin-1 and tumor necrosis factor alpha. *Biochim Biophys Acta* 1993;1182:57–63.

82. Campbell IK, Waring P, Novak U, et al: Production of leukemia inhibitory factor by human articular chondrocytes and cartilage in response to interleukin-1 and tumor necrosis factor alpha. *Arthritis Rheum* 1993;36:790–794.

Articular Cartilage:
Tissue Design and Chondrocyte-Matrix Interactions

Joseph A. Buckwalter, MD
Henry J. Mankin, MD

In 1892, Walt Whitman observed that "the narrowest hinge in my hand puts to scorn all machinery."[1] Despite remarkable advances in joint replacement, Whitman's observation stands unchallenged; no current prostheses come close to duplicating the function and durability of synovial joints. These complex structures, developed and progressively refined over hundreds of millions of years,[2] are formed by an arrangement of multiple distinct tissues, including joint capsule, ligament, meniscus, subchondral bone, synovial tissue, and hyaline articular cartilage. These tissues are self-renewing, respond to alterations in use, and provide stable movement with a level of friction less than that achieved by any prosthetic joint. The tissue that contributes the most to these extraordinary functional capacities is the hyaline articular cartilage.[3,4] It varies in thickness, cell density, matrix composition, and mechanical properties within the same joint, among joints, and among species;[5] however, in all synovial joints it consists of the same components, has the same general structure, and performs the same functions. Although it is at most only a few millimeters thick, it has surprising stiffness to compression and resilience; it also has an exceptional ability to distribute loads,[6,7] thereby minimizing peak stresses on subchondral bone. Perhaps

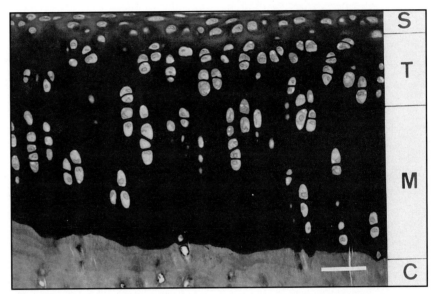

Fig. 1 Articular cartilage from the medial femoral condyle of an 8-month-old rabbit. The tissue is organized into four layers, or zones. These consist of a superficial zone (S); a transitional zone (T); a middle (radial), or deep, zone (M); and a calcified cartilage zone (C) (bar = 50 μm). (Reproduced with permission from Buckwalter JA, Hunziker EB, Rosenberg LC, et al: Articular cartilage: Composition and structure, in Woo SL-Y, Buckwalter JA (eds): *Injury and Repair of the Musculoskeletal Soft Tissues*. Park Ridge, IL, American Academy of Orthopaedic Surgeons, 1988, pp 405–425.)

most important, it has great durability; in most people, it provides normal joint function for 80 years or more. No synthetic material approaches this level of performance.

Grossly and histologically, adult articular cartilage appears to be a simple inert tissue. When examined from inside a synovial joint, normal articular cartilage appears as a slick firm surface that resists deformation. Light microscopy shows that it consists primarily of extracellular matrix, with only one type of cell, the chondrocyte, and that it lacks blood vessels, lymphatic vessels, and nerves (Fig. 1). Compared with tissues such as muscle or bone, cartilage has a low level of metabolic activity and appears to be less

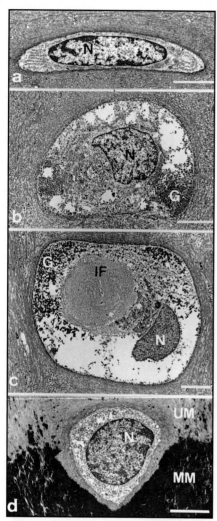

Fig. 2 Electron micrographs of chondrocytes from articular cartilage from the medial femoral condyle of a skeletally mature rabbit. **a**: superficial zone; **b**: transitional zone; **c**: middle (radial), or deep, zone; and **d**: calcified cartilage zone. N = nucleus, G = glycogen, IF = intermediate filaments, UM = unmineralized matrix, and MM = mineralized matrix (bar = 3 μm). (Reproduced with permission from Buckwalter JA, Hunziker EB, Rosenberg LC, et al: Articular cartilage: Composition and structure, in Woo SL-Y, Buckwalter JA (eds): *Injury and Repair of the Musculoskeletal Soft Tissues.* Park Ridge, IL, American Academy of Orthopaedic Surgeons, 1988, pp 405–425.)

responsive to changes in loading or to injury. Despite its unimpressive appearance and low level of metabolic activity, detailed study of the morphology and biology of adult articular cartilage shows

that it has an elaborate, highly ordered structure and that a variety of complex interactions between the chondrocytes and the matrix actively maintain the tissue.

This review covers the current understanding of the design of articular cartilage (the cell-and-matrix composition and the structure that make normal function of the cartilage possible) as well as the interactions between chondrocytes and their matrix that are necessary to maintain the tissue.

Composition of Articular Cartilage

Like other connective tissues, including tendon, ligament, and meniscus, articular cartilage consists of cells, matrix water, and a matrix macromolecular framework (Fig. 1), and like other connective tissues, articular cartilage derives its form and mechanical properties from its matrix.[3,4] The cells contribute little to the volume of the tissue, about 1% in adult human articular cartilage. (In other species, especially small animals such as mice, rats, and rabbits, which have thin articular cartilage, the cell density is many times greater than in humans).[8,9]

Chondrocytes

Within normal articular cartilage, there is only one type of cell: the highly specialized chondrocyte[4] (Fig. 2). Chondrocytes from different cartilage zones differ in size, shape, and probably metabolic activity,[10,11] but all of these cells contain the organelles necessary for matrix synthesis, including endoplasmic reticulum and Golgi membranes. They also frequently contain intracytoplasmic filaments, lipid, glycogen, and secretory vesicles, and at least some chondrocytes have short cilia extending from the cell into the matrix. These structures may have a role in sensing mechanical changes in the matrix. Chondrocytes surround themselves with their extracellular matrix and do not form cell-to-cell contacts. A spheroidal shape;

synthesis of type II collagen, large aggregating proteoglycans, and specific noncollagenous proteins; and formation of these molecules into cartilaginous matrix distinguish mature chondrocytes from other cells. Individual chondrocytes are surprisingly active metabolically (they have a glycolytic rate per cell similar to that of cells in vascularized tissues), but the total metabolic activity of the tissue is low because of the low cell density.

At first glance, chondrocytes seem to be observers rather than participants in the function of mature articular cartilage as a joint surface. They appear to remain unchanged in location, appearance, and activity for decades. The unique mechanical properties of articular cartilage—the types of macromolecules that form the framework of the matrix and the concentrations of water and macromolecules—seem to depend on the matrix.[3,4,6]

However, a matrix formed by mixing appropriate concentrations of water and cartilage macromolecules (collagens, proteoglycans, and noncollagenous proteins) will not duplicate the properties of articular cartilage. To produce a tissue that can provide normal function of the synovial joint, the chondrocytes must first synthesize appropriate types and amounts of macromolecules and then assemble and organize them into a highly ordered framework. Maintenance of the articular surface requires turnover of the matrix macromolecules, that is, continual replacement of degraded matrix components, and probably requires alterations in the macromolecular framework of the matrix in response to use of the joint. To accomplish these activities, the cells must sense changes in the composition of the matrix that are due to degradation of macromolecules as well as changes in the demands placed on the articular surface; the cells then must respond by synthesizing appropriate types and amounts of macromolecules.

In adult animals, chondrocytes derive their nutrition from nutrients in the synovial fluid, which, to reach the cell, must pass through a double diffusion barrier: first the synovial tissue and synovial fluid, and then the cartilage matrix. This latter barrier is restrictive not only with respect to the size of the materials but also with respect to their charges and to other features such as molecular configuration.[12] The nature of this system leaves chondrocytes with a low concentration of oxygen relative to most other tissues; therefore, they depend primarily on anaerobic metabolism.

The activity and function of articular cartilage chondrocytes during skeletal growth differ from those after completion of growth. In growing individuals, the chondrocytes produce new tissue to expand and remodel the articular surface; in skeletally mature individuals, they do not substantially change the volume of the tissue, but they replace degraded matrix macromolecules and they may remodel the articular surface.[13,14]

Cartilage first forms from undifferentiated mesenchymal cells that cluster together and synthesize cartilage collagens, proteoglycans, and noncollagenous proteins. The tissue becomes recognizable as cartilage under light microscopy when an accumulation of matrix separates the cells and they assume a spherical shape. During the formation and growth of articular cartilage, the cell density is high and the cells reach their highest level of metabolic activity, as the chondrocytes proliferate rapidly and synthesize large volumes of matrix. In growing mammalian articular cartilage, chondrocytes divide and produce new matrix in two zones: a peripheral zone, which enlarges and expands the articular surface, and a central zone, which also serves as the center of enchondral ossification of the epiphysis. With skeletal maturation, the rates of cell metabolic activity, matrix synthesis, and cell division decline. After completion of skeletal growth, most chondrocytes probably never divide but

rather continue to synthesize collagens, proteoglycans, and noncollagenous proteins. This continued synthetic activity suggests that maintenance of articular cartilage requires substantial ongoing internal remodeling of the macromolecular framework of the matrix. Enzymes produced by chondrocytes presumably are responsible for degradation of the matrix macromolecules, and chondrocytes probably respond to the presence of fragmented matrix molecules by increasing their synthetic activity to replace the degraded components of the macromolecular framework. Other mechanisms must also influence the balance between synthetic and degradative activity. For example, the frequency and intensity of joint loading influences chondrocyte metabolism. Immobilization of the joint or a marked decrease in joint loading alters chondrocyte activity so that degradation exceeds synthesis of at least the proteoglycan component of the matrix.[13,15] Persistent, increased use of the joint may also alter the composition and organization of the matrix, but this has not been demonstrated clearly in skeletally mature individuals.[13,15] With aging, the capacity of the cells to synthesize some types of proteoglycans and their response to stimuli, including growth factors, decrease.[16-20] These age-related changes may limit the ability of the cells to maintain the tissue and thereby contribute to the development of degeneration of the articular cartilage.[19]

Extracellular Matrix
The matrix of the articular cartilage consists of two components: the tissue fluid and the framework of structural macromolecules that give the tissue its form and stability. The interaction of the tissue fluid with the macromolecular framework gives the tissue its mechanical properties of stiffness and resilience.[6,21]

Tissue Fluid Water contributes as much as 80% of the wet weight of articular cartilage, and the interaction of the

water with the matrix macromolecules substantially influences the mechanical properties of the tissue.[3,6,22-25] This tissue fluid contains gases, small proteins, metabolites, and a high concentration of cations to balance the negatively charged proteoglycans. At least some of the water can move freely in and out of the tissue. The volume, concentration, and behavior of the water within the tissue depend primarily on its interaction with the structural macromolecules, particularly the large aggregating proteoglycans that help to maintain the fluid within the matrix and the concentrations of electrolytes in the fluid. Because these macromolecules have large numbers of negatively charged sulfate and carboxylate groups that attract positively charged ions and repel negatively charged ions, they increase the concentration of positive ions such as sodium and decrease the concentration of negative ions such as chloride. The increase in the total concentration of inorganic ions causes an increase in the osmolarity of the tissue; that is, it creates a Donnan effect. The collagen network resists the Donnan osmotic pressure caused by the inorganic ions associated with the proteoglycans.[6,21]

Structural Macromolecules The structural macromolecules of the cartilage, collagens, proteoglycans, and noncollagenous proteins, contribute 20% to 40% of the wet weight of the tissue.[3] The three classes of macromolecules differ in their concentrations within the tissue and in their contributions to the tissue properties. Collagens contribute about 60% of the dry weight of cartilage; proteoglycans contribute 25% to 35%; and noncollagenous proteins and glycoproteins, 15% to 20%. Collagens are distributed relatively uniformly throughout the depth of the cartilage, except for the collagen-rich superficial zone. The collagen fibrillar meshwork gives cartilage its form and tensile strength.[21] Proteoglycans and noncollagenous proteins bind to the collagenous meshwork or become mechanically

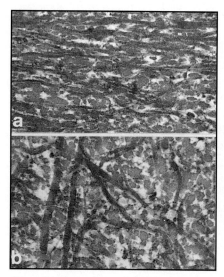
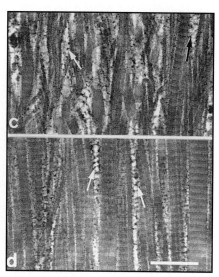

Fig. 3 Electron micrographs of the interterritorial matrix of articular cartilage from the medial femoral condyle of an 8-month-old rabbit. **a**: superficial zone; **b**: transitional zone; **c**: upper portion of the middle (radial), or deep, zone; and **d**: lower portion of the middle (radial), or deep, zone. The arrows indicate proteoglycans precipitated with ruthenium hexamine trichloride (bar = 0.5 μm). (Reproduced with permission from Buckwalter JA, Hunziker EB, Rosenberg LC, et al: Articular cartilage: Composition and structure, in Woo SL-Y, Buckwalter JA (eds): *Injury and Repair of the Musculoskeletal Soft Tissues.* Park Ridge, IL, American Academy of Orthopaedic Surgeons, 1988, pp 405–425.)

entrapped within it, and water fills this molecular framework. Some noncollagenous proteins help to organize and stabilize the macromolecular framework of the matrix, while others help chondrocytes to bind to the macromolecules of the matrix.

Collagens Articular cartilage contains multiple genetically distinct collagen types,[26-28] specifically types II, VI, IX, X, and XI. Types II, IX, and XI form the cross-banded fibrils seen with electron microscopy (Fig. 3). The organization of these fibrils into a tight meshwork that extends throughout the tissue provides the tensile stiffness and strength of articular cartilage and contributes to the cohesiveness of the tissue by mechanically entrapping the large proteoglycans. The principal collagen, type II, accounts for 90% to 95% of the collagen in articular cartilage and forms the primary component of the cross-banded fibrils. Type IX collagen molecules bind covalently to the superficial layers of the cross-banded fibrils and project into the matrix, where

they also can bind covalently to other type IX collagen molecules. Type XI collagen molecules bind covalently to type II collagen molecules and probably form part of the interior structure of the cross-banded fibrils. The functions of type IX and type XI collagens remain uncertain, but presumably they help to form and stabilize the collagen fibrils assembled primarily from type II collagen. The projecting portions of type IX collagen molecules may also help to bind together the collagen-fibril meshwork[26,27,29-31] and to connect the meshwork with proteoglycans.[31] Type VI collagen appears to form an important part of the matrix immediately surrounding the chondrocytes and to help chondrocytes attach to the matrix.[32,33] The presence of type X collagen only near the cells of the calcified cartilage zone of the articular cartilage and the hypertrophic zone of the growth plate (where the longitudinal cartilage septa begin to mineralize) suggests that it has a role in mineralization of the cartilage.

Proteoglycans Proteoglycans consist of a protein core and one or more glycosaminoglycan chains (long unbranched polysaccharide chains consisting of repeating disaccharides that contain an amino sugar).[31,34-36] Each unit of disaccharide has at least one negatively charged carboxylate or sulfate group, so the glycosaminoglycans form long strings of negative charges that repel other negatively charged molecules and that attract cations. Glycosaminoglycans found in cartilage include hyaluronic acid, chondroitin sulfate, keratan sulfate, and dermatan sulfate. The concentration of these molecules varies among sites within articular cartilage and also with age, injury to the cartilage, and disease.

Articular cartilage contains two major classes of proteoglycans: large aggregating proteoglycan monomers or aggrecans, and small proteoglycans including decorin, biglycan, and fibromodulin.[31,34-38] Because it may have a glycosaminoglycan component, type IX collagen is also considered a proteoglycan.[31] Aggrecans have large numbers of chondroitin-sulfate and keratan-sulfate chains attached to a protein core filament. Cartilage also contains large nonaggregating proteoglycans that resemble aggrecans in structure and composition and may represent degraded aggrecans.[16,36] Decorin has one dermatan-sulfate chain, biglycan has two dermatan-sulfate chains, and fibromodulin has several keratan-sulfate chains.[31] The tissue probably also contains other small proteoglycans that have not been identified. Aggrecan molecules fill most of the interfibrillar space of the cartilage matrix, contributing about 90% of the total cartilage matrix proteoglycan mass; large nonaggregating proteoglycans contribute 10% or less; and small nonaggregating proteoglycans contribute about 3%. Although the small proteoglycans contribute relatively little to the total mass of proteoglycans compared with the aggrecans, because of their small size they may be present in equal or higher molar amounts.

In the articular cartilage matrix, most aggrecans noncovalently associate with hyaluronic acid (hyaluronan) and link proteins (small noncollagenous proteins) to form proteoglycan aggregates[39-41] (Fig. 4). These large molecules have a central backbone of hyaluronan that can range in length from several hundred to more than 10,000 nanometers.[39,40] Large aggregates may have more than 300 associated aggrecan molecules.[40] Link proteins stabilize the association between monomers and hyaluronic acid and appear to have a role in directing the assembly of aggregates.[42,43] The formation of aggregates helps to anchor proteoglycans within the matrix, preventing their displacement during deformation of the tissue, and helps to organize and stabilize the relationship between proteoglycans and the collagen meshwork.

Centrifugation and biochemical and electron microscopy studies show two populations of proteoglycan aggregates within articular cartilage: a slow sedimenting population of aggregates with a low chondroitin sulfate-to-hyaluronate ratio and few monomers per aggregate, and a faster sedimenting population of aggregates with a higher chondroitin sulfate-to-hyaluronate ratio and more monomers per aggregate.[41,44-46] The superficial regions of articular cartilage contain primarily the smaller, slow-sedimenting aggregates, and the deeper regions contain both types of aggregates. Loss of the larger aggregates appears to be one of the earliest changes associated with osteoarthritis and immobilization of the joint. Increasing age is also associated with a loss of large proteoglycan aggregates from articular cartilage.[16,47]

The small nonaggregating proteoglycans have shorter protein cores than do aggrecan molecules; unlike aggrecans, they do not fill a large volume of the tissue or contribute directly to the mechanical behavior of the tissue. Instead, they bind to other macromolecules and probably influence cell function. Decorin and

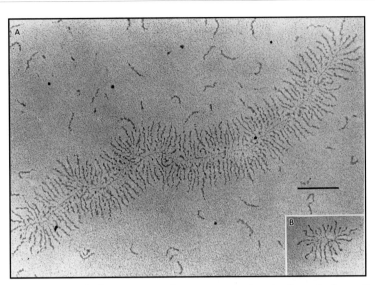

Fig. 4 Electron micrograph showing proteoglycan aggregates from bovine articular cartilage. The aggregates consist of central hyaluronan filaments and multiple attached aggrecan molecules. **A,** aggregate from a calf, and **B** (inset), aggregate from a steer. Aggregates from older animals have shorter hyaluronan filaments and fewer aggrecans; in addition, the aggrecans are shorter and vary more in length (bar = 500 μm). (Reproduced with permission from Buckwalter JA, Kuettner KE, Thonar EJ: Age-related changes in articular cartilage proteoglycans: Electron microscopic studies. *J Orthop Res* 1985;3:251-257.)

fibromodulin bind with type II collagen and may have a role in organizing and stabilizing the type II collagen meshwork.[31,48-50] Biglycan is concentrated in the pericellular matrix and may interact with type VI collagen.[31] The small proteoglycans also can bind transforming growth factor-β and may influence the activity of this cytokine in cartilage.[51]

Noncollagenous Proteins and Glycoproteins The noncollagenous proteins and glycoproteins are not as well understood as the collagens and proteoglycans. A wide variety of these molecules exist within normal articular cartilage, but thus far only a few of them have been studied. In general, they consist primarily of protein and have a few attached monosaccharides and oligosaccharides.[52,53] At least some of these molecules appear to help to organize and maintain the macromolecular structure of the matrix. Anchorin CII, a collagen-binding chondrocyte surface protein, may help to anchor chondrocytes to the collagen fib-

rils of the matrix.[54,55] Cartilage oligomeric protein, an acidic protein, is concentrated primarily within the territorial matrix of the chondrocyte and appears to be present only within cartilage and to have the capacity to bind to chondrocytes.[56,57] This molecule may have value as a marker of cartilage turnover and of the progression of cartilage degeneration in patients who have osteoarthrosis.[58-60] Fibronectin and tenascin, noncollagenous matrix proteins found in a variety of tissues, also have been identified within cartilage.[61-65] Their functions in articular cartilage remain poorly understood, but they may have roles in matrix organization, cell-matrix interactions, and the responses of the tissue in inflammatory arthritis and osteoarthritis.

Articular Cartilage Structure

To form articular cartilage, chondrocytes organize the collagens, proteoglycans, and noncollagenous proteins into a unique, highly ordered structure.[3] The

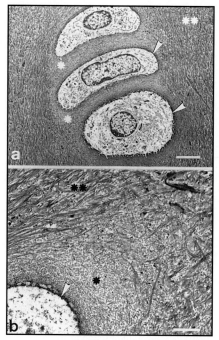

Fig. 5 Electron micrographs showing the matrix compartments of the articular cartilage of the medial femoral condyle of an 8-month-old rabbit. **a,**The image shows the pericellular matrix (arrowheads), the territorial matrix (asterisk), and the interterritorial matrix (double asterisk) (bar = 3 μm). **b,** Higher-magnification view of the compartments of the matrix, showing the relationship between the cell membrane and the pericellular matrix (bar = 1 μm). Note the short cell processes that extend through the pericellular matrix. (Reproduced with permission from Buckwalter JA, Hunziker EB, Rosenberg LC, et al: Articular cartilage: Composition and structure, in Woo SL-Y, Buckwalter JA (eds): *Injury and Repair of the Musculoskeletal Soft Tissues*. Park Ridge, IL, American Academy of Orthopaedic Surgeons, 1988, pp 405–425.)

composition, organization, and mechanical properties of the matrix; cell morphology; and, probably, cell function vary according to the depth from the articular surface (Figs. 1, 2, and 3). The composition, organization, and function of the matrix also vary according to the distance from the cell (Fig. 5).

Zones

The morphologic changes in chondrocytes and matrix from the articular surface to the subchondral bone make it possible to identify four layers, or zones. These consist of a superficial zone; a transitional zone; a middle (radial), or deep, zone; and a zone of calcified cartilage (Fig. 1).[4] The relative size and appearance of these zones vary among species and among joints within the same species; although each zone has different morphologic features, the boundaries between the zones cannot be sharply defined. Nonetheless, recent biologic and mechanical studies have shown that the zonal organization has functional importance.[3,10] The matrices differ with respect to concentrations of water, proteoglycan, and collagen and with respect to the size of the aggregates.[3] Cells in different zones differ not only in shape, size, and orientation relative to the articular surface (Fig. 2) but also in metabolic activity.[10] They may respond differently to mechanical loading, suggesting that the development and maintenance of normal articular cartilage depend in part on the differentiation of phenotypically distinct populations of chondrocytes.

Superficial Zone The unique structure and composition of the thinnest zone of articular cartilage, the superficial zone, give it specialized mechanical and possibly specialized biologic properties. This zone typically consists of two layers. A sheet of fine fibrils with little polysaccharide and no cells covers the joint surface. This portion of the superficial zone presumably corresponds to the clear film, often identified as the lamina splendens, which can be stripped from the articular surface in some regions. Deep to this acellular sheet of fine fibrils, flattened ellipsoid-shaped chondrocytes arrange themselves so that their major axes are parallel to the articular surface (Fig. 2). The chondrocytes synthesize a matrix that has a high concentration of collagen and a low concentration of proteoglycan relative to the other cartilage zones; studies of cultures of cells from the superficial zone have shown that these cells degrade

proteoglycans more rapidly and synthesize less collagen and proteoglycans than do cells from the deeper zones.[10] Concentrations of fibronectin and water are also highest in this zone.

The dense matrix of collagen fibrils lying parallel to the joint surface in the superficial zone (Fig. 3) helps to determine the mechanical properties of the tissue and affects the movement of molecules in and out of the cartilage. These fibrils give this zone greater tensile stiffness and strength than the deeper zones, and they may resist shear forces generated during use of the joint.[4,6,66] In vitro experiments have shown that the superficial zone also makes an important contribution to the compressive behavior of articular cartilage.[67] Removal of this zone increases the permeability of the tissue and probably increases loading of the macromolecular framework during compression; disruption or remodeling of the dense collagenous matrix of the superficial zone is one of the first detectable structural changes in experimentally induced degeneration of articular cartilage,[68] suggesting that alterations in this zone may contribute to the development of osteoarthrosis by changing the mechanical behavior of the tissue. The densely packed collagen fibrils also create a so-called skin for the articular cartilage that may limit the ingress of large molecules such as antibodies or other proteins and the egress of large cartilage molecules. By acting as a barrier to the passage of large molecules between the synovial fluid and the cartilage, the superficial zone may effectively isolate cartilage from the immune system. Thus, disruption of this zone not only may alter the structure and mechanical properties of articular cartilage, but also may release cartilage molecules that stimulate an immune or inflammatory response.

Transitional Zone As the name of this zone implies, the morphology and the matrix composition of the transitional zone are intermediate between the superficial zone and the middle (radial) zone. The transitional zone usually has several times the volume of the superficial zone. The cells have a higher concentration of synthetic organelles, endoplasmic reticulum, and Golgi membranes than do cells in the superficial zone (Fig. 2). Cells in the transitional zone assume a spheroidal shape and synthesize a matrix that has larger-diameter collagen fibrils, a higher concentration of proteoglycan, and lower concentrations of water and collagen than does the matrix of the superficial zone.

Middle (Radial) Zone The chondrocytes in the middle zone are spheroidal in shape and tend to align themselves in columns perpendicular to the joint surface (Figs. 1 and 2). This zone contains the largest-diameter collagen fibrils, the highest concentration of proteoglycans, and the lowest concentration of water. The collagen fibers pass into the tidemark, a thin basophilic line seen on light microscopic sections of decalcified articular cartilage that roughly corresponds to the boundary between calcified and uncalcified cartilage. The nature of the tidemark remains uncertain.[69] It may result from the concentration of basophilic calcified material at the interface between calcified and uncalcified matrix, possibly accentuated by tissue-processing, and thus may represent a so-called high water mark for calcification. Alternatively, one study revealed a band of fine fibrils corresponding to the tidemark,[70] suggesting that it represents a well-defined matrix structure.

Calcified Cartilage Zone A thin zone of calcified cartilage separates the radial zone (uncalcified cartilage) from the subchondral bone. The cells of the zone of calcified cartilage have a smaller volume than the cells of the radial zone, and they contain only small amounts of endoplasmic reticulum and Golgi membranes (Fig. 2). In some regions, these cells appear to be surrounded completely by calcified cartilage; that is, they are buried in individual calcific sepulchers, suggesting that the cells have an extremely low level of metabolic activity. However, recent work suggests that they may have a role in the development and progression of osteoarthritis.[69]

Matrix Regions

Variations in the matrix within zones allow the distinction of three compartments, or regions: a pericellular region, a territorial region, and an interterritorial region (Fig. 5).[3] The pericellular and territorial regions appear to serve the needs of chondrocytes, binding the cell membranes to the matrix macromolecules and protecting the cells from damage during loading and deformation of the tissue. They may also help to transmit mechanical signals to the chondrocytes when the matrix deforms during joint loading. The primary function of the interterritorial matrix (Fig. 3) is to provide the mechanical properties of the tissue.

Pericellular Region Chondrocyte cell membranes appear to attach to the thin rim of the pericellular matrix that covers the cell surface. This region is rich in proteoglycans and also contains noncollagenous proteins, such as the cell-membrane-associated molecule anchorin CII[54,55] and nonfibrillar collagens, such as type VI collagen.[32,33] It has little or no fibrillar collagen. Cytoplasmic extensions from the chondrocytes project into and through the pericellular matrix to the territorial matrix.

Territorial Region An envelope of territorial matrix surrounds the pericellular matrix of individual chondrocytes and, in some locations, pairs or clusters of chondrocytes and their pericellular matrices. In the radial zone, a territorial matrix surrounds each column of chondrocytes. The thin collagen fibrils of the territorial matrix nearest to the cell appear to adhere to the pericellular matrix. At a distance from the cell, they decussate and intersect at various angles, forming a fibrillar basket around the cells. This collagenous basket may provide mechanical protection for the chondrocytes during loading and deformation of the tissue. An abrupt increase in the diameter of the collagen fibril and a transition from the basket-like orientation of the fibrils to a more parallel arrangement marks the boundary between the territorial and interterritorial matrices. However, many collagen fibrils connect the two regions, making it difficult to identify precisely the boundary between them.

Interterritorial Region The interterritorial matrix makes up most of the volume of mature articular cartilage (Fig. 1) and contains the largest-diameter collagen fibrils. Unlike the collagen fibrils of the territorial matrix, these fibrils are not organized to surround the chondrocytes and they change their orientation relative to the joint surface 90° from the superficial zone to the radial zone (Fig. 3). In the superficial zone, the fibrils have a relatively small diameter and generally lie parallel to the articular surface; in the transitional zone, interterritorial fibrils assume more oblique angles relative to the articular surface; and, in the radial zone, they generally lie perpendicular (or radial) to the joint surface.

Chondrocyte-Matrix Interactions

The interdependence of the chondrocytes and the matrix makes possible the maintenance of the tissue throughout life. The relationship between the chondrocytes and the matrix does not end when the cells secrete the matrix macromolecules. The matrix protects the chondrocytes from mechanical damage during normal use of the joint, helping to maintain their shape and phenotype. Nutrients, substrates for the synthesis of matrix molecules, newly synthesized molecules, degraded matrix molecules, metabolic waste products, and molecules that help to regulate cell function, such as cytokines and growth factors, all pass through the matrix, and in some instances they may be stored in the matrix. The types of molecules that can pass through the matrix and the rate at which they can pass depend on the composition and organization of the matrix, primarily the concentration, composition, and organization of the large proteoglycans.

Throughout life, chondrocytes degrade and synthesize matrix macromolecules. The mechanisms that control the balance between these activities remain poorly understood, but cytokines with catabolic and anabolic effects appear to have important roles.[71-74] For example, interleukin-1 induces the expression of matrix metalloproteases that can degrade the matrix macromolecules, and it interferes with the synthesis of matrix proteoglycans at the transcriptional level. Other cytokines, such as insulin-dependent growth factor-I and transforming growth factor-β, oppose these catabolic activities by stimulating matrix synthesis and cell proliferation. In response to a variety of stimuli, chondrocytes synthesize and release these cytokines into the matrix, where they may bind to receptors on the cell surfaces (stimulating cell activity by either autocrine or paracrine mechanisms) or may become trapped within the matrix. The anabolic activities appear in large measure to be responses to structural needs of the matrix or other stimuli, possibly including mechanical loading of the tissue detected by the chondrocytes. The degradative response, on the other hand, appears to be the result of a complex cascade that includes the activation or inhibition of interleukin-1, stromelysin, aggrecanase, plasmin, and collagenase by factors such as prostaglandins, transforming growth factor-β, tumor necrosis factor, tissue inhibitors of metalloproteases, tissue plasminogen activator, plasminogen activator inhibitor, and other molecules.

The matrix also acts as a signal transducer for the chondrocytes. It transmits signals that result from mechanical loading of the articular surface to the chondrocytes, and the chondrocytes respond to these signals by altering the matrix, possibly through the expression of cytokines that act through autocrine or paracrine mechanisms. Experimental studies have shown that a persistent abnormal decrease in joint loading or immobilization of a joint decreases the concentration of proteoglycan in articular cartilage and the degree of proteoglycan aggregation and alters the mechanical properties of cartilage.[13,15,75] Resumption of use of the joint restores the composition and mechanical properties of the matrix toward normal; thus, maintenance of the normal composition of articular cartilage requires a minimum level of loading and motion of the joint.[14,15] Repetitive loading and motion of the joint at greater-than-normal levels may increase the synthetic activity of chondrocytes, but the chondrocytes have limited, if any, ability to expand the tissue volume in adults.

The details of how the mechanical loading of joints influences chondrocyte function remain unknown, but deformation of the matrix produces mechanical, electrical, and physicochemical signals that may have major roles in stimulating chondrocytes[14,76-78]. Compression of the articular surface deforms the matrix and may directly deform chondrocytes. Deformation of the matrix also produces electrical and physicochemical effects that may influence chondrocytes. It causes flow of the tissue fluid and the counter-ions relative to the fixed charged groups of the matrix macromolecules. This flow alters the charge density around the cells and produces a streaming potential. Changes in charge density within the matrix alter the Donnan osmotic pressure and the osmotic pressure gradients. Mechanically induced flow of the matrix fluid may also accelerate the flow of nutrients and metabolites through the matrix. Loading may also cause persistent changes in the molecular organization of the matrix, altering the

response of the chondrocytes to subsequent loading. Thus, the matrix may not only transduce and transmit signals, it may record the loading history of the tissue and alter the response of the cells on the basis of the loading history.

Summary
The unique biologic and mechanical properties of articular cartilage depend on the design of the tissue and the interactions between the chondrocytes and the matrix that maintain the tissue. Chondrocytes form the macromolecular framework of the tissue matrix from three classes of molecules: collagens, proteoglycans, and noncollagenous proteins. Type II, IX, and XI collagens form a fibrillar meshwork that gives the tissue its form and tensile stiffness and strength. Type VI collagen forms part of the matrix immediately surrounding the chondrocytes and may help the chondrocytes to attach to the macromolecular framework of the matrix. Large aggregating proteoglycans (aggrecans) give the tissue its stiffness to compression and its resilience and contribute to its durability. Small proteoglycans, including decorin, biglycan, and fibromodulin, bind to other matrix macromolecules and thereby help to stabilize the matrix. They may also influence the function of the chondrocytes and bind growth factors. Anchorin CII, a noncollagenous protein, appears to help to anchor chondrocytes to the matrix. Cartilage oligomeric protein may have value as a marker of turnover and degeneration of cartilage, and other noncollagenous proteins, including tenascin and fibronectin, can influence interactions between the chondrocytes and the matrix. The matrix protects the cells from injury due to normal use of the joint, determines the types and concentrations of molecules that reach the cells, and helps to maintain the chondrocyte phenotype.

Throughout life, the tissue undergoes continual internal remodeling as the cells replace matrix macromolecules lost through degradation. The available evidence indicates that normal matrix turnover depends on the ability of chondrocytes to detect alterations in the macromolecular composition and organization of the matrix, including the presence of degraded molecules, and to respond by synthesizing appropriate types and amounts of new molecules. In addition, the matrix acts as a signal transducer for the cells. Loading of the tissue due to use of the joint creates mechanical, electrical, and physicochemical signals that help to direct the synthetic and degradative activity of chondrocytes. A prolonged severe decrease in the use of the joint leads to alterations in the composition of the matrix and eventually to loss of tissue structure and mechanical properties, whereas use of the joint stimulates the synthetic activity of chondrocytes and possibly the internal tissue remodeling. Aging leads to alterations in the composition of the matrix and the activity of the chondrocytes, including the ability of the cells to respond to a variety of stimuli such as growth factors. These alterations may increase the probability of degeneration of the cartilage.

References

1. Whitman W: Leaves of grass (song of myself), in Kaplan J (ed): *Walt Whitman: Complete Poetry and Collected Prose.* New York, NY, Library of America, 1982.

2. Almquist EE: Evolution of the distal radioulnar joint. *Clin Orthop* 1992;275:5-13.

3. Buckwalter JA, Rosenberg LC, Hunziker EB: Articular cartilage: Composition, structure, response to injury, and methods of facilitating repair, in Ewing JW (ed): *Articular Cartilage and Knee Joint Function: Basic Science and Arthroscopy.* New York, NY, Raven Press, 1990, pp 19-56.

4. Buckwalter JA, Rosenberg LC, Hunziker EB, et al: Articular cartilage: Composition and structure, in Woo SL-Y, Buckwalter JA (eds): *Injury and Repair of the Musculoskeletal Soft Tissues.* Park Ridge, IL, American Academy of Orthopaedic Surgeons, 1988, pp 405-425.

5. Athanasiou KA, Rosenwasser MP, Buckwalter JA, et al: Interspecies comparisons of in situ intrinsic mechanical properties of distal femoral cartilage. *J Orthop Res* 1991;9:330-340.

6. Mow VC, Rosenwasser MP: Articular cartilage: Biomechanics, in Woo SLY, Buckwalter JA (eds): *Injury and Repair of the Musculoskeletal Soft Tissues.* Park Ridge, IL, American Academy of Orthopaedic Surgeons, 1988, pp 427-463.

7. Mow VC, Setton LA, Guilak F, et al: Mechanical factors in articular cartilage and their role in osteoarthritis, in Kuettner KE, Goldberg VM (eds): *Osteoarthritic Disorders.* Rosemont, Illinois, American Academy of Orthopaedic Surgeons, 1995, pp 147-171.

8. Stockwell RA: The cell density of human articular and costal cartilage. *J Anat* 1967;101:753-763.

9. Stockwell RA: Chondrocytes. *J Clin Pathol* 1978;12(suppl):7-13.

10. Aydelotte MB, Schumacher BL, Kuettner KE: Heterogeneity of articular chondrocytes, in Kuettner KE, Schleyerbach R, Peyron JG, et al (eds): *Articular Cartilage and Osteoarthritis.* New York, NY, Raven Press, 1992, pp 237-249.

11. Aydelotte MB, Michal LE, Reid DR, et al: Chondrocytes from the articular surface and deep zone express different, but stable, phenotypes in alginate gel culture. *Trans Orthop Res Soc* 1996;21:317.

12. Fischer AE, Carpenter TA, Tyler JA, et al: Visualisation of mass transport of small organic molecules and metal ions through articular cartilage by magnetic resonance imaging. *Magn Reson Imaging* 1995;13:819-826.

13. Buckwalter JA: Activity vs rest in the treatment of bone, soft tissue and joint injuries. *Iowa Orthop J* 1995;15:29-42.

14. Buckwalter JA, Lane NE: Aging, sports and osteoarthritis. *Sports Med Arthrosc Rev* 1996;4:276-287.

15. Buckwalter JA: Osteoarthritis and articular cartilage use, disuse, and abuse: Experimental studies. *J Rheumatol* 1995;43(suppl):13-15.

16. Buckwalter JA, Roughley PJ, Rosenberg LC: Age-related changes in cartilage proteoglycans: Quantitative electron microscopic studies. *Microsc Res Tech* 1994;28:398-408.

17. Buckwalter JA, Woo SL-Y, Goldberg VM, et al: Soft-tissue aging and musculoskeletal function. *J Bone Joint Surg* 1993;75A:1533-1548.

18. Guerne PA, Blanco F, Kaelin A, et al: Growth factor responsiveness of human articular chondrocytes in aging and development. *Arthritis Rheum* 1995;38:960-968.

19. Martin JA, Buckwalter JA: Articular cartilage aging and degeneration. *Sports Med Arthrosc Rev* 1996;4:263-275.

20. Martin JA, Buckwalter JA: Fibronectin and cell shape affect the age-related decline in chondrocyte synthetic response to IGF-I. *Trans Orthop Res Soc* 1996;21:306.

21. Buckwalter JA, Mow VC: Cartilage repair in osteoarthritis, in Moskowitz RW, Howell DS, Goldberg VM, et al (eds): *Osteoarthritis, Diagnosis and Medical/Surgical Management,* ed 2. Philadelphia, PA, WB Saunders, 1992, pp 71-107.

22. Lai WM, Mow VC, Roth V: Effects of nonlinear strain-dependent permeability and rate of compression on the stress behavior of articular cartilage. *J Biomech Eng* 1981;103:61-66.

23. Linn FC, Sokoloff L: Movement and composition of interstitial fluid of cartilage. *Arthritis Rheum* 1965;8:481-494.

24. Mankin HJ: The water of articular cartilage, in Simon WH (ed): *The Human Joint in Health and Disease.* Philadelphia, PA, University of Pennsylvania Press, 1978, pp 37-42.

25. Maroudas A, Schneiderman R: "Free" and "exchangeable" or "trapped" and "nonexchangeable" water in cartilage. *J Orthop Res* 1987;5:133-138.

26. Eyre DR: Collagen structure and function in articular cartilage: Metabolic changes in the development of osteoarthritis, in Kuettner KE, Goldberg VM (eds): *Osteoarthritic Disorders.* Rosemont, IL, American Academy of Orthopaedic Surgeons, 1995, pp 219-229.

27. Eyre DR, Wu JJ, Woods P: Cartilage-specific collagens: Structural studies, in Kuettner KE, Schleyerbach R, Peyron JG, et al (eds): *Articular Cartilage and Osteoarthritis.* New York, NY, Raven Press, 1992, pp 119-131.

28. Sandell LJ: Molecular biology of collagens in normal and osteoarthritic cartilage, in Kuettner KE, Goldberg VM (eds): *Osteoarthritic Disorders.* Rosemont, IL, American Academy of Orthopaedic Surgeons, 1995, pp 131-146.

29. Bruckner P, Mendler M, Steinmann B, et al: The structure of human collagen type IX and its organization in fetal and infant cartilage fibrils. *J Biol Chem* 1988;263:16911-16917.

30. Diab M, Wu JJ, Eyre DR: Collagen type IX from human cartilage: A structural profile of intermolecular cross-linking sites. *Biochem J* 1996;314:327-332.

31. Roughley PJ, Lee ER: Cartilage proteoglycans: Structure and potential functions. *Microsc Res Tech* 1994;28:385-397.

32. Hagiwara H, Schroter-Kermani C, Merker HJ: Localization of collagen type VI in articular cartilage of young and adult mice. *Cell Tissue Res* 1993;272:155-160.

33. Marcelino J, McDevitt CA: Attachment of articular cartilage chondrocytes to the tissue form of type VI collagen. *Biochim Biophys Acta* 1995;1249:180-188.

34. Hardingham TE, Fosang AJ, Dudhia J: Aggrecan, the chondroitin/sulfate/keratan sulfate proteoglycan from cartilage, in Kuettner KE, Schleyerbach R, Peyron JG, et al (eds): *Articular Cartilage and Osteoarthritis.* New York, NY, Raven Press, 1992, pp 5-20.

35. Rosenberg LC: Structure and function of dermatan sulfate proteoglycans in articular cartilage, in Kuettner KE, Schleyerbach R, Peyron JG, et al (eds): *Articular Cartilage and Osteoarthritis.* New York, NY, Raven Press, 1992, pp 45-63.

36. Rosenberg LC, Buckwalter JA: Cartilage proteoglycans, in Kuettner KE, Schleyerbach R, Hascall VC (eds): *Articular Cartilage Biochemistry.* New York, NY, Raven Press, 1986, pp 39-57.

37. Poole AR, Rosenberg LC, Reiner A, et al: Contents and distributions of the proteoglycans decorin and biglycan in normal and osteoarthritic human articular cartilage. *J Orthop Res* 1996;14:681-689.

38. Sandell LJ, Chansky H, Zamparo O, et al: Molecular biology of cartilage proteoglycans and link protein, in Kuettner KE, Goldberg VM (eds): *Osteoarthritic Disorders*. Rosemont, IL, American Academy of Orthopaedic Surgeons, 1995, pp 117-130.

39. Buckwalter JA, Rosenberg LC: Electron microscopic studies of cartilage proteoglycans: Direct evidence for the variable length of the chondroitin sulfate-rich region of proteoglycan subunit core protein. *J Biol Chem* 1982;257:9830-9839.

40. Buckwalter JA, Rosenberg L: Structural changes during development in bovine fetal epiphyseal cartilage. *Collagen Rel Res* 1983;3:489-504.

41. Buckwalter JA, Pita JC, Muller FJ, et al: Structural differences between two populations of articular cartilage proteoglycan aggregates. *J Orthop Res* 1994;12:144-148.

42. Buckwalter JA, Rosenberg LC, Tang LH: The effect of link protein on proteoglycan aggregate structure: An electron microscopic study of the molecular architecture and dimensions of proteoglycan aggregates reassembled from the proteoglycan monomers and link proteins of bovine fetal epiphyseal cartilage. *J Biol Chem* 1984;259:5361-5363.

43. Tang LH, Buckwalter JA, Rosenberg LC: Effect of link protein concentration on articular cartilage proteoglycan aggregation. *J Orthop Res* 1996;14:334-339.

44. Müller FJ, Pita JC, Manicourt DH, et al: Centrifugal characterization of proteoglycans from various depth layers and weight-bearing areas of normal and abnormal human articular cartilage. *J Orthop Res* 1989;7:326-334.

45. Pita JC, Manicourt DH, Müller FJ: Centrifugal and biochemical comparison of two populations of proteoglycan aggregates from articular cartilage of immobilized dog joints. *Trans Orthop Res Soc* 1990;15:17.

46. Pita JC, Müller FJ, Manicourt DH, et al: Early matrix changes in experimental osteoarthritis and joint disuse atrophy, in Kuettner KE, Schleyerbach R, Peyron JG, et al (eds): *Articular Cartilage and Osteoarthritis*. New York, NY, Raven Press, 1992, pp 455-469.

47. Buckwalter JA, Kuettner KE, Thonar EJ: Age-related changes in articular cartilage proteoglycans: Electron microscopic studies. *J Orthop Res* 1985;3:251-257.

48. Hedbom E, Heinegard D: Interaction of a 59-kDa connective tissue matrix protein with collagen I and collagen II. *J Biol Chem* 1989;264:6898-6905.

49. Hedbom E, Heinegard D: Binding of fibromodulin and decorin to separate sites on fibrillar collagens. *J Biol Chem* 1993;268:27307-27312.

50. Hedlund H, Mengarelli-Widholm S, Heinegard D, et al: Fibromodulin distribution and association with collagen. *Matrix Biol* 1994;14:227-232.

51. Hildebrand A, Romaris M, Rasmussen LM, et al: Interaction of the small interstitial proteoglycans biglycan, decorin and fibromodulin with transforming growth factor beta. *Biochem J* 1994;302:527-534.

52. Heinegård DK, Pimentel ER: Cartilage matrix proteins, in Kuettner KE, Schleyerbach R, Peyron JG, et al (eds): *Articular Cartilage and Osteoarthritis*. New York, NY, Raven Press, 1992, pp 95-111.

53. Heinegård D, Lorenzo P, Sommarin Y: Articular cartilage matrix proteins, in Kuettner KE, Goldberg VM (eds): *Osteoarthritic Disorders*. Rosemont, IL, American Academy of Orthopaedic Surgeons, 1995, pp 229-237.

54. Mollenhauer J, Bee JA, Lizarbe MA, et al: Role of anchorin CII, a 31,000-mol-wt membrane protein, in the interaction of chondrocytes with type II collagen. *J Cell Biol* 1984;98:1572-1579.

55. Pfaffle M, Borcher M, Deutzmann R, et al: Anchorin CII, a collagen-binding chondrocyte surface protein of the calpactin family. *Prog Clin Biol Res* 1990;349:147-157.

56. DiCesare PE, Morgelin M, Mann K, et al: Cartilage oligomeric matrix protein and thrombospondin 1: Purification from articular cartilage, electron microscopic structure, and chondrocyte binding. *Eur J Biochem* 1994;223:927-937.

57. Hedbom E, Antonsson P, Hjerpe A, et al: Cartilage matrix proteins: An acidic oligomeric protein (COMP) detected only in cartilage. *J Biol Chem* 1992;267:6132-6136.

58. Lohmander LS, Saxne T, Heinegård DK: Release of cartilage oligomeric matrix protein (COMP) into joint fluid after knee injury and in osteoarthritis. *Ann Rheum Dis* 1994;53:8-13.

59. Saxne T, Heinegård D: Cartilage oligomeric matrix protein: A novel marker of cartilage turnover detectable in synovial fluid and blood. *Br J Rheumatol* 1992;31:583-591.

60. Sharif M, Saxne T, Shepstone L, et al: Relationship between serum cartilage oligomeric matrix protein levels and disease progression in osteoarthritis of the knee joint. *Br J Rheumatol* 1995;34:306-310.

61. Chevalier X, Groult N, Larget-Piet B, et al: Tenascin distribution in articular cartilage from normal subjects and from patients with osteoarthritis and rheumatoid arthritis. *Arthritis Rheum* 1994;37:1013-1022.

62. Hayashi T, Abe E, Jasin HE: Fibronectin synthesis in superficial and deep layers of normal articular cartilage. *Arthritis Rheum* 1996;39:567-573.

63. Nishida K, Inoue H, Murakami T: Immunohistochemical demonstration of fibronectin in the most superficial layer of normal rabbit articular cartilage. *Ann Rheum Dis* 1995;54:995-998.

64. Salter DM: Tenascin is increased in cartilage and synovium from arthritic knees. *Br J Rheumatol* 1993;32:780-786.

65. Savarese JJ, Erickson H, Scully SP: Articular chondrocyte tenascin-C production and assembly into de novo extracellular matrix. *J Orthop Res* 1996;14:273-281.

66. Roth V, Mow VC: The intrinsic tensile behavior of the matrix of bovine articular cartilage and its variation with age. *J Bone Joint Surg* 1980;62A:1102-1117.

67. Setton LA, Zhu W, Mow VC: The biphasic poroviscoelastic behavior of articular cartilage: Role of the surface zone in governing the compressive behavior. *J Biomech* 1993;26:581-592.

68. Guilak F, Ratcliffe A, Lane N, et al: Mechanical and biochemical changes in the superficial zone of articular cartilage in canine experimental osteoarthritis. *J Orthop Res* 1994;12:474-484.

69. Oegema TR Jr, Thompson RC Jr: Histopathology and pathobiochemistry of the cartilage-bone interface in osteoarthritis, in Kuettner KE, Goldberg VM (eds): *Osteoarthritic Disorders*. Rosemont, IL, American Academy of Orthopaedic Surgeons, 1995, pp 205-217.

70. Redler I, Mow VC, Zimny ML, et al: The ultrastructure and biomechanical significance of the tidemark of articular cartilage. *Clin Orthop* 1975;112:357-362.

71. Lotz M, Blanco FJ, von Kempis J, et al: Cytokine regulation of chondrocyte functions. *J Rheumatol* 1995;43(suppl):104-108.

72. Morales TI: The role of signaling factors in articular cartilage homeostasis and osteoarthritis, in Kuettner KE, Goldberg VM (eds): *Osteoarthritic Disorders*. Rosemont, IL, American Academy of Orthopaedic Surgeons, 1995, pp 261-270.

73. Poole AR: Imbalances of anabolism and catabolism of cartilage matrix components in osteoarthritis, in Kuettner KE, Goldberg VM (eds): *Osteoarthritic Disorders*. Rosemont, IL, American Academy of Orthopaedic Surgeons, 1995, pp 247-260.

74. Trippel SB: Growth factor actions on articular cartilage. *J Rheumatol* 1995;(suppl 43):pp 129-132.

75. Buckwalter JA, Lane NE, Gordon SL: Exercise as a cause of osteoarthritis, in Kuettner KE, Goldberg VM (eds): *Osteoarthritic Disorders*. Rosemont, IL, American Academy of Orthopaedic Surgeons, 1995, pp 405-417.

76. Buckwalter JA: Editorial: Should bone, soft-tissue, and joint injuries be treated with rest or activity? *J Orthop Res* 1995;13:155-156.

77. Gray ML, Pizzanelli AM, Grodzinsky AJ, et al: Mechanical and physiochemical determinants of chondrocyte biosynthetic response. *J Orthop Res* 1988;6:777-792.

78. Grodzinsky AJ: Age-related changes in cartilage: Physical properties and cellular response to loading, in Buckwalter JA, Goldberg VM, Woo SL-Y (eds): *Musculoskeletal Soft-Tissue Aging: Impact on Mobility*. Rosemont, IL, American Academy of Orthopaedic Surgeons, 1993, pp 137-149.

Articular Cartilage: Degeneration and Osteoarthritis, Repair, Regeneration, and Transplantation

Joseph A. Buckwalter, MD

Henry J. Mankin, MD

Joint pain and loss of mobility are among the most common causes of impairment in middle-aged and older people.[1,2] In many instances, the degeneration of articular cartilage and alterations in other joint tissues that result from the loss of structure and function of articular cartilage cause the pain and the loss of motion.[3-8] This occurs most frequently in the clinical syndrome of idiopathic or primary osteoarthritis, but it may also result from joint injury or from developmental, metabolic, and inflammatory disorders that destroy the articular surface, causing secondary osteoarthritis.[3,4,7] An understanding of the degeneration of articular cartilage, osteoarthritis, and the potential for restoring an articular surface depends to a large extent on an appreciation of the biologic behavior and the responsiveness of articular cartilage to injury and disease. Of considerable importance is the observation, first reported centuries ago and confirmed by multiple investigators over the last 50 years, that adult articular cartilage lacks the capacity to repair structural damage resulting from injury or disease.[9-11]

This observation has contributed to the view that adult articular cartilage is an inert bearing surface, like high-density polyethylene or metal, and that degeneration of the articular surface with age is the result of mechanical wear with inevitable, irreversible loss of structure and mechanical performance resulting from joint use.[12] The implication of this view is that, other than limiting joint use or loading, little or nothing can be done to prevent the degeneration of articular cartilage, and the most appropriate treatment for advanced degeneration of cartilage leading to the clinical syndrome of osteoarthritis is replacement of the articular surface. Alternatively, if articular cartilage is not inert, in particular if it has the capacity to restore and remodel itself, then mechanical wear from joint use may not cause degeneration and osteoarthritis, and therapeutic approaches aimed at maintaining or restoring articular cartilage are appropriate for at least some patients. A determination of which view is correct is critical for developing and implementing methods of preventing and treating osteoarthritis.

This review covers the current understanding of the degeneration of articular cartilage (the alterations in composition and the deterioration in structure that lead to the loss of function of articular cartilage), the relationship between the degeneration of articular cartilage and osteoarthritis as well as that between degeneration of articular cartilage and joint use, and approaches to restoring the composition, structure, and function of articular cartilage.

Articular Cartilage Degeneration and Osteoarthritis

The degeneration, or the progressive loss of normal structure and function, of articular cartilage is an integral part of the clinical syndrome of osteoarthritis. Osteoarthritis, also referred to as degenerative joint disease, degenerative osteoarthritis, osteoarthrosis, and hypertrophic osteoarthritis, consists of a generally progressive loss of articular cartilage accompanied by attempted repair of the cartilage, remodeling and sclerosis of subchondral bone, and, in many instances, the formation of subchondral bone cysts and marginal osteophytes.[3,5-8,13-16] In addition to changes in the synovial joint, a diagnosis of osteoarthritis requires the presence of symptoms and signs that may include joint pain, restriction of motion, crepitus with motion, joint effusions, and deformity. Osteoarthritis occurs most frequently in the foot, knee, hip, spine, and hand joints,[2] but it can cause deterioration

Table 1
Known causes of joint degeneration (secondary osteoarthritis)

Cause	Presumed Mechanism
Intra-articular fracture	Damage to articular cartilage or incongruity of joint, or both
High-intensity-impact joint-loading	Damage to articular cartilage or subchondral bone, or both
Ligament injuries	Instability of joint
Dysplasia of joint and cartilage (developmental and hereditary)	Abnormal shape of joint or abnormal articular cartilage, or both
Aseptic necrosis	Bone necrosis leads to collapse of articular surface and incongruity of joint
Acromegaly	Overgrowth of articular cartilage produces incongruity of joint or abnormal cartilage, or both
Paget disease	Distortion or incongruity of joint due to bone-remodeling
Ehlers-Danlos syndrome	Instability of joint
Gaucher disease (hereditary deficiency of enzyme glucocerebrosidase, leading to accumulation of glucocerebroside)	Bone necrosis of pathological fracture leads to incongruity of joint
Stickler syndrome (progressive, hereditary arthro-ophthalmopathy)	Abnormal development of joint or articular cartilage, or both
Infection of joints (inflammation)	Destruction of articular cartilage
Hemophilia	Multiple joint hemorrhages
Hemochromatosis (excess deposition of iron in multiple tissues)	Mechanism unknown
Ochronosis (hereditary deficiency of enzyme homogentisic acid oxidase leading to accumulation of homogentisic acid)	Deposition of homogentisic acid polymers in articular cartilage
Calcium pyrophosphate deposition disease	Accumulation of calcium pyrophosphate crystals in articular cartilage
Neuropathic arthropathy (Charcot joints due to syphilis, diabetes mellitus, syringomyelia, myelomeningocele, leprosy, congenital insensitivity to pain, amyloidosis)	Loss of proprioception and joint sensation results in increased impact loading and torsion, instability of joint, and intra-articular fracture

of any synovial joint.

Osteoarthritis develops most commonly in the absence of a known cause (primary or idiopathic osteoarthritis). Less frequently, it develops as a result of a joint injury, infection, or one of a variety of hereditary, developmental, metabolic, and neurologic disorders; this group of conditions is referred to as secondary osteoarthritis (Table 1). The age of onset associated with secondary osteoarthritis depends on the underlying cause; thus, it may develop in young adults and even children as well as the elderly. In contrast, there is a strong association between the prevalence of primary osteoarthritis and increasing age. Efforts to determine the

exact prevalence of osteoarthritis have important limitations, including difficulty in defining and establishing the diagnosis and in evaluating more than a few synovial joints in each individual; however, studies of the percentage of people who have osteoarthritis as diagnosed on the basis of a medical history, examination, or radiographic evaluation uniformly confirm a striking increase in the prevalence of osteoarthritis of the hand, foot, knee, and hip joints with increasing age.[2,3,7,17,18] Studies of these joints have shown that the percentage of people who have mild, moderate, or severe radiographic changes indicative of osteoarthritis in at least one joint increases

progressively, from less than 5% of people younger than 25 years old to more than 80% of people more than 75 years old, and the percentage of people who have moderate or severe radiographic changes indicative of osteoarthritis in at least one joint increases progressively, from less than 5% of people younger than 45 years old to more than 40% of people more than 75 years old.[2] Despite this strong association between age and osteoarthritis, and despite the widespread view[12] that osteoarthritis results from normal wear and tear and eventually stiffens the joints of virtually everybody who lives past 65, the relationships between joint use, aging, and joint degeneration remain uncertain. Furthermore, the changes observed in articular cartilage from older individuals differ from those observed in articular cartilage from people who have osteoarthrosis[19] (Table 2), and normal lifelong joint use has not been shown to cause degeneration.[20,21] Thus, osteoarthritis is not simply the result of aging and mechanical wear from joint use, nor is primary osteoarthritis caused by inflammation. Unlike the joint destruction seen in joint diseases with a major inflammatory component, osteoarthritis consists of a retrogressive sequence of changes in the cells and matrix that result in the loss of structure and function of articular cartilage accompanied by cartilage repair and bone-remodeling reactions.[3,16] Because of the repair and remodeling reactions, the degeneration of the articular surface in osteoarthritis is not uniformly progressive, and the rate of degeneration varies among individuals and among joints. Occasionally, degeneration occurs rapidly, but in most joints it progresses slowly over many years, although it may stabilize or even decrease spontaneously, with at least partial restoration of the articular surface and a decrease in symptoms.

Osteoarthritis usually involves all of the tissues that form the synovial joint, including articular cartilage, subchondral and metaphyseal bone, synovial tissue, ligaments, joint capsule, and muscles that act across the joint; however, the primary changes consist of loss of articular cartilage, remodeling of subchondral bone, and formation of osteophytes.[3,8] The earliest histologic changes seen in osteoarthritis include fraying or fibrillation of the superficial zone of the articular cartilage, extending into the transitional zone; decreased staining for proteoglycans in the superficial and transitional zones; violation of the tidemark by blood vessels from subchondral bone; and remodeling of subchondral bone. Some investigators have postulated that stiffening of subchondral bone due to remodeling precedes and causes degeneration of articular cartilage and that progression of the degeneration requires stiffening of subchondral bone;[22] alternatively, loss of articular cartilage could increase peak stresses on subchondral bone, causing bone-remodeling. It is not clear which of these views is correct, or if either of them is entirely correct, but in most instances degeneration of articular cartilage and remodeling of subchondral bone are both present when symptoms develop, and it is the loss of articular cartilage that leads directly to the loss of joint function.

The earliest sign of osteoarthritis visible from the articular surface is localized fibrillation or disruption of the most superficial layers of the articular cartilage (Table 2). As the disease progresses, the surface irregularities become clefts, more of the articular surface becomes roughened and irregular, and the fibrillation extends deeper into the cartilage until the fissures reach subchondral bone. As the cartilage fissures grow deeper, the superficial tips of the fibrillated cartilage tear, releasing free fragments into the joint space and decreasing the thickness of the cartilage. At the same time, enzymatic degradation of the matrix further decreases the volume of the cartilage.[23-26] Eventually, the progressive loss of articular cartilage leaves only dense and often

Table 2

Differences between changes in articular cartilage due to aging and those due to degeneration in osteoarthritis[19,20]

	Aging	Osteoarthritis
Structure	Stable, localized, superficial fibrillation	Progressive, superficial fibrillation; fibrillation and fragmentation extending to subchondral bone; loss of tissue (decreased thickness of cartilage with complete loss in some regions); formation of fibrocartilaginous repair tissue
Cells	Decreased density of chondrocytes with skeletal growth, alteration in synthetic activity (smaller, more variable aggrecans), decreased response to growth factors, decreased synthetic activity	Initial increase in synthetic and proliferative activity, loss of chondrocytes, eventual decreased synthetic activity, increased degradative enzyme activity, appearance of fibroblast-like cells in regions of fibrocartilaginous repair tissue
Matrix	Decreased concentration of water, loss of large proteoglycan aggregates (decreased stability of aggregates), increased concentration of decorin, accumulation of degraded molecules (aggrecan and link protein fragments), increased collagen cross-linking, increased diameter of and variability in collagen fibrils, decreased tensile strength and stiffness in superficial layers	Initial increase in water content and, in some instances, in concentration of proteoglycans; disruption of collagenous macromolecular organization; progressive degradation and loss of proteoglycans, hyaluronan, and collagens; increased concentration of fibronectin; increased permeability and loss of tensile compressive stiffness and strength

necrotic eburnated bone.

Many of the mechanisms responsible for the progressive loss of cartilage in degenerative joint disease remain unknown, but the process can be divided into three overlapping stages: disruption or alteration of the cartilage matrix, the chondrocytic response to tissue damage, and the decline of the chondrocytic synthetic response and the progressive loss of tissue[3,27-32] (Table 3).

In the first stage, either before or with the appearance of fibrillation, the macromolecular framework of the matrix is disrupted or altered at the molecular level and the water content increases.[3,28,29,31,33,34] While the concentration of type-II collagen remains constant, decreases in the aggregation of proteoglycans, the concentration of aggrecans, and the length of the glycosaminoglycan chains usually accompany the increase in water content. At the

same time, alterations in the collagenous framework, including changes in the relationships between the minor collagens and the collagen fibrils, may allow swelling of the aggrecan molecules. Disruption or decreased organization of the macromolecular framework, decreased aggrecan concentration and aggregation, decreased length of the glycosaminoglycan chains, and increased water content all increase the permeability (the ease with which water and other molecules move through the matrix) and decrease the stiffness of the matrix; these alterations may increase the vulnerability of the tissue to additional mechanical damage. This first phase may occur as a result of a variety of mechanical insults, such as high-intensity impact or torsional loading of a joint; it may be due to accelerated degradation of matrix macromolecules as a result of joint inflamma-

Table 3
Stages in the development and progression of degeneration of articular cartilage in osteoarthritis[28,29,32,168]

Stage	Description
I. Disruption or alteration of cartilage matrix	Disruption or alteration of macromolecular framework of matrix associated with increase in concentration of water that may be caused by mechanical insults, degradation of matrix macromolecules, or alterations of chondrocyte metabolism. At first, concentration of type-II collagen remains unchanged, but collagen meshwork may be damaged, and concentration of aggrecans and degree of proteoglycan aggregation decrease.
II. Response of chondrocytes to disruption or alteration of matrix	When chondrocytes detect a disruption or alteration of their matrix, they can respond by increasing synthesis and degradation of the matrix and by proliferating. Their response may restore tissue, maintain tissue in an altered state, or increase volume of cartilage. They may sustain an increased level of activity for years.
III. Decline in response of chondrocytes	Failure of chondrocytic response to restore or maintain tissue leads to loss of articular cartilage accompanied or preceded by decline in chondrocytic response. The causes for this decline remain poorly understood, but they may partially result from mechanical damage to tissue with injury to chondrocytes and down-regulation of chondrocytic response to anabolic cytokines.

tion; or it may occur as a result of metabolic changes in the tissue that interfere with the ability of chondrocytes to maintain the matrix.

The second stage begins when chondrocytes detect the tissue damage or alterations in osmolarity, charge density, or strain and release mediators that stimulate a cellular response that is often quite brisk. The response consists of both anabolic and catabolic activity as well as chondrocyte proliferation.[3,15,19,28-30,32,35,36] Anabolic and mitogenic growth factors presumably have an important role in stimulating the synthesis of matrix macromolecules and the proliferation of chondrocytes; clusters or clones of proliferating cells surrounded by newly synthesized matrix molecules constitute one histologic hallmark of the chondrocytic response to the degeneration of cartilage.[3,19,28-30,32,36-38] Nitric oxide may have a role in the chondrocytic response, as chondrocytes produce this molecule in response to a variety of mechanical and chemical stresses.[39,40] It diffuses rapidly and can induce production of the cytokine interleukin-1, which stimulates the expression of metalloproteases that degrade the matrix macromolecules. Fibronectin fragments or other molecules present in damaged tissue may promote the continued production of interleukin-1 and the enhanced release of proteases.[41-44] Degradation of type-IX and type-XI collagens and other molecules may destabilize the type-II collagen-fibril meshwork, leaving many type-II fibrils intact initially but allowing expansion of aggrecans and increased water content. Disruption of the superficial zone, a decline in aggregation, and an associated loss of aggrecans due to enzymatic degradation increase the stresses on the remaining collagen-fibril network and chondrocytes with joint-loading. Enzymatic degradation also clears damaged and intact matrix components[24,25] and may release anabolic cytokines previously trapped in the matrix that stimulate the synthesis of matrix macromolecules and the proliferation of chondrocytes. In this second stage of the development of osteoarthritis, the repair response—the increased synthesis of matrix macromolecules and, to a lesser extent, cell proliferation—counters the catabolic effects of the proteases and may stabilize or, in some instances, restore the tissue. The repair response may continue for years, and in some patients it reverses the course of osteoarthritis at least temporarily. Furthermore, some therapeutic interventions have the potential for facilitating the repair response. For example, studies of osteoarthritic hips and knees after osteotomy have shown that altering the mechanical environment of the joint sometimes stimulates the restoration of an articular surface.[9,45-47]

Failure to stabilize or restore the tissue leads to the third stage in the development of osteoarthritis: a progressive loss of articular cartilage as well as a decline in the chondrocytic anabolic and proliferative response.[3,28,29,32,36] This decline could result from the mechanical damage and death of chondrocytes no longer stabilized and protected by a functional matrix, but it also appears to be related to, or initiated by, a down-regulation of the chondrocytic response to anabolic cytokines. This may occur as a result of synthesis and accumulation of molecules in the matrix that bind anabolic cytokines, including decorin, insulin-dependent growth-factor binding protein, and other molecules that can affect cytokine function. The loss of articular cartilage leads to the symptoms of osteoarthritis (pain and loss of joint function). This loss occurs more frequently with increasing age, possibly because age-related changes in the cartilage matrix and a decrease in the chondrocytic anabolic response compromise the ability of the tissue to maintain and restore itself.[19,48,49]

Alterations of the subchondral bone that accompany the degeneration of articular cartilage include increased density of the subchondral bone (subchondral sclerosis); formation of cyst-like bone cavities containing myxoid, fibrous, or cartilaginous tissue; and the appearance of regenerating cartilage within and on the subchondral bone surface. This response is usually most apparent on the periphery of the joint, where osseous and cartilaginous excrescences sometimes form sizable osteophytes. Increased density of subchondral bone resulting from formation of new layers of bone on existing trabeculae is usually the first sign of degenerative joint disease in subchondral bone, but in some joints subchondral cavities appear before a generalized increase in bone density. At the end stage of the disease, the articular cartilage has been completely lost, leaving thickened, dense subchondral bone articulating with a similarly denuded osseous surface. The bone-remodeling combined with the loss of articular cartilage changes the shape of the joint and can lead to shortening of the involved limb, deformity, and instability.

In most synovial joints, growth of osteophytes accompanies the changes in articular cartilage and in subchondral and metaphyseal bone. These fibrous, cartilaginous, and osseous prominences[50] usually develop around the periphery of the joint (marginal osteophytes), usually at the cartilage-bone interface, but they also may appear along the insertions of the joint capsule (capsular osteophytes). Intra-articular osseous excrescences that protrude from degenerating joint surfaces are referred to as central osteophytes.[51] Most marginal osteophytes have a cartilaginous surface that closely resembles normal articular cartilage, and they may appear to be an extension of the joint surface. In superficial joints they usually are palpable and may be tender, and in all joints they can restrict motion and contribute to pain with motion. Each joint has a characteristic pattern of osteophyte formation. Osteophytes in the hip usually form around the rim of the acetabulum and in the femoral articular cartilage. A prominent osteophyte along the inferior margin of the humeral articular surface commonly develops in degenerative dis-

ease of the glenohumeral joint. Presumably, osteophytes represent a response to the degeneration of articular cartilage and the remodeling of subchondral bone, including the release of anabolic cytokines that stimulate cell proliferation and the formation of osseous and cartilaginous matrices.[52,53]

The loss of articular cartilage leads to secondary changes in synovial tissue, ligaments, and capsules and in the muscles that move the involved joint. The synovial membrane often has a mild-to-moderate inflammatory reaction and may contain fragments of articular cartilage.[54] With time, the ligaments, capsules, and muscles become contracted. Decreased use of the joint and a decreased range of motion lead to muscle atrophy. These secondary changes often contribute to the stiffness and weakness associated with osteoarthritis.

Although the symptoms of osteoarthritis, primarily pain and stiffness of the joint, result from degeneration of the joint, the severity of the loss of articular cartilage is not necessarily closely related to the severity of the symptoms. Patients who have advanced joint degeneration may have relatively little pain and surprising mobility, while others who have moderate degeneration may have severe symptoms and limited motion. Furthermore, as with the degeneration of cartilage, the clinical syndrome of osteoarthritis may remain stable; may progress slowly over many years or even decades; may improve temporarily; or, occasionally, may progress rapidly to the point that the patient is completely disabled within a few years after the onset of the disease.

Joint Use and Joint Degeneration

An understanding of the relationships between joint use and joint degeneration forms a critical part of strategies to prevent and treat osteoarthritis.[20] Investigations of the effects that running has on animal and human joints indicate that moderate and possibly even strenuous

regular activity does not cause or accelerate the development of osteoarthritis in normal joints (those with normal articular surfaces, alignment, static and dynamic stability, innervation, and muscle control).[20,21,55] Furthermore, cyclic loading of cartilage stimulates matrix synthesis, whereas prolonged static loading or the absence of loading and motion causes degradation of the matrix and, eventually, degeneration of the joint.[55]

Despite the importance of regular activity for the maintenance of joints, some types of repetitive joint use apparently accelerate the development of degenerative joint disease.[20] Studies of individuals who have certain physically demanding occupations, including farmers, construction workers, metal workers, miners, and pneumatic-drill operators, have suggested that repetitive, intense joint-loading may lead to an early onset of joint degeneration.[20,21] Specific activities that have been associated with osteoarthritis include the repetitive lifting or carrying of heavy objects, an awkward work posture, vibration, continuously repeated movements, and a working speed that is determined by a machine; other studies have suggested that participation in sports or other activities that repetitively expose joints to high levels of impact or torsional loading may increase the probability of joint degeneration.[20,21,56-60]

Individuals who have an abnormal anatomy or function of the joint, including disruption or incongruity of the articular surface, dysplasia, malalignment, instability, disturbances of innervation of the joint or muscles, and inadequate muscle strength or endurance, probably have a greater risk of degenerative joint disease.[20] Subjecting the joints to loads greater than those that result from normal activities of daily living, especially activities that involve repetitive impact or torsion, presumably increases the risk further. These individuals and those who have early osteoarthritis can benefit from regular exercise, but they should have a detailed evaluation of their joint structure and function before beginning. In most instances, they would be best advised to select an exercise program that maintains joint motion and muscle strength with minimum loading.

Repair and Regeneration of Articular Cartilage

For at least 250 years, physicians and scientists have sought ways to repair or regenerate the articular surfaces of synovial joints after the loss or degeneration of articular cartilage.[10] (Repair refers to the restoration of a damaged articular surface with new tissue that resembles but does not duplicate the structure, composition, and function of articular cartilage; regeneration refers to the formation of new tissue indistinguishable from normal articular cartilage.[61-63]) They made little progress during most of this period, but in the last three decades clinical and basic scientific investigations have shown that implantation of artificial matrices, growth factors, perichondrium, periosteum, and transplanted chondrocytes and mesenchymal stem cells can stimulate the formation of cartilaginous tissue in osteochondral and chondral defects in synovial joints.[45,61,64-66] Other work has demonstrated that loading and motion of the joint can influence the healing of articular cartilage and joints[67-69] and that mechanical loading influences the repair process in all tissues that form parts of synovial joints.[62,70,71] In addition, review of several surgical procedures used to treat osteoarthritis, including osteotomy, penetration of subchondral bone, and joint distraction and motion, has shown that these procedures can stimulate the formation of new articular surfaces.[45] The apparent potential of these methods for stimulating the formation of cartilaginous articular surfaces has created great interest on the part of patients, physicians, and scientists; however, the wide variety of methods and

approaches for assessing the results has made it difficult to evaluate their relative success in restoring function of the joint and to define the most appropriate current clinical applications.

A better understanding of the lesions and degeneration of articular cartilage, and recognition of the limitations of current treatments, have also contributed to the recent interest in the repair and regeneration of cartilage.[3,9,10,45,72] Advances in the imaging of and the arthroscopic techniques for synovial joints have led to an increased understanding of the frequency and types of chondral defects and have made it possible for orthopaedic surgeons to diagnose and evaluate these lesions with great accuracy.[73] Age-related, non-progressive, superficial fibrillation of cartilage and focal lesions of the articular surface must be distinguished from degeneration of cartilage occurring as part of the syndrome of osteoarthrosis[74] (Table 2). Superficial fibrillation of articular cartilage occurs in many joints in association with increasing age and does not appear to cause symptoms or to affect the function of the joint adversely. Isolated defects of articular cartilage and osteochondral defects appear to result from trauma that often leaves most of the articular surface intact.[72,73] These defects commonly occur in adolescents and young adults who wish to maintain a high level of activity, and in some of these individuals they cause joint pain, effusions, and mechanical dysfunction. Although the natural history of isolated chondral and osteochondral defects has not been well defined,[66,75,76] clinical experience has shown that, if left untreated, these lesions fail to heal and that defects that involve a major portion of the articular surface may progress to symptomatic degeneration of the joint. Therefore, the treatment of selected isolated chondral and osteochondral defects may help to delay or prevent the development of osteoarthritis. Because debridement alone produces variable results,[45,73] inves-

tigators have sought better methods of treatment for these focal defects.

A variety of methods have the potential to stimulate the formation of a new articular surface, including penetration of subchondral bone, osteotomy, joint distraction, use of soft-tissue grafts, cell transplantation, use of growth factors, and use of artificial matrices. The available evidence indicates that the results vary considerably among individuals and that the tissue that forms after these treatments does not duplicate the composition, structure, or mechanical properties of normal articular cartilage (Fig. 1). However, the regeneration of normal articular cartilage may not be necessary in order for a procedure to be beneficial; in at least some instances, stimulating the formation of articular cartilage repair tissue may decrease symptoms and improve joint function.[45] Reports of the clinical results of procedures intended to restore a damaged or degenerated articular surface have documented clinical improvement for most (usually more than 75%) of the patients[47,64,73,77-91] (Table 4). However, these studies have serious limitations: the ages of the patients and the types of defects of the articular surface varied considerably; some series included patients who had advanced degenerative disease, while others included only those who had localized chondral defects in otherwise normal joints; and, as none of the studies were controlled or prospective, the durations of follow-up and the measures of outcome varied. Thus, it is difficult to compare the efficacy of the various approaches for the restoration of articular cartilage. Nonetheless, a review of the results of these procedures provides considerable insight into the potential for the restoration of articular surfaces.

Penetration of Subchondral Bone

Penetration of subchondral bone was the original method developed to stimulate the formation of a new articular surface,

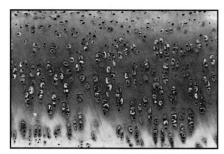 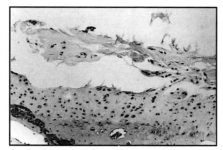 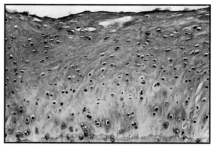

Fig. 1 Light micrographs of articular cartilage from rabbit patellae. The specimen was stained with safranin O to demonstrate the presence of glycosaminoglycans. **Left,** Normal articular cartilage. The matrix has a homogeneous, hyaline appearance. The matrix of the transitional and deep zones is stained diffusely with safranin O (dark regions), indicating a high concentration of glycosaminoglycans. **Center,** Well formed repair cartilage 6 months after the creation of an osteochondral defect. Compared with the normal articular cartilage, the zonal organization is less well defined, the matrix has a fibrous appearance, and safranin-O staining is concentrated near a few cells. The zone of calcified cartilage has re-formed. **Right,** Fibrillated repair cartilage 1 year after the creation of an osteochondral defect. Only a thin layer of fragmented tissue covers the subchondral bone, and the matrix lacks staining with safranin O.

and it is still the most commonly used[45,92] (Table 4). In regions with full-thickness loss or advanced degeneration of articular cartilage, penetration of the exposed subchondral bone disrupts subchondral blood vessels, leading to the formation of a fibrin clot over the bone surface.[45,62] If the surface is protected from excessive loading, undifferentiated mesenchymal cells migrate into the clot, proliferate, and differentiate into cells with the morphologic features of chondrocytes.[93] In some instances they form a fibrocartilaginous articular surface, but in others they do not[85,86] (Figs. 1 and 2).

Surgeons initially debrided degenerated articular cartilage and drilled into the subchondral bone through arthrotomies, and many patients reported a decrease in symptoms after this procedure.[94-97] Ficat and associates[81] excised damaged cartilage along with underlying subchondral bone for the treatment of degeneration of the articular surface of the patella; they referred to this procedure as spongialization. They reported a good or excellent result in 67 (79%) of 85 patients (Table 4). Surgeons have developed various other methods for the penetration of subchondral bone to stimulate the formation of a new cartilaginous surface, including arthroscopic abrasion of the articular surface and the creation of multiple small-

diameter defects or fractures with an awl or a similar instrument.[45,73,85,86,92]

Prospective, randomized, controlled trials of arthroscopic abrasion of osteoarthritic joints have not been reported, to our knowledge, but several authors have reviewed series of patients and have found that these procedures can decrease symptoms due to isolated defects of articular cartilage and osteoarthritis of the knee.[73,80,82,85,86,90] Baumgaertner and associates[98] reported less successful results with use of this method in 44 patients (49 knees); they noted early failure in 19 knees (39%), and 23 knees (47%) had had a failure at the latest follow-up examination. The excellent results decreased from 20 knees (41%) at the time of maximum improvement to 12 knees (24%) at the time of the latest follow-up.

Johnson[85,86] examined joint surfaces after arthroscopic abrasion and found that, in some individuals, this procedure resulted in the formation of a fibrocartilaginous articular surface that varied in composition, from dense fibrous tissue with little or no type II collagen to hyaline cartilage-like tissue with predominantly type II collagen. He also found that, in many patients who had either radiographic evidence of narrowing of the joint space or no radiographically demonstrable joint space, the joint space increased after

abrasion. Although the increase in the joint space presumably indicated the formation of a new articular surface, this new surface did not necessarily result in a decrease in the symptoms. Bert[99] and Bert and Maschka[100] found radiographic evidence of an increased joint space in 30 (51%) of 59 patients 2 years after abrasion arthroplasty; however, in 18 patients (31%), the symptoms were unchanged or more severe.

Some of the variability in the clinical results of attempts to restore an articular surface by penetration of subchondral bone may be the result of differences in the extent and quality of the repair tissue. However, to our knowledge, no study has documented a relationship between the extent and type of repair tissue and the result with regard to symptoms or function. This suggests that the formation of a new articular surface after the penetration of subchondral bone does not necessarily relieve pain.[45] The lack of a predictable clinical benefit from the formation of cartilage repair tissue may be due to variability among patients with respect to the severity of the degenerative changes, alignment of the joint, patterns of joint use, age, perception of pain, preoperative expectations, or other factors. It may also be attributable to the inability of the newly formed tissue to replicate

Table 4
Selected clinical reports of methods of restoring an articular surface

Authors	No. of Patients, Joints, or Defects	Results	Comments
Excision of damaged cartilage and underlying bone (spongialization)			
Ficat et al[81]	85 patients (patellae)	67 (79%) good or excellent	Used for treatment of patellar chondral lesions
Joint debridement and penetration of subchondral bone			
Ewing[80]	223 knees	163 (73%) improved	Increased severity of joint diseased decreased probability of good result
Friedman et al[82]	73 knees	44 (60%) improved, 25 (34%) unchanged, 4 (5%) worse	Patients < 40 years old had better results
Johnson[85,86]	> 400 knees	75% satisfactory	12% of patients were symptom-free at 2 years
Sprague[90]	69 knees	51 (74%) good, 7 (10%) fair, 11 (16%) poor	
Levy et al[73]	15 knees	6 excellent, 9 good, 0 fair or poor	All patients were competitive soccer players who had isolated chondral defects
Perichondrial grafts			
Seradge et al[89]	16 metacarpophalangeal joints	3 of 3 patients ≤ 20 years old, 3 of 4 21 to 30 years old, and 3 of 6 > 30 years old had good result	No patient > 40 years old had good result
	20 prox. interphalangeal joints	4 of 5 patients ≤ 20 years old, 4 of 6 21 to 30 years old, and 1 of 3 > 30 years old had good result	
Hommings et al[83]	25 patients (30 defects [knees])	Mean score on knee-function scale improved; 28 (93%) defects filled with cartilaginous tissue	Biopsy showed hyaline tissue; results not related to age
Distraction of joint			
van Valburg et al[91]	11 patients (11 ankles)	At average of 20 months, all patients had less pain and 5 were pain-free; 3 of 6 patients who had radiographs had increased joint space	No patient had arthrodesis
Osteotomy			
Weisl[47]	757 hips	Joint space increased immediately in approximately one third of patients and after 18 months in another one third; approximately two thirds had relief of pain for 5 years; after 10 years, only approximately one quarter had relief	Better results in patients with increased joint space and in those < 70 years old who had unilateral disease
Reigstad and Grønmark[88]	103 hips	70% had good result at 1 year; 51%, at 5 years; and 30%, at 10 years	
Bergenudd et al[77]	19 patients (knees)	Formation of new fibrocartilaginous surface in 9 patients, no change in 8, and deterioration of articular surface in 2	No correlation among histologic findings, radiographic appearance, postoperative varus-valgus angle, or clinical results
Insall et al[84]	95 knees	97% had good or excellent result at 2 years and 85%, at 5 years; 15% were pain-free at 9 years	
Carbon-fiber matrix			
Muckle and Minns[87]	47 patients (knees)	36 (77%) had satisfactory result at average of 3 years	No synovitis
Brittberg et al[78]	36 patients (knees)	30 (83%) had good or excellent result at average of 4 years	Good relief of pain, no adverse effects
Autologous chondrocyte transplantation			
Brittberg et al[79]	23 patients (knees)	14 of 16 patients who had femoral defect and 2 of 7 who had patellar defect had good or excellent result	Locking of joint eliminated, swelling and pain reduced
Buckwalter[64]	66 patients (knees)	47 (71%) improved	

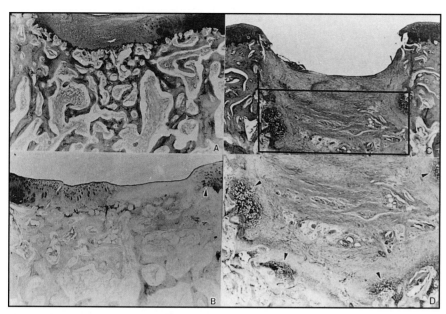

Fig. 2 Light micrographs showing the variability in osteochondral repair 4 to 6 weeks after the creation of osteochondral defects 4 mm in diameter and 3 mm deep in the medial femoral condyle of a rabbit. **A** and **B:** Osteochondral repair restored a fibrocartilaginous articular surface that nearly reaches the level of the adjacent cartilage surface (magnification × 20). The arrowhead in B indicates the right edge of the defect. **C:** Osteochondral repair failed to restore an articular surface (magnification × 20). **D:** Higher-magnification view from the lower portion of the repair tissue shown in C (magnification × 35). The arrowheads indicate cartilaginous repair tissue. (Courtesy of Dr. A.I. Caplan, Department of Biology, Case Western Reserve University, Cleveland, Ohio.)

the properties of articular cartilage.[9] Examination of the tissue that forms over the articular surface after the penetration of subchondral bone has shown that it lacks the structure, the composition, the mechanical properties, and in most instances the durability of articular cartilage[9,10,45,62,101] (Fig. 1). Therefore, even though this tissue covers the subchondral bone it may fail to distribute loads across the articular surface in a way that avoids pain with loading and additional degeneration of the joint.

Currently, it is not clear which method of penetration of subchondral bone produces the best new articular surface; differences in the selection of patients and the surgical technique among surgeons using the same method make it difficult to compare the efficacy of the different techniques. However, comparison of bone abrasion with subchondral drilling for the treatment of an experimental chondral defect in rabbits showed that, while neither treatment predictably restored the articular surface, drilling appeared to produce better long-term results than did abrasion.[102] This observation fits well with previous experimental work showing that chondral repair tissue that grows up through multiple drill-holes passing from the articular surface into vascularized bone spreads over exposed subchondral bone between the holes and forms a fibrocartilaginous articular surface.[101] It also suggests that small-diameter holes that leave the bone intact between defects lead to the formation of more stable repair tissue than do abraded bone surfaces.[102]

Despite evidence that the penetration of subchondral bone stimulates the for-

mation of fibrocartilaginous repair tissue, the clinical value of this approach remains uncertain. In contrast with reports of a decrease in symptoms in patients who had degeneration of cartilage and were managed with penetration of subchondral bone,[80,82,85,86,90] one investigator concluded that, while debridement of the joint can decrease symptoms in many patients, abrasion or drilling of subchondral bone does not benefit patients who have osteoarthritis of the knee and it may increase symptoms.[99] In addition, the short periods of follow-up; the lack of well-defined evaluations of outcome; the absence of randomized, controlled trials; and the possibility of a substantial placebo effect[103] or a decrease in the symptoms due to irrigation of the joint alone[104-107] make it difficult to define the indications for the penetration of subchondral bone.

Osteotomy

Clinical experience has led many surgeons to accept osteotomy as a method for the treatment of hip and knee joints with localized loss or degeneration of the articular surface.[45] Osteotomy has not been commonly used for the treatment of articular cartilage loss or degeneration in joints other than the hip and the knee, but in one study tibial osteotomy produced a good or excellent result in 15 of 18 patients who had primary osteoarthritis of the ankle, a rare condition in which osteoarthritis develops in the absence of any history of trauma.[108] Some surgeons have combined debridement of the joint and penetration of subchondral bone with osteotomy, but this approach is not widely used. In general, an osteotomy is planned in order to decrease loads on the most severely damaged regions of the joint surface, to bring regions of the joint surface that have remaining articular cartilage into opposition with regions that lack articular cartilage, or to correct malalignment that may contribute to symptoms and dysfunction of the joint.

Most hip and knee osteotomies performed to treat osteoarthritis alter the alignment of the joint in the coronal plane (varus and valgus osteotomies); however, some hip osteotomies are done to change the alignment of the joint in the sagittal plane (flexion and extension osteotomies) or to alter the relationship of the joint surfaces by rotation of the femoral head relative to the acetabulum (rotational osteotomies).

The optimum planes and degrees of realignment for specific osteoarthritic joints have not been defined; nonetheless, clinical experience has shown that osteotomies of the hip and the knee can decrease symptoms and stimulate the formation of a new articular surface.[45] The decrease in pain could result from a decrease in stresses on regions of the articular surface with the most advanced degeneration of cartilage, a decrease in intraosseous pressure, or the formation of a new articular surface, but the mechanisms of the improvement remain poorly understood.[45]

Most clinical studies have shown that, in at least some patients, osteotomy leads to a decrease in the radiographic signs of joint degeneration, with the improvement including the resolution of subchondral cysts or radiolucent lines, decreased density of subchondral bone, and increased radiographic joint space.[45] The latter change may result either from the altered relationship between the articular surfaces or from the formation of a new articular surface; that is, the osteotomy may alter the alignment of the joint to separate previously opposed joint surfaces, or it may rotate a cartilage-covered articular surface into opposition with a surface consisting of exposed bone, thus creating a radiographically visible cartilage space where, before the osteotomy, bone had opposed bone. In a series of 757 intertrochanteric osteotomies performed to treat osteoarthritis of the hip, the radiographic joint space increased immediately after the procedure in approximately one-third of the patients.[47] The increased joint space presumably resulted from alterations in the relationships between the joint surfaces. In another one-third of the patients, the joint space increased during the next 18 months, and these patients had better clinical results. This suggests that, over 18 months, a new articular surface developed in some areas of the joint as a result of the altered loading.[47] Evidence that hip osteotomy stimulates the formation of fibrocartilaginous tissue over articular surfaces that previously consisted of exposed bone supports this suggestion.[109,110]

The treatment of degenerative disease of the knee with osteotomy has also led to an increased radiographic joint space accompanied by decreased density of subchondral bone and, in some patients, the formation of a new fibrocartilaginous articular surface.[45] Bergenudd and associates[77] biopsied the articular cartilage of the medial femoral condyle at the time of the osteotomy and then again at an average of 2 years after the osteotomy in 19 patients who had degenerative disease of the medial side of the knee joint. The biopsies showed formation of a new fibrocartilaginous articular surface in nine patients, no change in eight patients, and deterioration of the articular surface in two patients (Table 4). Radiographs showed that six knees had improved, 11 had remained unchanged, and two had deteriorated. There was no correlation among the histologic findings, the radiographic appearance, the postoperative varus-valgus angle, or the clinical results.[77] In a similar study of 14 patients, proliferation of a new fibrocartilaginous surface was found on the tibial condyle in eight patients and on the medial femoral condyle in nine patients 2 years after the osteotomy.[46] The authors of that study also found no correlation between the restoration of an articular surface and the clinical outcome.

Long-term follow-up of patients who were managed with osteotomy for osteoarthritis of the hip or the knee have shown that the clinical results deteriorate with time.[47,84,88,111,112] Variables that appear to affect the results of knee osteotomy adversely include older age; obesity; severe degeneration, instability, or limited motion of the joint; surgical overcorrection or undercorrection; and postoperative loss of correction.[84,111-113] However, even patients who appear to be optimum candidates for osteotomy and who have a good initial outcome tend to have recurrent pain and evidence of progressive osteoarthritis with time.

Decreased Joint Loading Combined with Joint Motion

Several sets of observations suggest that decreased contact pressures of the articular surfaces combined with movement of the joint may stimulate the restoration of an articular surface on osteoarthritic joints. Before the development of artificial joints, surgeons found that resection of an osteoarthritic joint surface followed by decreased loading combined with motion of the joint resulted in the formation of fibrocartilaginous tissue over the osseous surfaces.[9,45,114] When the degenerated articular surfaces were resected along with some underlying bone, the space between the bone surfaces filled with a fibrin clot and then with granulation tissue. Decreased loading with motion of the resected joint facilitated the formation of opposing fibrocartilaginous surfaces, whereas immobilization and compression could lead to osseous or fibrous ankylosis. Reports have suggested that attempts to decrease loading of the joint by releasing the muscles that act across a degenerated hip joint can decrease symptoms and increase the radiographic cartilage space in some patients;[115-117] examination of osteoarthritic joints after osteotomy has shown formation of a new articular surface in some instances (as noted in the discussion of osteotomy).

These observations concerning the

effects of decreased contact pressures combined with motion of the joint have recently been supported by clinical studies of the effects of joint distraction and motion with use of external fixators. Aldegheri and associates[118] used distraction that allowed joint motion to manage 80 patients who had a variety of hip disorders. Twenty-four patients who either had inflammatory joint disease or were more than 45 years old had a poor result, and only four patients who were more than 45 years old had a good result; in contrast, 42 of 59 patients who were less than 45 years old and had osteoarthritis, dysplasia, osteonecrosis, or chondrolysis had a good result. These results suggest that, at least in patients who are younger than 45 years old, decreased contact pressures and motion of damaged hip-joint surfaces can decrease symptoms. In a recent preliminary report, van Valburg and associates[91] described encouraging results with use of distraction and motion of the joint in 11 patients who had advanced posttraumatic osteoarthritis of the ankle. After application of an Ilizarov device, the joint was distracted 0.5 mm each day for 5 days; the distraction of the articular surfaces was then maintained throughout the course of the treatment. The patients were allowed to walk a few days after the operation, active motion was started between 6 and 12 weeks postoperatively, and the distraction device was removed after 12 to 22 weeks. At an average of 20 months, none of the patients had had an arthrodesis. All 11 patients had less pain, and five were pain-free; six had more motion, and three of six who had radiographs had increased joint space[91] (Table 4). Although that study had important limitations,[119] the decrease in symptoms and the delay (if not the avoidance) of arthrodesis in all 11 patients indicates that distraction or other methods of decreasing joint contact forces combined with motion of the joint deserve additional evaluation.

Soft-Tissue Grafts

Treatment of osteoarthritic joints with soft-tissue grafts most often involves debridement of the joint and interposition of soft-tissue grafts consisting of fascia, joint capsule, muscle, tendon, periosteum, or perichondrium between debrided or resected articular surfaces.[45,120-125] The potential benefits include the introduction of a new cell population along with an organic matrix, a decrease in the probability of ankylosis before a new articular surface can form, and some protection of the graft or the host cells from excessive loading. The success of soft-tissue arthroplasty depends not only on the severity of the abnormalities of the joint and on the type of graft but also on postoperative motion to facilitate the generation of a new articular surface.[68,123,124]

Animal experiments and clinical experience have shown that perichondrial and periosteal grafts placed in articular cartilage defects can produce new cartilage.[45,68] Recently, encouraging results with use of periosteal grafts for the treatment of isolated chondral and osteochondral defects have been reported,[64] and other investigators have reported similar positive results with use of perichondrial grafts.[83,126] Seradge and associates[89] found that an older age of the patient adversely affected the results of soft-tissue grafts. They studied the results a minimum of 3 years after arthroplasty with a graft of rib perichondrium in 16 metacarpophalangeal joints and 20 proximal interphalangeal joints. Despite the small numbers in their series, the results suggested that increased age adversely affected the results in both groups of joints. Of the patients who had had an arthroplasty of the metacarpophalangeal joint and were available for evaluation, all three who were 20 years old or less, three of the four who were between 21 and 30 years old, and only three of the six who were more than 30 years old had a good result. Of the patients who had had an

arthroplasty of the interphalangeal joint and were available for evaluation, four of the five who were 20 years old or less, four of the six who were between 21 and 30 years old, and only one of the three who were more than 30 years old had a good result (Table 4). No patient who was more than 40 years old had a good result with either type of arthroplasty. Those authors concluded that arthroplasty with a perichondrial graft could be used for the treatment of posttraumatic osteoarthritis of the metacarpophalangeal joints and the proximal interphalangeal joints of the hand in young patients.

The clinical observation that perichondrial grafts produced the best results in younger patients[89] is in agreement with the concept that age may adversely affect the ability of undifferentiated cells or chondrocytes to form an articular surface or that, with age, the population of cells that can form an articular surface declines.[48] The age-related differences in the ability of cells to form a new articular surface may also help to explain some of the variability in the results of other procedures, including osteotomy or procedures that penetrate subchondral bone; younger people may have greater potential to produce a more effective articular surface when all other factors are equal.

Cell Transplantation

The limited ability of host cells to restore articular surfaces[9,10] has led investigators to seek methods of transplanting cells that can form cartilage into chondral and osteochondral defects. Experimental work has shown that both chondrocytes and undifferentiated mesenchymal cells placed in articular cartilage defects survive and produce a new cartilage matrix[45] (Fig. 3). Wakitani and associates[127] estimated that hyaline cartilage developed in 30 (75%) of 40 osteochondral defects in rabbits that had been treated with allograft articular chondrocytes embedded in collagen gels, while only fibrocartilage developed in 24 control defects. Other investigators have

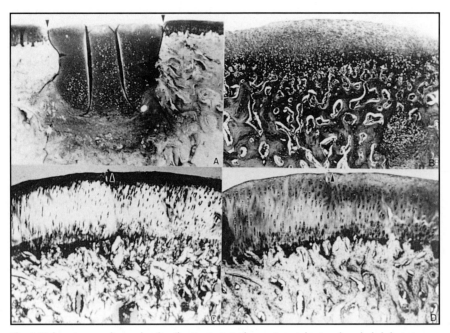

Fig. 3 Light micrographs made after the treatment of experimental osteochondral defects in rabbits with use of cell transplants. These micrographs are in contrast with those in Figure 2, showing untreated osteochondral defects. **A:** Osteochondral defect 6 months after transplantation of allogenic articular chondrocytes (magnification × 20). The arrowheads indicate the edges of the defect, which is filled with hyaline-like cartilage. **B:** Osteochondral defect 6 months after transplantation of autologous mesenchymal stem cells (magnification × 30). **C** and **D:** Higher magnification of osteochondral defect 6 months after transplantation of autologous mesenchymal stem cells (magnification × 100) (C is a polarized light image of D). The arrowheads mark the edge of the original defect, with repair tissue on the right and normal articular cartilage on the left. (Courtesy of Dr. I.A. Caplan, Department of Biology, Case Western Reserve University, Cleveland, Ohio.)

reported similar results with chondrocyte transplantation.[128-132] Recently, Brittberg[133] and Brittberg and associates[134] compared the results of the treatment of chondral defects in the articular surface of the patella in rabbits with use of periosteal grafts alone; with use of carbon-fiber scaffolds and periosteum; with use of autologous chondrocytes and periosteum; and with use of autologous chondrocytes, carbon-fiber scaffolds, and periosteum. They found that the addition of autologous chondrocytes improved the histologic quality and amount of repair tissue. Other studies have shown that mesenchymal cells aspirated from bone can produce cartilaginous tissue in goats[1] and that mesenchymal stem cells can repair large osteochondral defects in rabbits.[135,136]

Brittberg and associates[79] also described the use of transplants of autologous chondrocytes for the treatment of localized cartilage defects of the femoral condyle or the patella in 23 patients. Chondrocytes were obtained from the patients, cultured for 14 to 21 days, and then injected into the area of the defect and covered with a flap of periosteum. Two years or more after transplantation, 14 of the 16 patients who had a condylar defect and two of the seven who had a patellar defect had a good or excellent clinical result. Biopsy of the site of the defect showed hyaline-like cartilage in 11 of the 16 femoral and one of the seven patellar defects.[79] More recently, the results in a larger group of patients were reported.[64] More than 2 years after the

transplantation of chondrocytes for the treatment of chondral defects of the knee, 47 of 66 patients had improved function.

These results suggest that the transplantation of chondrocytes combined with the use of a periosteal graft can promote the restoration of an articular surface in humans. However, more work is needed to assess the function and durability of the new tissue, to determine if it improves joint function and delays or prevents joint degeneration, and to ascertain if this approach will be beneficial in the treatment of osteoarthritic joints.

Growth Factors

Growth factors influence a variety of cell activities, including proliferation, migration, matrix synthesis, and differentiation. Many of these factors, including fibroblast growth factors, insulin-like growth factors, and transforming growth factor-β, affect chondrocyte metabolism and chondrogenesis.[45,62] Bone matrix contains a variety of these molecules, including transforming growth factor-β, insulin-like growth factors, bone morphogenetic proteins, and platelet-derived growth factors.[62,137] In addition, mesenchymal cells, endothelial cells, and platelets produce many of these factors. Thus, osteochondral injuries and exposure of bone due to loss of articular cartilage may release these agents that affect the formation of cartilage repair tissue, and they probably have an important role in the formation of new articular surfaces after currently used surgical procedures, including resection arthroplasty, penetration of subchondral bone, soft-tissue grafts, and possibly osteotomy.

Local treatment of chondral or osteochondral defects with growth factors has the potential to stimulate the restoration of an articular surface that is superior to that formed after the penetration of subchondral bone alone, especially in joints with normal alignment and a normal range of motion and with limited regions of cartilage damage. A recent experimen-

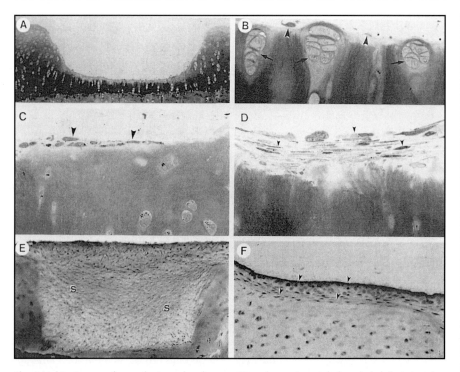

Fig. 4 Light micrographs made 4 weeks after creation of experimental chondral defects in rabbits (A through D) and minipigs (E and F). **A** and **B**: Untreated defects that have not healed. In B, the arrowheads indicate mesenchymal cells and the arrows indicate proliferating chondrocytes. **C**: Treatment with chondroitinase AC led to the removal of some of the matrix proteoglycans, thereby improving the adhesion of repair cells to the cartilage surface (arrowheads). **D**: Treatment with chondroitinase AC and the mitogenic factor interleukin growth factor-1 stimulated the formation of layers of mesenchymal cells and a fibrous matrix (arrowheads). **E**: Treatment with a fibrin matrix and the chemotactic-mitogenic factor transforming growth factor-β caused the defect to fill with mesenchymal tissue(s). **F**: The presence of layers of migrating mesenchymal cells (arrowheads) over normal cartilage suggests that these cells are chemotactically attracted to the defect from the synovial tissues. (Courtesy of E. Hunziker, University of Bern, Bern, Switzerland.)

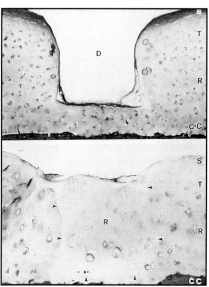

Fig. 5 Light micrographs showing chondral defects in the knee joints of minipigs. **Top:** untreated defect (D) in the articular surface. **Bottom:** new repair cartilage (R, edges marked by arrowheads) that formed in a chondral defect 6 weeks after treatment with free transforming growth factor-β and liposome-encapsulated transforming growth factor-β in a fibrin matrix. S, T, R, and CC = zones of articular cartilage (S = superficial, T = transitional, R = radial, and CC = calcified cartilage). (Courtesy of E. Hunziker, University of Bern, Bern, Switzerland.)

tal study of the treatment of partial-thickness cartilage defects with enzymatic digestion of proteoglycans that inhibit adhesion of cells to articular cartilage, followed by implantation of a fibrin matrix and timed release of transforming growth factor-β, showed that this growth factor can stimulate cartilage repair[138,139] (Figs. 4 and 5). The cells that filled the chondral defects migrated into the defects from the synovial tissue and formed a fibrous matrix. Despite the promise of this approach, the wide variety of growth factors, their multiple effects, their interactions, the possibility that the responsiveness of cells to growth factors may

decline with age,[48,49,140] and the limited understanding of their effects in osteoarthritic joints make it difficult to develop a simple strategy for the use of these agents to manage patients who have osteoarthritis. However, the development of growth-factor-based treatments for younger patients who have an isolated chondral or osteochondral defect and early degenerative changes of cartilage appears promising.

Artificial Matrices
The treatment of chondral defects with growth factors or cell transplants requires a method of delivering and, in most

instances, at least temporarily stabilizing the growth factors or cells in the defect. The success of these approaches therefore often depends on an artificial matrix (Figs. 4 and 5). In addition, an artificial matrix may allow and, in some instances, stimulate ingrowth of host cells, matrix formation, and binding of new cells and matrix to host tissue.[141] Investigators have found that implants formed from a variety of biologic and nonbiologic materials, including treated cartilage and bone matrices, collagens, collagens and hyaluronan, fibrin, carbon fiber, hydroxyapatite, porous polylactic acid, polytetrafluoroethylene, polyester, and other synthetic polymers, facilitate the restoration of an articular surface.[45] A lack of data makes it difficult to compare the relative merits of different types of artificial matrices and to evaluate the possibility that some implanted materials may cause synovitis;[142] however, the available evidence indicates that at least some types of artificial matrices can contribute to the restoration of an articular surface. In animal experiments, fibrous polyglycolic acid, collagen gels, and fibrin have proved to be effective matrices for the implantation of cells, and fibrin has been used to implant and allow timed release of a growth factor.[138,143-145] The treatment of osteochondral defects in rats and rabbits with carbon-fiber pads resulted in the restoration of a smooth articular surface consisting of firm fibrous tissue that filled the pads.[87] Use of the same approach to treat osteochondral defects of the knee in humans produced a satisfactory result in 36 (77%) of 47 patients who were evaluated clinically and arthroscopically 3 years after the operation.[87] Brittberg and associates[78] also studied the use of carbon-fiber pads for the treatment of articular surface defects; they noted a good or excellent result in 30 (83%) of 36 patients at an average of 4 years (Table 4).

Transplantation of Articular Cartilage

The transplantation of articular cartilage as part of an osteochondral graft has been shown to be a clinically effective method of replacing focal regions of damaged articular cartilage,[146-157] and experimental work has suggested that osteochondral grafts provide better restoration of articular surfaces than does the natural repair response to an acute osteochondral defect.[158] Compared with methods designed to repair or regenerate a new articular surface, osteochondral grafts have the advantage of providing a fully formed articular cartilage matrix and the potential for transplanting viable chondrocytes that are able to maintain the matrix.[149,159,160] Osteochondral grafts also can restore subchondral bone and the contour of the joint in patients who have

osteochondral defects or incongruity of the joint.

Autologous Grafts

Because of the small number of possible donor sites from which osteochondral autologous grafts may be obtained, use of these grafts has been limited to selected localized regions of damaged articular cartilage. In a small number of patients, surgeons have replaced damaged or lost articular surfaces with autologous grafts of articular cartilage obtained from the patella, the femoral condyle, and the proximal fibula,[147,156,157,161-164] and the results have shown that this technique can restore an articular surface. In two studies, osteochondral autologous grafts from the patella used to replace portions of the tibial articular surface healed and provided satisfactory function of the joint for more than a decade.[157,162] Outerbridge and associates[156] treated osteochondral defects of the femoral condyle with patellar osteochondral grafts in ten patients and found that function of the knee improved and symptoms were alleviated in all patients at an average of 6.5 years after transplantation.

Allografts

Because of their greater availability and because they can be prepared in any size, osteochondral allografts have been used more frequently than autologous surfaces.[146,148,150-155,165-167] Clinical experience with fresh and frozen osteochondral allografts has shown that they can heal to the host tissue and restore an articular surface. The use of fresh osteochondral allografts to replace portions of damaged tibial plateaus decreased pain and improved function in ten of 12 patients who were followed for more than 2 years.[167] Of 40 knees that had had transplantation of fresh osteochondral allografts because of localized degeneration of the articular surface, 31 had healing of the graft and nine had failure of the graft at 2 to 10 years.[155] Of the 31 successful transplants,

13 had an excellent result, 14 had a good result, and four had a fair result. The authors recommended use of fresh osteochondral allografts for the treatment of posttraumatic degenerative osteoarthritis of the patella, posttraumatic osteoarthritis, and traumatic defects of the tibial plateau as well as for osteochondritis dissecans and osteonecrosis of the femoral condyle. They advised against use of the grafts for the treatment of degenerative osteoarthritis of the knee involving both the femur and the tibia, and only three of these ten procedures succeeded.

Gross and associates[151] studied the results of 92 fresh osteochondral allografts used to treat posttraumatic osteoarticular defects of the knee. They reported a successful result in 69 knees (75%) at 5 years, in 59 knees (64%) at 10 years, and in 58 knees (63%) at 14 years. Flynn and associates[166] reported results with use of frozen osteochondral allografts that compared favorably with those with use of fresh allografts for the treatment of localized defects of the distal femoral articular surface. Those authors emphasized that use of frozen allografts permits the surgical reconstruction to be performed electively and allows time for more extensive testing of the donors for possible viral or bacterial infections.

Summary

The degeneration of articular cartilage as part of the clinical syndrome of osteoarthritis is one of the most common causes of pain and disability in middle-aged and older people. The strong correlation between increasing age and the prevalence of osteoarthritis, and recent evidence of important age-related changes in the function of chondrocytes, suggest that age-related changes in articular cartilage can contribute to the development and progression of osteoarthritis. Although the mechanisms responsible for osteoarthritis remain poorly understood, lifelong moderate use of normal joints does not increase the risk. Thus, the degeneration of normal articular cartilage is not simply the result of aging and mechanical wear. However, high-impact and torsional loads may increase the risk of degeneration of normal joints, and individuals who have an abnormal joint anatomy, joint instability, disturbances of joint or muscle innervation, or inadequate muscle strength or endurance probably have a greater risk of degenerative joint disease.

Recent work has shown the potential for the restoration of an articular surface. Currently, surgeons frequently debride joints and penetrate subchondral bone, as well as perform osteotomies, with the intent of decreasing symptoms and restoring or maintaining a functional articular surface. The results of these procedures vary considerably among patients. Clinical and experimental work has shown the important influence of loading and motion on the healing of articular cartilage and joints. Experimental studies have revealed that transplantation of chondrocytes and mesenchymal stem cells; use of periosteal and perichondrial grafts, synthetic matrices, and growth factors; and other methods have the potential to stimulate the formation of a new articular surface.

The long-term follow-up of small series of patients has shown that the transplantation of osteochondral autologous grafts and allografts can be effective for the treatment of focal defects of articular cartilage in selected patients. Thus far, none of these methods has been shown to predictably restore a durable articular surface to an osteoarthritic joint, and it is unlikely that any one of them will be uniformly successful. Rather, the available clinical and experimental evidence indicates that future optimum methods for the restoration of articular surfaces will begin with a detailed analysis of the structural and functional abnormalities of the involved joint and the patient's expectations for future use of the joint. On the basis of this analysis, the surgeon will develop a treatment plan that potentially combines correction of mechanical abnormalities (including malalignment, instability, and intra-articular causes of mechanical dysfunction), debridement that may or may not include limited penetration of subchondral bone, and applications of growth factors or implants that may consist of a synthetic matrix that incorporates cells or growth factors or use of transplants followed by a postoperative course of controlled loading and motion.

References

1. Butnariu-Ephrat M, Robinson D, Mendes DG, et al: Resurfacing of goat articular cartilage by chondrocytes derived from bone marrow. *Clin Orthop* 1996;330:234–243.

2. Praemer AP, Furner S, Rice DP: *Musculoskeletal Conditions in the United States*. Park Ridge, IL, American Academy of Orthopaedic Surgeons, 1992.

3. Buckwalter JA, Martin JA: Degenerative joint disease. *Clin Symp* 1995;47:11–32.

4. Dieppe P: Osteoarthritis: Management, in Klippel JH, Dieppe PA (eds): *Rheumatology*. St. Louis, MO, Mosby-Year Book, 1994, pp 8.1–8.8.

5. Dieppe P: The classification and diagnosis of osteoarthritis, in Kuettner KE, Goldberg VM (eds): *Osteoarthritic Disorders*. Rosemont, IL, American Academy of Orthopaedic Surgeons, 1995, pp 5–12.

6. Kuettner KE, Schleyerbach R, Peyron JG, et al (eds): *Articular Cartilage and Osteoarthritis*. New York, NY, Raven Press, 1992.

7. Moskowitz RW, Howell DS, Goldberg VM, et al (eds): *Osteoarthritis, Diagnosis and Medical/Surgical Management*, ed 2. Philadelphia, PA, WB Saunders, 1992.

8. Schiller AL: Pathology of osteoarthritis, in Kuettner KE, Goldberg VM (eds): *Osteoarthritic Disorders*. Rosemont, IL, American Academy of Orthopaedic Surgeons, 1995, pp 95–101.

9. Buckwalter JA, Mow VC: Cartilage repair in osteoarthritis, in Moskowitz RW, Howell DS, Goldberg VM, et al (eds): *Osteoarthritis, Diagnosis and Medical/Surgical Management*, ed 2. Philadelphia, PA, WB Saunders, 1992, pp 71–107.

10. Buckwalter JA, Rosenberg LC, Hunziker EB: Articular cartilage: Composition, structure, response to injury, and methods of facilitation repair, in Ewing JW (ed): *Articular Cartilage and Knee Joint Function: Basic Science and Arthroscopy*. New York, NY, Raven Press, 1990, pp 19–56.

11. Hunter W: On the structure and disease of articulating cartilages. *Phil Trans Roy Soc Lond* 1743;42:514–521.

12. Gorman C: Relief for swollen joints. *Time* 1996, Oct. 28, p 86.

13. Felson DT: The epidemiology of osteoarthritis: Prevalence and risk factors, in Kuettner KE, Goldberg VM (eds): *Osteoarthritic Disorders*. Rosemont, IL, American Academy of Orthopaedic Surgeons, 1995, pp 13–24.

14. Oddis CV: New perspectives on osteoarthritis. *Am J Med* 1996;100:10S–15S.

15. Poole AR, Rizkalla G, Ionescu M, et al: Osteoarthritis in the human knee: A dynamic process of cartilage matrix degradation, synthesis and reorganization. *Agents Actions* 1993;39(suppl):3–13.

16. Reimann I, Mankin HJ, Trahan C: Quantitative histologic analyses of articular cartilage and subchondral bone from osteoarthritic and normal human hips. *Acta Orthop Scand* 1977;48:63–73.

17. Lawrence RC, Hochberg MC, Kelsey JL, et al: Estimates of the prevalence of selected arthritic and musculoskeletal diseases in the United States. *J Rheumatol* 1989;16:427–441.

18. Peyron JG: Epidemiologic aspects of osteoarthritis. *Scand J Rheumatol* 1988;77:29–33.

19. Martin JA, Buckwalter JA: Articular cartilage aging and degeneration. *Sports Med Arthrosc Rev* 1996;4:263–275.

20. Buckwalter JA, Lane NE: Aging, sports and osteoarthritis. *Sports Med Arthrosc Rev* 1996;4:276–287.

21. Buckwalter JA, Lane NE, Gordon SL: Exercise as a cause of osteoarthritis, in Kuettner KE, Goldberg VM (eds): *Osteoarthritic Disorders*. Rosemont, IL, American Academy of Orthopaedic Surgeons, 1995, pp 405–417.

22. Radin EL, Rose RM: Role of subchondral bone in the initiation and progression of cartilage damage. *Clin Orthop* 1986;213:34–40.

23. Baici A, Lang A, Horler D, et al: Cathepsin B in osteoarthritis: Cytochemical and histochemical analysis of human femoral head cartilage. *Ann Rheum Dis* 1995;54:289–297.

24. Ehrlich MG, Armstrong AL, Treadwell BV, et al: The role of proteases in the pathogenesis of osteoarthritis. *J Rheumatol* 1987;14:30–32.

25. Martel-Pelletier J, McCollum R, Fujimoto N, et al: Excess of metalloproteases over tissue inhibitor of metalloprotease may contribute to cartilage degradation in osteoarthritis and rheumatoid arthritis. *Lab Invest* 1994;70:807–815.

26. Testa V, Capasso G, Maffulli M, et al: Proteases and antiproteases in cartilage homeostasis: A brief review. *Clin Orthop* 1994;308:79–84.

27. Lippiello L, Hall D, Mankin HJ: Collagen synthesis in normal and osteoarthritic human cartilage. *J Clin Invest* 1977;59:593–600.

28. Mankin HJ: The reaction of articular cartilage to injury and osteoarthritis: I. *N Engl J Med* 1974;291:1285–1292.

29. Mankin HJ: The reaction of articular cartilage to injury and osteoarthritis: II. *N Engl J Med* 1974;291:1335–1340.

30. Mankin HJ, Lippiello L: Biochemical and metabolic abnormalities in articular cartilage from osteo-arthritic human hips. *J Bone Joint Surg* 1970;52A:424–434.

31. Mankin HJ, Thrasher AZ: Water content and binding in normal and osteoarthritic human cartilage. *J Bone Joint Surg* 1975;57A:76–80.

32. Mankin HJ, Johnson ME, Lippiello L: Biochemical and metabolic abnormalities in articular cartilage from osteoarthritic human hips: II. Correlation of morphology with biochemical and metabolic data. *J Bone Joint Surg* 1971;53:523–537.

33. Eyre DR: Collagen structure and function in articular cartilage: Metabolic changes in the development of osteoarthritis, in Kuettner KE, Goldberg VM (eds): *Osteoarthritic Disorders.* Rosemont, IL, American Academy of Orthopaedic Surgeons, 1995, pp 219–227.

34. Farquhar T, Xia Y, Mann K, et al: Swelling and fibronectin accumulation in articular cartilage explants after cyclical impact. *J Orthop Res* 1996;14:417–423.

35. Cs-Szabo G, Roughley PJ, Plaas AH, et al: Large and small proteoglycans of osteoarthritic and rheumatoid articular cartilage. *Arthritis Rheum* 1995;38:660–668.

36. Mankin HJ, Johnson EM, Lippiello L: Biochemical and metabolic abnormalities in articular cartilage from osteoarthritic human hips: III. Distribution and metabolism of amino sugar-containing macromolecules. *J Bone Joint Surg* 1981;63A:131–139.

37. Middleton JF, Tyler JA: Upregulation of insulin-like growth factor I gene expression in the lesions of osteoarthritic human articular cartilage. *Ann Rheum Dis* 1992;51:440–447.

38. Trippel SB: Growth factor actions on articular cartilage. *J Rheumatol* 1995;43(suppl):129–132.

39. Amin AR, Di Cesare PE, Vyas P, et al: The expression and regulation of nitric oxide synthase in human osteoarthritis-affected chondrocytes: Evidence for up-regulated neuronal nitric oxide synthase. *J Exp Med* 1995; 182:2097–2102.

40. Blanco FJ, Ochs RL, Schwarz H, et al: Chondrocyte apoptosis induced by nitric oxide. *Am J Pathol* 1995;146:75–85.

41. Chevalier X: Fibronectin, cartilage, and osteoarthritis. *Semin Arthritis Rheum* 1993;22:307–318.

42. Homandberg GA, Hui F: Arg-Gly-Asp-Ser peptide analogs suppress cartilage chondrolytic activities of integrin-binding and nonbinding fibronectin fragments. *Arch Biochem Biophys* 1994;310:40–48.

43. Homandberg GA, Meyers R, Williams JM: Intraarticular injection of fibronectin fragments causes severe depletion of cartilage proteoglycans in vivo. *J Rheumatol* 1993;20:1378–1382.

45. Buckwalter JA, Lohmander S: Operative treatment of osteoarthrosis: Current practice and future development. *J Bone Joint Surg* 1994;76A:1405–1418.

46. Odenbring S, Egund N, Lindstrand A, et al: Cartilage regeneration after proximal tibial osteotomy for medial gonarthrosis: An arthroscopic, roentgenographic, and histologic study. *Clin Orthop* 1992;277:210–216.

44. Xie DL, Meyers R, Homandberg GA: Fibronectin fragments in osteoarthritic synovial fluid. *J Rheumatol* 1992;19:1448–1452.

47. Weisl H: Intertrochanteric osteotomy for osteoarthritis: A long-term follow-up. *J Bone Joint Surg* 1980;62B:37–42.

48. Buckwalter JA, Woo SL-Y, Goldberg VM, et al: Current concepts review: Soft-tissue aging and musculoskeletal function. *J Bone Joint Surg* 1993;75A:1533–1548.

49. Martin JA, Buckwalter JA: Fibronectin and cell shape affect the age-related decline in chondrocyte synthetic response to IGF-I. *Trans Orthop Res Soc* 1996;21:306.

50. Aigner T, Dietz U, Stoss H, et al: Differential expression of collagen types I, II, III, and X in human osteophytes. *Lab Invest* 1995;73:236–243.

51. Varich L, Pathria M, Resnick D, et al: Patterns of central acetabular osteophytosis in osteoarthritis of the hip. *Invest Radiol* 1992;28:1120–1127.

52. Middleton J, Arnott N, Walsh S, et al: Osteoblasts and osteoclasts in adult human osteophyte tissue express the mRNAs for insulin-like growth factors I and II and the type 1 IGF receptor. *Bone* 1995;16:287–293.

53. Van-Beuningen HM, van der Kraan PM, Arntz OJ, et al: Transforming growth factor-beta 1 stimulates articular chondrocyte proteoglycan synthesis and induces osteophyte formation in the murine knee joint. *Lab Invest* 1994;71:279–290.

54. Myers SL, Flusser D, Brandt KD, et al: Prevalence of cartilage shards in synovium and their association with synovitis in patients with early and endstage osteoarthritis. *J Rheumatol* 1992;19:1247–1251.

55. Buckwalter JA: Osteoarthritis and articular cartilage use, disuse, and abuse: Experimental studies. *J Rheumatol* 1995;43(suppl):13–15.

56. Radin EL, Paul IL: Response of joints to impact loading: I. In vitro wear. *Arthritis Rheum* 1971;14:356–362.

57. Radin EL, Schaffler M, Gibson G, et al: Osteoarthrosis as a result of repetitive trauma, in Kuettner KE, Goldberg VM (eds): *Osteoarthritic Disorders.* Rosemont, IL, American Academy of Orthopaedic Surgeons, 1995, pp 197–203.

58. Radin EL, Yang KH, Riegger C, et al: Relationship between lower limb dynamics and knee joint pain. *J Orthop Res* 1991;9:398–405.

59. Radin EL, Ehrlich MG, Chernack R, et al: Effect of repetitive impulsive loading on the knee joints of rabbits. *Clin Orthop* 1978;131:288–293.

60. Radin EL, Martin RB, Burr DB, et al: Effects of mechanical loading on the tissues of the rabbit knee. *J Orthop Res* 1984;2:.221–234.

61. Buckwalter JA, Mow VC, Ratcliffe A: Restoration of injured or degenerated articular cartilage. *J Am Acad Orthop Surg* 1994;2:192–201.

62. Buckwalter JA, Einhorn TA, Bolander ME, et al: Healing of the musculoskeletal tissues, in Rockwood CA Jr, Green DP, Bucholz RW, et al (eds): *Fractures in Adults,* ed 4. Philadelphia, PA, Lippincott-Raven, 1996, pp 261–304.

63. Woo SL-Y, Buckwalter JA: Preface, in Woo SL-Y, Buckwalter JA (eds): *Injury and Repair of the Musculoskeletal Soft Tissues.* Park Ridge, IL, American Academy of Orthopaedic Surgeons, 1988.

64. Buckwalter JA: Cartilage researchers tell progress: Technologies hold promise, but caution urged. *Bull Am Acad Orthop Surg* 1996;44:24–26.

65. Buckwalter JA: Regenerating articular cartilage: Why the sudden interest? *Orthop Today* 1996;16:4–5.

66. Messner K, Gillquist J: Cartilage repair: A critical review. *Acta Orthop Scand* 1996;67:523–529.

67. Moran ME, Kim HK, Salter RB: Biological resurfacing of full-thickness defects in patellar articular cartilage of the rabbit: Investigation of autogenous periosteal grafts subjected to continuous passive motion. *J Bone Joint Surg* 1992;74B:659–667.

68. Salter RB (ed): *Continuous Passive Motion (CPM): A Biological Concept for the Healing and Regeneration of Articular Cartilage, Ligaments, and Tendons From Origination to Research to Clinical Applications.* Baltimore, MD, Williams & Wilkins, 1993.

69. Salter RB, Simmonds DF, Malcolm BW, et al: The biological effect of continuous passive motion on the healing of full-thickness defects in articular cartilage: An experimental investigation in the rabbit. *J Bone Joint Surg* 1980;62A:1232–1251.

70. Buckwalter JA: Activity vs rest in the treatment of bone, soft tissue and joint injuries. *Iowa Orthop J* 1995;15:29–42.

71. Buckwalter JA: Editorial: Should bone, soft-tissue, and joint injuries be treated with rest or activity? *J Orthop Res* 1995;13:155–156.

72. Buckwalter JA: Mechanical injuries of articular cartilage, in Finerman GAM, Noyes FR (eds): *Biology and Biomechanics of the Traumatized Synovial Joint: The Knee as a Model.* Rosemont, IL, American Academy of Orthopaedic Surgeons, 1992, pp 83–96.

73. Levy AS, Lohnes J, Sculley S, et al: Chondral delamination of the knee in soccer players. *Am J Sports Med* 1996;24:634–639.

74. Mankin HJ, Buckwalter JA: Editorial: Restoration of the osteoarthritic joint. *J Bone Joint Surg* 1996;78A:1–2.

75. Maletius W, Messner K: The effect of partial meniscectomy on the long-term prognosis of knees with localized, severe chondral damage: A twelve- to fifteen-year followup. *Am J Sports Med* 1996;24:258–262.

76. Messner K, Maletius W: The long-term prognosis for severe damage to weight-bearing cartilage in the knee: A 14-year clinical and radiographic follow-up in 28 young athletes. *Acta Orthop Scand* 1966;67:165–168.

77. Bergenudd H, Johnell O, Redlund-Johnell I, et al: The articular cartilage after osteotomy for

medial gonarthrosis: Biopsies after 2 years in 19 cases. *Acta Orthop Scand* 1992;63:413–416.

78. Brittberg M, Faxén E, Peterson L: Carbon fiber scaffolds in the treatment of early knee osteoarthritis: A prospective 4-year followup of 37 patients. *Clin Orthop* 1994;307:155–164.

79. Brittberg M, Lindahl A, Nilsson A, et al: Treatment of deep cartilage defects in the knee with autologous chondrocyte transplantation. *N Engl J Med* 1994;331:889–895.

80. Ewing JW: Arthroscopic treatment of degenerative meniscal lesions and early degenerative arthritis of the knee, in Ewing JW (ed): *Articular Cartilage and Knee Joint Function: Basic Science and Arthroscopy.* New York, NY, Raven Press, 1990, pp 137–145.

81. Ficat RP, Ficat C, Gedeon P, et al: Spongialization: A new treatment for diseased patellae. *Clin Orthop* 1979;144:74–83.

82. Friedman MJ, Berasi CC, Fox JM, et al: Preliminary results with abrasion arthroplasty in the osteoarthritic knee. *Clin Orthop* 1984;182:200–205.

83. Homminga GN, Bulstra SK, Bouwmeester PS, et al: Perichondral grafting for cartilage lesions of the knee. *J Bone Joint Surg* 1990;72B:1003–1007.

84. Insall JN, Joseph DM, Msika C: High tibial osteotomy for varus gonarthrosis: A long-term follow-up study. *J Bone Joint Surg* 1984;66A:1040–1048.

85. Johnson LL: Arthroscopic abrasion arthroplasty: Historical and pathologic perspective. Present status. *Arthroscopy* 1986;2:54–69.

86. Johnson LL: The sclerotic lesion: Pathology and the clinical response to arthroscopic abrasion arthroplasty, in Ewing JW (ed): *Articular Cartilage and Knee Joint Function: Basic Science and Arthroscopy.* New York, NY, Raven Press, 1990, pp 319–333.

87. Buckle DS, Minns RJ: Biological response to woven carbon fibre pads in the knee: A clinical and experimental study. *J Bone Joint Surg* 1990;72B:60–62.

88. Reigstad A, Grønmark T: Osteoarthritis of the hip treated by intertrochanteric osteotomy: A long-term follow-up. *J Bone Joint Surg* 1984;66A:1–6.

89. Seradge H, Kutz JA, Kleinert HE, et al: Perichondrial resurfacing arthroplasty in the hand. *J Hand Surg* 1984;9A:880–886.

90. Sprague NF III: Arthroscopic debridement for degenerative knee joint disease. *Clin Orthop* 1981;160:118–123.

91. van Valburg AA, van Roermund PM, Lammens J, et al: Can Ilizarov joint distraction delay the need for an arthrodesis of the ankle? A preliminary report. *J Bone Joint Surg* 1995;77B:720–725.

92. Johnson LL: Arthroscopic abrasion arthroplasty, in McGinty JB (ed): *Operative Arthroscopy*, ed 2. Philadelphia, PA, Raven Press, 1996, pp 427–446.

93. Shapiro F, Koide S, Glimcher MJ: Cell origin and differentiation in the repair of full-thickness defects of articular cartilage. *J Bone Joint Surg* 1993;75A:532–553.

94. Bentley G: The surgical treatment of chondromalacia patellae. *J Bone Joint Surg* 1978;60B:74–81.

95. Haggart GE: The surgical treatment of degenerative arthritis of the knee joint. *J Bone Joint Surg* 1940;22:717–729.

96. Insall J: The Pridie debridement operation for osteoarthritis of the knee. *Clin Orthop* 1974;101:61–67.

97. Magnuson PB: Joint debridement: Surgical treatment of degenerative arthritis. *Surg Gynec Obstet* 1941;73:1–9.

98. Baumgaertner MR, Cannon WD Jr, Vittori JM, et al: Arthroscopic debridement of the arthritic knee. *Clin Orthop* 1990;253:197–202.

99. Bert JM: Role of abrasion arthroplasty and debridement in the management of osteoarthritis of the knee. *Rheum Dis Clin North Am* 1993;19:725–739.

100. Bert JM, Maschka K: The arthroscopic treatment of unicompartmental gonarthrosis: A five-year follow-up study of abrasion arthroplasty plus arthroscopic debridement and arthroscopic debridement alone. *Arthroscopy* 1989;5:25–32.

101. Mitchell N, Shepard N: The resurfacing of adult rabbit articular cartilage by multiple perforations through the subchondral bone. *J Bone Joint Surg* 1976;58A:230–233.

102. Frenkel SR, Menche DS, Blair B, et al: A comparison of abrasion burr arthroplasty and subchondral drilling in the treatment of full-thickness cartilage lesions in the rabbit. *Trans Orthop Res Soc* 1994;19:483.

103. Moseley JB Jr, Wray NP, Kuykendall D, et al: Arthroscopic treatment of osteoarthritis of the knee: A prospective, randomized, placebo-controlled trial. Results of a pilot study. *Am J Sports Med* 1996;24:28–34.

104. Chang RW, Falconer J, Stulberg SD, et al: A randomized, controlled trial of arthroscopic surgery versus closed-needle joint lavage for patients with osteoarthritis of the knee. *Arthritis Rheum* 1993;36:289–296.

105. Edelson R, Burks RT, Bloebaum RD: Short-term effects of knee washout for osteoarthritis. *Am J Sports Med* 1995;23:345–349.

106. Gibson JN, White MD, Chapman VM, et al: Arthroscopic lavage and debridement for osteoarthritis of the knee. *J Bone Joint Surg* 1992;74B:534–537.

107. Livesley PJ, Doherty M, Needoff M, et al: Arthroscopic lavage of osteoarthritic knees. *J Bone Joint Surg* 1991;73B:922–926.

108. Takakura Y, Tanaka Y, Kumai T, et al: Low tibial osteotomy for osteoarthritis of the ankle: Results of a new operation in 18 patients. *J Bone Joint Surg* 1995;77B:50–54.

109. Byers PD: The effect of high femoral osteotomy on osteoarthritis of the hip: An anatomical study of six hip joints. *J Bone Joint Surg* 1974;56B:279–290.

110. Itoman M, Yamamoto M, Yonemoto K, et al: Histological examination of surface repair tissue after successful osteotomy for osteoarthritis of the hip joint. *Int Orthop* 1992;16:118–121.

111. Berman AT, Bosacco SJ, Kirshner S, et al: Factors influencing long-term results in high tibial osteotomy. *Clin Orthop* 1991;272:192–198.

112. Matthews LS, Goldstein SA, Malvitz TA, et al: Proximal tibial osteotomy: Factors that influence the duration of satisfactory function. *Clin Orthop* 1991;272:192–198.

113. Coventry MB, Ilstrup DM, Wallrichs SL: Proximal tibial osteotomy: A critical long-term study of eighty-seven cases. *J Bone Joint Surg* 1993;75A:196–201.

114. Hass J: Functional arthroplasty. *J Bone Joint Surg* 1944;26:297–306.

115. Mensor MC, Scheck M: Review of six years' experience with the hanging-hip operation. *J Bone Joint Surg* 1968;50A:1250–1254.

116. Radin EL, Maquet P, Parker H: Rationale and indications for the hanging hip procedure: A clinical and experimental study. *Clin Orthop* 1975;112:221–230.

117. Scheck M: Roentgenographic changes of the hip joint following extra-articular operations for degenerative arthritis. *J Bone Joint Surg* 1970;52A:99–104.

118. Aldegheri R, Trivella G, Saleh M: Articulated distraction of the hip: Conservative surgery for arthritis in young patients. *Clin Orthop* 1994;301:94–101.

119. Buckwalter JA: Joint distraction for osteoarthritis. *Lancet* 1996;347:279–280.

120. Hoikka VE, Jaroma HJ, Ritsila VA: Reconstruction of the patellar articulation with periosteal grafts: 4-year follow-up of 13 cases. *Acta Orthop Scand* 1990;61:36–39.

121. Jensen LJ, Bach KL: Periosteal transplantation in the treatment of osteochondritis dissecans. *Scand J Med Sci Sports* 1992;2:32–36.

122. Niedermann B, Boe S, Lauritzen J, et al: Glued periosteal grafts in the knee. *Acta Orthop Scand* 1985;56:457–460.

123. O'Driscoll SW, Salter RB: The repair of major osteochondral defects in joint surfaces by neochondrogenesis with autogenous osteoperiosteal grafts stimulated by continuous passive motion: An experimental investigation in the rabbit. *Clin Orthop* 1986;208:131–140.

124. O'Driscoll SW, Keeley FW, Salter RB: Durability of regenerated articular cartilage produced by free autogenous periosteal grafts in major full-thickness defects in joint surfaces under the influence of continuous passive motion: A follow-up report at one year. *J Bone Joint Surg* 1988;70A:595–606.

125. Ostgaard SE, Weilby A: Resection arthroplasty of the proximal interphalangeal joint. *J Hand Surg* 1993;18B:613–615.

126. Engkvist O, Johansson SH: Perichondral arthroplasty: A clinical study in twenty-six patients. *Scand J Plast Reconstr Surg* 1980;14:71–87.

127. Wakitani S, Kimura T, Hirooka A, et al: Repair of rabbit articular surfaces with allograft chondrocytes embedded in collagen gel. *J Bone Joint Surg* 1989;71B:74–80.

128. Itay S, Abramovici A, Nevo Z: Use of cultured embryonal chick epiphyseal chondrocytes as grafts for defects in chick articular cartilage. *Clin Orthop* 1987;220:284–303.

129. Itay S, Abramovici A, Yosipovitch Z, et al: Correction of defects in articular cartilage by implants of cultured embryony chondrocytes. *Trans Orthop Res Soc* 1988;13:112.

130. Noguchi T, Oka M, Fujino M, et al: Repair of osteochondral defects with grafts of cultured chondrocytes: Comparison of allografts and isografts. *Clin Orthop* 1994;302:251–258.

131. Robinson D, Halperun N, Nevo Z: Regenerating hyaline cartilage in articular defects of old chickens using implants of embryonal chick chondrocytes embedded in a new natural delivery substance. *Calcif Tissue Int* 1990;46:246–253.

132. Shortkroff S, Barone L, Hsu HP, et al: Healing of chondral and osteochondral defects in a canine model: The role of cultured chondrocytes in regeneration of articular cartilage. *Biomaterials* 1996;17:147–154.

133. Brittberg M: *Cartilage Repair*. Göteborg, Sweden, Göteborg University, 1996. Thesis.

134. Brittberg M, Nilsson A, Lindahl A, et al: Rabbit articular cartilage defects treated with autologous cultured chondrocytes. *Clin Orthop* 1996;326:270–283.

135. Wakitani S, Goto T, Mansour JM, et al: Mesenchymal stem cell-based repair of a large articular cartilage and bone defect. *Trans Orthop Res Soc* 1994;19:481.

136. Wakitani S, Goto T, Pineda SJ, et al: Mesenchymal cell-based repair of large, full-thickness defects of articular cartilage. *J Bone Joint Surg* 1994;76A:579–592.

137. Buckwalter JA, Glimcher MJ, Cooper RR, et al: Bone biology: II. Formation, form, modeling, remodeling and regulation of cell function. *J Bone Joint Surg* 1995;77A:1276–1289.

138. Hunziker EB, Rosenberg L: Induction of repair in partial thickness articular cartilage lesions by timed release of TGF-beta. *Trans Orthop Res Soc* 1994;19:236.

139. Hunziker EB, Rosenberg LC: Repair of partial-thickness defects in articular cartilage: Cell recruitment from the synovial membrane. *J Bone Joint Surg* 1996;78A:721–733.

140. Pfeilschifter J, Diel I, Pilz U, et al: Mitogenic responsiveness of human bone cells in vitro to hormones and growth factors decreases with age. *J Bone Miner Res* 1993;8:707–717.

141. Paletta GA, Arnoczky SP, Warren RF: The repair of osteochondral defects using an exogenous fibrin clot: An experimental study in dogs. *Am J Sports Med* 1992;20:725–731.

142. Messner K, Gillquist J: Synthetic implants for the repair of osteochondral defects of the medial femoral condyle: A biomechanical and histological evaluation in the rabbit knee. *Biomaterials* 1993;14:513–521.

143. Freed LE, Grande DA, Lingbin Z, et al: Joint resurfacing using allograft chondrocytes and synthetic biodegradable polymer scaffolds. *J Biomed Mater Res* 1994;28:891–899.

144. Hendrickson DA, Nixon AJ, Grande DA, et al: Chondrocyte-fibrin matrix transplants for resurfacing extensive articular cartilage defects. *J Orthop Res* 1994;12:485–497.

145. Sams AE, Nixon AJ: Chondrocyte-laden collagen scaffolds for resurfacing extensive articular cartilage defects. *Osteoarthritis Cartilage* 1995;3:47–59.

146. Beaver RJ, Mahomed M, Backstein D, et al: Fresh osteochondral allografts for post-traumatic defects in the knee: A survivorship analysis. *J Bone Joint Surg* 1992;74B:105–110.

147. Bobic V: Arthroscopic osteochondral autograft transplantation in anterior cruciate ligament reconstruction: A preliminary clinical study. *Knee Surg Sports Traumatol Arthrosc* 1996;3:262–264.

148. Convery FR, Meyers MH, Akeson WH: Fresh osteochondral allografting of the femoral condyle. *Clin Orthop* 1991;273:139–145.

149. Czitrom AA, Keating S, Gross AE: The viability of articular cartilage in fresh osteochondral allografts after clinical transplantation. *J Bone Joint Surg* 1990;72A:574–581.

150. Garrett JC: Fresh osteochondral allografts for treatment of articular defects in osteochondritis dissecans of the lateral femoral condyle in adults. *Clin Orthop* 1994;303:33–37.

151. Gross AE, Beaver RJ, Mohammed MN: Fresh small fragment osteochondral allografts used for posttraumatic defects in the knee joint, in Finerman GAM, Noyes FR (eds): *Biology and Biomechanics of the Traumatized Synovial Joint: The Knee as a Model*. Rosemont, IL, American Academy of Orthopaedic Surgeons, 1992, pp 123–141.

152. McDermott AGP, Langer F, Pritzker KPH, et al: Fresh small-fragment osteochondral allografts: Long-term follow-up study on first 100 cases. *Clin Orthop* 1985;197:96–102.

153. Mahomed MN, Beaver RJ, Gross AE: The long-term success of fresh, small fragment osteochondral allografts used for intraarticular post-traumatic defects in the knee joint. *Orthopedics* 1992;15:1191–1199.

154. Meyers MH: Resurfacing of the femoral head with fresh osteochondral allografts: Long-term results. *Clin Orthop* 1985;197:111–114.

155. Meyers MH, Akeson W, Convery FR: Resurfacing of the knee with fresh osteochondral allograft. *J Bone Joint Surg* 1989;71A:704–713.

156. Outerbridge HK, Outerbridge AR, Outerbridge RE: The use of a lateral patellar autologous graft for the repair of a large osteochondral defect in the knee. *J Bone Joint Surg* 1995;77A:65–72.

157. Wilson WJ, Jacobs JE: Patellar graft for severely depressed comminuted fractures of the lateral tibial condyle. *J Bone Joint Surg* 1952;34A:436–442.

158. Dew TL, Martin RA: Functional, radiographic, and histologic assessment of healing of autogenous osteochondral grafts and full-thickness cartilage defects in the talus of dogs. *Am J Vet Res* 1992;53:2141–2152.

159. Ohlendorf C, Tomford WW, Mankin JH: Chondrocyte survival in cryopreserved osteochondral articular cartilage. *J Orthop Res* 1996;14:413–416.

160. Schachar N, McAllister D, Stevenson M, et al: Metabolic and biochemical status of articular cartilage following cryopreservation and transplantation: A rabbit model. *J Orthop Res* 1992;10:603–609.

161. Campanacci M, Cervellati C, Donati U: Autogenous patella as replacement for a resected femoral or tibial condyle: A report on 19 cases. *J Bone Joint Surg* 1985;67B:557–563.

162. Jacobs JE: Follow-up notes on articles previously published in the Journal: Patellar graft for severely depressed comminuted fractures of the lateral tibial condyle. *J Bone Joint Surg* 1965;47A:842–847.

163. Karpinski MR, Botting TD: Patellar graft for late disability following tibial plateau fractures. *Injury* 1983;15:197–202.

164. Yamashita F, Sakakida K, Suzu F, et al: The transplantation of an autogeneic osteochondral fragment for osteochondritis dissecans of the knee. *Clin Orthop* 1985;201:43–50.

165. Bayne O, Langer F, Pritzker KP, et al: Osteochondral allografts in the treatment of osteonecrosis of the knee. *Orthop Clin North Am* 1985;16:727–740.

166. Flynn JM, Springfield DS, Mankin HJ: Osteoarticular allografts to treat distal femoral osteonecrosis. *Clin Orthop* 1994;303:38–43.

167. Locht RC, Gross AE, Langer F: Late osteochondral allograft resurfacing for tibial plateau fractures. *J Bone Joint Surg* 1984;66A:328–335.

168. Mankin HJ: The response of articular cartilage to mechanical injury. *J Bone Joint Surg* 1982;64A:460-466.

The Treatment of Isolated Articular Cartilage Lesions in the Young Individual

David S. Menche, MD
C. Thomas Vangsness, Jr, MD
Mark Pitman, MD
Allan E. Gross, MD
Lars Peterson, MD, PhD

Introduction

Isolated articular cartilage defects occurring in the young individual present as a clinical dilemma. Accurate diagnosis prior to surgical intervention is extremely difficult. A clinician who is faced with an articular cartilage defect at the time of surgery cannot rely on data from the literature to support that any specific technique performed on a patient will result in a superior outcome. Therefore, the physician must have a knowledge of basic science studies and current clinical data in order to provide optimized individualized treatment.

For the purpose of this discussion, we will use the definition that partial thickness lesions are lesions that penetrate the articular cartilage but do not reach the subchondral bone. Full thickness articular cartilage lesions are lesions that reach but do not penetrate the subchondral bone. Osteochondral lesions are lesions that penetrate the subchondral bone. As detailed elsewhere, partial thickness and full thickness articular cartilage lesions have a minimal capacity for healing, whereas osteochondral defects may heal with a fibrocartilaginous repair tissue. This fibrocartilaginous repair tissue is suboptimal and most likely will degenerate over a period of time. In this chapter, we will discuss the treatment of isolated articular cartilage lesions and will focus on present day techniques and future trends.

Incidence

It is thought that the incidence of full thickness articular cartilage lesions is relatively high in sports-related injuries. However, very few studies in the literature document the incidence of these lesions. The incidence of articular cartilage defects in patients undergoing arthroscopy has varied in the literature.[1,2] In a Swedish study, surgeons performed 1,000 arthroscopies and found grade II or III chondral defects of a minimal diameter of 1 cm in only seven women and 21 men.[3] However, it is likely that the true incidence of chondral damage is grossly underestimated, because many times arthroscopists can overlook a chondral lesion, especially if it is in the posterior aspect of the femoral condyle.[2]

History

Patients who have isolated articular cartilage defects often complain of pain, catching, crepitation, locking, and/or swelling of the knee. They may also have symptoms of buckling and occasional giving way. Many times it is very difficult to differentiate a patient with chondral damage from a patient who has some other knee pathology, such as a meniscal tear.

Physical Examination

There is no physical sign that is pathognomonic for the diagnosis of an isolated articular cartilage defect. The examiner should palpate the joint for point tenderness along the medial and lateral femoral condyles and patella facet joints. With an articular cartilage injury, diffuse joint line tenderness, crepitation, and an effusion, with limitation of motion of the joint may be present. The knee should be carefully evaluated for ligamentous instability, varus or valgus malalignment and patella mobility and alignment, before considering the patient for surgical or nonsurgical treatment.

Diagnostic Tests

Routinely, radiographs will not show evidence of pure isolated articular cartilage lesions. Standing full leg-length radiographs are important in determining varus or valgus malalignment. Postero-anterior (PA) radiographs with the knee joint in 45° of flexion can demonstrate the presence of joint space narrowing that is not apparent on routine PA views with the knee in extension.[4] Studies evaluating magnetic resonance imaging (MRI) accuracy in identifying articular cartilage defects have revealed variable results.[5-8] Evaluation by MRI of partial thickness chondral injuries is even less reliable. Sensitivity for identifying full thickness articular cartilage lesions was significantly increased after postarthroscopic reinterpretation of the MRI. Clinically, we do not rely on MRI to make the diagnosis of a chondral defect. Possibly, the use of contrast to enhance MRIs will make this diagnostic test more accurate.[9] Arthro-

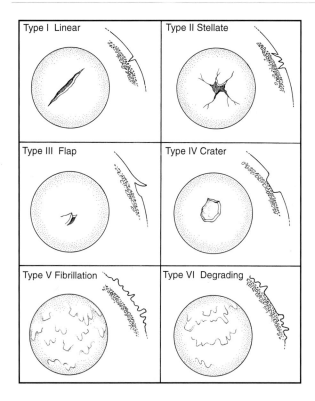

Type I Linear

Type II Stellate

Type III Flap

Type IV Crater

Type V Fibrillation

Type VI Degrading

Fig. 1 Bauer and Jackson classification of cartilage injury patterns. (Reproduced with permission from Bauer M, Jackson RW: Chondral lesions of the femoral condyles: A system of arthroscopic classification. *Arthroscopy* 1988;4: 97–102.)

scopy is the diagnostic test of choice in determining the presence of an articular cartilage lesion.

Grading Systems for Articular Cartilage Defects

Classification systems for grading articular cartilage defects began with the work surrounding "chondromalacia" of the undersurface of the patella. Original work by Outerbridge[10] in 1961 characterized the degenerative arthritic changes observed on the patella as grade I, softening with swelling; grade II, fragmentation and fissuring less than one-half inch in diameter; grade III, fragmentation and fissuring greater than one-half inch in diameter; and grade IV, subchondral bone exposed. Since this initial work, the advent of arthroscopy has further helped to clarify and develop other systems for grading articular cartilage lesions.

In 1976, Insall and associates[11] classified cartilage lesions of the patellae as I through IV. Characteristics of the four grades are: grade I, softening and swelling without any breaks on the cartilage surface; grade II, deep fissures extending to subchondral bone; grade III fibrillation; and grade IV, erosive changes and exposure of the subchondral bone.

In 1976, Goodfellow and associates[12] described the pathoanatomic differences of surface degeneration with flaking, which could progress to fibrillation, as opposed to the presence of basilar degeneration, which they believed would not affect the surface initially.

Ficat and Hungerford,[13] in their 1977 book, distinguished the characteristics of closed chondromalacia versus open chondromalacia. The closed chondromalacic lesion was about 1 cm^2 with a simple softening or a small blister seen macroscopically, but with an intact joint surface. They noted varying degrees of severity ranging from softening to pitting edema. They stated that an overall loss of elasticity of the cartilage could extend progressively in all directions. An open chondro-

malacic lesion had single or multiple fissures, which were either superficial or extended down to the subchondral bone. If there was ulceration, a localized loss of cartilage exposed the subchondral bone. Extensive exposed bone usually had a polished appearance, which they termed "eburnated." The authors also described chondrosclerosis, which is an abnormally hard cartilage surface, and tuft formation—the presence of multiple deep fronds of cartilage separated from one another by deep clefts that could extend down to the subchondral bone.

In 1984, Ogilvie-Harris and Jackson[14] further evaluated articular cartilage changes in a group of over 300 patients with patellar chondromalacia. In their classification, chondromalacia patellae was described as grade I, softening of the articular cartilage upon probing and minor surface fissuring with a closed blister lesion; grade II, major fasciculation of the articular cartilage confined to the patellae, ie, "crabmeat" appearance; and grade III, exposure of the subchondral bone of the patella with surface changes of the femoral groove. They felt that this grading system correlated with the pathoanatomic staging system of Outerbridge and that the clear cut-off points between each grade made it easy to use in clinical practice.

In 1984, Bentley and Dowd[15] classified cartilage lesions according to their size. In grade I, there is fibrillation or fissuring less than 0.5 cm. In grade II, fibrillation or fissuring is 0.5 to 1.0 cm in size. In grade III, there is an articular cartilage lesion 1 to 2 cm in size and in grade IV, there is a lesion greater than 2 cm, with or without exposed bone with fibrillation. No category was given to lesions that had an intact surface. In 1985, Johnson-Nurse and Dandy,[16] reviewed their arthroscopic finding in 76 knees. They noted fracture separations of the articular cartilage, and they provided a descriptive method for classifying articular cartilage lesions. In older patients, they found

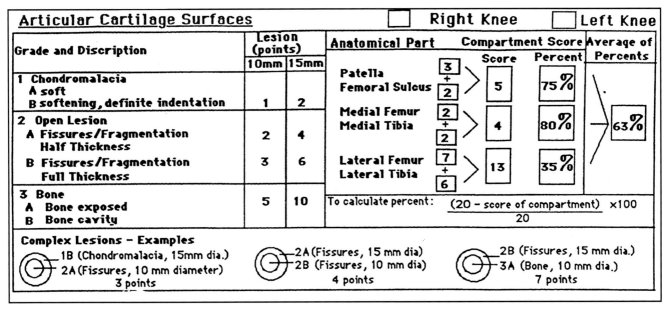

Fig. 2 Point scaling system for analysis of articular cartilage surface. (Reproduced with permission from Noyes FR, Stabler CL: A system for grading articular cartilage lesions at arthroscopy. *Am J Sports Med* 1989;17:505–513.)

fracture separations having either a full thickness separation of articular cartilage extending down to the subchondral bone or a partial thickness separation of articular cartilage, with the fragment attached at one edge as a flap without exposed subchondral bone.

Studies identified that many articular cartilage lesions that occur clinically were located between the calcified and noncalcified layer, ie, the separation of the tidemark.[16,17] Lesions that occurred at this calcified/noncalcified interface have been described as being partial thickness lesions. Those patients that did not have the protective layer of residual calcified cartilage overlying the bone did worse than patients who had partial thickness lesions. The author identified five other factors associated with a poor clinical outcome. These were patients who had large lesions, those with chronic degenerative changes with eburnated bone, patients who had full thickness lesions with loss of the tidemark, those with submeniscal weightbearing lesions, and patients who were older. This review showed that the

best prognosis was found with the small to medium acute partial thickness lesions on the weightbearing portion of the femoral condyles.[18]

In 1988, Bauer and Jackson[19] described a system based primarily on arthroscopic appearance (Fig. 1). The stellate lesion was found to be the most common followed by linear cracks. In their system, types I through IV were believed to be more traumatic in origin, and types V and VI were more degenerative in nature.

Terry and associates[2] described three distinct configurations of articular cartilage lesions. Type I was a flap type, in which a large flap of articular cartilage could be lifted off to expose the subchondral bone. Type II was a stellate lesion, with a compression fracture consisting of multiple small flaps. Type III was a crater lesion, in which a significant area of subchondral bone was visible with no overlying flaps. In their series, type II, the stellate type, was the most common.

The most comprehensive and specific grading system for articular cartilage

lesions was published by Noyes and Stabler[20] in 1989. The authors classified articular cartilage lesions by defining the surface description, the extent of the articular cartilage involvement, the diameter, the location of the lesion, and the degree of knee flexion that put the lesion in contact with the weightbearing area. They proposed a numbered scoring system in order to access objectively the extent of damage of an articular cartilage defect. This system enables the surgeon to thoroughly document and record articular cartilage injury. As with most classification systems, it is both subjective and qualitative in nature. However, this classification scheme is probably the most defined and accurate of all systems currently available for recording patient information and longitudinal studies (Fig. 2).

A generalized acceptance of this type of classification system will allow a more direct comparison of outcome studies on the future treatments of chondral defects. To date, it has been impossible to compare the results of different techniques,

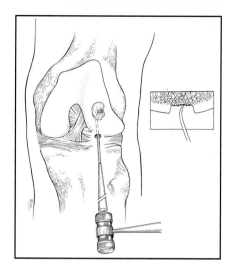

Fig. 3 Microfracture technique.

because various classification systems have been used. In addition, the grading of the cartilage lesion can vary, depending on whether it was based on the original defect or after debridement to a normal, healthy, stable articular cartilage border.

Overall, it should be understood that any grading system is based on visual observations without a good scientific understanding of the underlying cellular activity. There is always a subjective component for error. Any evaluation should incorporate the use of a mechanical device, such as a probe, to help gain more objective information about the texture and size of the macroscopic cartilage presentation.

Basic Science Research Studies

The natural history of articular cartilage healing has been studied extensively.[21-38] In basic science studies, classification of articular cartilage lesions has been based on the depth of the lesion. Primarily, this type of classification system has been used because the depth of the lesion dictates the biologic response of the tissue to spontaneous repair. Partial thickness cartilage lesions and full thickness cartilage lesions do not respond with any significant repair process. In contrast, osteo-chondral lesions will respond with a sub-optimal fibrocartilaginous repair.

In review of the basic science research studies on the effect of subchondral drilling in healing articular cartilage defects, several conclusions can be reached. Repair tissue forms routinely in the articular cartilage defect.[27] The repair is uniformly nonhyaline in nature.[39,40] Healing varies, depending on the size and location of the defect.[41] The repair tissue can potentially degenerate.[38,41] Continuous passive motion (CPM) appears to be beneficial.[42] The repair tissue did not result from chondrocytes adjacent to the articular cartilage, but from the mesenchymal cells in the marrow.[43]

A comparison of the results of the fibrocartilaginous healing obtained by performing subchondral drilling versus that obtained with burr arthroplasty was evaluated in a rabbit model. Both techniques resulted in suboptimal healing; however, in the animals undergoing subchondral drilling to heal articular cartilage defects, there was an increase in fibrocartilaginous healing and a decrease in degenerative changes. It is hypothesized that burring of the subchondral plate may cause an increase in the degenerative changes secondary to a mechanical breakdown of the joint surface.[44]

A significant amount of research has been done on the effect of perichondral transplantation in healing chondral defects. In the basic research studies on perichondral transplantation, the perichondrium has been shown to have an effective chondrogenic potential.[45-48] The transplants appear to produce biologically acceptable results morphologically, biochemically, and biomechanically, and the degradation of the repair tissue appears to be minimal.[49] Controversy exists about whether CPM will ultimately provide the best healing as it may affect graft fixation and ultimately cause early failure.[50] It appears that "hyaline-like cartilage formation" was seen in nonweightbearing areas after perichondral transplantation. In weightbearing areas, fibrocartilaginous formation was seen.[51]

A review of the literature on basic science studies evaluating the results of periosteal transplantation in the treatment of isolated articular cartilage defects indicates that cells from the cambium layer are derived from mesenchymal cells, which can ultimately differentiate into chondrocytes.[52] Controversy exists as to whether the cambium layer of the periosteum should be faced into the defect or outward, facing the joint. However, hyaline-like cartilage tissue was obtained in research models that treated articular cartilage defects with the cambium layer facing either outward into the joint[53] or inward, toward the defect.[54] Hyaline-like tissue can be obtained by using periosteal transplantation in conjunction with CPM.[55] The repair tissue appears to resemble hyaline cartilage. The cellular origin of the repair tissue may be from the mesenchymal cells in the subchondral bone as well as from the periosteum.[56] Incomplete bonding of adjacent cartilage on repair tissue often had a fibrillated superficial tangential zone. This incomplete bonding is of concern and may lead to early failures. Electron microscopic studies have confirmed that periosteum can alter its structure to resemble hyaline cartilage.[57] There appeared to be no statistically significant difference in the chondrogenic potential when comparing fresh and cryopreserved allografts.[58] Chondrocyte transplantation is not a new procedure. In 1965, Smith[59] isolated living chondrocytes from articular cartilage. Isolated chondrocytes were transplanted and created nodules of fresh cartilage.[60] Ia antigens, which have been shown to be important determinants in the rejection of tissue transplanted allografts, were detected on the surface of human chondrocytes.[61] The first experience of chondrocyte transplantation using a periosteal cover was performed in an experimental rabbit model at the Hospital for Joint

Diseases Orthopaedic Institute.[54] These initial data were presented in 1984 by Dr. Lars Peterson at the Orthopaedic Research Society Meeting in Atlanta, Georgia.[62] When comparing results of healing of 3 mm full-thickness articular cartilage defects created in the rabbit patella, the transplantation technique using periosteum and cells resulted in a significantly higher resurfacing of the surgically created defect than did the technique of covering the defect with periosteum alone.[54] Similar data, which established the benefits of the technique using cells with periosteum versus periosteum alone, were obtained in a later study performed in Sweden.[63]

The use of a matrix when performing chondrocyte transplantation has many theoretical advantages. Certain ideal matrix characteristics are important in order to achieve optimal repair. The matrix should act as a scaffold, retain its structural properties until intrinsic growth has occurred, and be degradable. Many experimental studies have been performed using matrices for resurfacing articular cartilage defects. Among these engineered devices are ones fabricated using demineralized bone (with perichondrium),[64] polylactic acid matrices,[65] polyglycolic acid matrices,[66] hydroxyapatite/Dacron composites,[67] fibrin,[68] collagen gels[54,69-72] and collagen fiber matrices.[73,74] One study that used a bilayer matrix in order to prevent fibrocartilaginous penetration into the defect revealed a clear advantage of cell-seeded implants over nonseeded implants in the treatment of isolated articular cartilage defects in the rabbit.[75]

In summary, in reviewing basic research studies involving chondrocyte transplantation, there appears to be chondrogenic potential using this technique. Cell-seeded matrices appear to provide a better repair than unseeded matrices. Basic science data support improved healing of articular cartilage defects with chondrocyte transplantation.

Treatment of Isolated Articular Cartilage Defects
Superficial Defects

Superficial injuries that do not violate the junction of the calcified zone and underlying osseous endplate demonstrate a lack of both inflammatory and repair components seen with more vascular tissue. Animal studies have shown ineffective healing.[26-28,76] Longer term follow-up of superficial lacerative injuries has demonstrated no further progression of healing over time and no evidence of progression to osteoarthritis.[32,39]

Ghadially and associates[29] used histology and electron microscopy to study tangential partial-thickness defects in rabbits. There was no repair even in the young animal. At 2 years the cartilage surfaces were almost identical to the initial appearance at the time of injury.[29] Clinically, single or multiple lacerations to the articular cartilage should cause little concern. A tangential slice of articular cartilage that is removed as a result of trauma, a surgeon's knife or an intra-articular shaver will remain as a defective area in the cartilaginous surface, with no evidence of repair.[38]

Full-Thickness Articular Cartilage Defects

Lavage The removal of intra-articular debris and/or other elements that can cause ongoing inflammatory reactions may be performed with or without arthroscopy. Generally, good short-term results have been described; however, these studies are not well controlled and do not have long-term follow-up.[77] Lavage most likely will not provide satisfactory pain relief for the athlete or the young active patient. Work by Moseley and associates[77] has demonstrated the difficulty in designing study protocols, especially with respect to controls and placebo effects.[77]

Arthroscopic Debridement and Abrasion Arthroplasty Abrasion arthroplasty pioneered by Lanny Johnson[78] in

the 1980s is the debridement of the articular cartilage defect to a normal stable tissue edge with superficial abrasion of the exposed subchondral bone. Abrasion arthroplasty initiates bleeding in the hope of forming a fibrocartilaginous scar over the exposed bone. This tissue has been demonstrated to be fibrocartilaginous in nature and is not true hyaline cartilage. The efficacy of the procedure is controversial, and results appear to be unpredictable, with limited clinical success. A significant failure rate was noted in patients who had undergone abrasion arthroplasty and who had a failed high tibial osteotomy.[79] More recently, one study revealed that 50% of patients who had undergone abrasion arthroplasty for degenerative arthritis underwent a total knee replacement at a mean of 3 years after abrasion.[80] In a retrospective review of patients who had undergone abrasion arthroplasty plus arthroscopic debridement versus arthroscopic debridement alone, the patients who had arthroscopic debridement alone did better.[81]

In contrast, other authors who had performed an abrasion arthroplasty reported favorable results.[78,82-84] To obtain satisfactory results, an intracortical rather than a cancellous abrasion should be performed.[78] An abrasion arthroplasty is contraindicated in patients who have inflammatory arthritis.

In evaluating the published studies using this technique there are multiple issues that are generally not addressed, including the degree of osteoarthritis, limb alignment, age and activity level of the patient, and durability of the fibrocartilage. Again, none of these studies have long-term follow-up.

Subchondral Drilling The biologic concept of drilling a full thickness articular cartilage defect is similar to abrasion arthroplasty. Multiple drill holes pass through the subchondral plate to bring in a blood supply, which will ultimately result in formation of a fibrocartilaginous covering over the exposed bone. Human

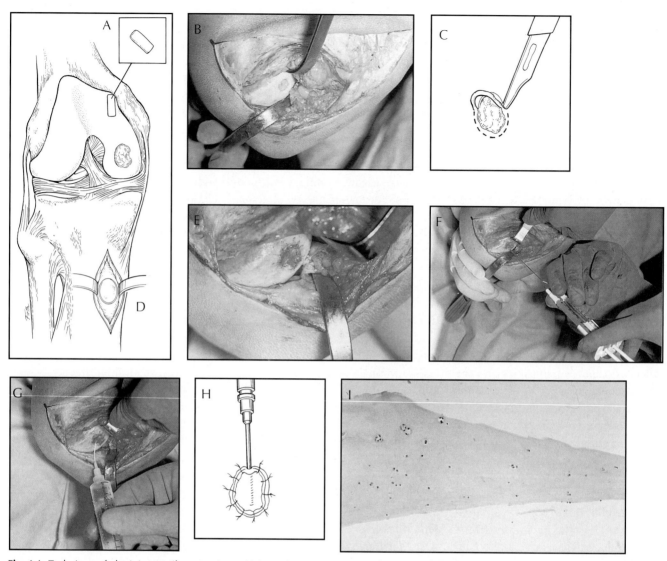

Fig. 4 A, Technique of obtaining cartilage specimen: Using a ring curette, a 5 mm by 12 mm full thickness articular cartilage specimen is obtained from the superior aspect of the medial femoral condyle and sent to the laboratory for culturing. **B** and **C,** Preparation of articular cartilage defect. **B,** Photograph of a prepared articular cartilage defect on the medial femoral condyle. **C,** It is imperative to resect all damaged articular cartilage until a healthy border of normal articular cartilage rim is obtained. When preparing the defect, be careful not to penetrate the subchondral bone. **D** and **E,** Periosteal patch. **D,** The periosteal patch is usually obtained from the superior medial aspect of the tibia just below the pes anserinus insertion. Careful attention must be made as to obtain the full thickness of the periosteum without damaging the tissue. **E,** The periosteal patch is sutured to the defect using 6-0 vicryl suture with the cambium layer facing the defect. **F,** Fibrin glue sealant is being placed around the margins of the sutured periosteum covering a medial femoral condylar defect. **G,** A saline trial injection is used to test for any leakage in the periosteal patch. **H,** Implantation of cells. Through the superior defect in the periosteum, the cells are injected in an even distribution over the entire surface of the defect. After completion of the cell implantation, the defect is closed with additional sutures and fibrin sealant. **I,** Biopsy. Photomicrograph of surgical biopsy obtained approximately 9 months after chondrocyte transplantation of a medial femoral condylar defect.

studies evaluating this method of treatment are uncontrolled and have no long-term follow-up.[85,86]

MicroFracture In this technique, the subchondral architecture is left intact except for the areas broached with small metal picks. The pick is used to bring in a blood supply from the subchondral area to the joint surface (Fig. 3). Again, studies are limited, and the tissue that evolves from this procedure is fibrocartilage.[87] Second-look arthroscopic procedures by Rodrigo and associates,[87] of patients who were placed on CPM machines after microfracture procedures showed visual improvement of the lesions and significant repair response. However, no histology was noted or presented in this short follow-up study.

Marrow or Stem Cell Techniques
These techniques involve debridement of the lesion followed by a packing of cancellous bone obtained from local or distant sites into the defect. Conceptually, the pleuripotential stem cells of cancellous bone marrow can differentiate into fibrocartilage or hyaline-like cartilage cells to help resurface damaged areas. No long-term studies have been done. Transplanting stem cells for possible differentiation into hyaline or hyaline-like articular cartilage is an exciting unproven concept.

Periosteal-Perichondral Grafts
Early animal studies have shown encouraging results in this area. Periosteal tissue or perichondral tissue is thought to be able to differentiate into hyaline-like tissue.[88] Long-term results have not been established and little work has been done in the human knee.[89,90] There is concern regarding the potential of increasing long-term failures with perichondrial transplantation as an increase in graft mineralization was noted in 20 of 25 knees and disruption of cartilage and bone was noted in two of three biopsies.[91]

Chondrocyte Transplantation
Since October of 1987, more than 400 patients who have had articular cartilage defects have been treated with autologous cultured chondrocytes in Gothenburg, Sweden. Those selected for surgery were patients between 15 and 50 years of age who had articular cartilage damage and symptoms of pain on weightbearing as well as pain after activities. On arthroscopic evaluation, chondral lesions that were treated with chondrocyte transplantation measured between 10 mm and 12 cm in diameter. These were full-thickness lesions, ie, lesions down to the subchondral bone. Cartilage was harvested from the upper medial femoral condyle in 98% of the patients. The cartilage harvests were subsequently sent to the labo-

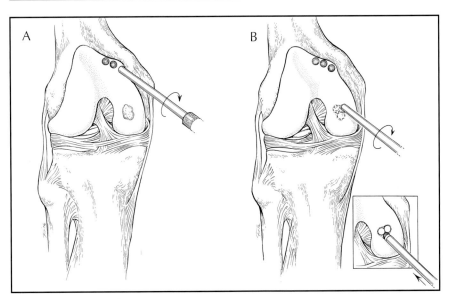

Fig. 5 A, Technique of obtaining osteochondral autograft: Using special cutting tools, osteochondral autografts are harvested from the articular cartilage rim. **B,** Similar-sized matching bony channels are made in the area of the articular cartilage defect, and the osteochondral autograft plugs are inserted into the previously made bony channels.

ratory and cultured. Transplants into the defects were performed several weeks later. The patients, initially treated with partial weightbearing, were full weightbearing at 6 weeks. Preliminary results of the first 100 patients who underwent chondrocyte transplantation with a minimal follow-up of 2 to 9 years revealed that approximately 90% were improved by the procedure. In patients who had osteochondritis dissecans, 85% considered themselves improved by the procedure. Results of a registry of patients undergoing this procedure in the United States revealed similar statistics.[92] No significant complications were reported.

If a surgeon has decided to perform chondrocyte transplantation, a specimen of articular cartilage is usually obtained from the superior medial femoral articular cartilage margin. It is important to obtain a full-thickness biopsy specimen approximately 12 mm in length and 5 mm wide. The articular cartilage specimen is sent to the laboratory for culturing (Fig. 4, A).

After the cells have been cultured, the

patient is scheduled for a second surgical procedure. At this time, an open arthrotomy is required for implantation of the cells. At the time of arthrotomy, the articular cartilage defect is assessed. It is extremely important to obtain a normal articular cartilage rim (Fig. 4, B and C). A periosteal patch is obtained from the superior medial aspect of the tibia, just below the pes anserinus (Fig. 4, D). The technique used to obtain the periosteal flap is extremely important to avoid damaging this tissue. A defect in the periosteum will allow leakage of the cells during implantation. The periosteum with the cambium layer facing into the defect is sutured into the margins of the articular cartilage using 6-0 vicryl suture (Fig. 4, E).

At the completion of the periosteal fixation, fibrin glue is placed as a sealant around the margins of the defect (Fig. 4, F). An opening is left along the superior aspect of the defect for installation of a trial saline injection to test the integrity of the periosteal patch (Fig. 4, G). If leakage is seen, additional sutures and/or more fibrin glue may be placed. The cells are subsequently injected through the superior opening of the periosteal patch (Fig 4, *H*). Sutures are placed as required and additional fibrin glue is used to seal this area. A superficial biopsy of tissue obtained approximately 9 months from the chondrocyte transplantation of the medial femoral condyle is seen in Figure 4, *I*.

Osteochondral Defects

Generally speaking, when an acute osteochondral fracture occurs in an adult, the ability of the lesion to heal is improved by surgical intervention. With either arthroscopy or arthrotomy, various techniques have been described to stabilize larger nonfragmented osteochondral defects. Screws or pins can be used to stabilize these fragments. Cannulated pin systems have been developed to help facilitate fixation. In addition, absorbable pins have been designed. Experimental fibrin glues have been used in European countries to stabilize osteochondral fragments. At the present time, synthetic fibrin glue does not have FDA approval for this indication. In general, smaller fragments are generally removed. If the fragment is large enough and fits anatomically, attempts should be made to replace the fragment and secure it in order to restore the articular surface contour.[93]

Osteochondral Transplantation

An osteochondral graft may prove to be effective for treatment of focal regions of damaged articular cartilage. Experimental work had suggested that osteochondral grafts may provide better restoration of articular surfaces than other modes of repair. The idea of providing a fully formed articular cartilage matrix with vital chondrocytes makes theoretical sense. The objective of osteochondral transplantation is to restore the subchondral bone and at the same time, to align the chondral surface of the joints. Dr. Lars Peterson has expressed concern regarding the potential for degeneration of the overlying articular cartilage after performing an osteochondral autograft. The violation of the subchondral plate may result in subchondral sclerosis, which has been described as the first reliable radiographic sign of arthrosis and can ultimately result in articular cartilage deterioration.[94]

Autografts

Recent work has demonstrated autograft techniques for filling articular cartilage defects. In the knee, cylindrical osteochondral plugs are harvested from other areas of the knee joint with special cutting tools (Fig. 5, *A*). Similar sized matching bony channels are made in the articular cartilage defect (Fig. 5, *B*). The new full thickness articular cartilage, subchondral bone, and cancellous bone plugs are inserted, thereby resurfacing the damaged area (Fig. 5, *C*). Limited published data regarding the results of this technique are available at the present time. Current reports limit its use to small chondral lesions ranging in size from 10 to 22 mm in diameter.[95]

Allografts

Studies have shown that osteochondral grafts work best in joints that had articular cartilage damage secondary to post-traumatic changes and osteochondritis dissecans.[96-99] Unicompartmental grafts have been shown to be more successful.[96-101] It is preferable to perform the operation before secondary changes occur on the other side of the joint. As in chondrocyte transplantation, if malalignment is present, an osteotomy must be performed in order to obtain satisfactory results.

One of the authors (A.E.G.) has had extensive experience using osteochondral allografts in the treatment of articular cartilage defects about the knee. Between 1972 and 1992, 123 patients had osteochondral defects reconstructed using fresh small fragment osteochondral allografts. At 5 years, 95% of patients demonstrated successful results. However, results deteriorated with time, with only 66% successful results at 20 years. There were minimal complications in the series, including three stiff knees, one wound hematoma, and one patella tendon rupture. After surgery, all grafts solidly united to the host bone at approximately 6 to 12 months, except for two cases in which there was a questionable union.[102]

When performing allograft transplantation, a mid-line approach is used. It is extremely important to excise the damaged articular surface completely, until a horizontal bed of bleeding bone is obtained. It must be emphasized that the graft should not be used to correct alignment but that an osteotomy should be performed if realignment of the limb is necessary (Fig. 6, *left*). After the graft is shaped, cancellous screws are used for rigid fixation (Fig. 6, *right*). Consideration should be given to performing a meniscal allograft if the meniscus is significantly damaged and does not appear to function biomechanically.

Future

In the treatment of isolated articular cartilage defects, the future holds many exciting horizons, which stem from the field of molecular biology. Manipulating the chondrocyte environment using extrinsic factors to stimulate and influence proliferation, migration, and differentiation of cartilage cells will require further investigation. Artificial matrices may allow binding of new cells and stimulation of cartilage matrix formation. Finally, low energy light stimulation may provide up regulation of any of these processes. Clearly defined parameters must be evaluated for any specific laser wavelength.

Summary

The treatment of isolated articular cartilage defects is an evolving field in orthopaedic surgery today. We have summarized the basic science and clinical data on the treatment of isolated articular cartilage defects. Further long-term controlled studies are required in order to compare definitively the efficacy of treatments in this difficult clinical area. In future studies, inclusion/exclusion criteria must be detailed, and classification systems need to be standardized. Comparative analysis can then be performed to assess the efficacy of various techniques.

Acknowledgements

The authors would like to acknowledge the technical assistance of Mrs. Natalie Varner and Mrs. Eudell Hayes in the preparation of this manuscript.

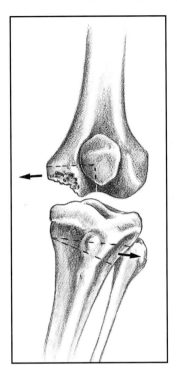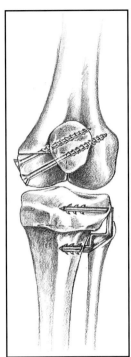

Fig. 6 Left, Preparation for allograft insertion. A resection of the damaged articular surface to a horizontal bed of cancellous bone is performed. Realignment of the lower extremity is achieved using a proximal tibial osteotomy. **Right,** Insertion of allograft. The graft is shaped to the defect and fixed rigidly using cancellous screws. (Reproduced with permission from Gross AE: Use of fresh osteochondral allografts to replace traumatic joint defects, in Citrom AA, Gross AE (eds): *Allografts in Orthopaedic Practice.* Baltimore, MD, Williams & Wilkins, 1992, p 71.)

References

1. Hopkinson WJ, Mitchell WA, Curl WW: Chondral fractures of the knee: Cause for confusion. *Am J Sports Med* 1985;13:309–312.

2. Terry GC, Flandry F, Van Manen JW, et al: Isolated chondral fractures of the knee. *Clin Orthop* 1988;234:170–177.

3. Messner K, Maletius W: The long-term prognosis for severe damage to weight-bearing cartilage in the knee: A 14-year clinical and radiographic follow-up in 28 young athletes. *Acta Orthop Scand* 1996;67:165–168.

4. Rosenberg TD, Paulos LE, Parker RD, et al: The forty-five-degree posteroanterior flexion weight-bearing radiograph of the knee. *J Bone Joint Surg* 1988;70A:1479–1483.

5. Wojtys E, Wilson M, Buckwalter K, et al: Magnetic resonance imaging of knee hyaline cartilage and intraarticular pathology. *Am J Sports Med* 1987;15:455–463.

6. Handelberg F, Shahabpour M, Casteleyn PP: Chondral lesions of the patella evaluated with computed tomography, magnetic resonance imaging, and arthroscopy. *Arthroscopy* 1990;6:24–29.

7. Karvonen RL, Negendank WG, Fraser SM, et al: Articular cartilage defects of the knee: Correlation between magnetic resonance imaging and gross pathology. *Ann Rheum Dis* 1990;49:672–675.

8. Speer KP, Spritzer CE, Goldner JL, et al: Magnetic resonance imaging of traumatic knee articular cartilage injuries. *Am J Sports Med* 1991;19:396–402.

9. Gylys-Morin VM, Hajek PC, Sartoris DJ, et al: Articular cartilage defects: Detectability in cadaver knees with MR. *Am J Roentgenol* 1987;148:1153–1157.

10. Outerbridge RE: The etiology of chondromalacia patellae. *J Bone Joint Surg* 1961;43B:752–757.

11. Install J, Falvo KA, Wise DW: Chondromalacia patellae: A prospective study. *J Bone Joint Surg* 1976;58A:1–8.

12. Goodfellow J, Hungerford DS, Woods C: Patello-femoral joint mechanics and pathology: 2. Chondromalacia patellae. *J Bone Joint Surg* 1976;58B:291–299.

13. Ficat RP, Hungerford DS (eds): *Disorders of the Patello-Femoral Joint.* Baltimore, MD, Williams & Wilkins, 1977, pp 194–243.

14. Ogilvie-Harris DJ, Jackson RW: The arthroscopic treatment of chondromalacia patellae. *J Bone Joint Surg* 1984;66B:660–665.

15. Bentley G, Dowd G: Current concepts of etiology and treatment of chondromalacia patellae. *Clin Orthop* 1984;189:209–228.

16. Johnson-Nurse C, Dandy DJ: Fracture-separation of articular cartilage in the adult knee. *J Bone Joint Surg* 1985;67B:42–43.

17. Levy AS, Lohnes J, Sculley S, et al: Chondral delamination of the knee in soccer players. *Am J Sports Med* 1996;24:634–639.

18. Dzioba RB: The classification and treatment of acute articular cartilage lesions. *Arthroscopy* 1988;4:72–80.

19. Bauer M, Jackson RW: Chondral lesions of the femoral condyles: A system of arthroscopic classification. *Arthroscopy* 1988;4:97–102.

20. Noyes FR, Stabler CL: A system for grading articular cartilage lesions at arthroscopy. *Am J Sports Med* 1989;17:505–513.

21. Mankin HJ: Localization of tritiated thymidine in articular cartilage of rabbits: II. Repair in immature cartilage. *J Bone Joint Surg* 1962:44A:688–698.

22. Mankin HJ: The reaction of articular cartilage to injury and osteoarthritis. *N Engl J Med* 1974;291:1285–1292.

23. Benefit GA, Bauer W: Further studies concerning the repair of articular cartilage in dog joints. *J Bone Joint Surg* 1935;17:141–150.

24. Bennett GA, Bauer W, Maddock SJ: A study of the repair of articular cartilage and the reaction of normal joints of adult dogs to surgically created defects of articular cartilage, "joint mice" and patellar displacement. *Am J Pathol* 1932;8:499–523.

25. Calandruccio RA, Gilmer WS Jr: Proliferation, regeneration, and repair of articular cartilage of immature animals. *J Bone Joint Surg* 1962;44A:431–455.

26. Campbell CJ: The healing of cartilage defects. *Clin Orthop* 1969;64:45–63.

27. DePalma AF, McKeever CD, Subin DK: Process of repair of articular cartilage demonstrated by histology and autoradiography with tritiated thymidine. *Clin Orthop* 1966;48:229–242.

28. Fuller JA, Ghadially FN: Ultrastructural observations on surgically produced partial–thickness defects in articular cartilage. *Clin Orthop* 1972;86:193–205.

29. Ghadially FN, Thomas I, Oryschak AF, et al: Long-term results of superficial defects in articular cartilage: A scanning electron-microscope study. *J Pathol* 1977;121:213–217.

30. Ito LK: The nutrition of articular cartilage and its method of repair. *Br J Surg* 1924;12:31–42.

31. Shands AR Jr: The regeneration of hyaline cartilage in joints: An experimental study. *Arch Surg* 1931;22:137–178.

32. Thompson RC Jr: An experimental study of surface injury to articular cartilage and enzyme responses within the joint. *Clin Orthop* 1975;107:239–248.

33. Meachim G: The effect of scarification on articular cartilage in the rabbit. *J Bone Joint Surg* 1963;45B:150–161.

34. Furukawa T, Eyre DR, Koide S, et al: Biochemical studies on repair cartilage resurfacing experimental defects in the rabbit knee. *J Bone Joint Surg* 1980;62A:79–89.

35. Mitchell N, Shepard N: Effect of patellar shaving in the rabbit. *J Orthop Res* 1987;5:388–392.

36. Kim HK, Moran ME, Salter RB: The potential for regeneration of articular cartilage in defects created by chondral shaving and subchondral abrasion: An experimental investigation in rabbits. *J Bone Joint Surg* 1991;73A:1301–1315.

37. Mitchell N, Shepard N: Healing of articular cartilage in intra-articular fractures in rabbits. *J Bone Joint Surg* 1980;62A:628–634.

38. Mankin HJ: The response of articular cartilage to mechanical injury. *J Bone Joint Surg* 1982;64A:460–466.

39. Meachim G, Roberts C: Repair of the joint surface from subarticular tissue in the rabbit knee. *J Anat* 1971;109:317–327.

40. Mitchell N, Shepard N: The resurfacing of adult rabbit articular cartilage by multiple perforations through the subchondral bone. *J Bone Joint Surg* 1976;58A:230–233.

41. Convery FR, Akeson WH, Keown GH: The repair of large osteochondral defects: An experimental study in horses. *Clin Orthop* 1972;82:253–262.

42. Salter RB, Simmonds DF, Malcolm BW, et al: The biological effect of continuous passive motion on the healing of full thickness defects in articular cartilage: An experimental investigation in the rabbit. *J Bone Joint Surg* 1980;62A:1232–1251.

43. Shapiro F, Koide S, Glimcher MJ: Cell origin and differentiation in the repair of full-thickness defects of articular cartilage. *J Bone Joint Surg* 1980;62A:1232–1251.

44. Menche DS, Frenkel SR, Blair B, et al: A comparison of abrasion burr arthroplasty and subchondral drilling in the treatment of full-thickness cartilage lesions in the rabbit. *Arthroscopy* 1996;12:280–286.

45. Tizzoni G: Sulla istologia normale e patologica delle cartilagina ialine. *Arch Sci Med Tonno* 1878;2:27–102.

46. Skoog T, Ohlsen L, Sohn SA: Perichondrial potential for cartilaginous regeneration. *Scand J Plast Reconstr Surg* 1972;6:123–125.

47. Ohlsen L: Cartilage formation from free perichondrial grafts: An experimental study in rabbits. *Br J Plast Surg* 1976;29:262–267.

48. Homminga GN, van der Linden TJ, Terwindt-Rouwenhorst EA, et al: Repair of articular defects by perichondrial grafts: Experiments in the rabbit. *Acta Orthop Scand* 1989;60:326–329.

49. Woo SL, Kwan MK, Lee TQ, et al: Perichondral autograft for articular cartilage: Shear modulus of neocartilage studied in rabbits. *Acta Orthop Scand* 1987;58:510–515.

50. Coutts RD, Amiel D, Woo SL, et al: Technical aspects of perichondrial grafting in the rabbit. *Eur Surg Res* 1984;16:322–328.

51. Bruns J, Kersten P, Lierse W, et al: Autologous rib perichondrial grafts in experimentally induced osteochondral lesions in the sheep-knee joint: Morphological results. *Virchows Arch A: Pathol Anat Histopathol* 1992;421:1–8.

52. Ham AW: A histological study of the early phases of bone repair. *J Bone Joint Surg* 1930;12:827–844.

53. Rubak JM: Reconstruction of articular cartilage defects with free periosteal grafts: An experimental study. *Acta Orthop Scand* 1982;53:175–180.

54. Grande DA, Pitman MI, Peterson L, et al: The repair of experimentally produced defects in rabbit articular cartilage by autologous chondrocyte transplantation. *J Orthop Res* 1989;7:208–218.

55. O'Driscoll SW, Salter RB: The repair of major osteochondral defects in joint surfaces by neochondrogenesis with autogenous osteoperiosteal grafts stimulated by continuous passive motion: An experimental investigation in the rabbit. *Clin Orthop* 1986;208:131–140.

56. Zarnett R, Salter RB: Periosteal neochondrogenesis for biologically resurfacing joints: Its cellular origin. *Can J Surg* 1989;32:171–174.

57. Curtin WA, Reville WJ, Brady MP: Quantitative and morphological observations on the ultrastructure of articular tissue generated from free periosteal grafts. *J Electron Microsc (Tokyo)* 1992;41:82–90.

58. Kreder HJ, Moran M, Keeley FW, et al: Biologic resurfacing of a major joint defect with cryopreserved allogeneic periosteum under the influence of continuous passive motion in a rabbit model. *Clin Orthop* 1994;300:288–296.

59. Smith AU: Survival of frozen chondrocytes isolated from cartilage of adult mammals. *Nature* 1965;205:782–784.

60. Chesterman PJ, Smith AU: Homotransplantation of articular cartilage and isolated chondrocytes: An experimental study in rabbits. *J Bone Joint Surg* 1968;50B:184–197.

61. Burmester GR, Menche D, Merryman P, et al: Application of monoclonal antibodies to the characterization of cells eluted from human articular cartilage: Expression of Ia antigens in certain diseases and identification of an 85-kD cell surface molecule accumulated in the pericellular matrix. *Arthritis Rheum* 1983;26:1187–1195.

62. Peterson L, Menche D, Grande D, et al: Chondrocyte transplantation: An experimental model in the rabbit. *Trans Orthop Res Soc* 1984;9:218.

63. Brittberg M, Nilsson A, Lindahl A, et al: Rabbit articular cartilage defects treated with autologous cultured chondrocytes. *Clin Orthop* 1996;326:270–283.

64. Dahlberg L, Kreicbergs A: Demineralized allogeneic bone martrix for cartilage repair. *J Orthop Res* 1991;9:11–19.

65. Chu CR, Coutts RD, Yoshioka M, et al: Articular cartilage repair using allogeneic perichondrocyte-seeded biodegradable porous polylactic acid (PLA): A tissue-engineering study. *J Biomed Mater Res* 1995;20:1147–1154.

66. Vacanti CA, Cima LG, Ratkowski D, et al: Tissue engineered growth of new cartilage. *Mater Res Soc Symp Proc* 1992;252:367–374.

67. Messner K, Gillquist J: Synthetic implants for the repair of osteochondral defects of the medial femoral condyle: A biomechanical and histological evaluation in the rabbit knee. *Biomaterials* 1993;14:513–521.

68. Hendrickson DA, Nixon AJ, Grande DA, et al: Chondrocyte-fibrin matrix transplants for resurfacing extensive articular cartilage defects. *J Orthop Res* 1994;12:485–497.

69. Kimura T, Yasui N, Ohsawa S, et al: Chondrocytes embedded in collagen gels maintain cartilage phenotype during long-term cultures. *Clin Orthop* 1984;186:231–239.

70. Wakitani S, Kimura T, Hirooka A, et al: Repair of rabbit articular surfaces with allograft chondrocytes embedded in collagen gel. *J Bone Joint Surg* 1989;71B:74–80.

71. Wakitani S, Ono K, Goldberg VM, et al: Repair of large cartilage defects in weight-bearing and partial weight-bearing articular surfaces with allograft articular chondrocytes embedded in collagen gels. *Trans Orthop Res Soc* 1994;19:238.

72. Yasui N, Osawa S, Ochi T, et al: Primary culture of chondrocytes embedded in collagen gels. *Exp Cell Biol* 1982;50:92–100.

73. Ben-Yishay A, Grande DA, Schwartz R, et al: Repair of articular cartilage defects with chondrocyte-collagen allograft. *Tissue Eng* 1995;1:119–133.

74. Pachence JM, Frenkel SR, Lin H: Development of a tissue analog for cartilage repair, in Cima LG, Ron ES (eds): *Tissue-Inducing Biomaterials*. Pittsburgh, PA, Materials Research Society, 1992, pp 125–130.

75. Frenkel SR, Pachence JM, Toolan BC, et al: A novel collagen bilayer matrix for articular cartilage repair. *Trans Orthop Res Soc* 1995;20:365.

76. Mankin HJ, Boyle CJ: The acute effects of lacerative injury on DNA and protein synthesis in articular cartilage, in Bassett CAL (ed): *Cartilage Degradation and Repair*. Washington, DC, National Research Council-National Academy of Sciences, National Academy of Engineering, 1967, pp 185–199.

77. Moseley JB Jr, Wray NP, Kuykendall D, et al: Arthroscopic treatment of osteoarthritis of the knee: A prospective, randomized, placebo-controlled trial. Results of a pilot study. *Am J Sports Med* 1996;24:28–34.

78. Johnson LL: Arthroscopic abrasion arthroplasty historical and pathologic perspective: Present status. *Arthroscopy* 1986;2:54–69.

79. Rand JA, Ritts GD: Abrasion arthroplasty as a salvage for failed upper tibial osteotomy. *J Arthroplasty* 1989;4(suppl):S45–S48.

80. Rand JA: Role of arthroscopy in osteoarthritis of the knee. *Arthroscopy* 1991;7:358–363.

81. Bert JM, Maschka K: The arthroscopic treatment of unicompartmental gonarthrosis: A five-year follow-up study of abrasion arthroplasty plus arthroscopic debridement and arthroscopic debridement alone. *Arthroscopy* 1989;5:25–32.

82. Aichroth PM, Patel DV, Moyes ST: A prospective review of arthroscopic debridement for degenerative joint disease of the knee. *Int Orthop* 1991;15:351–355.

83. Chandler EJ: Abrasion arthroplasty of the knee. *Contemp Orthop* 1985;11:21–29.

84. Friedman MJ, Berasi CC, Fox JM, et al: Preliminary results with abrasion arthroplasty in the osteoarthritic knee. *Clin Orthop* 1984;182:200–205.

85. Childers JC Jr, Ellwood SC: Partial chondrectomy and subchondral bone drilling for chondromalacia. *Clin Orthop* 1979;144:114–120.

86. Zorman D, Prezerowsitz L, Pasteels JL, et al: Arthroscopic treatment of posttraumatic chondromalacia patellae. *Orthopedics* 1990;13:585–588.

87. Rodrigo JJ, Steadman RJ, Silliman JF, et al: Improvement of full-thickness chondral defect healing in the human knee after debridement and microfracture using continuous passive motion. *Am J Knee Surg* 1994;7:109–116.

88. O'Driscoll SW, Keeley FW, Salter RB: Durability of regenerated articular cartilage produced by free autogenous periosteal grafts in major full-thickness defects in joint surfaces under the influence of continuous passive motion: A follow-up report at one year. *J Bone Joint Surg* 1988;70A:595–606.

89. Hoikka VE, Jaroma HJ, Ritsila VA: Reconstruction of the patellar articulation with periosteal graft. *Acta Orthop Scand* 1990;61:36–39.

90. Korkala O, Kuokkanen H: Autogenous osteoperiosteal grafts in the reconstruction of full-thickness joint surface defects. *Int Orthop* 1991;15:233–237.

91. Homminga GN, Bulstra SK, Bouwmeester PS, et al: Perichondral grafting for cartilage lesions of the knee. *J Bone Joint Surg* 1990;72B:1003–1007.

92. Cartilage Repair Registry: *Genzyme Tissue Repair.* Cambridge, MA, ABT Associates, 1997.

93. Johnson LL, Uitvlugt G, Austin MD, et al: Osteochondritis dissecans of the knee: Arthroscopic compression screw fixation. *Arthroscopy* 1990;6:179–189.

94. Radin EL, Parker HG, Pugh JW, et al: Response of joints to impact loading: III. Relationship between trabecular microfractures and cartilage degeneration. *J Biomech* 1973;6:51–57.

95. Bobic V: Arthroscopic osteochondral autograft transplantation in anterior cruciate ligament reconstruction: A preliminary clinical study. *Knee Surg Sports Traumatol Arthrosc* 1996;3:262–264.

96. McDermott AG, Langer F, Pritzker KP, et al: Fresh small-fragment osteochondral allografts: Long-term follow-up study on first 100 cases. *Clin Orthop* 1985;197:96–102.

97. Gross AE: Use of fresh osteochondral allografts to replace traumatic joint defects, in Czitrom AA, Gross AE (eds): *Allografts in Orthopaedic Practice.* Baltimore, MD, Williams & Wilkins, 1992, pp 67–82,

98. Zukor DJ, Paitich B, Oakeshott RD, et al: Reconstruction of post-traumatic articular surface defects using fresh small-fragment osteochondral allografts, in Aebi M, Regazzoni P (eds): *Bone Transplantation.* Berlin, Germany, Springer-Verlag, 1989, pp 293–305.

99. Oakeshott RD, Farine I, Pritzker KP, et al: A clinical and histologic analysis of failed fresh osteochondral allografts. *Clin Orthop* 1988;233:283–294.

100. Beaver RJ, Mahomed M, Backstein D, et al: Fresh osteochondral allografts for post-traumatic defects in the knee: A survivorship analysis. *J Bone Joint Surg* 1992;74B:105–110.

101. Zukor DJ, Oakeshott RD, Gross AE: Osteochondral allograft reconstruction of the knee: Part 2. Experience with successful and failed fresh osteochondral allografts. *Am J Knee Surg* 1989;2:182–191.

102. Ghazavi MT, Visram F, Davis AM, et al: Long term results of fresh osteochondral allografts for post traumatic osteochondral defects of the knee. *Orthop Trans* 1995;19:454.

Osteochondral Allografts
for Reconstruction of Articular Defects of the Knee

John C. Garrett, MD

Since 1972, osteochondral "minigrafts" have been used to patch full-thickness articular cartilage defects within the knee. These grafts, popularized by Gross, are typically used to patch defects 2 to 5 cm or greater in size, which have responded poorly to nonsurgical management, abrasion arthroplasty, or Pridie spongialization. Ideal cases are those in which there is a single, well-demarcated, full-thickness chondral defect in an otherwise normal knee, such as occurs in osteochondritis dissecans.[1] Select cases of fracture, specifically those of the tibial plateau or avulsion of a patellar facet, which may occur with patellar dislocation, are similarly reasonable choices. The aim is to ablate pain, buckling, and stiffness and, with a fully viable and robust graft, offset the tendency to arthritis, which otherwise might occur with less resilient replacement surfaces, such as the fibrocartilage that develops following abrasion arthroplasty.

When patching a full-thickness articular defect, the aim is to restore not only the overall congruence of the joint but also the microscopic structure of the articular cartilage. This structure is relatively complex. The surface, the lamina splendans, is responsible for gliding. It is made of a horizontally directed network of collagen with interspersed flattened chondrocytes. Beneath this veneer are arcades of collagen fibers, which arise from subchondral bone and function as "springs" in load bearing. The arcades are anchored to the subchondral bone at the tidemark and give firm fixation to the underlying skeleton. Articular segments vary in thickness and compliance as well as in the orientation of their surface rugae.

With minigrafts, the goal is long-term survival of a normal articular surface. Such success has been demonstrated histologically by Convery and associates[2] in a retrieved specimen of a fresh graft. Frozen grafts deteriorate with fissuring, delamination, fibrosis, or wholesale breakdown of the articular surface, which is unacceptable when minigrafts are used in otherwise pristine knees.

Transplantation of the articular surface is performed with an underlying segment of bone that acts as an "attachment vehicle" and secures the graft to the underlying bone. Eventually the bony segment is replaced by creeping substitution, a process that can require months to years.

Many scientists believe that, like heart valves and cornea, articular cartilage is "immunologically privileged."[3] Humoral and cell-directed antibodies are produced, but rejection is weak, presumably because antibodies are filtered by the ground substance and fail to reach their target, the chondrocyte.[4] This makes tissue typing and immunologic suppression unnecessary.[5] Similarly, transplantation of bone is associated with an immunologic response, but the reaction is slight and thought to be clinically insignificant. Zukor and associates[6] noted no indication of rejection in a series of 162 cases. A contrary view is held by some other physicians.[7]

Donors are screened with a schema delineated by the American Association of Tissue Banks.[8] Screening begins with a social history to rule out groups at high risk for human immunodeficiency virus (HIV) infection, including intravenous drug users, prostitutes, runaways, and homosexual persons. Screening continues with a medical history to rule out systemic disease, including infection, neoplasia, and arthritis. Blood is screened for types B and C hepatitis, syphilis, and HIV disease. Donor tissues are cultured for bacterial and fungal infection. Finally, autopsy with lymph node evaluation is performed (Table 1).

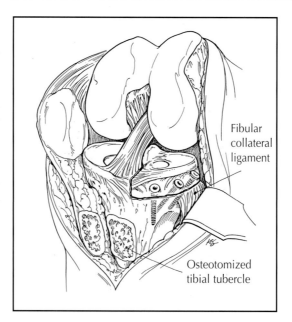

Fig. 1 Malunion after tibial plateau fracture reconstructed with an osteochondral allograft transplanted en bloc with an attached meniscus. (Reproduced with permission from Garrett JC: Osteochondral allografts for reconstruction of articular defects, in *Operative Arthroscopy*, ed 2. Philadelphia, PA, 1996, Lippincott–Raven, pp 395–403.)

It is important to match donors with recipients according to age and size. Tissue from a young donor is preferred. Donors are matched according to size as measured on anteroposterior radiographs. Discrepancies to 10% are reasonable. Isotopic transplantation with articular cartilage of similar contour, depth, and compliance is appealing, but subtleties in the transplantation process abound, especially in osteochondritis dissecans, in which the defective condyle often is enlarged and misshapen. Occasionally, a heterotopic graft that better matches the recipient site represents the best compromise.

After donor life support systems are terminated, the kidneys, heart, and lungs are removed; then orthopaedic grafts are obtained. Procedures are performed under sterile conditions, preferably within 12 hours of death. Specimens are pre-served in a tissue culture solution, containing antibiotics, at 4°C until transplantation, which is performed within 5 days.

Surgical Procedure
Tibial Plateau
Transplantation of the tibial plateau and adjoining meniscus may be indicated for severe malunion after fracture. The ideal case is an isolated tibial plateau fracture. Damage to the femoral condyles or rupture of the cruciate or collateral ligaments may compromise results. In my experience, the cases that have the best chance for success are those that are depressed 1 cm or less. Greater depression or devitalization of large segments of the proximal tibia as a result of the injury, surgery, bone grafting, or fibrous union may undermine the base of support and require extremely thick grafts, leaving patients at risk for significant collapse.

The lateral plateau is the one more commonly transplanted, and it may be approached through a lateral parapatellar incision. Osteotomy of the tibial tubercle permits medial reflection of the patella for exposure. External tibial guides used in total knee replacement are useful for resection of the tibia, which is cut parallel to the articular surface at the depth at which viable cancellous bone is encountered. The medial extent of the resection is the lateral margin of the anterior cruciate ligament. Fixation is achieved with the use of multiple 4.0-mm AO cancellous screws driven obliquely through the corner of the graft into the proximal tibia. Three or four screws are used in order to afford solid fixation and allow early range of motion (Fig. 1).

Femoral Condyles
Defects of the femoral condyles worthy of allograft transplantation are typically those greater than 2 cm in diameter. Such lesions are common in osteochondritis dissecans and in select cases of trauma. Although many surgeons customize grafts and use a "press-fit" technique of implantation,[9] lesions up to 3.0 cm in diameter can be replaced easily using commercially available instruments (Fig. 2).

With standard lesions the aim is to drill a cylindrical hole and to remove all fibrous tissue and sclerotic bone in order to leave a biologically viable bed. The defect is replaced with a plug of bone and articular cartilage of similar dimensions. The orientation of the axis of the cylin-

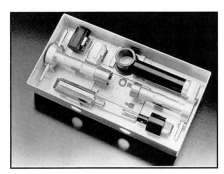

Fig. 2 Instruments designed by the Linvatec Corporation for use with osteochondral transplantation for defects from 2 to 3 cm in diameter. (Reproduced with permission from Garrett JC: Osteochondral allografts for reconstruction of articular defects, in *Operative Arthroscopy*, ed 2. Philadelphia, PA, 1996, Lippincott–Raven, pp 395–403.)

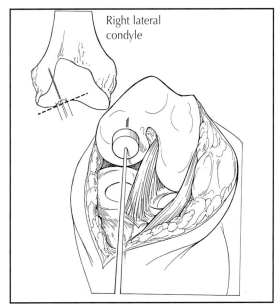

Fig. 3 Cylindrical guide placed over the defect to guide insertion of a Kirschner wire perpendicular to the surface of the defect. (Reproduced with permission from Garrett JC: Osteochondral allografts for reconstruction of articular defects, in *Operative Arthroscopy*, ed 2. Philadelphia, PA, 1996, Lippincott–Raven, pp 395–403.)

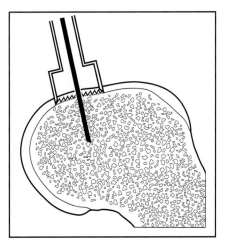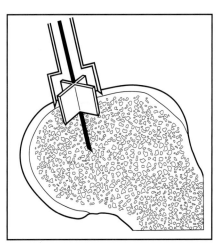

Fig. 4 Devices used to prepare the recipient graft site. **Left**, Hand–driven device used to cut the articular cartilage. **Right**, Power-driven device used to cut the subchondral bone. (Reproduced with permission from Garrett JC: Osteochondral allografts for reconstruction of articular defects, in *Operative Arthroscopy*, ed 2. Philadelphia, PA, 1996, Lippincott–Raven, pp 395–403.)

drical hole is matched with that of the donor plug by placing a cylindrical guide over the defect. A guide wire is driven through the guide into the center of the defect (Fig. 3). A hand-powered device is used to cut sharply through the articular cartilage (Fig. 4). The bony base is penetrated with an auger until normal trabeculae and punctate hemorrhage, both indicative of viable bone, appear. The resulting defect is usually 4 to 5 mm deep.

The defect is matched with the corresponding portion of the donor femoral condyle (Fig. 5). In some cases of osteochondritis dissecans distortion of the recipient femur creates disparity between the size of donor and recipient condyles and necessitates the use of a heterotopic donor site. A segment of the donor femur including the specific portion to be used in the transplant is removed and steadied in a jig (Fig. 5). Proper orientation to the articular surface is established with the use of a second cylindrical guide. In order to minimize shear between the articular cartilage and the underlying bone, the articular surface is first cut with a hand-powered instrument. A plug cutter is then used to cut the subchondral bone. The result is a composite, cylindrical specimen of articular cartilage and under-

lying bone (Fig. 5).

The donor plug is matched with the defect according to depth (Fig. 6). Typically, the plug is 5 to 6 mm in height. Often it is inserted several times in order to evaluate the fit. If the graft is proud, the bone at the base of the plug can be shaved with an oscillating saw. If excess bone has been removed, height can be regained by packing bone shavings

beneath the graft. The graft is secured with 4-mm Acumed screws, which afford excellent fixation and compression yet are more easily removed arthroscopically than Herbert screws. In my experience, resorbable pins yield inadequate fixation and compression. Invariably there is a 1 or 2 mm difference between one segment of the graft and the surrounding femoral condyle. This differ-

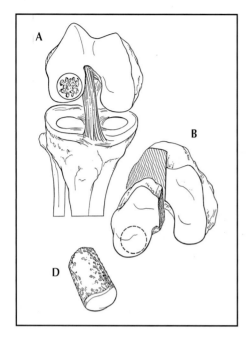

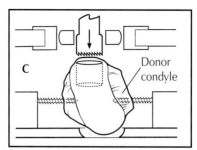

Fig. 5 A, Defect in the recipient condyle. **B,** Defect matched to donor condyle. **C,** Transplant condyle in jig, oriented to articular surface. Hand–powered cutter. **D,** Cylindrical graft of articular cartilage and underlying bone. (Reproduced with permission from Garrett JC: Osteochondral allografts for reconstruction of articular defects, in *Operative Arthroscopy*, ed 2. Philadelphia, PA, 1996, Lippincott–Raven, pp 395–403.)

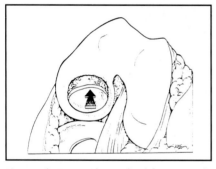

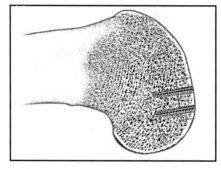

Fig. 6 Left, Donor plug graft. **Right,** Acumed screw placement. (Reproduced with permission from Garrett JC: Osteochondral allografts for reconstruction of articular defects, in *Operative Arthroscopy*, ed 2. Philadelphia, PA, 1996, Lippincott–Raven, pp 395–403.)

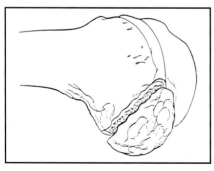

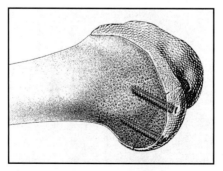

Fig. 7 With large lesions of the posterior aspect of the lateral femoral condyle full width segment grafts may be required. (Reproduced with permission from Garrett JC: Osteochondral allografts for reconstruction of articular defects, in *Operative Arthroscopy*, ed 2. Philadelphia, PA, 1996, Lippincott–Raven, pp 395–403.)

ence can be minimized with the compressive effect of the screws, which effectively warp a thin graft and depress an otherwise proud edge. The screws are countersunk sufficiently to permit early range of motion without compromising later removal (Fig. 6).

For lesions of greater dimensions, especially giant lesions of osteochondritis dissecans of the far posterior aspect of the lateral femoral condyle, custom-designed, full-width segments of a condyle may be required (Fig. 7).

Patella

Large defects in the medial facet of the patella can occur as the result of patellar dislocation. If the extensor mechanism alignment is reasonable or easily corrected, articular defects can be reconstructed with the use of osteochondral allografts. The knee is approached via a medial parapatellar arthrotomy. The patella is everted and the articular defect replaced using commercially available instruments or, more commonly, by removing the medial facet with a sagittal cut through the keel of the patella and a second perpendicular cut through the subchondral bone (Fig. 8). The matched portion of the graft is inserted and fixed with 4-mm Acumed screws, which are driven through the articular surface into the cortical bone and deeply countersunk.

Adjunct Procedures

In some cases, osteochondral grafts may be exposed to adverse compression forces because of malalignment. Minimal degrees of excess varus or valgus may be tolerated, but when angulation deviates greater than 10° from normal, osteotomy should be considered. In order to maximize vascularity of the recipient bone, Beaver and Gross[10] suggest that femoral osteotomy be performed when the lesion is in the tibia and vice versa. However, the goal of finishing with a horizontal joint surface often necessitates osteotomy of the femur in cases of valgus and of the tibia in cases of varus irrespective of the site grafted.

Rehabilitation

Range-of-motion exercises are begun immediately following surgery. The aim is proper nutrition of the articular cartilage as well as restoration of a normal arc of motion. Weightbearing is avoided until there is union between graft and host, which usually is achieved by 6 weeks with small plug grafts and by 4 months with grafts of the tibial plateau. With patellar resurfacing, weightbearing is permitted, but vigorous resisted exercise is withheld for 2 months to prevent the graft from being dislodged by excessive shear forces.

Results

For long-term survival, the bony portion of a graft must heal to the recipient bed and then revascularize without crumbling or collapsing.[11] Subsidence of 1 to 3 mm has been noted in up to 70% of tibial plateau grafts.[12] The chondrocytes of the cartilaginous cap must remain viable and continue to produce glycoproteins and collagen, thus assuring maintenance of the microarchitecture of the articular surface. Chondrocyte viability has been assessed with $^{35}SO_4$ and ^3H-cytidine autoradiography. The percentage of viable chondrocytes ranged from 69% to 99% in three grafts studied at 12, 24, and 41 months. Even when failure occurred, 66% of the failed grafts had viable chondrocytes.[13] Grafts that replace either the femur or tibia alone have a much higher survival rate than do those in which both surfaces are replaced (70% versus 25% at 10 years).[10,14]

The fit of a graft transplanted into a condyle is easy to appreciate visually but difficult to quantify precisely. Creating flush margins minimizes abrasive wear, cutting, ploughing, and filing. Restoring normal congruence of the femoral condyle with material of similar stiffness optimizes weightbearing characteristics.

Realigning the microscopic rugae of the graft with those of the recipient femoral condyle enhances gliding. Grafts undoubtedly work best in compartments blessed with a meniscus and a normal opposing articular surface. When necessary, menisci can be transplanted concomitantly with osteochondral allografts.

Gross malalignment, which might adversely affect the graft, should be corrected with osteotomy. Grafts buried within a femoral condyle are protected by the surrounding rim of the condyle. If collapse begins, the majority of the force is subsequently applied to the surrounding condyle, thereby minimizing collapse and avoiding the development of angulation. In contrast, collapse of a graft that does not have a surrounding protective collar, as in the case of a tibial plateau, can lead to adverse angulation, which increases forces on the graft, thereby accelerating collapse.

Success with osteochondral allografts is measured clinically in terms of elimination of pain, swelling, and buckling; radiographically in terms of bony healing and maintenance of joint space and congruence; and arthroscopically in terms of a normal articular surface as visualized and probed (Fig. 9). Today, osteochondral allografts are used in the United States, Canada, and Europe. With isolated lesions, Meyers and associates[15] reported a 77.5% success rate at 2 to 10 years. In a similar series, the team working with Gross reported a 72% success rate at 14 years.[10,16] With transplants of the tibial plateau followed up for longer than 2 years, Gross reported less than 3 mm collapse and clinical improvement in ten of 12 cases. In an expanded series, 21 of 28 cases were noted to be a success and the benefit of osteotomy to correct alignment was noted.[6] I have noted similar favorable outcomes in allograft surgery of large articular defects in cases of osteochondritis dissecans in which osteochondral fragments have been removed. In an expanded series, success, as measured by healing

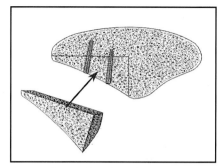

Fig. 8 Technique for allograft replacement of a patella facet. (Reproduced with permission from Garrett JC: Osteochondral allografts for reconstruction of articular defects, in *Operative Arthroscopy*, ed 2. Philadelphia, PA, 1996, Lippincott-Raven, pp 395–403.)

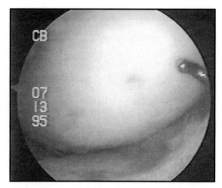

Fig. 9 Osteochondral allograft medial femoral condyle 1 year postoperative.

of the transplant with resolution of pain and swelling, was noted with 16 of 17 grafts of the lateral femoral condyle and 48 of 53 grafts of the medial femoral condyle.[17] With patellar grafts alone, Convery and associates[14] noted success in three of four grafts. Grafts of both the patella and trochlea yielded success in five of eight cases.

Conclusion

Osteochondral "minigrafts" can be used to patch full-thickness articular defects resulting from trauma and osteochondritis dissecans. Ideal cases are those in which there is a single, well-demarcated, full-thickness defect that is 2 to 5 cm in diameter.

References

1. Garrett JC: Osteochondritis dissecans. *Clin Sports Med* 1991;10:569–593.

2. Convery FR, Akeson WH, Amiel D, et al: Long-term survival of chondrocytes in an osteochondral articular cartilage allograft. *J Bone Joint Surg* 1996;78A:1082–1088.

3. Langer F, Gross AE: Immunogenicity of allograft articular cartilage. *J Bone Joint Surg* 1974;56A:297–304.

4. Elves MW: Newer knowledge of the immunology of bone and cartilage. *Clin Orthop* 1976;120:232–259.

5. Langer F, Czitrom A, Pritzker KP, et al: The immunogenicity of fresh and frozen allogeneic bone. *J Bone Joint Surg* 1975;57A:216–220.

6. Zukor DJ, Oakeshott RD, Gross AE: Osteochondral allograft reconstruction of the knee: Part 2. Experience with successful and failed fresh osteochondral allografts. *Am J Knee Surg* 1989;2:182–191.

7. Rodrigo JJ, Schnaser AM, Reynolds HM Jr, et al: Inhibition of the immune response to experimental fresh osteoarticular allografts. *Clin Orthop* 1989;243:235–253.

8. *Standards for Tissue Banking.* McLean, VA, American Association of Tissue Banks, 1993.

9. Convery FR, Meyers MH, Akeson WH: Fresh osteochondral allografting of the femoral condyle. *Clin Orthop* 1991;273:139–145.

10. Beaver RJ, Gross AE: Fresh small-fragment osteochondral allografts in the knee joint, in Aichroth PM, Cannon WD Jr (eds): *Knee Surgery: Current Practice.* London, England, Martin Dunitz, 1992, pp 464–471.

11. McDermott AGP, Langer F, Pritzker KPH, et al: Fresh small-fragment osteochondral allografts: Long-term follow-up study on first 100 cases. *Clin Orthop* 1985;197:96–102.

12. Locht RC, Gross AE, Langer F: Late osteochondral allograft resurfacing for tibial plateau fractures. *J Bone Joint Surg* 1984;66A:328–335.

13. Czitrom AA, Keathing S, Gross AE: The viability of articular cartilage in fresh osteochondral allografts after clinical transplantation. *J Bone Joint Surg* 1990;72A:574–581.

14. Convery FR, Botte MJ, Akeson WH, et al: Chondral defects of the knee. *Contemp Orthop* 1994;28:100–107.

15. Meyers MH, Akeson W, Convery FR: Resurfacing of the knee with fresh osteochondral allograft. *J Bone Joint Surg* 1989;71A:704–713.

16. Beaver RJ, Mahomed M, Backstein D, et al: Fresh osteochondral allografts for post–traumatic defects in the knee: A survivorship analysis. *J Bone Joint Surg* 1992;74B:105–110.

17. Garrett JC: Osteochondral allografts, in Heckman JD (ed): *Instructional Course Lectures 42.* Rosemont, IL, American Academy of Orthopaedic Surgeons, 1993, pp 355–358.

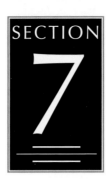

SECTION 7

Bone Grafting

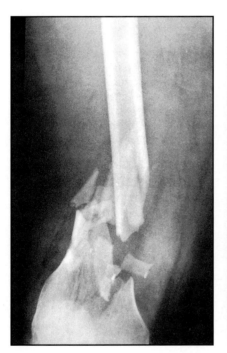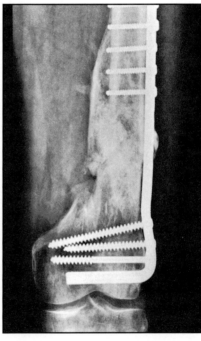

57 Bone Grafting and New Composite Biosynthetic Graft Materials

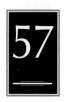

Bone Grafting and
New Composite Biosynthetic Graft Materials

Joseph M. Lane, MD
Mathias P.G. Bostrom, MD

Over the last decade, the desire to incorporate the favorable properties of different materials into an effective bone graft compound has led to the manipulation and development of a number of new synthetic bone grafting products. These composite grafts can be defined as combinations of osteoconductive matrices, osteogenic cells, and/or osteoinductive materials. In discussing their efficacy as alternatives to autogenous or allogeneic bone grafts, the various components of these new grafts will be described, and practical experience both in animals and in humans will be reported.

Autogenous Bone Graft

Bone grafting is commonly used to augment bone healing throughout a broad spectrum of orthopaedic musculoskeletal disorders. Bone grafts have been used to reconstruct or replace skeletal defects, augment fracture repair, and stimulate arthrodeses following oncologic surgery, trauma, growth defects, and arthritis. Over many years of experience, autologous cancellous bone grafting has represented the "gold standard" for grafting.

The ideal bone graft or bone graft substitute should provide three elements: (1) an osteoconductive matrix to provide a scaffolding amenable to bone ingrowth; (2) osteoinductive factors to provide chemical or physical components that induce the various stages of the bone

repair process; and (3) osteogenic cells that will differentiate to carry forth the various stages of bone regeneration. Autogenous cancellous bone graft, the "gold standard," contains all three of these components: (1) hydroxyapatite and collagen, which are well suited to serve as an osteoconductive framework; (2) numerous stromal cells within the cavity lining, which have osteogenic potential; and (3) cancellous bone and the adjacent hematoma, which contain a family of growth factors, most notably bone morphogenetic proteins (BMP) and transforming growth factor-β (TGF-β), which have the ability to induce the regenerative processes as well as to augment the process. While autogenous cancellous bone grafts have all these of these elements, in autogenous cortical bone these elements are present to a more limited extent. Fewer than 5% of cortical bone cells survive grafting. The advantage of cortical grafts, however, is that their structure confers compressive strength, thus providing mechanical support. In addition to the osteoinductive, osteoconductive, and osteogenic properties of these autogenous grafts, they are histocompatible, do not transport disease, and retain viable osteoblasts that participate in the formation of bone.

Although autogenous bone grafting is effective, it is associated with several shortcomings and potential complica-

tions. Its disadvantages are that a limited quantity of bone is available for harvest and that there is significant donor site morbidity, with rates as high as 25% including donor site infections and pain, increased anesthesia time, and significantly increased blood loss.[1]

The bone regeneration that is initiated with autogenous cancellous bone occurs in three major steps.[2-5] First the undifferentiated osteoprogenitor cells are recruited, both from the host bed and from the living cells within the autograft bone marrow cavity. Then, by osteoinduction these cells differentiate to give rise to osteoblasts and chondrocytes. Finally, a simple scaffolding is established upon which active osteoprogenitor cells can produce new bone. Bony continuity is achieved across the desired space, and the new bone is remodeled along the lines of stress according to the rules of Wolf.

Osteoinduction is mediated by numerous growth factors provided by bone matrix itself. Most notable of these are the BMPs, low molecular weight proteins that initiate endochondral bone formation, presumably by stimulating local progenitor cells of osteoblast lineage and by enhancing bone collagen synthesis. BMP is produced by the differentiating stem cells. TGF-β, closely related to BMPs by sequence of homology, is present in the graft hematoma after release by the platelets, and is further synthesized by the mesenchymal cells. TGF-β stimulates cell proliferation and matrix formation. Other growth factors present during the grafting process include fibroblast growth factors (FGF), which are angiogenic factors that promote neo-vascularization and wound healing, and platelet-derived growth factor (PDGF), which acts as a local tissue-growth regulator. PDGF was initially isolated in blood platelets, underscoring one of the important roles of the clot after a fracture, but recently other tissues, including bone, seem to synthesize it as well. Insulin-like growth factors and micro-globulin-β are examples of other bone matrix synthesizing growth factors important in bone healing.

Cancellous bone initially has little structural integrity, but this weakness changes rapidly secondary to bone augmentation and union with preexisting osteostructures. Bone strength increases as bone mass accumulates and the construct is remodeled along the line of stress. The converse occurs with cortical bone. It initially conveys structural strength to the graft as it undergoes osteointegration across the bone gap. It then undergoes a remodeling phase in which nonviable bone is removed by osteoclastic tunneling and resorption. During the resorptive phase, which continues for 18 months in dogs and presumably longer in humans, the bone strut loses approximately one third of its strength before enhanced strength recurs. Cortical bone graft retains significant islands of nonreplaced, nonviable bone throughout the life of the individual.

Free vascularized cortical grafts most commonly involve the fibula, although other bones, such as the ribs and the iliac crest, have been used for this purpose.[4,6–11] Because the bone does not undergo significant cell necrosis, but remains viable through its arterial and venous anastomoses, some of the problems associated with nonvascularized cortical bone are avoided. Biomechanical

studies have demonstrated that it is superior to nonvascularized cortical graft for approximately 6 months, after which time no difference can be demonstrated in terms of torque, bending, and tension strength. The disadvantages of vascularized graft include donor site morbidity, which is minor in most cases, increased surgical time, and greater utilization of resources. It is clearly superior to nonvascularized cortical bone graft when the bridging defect is over 12 cm.[4] Reported stress fracture rates for this distance in nonvascularized cortical bone exceed 50%; the rate of fracture for vascularized grafts is less than 25%.[4] In addition, vascularized grafts have a greater ability to heal stress-related fractures and to increase the girth of the grafted area than does nonvascularized cortical bone.

Allografts

Sterilely harvested allografts are available as fresh, frozen, and freeze-dried. With fresh allografts no preservation is required; however, the limited time by which the grafting transfer must be performed provides a short period to test for donor disease. In addition, in clear contradistinction to autografts, fresh allografts induce an intense immune response. Thus fresh allografts currently are not a mainstay in grafting. Their applications are limited to joint resurfacing, in which success reflects maintenance of viable transplanted chondrocytes.

The majority of allografts today are either frozen or freeze-dried. Frozen allografts are maintained at temperatures below –60°C to diminish degradation by enzymes and to afford decreased immunogenicity without altering their biomechanical properties. Osteochondral allografts undergo a much more controlled slow freeze that includes use of a cyropreservative, for the cartilage, in the form of glycerol or dimethylsulfoxide so as to prevent ice crystal formation within cells. There is controversy regarding the viability of the cartilage, and studies have

demonstrated values ranging from 20% to 70% viability using these preservation techniques.[12,13] Freeze-drying involves removal of tissue water from the frozen tissue, after which the tissues are vacuum-packed and can be stored at room temperature for as long as 5 years. These allografts have a further decrease in antigenicity, almost no biochemical changes, and no changes in limited osteoconductive properties. Freeze-dried grafts, however, do undergo biomechanical alteration, with loss of hoop strength and compressive strength upon rehydration. In all these techniques, while the osteoprogenitor cells are destroyed, the osteoconductive properties are largely retained in terms of the cancellous and cortical structure. Furthermore, the deeply bound, limited osteoinductive material present in the graft may be only partially retained.

Allografts can be used for nonstructural purposes, such as reconstructing defects after curettage of a benign neoplasm and periarticular bone cysts. In addition, osteolytic cavities at time of joint arthroplasty revision can be filled with allograft. Morcellized cancellous and cortical chips can be used for these purposes. Some clinicians recommend mixing allograft bone with autogenous tissue to enhance osteoinduction and/or mixing it with bone marrow to reintroduce osteoprogenitor cells. Data as to the efficacy of this process are not available.

In terms of their structural roles, allografts can be used as an intercalary segment to reconstruct a diaphyseal defect of long bone. Large segments can be modeled to replace acetabular, femoral, and tibia defects during arthroplasty, and allografts can be implemented to facilitate arthodesis about the ankle, hip, and spine. Osteochondral allografts have also been used for the dual purposes of replacing resected bone and providing a biologic joint surface.[14,15]

The various allograft structures available include ilial bicortical and tricortical strips, patellae, cancellous cortical dowels, fibular shafts and wedges, femoral cross-sections, and ribs. Large frozen bone segments include whole or partial tibia, humerus, femur, talus, acetabulum, ilium, and hemipelvis. Complications of large allografts, when used structurally, include nonunion (10%), fractures (5% to 15%), and infection (10% to 15%).[16-19] Morcelized allograft lacks the osteoinduction and osteoprogenitor cells of autologous bone graft and has been used largely as a filler or extender of autogenous graft. In individuals, such as children, who have a very high potential for bone regeneration, allografts can be used without autologous augmentation.

One of the main concerns of allograft bone is the transmission of infection, most notably hepatitis or AIDS. Since 1976, most of the tissue banks in the United States are members of the American Association of Tissue Banks (AATB), which evaluates member banks for compliance with a comprehensive set of standards. Strict donor screening and tissue testing techniques have significantly lowered the risk of disease transmission. AATB records indicate that of three million tissue transplants, only two donors' tissues have been linked with documented transmission of AIDS virus. Both cases involved transplantation of unprocessed, fresh-frozen allografts. On December 14, 1993, the FDA mandated that every national tissue bank comply with governmental regulations that essentially parallel the AATB's comprehensive screening program. These regulations include donor screening, repeated infectious disease testing, labeling requirements, long-term tracking of the graft, and inspections of such facilities. Although local in-hospital bone banks may have difficulty in fulfilling these obligations, they now are required by law to comply. The risk of HIV infection from allografts is calculated at less than one per million if all these steps are performed.[20]

Sterilization of allografts compromises the tissue. Ethylene oxide and radiation alter some of the structural properties as well as the biochemical properties of the graft. In the one well-documented incidence of a donor with AIDS, which occurred in 1985, grafts from this individual that were lyophilized and irradiated did not give rise to AIDS; fresh frozen grafts from the same source gave rise to AIDS. Thus, there is a suggestion that processing may destroy the AIDS virus. In addition, testing for transmissible diseases has improved substantially. Most investigators to date have dealt largely with intact or large segmental allografts. Little is known about the effect of partial demineralization, surface alteration, and choice of appropriate particle size to enhance the grafting potential.

Demineralized Bone Matrix

Demineralized bone matrix (DBM), which represents the other extreme of processing attempts to completely remove the mineral phase of bone. DBM is produced by acid extraction of bone, leaving noncollagenous proteins, bone growth factors, and collagen. Demineralized materials have no structural strength, but they have enhanced osteoinductive capability, afforded most notably by BMP. DBM is currently prepared by bone banks and is pathogen free by virtue of donor selection. DBM has been used in clinical maneuvers to promote bone group regeneration, mainly in well-supported, stable skeletal defects. Excellent results from clinical trials have been reported. Despite the enhanced osteoinductive potential, the actual functionally accessible BMP within these demineralized grafts is exponentially lower than that used in recombinant BMP studies.

The actual amounts of BMP available from the various graft preparations have not been determined by the banks. Some commercially available DBM preparation could not induce bone in the Urist bio-

logic mouse muscle test. All the DBMs are easy to mold intraoperatively; however, they do not provide intrinsic strength. The clinical applications of DBMs include augmentation of traditional autogenous bone grafts in repairing cysts, fractures, nonunions, and stable fusions.

At this time the FDA requires sterilization of the DBM as prepared by bone banks, and this sterilization may decrease the viability of some of the available BMP. DBM does afford the potential of enhanced osteoinduction, and to date it has been used as an adjunct to more traditional grafting materials. When successful in achieving union, DBM develops bone with mechanical strength comparable to that of autograft. DBM is currently available freeze-dried and processed from cortical/cancellous bone in the form of powder, chips, or as a gel.

Some of the DBM is processed from human bone by a patented technique that incorporates a permeation treatment that does not expose tissue to ethylene oxide or gamma radiation, thus possibly protecting larger amounts of native BMP. It is processed into a gel consistency and is packaged in a syringe, from which it can be applied directly intraoperatively. It has no structural strength, and has been most successfully used in conjunction with internal fixation or as an adjunct of other grafting materials. Two additional types of gel formulation are available. One is in the form of a collagen mat that retains the noncollagenous proteins; the other is a woven collagen mass that has the appearance of steel wool.

Bone Marrow

The osteogenic capabilities of bone marrow have been well known since it was first observed in 1869 by Boujon, as reported by Burwell[21] and Burwell and associates.[22] Bone marrow contains osteoprogenitor cells on the order of 1 per 50,000 nucleated cells in the young to 1/2,000,000 in the elderly, and certain concentration techniques have increased that number fivefold.[23] Burwell, Salama, and Weismann all have used bone marrow, either by itself or in combination with an inorganic matrix, for clinical application.[21-26] Bone marrow, when grown in porous ceramic, can bring osteoprogenitor cells to a deficient grafting bed.[27] Werntz and associates[28] used a rat model of a femoral segmental defect to test the hypothesis that autogenous marrow has the osteogenic capability to heal a bone defect. Following bone marrow implantation, woven bone was produced initially, and this progressed to early lamellar bone and subsequently molded in a volumetric fashion. The bone marrow, when placed in a fresh femoral defect and given in sufficient amounts, produced a rate of union comparable to that of autogenous bone graft. The bone formed by marrow demonstrated biomechanical properties comparable to those of a cancellous bone graft. Significant bone formation occurred when the marrow was injected percutaneously into femoral nonunions. These studies as well as those by other investigators indicate that bone marrow can lead to structurally competent bone regeneration in an orthotopic location.

Clinically, Connolly and associates[29-31] have demonstrated that bone marrow can be used to treat nonunions in patients when provided in adequate amounts. Bone marrow should be harvested in aliquots of approximately 2.5 ml per site. If gathered in larger amounts, the marrow would be diluted with blood. The marrow should be used immediately to maintain its viability. Although it has had only limited reported clinical use, bone marrow offers the ability to augment all the synthetic grafts and allografts that are currently used as well as to reestablish a more normal fracture hematoma following extensive irrigation. There is essentially no morbidity from obtaining bone marrow. It is desirable if the osteoprogenitor cells could be easily increased in number and in concentration so as to

allow a smaller volume of stem cells to be used clinically. Bruder and associates[32] have isolated bone marrow and grown it under special culture conditions to specifically expand mesenchymal stem cells. These cells, when given in an appropriate composite mixture including ceramics and collagens, have been able to heal osseous defects in a series of animal models. Although they are still in preclinical trials at this time, these techniques offer further opportunities for the use of an expanded marrow stem cell population.

Biosynthetic Graft Materials
Ceramics
Ceramics have been used solely as osteoconductive bone graft matrices. Most calcium phosphate ceramics currently under investigation are synthetic, composed of hydroxyapatite, tricalcium phosphate, or a combination of the two. These biomaterials are commercially being produced as porous implants, nonporous dense implants, or granular particles with pores. Most calcium phosphate ceramics are created using a high-temperature process, called sintering, along with high-pressure compaction techniques. Another form of ceramics, replamineform, is produced from marine coral specimens using hydrothermal exchange methods that replace the original calcium carbonate of the coral with a calcium phosphate replicate. In contrast to the random pore structure created in totally synthetic porous materials, the pore structure of the coralline calcium phosphate implants is highly organized, and is similar to that of human cancellous bone.

Cancellous bone itself has a complex trabecular pattern in which approximately 20% of the total matrix is bone and the remaining area is marrow space interconnected through pores. Synthetic ceramics have pores of various sizes, but lack pore interconnectivity. Therefore, when used as graft material, the ingrowing osteo-

genic process must resorb the synthetic ceramic to gain access to the interior pores. The exceptions are ceramics derived from materials such as coral that have biologic pore interconnectivity mesh networks. There are some new materials currently under development in which a collagen matrix mesh network is initially established, and is then lightly covered with a carbonate-enriched hydroxyapatite ceramic so that the pores remain interconnected.

The chemical composition of ceramic profoundly affects its rate of bioresorption. Tricalcium phosphate (TCP) undergoes biologic resorption 10 to 20 times faster than hydroxyapatite. In some clinical trials, TCP has been reported to have been totally resorbed, but in most others it persists for years. Once in the body, TCP is in part converted chemically to hydroxyapatite, which is degraded slowly. The resorbing cell for hydroxyapatite is the foreign body giant cell and not the osteoclast. It resorbs 2 to 10 mm of hydroxyapatite and then ceases further resorption. Consequently, segments of hydroxyapatite ceramic will remain in place in the body for periods of as long as 7 to 10 years. In clinical applications, TCP remodels more readily due to its porosity, but it is weaker. It provides significantly less compressive strength than hydroxyapatite. The combination of the two is used clinically to offer both advantages. Material factors, such as surface area, affect the biologic degradation and, in general, the larger the surface area the greater the bioresorption. Dense ceramic blocks with small surface areas biodegrade slowly, compared with porous implants. Thus, the shape and architecture of the ceramic have a profound effect on resorption rates.

The ceramics are brittle and have very little tensile strength. Use of ceramics in applications that require significant torsion, bending, or shear stress seems impracticable at present. However, mechanical properties of porous calcium phosphate materials are comparable to cancellous bone once they have been incorporated and remodeled. Ceramics must be shielded from loading forces until bony ingrowth has occurred. Rigid stabilization of surrounding bone and nonweightbearing are required during this period because the ceramics can tolerate minimal bending and torque load before failing unless used in sites of relatively low mechanical stress or when forces are basically compressive.

The optimal osteoconductive pore size for ceramics appears to be between 150 and 500 μm. Ceramics appear to have no early adverse effects, such as inflammation, and foreign body responses to ceramics are practically nonexistent when the ceramics are in a structural block arrangement. However, small granules of material have been shown to elicit a foreign body giant cell reaction. When ceramics are used, the radiographic findings demonstrate a continued presence of the ceramic for a prolonged period of time due to the failure of complete remodeling. Persistent dense radiographic imagery makes it difficult to determine the degree of bony growth and incorporation into the implant. Tricalcium phosphate, which is more biodegradable, loses more of its radiodensity and appears to be more fully incorporated into the bone.

The replamineform ceramics are a porous hydroxyapatite material derived from the calcium carbonate skeletal structure of sea coral. The pore size of these is determined by the genus of coral used. The coral genus *Gonipora* exhibits a microstructure similar to that of human cancellous bone. The coralline hydroxyapatite derived from *Gonipora* has large pores measuring from 500 to 600 μm in diameter with interconnections of 220 to 260 μm. The coral genus *Porites* has a microstructure that appears similar to that of interstitial cortical bone, with a smaller pore diameter of 200 to 250 μm, parallel channels interconnected by 190 μm fenestrations, and a porosity of 66%.

A porous ceramic consisting solely of tricalcium phosphate is available. It has a 36% porosity and contains a uniform distribution of large interconnecting pores ranging from 100 to 300 μm in size. The initial compressive and tensile strength have been shown to decrease by 30% to 40% after 4 months in situ.

A ceramic that forms in vivo has been created. This ceramic has a high carbonate substitution within the hydroxyapatite.[33] When injected or placed in a bony cavity it creates a very firm ceramic mass within hours, and most of its compressive strength is achieved within 24 hours. There is little control, however, over the porosity of this material. There is some demonstration that extraosseous forms can be resorbed. However, within bony cavities this low-porosity ceramic remains stable for long periods of time due to its high density. This injectable ceramic is under clinical trial for use in metaphyseal fractures.

Other forms of calcium products have been used in the past, most notably calcium sulfate or plaster of Paris. This material, which solidifies within the site, has been used clinically for more than 30 years.[34] It has a very rapid turnover; most of it is resorbed within weeks to months. New forms of commercially available calcium sulfate are currently being introduced to the market.

Experimental animal studies have consistently indicated superior performance of autologous bone graft when compared to ceramic implants alone. However, some studies have yielded promising results when certain specific conditions are met. In canine proximal tibial defects, coralline hydroxyapatite fares quite favorably as compared to cortical cancellous autogenous graft.[35–37] Clinically, the first successful results with ceramics were reported by dentistry and reconstructive craniofacial surgery. In orthopaedics, Bucholz and associates[38] have demonstrated a similar efficacy of coralline hydroxyapatite ceramics and

autogenous grafts for certain applications, particularly tibial plateau fractures that are under compression. In a random trial using coralline hydroxyapatite versus cancellous bone in the tibia, they reported no differences in functional outcome. Histologic analysis of the newly formed bone at the time of hardware removal revealed bony growth into and around the ceramic with both cortical and cancellous bone in appropriate locations. Bucholz has also studied tricalcium phosphate and found it comparable to autogenous bone for filling defects secondary to trauma and benign tumors. Because of their brittle nature, when they are placed in a structural position, such as anterior vertebral body fusions, the ceramics must be protected by the orthopaedic implant fixation or they can shatter.

An advantageous property of ceramics is that, when used as filling to restore volume in cavities, the osteoconductive hydroxyapatite bonds well to bone. Bone ceramics alone lack osteoinductive property. However, there is some suggestion that hydroxyapatite has sufficient affinity for the local growth factors that promote regeneration. Coralline hydroxyapatite, when placed in a muscle pouch, will in fact demonstrate onlay bone growth. Nakahara and associates[27] have indicated in animal studies that ceramics can be filled with bone marrow prior to use, and that bone marrow grows well within the ceramics and results in a composite. Bruder and associates[32] have also demonstrated that, when used in animal models, the mesenchymal stem cells work best when used in conjunction with ceramic hydroxyapatite. Composites of ceramics and bone marrow have not been reported in human trials to date. It can be concluded that ceramics can serve as a bone graft expander and/or filler material, particularly in compressive application. Because ceramic is brittle and has no initial hoop strength or sheer strength, the bone must be protected while the ceramic is being incorporated.

Composite Grafts

A composite consisting of suspended deantigenated bovine fibrillar collagen and porous calcium phosphate ceramic, of which 65% is hydroxyapatite and 35% is tricalcium phosphate, has been introduced. The mixture is nonosteoinductive, and the addition of autogenous bone marrow provides osteoprogenitor cells and a limited amount of growth factors, such as platelet-derived growth factor (PDGF) and TGF-β, within the bone marrow clot. The calcium phosphate consists of granules having 70% porosity and a pore diameter ranging from 500 to 1,000 μm. The collagen is purified from bovine dermis and is 95% type-I collagen and 5% type-III collagen. Cornell and associates,[39] in a prospective randomized multicenter trial, compared the composite graft with a cancellous iliac bone graft in acute long bone fractures. The composite graft plus autogenous marrow showed no significant differences in functional result or radiographic appearances as compared to autogenous bone graft. The use of the composite significantly shortened the surgical time and avoided the complications and morbidity of autograft harvesting. However, the study did not include a control group treated without any grafting, and additional trials with such controls are needed, particularly in the face of markedly improved trauma instrumentation and methodology.

The composite, because it is currently available only as a paste or in soft strips, provides no structural strength. In addition, it has a tendency to flow if bleeding continues at the site of the fracture. Care must be taken to maintain the strip's location until the clot has formed. Biopsies of patients with the composite demonstrated slight inflammation at the site of the granules, but the 130 patients treated with the composite had no infections. Five of the patients treated with autogenous graft had infections and none of the patients treated with ceramics had infections. This composite appears to be a material that can be used as a bone graft expander or a graft substitute for stabilized fractures that are protected for internal fixation but require grafting to correct extensive comminution or segmental bone loss. Its use is contraindicated in intra-articular fractures because of the potential for migration of granules into the joint.

Osteoinductive Growth Factors

Growth factors, which are another important area of investigation, are used to enhance fracture healing, which requires a complex interaction of many local and systemic regulatory factors.[40–50] This complex interaction of local mediators causes primitive undifferentiated mesenchymal cells to migrate, proliferate, and differentiate at the fracture site. These local mediators, along with the microenvironment, also influence the genetic coding that determines the type of matrix that the repair cells will form.[41] As recent studies have furthered the knowledge of cellular proliferation, chondrogenesis, and osteogenesis, a number of mediators have been implicated as the predominant growth factors in fracture healing. Some of these factors include acidic and basic fibroblast growth factor, PDGF, TGF-β, and bone morphogenetic protein (BMP).[40–51]

Bostrom and associates[40] used immunolocalization to identify the expression of BMP-2 and -4 in fracture healing. In their studies they define and characterize the physiologic presence, localization, and chronology of BMP in both endochondral and membranous fracture healing. During the early stages of fracture healing, only a small number of primitive cells stained positively in the fracture's callus. As the process of endochondral ossification proceeded, the presence of BMP-2 and -4 increased significantly, especially in the primitive mesenchymal and chondrocytic cells. As the cartilage component of the callus matured, with a concomitant decrease in the number of primitive cells, there was a concomitant decrease in both the intensity and number of the positively staining cells with BMP. As osteoblasts started to lay down woven bone on the chondroid matrix, these osteoblastic cells exhibited a strong positive staining for BMP. The intensity of the staining decreased, however, as lamellar bone replaced the primitive bone. A similar observation was noted for areas undergoing intramembranous ossification. Initially, within several days after the fracture, periosteal cells and osteoblasts exhibited intense staining for BMP. As woven bone was replaced with lamellar bone, the staining increased. The data from these authors, as well as others, suggest that BMPs are important regulators in osteogenic differentiation during fracture repair.[50]

The BMPs are low molecular weight glycoproteins that function as morphogens.[52] The BMPs belong to an expanding TGF-β super family. The BMPs have a pleomorphic function that ranges from extracellular and skeletal organogenesis to bone generation and regeneration.[52] BMP-induced bone in postfetal life recapitulates the process of embryonic and endochondral ossification. Through recombinant gene technology, BMP is available in large amounts for basic research and clinical trials.[53] Recombinant human BMP (rhBMP) induces structurally sound orthotopic bone in a variety of experimental systems, including porous ingrowth in rats, femoral defects in rats, femoral defects in rabbits, femoral and mandibular defects in sheep, defects in spine fusions in dogs, and long-bone defects and spine fusions in monkeys.[54–58]

BMP has been used successfully under the guidance of Drs. Urist, Johnson, and Dawson for the treatment of established nonunions and spine fusions.[59–62] In 70 patients, they have not reported any instances of tumor genesis or other untoward events. Urist's clinical

BMP preparation represents a mixture of BMPs, though it is highly concentrated (300,000 ×). To date, it has resulted in a success rate of over 93% in failed nonunions, and 100% in spine fusions. Urist's product, however, is not recombinant BMP and in addition contains a number of different BMPs. Urist's mixture also contains osteocalcin.

Most studies reported to date with rhBMPs have been animal studies, although clinical trials are currently underway in the United States and Europe. Kirker-Head and associates[63] evaluated the long-term healing of bone using rhBMP-2 in adult sheep. By 12 months all the defects were structurally intact and were rigidly healed. Both woven and lamellar bone bridged the defect site, and apparently the normal sequence of ossification, modeling, and remodeling events had occurred. These reports using rhBMP-2 confirm prior reports by Toriumi and associates,[57] Gerhart and associates,[56] and Yasko and associates,[58] that BMP-2 can indeed heal skeletal defects in a wide range of animals. Cook and associates[54,55,64,65] have used BMP-7 to heal large segmental defects in rabbits, dogs, and primates. In their latter studies, five of six ulnas and four of five tibias treated with BMP-7 in African green monkeys exhibited complete healing in 6 to 8 weeks, with bridging of the defect and new bone formation in 4 weeks. Two unhealed defects both exhibited new bone formation. In their studies, all the tibial defects and all the ulnar defects that had been treated with autogenous bone graft developed fibrous union with little new bone formation. Thus, these studies demonstrated the efficacy of rhBMP in a nonhuman primate.

In a similar fashion, attention has been directed toward using rhBMPs in spine fusion procedures. Spine fusions play a very important role in the treatment of a number of pathologic conditions, including spine trauma, congenital anomalies,

degenerative diseases, and tumors. It is estimated that more than 180,000 spine fusions were performed in the United States in 1983. Boden, Sandhu, and Muschler have developed spine models that can be used to test recombinant factors.[66–71] Sandhu and associates[69] performed a number of studies using BMP-2 in a canine spine intraspinous process model. They found that the dosage of BMP was the critical element, and that this was unrelated to whether or not there was decortication of the fusion model. They further showed that rhBMP-2 with polylactic acid carrier is clearly superior at both higher and lower doses to autogenous iliac crest bone for inducing transverse process arthrodesis in a canine. BMP-2 doses ranging from 57 μg to 2.3 mg resulted in 100% clinical fusion and 85% radiologic fusion by 3 months as compared to no autogenous fusions at that time point. Radiologically delayed union occurred with lower doses, although differences were not significant. Fusions achieved with higher doses were mechanically stiffer in the axial plane than those with low doses, and BMP-dosed fusions were stiffer than autograft fusions in all planes. These studies clearly have demonstrated the efficacy of higher doses of rhBMP-2 for inducing posterolateral lumbar fusion in a canine model. Muschler and associates[68] also studied spine fusions in dogs, and they confirm that the use of rhBMP-2 in their experimental models demonstrated a fusion rate of 100% for a single-level lumbar arthrodesis without adverse neurologic or systemic sequelae. They felt that these results confirmed the use of this agent for spine fusions.[47] Boden and associates,[66,67] in a similar set of experiments performed on rabbits, further confirmed the use of rhBMP-2 as an excellent agent for spine fusion.

Cook and associates[64] tested the effect of rhBMP-7 or osteogenic protein-1 in the spine of mongrel dogs. Their agent was an effective bone graft substitute for

achieving stable posterior spine fusion in a significantly more rapid fashion than can be achieved by autogenous graft in the same spinal application. There now appears to be adequate evidence that both rhBMP-2 and -7, used in pharmacologic doses in various animal models, are quite efficacious and are superior to autogenous grafts in achieving spine fusion.

Other growth factors have been evaluated as to their efficacy in the treatment of biologic enhancement. Critchlow and associates[72] evaluated the effect of exogenous TGF-β in a rabbit fracture model. The investigators injected the TGF-β into the developing callus of the rat tibial fractures healing under stable or unstable mechanical conditions 4 days after fracture. The fractures were examined for 4 to 14 days after fracture. A large amount of edema developed around the injection site. The fractures that were healing under stable mechanical conditions consisted almost entirely of bone. The effects of 16-μg injections of TGF-β were minimal, but the 600-μg dose led to a small increase in the size of the callus. Fractures that were healing under unstable mechanical conditions had a large area of cartilage over the fracture site with bone on each side. The effects of TGF-β on unstable fractures were to retard and reduce bone and cartilage formation in the callus. The overall size of the callus was not affected. In conclusion, it was felt by these authors that TGF-β does not stimulate fracture healing under either stable or unstable mechanical conditions during the initial healing phase. It was further argued that agents that stimulate callus proliferation may retard bone remodeling.

Andrew and associates[73] evaluated the effect of platelet-derived growth factor (PDGF), especially in normally healing human fracture. PDGF has been shown to have effects on bone and cartilage cells. However, its role in fracture healing is not clearly identified. Biopsy materials from 16 normally healed fractures were obtained at various times after injury and were evaluated for PDGF by chemistry and in-situ hybridization. PDGF-α chain was found to be expressed by many cell types over a prolonged period during fracture healing. These cells include the endothelial and mesenchymal cells, and granulation tissue in the osteoblast, chondroblast sites, and osteoclasts later during fracture healing. In contrast, PDGF-β chain gene expression was more restricted, being directed principally in osteoclasts at the stage of bone formation. Because PDGF was detected using immunochemistry in various cell types during the fracture repair, the authors consider it to play an important role in the regulation of this process.

Currently, none of the recombinant growth factors have been approved for use by the FDA, and human trials are ongoing. However, the clot associated with bone marrow and the noncollagenous mixture in demineralized bone available from the bone bank and from processed allografts do contain small amounts of biologically active factors. More comprehensive studies are warranted to demonstrate the actual efficacy of these factors as providing true augmentation to the healing process.

Conclusion

For the orthopaedic surgeon, a number of grafting materials are available as alternatives to autogenous bone graft for use in a wide range of clinical applications. Allografts can provide structure and osteoconduction; however, they offer limited osteoinduction and no osteoprogenitor cells. Indications for their use are similar to those for autogenous graft, including repair of nonunions, promotion of arthrodesis, and segmental replacements of long bones. However, if the grafting bed is unfavorable, the allograft bone must be augmented with either autograft or other graft substitutes that provide growth factors and osteoprogenitor cells. Particularly in compro-

mised beds, immediately revascularized bone autografts offer distinct advantages over traditional grafts. Concerns regarding allografts include fracture, osteointegration, transmission of disease, and infection.

Ceramics are available in powders, granules, and blocks. The ceramic blocks provide compressive strength and can confer critical structural support. However, they are brittle and until they are incorporated into the existing adjacent bone they are mechanically weak when exposed to shear and tension forces. Because ceramics are exclusively osteoconductive, they must be combined with autograft or have access to a rich bone marrow and, as such, are effective graft fillers or expanders.

DBM offers a limited source of BMP and can be used as an adjunct in the regeneration process due to its limited osteoconductive potential. DBM provides no immediate torque or compressive strength. It must be supplemented by appropriate instrumentation when grafting large cortical segmental defects. Its clinical applications include augmentation of autogenous and allograft bone for repairing fracture, packing cysts, and promoting arthrodesis, including both posterolateral lumbar fusions and hip fusions with instrumentation.

Bone marrow is best used as an adjunct to existing allograft or biosynthetic ceramics to provide osteoprogenitor cells to compromised grafting beds. It provides no structural strength, and it is strictly an adjunct to other grafts and works well as a treatment to correct nonunions.

Composite grafts, including ceramic, collagen, and bone marrow, have been used successfully, but again they lack structure and must be protected until they are osteointegrated. They have a role in augmenting limited autogenous bone grafting.

BMP is not currently available in highly purified or recombinant form, but

the closest alternative, DBM, is readily available from bone banks. The use of rhBMP is still in clinical trials, but it is anticipated that it will be readily available to orthopaedic surgeons in the near future. In settings in which the grafting site is compromised and all three components of osteoconduction, osteoinduction, and osteoprogenitor cells are required, then autogenous graft is probably superior. However, a composite of particulate, ceramic, bone marrow, and DBM, which incorporates all three regenerative components, may be just as effective. Clinical trials will be needed to further define the relative efficacy of these components.

References

1. Younger EM, Chapman MW: Morbidity at bone graft donor sites. *J Orthop Trauma* 1989;3:192–195.

2. Burchardt H: The biology of bone graft repair. *Clin Orthop* 1983;174:28–42.

3. Burchardt H, Busbee GA III, Enneking WF: Repair of experimental autologous grafts of cortical bone. *J Bone Joint Surg* 1975;57A:814–819.

4. Enneking WF, Eady JL, Burchardt H: Autogenous cortical bone grafts in the reconstruction of segmental skeletal defects. *J Bone Joint Surg* 1980;62A:1039–1058.

5. Wilson PD Jr: A clinical study of the biomechanical behavior of massive bone transplants used to reconstruct large bone defects. *Clin Orthop* 1972;87:81–109.

6. Buncke HJ, Furnas DW, Gordon L, et al: Free osteocutaneous flap from a rib to the tibia. *Plast Reconstr Surg* 1977;59:799–804.

7. Han CS, Wood MB, Bishop AT, et al: Vascularized bone transfer. *J Bone Joint Surg* 1992;74A:1441–1449.

8. Lee EH, Goh JC, Helm R, et al: Donor site morbidity following resection of the fibula. *J Bone Joint Surg* 1990;72B:129–131.

9. Shaffer JW, Field GA, Goldberg VM, et al: Fate of vascularized and non-vascularized autografts. *Clin Orthop* 1985;197:32–43.

10. Taylor GI, Miller GD, Ham FJ: The free vascularized bone graft: A clinical extension of microvascular techniques. *Plast Reconstr Surg* 1975;55:533–544.

11. Weiland AJ, Moore JR, Daniel RK: Vascularized bone autografts: Experience with 41 cases. *Clin Orthop* 1983;174:87–95.

12. Ohlendorf C, Tomford WW, Mankin HJ: Chondrocyte survival in cryopreserved osteochondral articular cartilage. *J Orthop Res* 1996;14:413–416.

13. Tomford WW, Springfield DS, Mankin HJ: Fresh and frozen articular cartilage allografts. *Orthopedics* 19923;15:1183–1188.

14. Mankin HJ, Doppelt S, Tomford W: Clinical experience with allograft implantation: The first ten years. *Clin Orthop* 1983;174:69–86.

15. Mnaymneh W, Malinin TI, Makley JT, et al: Massive osteoarticular allografts in the reconstruction of extremities following resection of tumors not requiring chemotherapy and radiation. *Clin Orthop* 1985;197:76–87.

16. Berrey BH Jr, Lord CF, Gebhardt MC, et al: Fractures of allografts: Frequency, treatment, and end-results. *J Bone Joint Surg* 1990;72A:825–833.

17. Flynn JM, Springfield DS, Mankin HJ: Osteoarticular allografts to treat distal femoral osteonecrosis. *Clin Orthop* 1994;303:38–43.

18. Mankin HJ, Sringfield DS, Gebhardt MC, et al: Current status of allografting for bone tumors. *Orthopedics* 1992;15:1147–1154.

19. Tomford WW, Thongphasuk J, Mankin HJ, et al: Frozen musculoskeletal allografts: A study of the clinical incidence and causes of infection associated with their use. *J Bone Joint Surg* 1990;72A:1137–1143.

20. Buck BE, Malinin TI, Brown MD: Bone transplantation and human immunodeficiency virus: An estimate of risk of acquired immunodeficiency syndrome (AIDS). *Clin Orthop* 1989;240:129–136.

21. Burwell RG: The function of bone marrow in the incorporation of a bone graft. *Clin Orthop* 1985;200:125–141.

22. Burwell RG, Friedlaender GE, Mankin HJ: Current perspectives and future directions: The 1983 Invitational Conference on Osteochondral Allografts. *Clin Orthop* 1985;197:141–157.

23. Morrison SJ, Wandycz AM, Akashi K, et al: The aging of hematopoietic stem cells. *Nat Med* 1996;2:1011–1016.

24. Morrison SJ, Uchida N, Weissman IL: The biology of hematopoietic stem cells. *Ann Rev Cell Dev Biol* 1995;11:35–71.

25. Salama R, Burwell RD, Dickson IR: Recombined grafts of bone and marrow: The beneficial effect upon osteogenesis of impregnating xenograft(heterograft) bone with autologous red marrow. *J Bone Joint Surg* 1973;55B:402–417.

26. Salama R, Weissman SL: The clinical use of combined xenografts of bone and autologous red marrow: A preliminary report. *J Bone Joint Surg* 1978;60B:111–115.

27. Nakahara H, Goldberg VM, Caplan AI: Culture-expanded periosteal-derived cells exhibit osteochondrogenic potential in porous calcium phosphate ceramics in vivo. *Clin Orthop* 1992;276:291–298.

28. Werntz J, Lane J, Piez K, et al: The repair of segmental bone defects with collagen and marrow. *Orthop Trans* 1986;10:262–263.

29. Connolly J, Guse R, Lippiello L, et al: Development of an osteogenic bone-marrow preparation. *J Bone Joint Surg* 1989;71A:684–691.

30. Connolly JF, Guse R, Tiedeman J, et al: Autologous marrow injection as a substitute for operative grafting of tibial nonunions. *Clin Orthop* 1991;266:259–270.

31. Tiedeman JJ, Connolly JF, Strates BS, et al: Treatment of nonunion by percutaneous injection of bone marrow and demineralized bone matrix: An experimental study in dogs. *Clin Orthop* 1991;268:294–302.

32. Bruder SP, Fink DJ, Caplan AI: Mesenchymal stem cells in bone development, bone repair, and skeletal regeneration therapy. *J Cell Biochem* 1994;56:283–294.

33. Constantz BR, Ison IC, Fulmer MT, et al: Skeletal repair by in situ formation of the mineral phase of bone. *Science* 1995;267:1796–1799.

34. Peltier LF: The use of plaster of Paris to fill defects in bone. *Clin Orthop* 1961;21:1–31.

35. Holmes RE, Bucholz RW, Mooney V: Porous hydroxyapatite as a bone-graft substitute in metaphyseal defects: A histometric study. *J Bone Joint Surg* 1986;68A:904–911.

36. Holmes RE, Bucholz RW, Mooney V: Porous hydroxyapatite as a bone graft substitute in diaphyseal defects: A histometric study. *J Orthop Res* 1987;5:114–121.

37. Sartoris DJ, Holmes RE, Bucholz RW, et al: Coralline hydroxyapatite bone graft substitutes in a canine diaphyseal defect model: Radiographic features of failed and successful union. *Skeletal Radiol* 1986;15:642–647.

38. Bucholz RW, Carlton A, Holmes R: Interporous hydroxyapatite as a bone graft substitute in tibial plateau fractures. *Clin Orthop* 1989;240:53–62.

39. Cornell CN, Lane JM, Chapman M, et al: Multicenter trial of Collagraft as bone graft substitute. *J Orthop Trauma* 1991;5:1–8.

40. Bostrom MP, Lane JM, Berberian WS, et al: Immunolocalization and expression of bone morphogenetic proteins 2 and 4 in fracture healing. *J Orthop Res* 1995;13:357–367.

41. Canalis E, McCarthy T, Centrella M: Growth factors and the regulation of bone remodeling. *J Clin Invest* 1988;81:277–281.

42. Celeste AJ, Iannazzi JA, Taylor RC, et al: Identification of transforming growth factor beta family members present in bone-inductive protein purified from bovine bone. *Proc Natl Acad Sci USA* 1990;87:9843–9847.

43. Jingushi S, Heydemann A, Kana SK, et al: Acidic fibroblast growth factor (aFGF) injection stimulates cartilage enlargement and inhibits cartilage gene expression in rat fracture healing. *J Orthop Res* 1990;8:364–371.

44. Joyce ME, Jingushi S, Bolander ME: Transforming growth factor-beta in the regulation of fracture repair. *Orthop Clin North Am* 1990;21:199–209.

45. Joyce ME, Jingushi S, Scully SP, et al: Role of growth factors in fracture healing. *Prog Clin Biol Res* 1991;365:391–416.

46. Joyce ME, Terek RM, Jingushi S, et al: Role of transforming growth factor-beta in fracture repair. *Ann N Y Acad Sci* 1990;593:107–123.

47. Noda M, Camilliere JJ: In vivo stimulation of bone formation by transforming growth factor-beta. *Endicrinology* 1989;124:2991–2994.

48. Simmons DJ: Fracture healing perspectives. *Clin Orthop* 1985;200:100–113.

49. Triffitt JT: Initiation and Enhancement of bone formation: A review. *Acta Orthop Scand* 1987;58:673–684.

50. Yang LJ, Jin Y: Immunohistochemical observations on bone morphogenetic protein in normal and abnormal conditions. *Clin Orthop* 1990;257:249–256.

51. Sporn MB, Roberts AB: Transforming growth factor-beta: Multiple actions and potential clinical applications (clinical conference). *JAMA* 1989;262:938–941.

52. Wozney JM: The bone morphogenetic protein family and osteogenesis. *Mol Reprod Dev* 1992;32:160–167.

53. Hahn GV, Cohen RB, Wozney JM, et al: A bone morphogenetic protein subfamily: Chromosomal localization of human genes for BMP5, BMP6, and BMP7. *Genomics* 1992;14:759–762.

54. Cook SD, Baffes GC, Wolfe MW, et al: Recombinant human bone morphogenetic protein-7 induces healing in a canine long-bone segmental defect model. *Clin Orthop* 1994;301:302–312.

55. Cook SD, Baffes GC, Wolfe MW, et al: The effect of recombinant human osteogenic protein-1 on healing of large segmental bone defects. *J Bone Joint Surg* 1994;76A:827–838.

56. Gerhart TN, Kirker-Head CA, Kirz MJ, et al: Healing of large mid-femoral segmental defects in sheep using recombinant human bone morphogenetic protein (BMP-2). *Trans Orthop Res Soc* 1991;16:172.

57. Toriumi DM, Kotler HS, Luxenberg DP, et al: Mandibular reconstruction with a recombinant bone-inducing factor: Functional, histologic, and biomechanical evaluation. *Arch Otolaryngol Head Neck Surg* 1991;117:1101–1112.

58. Yasko AW, Lane JM, Fellinger EJ, et al: The healing of segmental bone defects, induced by recombinant human bone morphogenetic protein (rhBMP-2): A radiographic, histological, and biomechanical study in rats. *J Bone Joint Surg* 1992;74A:659–670.

59. Johnson EE, Urist MR, Finerman GA: Repair of segmental defects of the tibia with cancellous bone grafts augmented with human bone morphogenetic protein: A preliminary report. *Clin Orthop* 1988;236:249–257.

60. Johnson EE, Urist MR, Finerman GA: Bone morphogenetic protein augmentation grafting of resistant femoral nonunions: A preliminary report. *Clin Orthop* 1988;230:257–265.

61. Johnson EE, Urist MR, Finerman GA: Resistant nonunions and partial or complete segmental defects of long bones: Treatment with implants of a composite of human bone morphogenetic protein (BMP) and autolyzed, antigen-extracted, allogeneic (AAA) bone. *Clin Orthop* 1992;277:229–237.

62. Johnson EE, Urist MR, Schmalzried TP, et al: Autogeneic cancellous bone grafts in extensive segmental ulnar defects in dogs: Effects of xenogeneic bovine bone morphogenetic protein without and with interposition of soft tissues and interruption of blood supply. *Clin Orthop* 1989;243:254–265.

63. Kirker-Head CA, Gerhart TN, Schelling SH, et al: Long-term healing of bone using recombinant human bone morphogenetic protein 2. *Clin Orthop* 1995;318:222–230.

64. Cook SD, Dalton JE, Tan EH, et al: In vivo evaluation of recombinant human osteogenic protein (rhOP-1) implants as a bone graft substitute for spinal fusions. *Spine* 1994;19:1655–1663.

65. Cook SD, Wolfe MW, Salkeld SL, et al: Effect of recombinant human osteogenic protein-1 on healing of segmental defects in non-human primates. *J Bone Joint Surg* 1995;77A:734–750.

66. Boden SD, Schimandle JH, Hutton WC: The use of an osteoinductive growth factor for lumbar spinal fusion: Part II. Study of dose, carrier, and species. *Spine* 1995;20:2633–2644.

67. Boden SD, Schimandle JH, Hutton WC, et al: The use of an osteoinductive growth factor for lumbar spinal fusion: Part I. Biology of spinal fusion. *Spine* 1995;20:2626–2632.

68. Muschler GF, Hyodo A, Manning T, et al: Evaluation of human bone morphogenetic protein-2 in a canine fusion model. *Clin Orthop* 1994;308:229–240.

69. Sandhu HS, Kanim LE, Kabo JM, et al: Evaluation of rhBMP-2 with an OPLA carrier in a canine posterolateral (transverse process) spinal fusion model. *Spine* 1995;20:2669–2682.

70. Schimandle JH, Boden SD: Spine update: The use of animal models to study spinal fusion. *Spine* 1994;19:1998–2006.

71. Schimandle JH, Boden SD, Hutton WC: Experimental spinal fusion with recombinant human bone morphogenetic protein-2. *Spine* 1995;20:1326–1337.

72. Critchlow MA, Bland YS, Ashhurst DE: The effect of exogenous transforming growth factor-beta 2 on healing fractures in the rabbit. *Bone* 1995;16:521–527.

73. Andrew JG, Hoyland JA, Freemont AJ, et al: Platelet-derived growth factor expression in normally healing human fractures. *Bone* 1995;16:455–460.

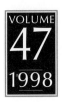

Cumulative Index
1997-1998

Agonist/antagonist activity, 46: 40
AIDS transmission
  and allograft sterilization, **47: 380, 385, 527**
  and osteochondral allografts, **47: 517–518**
Akin procedure, 46: 366–*367, 368*
Alcoholism in elderly, 46: 413–*414*
Algorithm
  for anterior knee pain, **47: 339–343**
  for failed lateral epicondylitis surgery, **47:** *171*
  for malunited proximal humerus fractures, **47: 140**
  for osteolysis after total hip arthroplasty, **47:** *322, 323, 325*
  for periprosthetic patellar fractures, **47:** *457*
  for supracondylar periprosthetic fractures, **47:** *452*
Allograft bone, defined, 46: 230–231
Allografts, **47: 526–527**
  for acetabular revision arthroplasty, **47: 265–273**
    clinical results of, **47: 271–273**
    surgical technique, **47:** *268–269*
  composite, 46: *233,* 234
  for knee ligaments and meniscal reconstruction, **47: 379–394**
    ACL reconstruction, **47: 385–388**
    LCL reconstruction, **47: 389–391**
    meniscal allografts, **47: 392–393**
    PCL reconstruction, **47: 388–389**
  osteochondral allografts for the knee, **47: 500, 517–***521*
    results of, **47: 512**
    screening for donors, **47: 517–518**
    surgical procedure, **47:** *518–521*
  in periprosthetic femoral fracture treatment, **47: 257–***263*
    advantages and disadvantages of, **47: 262**
    technique, **47: 257–259**
  in revision knee arthroplasty, 46: 231–234
  sterilization of, **47: 380–385**
    and disease transmission, **47: 385, 527**
  in total knee arthroplasty, 46: 234–236
Allogrip, 46: 233
Alzheimer's disease, 46: 423
American Association of Tissue Banks, **47: 385, 527**
American Spinal Injury Association (ASIA) impairment scale, 46: 117
Amitriptyline and aging, 46: 415
Amputation
  for infected knee arthroplasty, 46: 217
  versus limb salvage, 46: 511–517
    cost of, 46: 517
    factors affecting outcome, 46: 513–517
    factors affecting salvage, 46: 511–512
    scoring systems, 46: 512–513
    which injuries, 46: 511
  surgery in peripheral vascular disease, 46: 501–508
    cognitive and psychological requirements for walking in amputees, 46: 502
    functional levels, 46: 505–508
    joints as energy couples, 46: *501*–502

    load transfer, 46: *502–503*
    rehabilitation, 46: 508
    selection of level, 46: 504–505
    wound healing, 46: 503–*504*
Analgesics in treating loxoscelism, 46: 71
Anatomy
  Achilles tendon, **47: 419**
  ankle, 46: *323–324*
  arthroscopic anatomy of lumbar spine, 46: 148–151
  distal radioulnar joint, **47: 209**
  elbow, **47: 151–***152*
  foot, 46: *324–325, 358–364*
  hindfoot, **47: 421–422**
  intrapelvic vascular structures, **47: 280**
  knee, **47: 345–***346, 370*; 46: *165*
  posterior tibial tendon, 46: 393
  radius, distal, **47: 191, 193**
  shoulder, **47: 97–100**
  wrist, **47: 219–220**
Anconeus compartment syndrome, **47: 170**
Anderson Orthopaedic Research Institute (AORI) bone defect classification, 46: 229–230
Angiofibroblastic hyperplasia, 46: 572
Ankle, imaging of, 46: 524–526
Ankle arthrodesis, 46: 348–351
Ankle/brachial pressure index, 46: 183
Ankle disarticulation, 46: 506
Ankle fractures, 46: 311–318
  anatomy and biomechanics, 46: 311–*312*
  association of tibial shaft fractures with ipsilateral, 46: 276–277
  classification of, 46: 312–315
  current issues in, 46: 315
  deltoid ligament injuries, 46: 315–316
  isolated lateral malleolar, 46: 315
  posterior malleolar, 46: 316
  postoperative and post-injury management, 46: 318
  radiographic evaluation, 46: 312, *313*
  syndesmotic injuries, 46: 316–318
Ankle fusion with bone loss, 46: 354
Ankylosing spondylitis, 46: 394
Anterior cruciate ligament
  allograft reconstruction, **47: 385–388**
  bioresorbable implants in ACL reconstruction, 46: *541–542*
  injuries in skeletally immature patients, **47: 351–358**
    diagnosis, **47: 351**
    tibial eminence fractures, **47: 352–***354*
    treatment for, **47: 354–358**
  loss of motion following surgery on, **47: 361;** 46: *251–259*
    literature review, 46: 252–256
  revision ACL reconstruction, **47: 361–366**
    causes of reconstruction failure, **47: 361–364**
Anterior-inferior subluxation as complication in humeral head replacement, 46: 19
Anterior release for spinal deformity, 46: 135

Osteochondritis dissecans, 46: 572
Osteogenesis, distraction, 46: 284
Osteoinductive growth factors, **47: 530–532**
Osteolysis, **47: 307–317**
 and aseptic loosening, **47: 307, 309–*310***
 diagnosis of, **47: 309–*310***
 epidemiology
  after total hip arthroplasty, **47: 314–317**
  after total knee replacement, 46: 210-*211*
 and fractures, **47: 239, 254**
 pathophysiology of, **47: 307–309**; 46: 211
 prevention of, 46: 212
 radiographic appearance of, **47: 310–314**
 and resorbable implants, 46: 537
 risk factors for, **47: 317**
 treatment, **47: 321–328**; 46: 211-*212*
  for acetabular defects, **47: 324–328**
  for femoral defects, **47: 321–324**
 in weight lifters, **47: 37**
Osteolytic defects, debris-generated, 46: 227–228
Osteomyelitis, imaging of, 46: 525–526
Osteonecrosis
 as complication of internal fixation of proximal humeral
  fractures, 46: 30–31
 as complication of talar injuries, 46: 324
 magnetic resonance imaging of, **47: 16–*17***
 shoulder arthroplasty for, **47: 132**
 in talar body, 46: 337, 350
 in talar neck fractures, 46: 328–329, 331–332
Osteopenia in elderly, 46: 424
Osteophytes, **47: 491**
Osteoporosis
 bone biomechanics, 46: 447
  physical activity, 46: 448
 bone metabolism in, 46: 445
  calcitropic hormones, 46: *446–447*
  calcium, 46: 445–446
 in elderly, 46: 424
 evaluation of, 46: *448–449*
  bone histomorphometry, 46: 451
  history, 46: 449–450
  imaging studies and measurement of bone mineral density, 46: 450
  laboratory studies, 46: 450–451
 growth factors as potential therapeutic agents in, 46: 495–497
 treatment of, pharmacologic therapy, 46: 451–454
Osteoporotic bone, biomechanical considerations of hip and spine fractures in, 46: 431–437
Osteoporotic fractures, 46: 7
Osteosynthesis, 46: 544
Osteotomy
 arthrodesis with, 46: 343–344
 arthrodesis without, 46: 344–345
 and articular cartilage regeneration, **47: 495–496**

calcaneal, 46: 397–*398*
chevron, 46: 370–*372, 373*
corrective, of radius, 46: 107
distal femoral varus, **47: 434**
distal metatarsal, 46: 372–*375*, 385–386
Dwyer-type, 46: 343
fibular, **47: 433**
of first cuneiform, 46: 386
of first metatarsal, distal soft-tissue reconstruction of, 46: 374–378
of the knee, **47: 429–434**
 and articular cartilage regeneration, **47: 496**
 indications for, **47: 430–431**
 patient assessment, **47: 431–432**
medial transfer of tibial tubercle by, 46: 172–173
multiple, 46: 385–387
olecranon, **47: 155**
pediatric, 46: 540
proximal phalangeal, 46: 366–367
rotational, of first metacarpal, 46: 108
simple, 46: 343
through previous ankle fusion, 46: 356
through triple arthrodesis, 46: 356
tibial
 proximal tibial osteotomies, **47: 432–434**
 tubercle, 46: 222–*224*, 246
Outcome assessment after fracture in the elderly, 46: 439–443
Oxidative degradation of ultra-high molecular weight polyethylene, 46: 207
Oxygenated blood as prerequisite to wound healing, 46: 503–504
Oxygen free radical scavengers in treating spinal cord injuries, 46: 118

P

Paget's disease, pathologic fractures in, 46: 426, *427*
Pain, anterior knee, **47: 339–343**
 algorithm, **47: *340–341***
Pain dysfunction syndrome
 definition of, 46: 262
 primary components of, 46: 262
 secondary components of, 46: 262
Palindromic arthritis, 46: 78
Palsy, peroneal nerve, 46: 181
Pantalar arthrodesis, 46: *353*, 354–355
Parathyroid hormone in osteoporosis, 46: 446
Parathyroid hormone-related protein (PTHrP)
 as autocrine/paracrine growth factor in cartilage, **47: 465, 472**
 and Jansen-type chondrometaphyseal dysplasia, **47: 466**
Paravertebral blockade, 46: 264
Parkinson's disease, 46: 423
Patella facet, allograft replacement of, **47: 520, *521***
Patella infera contracture syndrome, 46: 251–259
Patella infera syndrome, 46: 241–249

Index

W

Walking
 biomechanics of forward human locomotion
  demarcation between walking and running, **47: 397**–*398*
  gait cycle, **47: 398,** *399*
  potential and kinetic energy in, **47: 398,** *400*
 energy demands in amputees for, 46: *501*–502
 psychological requirements in amputees, 46: 502
Warfarin
 as prophylactic agent after total knee replacement, 46: 186
 for thromboembolic disease, **47: 332–333;** 46: 188
Weber classification system for ankle injury, 46: 313
Weight lifter's shoulder, **47: 37**
Werner syndrome, 46: 497
Wound healing, amputation, 46: 503–*504*
Wound treatment in tibial shaft fractures, 46: 298–299
Wright test, **47: 87**
Wrist
 anatomy, **47: 219–220**
 imaging of, 46: 523–524
  for carpal instability, **47: 222–224**
 mechanics, **47: 220–221**

Wrist instability, **47: 203–208**
 classification scheme for, **47: 203–204**
 distal radioulnar joint instability, **47: 199–201, 209–213**
  acute, **47: 210**
  chronic, **47: 210–213**
 midcarpal (MCI), **47: 204–208**
  diagnosis of, **47: 204–205**
  Lichtman's classification for, **47: 205–206**
 radial-sided, **47: 219–227**
  diagnosis of, **47: 221–222**
  imaging for, **47: 222–224**
  treatment for scapholunate instability, **47: 224–227**
 ulnar-sided, **47: 215–218**

Y

Yergason test, **47: 88**

Z

Zanca radiographic view of acromioclavicular joint, **47: 23,** *36*
 after failed rotator cuff repair, **47: 88**
 postoperative heterotopic ossification, **47:** *92*
 for weight lifter's shoulder, **47: 37**
Zickel supracondylar rods, **47: 439–440**
Zones, articular cartilage, **47: 477–478**
 calcified cartilage zone, **47: 483**
 middle zone, **47: 483**
 superficial zone, **47: 482**
 transitional zone, **47: 482–483**